PEDIATRIC GASTROINTESTINAL IMAGING AND INTERVENTION

Second Edition

PEDIATRIC GASTROINTESTINAL IMAGING AND INTERVENTION

Second Edition

DAVID A. STRINGER

BSc, MBBS, FRCR, FRCPC

President, DC DiagnostiCare Inc
Edmonton, Alberta

PAUL S. BABYN, MDCM

Associate Professor in Medical Imaging
University of Toronto
Radiologist-in-Chief
The Hospital for Sick Children
Toronto, Ontario

2000
B.C. Decker Inc.
Hamilton • London

B.C. Decker Inc.
4 Hughson Street South
P.O. Box 620, L.C.D. 1
Hamilton, Ontario L8N 3K7
Tel: 905-522-7017; 1-800-568-7281
Fax: 905-522-7839
E-mail: info@bcdecker.com
Website: http://www.bcdecker.com

BC Decker

ISBN 1–55009–079–8

Printed in Canada by the University of Toronto Press

Sales and Distribution

United States
B.C. Decker Inc.
P.O. Box 785
Lewiston, NY U.S.A. 14092-0785
Tel: 905-522-7017/1-800-568-7281
Fax: 905-522-7839
e-mail: info@bcdecker.com
website: http://www.bcdecker.com

Canada
B.C. Decker Inc.
4 Hughson Street South
P.O. Box 620, L.C.D. 1
Hamilton, Ontario L8N 3K7
Tel: 905-522-7017/1-800-568-7281
Fax: 905-522-7839
e-mail: info@bcdecker.com
website: http://www.bcdecker.com

Japan
Igaku-Shoin Ltd.
Foreign Publications Department
3-24-17 Hongo, Bunkyo-ku,
Tokyo 113-8719, Japan
Tel: 3 3817 5676
Fax: 3 3815 6776
e-mail: fd@igaku.shoin.co.jp

U.K., Europe, Scandinavia, Middle East
Blackwell Science Ltd.
Osney Mead
Oxford OX2 0EL
United Kingdom
Tel: 44-1865-206206
Fax: 44-1865-721205
e-mail: info@blackwell-science.com

Australia
Blackwell Science Asia Pty, Ltd.
54 University Street
Carlton, Victoria 3053
Australia
Tel: 03 9347 0300
Fax: 03 9349 3016
e-mail: info@blacksci.asia.com.au

South Korea
Seoul Medical Scientific Books Co.
C.P.O. Box 9794
Seoul 100-697
Seoul, Korea
Tel: 82-2925-5800
Fax: 82-2927-7283

South America
Ernesto Reichmann, Distribuidora
de Livros Ltda.
Rua Coronel Marques
335-Tatuape, 03440-000
Sao Paulo-SP-Brazil
Tel/Fax: 011-218-2122

Foreign Rights
John Scott & Co.
International Publishers' Agency
P.O. Box 878
Kimberton, PA 19442
Tel: 610-827-1640
Fax: 610-827-1671

Notice: The authors and publisher have made every effort to ensure that the patient care recommended herein, including choice of drugs and drug dosages, is in accord with the accepted standard and practice at the time of publication. However, since research and regulation constantly change clinical standards, the reader is urged to check the product information sheet included in the package of each drug, which includes recommended doses, warnings, and contraindications. This is particularly important with new or infrequently used drugs.

CONTRIBUTORS

PAUL S. BABYN, MDCM
Department of Diagnostic Imaging
The Hospital for Sick Children
University of Toronto
Toronto, Ontario
Pediatric Biliary Imaging, The Liver,
The Pancreas, The Spleen

KEVIN M. BASKIN, MD
Centre for Image Guided Therapy
Centre for Research in Education
The Hospital for Sick Children
University of Toronto
Toronto, Ontario
Pediatric Gastrointestinal Interventions

SHEILA C. BERLIN, MD
Division of Pediatric Radiology
Rainbow Babies and Children's Hospital
Cleveland, Ohio
Large Bowel

PETER CHAIT, MB, ChB
Department of Diagnostic Imaging
The Hospital for Sick Children
University of Toronto
Toronto, Ontario
Pediatric Gastrointestinal Interventions

CATHERINE CHEN, MD
Division of General Surgery
The Hospital for Sick Children
University of Toronto
Toronto, Ontario
Gastrointestinal Imaging in Pediatric Surgery

BAIRBRE CONNOLLY, MB, ChB
Interventional Radiology, Diagnostic Imaging
The Hospital for Sick Children
University of Toronto
Toronto, Ontario
Pediatric Gastrointestinal Interventions

CHEE HIEW, MB, BS, FRACR
Department of Radiology
Austin and Repatriation Medical Centre
Heidelberg, Victoria
Melbourne, Australia
Pediatric Biliary Imaging, The Liver

DOUG JAMIESON, MB, ChB, FRCPC
Department of Radiology
British Columbia Children's Hospital
University of British Columbia
Vancouver, British Columbia
Small Bowel

PETER C.W. KIM, MDCM, PhD, FRCS(C)
Division of General Surgery
The Hospital for Sick Children
University of Toronto
Toronto, Ontario
Gastrointestinal Imaging in Pediatric Surgery

SAMBASIVA R. KOTTAMASU, MD
Department of Pediatric Imaging
Wayne State University School of Medicine
Nuclear Medicine
Children's Hospital of Michigan
Detroit, Michigan
Pharynx and Esophagus, Diaphragm and
Esophagogastric Junction, The Stomach

MARGARET A. MARCON, MD, FRCPC
Division of Gastroenterology and Nutrition
The Hospital of Sick Children
University of Toronto
Toronto, Ontario
Upper and Lower Gastrointestinal Endoscopy

HELEN NADEL, MD, FRCPC (Nuclear Medicine)
Department of Radiology
British Columbia Children's Hospital
University of British Columbia
Vancouver, British Columbia
Techniques for Investigation of the Pediatric
Gastrointestinal Tract

MARILYN RANSON, BSc, MD, FRCPC
Department of Diagnostic Imaging
The Hospital for Sick Children
University of Toronto
Toronto, Ontario
Pediatric Biliary Imaging

BRUCE M. SHUCKETT, MD, FRCPC
Gastrointestinal Imaging
The Hospital for Sick Children
University of Toronto
Toronto, Ontario
The Liver

CARLOS J. SIVIT, MD
Division of Pediatric Radiology
Rainbow Babies and Children's Hospital
Cleveland, Ohio
Large Bowel

DAVID A. STRINGER, BSc, MBBS, FRCR, FRCPC
DC DiagnostiCare Inc
Edmonton, Alberta
Previously: University of British Columbia
Divisions of General Radiology and Ultrasound
The Hospital for Sick Children Toronto, Ontario and
The British Columbia Children's Hospital Vancouver,
British Columbia
*Techniques for Investigation of the Pediatric
Gastrointestinal Tract, Pharynx and Esophagus,
Diaphragm and Esophagogastric Junction,
The Stomach, Small Bowel, Large Bowel,
The Liver, The Spleen*

JONATHAN E. TEITELBAUM, MD
Department of Pediatrics
Monmouth Medical Center
Long Beach, New Jersey
Gastrointestinal Imaging in Pediatric Gastroenterology

MICHAEL TEMPLE, MD
Interventional Radiography
The Hospital for Sick Children
University of Toronto
Toronto, Ontario
Pediatric Gastrointestinal Interventions

W. ALLAN WALKER, MD
Division of Nutrition
Harvard School of Medicine
Pediatric Gastroenterology and Nutrition
Massachusetts General Hospital and
Children's Hospital
Boston, Massachusetts
Gastrointestinal Imaging in Pediatric Gastroenterology

CHRISTEL WIHLBORG, MD
Department of Diagnostic Imaging
The Hospital for Sick Children
University of Toronto
Toronto, Ontario
The Liver

TARA WILLIAMS, MD
Department of Diagnostic Imaging
The Hospital for Sick Children
University of Toronto
Toronto, Ontario
The Liver, The Pancreas

KATHERINE A. ZUKOTYNSKI, BASc
The University of Toronto Medical School
Toronto, Ontario
The Liver

PREFACE

The burgeoning of new modalities and their subsequent clinical application over the last decade has necessitated another reappraisal of the imaging required for every organ system in children, and the gastrointestinal tract is no exception in this regard. Hence, the need for updating this book from its first edition in 1989. The gastrointestinal tract can now be imaged by a wide variety of radiological modalities and techniques, including sonography, plain films, fluoroscopy, computed tomography (CT), nuclear medicine, angiography, interventional studies, and magnetic resonance (MR). In most pediatric hospitals, all of the latest imaging modalities are available, including modern fluoroscopic units with digital hard or soft copy, sonography with colour Doppler, SPECT Nuclear Medicine Imaging Cameras, spiral CT scanners, MR scanners, and digital angiographic units.

In this text the gastrointestinal tract refers to all intraabdominal structures excluding the genitourinary tract and adrenal glands. Our purpose is to review the clinical and radiological features across the spectrum of imaging modalities for each clinical diagnosis affecting the gastrointestinal tract, and to consider the most appropriate imaging modality for each situation. The information in this book constitutes a distillate of our combined knowledge, and also reflects the great assistance of many other experts as contributing authors here as well as those cited in the literature. We are deeply indebted to both groups.

The first two chapters, kindly provided by Drs. Catherine Chen, Peter Kim, Jonathan Teitelbaum, and Allan Walker, provide an introductory overview of the common clinical findings related to the gastrointestinal tract as encountered by pediatric gastroenterologists and pediatric surgeons. In Chapter 3, we have provided an overview of the different techniques of examination that we and others use with a section provided by Dr. Helen Nadel on Nuclear Medicine. Many techniques are markedly different from those performed in adults, and this section should be particularly helpful to residents, fellows, and adult radiologists that perform examinations in children. Pediatric radiologists may also find it interesting to compare these techniques with their own.

In the next two chapters, new additions to this edition, two experts in their fields, namely Drs. Margaret Marcon and Peter Chait, review the current applications of endoscopy and interventional radiology respectively. These areas are rapidly changing and should be of great interest to all in this field.

In the remaining nine chapters, each region of the gastrointestinal tract, from esophagus to spleen, is discussed in turn, with respect to normal and abnormal radiological findings. Common and rare abnormalities are illustrated by various modalities, and for each condition the modality of choice is discussed. Which modality to use will depend, of course, on the available equipment and expertise as well as the clinical problem itself. These sections are the core of the book and cover the broad range of diseases likely to be met by radiologists, gastroenterologists, pediatric surgeons, and pediatricians.

For the purposes of this book, the ideal modality is defined as that which provides sufficient information rapidly enough to ensure proper patient management with minimum patient discomfort, radiation exposure, and cost. This is based primarily upon our experience at the Hospital for Sick Children in Toronto, the British Columbia Children's Hospital in Vancouver, and other pediatric hospitals listed for the remaining contributors.

This book should be useful to residents, fellows, and adult and pediatric radiologists and interventional radiologists as well as of interest to many other physicians caring for children including pediatricians, gastroenterologists, hepatologists, pediatric surgeons, and paediatric oncologists. For those so inclined, an extensive bibliography is included to serve as a basis for further study. Our aim is to assist a varied group of clinicians and radiologists in making safe, accurate, and rapid diagnoses that result in expeditious management of pediatric patients.

DAS

PSB

ACKNOWLEDGMENTS

We are grateful to the many colleagues and friends who supported us while this second edition was in progress. Many other authors have helped with this second edition and we are grateful to them all for their valuable contributions as listed in their respective chapters. Any omissions in the text are not due to their considerable efforts but must be shouldered by us.

Without the current and former members of the general divisions of radiology and ultrasound in our hospitals who performed many of the studies that make up our total experience, this book would not have been possible. These radiologists include many of the new authors within this edition and also Drs. Doug Alton, Pat Burrows, Alan Daneman, Robyn Cairns, Peter Liu, David Manson, Don Newman, Bernard Rielly, Michael Sargent, and Dan Wilmot. A special mention should be made of all the students and fellows who provided the inspiration to delve more deeply into many areas with their continual enthusiasm. We value their friendship, helpful advice and encouragement. In addition, Dr. Derek Harwood-Nash was always so encouraging to academic endeavor that he helped form our method of practice. It was a very sad day indeed when we lost such a mentor in such an early and unexpected way.

Many support staff have been involved. We are particularly grateful to Kerri Detz, Abby MacInnes, Cheryl Wattam, Linda Halpert, and Lori Fearon, and most recently Laurie Taylor. The Visual Education Department of The Hospital for Sick Children, Toronto, and in particular Lou Scaglione and Mary Casey, prepared many of the illustrations.

A very special mention must go to Debbie Kerrigan, our contrast procedure nurse at The Hospital for Sick Children, Toronto. Debbie helped organize a teaching file collection, from which many of the illustrations have been taken. In addition, she labelled all the pictures and accompanying slides—a Herculean task, which she performed not only efficiently, but with an excellent sense of humor and remarkable cheerfulness. It is a real pleasure to know her and her husband Alasdair and to be their friends.

We would also like to thank the staff at BC Decker, and especially Diane Dent, Paul Donnelly, Drew McCarthy, and Jennifer Therriault, for all their help and understanding in bringing this book to a conclusion.

Finally, a deep thank you for our long-suffering families, our wives Judy and Elizabeth, and our children, Charles, Rosemary, Henry, André, Laura, Michael and Jonathan who had to live through the rebirth of this book, the second edition.

"At last the albatross is no longer around our necks."

To Judy, Charles, Rosemary, Henry
and my parents, without whose support
neither edition would have been possible.

DAS

To Elizabeth, André, Laura, Michael and
Jonathan—the inspiration for all I do.

PSB

CONTENTS

1

GASTROINTESTINAL IMAGING IN PEDIATRIC GASTROENTEROLOGY

Jonathan E. Teitelbaum, MD, and W. Allan Walker, MD

Because children are not merely smaller versions of adults, the practice of pediatric gastroenterology and nutrition has evolved into a unique subspecialty. Early in the twentieth century, gastroenterologists were limited in their access to the digestive tract as well as to diagnostic tests and therapeutic modalities. Chronic gastritis was diagnosed by scrutinizing gastric aspirates, and treatment involved special diets and gastric lavage. For this reason, many feel the discovery of the x-ray by Wilhelm Roentgen in 1895 contributed greatly to the transformation of clinical gastroenterology (Kirsner, 1998). Thus, although the history and physical examination of the patient remain vital tools for the clinician, traditional descriptive terms such as succussion splash, fluid wave, and borborygmi are replaced by terms such as T2-weighted image, echotexture, and technetium scan. Indeed, with the increased availability and accuracy of prenatal ultrasonography, some patients present to the gastroenterologist shortly after birth and before the onset of signs or symptoms (i.e., choledochal cyst, gallstones, meconium peritonitis). However, these technologic advances do not replace the history and the physical examination but rather supplement them. The clinician must work closely with the radiologist to select and interpret those tests useful in answering the questions the patient's signs and symptoms pose. A guide to the use of radiographic tests for identifying gastrointestinal disease by age group is given in Table 1–1 and discussed below.

There is a tremendous emphasis on the gastrointestinal tract of infants because parents focus on those functions they can observe: ingestion, growth, and the passage of stool and flatus. As children change from infants to young adults, the types of gastrointestinal disease from which they might suffer also change. In addition, a young child who is unable to clearly express discomfort to the caregiver or physician presents a unique challenge to the pediatric specialist, who gathers information secondhand from parents who offer their interpretation of their child's signs and symptoms.

DISORDERS OF INGESTION

Normal feeding is an important factor in a child's growth, in the development of normal swallowing patterns and oromotor reflexes, and in parent-child bonding. Many potential obstacles can interfere with this process, including prematurity, congenital anatomic anomalies, alterations in metabolism, and socioeconomic factors. At times, children are unable to accomplish normal nutritive feeding, and enteral tube feeding and parenteral feeding have surfaced as alternate means of providing nutrition.

Transfer Dysphagia

Deglutination of amniotic fluid can be demonstrated at 16 to 17 weeks of gestation (Humphrey, 1967), and subsequent coordination of sucking, swallowing, and breathing is well established in the term infant. Difficulties with this process can be due to grossly apparent congenital anomalies including choanal atresia (in which the child cannot inspire

TABLE 1–1.   Radiographic Tests for Identifying Gastrointestinal Disease by Child Age

Test	Age (Growth Stage)		
	Infant	*Child*	*Adolescent*
Barium swallow and esophagraphy	Esophageal stenosis Tracheoesophageal fistula Oropharyngeal dysphagia Hiatus hernia Congenital web	Foreign body ingestion Caustic ingestion Hiatus hernia Achalasia	Schatzki's ring Hiatus hernia Peptic stricture Achalasia
Upper GI / SBFT	Intestinal malrotation Pyloric stenosis Duodenal atresia Annular pancreas	Intestinal malrotation Hiatus hernia Duodenal / gastric ulcer Ménétrier's disease Crohn's disease	Intestinal malrotation Hiatus hernia Duodenal ulcer Crohn's disease
Barium enema	Hirschsprung disease Intussusception	Intussusception Hirschsprung disease Sigmoid volvulus	Intussusception Sigmoid volvulus

Abdominal US	Pyloric stenosis
	Choledochal cyst
	Gallstones
		Uretero-pelvic junction
		  obstruction
		Biliary obstruction, gallstones
		Pancreatitis, pseudocyst
		Portal hypertension
		  (with Doppler)
		Appendicitis
			Uretero-pelvic junction
			  obstruction
			Biliary obstruction, gallstones
			Pancreatitis, pseudocyst
			Portal hypertension
			  (with Doppler)
			Ovarian torsion
			Appendicitis

Nuclear medicine	Biliary atresia (DISIDA) Delayed gastric emptying Aspiration	Meckel's diverticulum Occult GI bleeding	Occult GI bleeding Biliary dyskinesis Gastroparesis

GI, gastrointestinal series; SBFT, small bowel follow through; US, ultrasonography; DISIDA, diisopropyl iminodiacetic acid.

nasally while sucking) or cleft lip (in which the infant cannot properly form a seal around the nipple). Painful infectious stomatitis (i.e., herpes virus or Coxsackie virus) is a more common cause of transient refusal to eat. These and other difficulties with the oral phase of swallowing can be assessed at the bedside by the trained physician or speech pathologist. However, the complex array of coordinated actions that occur in the veiled space beyond the lips and that define the pharyngeal and esophageal portions of the swallow can only be inferred by the clinician. Specialized tests have been developed to reveal these functions, including videofluoroscopy, ultrasonography (US), radionuclide

imaging, fiber-optic endoscopy of swallowing, and cervical auscultation (Lefton-Greif and Loughlin, 1996). Indeed, without videofluoroscopy, clinicians have been shown to miss as much as 40% of aspiration events or subtle findings involving incoordination of swallow that vary with the viscosity of the solid or liquid (Logeman, 1983; Zerilli et al., 1990).

True Dysphagia

Although true dysphagia is rare in children, the sensation of food being "stuck" can be a manifestation of a congenital anatomic obstruction or impingement upon the esophagus, as with aberrant vascular structures, incomplete recanalization of the esophagus (i.e., esophageal atresia, stenosis, or web), or dynamic pathology such as a Schatzki's ring. These are best demonstrated by contrast studies of the esophagus. Alternatively, dysphagia may be the presenting symptom of reflux esophagitis in the absence of a suggestive history or peptic stricture. This often resolves with empiric treatment with anti-reflux or acid blockade therapy (Catto-Smith et al., 1991). One must consider the ingestion of a foreign body as a potential etiology as well, particularly in toddlers and young infants who are first developing their oromotor skills. Etiologies of dysphagia can be further elucidated by esophagoscopy (to detect eosinophilic esophagitis) and manometry (to detect achalasia).

Esophagitis

Inflammation of the esophagus may be due to regurgitation of acidic gastric contents onto the squamous epithelium. Most gastroesophageal reflux is thought to be secondary to inappropriate relaxation of the lower esophageal sphincter. The discovery of effective acid-blocking agents (H_2 blockers and proton pump inhibitors) has dramatically improved the gastroenterologist's ability to treat acid-related injury. Patients with symptoms of epigastric pain, heartburn, dysphagia, and halitosis often improve with empiric therapy and warrant no further investigation. Rarely, a child with persistent symptoms despite treatment may have a hiatus hernia demonstrated by contrast esophagography. Other causes of esophagitis can be seen in susceptible hosts, including infection with *Candida*, cytomegalovirus (CMV), or herpes in the immunocompromised host, or eosinophilic infiltration in the atopic individual. In these instances, acid blockade typically does not provide symptomatic relief, and esophagoscopy and biopsy are required to establish the diagnosis.

Regurgitation

The effortless regurgitation of gastric contents is characteristic of infants who have inappropriate relaxation of the lower esophageal sphincter and/or delayed gastric emptying. This can be exacerbated by any process that affects gastrointestinal motility. Because most infants will outgrow this tendency as they are introduced to solid foods and begin to sit and stand erect, further investigation or treatment is not typically warranted. However, treatment is indicated if the regurgitation is thought to be contribut-

ing to poor weight gain (through loss of nutrients), respiratory problems (i.e., aspiration pneumonia, reactive airways disease, or apnea), or pain due to esophagitis. Continuous pH monitoring of the esophagus can quantify the amount of gastroesophageal reflux and help to establish temporal relationships between reflux and apnea (Spitzer et al., 1984). Radiographic studies including contrast esophagography (to evaluate for hiatus hernia) or radionuclide milk scan (to quantify the rate of gastric emptying) may be helpful.

Anorexia

Anorexia is a symptom resulting from various cytokines' (i.e., tumor necrosis factor [TNF]-alpha and interleukin-1 [IL-1] beta) modulation of hypothalamic feeding-associated sites, prostaglandin-dependent mechanisms, modification of neurotransmitter systems, and gastrointestinal, metabolic, and endocrine factors. It is associated with acute and chronic states of inflammation, infection, bacterial toxin-mediated injury, malignancy, and necrosis. Long-term anorexia is deleterious and can result in cachexia (Plata-Salaman, 1996). This is of particular concern to the pediatrician, who follows a child's growth and development and who strives to realize the child's potential. Underlying abnormalities rarely manifest as anorexia alone, and the clinician is often aided by localized abdominal pain, relevant medical history, palpable masses, or serologic abnormalities. Inflammation of the proximal intestinal tract is often implicated and is associated with diseases such as celiac sprue, Crohn's disease, and gastroparesis. Contrast radiography of the intestine is often helpful, supplemented by examination of biopsy samples obtained at endoscopy. Various medications or unpalatable elimination diets represent iatrogenic etiologies of anorexia. One must also consider anorexia nervosa as a diagnosis, particularly in adolescents.

ACUTE ABDOMINAL PAIN

Acute abdominal pain can be associated with several life-threatening conditions. Large clinical series reveal that surgical emergencies account for 30 to 38% of cases, medical conditions for 20 to 36%, and nonspecific abdominal pain for 30 to 38% (Jones, 1976). For this reason, the clinician's gathering of history must focus on the age of the patient, recent trauma, prior medical or surgical conditions, and the association of the pain with emesis, bowel movements, and ingestion of food.

Age-related illnesses must be considered, including intussusception and volvulus in children less than 2 years of age; appendicitis and urinary tract infections in school-age children; and appendicitis, urinary infections, pelvic inflammatory disease, and endometriosis in adolescents. Technologic advances and the adaptation of radiographic techniques as adjuncts in these situations have been the subject of many studies. One emergency room study of 354 children aged less than 15 years used plain abdominal radiography and identified 17% of the patients as having potentially life-threatening diseases or conditions (i.e., appendicitis, a foreign body, intussusception) whereas the remaining 83% had minor viral illnesses. Of those with major illness, 93% had at least one of the following five features: prior abdominal surgery, foreign body ingestion, abnormal bowel sounds, abdominal distention, or peritoneal signs (Rothrock et al., 1992). A similar study looked at the use of ultrasonography in 182 pediatric patients with suspected appendicitis. Ultrasonography successfully diagnosed appendicitis in 31 of 38 (82%) of these patients and identified an etiology for the pain in 34 of the 58 children who had other disease processes including ovarian cysts, adnexal torsion, intrauterine pregnancy, intussusception, gallbladder disease, pancreatitis, and pylonephritis (Siegel et al., 1991). Other radiographic modalities are usually reserved for specific settings, as in the use of computed tomography (CT) for abdominal trauma, or the use of air enema for the reduction of iliocolic intussusception.

CHRONIC ABDOMINAL PAIN

Recurrent abdominal pain is one of the most common complaints in childhood. Epidemiologic studies reveal that this is particularly true between the ages of 5 and 15 years, with an overall incidence of 10.8% and with a higher incidence in girls (12.3%) than in boys (9.5%) (Apley and Naish, 1957). Further studies suggest that the vast majority of these children have no identifiable etiology for pain that is typically periumbilical, exacerbated in the setting of stress, and more prevalent in families whose other members suffer from nonspecific abdominal pain. However, 10% of these children are found to have organic etiologies for their pain (Apley, 1975). Clin-

icians therefore try to separate those with organic disease from those without organic disease by history and by physical examination.

Historical clues more commonly seen in children with organic disease include an age of less than 5 years, localization of the pain to a site other than periumbilical, pain that awakes the child from sleep, and persistent emesis or fever. Although many of the organic etiologies can be attributed to lesions in the gastrointestinal tract (including intermittent intussusception, gastritis, esophagitis, inflammatory bowel disease, and constipation), many (such as pancreatitis, gallstones, renal stones, hydronephrosis, ovarian cysts, and mesenteric cysts) cannot be so attributed. Clinicians typically treat children empirically with acid-blocking agents for suspected esophagitis or gastritis or with laxatives for suspected constipation. Intestinal infection with parasites, such as *Giardia*, or carbohydrate malabsorption associated with lactose intolerance (particularly among the black and Asian population) must also be considered. If the history does not suggest these entities or if treatment is unsuccessful, US is often considered as an imaging modality for its ability to inspect all the intra-abdominal organs. However, a study of 106 children aged 5 to 12 years with over 6 months of nonspecific abdominal pain and who were referred to US found that none had an identifiable cause for the pain (van der Meer et al., 1990). A negative finding on an imaging study is often reassuring to the physician and parent, emphasizing that serious organic pathology is not present.

VOMITING

The forceful evacuation of gastric contents is never normal. Of concern in children is the possibility of an anatomic obstruction within the lumen of the gastrointestinal tract. Initial evaluation focuses on identifying the level of obstruction; here, plain-film radiography is very useful. Patients with esophageal obstruction, as seen with achalasia, typically vomit undigested food that is acidic in neither odor nor taste, and chest films may reveal a dilated esophagus with an air-fluid level. Obstruction at the level of the gastric outlet, as seen with pyloric stenosis or duodenal ulcer, presents as nonbilious emesis in which partially digested foodstuff may be present hours after ingestion. Plain abdominal films may reveal a dilated stomach, and contrast films and US have proved to be diagnostic as well. The bilious emesis present with midgut volvulus associated with intestinal malrotation heralds a surgical emergency. Abdominal radiography may reveal a gasless abdomen, and contrast studies and US can be diagnostic. Distal obstructions of the intestine are typically associated with abdominal distention and pain and also have a characteristic pattern on plain radiographs, with multiple air-fluid levels and distended loops of bowel.

Inflammation of the intestinal tract is also a common cause of emesis, particularly secondary to bacterial or viral pathogens that trigger the release of various cytokines that act as proemetics. Metabolic derangements including acidosis as seen in diabetes mellitus or inborn errors of metabolism can also result in emesis. Vomiting can also be present when there is distention of other hollow viscera, including ureters and the biliary tree. In these instances, the associated pain may aid in localizing the affected area, and US may be diagnostic. Finally, one needs to consider central causes of emesis, including brain tumors. Historically, a brain tumor typically results in morning emesis, and there may be abnormalities in the patient's neurologic examination. Computed tomography or MR of the head is used in confirming this diagnosis.

DIARRHEA

Infections are by far the most common causes of acute diarrhea throughout the world. Acute diarrhea remains one of the leading causes of childhood morbidity and mortality in developing nations with an estimated 3 to 5 billion cases per year worldwide and 5 to 18 million deaths per year (Snyder and Merson, 1982). Stool cultures and viral studies are helpful in identifying common pathogens. Infectious causes are typically self-limited, and the diarrhea lasts less than 2 weeks. Radiographic studies may reveal interhaustral indentations or thickening of the small bowel mucosal folds. However, radiography is typically not needed in the diagnosis or management of these entities.

Chronic diarrhea is typically classed as osmotic or secretory, the former being more common. Carbohydrate malabsorption and the subsequent generation of osmotically active particles by colonic bacteria is a common cause of osmotic diarrhea. Deficiency of disaccharidases such as lactase or sucrase-isomaltase can be diagnosed by hydrogen

breath testing after carbohydrate ingestion or by quantification of the enzyme from biopsy samples. Secondary loss of disaccharidases can result from intestinal inflammation as in Crohn's disease, eosinophilic or allergic enteritis, or celiac sprue. Contrast radiographic studies may help to demonstrate thickening of the intestinal folds and flocculation of contrast material due to increased intestinal fluid. However, a tissue diagnosis is required for a specific diagnosis.

Diarrhea of lower volume may also be due to fat malabsorption as seen in patients with the pancreatic insufficiency of cystic fibrosis or Shwachman-Diamond syndrome. These patients often exhibit poor weight gain and may suffer from deficiencies of fat-soluble vitamins. Radiographic studies may demonstrate chronic lung disease in patients with cystic fibrosis, and a lipomatosis pancreas may show on US, or epiphyseal dysplasia in the child with Shwachman-Diamond syndrome. Toddlers may suffer from a nonspecific diarrhea of childhood due to excessive juice intake coupled with decreased fat intake. Secretory diarrheas persist despite the lack of oral intake and often are associated with neuroendocrine tumors most commonly found in the head of the pancreas. Medicines, including prokinetics, may also contribute to diarrhea.

CONSTIPATION

The normal passage of stools typically begins during the first 24 to 36 hours of life with the passage of meconium. This can be significantly delayed in a number of situations. Anatomic abnormalities including imperforate anus or anterior displacement of the anus should be detected early in the child's life. Radiographic studies including contrast studies through fistulas, urethrograms, or ultrasound are often used to guide the surgeon. Hirschsprung disease also results in delayed passage of meconium although the diagnosis is often missed in the neonatal period, with 15% of affected individuals being diagnosed in the first month, 64% by the third month, and 82% by the end of the first year of life (Kleinhaus et al., 1979). Persistent constipation, poor weight gain, and even bloody stools due to enterocolitis may ensue before the proper diagnosis is made. The history is often suggestive, and a tight anal sphincter and colon and absence of stool in the rectal vault on physical examination often help guide the clinician to a diagnosis. A contrast enema that demonstrates a nondistensible rectum, irregular peristaltic contractions, and transition to a dilated proximal colon or manometric evidence of the absence of normal anal reflexes suggests this diagnosis, which is then confirmed by rectal biopsy. Other neonatal patients who have delayed passage of meconium include the premature infant and the ill child.

Toddlers who present with constipation are often of concern to the parent attempting to initiate toilet training. The majority of these patients suffer from functional constipation rather than anatomic abnormalities. However, one should consider hypothyroidism and hypercalcemia as potential metabolic derangements, as well as medicines that could be contributing to the altered colonic motility. The child with functional constipation often has stool-withholding behaviors such as crossing the legs or squatting. Physical examination may reveal palpable stool in the abdomen and a dilated rectum with hard stool palpable at the anal verge. When the history and physical examination are as described here, there appears to be no role for radiographic imaging. Treatment usually involves a laxative, a dietary increase in fiber, and/or behavioral modification. However, radiology can be useful in identifying those patients with fecal loading in a difficult examination (i.e., due to obesity) or when the clinician is concerned about colonic motility disorders (i.e., colonic inertia). In these instances, radiopaque markers are used to assess colonic transit and colonic segmental dysfunction (Zaslavsky et al., 1998). Some literature also exists on the use of evacuating proctography (Fotter, 1998) although this is not a universally excepted technique for evaluating pediatric constipation. Finally, disorders of the spinal cord and associated reflexes involved in normal defecation may present as constipation. A careful neurologic examination and questions concerning urinary function are essential. Patients with histories or physical examinations of concern can be assessed by spinal MR or CT.

GASTROINTESTINAL HEMORRHAGE

Bleeding from the intestinal tract is often categorized by blood loss (occult versus gross blood loss) and by the site of bleeding (upper gastrointestinal tract versus lower intestinal tract, as demarcated by the duodenojejunal junction). Differentiation of upper tract bleeding is often aided by gastric lavage to detect the presence of blood. As with most signs in the pediatric age group, the various etiologies change according to the patient's age.

Upper gastrointestinal bleeding can present as gross hematemesis, "coffee-ground" emesis, or melena. A newborn with hematemesis often can be shown by Apt-Downey test to be vomiting maternal blood swallowed during the birthing process or while breast-feeding. Vomiting of the child's own blood may be secondary to stress-related ulcers, esophagitis, or intraluminal arteriovenous malformations. These are best appreciated by endoscopy once the patient is stabilized. Older children may also suffer from ulcers or, in those patients with portal hypertension, esophageal varices. In these instances, endoscopy again offers the opportunity to identify the source of bleeding and perform invasive maneuvers such as sclerotherapy or banding to stop the bleeding and/or to prevent future bleeding. When the cause of the portal hypertension is unknown, radiographic tests including CT, MRA, (Magnetic Resonance Angiography) or US with Doppler flow often identify the underlying etiology.

Colonic bleeding often occurs secondary to inflammation of the colon. Acute inflammation can be secondary to invasion by bacteria as detected by stool culture. In infants, colitis is often due to milk protein allergy, and empiric formula changes often resolve the colitis, thus obviating the need for further investigation. Infants with Hirschsprung enterocolitis may also present with rectal bleeding. These children typically appear ill, and history will often aid the diagnosis. Older children with rectal bleeding commonly show small amounts of blood after the passage of a painful stool. Physical examination may reveal a rectal fissure, and laxatives often resolve the bleeding and constipation. Painless hematochezia in toddlers and young children is commonly due to either benign juvenile polyps or a Meckel's diverticulum. The polyps are typically inflammatory and sometimes can be palpated on rectal examination. Colonoscopy allows for identification and removal of these lesions. A Meckel's diverticulum that contains ectopic gastric mucosa results in small bowel ulceration and bleeding. This lesion is often difficult to appreciate on contrast studies of the small intestine and too distant to be visualized by endoscopy. Scintigraphic studies using Tc 99m pertechnetate have been developed to detect ectopic gastric mucosa, and allow for diagnosis when seen in the proper clinical setting. Idiopathic colitis associated with either Crohn's disease or ulcerative colitis can also be seen in the pediatric patient. The diagnosis is supported by colonoscopy and biopsy, with histologic evidence of chronic inflammation and granulomas (in Crohn's disease). Radiographic studies including contrast radiography of the small intestine may help differentiate these two entities.

Sources of occult gastrointestinal blood loss may be difficult to identify if they are located in portions of the small intestine that are inaccessible to the endoscope. In these instances, and particularly if the rate of bleeding is brisk, technetium-99m-labeled red-blood-cell scans or angiography are used to localize the site of bleeding. In a study of 11 children with chronic gastrointestinal blood loss but unrevealing endoscopy, 6 had normal angiograms even in the absence of active bleeding (Meyerovitz and Fellows, 1984).

REFERENCES

Apley J, Naish N. Recurrent abdominal pains: a field survey of 1000 school children. Arch Dis Child 1957;33:165–70.

Apley J. The child with abdominal pains. 2nd ed. Oxford: Blackwell; 1975.

Catto-Smith AG, Machida H, Butzner JD, et al. The role of gastroesophageal reflux in pediatric dysphagia. J Pediatr Gastroenterol Nutr 1991;12(2):159–65.

Fotter R. Imaging of constipation in infants and children. Eur Radiol 1998;8(2):248–58.

Humphrey T. Reflex activity in the oral and facial arch of the human fetus. In: Bosma JF, editor. Second symposium on oral sensation and perception. Springfield: Charles C. Thomas; 1967. p. 195.

Jones PF. Active observation in management of acute abdominal pain in childhood. BMJ 1976;2(6035):551–3.

Kirsner JB. The origin of 20th century discoveries transforming clinical gastroenterology. Am J Gastroenterol 1998;93(6):862–71.

Kleinhaus S, Boley SJ, Sheran M, Sieber WK. MR disease: a survey of the members of the surgical section of the American Academy of Pediatrics. J Pediatr Surg 1979;14:588–97.

Lefton-Greif MA, Loughlin GM. Specialized studies in pediatric dysphagia. Semin Speech Lang 1996;17(4):311–29.

Logeman JA. Evaluation and treatment of swallowing disorders. San Diego: College Hill Press; 1983.

Meyerovitz MF, Fellows KE. Angiography in gastrointestinal bleeding in children. Am J Roentgenol 1984;143:837–40.

Plata-Salaman CR. Anorexia during acute and chronic disease. Nutrition 1996;12(2):69–78.

Rothrock SG, Green SM, Hummel CB. Plain abdominal radiography in the detection of major disease in children: a prospective analysis. Ann Emerg Med 1992;21(12):1423–9.

Siegel MJ, Carel C, Surrat S. Ultrasonography of acute abdominal pain in children. JAMA 1991;266:1987–9.

Snyder JD, Merson MH. The magnitude of the global problem of acute diarrheal disease: a review of acute surveillance data. Bull World Health Organ 1982;60:605–13.

Spitzer AR, Boyle JT, Tuchman DN, Fox WW. Awake apnea associated with gastroesophageal reflux: a specific clinical entity. J Pediatr 1984;104(2):200–5.

van der Meer SB, Forget PP, Arends JW, et al. Diagnostic value of ultrasound in children with recurrent abdominal pain. Pediatr Radiol 1990;2:501–3.

Zaslavsky C, da Silveira TR, Maguilnik I. Total and segmental colonic transit time with radio-opaque markers in adolescence with functional constipation. J Pediatr Gastroenterol Nutr 1998;27(2):138–42.

Zerilli KS, Stefans VA, DiPietro MA. Protocol for the use of videofluoroscopy in pediatric swallowing dysfunction. Am J Occup Ther 1990;44(5):441–6.

2

GASTROINTESTINAL IMAGING IN PEDIATRIC SURGERY

Catherine Chen, MD, and Peter C.W. Kim, MDCM, PhD, FRCS(C)

GENERAL CONSIDERATIONS

Children and adults differ greatly in their physiologic responses to illness as well as in the spectrum of disease. The constellation of signs and symptoms that suggest gastrointestinal (GI) disease usually prompts consultation with the pediatric general surgeon. To aid in diagnosis, a thorough history and physical examination should begin every clinical evaluation of the patient. If the patient is a newborn infant or a young child, the parent or guardian becomes a vital source of information. Pertinent questions regarding the acute symptoms should be asked as well as details of prenatal care, nutrition, and environmental or social issues. Further diagnostic and therapeutic investigations often require the expertise of a pediatric radiologist. The timing and type of radiologic study are based on the differential diagnosis at hand after evaluation of all available data. A close working relationship between the pediatric surgeon and the pediatric radiologist ensures timely diagnosis and treatment for the child requiring surgery for GI disease. In this chapter, we aim to provide general guidelines—rather than a comprehensive review of radiologic studies—that can aid in the diagnosis of pediatric surgical problems (Polley et al., 1985) based on clinical presentation (summarized in Table 2–1).

SIGNS AND SYMPTOMS OF GASTROINTESTINAL DISEASE IN CHILDHOOD

Vomiting

Vomiting, or the forceful extrusion of gastric contents, is a common symptom that is never normal. When associated with abdominal pain, the pediatric surgeon must diligently seek a cause of partial or complete obstruction of the intestinal tract anywhere from stomach to cecum. Vomiting in any child with a previous abdominal incision is suggestive of bowel obstruction unless proved otherwise. The color of the emesis can be diagnostic. Bile-stained emesis in a neonate should be immediately evaluated by a pediatric surgeon and usually indicates obstruction distal to the second part of the duodenum. The more distal the obstruction, the greater is the likelihood of abdominal distention.

Congenital defects often presenting with bilious emesis in the newborn include bowel atresia, intestinal web, malrotation with possible midgut volvulus, Hirschsprung disease, and meconium ileus. Plain-film radiography can help delineate proximal or distal bowel obstruction. Contrast enema is the next study of choice and may demonstrate a microcolon with distal small bowel atresia, an abnormally located cecum in malrotation, a transition zone in colon suggestive of Hirschsprung disease, or inspissated meconium plugs within a microcolon in meconium ileus. If malrotation is suspected, an upper gastrointestinal (UGI) contrast study can also be done to confirm abnormal location of the duodenal-jejunal junction.

Nonbilious emesis in the young infant should prompt a work-up for gastric outlet obstruction. In the first 2 months of life, the most common cause is pyloric stenosis. If the pathognomonic olive is not palpable, abdominal ultrasonography can accurately diagnose the thickness of the pyloric muscle with measurements of length and wall thickness. Upper GI series can also be obtained if ultrasonography is

TABLE 2–1.   Summary of Useful Radiologic Modalities Based on Presenting Clinical Symptoms

Symptom	Radiologic Imaging
Vomiting	
Bilious	AXR 2 views
	Ba enema
	UGI
Nonbilious	Abd US
	UGI
Dysphagia	CXR 2 views
	UGI
Abdominal Pain	
Acute	AXR 2 views
	Abd US
	ACE (intussusception)
	UGI (malrotation)
Chronic	AXR 2 views
	UGI, Ba enema, Abd US, Abd CT as indicated
Constipation	AXR 2 views
	Ba enema
GI hemorrhage	Abd US (intussusception, enteric cyst)
	Ba enema (Hirschsprung)
	Tc-99m pertechnetate scan (Meckel's diverticulum)
Jaundice	Abd US
	DISIDA or Tc-99m scan
Trauma	Cspine views, CXR, pelvis x-ray
	Abd CT

Abbreviations: Abd CT = abdominal CT scan; Abd US = abdominal ultrasound; ACE = air contrast enema; AXR = abdominal x-ray; Ba enema = barium or contrast enema; Cspine = cervical spine; CXR = chest x-ray; DISIDA = disopropyl iminodiacetic acid; UGI = upper gastrointestinal series.

not definitive and may show the "string sign" consistent with an elongated and narrow pyloric channel. The upper GI series may demonstrate other causes of nonbilious emesis, such as gastroesophageal reflux (GER) or pylorospasm.

The syndrome of GER was originally described in 1935. Various methods of operative repair of the hiatus to correct GER have been popular since the 1940s. In normal patients, the anatomy and physiol-ogy of the gastroesophageal (GE) junction act to prevent reflux of the gastric juice into the esophagus. Anatomic factors include the phrenoesophageal ligament, the angle of His, and the properties of the gastric mucosa at the GE junction. Important physiologic factors include the lower esophageal sphincter, the length of intra-abdominal esophagus, the difference between intra-abdominal and intrathoracic pressures, and mediators of gastric acid secretion, such as gastrin, prostaglandins, and catecholamines.

Vomiting is the most common clinical symptom of GER. A spectrum of disease can result, ranging from gradual resolution of symptoms over the first 2 years of life as children resume a more upright posture to progressive failure to thrive and aspiration pneumonia. Vomiting may be subtle and present only as bronchospasm, often confused with asthma. Significant GER may be associated with esophagitis and subsequent development of diffuse esophageal spasm, chronic anemia, and stricture formation. Factors that contribute to the development of GER include delayed gastric emptying, gastric outlet obstruction, intestinal obstruction, and central nervous system disorders. Gastroesophageal reflux is also frequently seen in children with esophageal atresia and tracheoesophageal fistula or congenital diaphragmatic hernia.

The diagnosis of GER usually begins with a barium swallow and UGI series. These studies can document GER with the aid of fluoroscopy and can also demonstrate associated findings of esophageal dysmotility, hiatus hernia, mucosal inflammation with esophagitis, and stricture. Therapeutically, it is important to distinguish GER from other esophageal neuromotor disorders such as achalasia, diffuse esophageal spasm, and scleroderma. Mentally retarded children have a significant incidence of delayed gastric emptying and GER, which can be diagnosed by UGI series or, more accurately, by technetium-99m pertechnetate nuclear scan. If the barium swallow and UGI series are normal but GER is suspected clinically, a 24-hour pH monitoring study can most accurately diagnose GER. Esophagoscopy and distal esophageal biopsy may be helpful for the diagnosis of esophagitis and Barrett's esophagus, and esophageal manometry can evaluate esophageal motility and lower esophageal sphincter pressure.

Treatment of GER should begin with non-operative therapy. Medical therapy includes upright positioning, thickened feedings, a prokinetic agent such as metoclopramide, and an H_2 blocker. Over 80% of infants respond to medical therapy and do not require a fundoplication. Some authors do not recommend surgery in any patient less than 6 months of age because of the potential for spontaneous resolution of symptoms. Medical treatment is continued for a few months in infants and for 6 to 8 weeks in older children after which the risk of esophagitis and stricture increases. Indications for fundoplication include failure of medical therapy and development of complications such as severe esophagitis, Barrett's metaplasia, stricture, and significant bleeding. Operative management of GER includes a fundoplication, most commonly the Nissen 360° complete wrap or the anterior 270° partial wrap. If significant delayed gastric emptying is present, some authors recommend adding a gastric emptying procedure, such as pyloroplasty, to the fundoplication as well as gastrostomy. Neurologically impaired children with GER have also been managed by radiologic placement of gastrostomy and jejunal tubes.

Dysphagia

True dysphagia is uncommon in children. However, in newborns, the most common anatomic cause is esophageal atresia (EA). Infants with EA tend to drool and often have episodes of choking, coughing, and cyanosis related to difficulties in managing pharyngeal secretions. The diagnosis is usually entertained when there is difficulty passing a nasogastric tube through the mouth or nose into the stomach. Plain chest radiographs often confirm the atresia with a proximal pouch. On the abdominal portions of the plain films, a gasless abdomen confirms the presence of EA without tracheoesophageal fistula (TEF). Contrast studies are not generally necessary for diagnosis and carry a risk of contrast-medium aspiration.

In older children, ingestion of foreign bodies can cause dysphagia if the objects lodge in the esophagus at the level of the cricopharyngeus or the diaphragmatic hiatus. Plain chest radiographs confirm the type, size, and location of the esophageal foreign body, which is then removed by rigid esophagoscopy if the object has not passed into the stomach. Corrosive damage to the esophagus can be a devastating consequence of ingestion of lye or acid. Plain chest radiographs may demonstrate severe edema of the soft tissues of the neck and mediastinum. If perforation has occurred, mediastinal emphysema or pneumoperitoneum may be evi-

dent. Esophagoscopy is usually performed within the first 24 hours for diagnosis. A barium swallow within the first 48 hours following injury can assess esophageal motility. Subsequent follow-up contrast studies are often obtained in severe cases to diagnose stricture formation. Contrast studies are also helpful in children who have undergone prior repair of EA or TEF and who present with dysphagia. Stricture formation from persistent GER or the presence of a foreign body or food bolus at the anastomosis can be diagnosed.

Perforation of the esophagus after traumatic injury or after endoscopic instrumentation is suspected in a child with fever, dysphagia, and anterior chest pain. Plain-film radiography may document mediastinal emphysema; water-soluble contrast studies are often confirmatory.

Acute Abdominal Pain

Children with acute abdominal pain often present with associated symptoms of fever, vomiting, diarrhea, or GI bleeding. The history and physical examination are of paramount importance for diagnosis. Causes of acute abdominal pain vary according to the age of the patient. Likely diagnoses to consider in children less than 2 years of age include intestinal obstruction from intussusception or malrotation with midgut volvulus. Appendicitis is less common in the very young child. Other causes of acute abdominal pain in young children include gastroenteritis, urinary infections, and pneumonia. Plain-film radiography followed by ultrasonography is helpful in the diagnosis of intussusception or appendicitis. If an intussusception is seen on ultrasonography, an attempt should be made at reduction, using air contrast or barium enema. If reduction does not occur immediately, several more attempts should be made before abandoning the procedure. Therapeutic enema studies should only be performed at pediatric centers where pediatric surgeons are available to take a child to the operating room if a perforation occurs or if repeated reduction is not successful. Children presenting with bilious emesis and bowel obstruction should undergo plain-film radiography followed by UGI contrast study to assess the location of the duodenal-jejunal flexure. The UGI series remains the gold standard for the diagnosis of malrotation. Critically ill patients with a bowel obstruction should proceed directly to operative abdominal exploration rather than further radiologic investigation.

In children older than 2 years of age, acute appendicitis remains the most common cause of acute abdominal pain. Other causes include constipation, acute pancreatitis, inflammatory bowel disease, diabetic ketoacidosis, and cholelithiasis. Adhesive bowel obstruction should be considered in any child presenting with bilious emesis and a prior abdominal incision. Plain-film radiography and ultrasonography are most helpful if acute appendicitis is not definitively diagnosed by history and physical examination.

Chronic Abdominal Pain

Recurrent chronic abdominal pain is often difficult to diagnose and frustrating to treat for the pediatrician or pediatric surgeon. History of onset of pain, characteristics of pain, and family history are important to elicit. In older children between ages 7 and 12 years, an organic cause for chronic abdominal pain is not found in 90 to 95% of patients. The differential diagnosis should include mechanical bowel obstruction, postoperative adhesions, lactose intolerance, peptic ulcer disease, inflammatory bowel disease, and chronic functional constipation. Meconium ileus equivalent should be considered in children with cystic fibrosis. Depending on the symptomatology, plain-film radiography, UGI and enema contrast studies, endoscopy, ultrasonography, and abdominal computed tomography (CT) may be revealing. Investigations should be kept to a minimum, unless specifically indicated. If no organic cause is found, patients and families should be reassured and encouraged to continue regular school and extracurricular activities.

Constipation

Constipation is defined as difficulty or delay in the passage of stool. In newborn infants, failure to pass meconium within the first 48 hours of life is highly suggestive of Hirschsprung disease and virtually diagnostic in several large series (Rowe et al., 1995; Scherer, 1995). Other clinical presentations can include low intestinal obstruction with or without sepsis and associated enterocolitis. The age at diagnosis of Hirschsprung disease is variable, and approximately half the patients in the United States are diagnosed in the neonatal period. In older children or adults, the diagnosis is usually made during evaluation for chronic constipation. Chronic abdominal distention is a characteristic finding in older children. Malnutri-

tion and failure to thrive may be seen but is less common in the developed nations.

The differential diagnosis of functional constipation in older children should include severe chronic dehydration, idiopathic hypocalcemia, diabetes insipidus, cystinosis, hypokalemia, hypermagnesemia, and hypothyroidism. Children with chronic disabilities resulting from cerebral palsy, spinal cord lesions that cause sphincter dysfunction, delayed development, cancer, or chronic malnutrition are frequently constipated. Diagnostic studies usually include plain-film radiography of the abdomen, barium enema, and confirmation by full-thickness rectal biopsy.

Gastrointestinal Hemorrhage

Gastrointestinal hemorrhage can present with melena and/or hematemesis. Initial assessment of any child with presumed GI bleed should include large bore intravenous access, coagulation studies, blood type and screen, and a nasogastric tube to assess gastric aspirates. Blood in gastric aspirates and/or passage of melena imply an upper source of GI hemorrhage. The differential diagnosis of GI bleed in childhood varies with age. In the newborn period, true hematemesis should be distinguished from vomiting of swallowed maternal blood. A generalized bleeding diathesis and stress gastritis may follow birth asphyxia or sepsis and present with upper intestinal bleeding. Other causes include congenital lesions such as hemangiomas, arteriovenous malformations, or GI duplication cysts. Rectal bleeding in a newborn infant may be due to necrotizing enterocolitis, bacterial or milk-induced enterocolitis, malrotation with midgut volvulus, or enterocolitis associated with Hirschsprung disease.

In older children, hematemesis and melena are uncommon. Upper GI causes include peptic ulcer disease or diffuse gastritis, esophagitis from severe GE reflux, and esophageal varices in children with portal hypertension. Bleeding disorders associated with leukemia or thrombocytopenia, Henoch-Schönlein purpura, and hemolytic uremic syndrome can present with upper or lower GI bleeding. Fresh blood per rectum should prompt a work-up for Meckel's diverticulum, colonic juvenile polyps, ulcerative colitis, or anal fissure. Acute abdominal pain with blood per rectum is seen in 95% of infants with idiopathic intussusception.

Most episodes of upper GI bleeding are self-limited and cease when correction of coagulopathy is achieved or acid-reducing agents are begun for stress gastritis. Radiologic studies are indicated if the differential diagnosis includes surgical conditions, such as Hirschsprung disease with enterocolitis, gut duplication cysts, intussusception, or Meckel's diverticulum. Ultrasonography is helpful for diagnosis of duplication cysts and intussusception; the contrast enemas with barium are diagnostic for Hirschsprung disease, and air contrast enemas are therapeutic for reduction of intussusception. A bleeding Meckel's diverticulum can be diagnosed by a technetium-99m pertechnetate isotope scan, which images the gastric mucosa often found within the diverticulum. Occasionally, endoscopy may be necessary to confirm the presence of esophageal varices or biopsy for the suspected colonic polyps or inflammatory bowel disease.

Jaundice

Neonatal jaundice is common and is most often due to immaturity of the enzyme glucuronyl transferase. Hyperbilirubinemia in physiologic jaundice is therefore predominantly due to an increase in the indirect unconjugated fraction. Initiation of enteral feeds stimulates the enzyme system and usually leads to the resolution of jaundice within 7 to 10 days. Jaundice persisting more than 2 weeks is pathologic and should prompt further investigation.

The differential diagnosis for persistent neonatal jaundice is wide and varied. Nonsurgical causes include Rh and ABO incompatibility, breast feeding, hemolytic disease (spherocytosis), Gilbert disease, and Crigler-Najjar syndrome. Infants in whom more than 20% of the total bilirubin is direct should be evaluated for cholestasis or biliary obstruction. A number of conditions can cause cholestasis or obstruction: systemic infections (bacterial, viral, Toxoplasma), genetic or metabolic disorders (alpha1-antitrypsin deficiency, galactosemia, tyrosinemia, cystic fibrosis, Gaucher's disease, iron storage disease), neonatal hepatitis, biliary atresia, choledochal cyst, inspissated bile plug syndrome, bile duct compression, parenteral alimentation cholestasis, bile duct stricture, spontaneous perforation of the bile duct, and intrahepatic cholestasis from arteriohepatic dysplasia (Alagille syndrome) and Byler's disease.

Most nonsurgical causes of neonatal jaundice can be excluded within the first month of age. The pediatric gastroenterologist or surgeon is often faced with a difficult diagnosis of biliary atresia or neonatal jaundice, which are often clinically difficult to distinguish. Helpful diagnostic studies include abdominal ultrasonography, which may demonstrate a choledochal cyst or absence of the gallbladder suggestive of biliary atresia. A technetium-99m or disopropyl iminodiacetic acid (DISIDA) scintiscan will demonstrate failure of hepatic clearance of the isotope in complete biliary obstruction, also suggestive but not diagnostic of biliary atresia. Percutaneous liver biopsy followed by a limited exploratory laparotomy with direct cholangiography by 10 weeks of age is often needed to confirm or exclude the diagnosis of biliary atresia. If biliary atresia is documented, the porta hepatis is explored, and a bypass is performed with a Kasai hepatic portoenterostomy.

TRAUMATIC INJURY IN THE PEDIATRIC PATIENT

Management of the critically injured pediatric trauma patient requires prompt recognition and treatment of life-threatening injuries. Radiographic evaluation plays a key role in the assessment of the trauma patient after standard Advanced Trauma Life Support (ATLS) procedures are followed to secure an airway and adequate circulation with intravenous access. After immediate plain-film evaluation of the cervical spine, chest, and pelvis, the patient is stabilized and may require CT of the abdomen to further evaluate abdominal injuries. Children with penetrating abdominal injuries that violate the peritoneum, those with blunt injuries remaining hemodynamically unstable after resuscitation, and those with peritonitis on physical examination should forego abdominal CT evaluation and should be taken directly to the operating room.

Computed tomography is the most frequently used imaging modality to assess traumatic abdominal injuries and has replaced diagnostic peritoneal lavage as the procedure of choice in hemodynamically stable children. Intravenous and GI contrast enhancement should be used. In addition to detection of solid organ injury, especially to liver, spleen, pancreas, and kidneys, CT can identify intraperitoneal or retroperitoneal blood, fluid, or air and bony abnormalities of the pelvis. Hollow-organ injuries to the bowel may be suggested by subtle findings such as free intraperitoneal fluid or bowel wall thickening. Bladder injuries may not be apparent on abdominal CT unless the bladder is fully distended by clamping a Foley catheter. More commonly, bladder injuries are confirmed by multiple-view cystography. Ultrasound examinations of the abdomen in the emergency department have been used in Europe to detect intraperitoneal fluid and solid-organ injury but remain controversial in the United States. Current recommendations for abdominal CT in trauma include children with physical signs and symptoms of abdominal injury, multisystem injuries including head trauma, gross hematuria, and known high-energy mechanism of injury (Swenson et al., 1975).

REFERENCES

Polley TZ, Coran AG, Wesley JR. A ten-year experience with 92 cases of Hirschsprung disease. Ann Surg 1985;202:349–55.

Rowe MI, O'Neill JA Jr, Grosfeld JL, et al. Essentials of pediatric surgery. St. Louis: Mosby;1995.

Scherer LR III. Diagnostic imaging in pediatric trauma. Semin Pediatr Surg 1995;4:100–8.

Swenson O, Sherman JO, Fisher JH, Cohen E. The treatment and postoperative complications of congenital megacolon: a twenty-five year follow-up. Ann Surg 1975; 182:266–73.

3

TECHNIQUES FOR INVESTIGATION OF THE PEDIATRIC GASTROINTESTINAL TRACT

David A. Stringer, BSc, MBBS, FRCR, FRCPC, and
Helen Nadel, MD, FRCPC (Nuclear Medicine)

GENERAL CONSIDERATIONS

The indications and techniques for examining the gastrointestinal tract in children, particularly in infants, are often different from those of adults. Significant morbidity and mortality can result from a carelessly or improperly performed technical procedure. Inability to complete a procedure because of poor patient cooperation is often due to the failure of the examiner rather than the child. Children usually cooperate if the approach is considerate and confident. Great care must be taken to inform the child of the exact nature of each procedure in an appropriate, friendly, and reassuring manner. For invasive procedures in infants and young children, sedation may be necessary but it is rarely if ever indicated for noninvasive techniques.

There is no substitute for a careful history and physical examination in the clinical evaluation of patients. The subsequent investigation of the child depends on these findings, and a good rapport between referring physician and radiologist ensures expeditious and safe radiologic tests with a minimum of distress or harm to the patient. Ionizing radiation is potentially harmful and can cause chromosomal anomalies especially to cells undergoing mitosis. In addition, the risk of neoplasia is of concern in children due to their long life expectancy. Ultrasonography (US) is therefore the initial modality of choice in the investigation of many pediatric abdominal conditions. Bowel gas in the gastrointestinal tract reduces the usefulness of US, so contrast studies are often used instead. The subsequent investigation depends on these findings in conjunction with the clinical assessment. The value of each modality and the techniques involved are discussed in this chapter.

ULTRASONOGRAPHY

Ultrasonography should be considered the first choice in the radiologic investigation of any child, as US is a radiation-free procedure that requires little or no preparation. As far as is known, it is completely safe when used for diagnosis. In children, lack of fat planes and smaller size make US generally easier to perform and more reliable than in adults (Cremin, 1985). Ultrasonography is not organ-dependent, as it can view many organs simultaneously. In children, we have found it better than computed tomography (CT) or magnetic resonance imaging (MR) for investigating cystic or other benign lesions. Ultrasonography is our first choice for investigating many lesions in infants or small children as they have less intra-abdominal fat to degrade the ultrasonography and not enough to

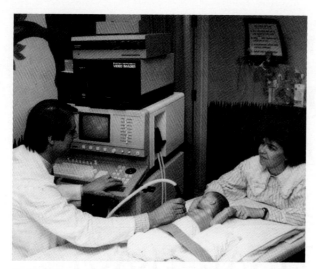

FIGURE 3–1. Sonography of an infant. The infant's legs are restrained by wrapping them in a towel. An assistant provides minimal restraint to the arms.

enhance the CT. However, in many other instances, US and CT are complementary and together give a high diagnostic accuracy (Brasch, 1980). Generally, US is the first cross-sectional imaging modality used, with CT and MR reserved for situations where US fails to provide the diagnosis or when more complete information is required (Holm, 1977).

Ultrasonography may be performed without sedation; minimal restraint may be necessary for infants and small children (Figure 3–1). Feeding an infant by bottle prior to or during an investigation often settles a baby and permits a satisfactory examination. Explanation and demonstration of US are usually sufficient to allay the fears of older children.

Preparation of the Patient

To evaluate the upper abdomen including the gallbladder, the child should be fasting. The length of the fast depends on the age and clinical status of the child but the following times are commonly used: 4 hours for infants (under 1 year of age), 6 hours for young children (1 to 2 years of age), and 8 hours for older children. To fill the bladder, which is necessary for pelvic examinations, water is given to older children. In infants and young children there is a certain amount of luck involved in catching the bladder full. The presence of a suprapubic transducer often stimulates urination, and only patience, perseverance, and a modicum of luck will permit a successful examination. Catheterization of the bladder is rarely if ever indicated.

The stomach can have a variable appearance depending on its contents (Figure 3–2). To exclude hypertrophic pyloric stenosis in young infants, the stomach should be filled with a glucose solution either by feeding from a bottle or via a nasogastric tube. Only by adequately distending the stomach in this way can gastric hyperperistalsis, pyloric tumor, and inadequate gastric emptying be fully appreciated (Figure 3–3).

To evaluate the gastric wall or gastroesophageal reflux in an older child, the stomach also needs to be full of fluid. The child is instructed to drink water prior to these examinations.

Fetal Ultrasonography

Open neural tube defects such as spina bifida or anencephaly can be diagnosed by US. The clinician is alerted to the possibility of these conditions by finding a raised alpha-fetoprotein level in maternal serum at about 15 weeks' gestation. Alpha-fetoprotein is produced in the fetal liver, gastrointestinal tract, and yolk sac and is excreted in the urine, reaching a maximum concentration in the amniotic fluid at approximately 15 weeks' gestation, falling

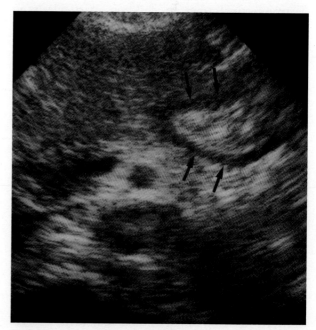

FIGURE 3–2. Normal gastric sonography. The stomach is full of echogenic food and the gastric antral muscle (*arrows*) is normal. To exclude hypertrophic pyloric stenosis in young infants, the stomach may be filled with a glucose solution either by bottle-feeding or via a nasogastric tube.

thereafter. Excessively high alpha-fetoprotein levels are detected in maternal serum and amniotic fluid when there is an open neural tube defect or an esophageal or duodenal atresia. Fetal US can detect all these conditions.

Dilated loops of bowel are easily seen by US and usually indicate the need for surgery (Estroff, 1992). There is also some evidence of an increased incidence of cystic fibrosis in this group of patients (Estroff, 1992). Polyhydramnios is associated with serious congenital abnormalities in about 20% of cases (Alexander, 1982), and these should be sought diligently. Ultrasonography is increasingly used to diagnose a variety of antenatal disorders associated with polyhydramnios, such as diaphragmatic hernia (Bennacerraf, 1986), duodenal (Farrant, 1981) or jejunal atresia, meconium ileus and peritonitis (Lince, 1985; McGahan, 1983; Denholm, 1984) omphalocele (Brown, 1985; Nelson, 1982; Grignon, 1986), and gastroschisis (Chinn, 1983; Grignon, 1986; Emmanuel, 1995), as well as associated renal, cardiac, or skeletal abnormalities. Thus, time and place of delivery can be planned so that the abnormality can be dealt with expeditiously after birth.

Neonatal and Young Infants

In the neonate and young infant, excellent visualization of many abdominal organs is possible because of the lack of fat and the small size of the patient. Ultrasonography is particularly useful in diagnosing hypertrophic pyloric stenosis (Pilling, 1983), gallstones (Brill, 1982), and eventration. Ultrasonography can also show the situs of abdominal and, occasionally, thoracic structures and can demonstrate vascular

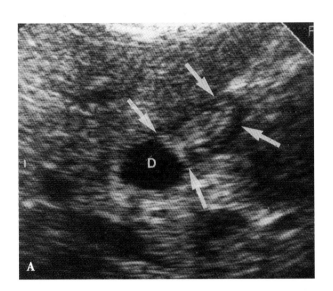

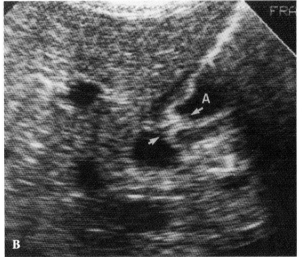

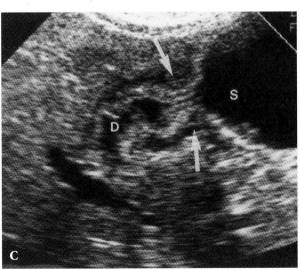

FIGURE 3–3. Normal gastric sonography. *A*, An initial image shows a somewhat long gastric antrum and pylorus (*between arrows*) proximal to a fluid-filled duodenal cap (D). *B*, With more fluid instilled into the stomach the antrum fills (A) and the short pyloric canal can be seen (*arrows*). *C*, With further filling of the stomach, waves of peristalsis (*between arrows*) can be seen passing from the body of the stomach (S) into the antrum, pushing fluid on into the duodenal cap (D).

anomalies or occlusion (Oppenheimer, 1982). In addition, US may show the defect in anorectal malformations as well as any associated renal anomalies.

Older Infants and Children

In older infants and children, US is particularly useful in evaluating the liver, biliary tree (McGahan, 1982), pancreas, spleen, and mass lesions. Ultrasonography can differentiate between cystic and solid lesions with great accuracy. Abscesses can be localized and drained under ultrasonographic guidance; this is the commonest interventional procedure in children at our hospital. Even the bowel can be evaluated to some extent (Stringer, 1986). The gastric wall can easily be examined and mass lesions, inflammatory bowel disease, and intussusceptions can all be visualized in the more distal portions of the bowel.

The value of range-gated duplex Doppler US is still being assessed but early findings indicate that it can be useful in demonstrating presence and direction of flow and flow profiles in the major abdominal vessels. We have found it most helpful in evaluating portal hypertension by showing abnormal or absent portal vein flow and the presence of any collateral circulation (Stringer, 1985). It is also helpful in managing the post-liver transplant patient, especially as the procedure can be performed at the intensive care bedside of these often very sick children (Stringer, 1985).

RADIOGRAPHY: PLAIN FILMS

The aim in pediatric radiology is to keep radiation dosage to the minimum needed to obtain the required diagnostic information. This is achieved by using fast film-screen combinations, no grid in smaller children, and preferably Kevlar or carbon fiber cassettes when plain films are taken. Digital radiographic techniques can further reduce radiation dosage (Stringer, 1994; Kottamasu, 1997), and the most available and economic at present are the stimulable phosphor systems where a latent image is captured on a europium-doped phosphor plate and subsequently read by a laser reader (Stringer, 1994; Kottamasu, 1997).

Gas patterns in the abdomen can be used to assess gut anatomic and functional status. Gas is usually present in the stomach within 10 to 15 minutes of birth. If the stomach does not contain gas after 1 hour, esophageal obstruction should be suspected. The presence of gas in the stomach has been advocated as proof that respiration occurred after birth (Dillon, 1942); however, it has been shown that in the first minute of life some normal neonates do not have air in the stomach (Boreadis, 1956). Gas normally reaches the proximal small bowel within an hour and has filled most of the small bowel by 6 hours. The large bowel is filled by 13 to 14 hours (Frimann-Dahl, 1954; Hajdu, 1955), often with passage of meconium within the same period of time.

In neonates with respiratory distress, a chest radiograph is taken to assess the lungs and to exclude extrapulmonary causes such as diaphragmatic hernia and to assess for esophageal atresia, tracheoesophageal fistula, and mass lesions.

Abdominal plain films are helpful in the neonate with bowel obstruction and are often sufficient to make the diagnosis or at least indicate the next investigation. Duodenal and proximal jejunal atresia have a characteristic plain-film appearance. In more distal obstruction, the large bowel mimics the appearance of the small bowel in the neonatal period. Large and small bowel may be differentiated on lateral views, as the ascending and descending parts of the colon overlie the spine whereas the small bowel is located more anteriorly. The level or cause of the obstruction may be suspected by associated findings such as the bubbly pattern produced by meconium ileus, calcification following meconium peritonitis, gas within a hernial sac, or gas in the bladder from a high anorectal malformation. Plain films are also crucial in the early diagnosis and management of neonatal necrotizing enterocolitis.

In older children, plain films help in the assessment of foreign bodies, obstruction, and intra-abdominal gas, fluid, or calcification. The appearances on film of these conditions in children are similar to those in adults. (Detailed descriptions of plain-film findings can be found in subsequent chapters.)

RADIOGRAPHY: CONTRAST EXAMINATIONS

General Principles

In children, the indications for, and techniques of, the examinations are different from those in adults. The type of examination depends on clinical circumstances more so than in adults. In children, congenital abnormalities, such as malrotation, occur much more frequently than ulcers or tumors, which are rare. There is more risk in the procedures, particularly in the neonatal period, and a number of fatalities have occurred. Therefore, contrast examinations should not be performed on infants or young children by radiologists who are inexperienced in pediatric examinations.

Radiation dosages should be kept to a minimum. A grid should be used only for the largest patients on spot or overhead tube films when extra detail is required as in double-contrast examinations. Otherwise, films taken without a grid are sufficiently diagnostic. The 100- or 105-mm spot films give a lower dosage than full-size radiography (Soini, 1983) but if these are not available, the fastest film-screen combination that will give adequate diagnostic information should be used, preferably with Kevlar or carbon fiber cassettes. Videorecording the procedures is relatively cheap and often obviates the need for repeat fluoroscopy.

Further dosage reduction is possible by using a digitized last-image hold to reduce fluoroscopy time (Hynes, 1985; Stringer, 1986). Digital photospot technology is opening the way to further dosage reduction by soft copy or by hard copy stored images, obviating the need for additional exposures as well as allowing manipulation and edge enhancement of images.

Cleanliness in the fluoroscopy suite is essential. Neonates are fed only sterile food in the nursery, and ideally they should receive only canned, sterile contrast media when in the radiology department. Water-soluble contrast media are usually sterile but many barium preparations are not. Fortunately, many of these barium preparations are acceptable, as they have extremely low bacterial counts and are cheaper. The decision as to which barium to use will vary from country to country, but the avoidance of infection is the universal guiding principle.

Choice of Contrast Media

There are a number of available contrast media, which may be divided into three main groups: barium sulfate, water-soluble contrast media, and gas (usually air). Which contrast medium to use will depend on the diagnostic problem and procedure. Some general principles are discussed below.

Barium Sulfate
Barium sulfate is the most common contrast medium and is used unless there is a contraindication

such as a suspected perforation. Barium in the retroperitoneum or mediastinum can result in granuloma formation and fibrotic scarring. Barium sulfate is almost insoluble and is ingested by the body's phagocytes, which try to digest the particles. The soluble salts created in the phagocytes appear to cause few problems for adults; however, children have a longer life expectancy, and so, for children, special care to avoid leaks is recommended. In view of the possible risks it is surprising how few complications resulting from barium leakage are seen in children, provided the leak is recognized and measures are taken to prevent infection.

Possible lung aspiration should be considered a contraindication even though barium sulfate has been advocated as a bronchographic contrast medium (Sauvegrain, 1969; Meradji, 1980) and is relatively well tolerated with only temporary respiratory embarrassment. However, more severe effects with cyanosis can last for several hours and even result in death (Nice, 1964; Nelson, 1964). Modern barium preparations have many additives, which may increase lung toxicity. However, even pure barium sulfate suspension has been shown to cause atelectasis and an inflammatory reaction possibly due to plugging of the bronchi (Willson, 1959; Ginai, 1984) but experimental evidence of production of fibrosis in the lungs with foreign body reaction is inconclusive (Arrigoni, 1933; Huston, 1952). Until recently anaphylaxis was not considered a possible complication of barium preparations; however, there have been reports of reactions in both adults and children (Stringer, 1993), probably related to proprietary additives to barium preparations. This rare complication probably occurs mostly in patients who have allergies.

In infants, if a contrast enema is indicated, barium is often contraindicated because it may exacerbate a meconium obstruction, while a small bowel atresia may be associated with a distal bowel defect or perforation (Wolfson, 1970).

Water-Soluble Contrast Media
The water-soluble contrast media include conventional hyperosmolar contrast media, bronchographic media, and the low osmolar contrast media. Iso-osmolar water-soluble contrast media are the safest but are expensive. Each of the types is discussed below.

Conventional Hyperosmolar Water-Soluble Media. Conventional hyperosmolar water-soluble media include iothalamate and diatrizoate in a variety of hyperosmolar proprietary preparations such as Gastrografin, Renografin, Hypaque, Conray, and Cystoconray. These contrast media should be used only in the large bowel for reasons given below.

In the upper gastrointestinal tract, these conventional hyperosmolar water-soluble media should not be used because of the risk of lung toxicity and pulmonary edema, possibly leading to death if the lungs are aspirated (Chiu, 1974; Reich, 1969). Gastrografin (a solution of diatrizoate meglumine and diatrizoate sodium with polysorbate 8, Tween 80) is particularly toxic to the lungs as it is very hyperosmolar and can precipitate gross pulmonary edema. Even instilling one of these contrast media into the stomach directly by nasogastric tube or by gastrostomy does not preclude gastroesophageal reflux and secondary lung aspiration with potentially fatal effect. Also, these media are absorbed by the normal gastrointestinal tract and are therefore useless for small bowel examination (Hay, 1990).

Conventional water-soluble contrast media have pharmacologic effects even when diluted to iso-osmolar levels. These include cholinesterase inhibition, release of histamine and, in the bowel, release of a serotonin-like substance (Ratcliffe, 1985). Hence, they should never be used in the upper gastrointestinal tract in children.

The conventional hyperosmolar contrast media are used most commonly in the evaluation of the neonatal large bowel. Water-soluble contrast material is preferred, as many neonatal conditions are amenable to treatment with these media, and the risk of perforation is relatively high in this group especially if a complicated atresia is present. In particular, water-soluble contrast material facilitates the expulsion of meconium (Cohen, 1982) and is of use in neonates with meconium ileus or when bowel obstruction is due to plugging of the bowel by meconium pellets. A theoretical disadvantage of using a water-soluble contrast medium is that Hirschsprung disease may be more difficult to detect as delayed films cannot be taken (Poole, 1976b) but we have not found this to be a practical problem.

A 17% solution of diatrizoate (Cystoconray or Hypaque) is a preferable medium and has a relatively low osmolality. This can be mixed with N-acetylcysteine, a mucolytic agent, if a meconium obstruction is suspected or found; this may be an effective treatment (Shaw, 1969) although far from proven

(CF Consensus Conference, 1991). If perforation occurs, electrolyte/fluid imbalance is possible but is not a concern if the contrast medium has been diluted sufficiently to give a low osmolar concentration. An added advantage of these media is that they are much cheaper than the iso-osmolar water-soluble contrast media.

In the past, Gastrografin has been advocated for the treatment of meconium ileus partly for its hyperosmolar hygroscopic effect and partly for the effect of the polysorbate wetting agent that it used to contain (Noblett, 1969; Bowring, 1970). Both of these effects were felt to be important in drawing fluid into the bowel and lubricating the passage of the sticky meconium. The disadvantage of Gastrografin is that it can cause serious dehydration by drawing fluid into the bowel lumen (Harris, 1964). In addition, Gastrografin may be absorbed in sufficient quantities to exacerbate the dehydration by affecting bowel osmolality (Poole, 1976a). To prevent this, the baby has to be continuously hydrated intravenously. The high osmolality draws excessive fluid into the gut, which, in addition to causing dehydration, may distend the bowel proximal to the obstruction, resulting in bowel perforation. In adults, these contrast media have also been implicated in gut perforation proximal to an obstructing lesion (Seltzer, 1978).

Gastrografin or other hyperosmolar contrast media such as Renografin may cause serious inflammation to the mucosa (Leonides, 1976; Lutzger, 1976; Grantmyre, 1981). Tween 80 has been implicated as the most irritant component (Lutzger, 1976). There is some evidence that these contrast media cause no harmful effects on the colon if there is no overdistension, but that overdistension results in severe changes (Wood, 1978). Finally and most importantly, there is no convincing evidence that the effectiveness of the high osmolar media is any more than that of the safer media and some evidence that their respective results are similar (Franken, 1993; CF Consensus Conference, 1991).

For the above reasons, Gastrografin and other very hyperosmolar solutions are not used even in the large bowel by our hospital.

In older children, water-soluble contrast media are usually reserved for the few instances in which perforation is possible. The majority of these examinations are loopograms, which are discussed later in this chapter. The value of water-soluble contrast media in intussusception is controversial (Campbell,

1986) and is discussed in Chapter 10. In our hospital, air is used as the contrast medium of choice for intussusception. Water-soluble contrast media have also been advocated for treating cystic fibrosis patients who develop distal intestinal obstruction syndrome (DIOS or meconium ileus equivalent). However, other methods of treatment using a balanced electrolyte solution containing polyethylene glycol (Golytely) are now recommended (Cleghorn, 1986) (see Chapter 10) and will probably obviate the need for water-soluble contrast enemas for these patients.

Bronchographic Contrast Media. Bronchographic contrast media such as Hytrast and Dionosil can be obtained in oily and aqueous solutions, only the aqueous should be used in the gut. These media used to be used occasionally if an esophageal leak into the mediastinum or lungs was clinically suspected but they are expensive and so unpalatable as to reduce patient cooperation. Hence, these media have now been replaced by the iso-osmolar water-soluble contrast media.

If the iso-osmolar water-soluble contrast media are not available, then aqueous bronchographic contrast media are the safest media in the lungs (Sauvegrain, 1969) and hence can be used in those gastrointestinal examinations where there is a risk of aspiration. However, serious effects may occur if there is an intraperitoneal leak. An animal study showed that bronchographic contrast media were rapidly fatal when injected into the peritoneum (Ginai, 1985).

Iso-Osmolar Water-Soluble Contrast Media. The low osmolar water-soluble contrast media include the nonionic iopamidol (Niopam in Europe or Isovue in North America) and iohexol (Omnipaque) or the ionic ioxaglate (Hexabrix). Metrizamide (Amipaque) was the first low osmolar water-soluble contrast medium to be used in North America (Cohen and Smith, 1982; Cohen and Weber, 1982). It has the disadvantage of being a solid requiring mixing and so has been replaced by others that are less expensive and obtainable already mixed as isotonic solutions. In addition, metrizamide may not be stable in an acid environment such as the stomach and hence probably should not be used.

The iso-osmolar water-soluble contrast media fulfill the criteria for the ideal media except that they are expensive. They have no known effect on the

lungs or peritoneum and are not absorbed by the bowel (Figure 3–4). At isotonic concentrations excellent single-contrast visualization is possible (Figure 3–5). These media are being used with increasing regularity to evaluate the gastrointestinal tract in pediatric patients in North America and have been so used extensively in Europe. The advantages of these media are many. So little contrast medium is absorbed that the gut can be clearly visualized for prolonged periods, an advantage when delayed films are required as in the diagnosis of Hirschsprung disease. Indeed, nonionic media (iopamidol and iohexol) are usually not absorbed at all from the pediatric gut (Ratcliffe, 1985), and hence pyelography will indicate a perforation even if the leak itself is not visible. An exception to this rule occurs when the bowel mucosa is abnormal as some absorption can then occur, and this should be remembered when interpreting results. Ioxaglate is ionic although of low osmolality and hence may be absorbed in small quantities through damaged mucosa to produce a pyelogram (Ratcliffe, 1985). Despite this, ioxaglate has been useful in a number of children (Ratcliffe, 1983, 1985). Ioxaglate has been shown to cause little effect on the peritoneum in experimental animals

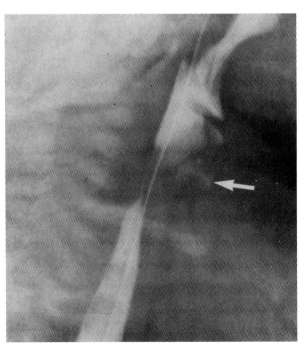

FIGURE 3–4. New iso-osmolar water-soluble contrast media. There is aspiration into the proximal portion of trachea (*arrow*). No sequelae have been seen from this occurrence in our hospital.

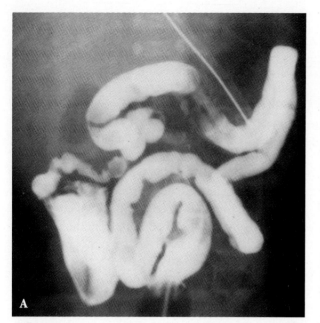 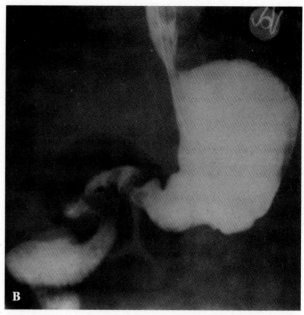

FIGURE 3–5. New iso-osmolar water-soluble contrast media. Isotonic ioxaglate (Hexabrix) gives good opacification of the infant colon (*A*) and upper gastrointestinal tract (*B*). The contrast meal shows type I malrotation (nonrotation) (see Chapter 9).

(Ginai, 1985) whereas some of the intraperitoneal bronchographic media caused rapid death in these same animals (Ginai, 1985). In our experience, ioxaglate has been a safe contrast medium with no sequelae in the lungs or peritoneum when aspiration (Figure 3–4) or perforation has occurred.

The indications for using the iso-osmolar water-soluble contrast media in the gut are summarized in Table 3–1 (Ratcliffe, 1985). The major disadvantage is the expense, and so at our hospital they are generally reserved for procedures when perforation or aspiration is known or suspected, or for use in the most fragile premature neonates.

Air and Other Gases

Air is rarely regarded as a contrast medium but in pediatrics it can be safe and useful in specific situations. Air is an excellent safe contrast medium for diagnosing esophageal, duodenal, jejunal, or large bowel atresia. The diagnosis is generally possible on plain films but the injection of air into the large or small bowel may facilitate the delineation of obstruction. Air enemas have been used in the diagnosis and treatment of intussusception. The air enema is now the contrast medium and technique of choice in our hospital but is not universally accepted. (This is discussed in more detail in Chapter 10.)

Barium Examinations of the Upper Gastrointestinal Tract

Single-Contrast Barium Meal

Infants and Young Children. The clinical problems of infants and young children differ from those of adults. They are often related to congenital anomalies such as malrotation and duodenal web, to conditions peculiar to childhood such as hypertrophic pyloric stenosis, or to functional problems such as achalasia and infantile chalasia. Hence, single-contrast examinations are usually more than adequate for infants and for many older children.

Barium sulfate is a relatively safe contrast medium. It is relatively nontoxic, not highly osmolar, and it mimics milk more closely than do water-soluble media. A mixture of one part 58% wt/wt barium sulfate to two parts sterile 5% dextrose water (250 mmol glucose per liter) is used in our hospital.

Infants are generally willing to drink this barium if they have not been fed during the previous 3 to 4 hours. Children between 1 and 2 years of age should not eat or drink for 6 hours prior to the examination. Over 2 years of age, the children should fast for 8 hours. The length of fast will depend on the size and clinical status of the patient.

TABLE 3–1.   Criteria For Use of Low Osmolality Contrast Media in the Pediatric Gut

Risk of lung aspiration
    Laryngopharyngeal dyskinesia
    H-type fistula
    Vomiting or refluxing child
Risk of bowel leak
    Recent surgery on bowel
    To demonstrate site of leak
    To demonstrate fistula(e)
Risk of barium inspissated
    Cystic fibrosis
    Blind loop of bowel
    Hirschsprung disease
Neonatal obstruction/meconium ileus
Endoscopy or biopsy immediately following examination

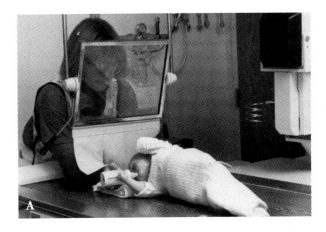

In older children, the concentration of barium (58% wt/wt mixed with two parts water) is the same as for infants but proportionately more is given to fill the stomach. Flavorings can be used and are easily mixed in a blender.

Barium can be fed to infants from a bottle (Figure 3–6A). This is the most physiologic method, but for the lateral view of the esophagus it may be difficult to keep the bottle above the horizontal when the infant lies on the side. When difficulty is encountered, contrast can be injected via an orogastric tube inserted through a teat (Poznanski, 1969; Hyde, 1980; Becker, 1972). Older children generally find it easier to drink barium through a straw if lying but if erect may find it easier to drink directly from a cup.

The method of examining the esophagus, stomach, and duodenum in an infant differs from an adult examination. Particular attention is paid both to the midesophagus, which is the site of many congenital anomalies such as vascular rings and H-type tracheoesophageal fistulae, and to the position of the duodenojejunal junction, which should be identified to exclude malrotation on all initial upper gastrointestinal examinations.

The infant is fed while lying on the right side (Figure 3–6A) so that the lateral fluoroscopic view of the esophagus puts particular emphasis on the region around the carina, which is where most anomalies occur (Figure 3–6B). If enough barium has passed into the stomach with the infant in this

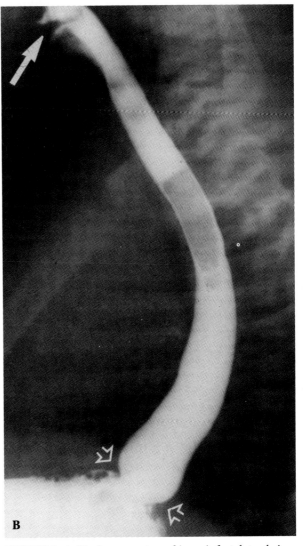

FIGURE 3–6. Single-contrast meal in an infant, lateral view. *A,* The infant is fed while lying on the right side. *B,* The esophagus is distended with barium and bubbles of air as the infant swallows. In this projection, with a 9-inch image intensifier, a full view from epiglottis (*white arrow*) to esophagogastric junction (*open arrows*) should be possible.

position, the pylorus and duodenal loop can be screened (Figure 3–7). As soon as the third part of the duodenum appears to fill, the infant is quickly turned supine, briefly on to the left side to drain the barium out of the antrum and into the fundus and then quickly back to the supine position (Figure 3–8A) so that the position of the duodenojejunal

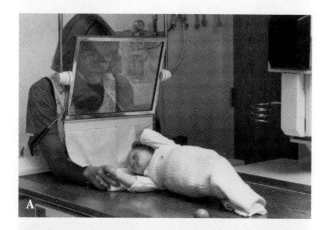

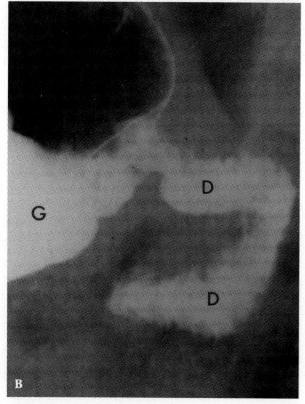

FIGURE 3–7. Single-contrast meal in an infant, lateral view. *A,* After approximately 30 mL of contrast medium the feed is stopped and the patient is maintained in the lateral position. *B,* Contrast media fills the gastric antrum (G) and duodenal loop (D) as far as the third part of the duodenum.

flexure can be accurately delineated through the air-filled gastric antrum (Figure 3–8B). Malrotation can be excluded confidently on a barium meal examination only by showing a normally positioned duodenojejunal junction in the true frontal projection (see Chapter 9). Occasionally, the duodenal loop, especially in the second part, may be tortuous (Figure 3–9), and this should not be mistaken for an abnormality. Careful judgment is needed with close correlation with the clinical findings and with close consultation with the appropriate clinicians. In particular, the presence of bilious vomiting, even if intermittent, should be treated as a serious indicator of significant disease such as malrotation (see Chapter 9).

With further swallows, the esophagus can now be assessed in the anteroposterior projection (Figure 3–10). When the stomach is full of barium, a test for gastroesophageal reflux may be carried out by gently rocking the child in the supine position. Prior to testing for reflux, it is necessary to burp the child to remove excess swallowed air (see Chapter 7). Further spot films are taken as necessary. The antrum and duodenum may be further assessed in the oblique projections; the pyloric canal may best be visualized in lateral or oblique projections. Delayed films may occasionally be necessary if hypertrophic pyloric stenosis is suspected.

To prevent aspiration when there is delayed or obstructed gastric emptying or if gross gastroesophageal reflux occurs, the stomach contents should be drained and/or the infant should be nursed erect after the procedure.

Older Children. Single-contrast studies may be necessary in an older child to exclude obstruction, varices, and gastroesophageal reflux or may be performed as part of a small bowel follow-through examination. The technique is similar to that described above except that the patient initially lies semiprone to swallow the barium (Figure 3–11), and the fluoroscopic time and the number of spot films are kept to the minimum necessary to answer the clinical problem.

Video Prone Esophagography

When H-type or recurrent tracheoesophageal fistula is suspected, an 8 or 10 French feeding tube is positioned in the esophagus, and contrast media—usually barium, as it is well visualized in small fistulae—is injected with the patient lying prone on the footstep of an erect fluoroscopic table (Figure 3–12A) (Stringer, 1984). The barium will layer on the anterior surface, and air bubbles will rise to the posterior aspect of the esophagus (Figure 3–12B). The position of the feeding tube is then altered so that each level of the esophagus can be distended

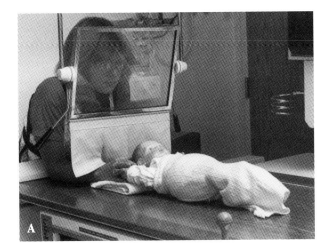

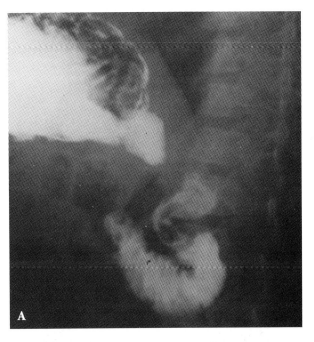

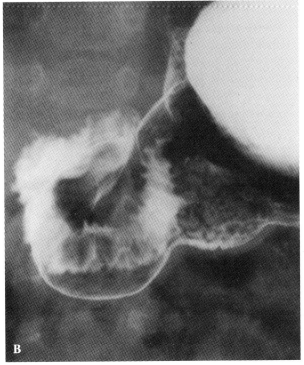

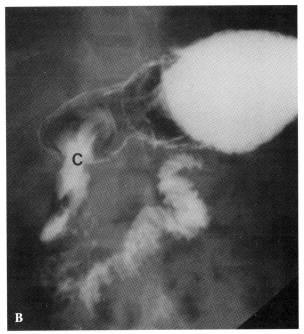

FIGURE 3–8. Single-contrast meal in an infant, frontal view. *A,* As soon as the third part of the duodenum appears to fill, the infant is quickly turned supine, briefly onto the left side to drain the barium out of the antrum and into the fundus and then quickly back to the supine position. *B,* The location of the entire duodenal loop and in particular the duodenojejunal flexure is delineated through the air-filled gastric antrum. Note the position of the duodenojejunal flexure to the left of the left vertebral pedicles and near the same level as the duodenal cap.

FIGURE 3–9. Single-contrast meal in an infant, frontal view. The duodenal loop is tortuous especially in its second portion as shown on lateral (*A*) and frontal (*B*) projections. Note that the fourth part of the duodenum coming up to the duodenojejunal junction lies in a normal position to the left of the vertebral pedicles and almost at the height of the duodenal cap (C).

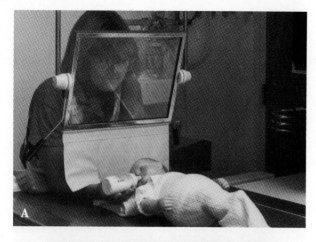

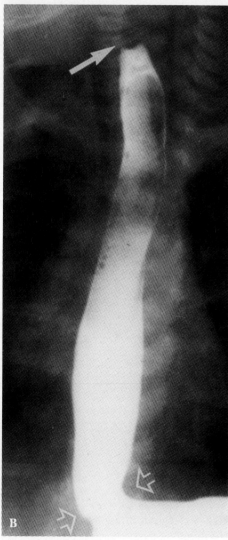

FIGURE 3–10. Single-contrast meal in an infant, frontal view. *A,* The infant's head is turned to the side and further feed can be given in the supine position. *B,* The esophagus is again outlined by barium and air from cricopharyngeus (*arrow*) to esophagogastric junction (*open arrows*).

with barium at least twice during the examination. The complete procedure is recorded on videotape.

If reflux is suspected, at the end of the procedure barium should be aspirated via the tube or the infant should be nursed erect. Aqueous bronchographic media can be used instead of barium (Thomas, 1969) although the low osmolar contrast media are preferable if there is concern that large quantities will pass into the lungs.

Double-Contrast Barium Meal

Double-contrast examinations are more difficult to perform in children than in adults, and the radiation dosage is higher than for single-contrast examinations because there is more fluoroscopy and because more images are taken. Hence, double-contrast barium meal examinations are generally reserved for children over 7 years of age when looking for esophagitis, erosions, ulcers, or mass lesions. Under 5 years of age it is rare for a child to be cooperative enough for a satisfactory examination, which should include the use of an effervescent agent and high-density barium. If a double-contrast examination is essential under this age (a rare eventuality) and no substitute test is possible, then it is often best to use a nasoesophageal or nasogastric tube to perform a diagnostic examination. In the few patients of this age who pose a real diagnostic dilemma, the value of a low-density barium meal using swallowed air is dubious. It may be better to use other tests such as endoscopy even though these require a general anesthetic in this age group. Between the ages of 5 and 10 years, cooperation improves so that while it is unusual at 5 years to obtain a satisfactory examination, by 10 years it is unusual to fail.

Varices can be detected by single- and double-contrast studies but are often difficult to visualize when small. Also, if US and Doppler have not been helpful, a biphasic double- and single-contrast examination may be required.

The method of double-contrast examination depends on the degree of patient cooperation. Children generally have more difficulty swallowing the effervescent agent than adults do, especially if given with barium. It is usually easier to give them effervescent tablets and 10 to 20 mL water. (The granules tend to froth in the mouth, an alarming phenomenon for most children.) Injections of glucagon or other agents to produce hypotonia also decrease patient cooperation and hence are rarely, if ever, indicated.

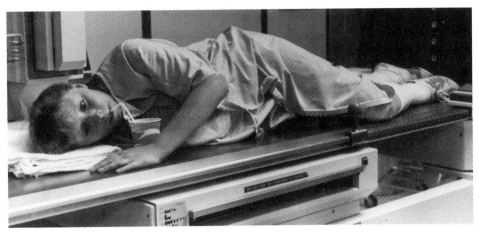

FIGURE 3–11. Single-contrast meal in an older child, oblique view. The patient lies semi-prone to swallow the contrast material and the fluoroscopic time and number of spot films are kept to the minimum necessary to answer the clinical problem.

The preparation is the same as for a single-contrast examination. High-density low viscosity barium gives the best results (Hyslop, 1982) and should be used to the manufacturer's specifications without additional flavoring as this interferes with the coating properties. Unfortunately these preparations are less palatable and children tend to dislike their chalky consistency. We use an 85% wt/wt, 250% wt/vol barium sulfate suspension with excellent coating properties, and we find that with coaxing, children will take enough for a satisfactory examination.

The examination is best started erect with gas tablets and 15 mL water followed quickly by high-density barium (Figure 3–13A). Gas granules are tolerated less well as they effervesce quickly. A double-contrast view of the esophagus is obtained (Figure 3–13B, C). The patient then faces the table-top, which is rotated to the horizontal, the child turns onto their left side and then onto their back (Figure 3–14A). Good barium coating is obtained by rolling the patient 360 degrees in each direction, and images are taken when the coating is adequate and when the region of interest is best displayed. Views of the air-filled gastric antrum (Figure 3–15A), duodenal cap (Figure 3–15B), and fundus (Figure 3–16A, B) are obtained as is a supine view (Figure 3–14B) to localize the duodenojejunal junction. As in a single-contrast study, reflux is looked for after filling the stomach with more dilute barium. Radiation dosages are kept to a minimum by not using a grid and by reducing fluoroscopy time as much as possible. Average fluoroscopy time for the procedure should be approximately 1 to 1$^{1}/_{2}$ minutes. To further reduce radiation dosage, fewer images are taken than in an examination of an adult.

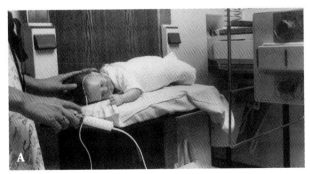
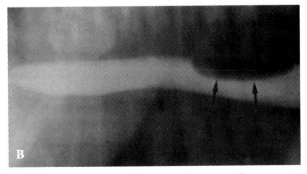

FIGURE 3–12. Normal video prone esophagogram. *A,* The infant lies prone on the footstep of an erect fluoroscopic table, and contrast is injected via an 8 or 10 French feeding tube positioned in the esophagus. *B,* Injected barium distends the esophagus. Ingested gas (*arrows*) rises to the posterior aspect of the esophagus.

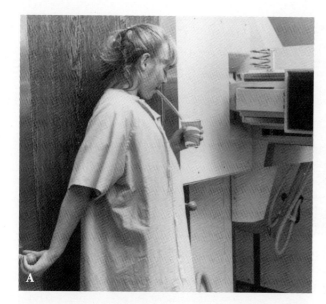

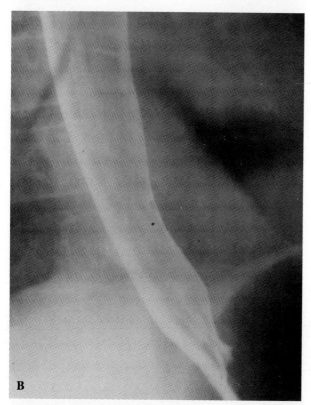

FIGURE 3–13. Double-contrast meal in an older child, normal esophagus. *A,* With the patient erect, following ingestion of gas tablets, high density barium is swallowed. Double-contrast views of the esophagus are shown taken with a 9-inch image intensifier (*B*) and an 11-inch image intensifier (*C*). The 11-inch intensifier covers a larger portion of the esophagus in these older patients.

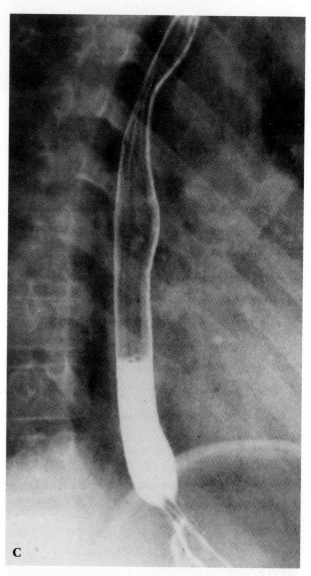

Small Bowel Examinations

The small bowel follow-through examination is generally considered to be the most appropriate initial technique for examining the small bowel. When the terminal ileum is difficult to visualize or if the evidence for fistulae is equivocal, a peroral pneumocolon can be performed (Stringer, Sherman, et al., 1986). Occasionally when the peroral pneumocolon is not helpful, the terminal ileum may then be shown by reflux of air and barium on a double-contrast barium enema if this is being performed for large bowel evaluation. The small bowel enema is more invasive and so is reserved for those few patients in whom the small bowel follow-through examination and peroral pneumocolon have failed to solve a diagnostic dilemma (Stringer, Cloutier, et

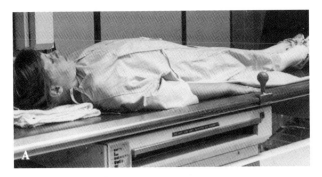

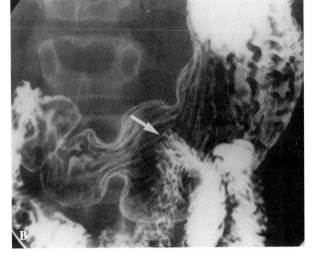

FIGURE 3–14. Double-contrast meal in an older child, normal duodenojejunal junction. The patient is supine (*A*), and on double-contrast views (*B*) the location of the duodenojejunal junction (arrows) is well outlined lateral to the left vertebral pedicles on this supine view.

al., 1986). This occurs most commonly in the terminal ileum. In addition, if there is a mass effect from possible Crohn's disease or lymphoma, if small mass lesions are suspected, or if fine detail is required, the more invasive small bowel enema can be performed (Stringer, Cloutire, et al., 1986).

Small Bowel Follow-Through Examination

In children, small bowel pathology will usually be well shown if the passage of barium is followed through the small bowel by both overhead radiograph and fluoroscopy with compression spot films where necessary. The examination is best performed following a single-contrast barium meal as the gas and high-density barium used in double-contrast examinations degrade the small bowel delineation. At our hospital, the small bowel follow-through examination consists of a meal of 58% wt/wt barium sulfate diluted in two parts of water, with prone abdominal films taken every half hour for up to 90 minutes or

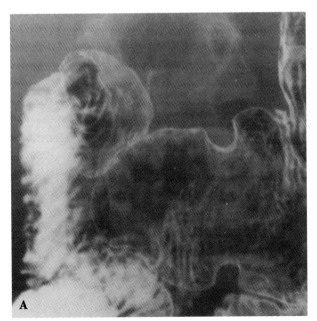

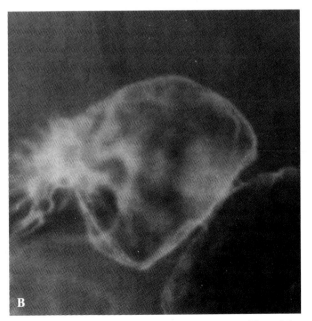

FIGURE 3–15. Double-contrast meal in an older child, normal antrum and duodenal cap. *A*, A supine spot film of the gastric antrum shows most but not all of the duodenal cap. *B*, An oblique view demonstrates a normal duodenal cap and short pyloric canal.

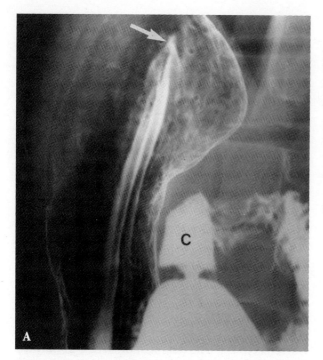
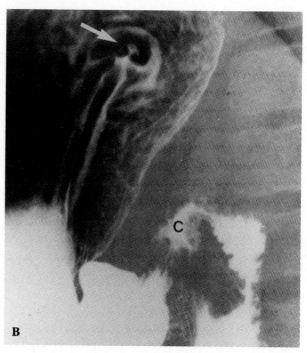

FIGURE 3–16. Double-contrast meal in an older child, normal fundus and duodenal cap. With the patient lying on the right side the duodenal cap (C) is filled with barium and often distends well (*A*). A double-contrast view of the fundus is obtained. The esophagogastric junction may have a linear appearance (*A*) with folds originating at the esophagogastric junction (*arrow*) or may have a rounded appearance (*B*) with an elevated ring around the junction (*arrow*) and linear folds radiating inferiorly.

until the barium has reached the large bowel (Figure 3–17). The prone position gives better separation of bowel loops. If transit of barium is slow, delayed films are taken at intervals as decided by the attending radiologist. Fluoroscopy with one to four spot films is performed to delineate the terminal ileum or any abnormalities seen on the plain films. Average total fluoroscopic time is about 1¹/₂ to 2 minutes.

In children, the normal terminal ileum often shows a lymphoid follicular pattern which can be very striking (Figure 3–18) and must not be confused with pathology such as Crohn's disease (see Chapter 9).

Peroral Pneumocolon

General Considerations and Indications. In adults, the peroral pneumocolon has been advocated for the delineation of the proximal large bowel (Heitzman, 1961; Pochaczevsky, 1974) and, more recently, the terminal ileum when these areas are not well visualized on conventional small bowel follow-through examination (Kelvin, 1982; Kellett, 1977; Laufer, 1979; Kressel, 1982; Stringer, Sherman, et al., 1986).

In adults and children, the indications for the peroral pneumocolon examination at the end of a small bowel follow-through examination include (1) a poorly seen terminal ileum (Figure 3–19A), (2) clinically suspected inflammatory bowel disease with an apparently normal terminal ileum, and (3) an abnormal terminal ileum with equivocal fistula (Kressel, 1982; Stringer, Sherman, et al., 1986).

In children, visualization of the terminal ileum is important primarily to diagnose or exclude Crohn's disease, or to evaluate the extent of the disease preoperatively. Since Crohn's disease is extremely rare under the age of 8 years, peroral pneumocolon is rarely necessary in younger children. The peroral pneumocolon is well tolerated in children, requires no patient preparation, and requires little additional radiation (Stringer, Sherman, et al., 1986).

Technique Employed. The procedure entails insufflation of air per rectum (Figure 3–20) when barium from a conventional follow-through examination has reached the terminal ileum (Figure 3–19B). The technique can easily be incorporated into the routine follow-through examination as an extra method of spot filming the terminal ileum when this region is not clearly delineated by standard spot images. The terminal ileum can be a difficult portion of the small bowel to examine satisfactorily on a conventional small bowel barium follow-through examination, especially if the cecum lies deep in the pelvis. In this situation the peroral pneumocolon can provide diagnostic information and obviate further, more invasive investigation (Stringer, Sherman, et al., 1986).

Small Bowel Enema

General Considerations and Indications. Since the introduction in 1929 of the small bowel enema,

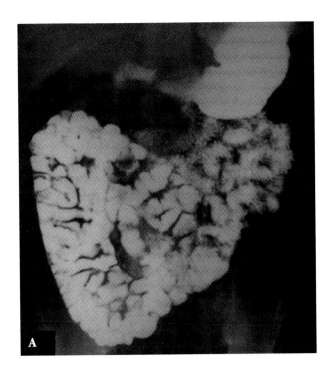

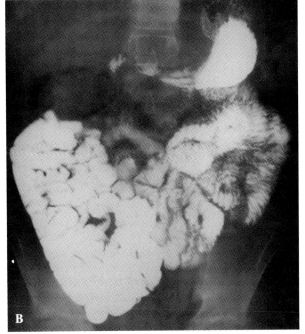

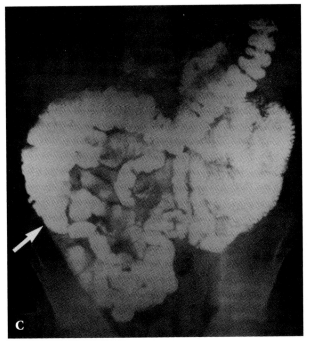

FIGURE 3–17. Normal small bowel follow-through examination in an older child. The small bowel follow-through examination shows good filling of proximal small bowel at 30 minutes (*A*), more filling of distal bowel at 60 minutes (*B*), and filling of cecum (*arrow*) (*C*) at 90 minutes.

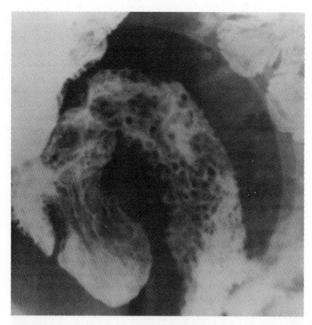

FIGURE 3–18. Normal lymphoid follicles in the terminal ileum of an older child. A spot compression film of a terminal ileum during a conventional small bowel follow-through examination shows multiple small symmetrical nodules indicating lymphoid follicles.

otherwise known as enteroclysis, (Pesquera, 1929) the intubation technique has been simplified (Bilbao, 1967; Sellink, 1974). This examination has shown excellent diagnostic correlation in adult series (Sanders, 1976; Vallance, 1980; Vallance, 1981) but there have been few reports of its indications and usefulness in children (Eklof, 1978; Ratcliffe, 1983; Stringer, Cloutier, et al., 1986).

In adults, the small bowel enema has been advocated for the investigation of early or preoperative Crohn's disease (since it is superior to the small bowel follow-through in demonstrating skip lesions) as well as bowel wall abnormalities, small bowel obstruction, or suspected tumor or radiation damage (Herlinger, 1979). The majority of children with Crohn's disease do not need a small bowel enema for a definitive diagnosis (Stringer, Cloutier, et al., 1986). The extent of the disease is better shown by small bowel enema in adults (Vallance, 1981; Ekberg, 1977a; Herlinger, 1982) but this additional information is not required unless surgical intervention is being considered. The decision to operate is dependent on the clinical status of the patient, and radiology is most useful in the initial diagnosis and in indicating the location of severe disease. If surgery is performed, most surgeons will be guided by operative rather than radiologic findings. Therefore, in most patients with Crohn's disease, a small bowel follow-through examination, which is better tolerated, less invasive, and requires less radiation, would be sufficient (Stringer, Cloutier, et al., 1986).

The major indication for using the small bowel enema is the failure of the small bowel follow-through

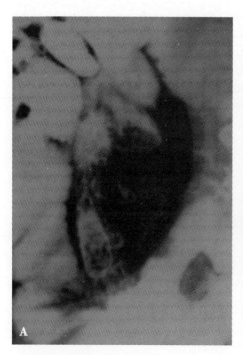

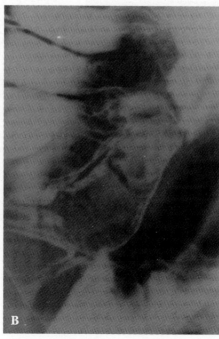

FIGURE 3–19. Normal terminal ileum on peroral pneumocolon. *A,* The terminal ileum is poorly seen during a conventional small bowel follow-through examination despite compression. *B,* A peroral pneumocolon performed within minutes of (*A*) demonstrates a normal terminal ileum.

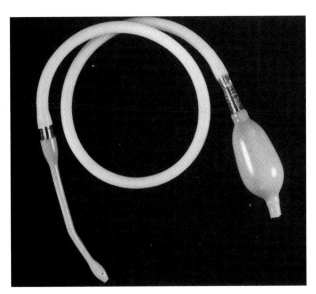

FIGURE 3–20. Peroral pneumocolon insufflator. An insufflator for peroral pneumocolon can be easily made using an enema tip, an insufflator bulb, tubing, and connectors.

examination to solve a diagnostic problem (Stringer, Cloutier, et al., 1986). In particular, the small bowel enema can be helpful in examining mass lesions, a poorly seen terminal ileum, as well as in differentiating between normal and abnormal small bowel when this is unclear from the small bowel follow-through examination (Table 3–2) and if other studies such as US or CT are either unsuitable or unhelpful.

The presence of a mass found on a barium follow-through examination raises the possibility of lymphoma but may be the result of intestinal spasm with or without bowel wall thickening in Crohn's disease. While these conditions often cannot be differentiated on a small bowel follow-through (Sartoris, 1984), laparotomy is to be avoided if possible, especially in Crohn's disease. In our experience with a mass on small bowel follow-through, small bowel enema clearly demonstrates skip lesions or overcomes intestinal spasm sufficiently to help make a more confident diagnosis of Crohn's disease, thereby obviating laparotomy (Stringer, Cloutier, et al., 1986).

The terminal ileum is sometimes an elusive part of the bowel to examine on small bowel follow-through, especially when it is positioned deep within the pelvis, and it may not be seen well enough to allow a confident diagnosis. In this case, and if the peroral pneumocolon is inconclusive and a double-contrast barium enema is not scheduled or does not reflux into the terminal ileum, then the small bowel enema is useful in demonstrating a definite abnormality or confirming normality of the terminal ileum (Stringer, Cloutier, et al., 1986). However, occasionally the small bowel enema still may not show the distal portion satisfactorily (Kelvin, 1982).

Technique Employed. The small bowel enema examination is relatively well tolerated in children as young as 1 year of age and produces no complications. Although sedation has been recommended (Ratcliffe, 1983), we do not use it because of the risk of reflux of barium back into the stomach from the small bowel, inducing emesis and possibly aspiration. In adults, dilute barium or more dense barium followed by air, water, or methyl cellulose may be used (Sartoris, 1984; Ekberg, 1977b; Herlinger, 1982). We have found that dilute barium followed by cool water gives satisfactory visualization of all parts of the bowel.

The technique varies according to the age of the patient. In a large cooperative adolescent the adult technique can be used. In children over 5 years of age we give a detailed explanation together with active encouragement during the procedure, resulting in excellent tolerance and cooperation. A torque control guide wire and either a 12 or 14 French Bilbao Dotter tube are used in older patients, depending on their size. In an infant or young child, an 8 or 10 French end-holed tube is passed into the proximal jejunum with the aid of a floppy-ended guide wire, the procedure of tube placement being similar to that of any usual nasojejunal feeding tube placement. The nasal route is used to pass the tube as it is better tolerated than the oral route (Maglinte, 1986).

TABLE 3–2. Investigation of the Small Bowel

Conventional small bowel follow-through examination
If terminal ileum is poorly seen
↓
Peroral pneumocolon
If terminal ileum is still poorly seen
↓
(Double-contrast barium enema,
if being performed for other reasons,
with reflux into terminal ileum)
If terminal ileum is still poorly seen
or if there is still a diagnostic dilemma
↓
Small bowel enema

Constant reassurance of the patient is necessary while the tip of the tube is positioned with a guide wire at or preferably just beyond the duodenojejunal junction. The rest of the examination appears to cause no undue symptoms (Stringer, Cloutier, et al., 1986; Herlinger, 1979) although some discomfort may be felt if infusion is too fast.

The concentration of barium and the diluting fluid vary from radiologist to radiologist. Some use concentrated barium followed by methylcellulose. We prefer dilute barium (1 to 7 dilution of 56% wt/wt Polibar) followed by cool water. The barium is instilled into the jejunum by gravity. Cool water is then instilled into the system through a Y-connector (Figure 3–21) to dilute the barium further if it appears too dense for a see-through effect on fluoroscopy and to advance the barium column once the proximal small bowel has been examined (Figure 3–22). During the procedure, great care must be

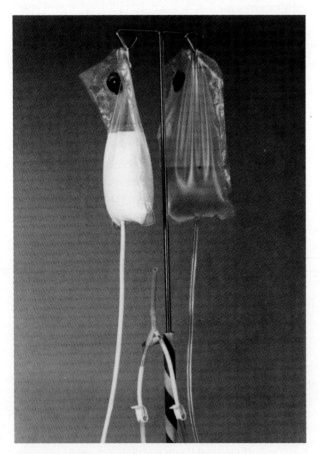

FIGURE 3–21. Normal small bowel enema equipment. A dilute barium sulfate solution and cool water are connected via a Y connector. Note the clamps on each enema bag tube enabling either water or barium to be instilled.

taken to avoid the retrograde passage of barium into the stomach as this can induce vomiting with aspiration. On average, intermittent fluoroscopy totaling 3 to 5 minutes is required during the approximately 20 minutes that the barium takes to reach the terminal ileum. About five to ten spot films are taken with occasionally one or two full abdominal films, depending on the size of the patient.

Plasma electrolyte status remains satisfactory in larger patients who initially have normal electrolyte status (Barloon, 1986). In smaller patients or patients with pre-existing electrolyte disturbances, normal saline could be substituted for water. This decision is best made in consultation with the clinician.

Barium Examinations of the Large Bowel

Single-Contrast Barium Enema

General Considerations and Indications. A single-contrast barium enema is much more commonly performed than a double-contrast examination, and no preparation is required. It can be used to exclude intussusception, demonstrate the gross anatomy of the large bowel, show the position of the cecum, and occasionally investigate Hirschsprung disease or other causes of constipation. As with a double-contrast examination, it is contraindicated in toxic megacolon, following a recent noncolonoscopic biopsy, or if there is a risk of perforation. In those few children with possible Hirschsprung disease who need a diagnostic enema, care should be taken not to overfill the colon proximal to the zone of transition as this may precipitate obstruction or fluid imbalance.

Technique Employed. To examine the bowel, barium is instilled with the patient lying on the left side, and a lateral film of the rectum to include the rectosigmoid is taken (Figure 3–23A). The patient then rolls to the prone position while the rest of the large bowel is filled, as shown by appendiceal or terminal ileum filling. A spot film of the cecum is taken to show its position relative to the right iliac wing (Figure 3–23B). The patient may have to lie in an oblique position to obtain a satisfactory view. An overhead abdominal film is taken (Figure 3–23C), the patient is allowed to evacuate the barium, and a post-evacuation film is taken at least 10 minutes later (Figure 3–23D). Evacuation will be aided if 10 mL of bisacodyl (Dulcolax) is mixed per liter of barium but

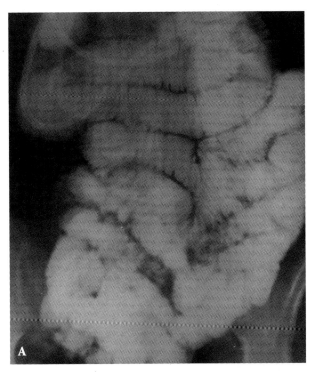 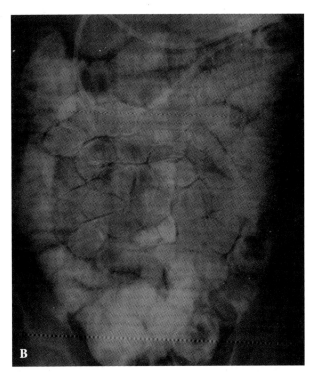

FIGURE 3–22. Normal small bowel enema. *A,* Dilute barium has been instilled into the jejunum. *B,* Instilling cool water dilutes the barium further, giving a see-through effect in the small bowel and advancing the barium column into the large bowel.

bisacodyl should not be used if the patient is generally unwell or if either colitis or rectal bleeding is present.

A separate technique is used for the diagnosis and reduction of intussusception (see Chapter 10).

Double-Contrast Barium Enema

General Considerations and Indications. In both adults and children, findings of colonic mucosal lesions on colonoscopy correlate poorly with those demonstrated on single-contrast examination (Gans, 1975; Cadranel, 1977; Thoeni, 1977; Tedesco, 1978; Habr-Gama, 1979; Chong, 1982; Williams, 1982). In adults, double-contrast barium enemas are more successful than single-contrast studies at detecting mucosal lesions or polyps (Thoeni, 1977; Williams, 1982; Laufer and Hamilton, 1976) and correlate better with lesions noted at colonoscopy and sigmoidoscopy (Simpkins, 1972).

Likewise in children, the double-contrast technique is more sensitive than a single-contrast examination at detecting the presence of early ulcerative or granulomatous colitis (Winthrop, 1985). When a high-density low-viscosity barium sulfate suspen-sion is used, there is excellent correlation with colonoscopic and histologic findings (Stringer, 1986). The barium preparation should be at least 100% wt/vol with irregular particles of barium sulfate in suspension. The lymphoid follicular pattern is a good indicator of how well the barium is coating the mucosa. Lymphoid follicles are always present pathologically in children and can be reliably detect-ed in nearly all children if such a high-density low-viscosity barium sulfate containing irregular par-ticles is used (Figure 3–24) (Miller, 1987).

For the above reasons, we recommend undi-luted Polibar in 100% or 105% wt/vol concentration for our double-contrast examinations that we per-form if there is rectal bleeding, evidence of colitis, or suspicion of a mass lesion. Undiluted Polibar is vis-cous, and filling of the large bowel is slow. This has the advantage that no discomfort is felt during the filling phase. In order to speed up the process, ¹/₂-inch tubing is advisable.

Technique Employed. The technique used is similar to that described for adults (Laufer, 1979; Franken, 1982; Stringer, 1986) but less air and barium are used, the amount varying according to the patient's size. As large bowel malignancy and malignant change in small isolated polyps are rare in children, shorter fluoroscopy times and fewer films are required, resulting in less radiation than for an equivalent adult study.

Prior to the examination, colonic evacuation of retained stools is induced by administering a clear

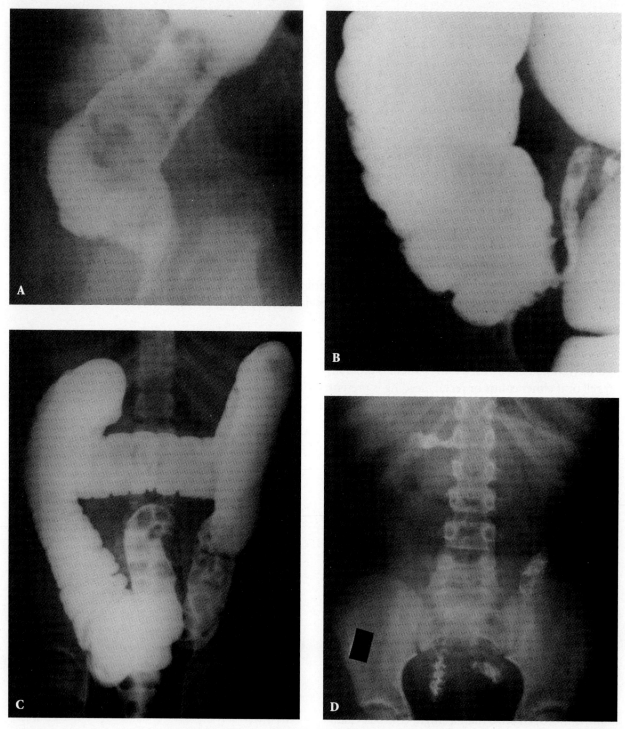

FIGURE 3–23. Normal single-contrast barium enema. *A,* The rectum and rectosigmoid junction are outlined by barium in the lateral projection. *B,* The barium-filled cecum lies over the right iliac wing in the right iliac fossa. *C,* Barium fills the entire large bowel and shows minor fecal residue. *D,* Post evacuation. The large bowel has almost completely emptied.

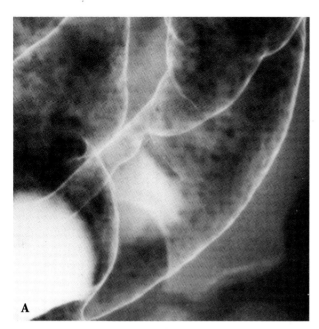 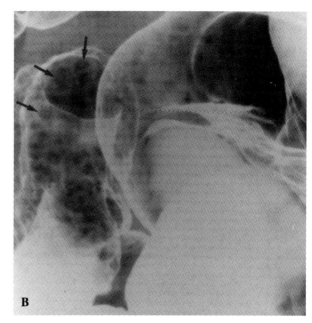

FIGURE 3–24. Normal lymphoid follicles on double-contrast barium enema. *A,* Double-contrast barium enema shows lymphoid follicles as faint, smooth, well-demarcated lucencies. *B,* Some follicles have an umbilicated appearance with a small central fleck of barium (*arrows*). Lymphoid follicles are a normal finding in the large bowel and indicate good coating with barium. (Reprinted with permission from Miller M, Stringer DA, Chui-Mei T, et al. Lymphoid follicular pattern in the colon: an indicator of barium coating. J Can Assoc Radiol 1987;38:256–8.)

liquid diet for 36 hours followed by magnesium citrate or castor oil (1 mg per kg of body weight) the afternoon prior to the examination and by administering fleet or saline enemas the evening before and morning of the examination. Purgatives are withheld only from patients with suspected active colitis. This preparation is similar to that for a colonoscopy, so if both tests are needed, the double-contrast barium enema can be performed within 24 hours of the colonoscopy as long as only superficial colonoscopic biopsies have been taken (Maglinte, 1982; Harned, 1982; Lappas, 1983; Harned, 1985).

The procedure is explained to the child and parents. With the patient prone, high-density barium sulfate is instilled per rectum until the splenic flexure or midtransverse colon is reached. The prone position is preferred as the barium can run downhill into the transverse colon. Then the patient turns onto his or her right side, facilitating filling of the right hemicolon while at the same time some of the barium is drained from the rectum to prevent overfilling. The patient sits up or the table is elevated with the patient now in the supine position. This ensures that barium will reach the cecum *before* any air is instilled. This is different from the usual adult procedure and is because the painful part of the test is the insufflation of air, which should be performed slowly and close to the end of the examination. In this way it is possible to obtain good patient cooperation. In adults, carbon dioxide is preferable to air as it causes less discomfort (Coblentz, 1985; Grant, 1986) but this is not routine in children.

As soon as the air has been instilled, the child turns 360 degrees twice in both directions. Spot images of the air-filled lateral rectum (Figure 3–25) and an oblique view of the air-filled cecum to include any reflux into the terminal ileum (Figure 3–26) are taken. Overhead views are then taken and expeditiously checked, and the child is then sent to the washroom to relieve the discomfort.

Radiation dosage is greater for a double-contrast examination than for a single-contrast examination; fluoroscopy and the number of additional spot films should be curtailed as far as possible. We routinely take a total of six images: lateral rectum, right anterior oblique spot film of the cecum, a supine, prone, and both decubitus films (Figures 3–25 and 3–27). Further films are taken as deemed necessary by the radiologist at the time of the examination. Occasionally the lateral view of the rectum

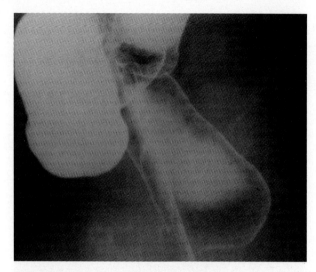

FIGURE 3–25. Normal rectum in an infant. The rectum is well distended with air on this double-contrast barium enema examination. Some barium is pooling on the dependent side of the rectum. Around this, faint lucencies are seen due to lymphoid follicles. The Foley catheter has been placed too high in this infant.

is obscured by barium in both decubitus positions, in which case a cross-table lateral shoot through film may be helpful (Figure 3–28).

In infants the technique can be modified to suit the clinical indication, which in this age group is most often rectal bleeding. The examination is easiest to control if the barium and air are injected by syringe and spot films are taken expeditiously to visualize all parts of the gut (Figure 3–29). The lymphoid follicular pattern is particularly prominent in this age group.

Double-Contrast Barium Enema versus Colonoscopy. Colonoscopy and double-contrast barium enema are complementary techniques in children, and any one patient may be more sensitive to one than to the other (Stringer, 1986). Colonoscopy provides direct vision, permits biopsies, and allows polypectomies. However, colonoscopy is a more invasive procedure than double-contrast barium enema. Colonoscopy often requires significant sedation in children and has been associated with a small incidence of serious complications such as bleeding, perforation, or even explosion if polypectomy is performed (Geenen, 1975; Burdelski, 1978; Bigard, 1979; Kozarek, 1980). Double-contrast barium enema is less invasive, does not require sedation, permits easy and rapid

visualization of the entire large bowel and often the terminal ileum, and has negligible complications in a viable large bowel.

The extent of colitis may be underestimated by either procedure (Stringer, 1986). Infrequently both double-contrast barium enema and colonoscopy will fail to detect small polyps in adults and children (Gans, 1975; Stringer, 1986; Laufer and Smith, 1976; Williams, 1974). More polyps could probably be shown on double-contrast barium enema in children by taking multiple spot films of overlying loops of bowel; but the benign nature of juvenile polyps, unlike the adenomatous polyps of adults, makes the routine use of spot films and the resulting increase in radiation dosage unacceptable. Colonoscopy may also fail to detect polyps if a haustral fold or Houston's valve hides them or if they are located in a region of sharp angulation (Laufer and Smith, 1976). Occasionally histology will detect an abnormality unsuspected on

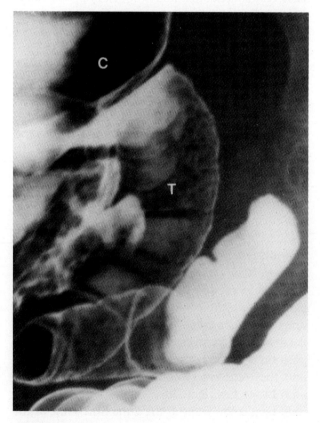

FIGURE 3–26. Normal terminal ileum on double-contrast barium enema. Barium and air have refluxed from the cecum (C) back into the terminal ileum (T), which shows some regular nodularity due to lymphoid follicles. The cecum was included on another spot film.

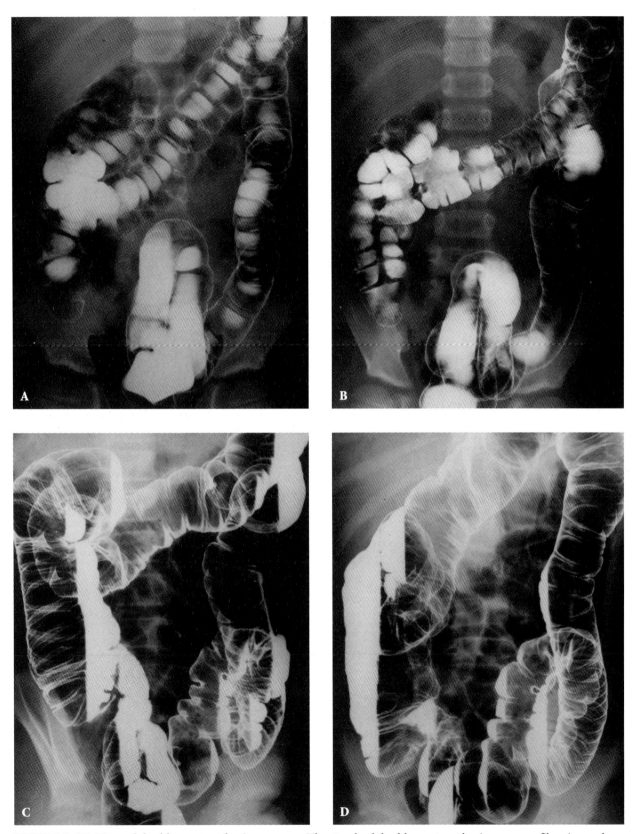

FIGURE 3–27. Normal double-contrast barium enema. The standard double-contrast barium enema films in our hospital are supine (*A*), prone (*B*), and left- (*C*) and right- (*D*) side-down decubitus films. Some top and bottom cropping has occurred in this reproduction.

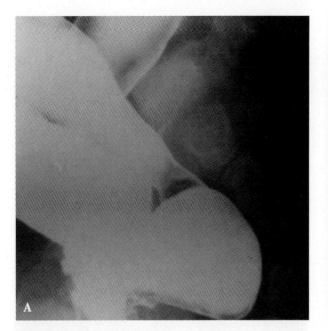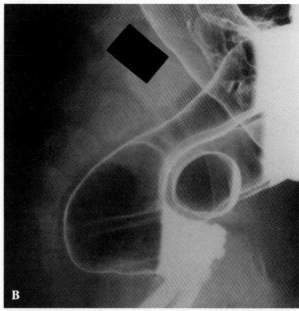

FIGURE 3–28. Normal rectum on double-contrast barium enema. *A,* The rectum is obscured by barium on this lateral view. *B,* A cross-table lateral shoot through film enabled good visualization of the rectum in this patient.

colonoscopy or double-contrast barium enema—the so-called "microscopic colitis," whose existence, however, is controversial (Stringer, 1986; Bo-Linn, 1985).

The most common failure of double-contrast barium enema is in the detection of early mild distal colitis when the only colonoscopic findings are of

loss of the normal vascular mucosal pattern due to edema (Stringer, 1986). See also Chapter 4.

Defecography
Defecography may occasionally be helpful in the assessment of constipation (Nussle, 1976; Mahieu,

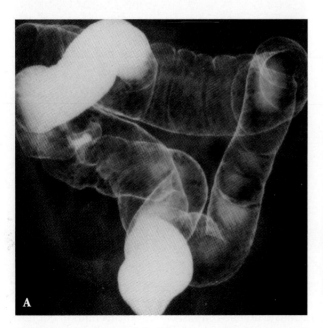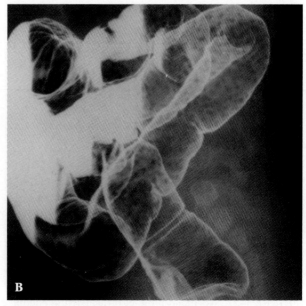

FIGURE 3–29. Normal double-contrast barium enema in an infant. *A* and *B,* 105-mm spot films can cover all areas of the large bowel and in this patient show a prominent lymphoid follicular pattern common in infants.

1984; Ekberg, 1985). A video recording of defecation following a limited barium enema is performed with the patient in the lateral position. The examination requires no patient preparation apart from an explanation of what is involved. Barium is instilled into the rectum and distal large bowel in the same way as at the start of a single-contrast barium enema. Then, with the fluoroscopic table erect, the patient sits on a suitable receptacle or commode so that lateral views of the rectum and anus can be taken. The entire procedure should be recorded on videotape. Ideally, films should be taken with the patient at rest (Figure 3–30A), squeezing and lifting, straining, evacuating (Figure 3–30B), and after evacuating; however, this is not possible with younger patients.

From the examination the anorectal angle, puborectalis sling, and anal closure can be assessed. The value of this information in children is still being elucidated. However, in our experience it has been occasionally helpful to the surgeons in managing patients with chronic constipation, especially following operations for Hirschsprung disease.

Water-Soluble Contrast Media

Examination of the Upper Gastrointestinal Tract
Water-soluble contrast examinations of the upper gastrointestinal tract in children are rarely neces-

sary. If there is a perforation, water-soluble contrast media are indicated but care must be taken to prevent aspiration; hyperosmolar contrast media should never be used (see previous section).

The indications for the expensive low osmolar contrast media are shown in Table 3–1 and are discussed above. The major indications include patients at risk of lung aspiration (see Figure 3–4), suspected malrotation (see Figure 3–5B), bowel perforation, barium inspissation, neonatal obstruction (especially meconium ileus), and contrast examination prior to endoscopy or biopsy. The technique of examination is similar to that described for barium examinations.

Examination of the Lower Gastrointestinal Tract

In the Newborn. A water-soluble contrast enema in the newborn infant is usually performed to investigate obstruction or to show the anatomic position of the gut. In addition, conditions such as meconium ileus and meconium plug syndrome, also known as functional immaturity of the large bowel, can be both diagnosed and treated. The indications are discussed in the previous section and listed in Table 3–1.

There is no preparation for a large bowel study in the newborn but supine and erect films of

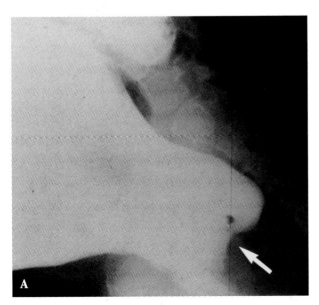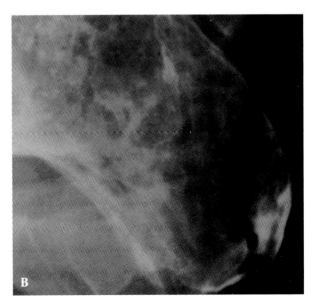

FIGURE 3–30. Defecograph. *A,* During the filling phase, the grossly dilated rectum and distal large bowel fills with barium. There is a prominent anorectal angle due to the puborectalis sling (*arrow*). *B,* The evacuation film shows a change in the anorectal angle which becomes less acute and the anus opens.

the abdomen should be taken to exclude the presence of intraluminal intraperitoneal gas, which would contraindicate the examination. A soft catheter should be inserted gently until its tip is just inside the rectum. Great care should be taken as the rectosigmoid junction is very near to the anus in infants, and too vigorous an insertion or too rigid or long a tube may result in perforation. The buttocks are taped, and the large bowel is filled by gentle injection of contrast from a syringe. The child may need to be turned prone and the buttocks squeezed by hand to prevent leakage. The hand can be protected by a lead glove or by lead positioned on the tabletop. Fluoroscopic monitoring and number of spot films should be kept to a minimum. The minimum number of films should include a lateral view of the rectum to include the rectosigmoid junction and a frontal view to show the relationship of the cecum to the right iliac wing (see Figure 3–5A). The cecum may be obscured by redundant loops of sigmoid colon; this can be avoided by first examining the distal large bowel with barium and then pushing this distal barium proximally with water so that the cecum can be seen through the water-filled sigmoid colon.

Older Infants and Children. Water-soluble contrast media are rarely used, being reserved for cases where perforation is possible. The technique in older children is the same as that of single-contrast barium enema.

Loopography

Loopography is performed to examine the bowel distal to an enterostomy for patency or extravasation. A water-soluble contrast medium is therefore the medium of choice.

Prior consultation with the surgeon helps ensure a safe and useful examination. Sometimes contrast material can be instilled via the anus but if rectal surgery has been performed, this route is invariably contraindicated. Catheters should be inserted carefully to prevent trauma; contrast material should be injected cautiously, especially initially. Foley balloon catheters should not be inflated in the enterostomy as perforation is easy to produce. This is more likely to occur in children than in adults as the diameter of the bowel varies, depending not only on the age and size of the patient but also on the degree of use of that portion of the gut.

Anorectal Atresia Examination

It is of paramount importance to recognize preoperatively whether an anorectal atresia is high or low. A high atresia mistaken for a low atresia can lead to an inappropriate operation which can result in permanent incontinence. Hence, in many hospitals, if there is any doubt over whether a lesion is high or low, a colostomy is performed.

Inverted abdominal radiography has been used to aid localization of the rectum. However, this technique can give misleading results; a crying child can give a result of low atresia, and impacted meconium can mimic a high atresia (see Chapter 10). Hence we no longer recommend this approach. Cystourethrography or loopography following colostomy, using water-soluble contrast media, may be helpful in demonstrating the anatomy (see Chapter 10). Percutaneous punctures are rarely if ever performed in our hospital as these patients invariably require colostomy and can be investigated electively later by loopography.

Peritoneography and Herniography

Water-soluble contrast media injected directly into the peritoneal cavity have been used in the identification of patent processus vaginalis, hernia, communicating hydrocele, or undescended testis in an infant (Oh, 1973) or child but this technique is rarely if ever required today.

Air Techniques

Air is rarely regarded as a contrast medium but in pediatrics it is an excellent and safe contrast medium for diagnosing esophageal, duodenal, or jejunal atresia.

Frontal and lateral views of the chest with a catheter in position are usually sufficient to delineate the extent of an esophageal atresia, whereas the presence of gas in the stomach indicates the presence of a distal fistula.

The proximal pouch may be further delineated by injecting air via a nasogastric tube. The distension of the air-filled esophageal pouch may be associated with profound bradycardia, presumably secondary to a vagal reflex, or may compromise the trachea and cause respiratory difficulties. If such complications occur, the air should be quickly aspirated from the pouch. It follows, therefore, that distension of an esophageal pouch is a procedure that should not be performed unless absolutely necessary and then preferably under fluoroscopic control and with heart rate monitoring.

Duodenal or proximal jejunal atresia is usually obvious from the plain films. Occasionally, when minimal bowel gas is present, the diagnosis may be confirmed by injecting air through a nasogastric tube under fluoroscopic control. Under these circumstances, air is the safest contrast medium.

In the large bowel, bowel gas in a dilated colon is useful in the assessment of anorectal malformations. Gas may be seen in the bladder if there is a fistulous communication confirming that the large bowel ends high up (see Chapter 10).

Air (and occasionally carbon dioxide) enemas have been extensively used in the diagnosis and treatment of intussusception, and air is now the contrast medium and technique of choice for intussusception reduction in many hospitals (Gu, 1988). Air is insufflated per rectum outlining the intussusception, which with practice is easily visualized as a typical filling defect in the bowel. Once delineated, further gas is insufflated to reduce the intussusception. It is particularly important to keep the pressure to a maximum of 120 mm Hg initially and never to exceed 140 mm Hg (Gu, 1988; Shiels, 1990, 1991, 1993, 1995). For the inexperienced, a pressure release valve is helpful to prevent persistent inadvertent high pressure rises (Shiels, 1990). Transitory rises in pressure occur in struggling children who are subjected to Valsalva's effect but this does not cause any increased risk because intra-abdominal pressure as well as intraluminal bowel pressure rises so there is no additional risk of perforation (Shiels, 1995). Air enema is even a safe enough technique to undertake repeated delayed reduction attempts under certain circumstances which may aid reduction (Connolly, 1995). If perforations occur, they are usually easily repaired surgically without complication because there is no soiling of the peritoneum by barium (Daneman, 1995, 1996).

The reduction rate is better with air than barium probably because air fills any viscus it is put into, giving an even pressure over the intussusceptum and potentially aiding reduction whereas barium, as with any fluid, will layer on the dependent surface of the bowel. Reduction occurs more quickly, and there are some reports that recurrence rate is lower with air reduction (Daneman, 1995, 1996). (For a further description and discussion of the technique of air reduction of intussusception see Chapter 10.)

MISCELLANEOUS TECHNIQUES

Intestinal Tube Placement

Gastrojejunal tubes, nasojejunal tubes, small bowel biopsy capsules, and pancreatic enzyme aspiration tubes often require fluoroscopy for accurate placement. However, by allowing plenty of time for tubes to pass into the small bowel without screening, fluoroscopy can be kept to a minimum.

The most commonly positioned tubes are nasojejunal feeding tubes in small infants. These infants have an increased risk of bowel perforation (Cheek, 1973; Boros, 1974; Chen, 1974; Sun, 1975; Rhea, 1975; Siegle, 1976; Perez-Rodrigues, 1978; Merten, 1980; McAlister, 1985); hence, a soft tube such as a silastic or Erythrothane tube should be used but even these may cause perforation (McAlister, 1985). Few of the many types of nasojejunal tubes permit the use of conventional guide wires. Some of the tubes contain a polymer guide wire, which can be removed but not reinserted. Familiarity with the type of tube to be inserted is essential before starting the procedure.

When a gastrostomy is present and gastroesophageal reflux prevents gastrostomy feeding, a feeding tube can be positioned via the gastrostomy into the jejunum (McLean, 1982; Strife, 1985). To facilitate tube placement, an endotracheal tube can be used as a guide to steer the tube through the pylorus (Strife, 1985). A gastrojejunal tube has two advantages: it is easier to secure to the body to prevent removal of the tube by the child, and it avoids trauma to the esophagus and nasal air passages.

Percutaneous gastrostomy obviates the need for endoscopy or surgery (Ho, 1983, 1985) and may be suitable for some pediatric patients. These and other interventional techniques are considered in Chapter 5.

Video Velopharyngeal Examination

General Considerations and Indications
The assessment of speech disorders related to velopharyngeal function depends on clinical, investigative, and endoscopic evaluation as well as radiologic examination. Therefore, an interdisciplinary study team, including a speech pathologist, is essential in the radiologic study of speech disorders (Skolnick, 1977). The examination may be combined with nasoendoscopy to assess the velopharyngeal portal (Croft, 1981; Sinclair, 1982).

Children generally need to be over 5 years of age to cooperate sufficiently for the analysis and to be eligible for pharyngoplasty. Pharyngoplasty consists of bridging the velopharyngeal portal with a flap of tissue which is taken from the posterior wall of the pharynx and inserted into the posterior aspect of the soft palate. The aim is to ensure closure of a persistent velopharyngeal portal opening during speech. This technique is used in the treatment of hypernasal speech.

Real-time ultrasonography has been used to evaluate lateral pharyngeal wall movement, to assess velopharyngeal movement, and to predict surgical success in velopharyngeal insufficiency (Skolnick, 1985; Kelsey, 1982). This technique requires further evaluation.

Fluoroscopy is useful in the assessment of speech disorders; since radiation dosage must be minimized, video rather than cine recording is used (Skolnick, 1969). Fluoroscopy is used to assess velopharyngeal function during speech (Skolnick, 1970). Most commonly the speech disorder is idiopathic or secondary to cleft palate. Video velopharyngeal analysis may also be useful prior to or following adenoidectomy in the assessment of hypernasal speech. Other indications include a variety of syndromes (e.g., velocardiofacial syndrome) or before and after facial reconstruction surgery.

Techniques Employed

Whatever the indication, the technique is similar. With the patient supine, 1 to 2 mL 56% wt/wt barium is instilled into each nostril. The patient then sniffs to coat the palate and nasopharynx. Soft palate movement can then be observed using videofluoroscopy in lateral (Figure 3–31), frontal (Figure 3–32), Waters' (Figure 3–33), Towne's (Figure 3–34), and basal projections (Figure 3–35) (Skolnick, 1970; Stringer, 1985, 1986).

A series of phrases is repeated by the patient in each projection to assess velopharyngeal closure in a variety of speech tasks. Each patient repeats the sentences, "Put the baby in the buggy," "Give Gary the chocolate cake," "Susie sees the sun in the sky," and "My name is _____." The patient also makes the sounds, "s," "sh," and "ooh" and counts from one to ten. The entire examination is recorded on videotape with sound.

The radiologic appearances in each projection during quiet respiration and during phonation are shown in Figures 3–31 to 3–35. The types of small defects visible on phonation in velopharyngeal insufficiency using the Towne's and basal views are demonstrated in Figures 3–34 and 3–35, respectively.

The lateral view shows the anatomy of the soft palate and provides information on the movement of the tongue, palate, and posterior pharyngeal wall as well as demonstrating any Passavant's ridge (Figure 3–36) or eustachian tube opening (Figure 3–37). Passavant's ridge, originally described in 19th-century cleft palate patients, is not uncommon in patients with hypernasality and may also be seen in normal subjects. It seems to help complete closure of the velopharyngeal portal although the functional significance of a Passavant's ridge is not well understood (Glaser, 1979). The examination should be performed in the presence of a speech pathologist (Skolnick, 1977). Unfortunately, the lateral view may miss some essential information (Stringer, 1986). Small defects are difficult to see if there is too little barium in the portal to demonstrate bubbling or if the adenoids are irregular, giving multiple lines of barium. In addition, the lateral view cannot demonstrate movement of the lateral pharyngeal walls or the sphincteric movement of the velopharynx. Lateral pharyngeal walls can move incongruously with respect to the velum (Sphrintzen, 1974). Further, some authors believe that the extent of lateral wall movement is a reliable predictor of surgical success in velopharyngeal insufficiency (Kelsey, 1982). Others think that the site and shape of the velopharyngeal portal defect are important, since central defects do well surgically but lateral defects may not (Quattromani, 1977).

Lateral wall movement can be assessed by a variety of views. The frontal view was the first to be described and in many patients gives adequate information, even though the data may be difficult to assess because of overlapping structures. The Waters' view may be easier to assess as the mandible acts as a window through which the walls can be more easily seen than in the frontal view (Stringer, 1985) (compare Figures 3–32 and 3–33). However, neither the frontal nor Waters' views, even when supplemented by oblique views, give full information about the sphincteric closure of the velopharyngeal portal, which some surgeons and speech pathologists argue is important in full speech assessment (LaRossa, 1980). For this, another view such as the basal or Towne's projection is necessary (Stringer, 1986).

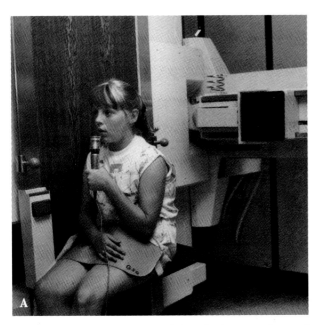
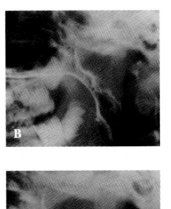
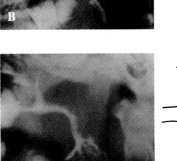
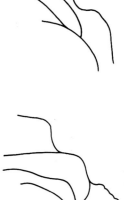

FIGURE 3–31. Lateral view of the velopharyngeal portal. *A*, The patient sits on the footstool. The velopharyngeal portal is shown open at rest (*B*) and closed during phonation of sibilants (*C*). The superior surface of the normal soft palate and posterior pharyngeal walls are coated with barium. (Reprinted with permission from Stringer DA, Witzel MA. Velopharyngeal insufficiency on multiview videofluoroscopy: a comparison of projections. AJR 1986;146:15–9.)

Neither the basal nor the Towne's view can be performed on standard fluoroscopic equipment without neck extension or flexion. The basal view, which is more widely used, requires marked hyperextension of the neck (see Figure 3–35), which may exaggerate the degree of incompetence seen during speech (McWilliams, 1968). Conversely, the Towne's view is performed with the neck well flexed (see Figure 3–34), which may decrease the degree of incompetence seen during speech (McWilliams, 1968). In our opinion, the Towne's view was more effective at detecting incompetence than the basal or lateral projection, and it never missed a defect seen on the other views (Stringer, 1986). The Towne's view was especially helpful when the adenoids were large whereas a satisfactory basal view has been difficult to obtain in patients with large adenoids (Stringer, 1986). We also found that the position for the Towne's view was easier for children to maintain than that for the basal view (Stringer, 1986). In addition, the Towne's view has the advantage of avoiding primary-beam irradiation of the thyroid gland. Although the eyes may be irradiated, they can often be excluded from the primary beam by careful coning. Radiation dosage is minimized during the procedure by careful coning, keeping the fluoroscopy to the shortest time necessary for the study, and using video recording rather than cineradiography.

Nasopharyngoscopy is used by some clinicians to investigate suspected velopharyngeal incompetence. The shape and movement of the velopharynx seen with flexible nasopharyngoscopes compares better with that seen on the Towne's view than on the basal view (Stringer, 1988).

In summary, in our opinion the lateral view alone is insufficient to assess the velopharyngeal portal. The Towne's view gives the best visibility, especially if there are large adenoids. It is performed with the patient in a comfortable, easily maintained position and the view of the portal is most similar to that shown by a flexible nasopharyngoscope. The basal view can be reserved for the few cases where the Towne's view has not given sufficient diagnostic information.

Sialography

Sialography may be performed on the submandibular and parotid glands in children with suspected calculi or swollen salivary glands of uncertain etiology. Sialography should not be performed if acute infection is present.

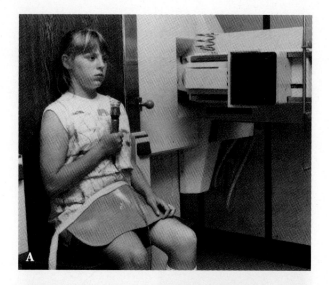

FIGURE 3–32. Frontal view of the velopharyngeal portal. *A,* The patient sits on the footstool facing the x-ray tube. *B,* The lateral pharyngeal walls (*arrows*) are shown at rest. *C,* The walls move medially during phonation. The posterior aspect of the soft palate and posterior pharyngeal walls are coated with barium. (Reprinted with permission from Stringer DA, Witzel MA. The Waters projection for evaluation of the lateral pharyngeal wall movement in speech disorders. AJR 1985;145:409–10.)

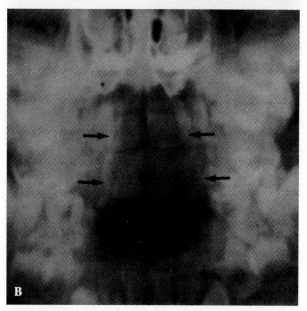

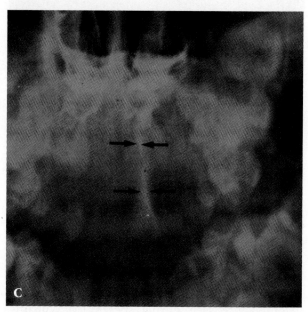

Sialography is a relatively easy technique to perform on cooperative children over the age of 5 years. When time is taken to explain to the child what is involved and that no sharp needles are used, only the exceptional child is uncooperative. The various types of flexible sialogram catheters are preferable to the rigid lacrimal needles, as they allow some patient movement (Rabinov, 1969; Manashil, 1977).

Submandibular cannulas (0.3 to 0.57 mm diameter) are usually needed to cannulate the parotid duct in young children, as a parotid duct cannula (0.81 mm diameter) is too large. This allows the parotid duct to be cannulated without dilatation. The submandibular duct is occasionally too

small to cannulate in very young children, and the procedure should be abandoned promptly before the duct is traumatized. A high-density (75%) water-soluble contrast medium gives satisfactory results and avoids any possible complications such as foreign body reactions which may occur if oily contrast media are used and if there is extravasation. The rest of the technique is similar to that used in adults (Manashil, 1977; Yune, 1972).

We take anteroposterior and lateral plain films looking for calcific stones before contrast injection. Filling of the gland is best performed under fluoroscopy with spot films taken in frontal and lateral projections. Fluoroscopy allows radiation and repeat films to be kept to a minimum. We no longer

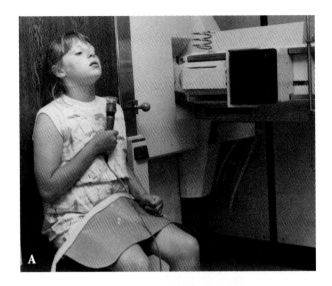

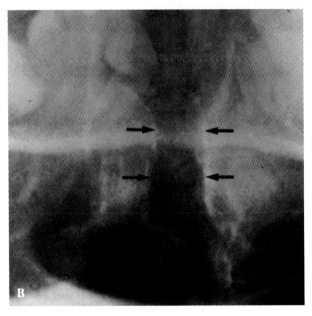

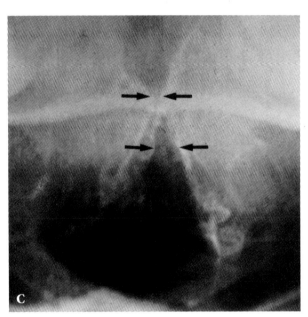

FIGURE 3–33. Waters' view of the velopharyngeal portal. *A,* The patient sits facing the x-ray tube, with the chin elevated. *B,* The lateral pharyngeal walls (*arrows*) are shown at rest and move medially during phonation (*C*). The posterior aspect of the soft palate and posterior pharyngeal walls are coated with barium. (Reprinted with permission from Stringer DA, Witzel MA. The Waters projection for evaluation of lateral pharyngeal wall movement in speech disorders. AJR 1985;145:409–10.)

take the postevacuation film 5 minutes after administering a sialogogue such as citric acid or lemon juice (Rubin, 1957), as in a prospective study of 80 patients at our hospital these views failed to give us any extra information.

When the ducts are filled some discomfort is often experienced by the patient but this is seldom a problem if the patient has been forewarned that discomfort will be felt when the ducts are full but that this discomfort will rapidly abate when the injection stops. The patient should also be advised to stay very still at this stage so that the test can be quickly finished without further injections.

The technique of enhancing the salivary glands by sialography during computed tomography (CT sialography), is useful in adults when space-occupying lesions are present (McGahan, 1984; Evers, 1985) and can be incorporated into a diagnostic aspiration procedure. However, there is some controversy over whether this affects patient management (Stacey-Clear, 1985). Sialography without CT is often unhelpful in space-occupying lesions but valuable in infective conditions (McGahan, 1984).

Rectal Manometry

Reflex relaxation of the internal sphincter, which is dependent on the presence of intact ganglion cells (Mahboubi, 1979), occurs when a balloon is inflated in the rectum. Failure of relaxation suggests Hirschsprung disease.

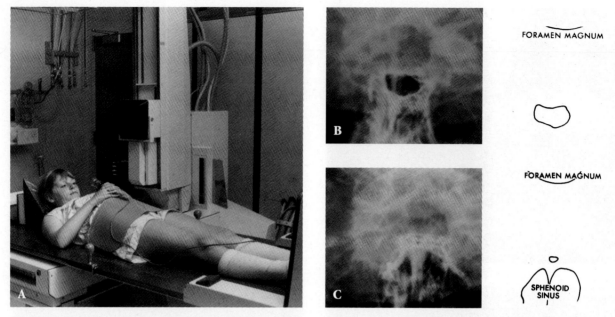

FIGURE 3–34. Towne's view of the velopharyngeal portal, prone position. *A,* The patient lies supine with the neck extended on a foam bolster. *B,* The velopharyngeal portal is shown open at rest, and (*C*) during phonation of sibilants, a small defect is present. The velopharyngeal portal is coated with barium. (Reprinted with permission from Stringer DA, Witzel MA. Velopharyngeal insufficiency on multiview videofluoroscopy: a comparison of projections. AJR 1986;146:15–9.)

COMPUTED TOMOGRAPHY

Computed tomography is a useful modality for visualizing structures in the pediatric abdomen (Daneman, 1986), particularly in malignant disease, complex lesions, and older children. However, CT is an invasive procedure in that oral and/or intravenous contrast media are usually required and that rectal or intravaginal contrast may sometimes be needed. There are many oral contrast media available; a typical one would be 5 mL of Gastrografin in 200 mL of flavored drink for older children or 5 mL of Iohexol in 200 mL of water for sedated younger children. Low osmolar contrast media (2 to 3 mL per kg body weight) are given for intravenous enhancement.

Some children find that being placed into the aperture of a CT unit is a frightening experience. Sedation is often required for children under 4 years of age, despite fast scan times (Kirks, 1983).

The invasiveness and cost of the procedure along with the added disadvantage of sedation means that we reserve CT for problems that cannot be solved adequately by other safer and less invasive modalities such as US. In adults, fat planes and the size of the patient aid CT imaging but degrade US images; the converse is true in children.

Indications

Computed tomography is particularly useful in blunt abdominal trauma (Kuhn, 1981) as multiple organs such as the liver (see Chapter 11), spleen (see Chapter 14), pancreas (see Chapter 13), and adjacent bones are quickly and accurately visualized. Computed tomography is now the procedure of choice in the investigation of significant trauma at our hospital. Intra-abdominal abscesses can be well demonstrated (Afshani, 1981) if US has failed to delineate them satisfactorily. Computed tomography is very useful in investigating the retroperitoneum (Kuhns, 1981).

Computed tomography can image thickened bowel wall (see Chapter 9) but is rarely indicated for this purpose in children unless there is a diagnostic dilemma, such as may occur in patients with Crohn's disease with possible abscess formation (see Chapter 9). Tumors of the gut are uncommon in children and therefore often cause diagnostic difficulty; CT can then be helpful (see Chapters 8 and 9).

Computed tomography can help to investigate thoracic mass lesions, such as foregut malformations, although other methods already discussed are usually sufficient (Kirks and Korobkin, 1981).

Abdominal masses can be investigated by CT (Kirks and Merton, 1981), but for children this method should be reserved for the patients in whom US has failed to demonstrate the anatomy sufficiently. In this regard CT is particularly helpful in malignant primary tumors of the liver (see Chapter 11). Metastases are also well seen (see Chapter 11). Benign masses of the liver can be visualized well but may be difficult to differentiate from malignant lesions unless they are cystic or have a vascular etiology, such as hemangioma or aneurysm, as these may have characteristic patterns of enhancement (see Chapter 11).

Computed tomography can accurately show calcification in the biliary tree (see Chapter 11) or pancreas (see Chapter 13) and may also be used to investigate hepatic parenchymal disease by demonstrating enhancing nodules in cirrhosis, dilated intrahepatic ducts, or fat and iron deposition (see Chapter 11). Fat is characteristically found in the pancreas in older patients with cystic fibrosis and is well shown by CT (see Chapter 13).

Splenic cysts may be difficult to diagnose confidently with US as they may display multiple echoes due to cholesterol crystals, and so CT may occasionally be used in this case (see Chapter 14). Solid masses within the spleen are rare but can also be accurately delineated with CT (see Chapter 14).

MAGNETIC RESONANCE IMAGING

Magnetic resonance imaging is a body-section-imaging modality that does not use ionizing radiation. It has no significant complications and causes no discomfort to the child, although the enclosed space and noise of the equipment may cause problems due to fright or claustrophobia. It is less invasive than CT as intravenous contrast media are not presently required. However, as in CT, sedation is usually necessary in children aged 1 to 8 years (Cohen, 1986c). Magnetic resonance imaging has certain other advantages over CT and US, namely, the ability to image in different planes, better delineation of soft tissues, and nonproduction of artifacts from bone or nonferromagnetic implanted metal. In the future, characterization may be possible by spectroscopic analysis (Cohen, 1986a) although results so far are unpromising.

The relative disadvantages include the cost of the equipment and the length of time of examination (30 to 90 minutes). The signals detected are weak and movement such as respiration and peristalsis will degrade the image. Respiratory gating will

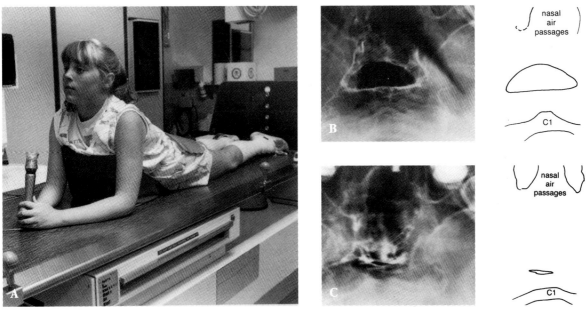

FIGURE 3–35. Basal view of the velopharyngeal portal, supine position. *A,* The patient lies prone with the head vertical by resting on the arms and foam bolster. *B,* The velopharyngeal portal is shown open at rest. *C,* During phonation of sibilants a small defect is present. The velopharyngeal portal is coated with barium. (Reprinted with permission from Stringer DA, Witzel MA. Velopharyngeal insufficiency on multiview videofluoroscopy: a comparison of projections. AJR 1986;146:15–9.)

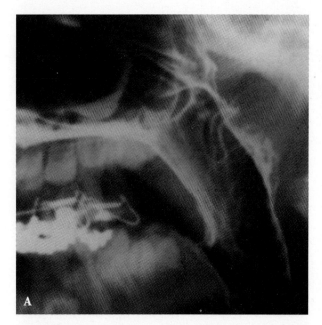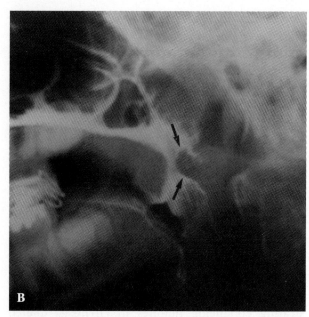

FIGURE 3–36. Lateral view of nasopharynx. *A,* At rest the posterior aspect of the soft palate and posterior pharyngeal walls coated with barium are seen with the portal open. *B,* During phonation of sibilants the portal is closed. A Passavant's ridge (*arrows*) is seen.

overcome one of these problems (Johnston, 1985) and signal averaging can be used to improve image quality despite motion; however, both increase the time of the examination (Cohen, 1990). Calcium and bone are not directly seen with MR and so calcium deposition and subtle bone destruction may be missed (Bydder, 1982; Brant-Zawadski, 1984). Sick infants and children often need close monitoring, and equipment may malfunction due to the magnetic field (Hope, 1985). These problems can be alleviated by using nonferrous electrodes, monitoring respiration by a pneumonic tube taped to the abdomen, and using Doppler probes to monitor blood pressure and heart rate (Hope, 1985; Roth, 1985).

When an MR examination has been decided upon, the older child has a full explanation and demonstration of the equipment to allay fears. The repetitive loud tapping noise due to gradient coil switching is explained to the child. The child is asked to evacuate the bladder (and if necessary, bowels) prior to being positioned comfortably on the table. A parent is encouraged to remain with the child for comforting. Both child and parent should have no magnetic material in their possession and should be carefully screened before the examination begins.

In younger children, usually aged 1 to 8 years, sedation similar to that given for CT is necessary.

In many institutions this is performed by anesthetists, and if available they can certainly help improve the quality of the examination as well as give the best service to the child. Infants usually fall asleep for the examination if they are fed in the hour prior to scanning.

The smallest coil size possible is selected for maximum resolution. The "head" coil usually fits children under 8 years of age.

The pulse sequence is then selected depending on the area and condition of interest. Usually a T1-weighted spin echo sequence is satisfactory for anatomy but if maximum contrast between pathologic and nonpathologic conditions is required, a T2-weighted spin echo pulse sequence may be used. Gradient echo, inversion recovery, and fat saturation sequences can also be useful (Cohen, 1990).

In the abdomen in children, MR is most commonly used to evaluate hepatic and other masses but increasingly other indications for MR are being evaluated. Gadolinium contrast medium is generally used to investigate mass lesions.

General and Bowel. Unfortunately, peristalsis interferes with intestinal imaging. Respiratory gating, fast sequences, and signal averaging help to some extent. More recently, image sequences using very long T1-weighted sequences and water as bowel contrast have been used with significant success. Further refinements may well change how we image the bowel in the future.

In the gastrointestinal tract, MR can at present detect inflammatory disorders such as inflammatory bowel disease and necrotizing enterocolitis (Cohen, 1986b). Tumors such as lymphoma of the small bowel can be identified. Bowel wall hematomas from trauma or Henoch-Schönlein purpura can be seen (Cohen, 1986b; Hahn, 1986). Duplication cysts (Rhee, 1988) and diaphragmatic hernias can all be seen well but other methods of investigation are just as effective and are easier and cheaper (Cohen, 1990). Anorectal anomalies and anatomy are superbly outlined by MR (Cohen, 1990).

Abdominal abscesses may be visualized but these are best detected adjacent to the liver (Cohen 1986b, Cohen, 1990). Elsewhere in the abdomen, abscesses are difficult to distinguish from bowel loops, similar to CT (Wall, 1985).

Liver and Biliary Tree. The normal liver is well contrasted against adjacent structures except when motion degrades the image. The liver has relatively short T1 and T2 relaxation times, and therefore, has a higher signal intensity than the spleen on T1-weighted images and a lower signal intensity on T2-weighted images. Portal and intrahepatic vessels are well seen but the intrahepatic biliary tree is not visualized (Cohen, 1985, 1990).

Liver MR is sensitive for detecting liver lesions (Davis, 1984) but is often not specific even between tumors and infection, as both can give prolonged T1 and T2 times (Boechat, 1988; Li, 1988; Ros, 1987). Cavernous hemangiomas often appear different from malignant liver tumors but these signs are not always reliable (Cohen, 1990) (see Chapter 10). Cavernous hemangiomas appear similar to multilocular cysts and have significantly longer T2 relaxation times than malignant liver tumors (Ohtomo, 1982). Indeed, even small cavernous hemangiomas can be detected more accurately by MR than by US or CT (Itai, 1985) or even selective hepatic angiography (Glaser, 1985). Cystic lesions are usually hypointense on T1-weighted images and hyperintense on T2-weighted images.

Diffuse hepatic fatty infiltration is difficult to detect by MR, which is less sensitive than CT (Buonocore, 1983); however, focal fat, diffuse hepatitis, or iron deposition (Brasch, 1984) can be

more easily differentiated in MR. The liver can also be examined in the fetus, but the value of this is not yet determined (Weinreb, 1985).

The gallbladder is seen when present and has a variable signal intensity depending on the age of the bile (Cohen, 1990). Gallstones are not detectable as they produce a very weak signal and hence are only appreciated as negative defects if the bile is of a concentration to be visible. Choledochal cysts can be seen but US is preferable for their investigation. Promising new imaging techniques with very long T1 sequences can show the biliary tree in fine detail but are not yet routinely used.

Spleen. The signal intensity of the spleen is variable but longer than the liver (Cohen, 1990). In the spleen, abscesses, cysts, and tumors can all be identified but this is of minor importance as other modalities can be used.

Pancreas. The signal intensity of the pancreas is variable and generally between that of the liver and the spleen (Cohen, 1990). Cystic fibrosis with fat deposition in a small pancreas can be detected as in US and CT. Pancreatitis gives a larger, less well-defined pancreas (Davis, 1984), and pseudocysts are also

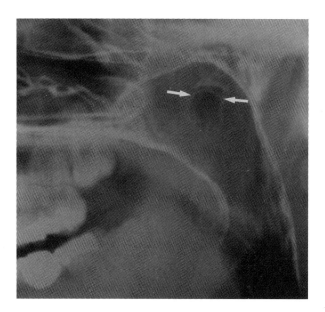

FIGURE 3–37. Lateral view of nasopharynx. At rest the posterior aspect of the soft palate and posterior pharyngeal walls coated with barium are seen with the portal open, and there is excellent visualization of the eustachian tube (*between arrows*).

distinguishable. Pancreatic ducts are less well seen than with CT but the splenic artery, and to a lesser extent the splenic vein, can be distinguished without intravenous enhancement (Davis, 1984). Surface coils may give better delineation of pancreatic lesions (Simeone, 1985). The bowel loops are also difficult to distinguish from pancreas that is further obscured by respiratory movement. The advent of oral iron as a contrast media may help the visualization of the pancreas. The oral iron is usually given as 3.38 mg of ferric iron per mL, given as a dilute solution of Geritol or 25 mg per mL of ferrous iron given as a dilute solution of Fer-In-Sol (Cohen, 1986b).

New imaging techniques with very long T1 sequences can show the pancreatic ducts in fine detail. These techniques show promise for the future but are not yet routinely used.

The Future. With improvements in technology, MR will probably become as important as US in the investigation of childhood abdominal disorders. The future is most exciting in this area.

ANGIOGRAPHY

The advent of high-quality US, CT, nuclear scintigraphy, and MR has led to a continuing reassessment of the role of angiography. Angiography is now mostly used in the pediatric gastrointestinal tract to assess solid hepatic mass lesions and in gastrointestinal bleeding (Moore, 1982).

In solid hepatic mass lesions, angiography can be useful in patients where partial hepatectomy is contemplated as it gives detailed information of the hepatic arterial, hepatic venous, and portal venous anatomy; however, many surgeons do not require this detailed information. A histologic diagnosis based on angiographic appearance is fraught with problems and is usually inadvisable (see Chapter 11) (Moore, 1982). The extent of involvement of the inferior vena cava is usually seen on CT or US, with or without Doppler; however, cavography may be helpful in the few cases where there is a diagnostic dilemma.

Arterial chemotherapy infusion may use angiographic techniques, and arterial occlusion with embolization is possible in malignant tumors, especially hemangioendotheliomas (Moore, 1982).

The other major indication for abdominal angiography is massive bleeding of the gastrointesti-

nal tract. Of course, endoscopy is the procedure of choice in the investigation of bleeding in the upper gastrointestinal tract. Barium meal examinations are also useful, especially in children when hemorrhage occurs from esophageal varices secondary to portal hypertension (Buonocore, 1972). It should be remembered that peptic ulceration is less common in children. Angiography is helpful when these other modalities have failed to give adequate information or where there is insufficient time for these investigations. For angiography to be successful at showing the bleeding site, the rate of blood loss must be at least 0.5 mL per minute (Whitley, 1979).

Angiography of the upper gastrointestinal tract may show varices, a bleeding site such as an ulcer, focal areas of contrast medium extravasation in stress ulceration, or focal or diffuse gastric hyperemia in hemorrhagic gastritis (Franken, 1982). In the small bowel, a bleeding Meckel's diverticulum may be identified by the extravasation of contrast. In the large bowel, endoscopy and double-contrast barium examinations are usually sufficient to demonstrate a cause for bleeding but occasionally angiography may be useful.

Angiographic techniques similar to those used in adults such as the use of gelfoam with or without Pitressin infusion are occasionally used to stop hemorrhage from the gut.

NUCLEAR MEDICINE

General Principles and Sedation

The effective practice of nuclear medicine in children is technically demanding due to the unique needs of the young patient. Technical advances in radiopharmaceutical and instrumentation technology have made the clinical use of nuclear medicine in children more rewarding in allowing greater investigation of physiology instead of anatomy (Nadel, 1995). This shift is ideally suited to the investigation of gastrointestinal problems where quantification of many functions is important and thus the use of nuclear medicine techniques is growing rapidly, offering the clinician important information not previously easily accessible in daily practice.

Immobilization and care of the child during nuclear medicine examinations are important factors in producing high-quality studies in children. It is routine in many departments to allow parents and/or siblings to remain in the imaging room to provide a sense of security and safety for the child. Similarly, the patient is allowed to hold a favorite toy or a prized possession and parents are instructed to bring such items with them for the test.

For neonates up to 2 years of age, bundling in a papoose-type holder, sleep deprivation, and feeding the child while on the imaging table can be all that is required for immobilization. Immobilization and cooperation of children aged 4 to 5 years can be achieved with entertainment, including videos, music, stories, or distraction techniques such as bubble-blowing. Older children are usually reassured by a calm manner and simple explanation of the procedure involved. Children between the ages of 2 to 5 years or who are mentally retarded or have severe attention deficit problems are more likely to require sedation. Sedation is more the exception than the rule to assure a good study in our laboratory. If sedation is necessary, guidelines for the safe and effective sedation of children are well-established in the literature (Pintelon, 1994; Weiss, 1993).

Radiopharmaceutical Dosages

The dosage of radiopharmaceuticals used in gastrointestinal scintigraphic examinations is listed in Table 3–3 and is usually based on either body surface area or the weight of the child with minimum and maximum values. Pediatric GI scintigraphic procedures are considered safe and good quality can be obtained with acceptable radiation dosages. The absorbed radiation dosages for the radiopharmaceuticals used for these evaluations in children can be found in standard pediatric nuclear medicine textbooks (Miller, 1994; Treves, 1995).

Multiple functions at different sites in the gastrointestinal tract may be altered in a symptom or set of symptoms. Nuclear medicine offers the ability to describe and quantify these functions. A list of nuclear medicine examinations which can be used in children to evaluate disorders involving the gastrointestinal tract are listed in Table 3–4. Some of these are discussed below in more detail. In-depth details of these examinations can be found in standard nuclear medicine textbooks.

Types of Examination

Gastroesophageal Dysfunction and Reflux
Although gastroesophageal reflux is physiologic when infrequent, it may be associated with significant morbidity and even life-threatening events in children. Generally the diagnosis can be established using three commonly available noninvasive tests each having their own advantages.

Prolonged pH monitoring with an indwelling esophageal probe is the recognized "gold standard" for establishing the frequency and severity of reflux in children with detection rates of 90 to 100%. Although technically challenging and not always successful, the probe can be used for simultaneous detection of apnea and bradycardia. There remains some disagreement regarding diagnostic criteria using this technique and concern that it is too sensitive. Upper GI series have the advantage of being able to assess swallowing and morphology of the upper tract but has lower reported sensitivity in the range of only 50% and can result in heavy exposure to radiation during prolonged fluoroscopy.

TABLE 3–3.   Administered Minimum/Maximum Doses of Common Radiopharmaceuticals Used in Pediatric Gastrointestinal Scintigraphy

Study	Radiopharmaceutical	Administration	
		Minimum MBq	*Maximum*
Visceral heterotaxy	Tc 99m denatured red blood cells	37–74	1–2
Biliary scan	Tc 99m mebrofenin	9.25–111	0.25–3.0
Gastroesophageal reflux and aspiration	Tc 99m phytate colloid	20	20
or gastric emptying scan	Tc 99m-labeled-RBC bleeding scan	75–370	2–10
Meckel scan	Tc 99m pertechnetate	75–370	2–10
Liver/spleen scan	Tc 99m phytate colloid	75–220	2–6

*Ranges shown are for minimum/maximum dose based on child's weight.

TABLE 3–4.   Indication for Pediatric Gastrointestinal Scintigraphy

Examination	Indication
Gastroesophageal reflux and aspiration scan	Suspected gastroesophageal reflux and/or aspiration
Sialography	Suspected aspiration of saliva
Esophageal motility	Esophageal dysfunction
Gastric emptying	Suspected dysmotility
C-14 breath test	Suspected bacterial overgrowth of *Helicobacter pylori*
Schilling test	Suspected malabsorption or pernicious anemia
Biliary scintigraphy	Neonatal jaundice
	Choledochal cyst
	Cystic fibrosis
	Bile leak
	Bile duct obstruction
	Gallbladder dysfunction
	Transplant and postoperative evaluation
Colloid liver/spleen scan	Parenchymal liver disease
	Visceral heterotaxy
	Functional hyposplenism
Labeled-white-cell scan	Inflammatory bowel disease
Ectopic gastric mucosa scan	Detection of Meckel's diverticulum
Red-blood-cell bleeding scan	Acute GI bleed
	Fever of unknown origin
Radiolabeled MIBG	Neuroendocrine tumors
Octreotide scan	Gastrointestinal endocrine tumors

Scintigraphic studies for reflux, on the other hand, are physiologic, sensitive, and relatively easy to perform, allowing continuous monitoring over several hours with sensitivities of 60 to 80% (Arasu, 1980; Schatzlein, 1979; Guillet, 1984). They offer the opportunity to assess esophageal transit during the same study. Analysis of the swallowed bolus allows quantitation of esophageal transit times in motility disorders, and delays in transit can be localized to different regions of the esophagus (Malmud, 1982; Klein, 1984; Heyman, 1985, 1998). Gastric emptying and aspiration can be assessed with this examination as well. It has been suggested that the reported incidence of aspiration is too low and that results correlate poorly with delayed gastric emptying (Cleveland, 1995).

Oral technetium 99m sulfur colloid or phytate colloid is used since the colloid is not absorbed from the gastrointestinal tract. Also, if it is aspirated into the lungs, it remains as a localized area which is readily detectable and is eventually cleared by action of the cilia. Technetium 99m colloid is given orally with milk or formula to an infant.

The patient is given the feed orally and is imaged under the camera in the supine position. Once the feeding is complete, the patient is imaged continuously for 1 hour. Dynamic images are acquired into the computer every 10 seconds. The physician then is able to view the images dynamically at the computer terminal and adjust the contrast as required (Figure 3–38).

If aspiration is also being considered, images of the thorax to visualize the lungs are taken at approximately 1 hour and 4 hours after the dynamic reflux images. A relatively simple way to assess direct aspiration of saliva is to perform a salivagraphic examination (Heyman, 1989). A small amount of radiocolloid similar to that used for reflux scan is placed on the tongue and allowed to mix with oral secretions. Anterior images of the thorax with the patient supine are collected in the computer at 30 second intervals to 1 hour or terminated earlier if aspiration with visualization of the tracheobronchial tree is obtained (Figure 3–39).

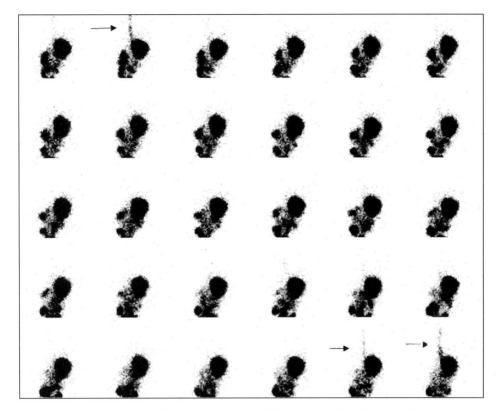

FIGURE 3–38. Gastroesophageal reflux scan. The arrows identify multiple episodes of reflux into the upper esophagus visualized over the course of dynamic scanning. Each image represents a 1-minute time interval.

Gastric Emptying

Abnormalities of gastric emptying occur in a variety of disorders and may cause either accelerated or delayed emptying which is easily measured using scintigraphic techniques. Just as in reflux studies, these examinations compare favorably to conventional barium studies and more invasive manometric techniques in that they are physiologic, noninvasive, and offer favorable dosimetry. Scintigraphic evaluation of gastric emptying time is the current gold standard for quantitatively assessing abnormal gastric motility.

Normally in the newborn stomach there are no peristaltic movements for the first few days of life. The normal receptive relaxation of the fundus which occurs when food enters the stomach is also absent in newborns and has been postulated to be partly responsible for the increased frequency of reflux in that population (Heyman, 1985).

The physiology of gastric emptying is known to be biphasic with liquids being emptied predominately but not exclusively by fundal action and solids being more influenced by antral contraction. The so-called "lag phase" is the time required for solid food to be broken to an acceptable size to pass through the pylorus (Heyman, 1995). Scintigraphic techniques ideally should reflect this physiology and use radiolabeled standard meals including both solids and liquids although this is not always possible in infants who are ill. If only one material is used, solids should be chosen as they will demonstrate more subtle alterations.

The evaluation of gastric emptying can be and is frequently performed in conjunction with investigation for gastroesophageal reflux. Gastric emptying time studies are technically challenging and require careful attention to preparation of the patient and radiolabeled meals as well as the actual examination and subsequent calculations which require mathematical modeling and assessment of depth changes of the bolus during the examination (Urbain, 1995). Infants are fed formula or cereal labeled with technetium Tc 99m phytate or sulfur colloid in their usual meal volume. Children older than 1 year of age are fed a meal with a radiolabeled egg, or with yogurt if allergic to egg.

There is a wide variation in normal values and the results are influenced by, among other factors, meal sugar and protein content, time of day, medications, age, and gender of the patient. Normal values in infants and children vary with age and size and each lab must ensure that they develop meaningful ranges for these values, generally a T1/2 of 90 ± 30 minutes (Heyman, 1998). Results can be expressed as a T1/2 or percent residual at 60 or 90 minutes or both. In infants and children in whom milk is used as the meal, it has been recommended that percent residual at 60 minutes be used as emptying of milk is biexponential (Notghi, 1995). Ideally 50% should be emptied by 90 minutes (Figure 3–40).

Ectopic Gastric Mucosa Study

The usual indication of this study is to look for Meckel's diverticulum in a child with painless rectal bleeding, using technetium Tc 99m pertechnetate with highly accurate results (Sfakianakis, 1981). Ectopic gastric mucosa can be found in duplications and enteric cysts. Barrett's esophagus can also give a positive test.

Technetium Tc 99m pertechnetate is given intravenously according to the dosage schedule, and localizes in gastric mucosa. The exact site of histologic localization is still controversial. Initially, data supported the theory that pertechnetate primarily localizes in the parietal cells. However, subsequent data indicates that parietal cells are not necessary for pertechnetate uptake by the stomach (Chaudhuri, 1977) and that it is taken up primarily in superficial mucous secreting cells (Williams, 1983).

To prevent secretion of pertechnetate into the gastric lumen and further passage throughout the small bowel which could obscure the abdomen, the patient should fast for 8 hours prior to the study. However, in a young infant, fasting time is reduced to 4 hours because of the baby's vulnerability to dehydration and electrolyte imbalances. For an optimal study, the patient should not have ingested a laxative or aspirin (ASA) which can cause bowel inflammation for 5 days prior to the scan. A barium study should not be performed for at least 48 hours prior to the scan as retained barium can interfere with visualization of the gastric mucosa.

More recently, pharmaceuticals such as pentagastrin, glucagon, and cimetidine (Yeker, 1984) have been given to augment the sensitivity of the study. Pentagastrin increases the gastric excretion of radionuclide and is given in a dose of 6 µg per kg subcutaneously. Glucagon decreases intestinal peristalsis and therefore prevents spillage of gastric contents into the bowel and so can be useful; the dose is 0.5 to 1.0 mg given intramuscularly or intravenously. Cimetidine is an H_2 receptor antagonist that decreases gastric output by approximately 50% in the resting state and also decreases the volume of secreted gastric juice and pepsin. The clinical effect of cimetidine is to inhibit the secretion of pertechnetate into the gastric lumen; it is usually given in a dose of 300 mg orally for 2 days prior to the study. However, many of the patients present as emergencies with lower gastrointestinal tract bleeding, and the cimetidine may have to be given more quickly. It can be given at a dose of 5 mg per kg intravenously (maximum 300 mg) in a slow bolus 20 minutes prior to the scan.

A flow study is performed at the time of the injection and is useful for detecting vascular lesions as the cause of bleeding, such as hemangiomas. Anterior views of the abdomen are acquired

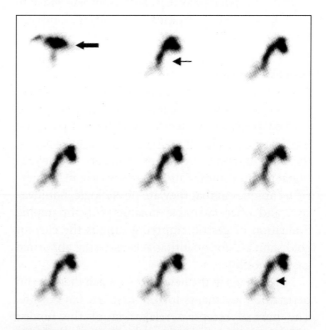

FIGURE 3–39. Salivagram. Salivagram examination in a child with cerebral palsy identifying aspiration of the child's own saliva. The large arrow points to radioactivity pooled on the tongue. The smaller arrow identifies activity in the trachea, and the arrow head shows activity in the trachea bifurcating into the right and left mainstem bronchus on further sequential images.

approximately every minute after an initial 2-minute dynamic flow phase for 15 minutes following injection. Lateral and posterior views are also taken 15 minutes post injection. Repeat delayed views (i.e., anterior, posterior, right lateral) at 30 minutes are sometimes useful but later imaging does not add to the study. It is important that the patient empty the bladder both prior to and at 30 minutes into the study, as there is renal excretion of pertechnetate into the bladder which can obscure a small Meckel's diverticulum lying behind the bladder (Figure 3–41).

Uptake in the diverticulum usually parallels the course of uptake in the stomach but is of less intensity due to the smaller amount of gastric mucosa in the diverticulum compared with the stomach. Diverticula are mobile and, although most often located in the right lower quadrant, can move about the abdomen during the examination. Transit of contents of the diverticulum, dilution of radiopharmaceutical by bowel content, insufficient gastric mucosa, impaired vascular supply, and poor positioning can be potential causes for uncommon false-negative studies. Careful positioning to ensure that the entire bladder is included on the images and the use of additional positional and postvoid images will minimize false-negative studies. We routinely image the thorax in young infants and children who may not be able to adequately localize their symptoms, to look for other sites of potential ectopic gastric mucosa. Bowel ulceration and inflammation and renal activity may also cause false-positive results (see Figure 3–43).

Because pertechnetate is also taken up by the thyroid gland, choroid plexus, and salivary glands, potassium perchlorate at 10 mg per kg is administered after the study is completed, to competitively inhibit the uptake and thereby reduce radiation to the thyroid.

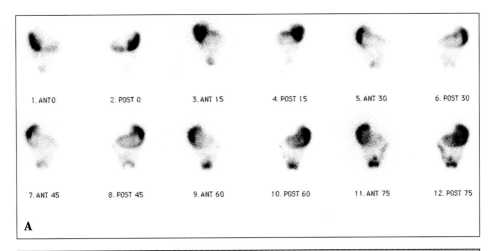

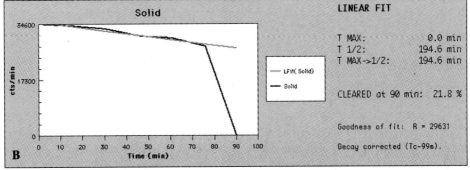

FIGURE 3–40. Gastric emptying study. *A,* Sequential images taken in anterior and posterior projections at 15-minute intervals for the assessment of gastric emptying. At 75 minutes, there is visually still a considerable amount of activity in the stomach. *B,* Quantitative assessment shows delayed gastric emptying with the T1/2 considerably prolonged and less than 50% emptying at 90 minutes.

Bleeding Studies

In pediatrics, the Meckel scan as described previously is usually the study of choice for gastrointestinal bleeding. However, if other bleeding sites are suspected or if the bleeding is acute, technetium 99m-labeled red blood cells (Tc 99m RBCs) (Figure 3–42) or technetium 99m sulfur colloid (Tc 99m-SC) is used.

The patient's red blood cells should be labeled with technetium-99m using a technique to visualize the vascular compartment and active extravasation at an active bleeding site. Detection rates are excellent when the patient is bleeding with a minimum rate of 0.1 to 0.5 mL/min to visualize the bleeding lesion, depending on the actual site, although slower rates have been visualized experimentally (see Figure 3–44). Imaging must be performed at the time the patient is actively bleeding. Technetium 99m RBC study allows intermittent surveillance of the abdomen over a 24-hour period. Initial angiographic images and static computer images are obtained for 2 hours. Delayed imaging at 3 to 4 and up to 6 to 8 hours can be obtained

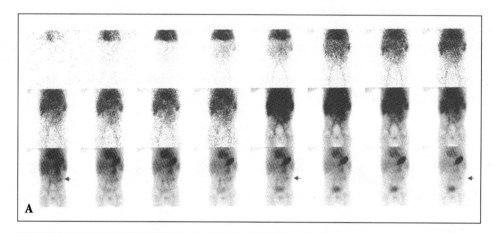

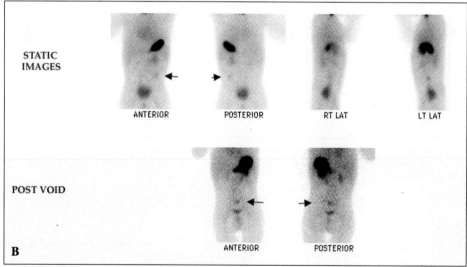

FIGURE 3–41. Meckel's diverticulum study. *A,* Tc-99m pertechnetate scan for detection of Meckel's diverticulum. Initial dynamic images show activity in the stomach, and faintly on dynamic sequential images there is activity in the left midabdomen in this child who presented with rectal bleeding. *B,* Further static images at 15 minutes after the injection of radiotracer identify a persistent focus in the left midabdomen (*arrow*). Following voiding with an empty bladder, this abnormal focus of radioactivity is noted to fall down into the lower pelvis in the usual location for an expected Meckel's diverticulum, which was confirmed at surgery. The examination was done with cimetidine premedication.

if the bleeding site is not visualized initially. Colonic activity will be noted at 24 hours in the presence of an upper GI bleeding site, with no significant colonic activity if there has not been bleeding in the previous 24 hours. Dynamic cine viewing of the continuously acquired imaging is essential to assess for small areas of activity that show rapid intestinal transit. Barium and contrast can interfere with visualization on scintigraphic examination; therefore, a Meckel scan or a Tc-99m RBC study should be performed before barium GI examination or angiography, and a Meckel scan should be done before a Tc-99m RBC study.

When Tc-99m-SC is used to detect bleeding sites, it will circulate in the vascular compartment with a half-life of 2.5 to 3.5 minutes and will extravasate at actively bleeding sites before it is cleared by the reticuloendothelial system. Because of this rapid background clearance, a Tc-99m-SC scan will detect even smaller bleeding volumes between 0.05 and 0.1 mL per minute (Alavi, 1977; Berger, 1983). However, the bleeding site must be visualized early in the study due to the rapid liver uptake of radionuclide from the blood. In spite of this, it is a useful screening procedure in the detection of bleeding and has been reported as superior to contrast angiography (Alavi, 1981).

Following intravenous injection of either Tc-99m RBCs or Tc-99m-SC, serial images are taken (see Figure 3–44). In the case of a red blood cell study, the patient is imaged in the anterior position for up to an hour with lateral or posterior views as necessary. The Tc-99m-SC study requires images for only approximately 30 minutes due to rapid liver clearance of the radiotracer. Views in multiple projections may be necessary to clarify areas obscured by liver radioactivity.

Liver and Spleen Scintigraphy

Radionuclide liver/spleen scanning has been a well-established method to assess both congenital and acquired disease. It readily shows normal variations in position such as low-lying liver and in anatomy such as Riedel's lobe, which may be confused clinically with an enlarged liver. With the increased use of ultrasonography and other noninvasive anatomic imaging studies, liver/spleen single photon emission computed tomography (SPECT) scintigraphy is now used mainly to assess visceral heterotaxy and functional hyposplenism.

Technetium 99m sulfur colloid is phagocytosed by Kupffer's cells in the reticuloendothelial system and so can be used to image the spleen and liver. Particle size and blood flow patterns as well as Kupffer's cell function will alter the distribution and uptake of sulfur colloid.

Visceral heterotaxy syndromes include asplenia and polysplenia. Children with asplenia are at risk for overwhelming bacterial infections. Prompt identification of asplenia can ensure the patient will obtain the necessary prophylaxis to prevent sepsis. In infants with suspected visceral heterotaxy who have equivocal ultrasound examinations, liver/spleen scintigraphy with Tc 99m colloid alone or combined with heat-damaged red-blood-cell

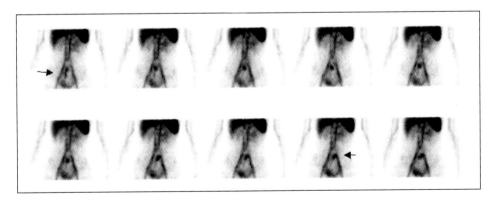

FIGURE 3–42. Labeled-red-blood-cell-scan. Labeled-red-blood-cell scan to assess for bleeding focus in a child presenting with acute rectal bleeding. Selected images in the dynamic sequence of this scan show a focus in the right abdomen which demonstrates colonic transit over time (*arrows*). At surgery, the bleeding focus was found to be a Meckel's diverticulum with ulceration.

scintigraphy can demonstrate position of the liver and the presence or absence of the spleen and will show the presence of any accessory spleen (Armas, 1985; Oates, 1997; Waldman, 1977) (Figure 3–43).

Functional hyposplenism may be clinically manifested by the presence of circulating Howell-Jolly bodies. In children with polysplenia, the multiple spleens may not have adequate reticuloendothelial cell function. Other causes of functional asplenia include vascular occlusion, hemoglobinopathies, infiltrative disorders including tumor and amyloid, celiac sprue, systemic lupus erythematosus, previous radiotherapy and chemotherapy, and immunodeficiency syndromes (Armas, 1985; Malleson, 1988). In children found by other anatomic imaging to have a spleen, the nonvisualization of splenic activity on a Tc-99m colloid liver/spleen scan based on reticuloendothelial system (RES) phagocytosis will confirm significant functional asplenia.

Selective spleen scintigraphy visualizes the spleen alone without interfering activity from the liver (Armas, 1985) (Figure 3–43B). This is most useful in suspected asplenia or when a midline centrally placed liver is present which could obscure an abnormally sited spleen (Ota, 1997). Functional asplenia and suspected splenic hypoplasia may also be indications, although assessment by Tc-99m sulfur colloid scan based on RES phagocytosis is usually adequate (Sty, 1985).

By damaging the patient's red blood cells with heat and reinjecting them labeled with 99m-technetium, the spleen alone can be visualized. Normally the spleen avidly sequesters damaged RBCs and appears hot on scan with only faint hepatic visualization. If no functioning spleen is present, there will be marked liver localization secondary to RES phagocytosis and some excretion of free pertechnetate by the kidneys.

Between 3 and 8 mL of blood are taken from the patient, depending on age. Lesser volumes have been used (Erhlich, 1982) but with decreased labeling efficiency. These are labeled with technetium

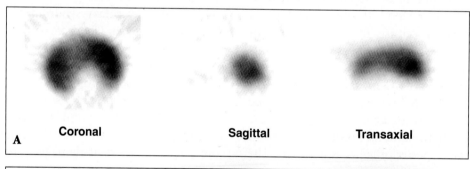

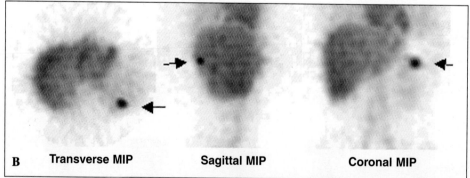

FIGURE 3–43. Spleen study. *A,* Infant with visceral heterotaxy syndrome. Howell-Jolly bodies were found in the circulating blood. Asplenia was suspected. Colloid liver/spleen scan identifies a transverse liver which is symmetric. No splenic tissue is seen, confirming the diagnosis of asplenia. The child was given Pneumovax for prophylaxis. *B,* Heat-damaged red-cell-scan in a child who had a previous splenectomy for chronic idiopathic thrombocytopenic purpura. The tomographic maximal intensity projection (MIP) images identify a residual amount of splenic tissue felt to be an accessory spleen.

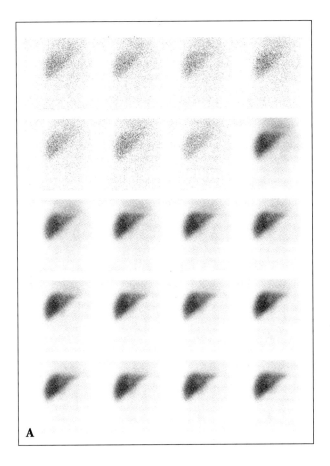

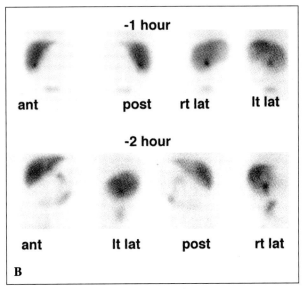

FIGURE 3–44. Biliary scan. *A*, Newborn with jaundice. Initial dynamic images of a Tc 99m mebrofenin biliary scan show normal hepatic extraction but no visualization of activity in the gastrointestinal tract. *B*, Subsequent delayed images at 1 hour show the presence of activity in the gallbladder. On the 2-hour images, after the infant was fed a fatty meal (formula), excretion into the gastrointestinal tract is noted, thereby ruling out biliary atresia.

99m pertechnetate and heated in a water bath at 50°C for 10 minutes under sterile conditions. The radioactive damaged red blood cells are then re-injected into the infant or child. After this, static planar images followed by SPECT imaging are taken at 1 to 1.5 hours to allow for adequate localization.

Biliary Scan

Imaging of the patency and function of the biliary tree is possible using one of the iminodiacetic acid (IDA) derivatives which is actively taken up by the hepatocytes and excreted into the bile canaliculi. Hepatobiliary scintigraphy using iminodiacetic radiopharmaceuticals provides clinically useful information on function of the biliary tract in a variety of pathologic processes in children, including neonatal jaundice, gallbladder dysfunction, trauma, and liver transplantation. In children, the commonest iminodiacetic compounds used are diisopropyliminodiacetic acid (DISIDA) and methyltribroiminodiacetic acid (mebrofenin). These agents have the greatest hepatocyte uptake and lowest renal excretion.

A minimum fast of 4 hours in young infants and children and 6 to 8 hours in older children is required for patient preparation. Prolonged fasting greater than 24 hours should be avoided as should hyperalimentation as either may cause nonvisualization of the gallbladder due to the presence of viscous bile in the gallbladder.

If the indication for the examination is to distinguish neonatal hepatitis from atresia, the patient is premedicated with phenobarbital orally, 5 mg per kg daily in divided doses each day for 5 days prior to the scan, to enhance enzymatic excretion of bile and thereby reduce false-positive interpretations of biliary obstruction when cholestasis is present (Majd, 1981).

The Tc-99m-IDA is injected intravenously within the dosage range as noted in Table 3–3. The patient is imaged sequentially in the anterior position for approximately 30 minutes. At this time lateral and posterior views are taken. Further images are taken depending whether there has been excretion into the small bowel. If there has been none, images are usually taken at 60 minutes in the anterior,

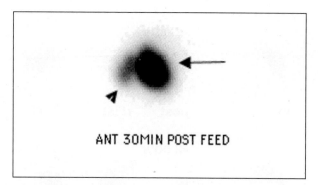

ANT 30MIN POST FEED

FIGURE 3–45. Biliary scan. A child with a cystic mass noted on ultrasound examination in the region of the porta hepatis. The intense focus of activity (*arrow*) is uptake in a type 1 choledochal cyst. The lateral activity (*arrowhead*) is activity in the gallbladder.

right lateral and posterior projections, and thereafter as necessary at 2, 4, and even 24 hours. In neonatal hepatitis, excretion may occur so slowly that images at 24 hours are necessary.

One common specific indication is to distinguish neonatal hepatitis from biliary atresia as a cause of neonatal jaundice by assessing hepatocyte clearance and biliary excretion into the intestine. Biliary atresia can be ruled out in an infant if a patent biliary tree is demonstrated with passage of activity into the bowel (Figure 3–44). If no radiopharmaceutical is seen in the bowel on imaging up to 24 hours, distinction between severe hepatocellu-

lar disease and biliary atresia cannot be made and investigation with open liver biopsy and operative cholangiography is usually the next procedure. A sensitivity and specificity of 97% and 82% respectively has been achieved for hepatobiliary imaging in the diagnosis of biliary atresia (Gerhold, 1983). However, the study is less accurate in infants older than 3 months in whom hepatic parenchymal damage has developed secondary to biliary atresia.

Following the Kasai procedure for biliary atresia, hepatobiliary scanning is useful to assess the patency of the hepatoenteric anastomosis. Bile leak following this procedure and in liver transplantation and trauma is also readily identified. Cholescintigraphy in suspected bile leak provides information generally not available with other techniques except direct cholangiography. If the amount of intraperitoneal accumulation of tracer is greater than that entering the gastrointestinal tract, surgery is usually indicated (Lette, 1990).

Biliary scintigraphy readily establishes the diagnosis of choledochal cyst in all age groups and differentiates this from other causes of cystic masses in the right upper quadrant (Figure 3–45). In this respect, it is complimentary to US and CT. The differential diagnosis of choledochal cyst includes pancreatic pseudocyst, duodenal diverticulum, hydatid disease, hepatic artery aneurysm, and simple hepatic cysts. Occasionally ovarian cysts, mesenteric cysts, bowel duplication cysts, and renal cysts, by virtue of their location, can

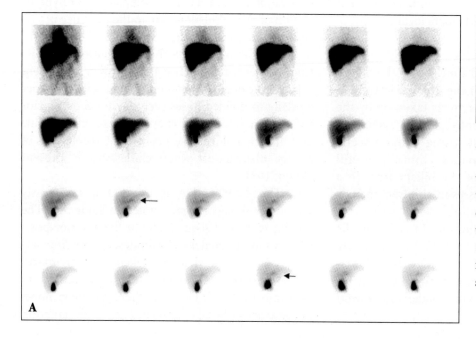

A

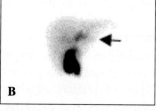

B

FIGURE 3–46. Biliary scan in cystic fibrosis. *A* and *B*, Child with cystic fibrosis showing the characteristic appearance of stasis of the radioactivity in the left hepatic duct (*arrow*) on (*A*) initial sequential dynamic images and (*B*) subsequent static delayed image.

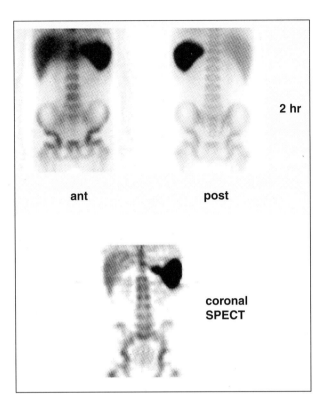

2 hr

ant   post

coronal
SPECT

FIGURE 3–47. White-blood-cell-scan. Images from a Tc 99m HMPAO labeled-white-blood-cell scan for detection of inflammatory bowel disease. No abnormal activity is seen in the abdomen at 2 hours or on the coronal SPECT examination. This is a normal examination.

mimic choledochal cyst. Combined anatomic and physiologic imaging will make the diagnosis of choledochal cyst. Computed tomography and US can demonstrate the cystic lesion but hepatobiliary scintigraphy confirms the biliary origin of the cystic lesion if this information is required preoperatively (Camponovo, 1989; Nadel, 1996).

The impairment of both intra- and extrahepatic biliary drainage is an important cause of liver disease in cystic fibrosis. More than 50% of patients with cystic fibrosis have sonographic and scintigraphic abnormalities of the gallbladder and cystic duct. Hepatobiliary scintigraphy in cystic fibrosis has shown characteristic patterns of dilatation of mainly the left hepatic duct, narrowing of the distal common bile duct, gallbladder dysfunction, and delayed bowel transit (Dogan, 1994; Gaskin, 1988; Nagel, 1989; O'Brien, 1992) (Figure 3–46).

Cholecystitis in children may be acalculous and a complication of prolonged illness, infection, or trauma (Paret, 1994; Ternberg, 1975). Sensitivity

and specificity for the scintigraphic diagnosis of acute acalculous cholecystitis is reported to range from 68 to 93% and 38 to 93%, respectively. The combined ultrasonography and hepatobiliary scintigraphy findings are helpful in establishing the diagnosis. Ultrasonographic findings include a thickened gallbladder wall, gallbladder distention, pericholecystic collection of fluid, subserosal edema without ascites, intramural gas, and a sloughed mucosal membrane (Cornwell, 1989). Hepatobiliary scintigraphy may show the characteristic scintigraphic pattern in adults of nonvisualization of the gallbladder. The gallbladder can, however, be visualized in the presence of acalculous cholecystitis and toxic cholecystitis (Coughlin, 1990; Mirvis, 1986; Nora, 1984; Weissmann, 1981).

Hepatobiliary imaging in children who have undergone liver transplantation will assess graft vascularity, parenchymal function, biliary drainage, presence of a leak, and obstruction (Gelfand, 1992; Kim, 1994; Shah, 1995; Westra, 1993).

Imaging of Inflammation

The demonstration of intra-abdominal sources of infection remains a challenging imaging and clinical problem. The frontline imaging techniques of US, CT, and MR provide structural detail but cannot always differentiate adequately treated residual morphologic alterations. A variety of scintigraphic studies can provide physiologic information not available through other means. These studies make a significant contribution to the clinical problems of whether active infection exists in the abdomen, and of the location, extent, and response to therapy over time of such infection. While gallium has a time-honored place in the visualization of infection, recent radiopharmaceutical innovations allow more specific and sensitive delineation of a variety of infectious processes.

One relatively recent innovation is the use of radiolabeled autologous white blood cells (labeled WBCs). Radiolabeled WBCs will leave the circulation at sites of infection and migrate into the infected tissues as part of the normal host response. Scanning with labeled WBCs (In-111-WBC scanning) has been used extensively, and the recent addition of Tc 99m hexamethylpropylene amine oxime (HMPAO) as a practical label for autologous white blood cells offers high-quality images with more favorable dosimetry.

Normal distribution of WBCs occurs in the spleen and liver with faint marrow activity. Transient WBC sequestration in the lungs may occur in the first few hours. Imaging of the abdomen is usually performed at 24 hours, but early images at 2, 4, or 6 hours may reflect sites of involvement more accurately because of later migration of white cells into and throughout the bowel lumen which may by 24 hours cause false-positive results (Figure 3–47).

Other new radiopharmaceuticals employ radiolabeled nonspecific IgG, and radiolabeled antigranulocyte antibodies can demonstrate inflammatory processes although the mechanism is less specific for infection than that of labeled white blood cells since it is dependent on increased vascular permeability. Work continues in the development of radiolabeled chemotactic peptides and liposomes (Oyens, 1995).

With respect to the use of readily available labeled white blood cells, there have been concerns expressed regarding putative permanent radiation-induced chromosomal aberrations occurring in the re-injected lymphocytes, although such cells are short-lived and the risk of malignancy is small. The relatively high splenic radiation dose associated with the technique is cause for its limited use in children (Papos, 1996). In addition, the labeling procedure is somewhat tedious and requires a comparatively large volume of blood in infants and young children (Oyens, 1995).

Nevertheless, in appropriate clinical settings this technique is advocated for use in children, for example in inflammatory bowel disease (Jobling, 1996; Papos, 1996). For pediatric use the optimum label for white blood cells is Tc-99m-HMPAO when directly compared with indium in the same patients. Neither agent requires bowel preparation or cleansing (Mansfirel, 1995).

Labeled white blood cells can be used to determine whether there is active inflammation in the colon with good sensitivity, specificity, and diagnostic accuracy compared to endoscopy and radiology, which patients dislike (Papos, 1996). This technique can be used in the initial diagnosis of inflammatory bowel disease, especially in the small bowel, which is more difficult to assess than the colon (Shah, 1997; Kenan, 1992) and in the assessment of exacerbation or recurrence. Scanning with labeled white blood cells is effective as a screening examination in children in whom the diagnosis of inflammatory bowel disease should be considered, as it has the advantage of being able to assess both the large and small bowel in one easy, comfortable, and sensitive examination (Shah, 1997; Jobling, 1996; Jewell, 1996; Charron, 1998).

This study can be particularly helpful in patients with known Crohn's disease presenting with a clinical picture of small bowel obstruction when it is desirable to differentiate between obstruction from fibrotic stricture and from inflammatory stricture, thus permitting appropriate therapy.

When assessing patients with Crohn's disease for the presence of extraintestinal complications such as sepsis, abscess, or fistulae, studies with labeled white blood cells are best used as complementary tools to ultrasonography and CT. Abscesses will be visualized as intensely abnormal focal accumulations of white blood cells on late images at 24 hours.

Gastrointestinal Tumors

Neuroendocrine tumors or apudomas can involve the intestinal tract and pancreas and are divided into two groups, carcinoid tumors and endocrine pancreatic tumors, which are described by their hormone production and include vipomas, gastrinomas, insulinomas, somatostatinomas, and nonfunctioning islet cell tumors. The best radiopharmaceutical for imaging these tumors depends on the metabolic characteristics of the tumor. Recent advances now allow for use of many radiopharmaceuticals including radiolabeled metaiodobenzylguanidine (MIBG), vasointestinal peptide, and indium-111 pentetreotide (Seregni, 1998). In many cases, unexpected lesions not seen on CT and MR can be localized, which can indicate whether treatment with somatostatin analogues or other specific radiotherapy may be helpful (Shi, 1998; Savelli, 1998; Oberg, 1996).

REFERENCES

ULTRASONOGRAPHY

Alexander ES, Spitz HB, Clark RA. Sonography of polyhydramnios. Am J Roentgenol 1982;138:343–6.

Benacerraf BR, Greene MF. Congenital diaphragmatic hernia: US diagnosis prior to 22 weeks gestation. Radiology 1986;158:809–10.

Brasch RC, Abols IB, Gooding CA, et al. Abdominal disease in children: a comparison of computed tomography and ultrasound. Am J Roentgenol 1980;134:153–8.

Brill PW, Winchester P, Rosen MS. Neonatal cholelithiasis. Pediatr Radiol 1982;12:285–8.

Brown B St.J. The prenatal ultrasonographic features of omphalocele: a study of 10 patients. J Assoc Can Radiol 1985;36:312–5.

Chinn DH, Filly RA, Callen PW, et al. Congenital diaphragmatic hernia diagnosed prenatally by ultrasound. Radiology 1983;148:119–23.

Cremin BJ. Real time ultrasonic evaluation of the paediatric abdomen: technique and anatomical variations: a personal view. Br J Radiol 1985;58:859–68.

Denholm TA, Cros HC, Edwards WH, et al. Prenatal sonographic appearance of meconium ileus in twins. Am J Roentgenol 1984;143:371–2.

Emmanuel PG, Garcia GI, Angtuaco TL. Prenatal detection of anterior abdominal wall defects with US. Radiographics 1995;15:517–30.

Estroff JA, Parad RB, Benacerraf BR. Prevalence of cystic fibrosis in fetuses with dilated bowel. Radiology 1992;183:677–80.

Farrant P, Dewbury KC, Meire HB. Antenatal diagnosis of duodenal atresia. Br J Radiol 1981;54:633–5.

Grignon A, Filiatrault D, Yasbeck S. Gastroschisis and omphalocele: prenatal ultrasonographic diagnosis and portnatal evolution. Presentation at the 29th Annual Meeting of the Society for Pediatric Radiology; 1986 April 9–13; Washington, D.C.

Holm HH, Smith EH, Bartrum RJ. The relationship of computed tomography and ultrasonography in diagnosis of abdominal disease. J Clin Ultrasound 1977;5:230–7.

Lince DM, Pretorius DH, Manco-Johnson ML, et al. The clinical significance of increased echogenicity in the fetal abdomen. AJR 1985;145:683–6.

McGahan JP, Phillips HE, Cox KL. Sonography of the normal pediatric gall bladder and biliary tract. Radiology 1982;144:873–5.

McGahan JP, Hanson F. Meconium peritonitis with accompanying pseudocyst: prenatal sonographic diagnosis. Radiology 1983;148:125–6.

Nelson PA, Bowie JD, Filston HC, et al. Sonographic diagnosis of omphalocele in utero. AJR 1982;138:1178–80.

Oppenheimer DA, Carroll BA, Garth KE. Ultrasonic detection of complications following umbilical arterial catheterization in the neonate. Radiology 1982;145: 667–72.

Pilling DW. Infantile hypertrophic pyloric stenosis: a fresh approach to diagnosis. Clin Radiol 1983;344:51–3.

Stringer DA, Daneman A, St. Onge O. Doppler assessment of abdominal and peripheral vessels in children. Presented at the 71st meeting of the Radiological Society of North America; 1985; Chicago.

Stringer DA, Daneman A, Brunelle F, et al. Sonography of the normal and abnormal stomach (excluding hypertrophic pyloric stenosis) in children. J Ultrasound Med 1986;5:183–8.

RADIOGRAPHY: PLAIN FILMS

Boreadis AG, Gershon-Cohen J. Aeration of the respiratory and gastrointestinal tracts during the first minute of neonatal life. Radiology 1956;67:407–9.

Dillon JG. The respiratory function of the digestive tract as the basis of roentgenographic life test. AJR 1942;48: 613–24.

Frimann-Dahl J, Lind J, Wigelius C. Roentgen investigations of the neonatal gaseous content of the intestinal tract. Acta Radiol 1954;41:256–68.

Hajdu N. Plain radiography of the abdomen in paediatric practice. Part I. Neonatal period. Br J Radiol 1955;28:590–7.

Kottamasu S, Kuhns L, Stringer DA. Pediatric musculoskeletal computed radiography. Pediatr Radiol 1997;27: 563–75.

Stringer DA, Cairns R, Poskitt K, et al. Comparison of stimulable phosphor technology and conventional film-screen technology in pediatric scoliosis. Pediatr Radiol 1994;24:1–5.

RADIOGRAPHY: CONTRAST EXAMINATIONS

General Principles

Hynes DM, Edmonds EW, Rowlands JA, et al. Videofluorography pulsed fluoroscopy using a 512 × 512-pixel digital image system. Radiology 1985;155:519–23.

Soini I, Kiwru A, Makela PJ, et al. Double contrast examination of the stomach: 100 mm fluorography vs full size radiography. Radiology 1983;148:627–31.

Stringer DA, Gough L, Schulenburg K, et al. Preliminary experience with a high resolution digital image store for pediatric radiology. Presented at the 72nd Annual Assembly of the Radiological Society of North America; 1986 November 30–December 5; Chicago.

Choice of Contrast Media

Arrigoni A. Pneumoconiosi da bario. Clin Med Ital 1933;64:299–324.

Ginai AZ, Kate FJW, Berg RGM, et al. Experimental evaluation of various available contrast agents for use in the upper gastrointestinal tract in case of suspected leakage. Effects on lungs. Br J Radiol 1984;57:895–901.

Huston J, Wallach DP, Cunningham GJ. Pulmonary reaction to barium sulphate in rats. Arch Pathol 1952;54:430–8.

Meradji M. Radiological approach to the upper digestive tract in infants and young children. J Belge Radiol 1980; 63:25–32.

Nelson SW, Christoforidas AJ, Pratt PC. Further experience with barium sulfate as a bronchographic contrast medium. AJR 1964;92:595–614.

Nice CM, Waring WW, Killelea DE, et al. Bronchography in infants and children. Barium sulfate as a contrast agent. AJR 1964;91:564–70.

Sauvegrain J. The technique of upper gastro-intestinal investigation in infants and children. In: Karger S, editor. Progress in pediatric radiology. New York: Basel; 1969. p. 26–51.

Stringer DA, Hassall E, Ferguson AC, et al. Hypersensitivity reaction to pediatric single contrast barium meal studies. Pediatr Radiol 1993;23:587–8.

Willson JKV, Rubin PS, McGee TM. The effects of barium sulphate on lungs. A clinical and experimental study. AJR 1959;82:84–9.

Wolfson JJ, Williams H. A hazard of barium enema studies in infants with small bowel atresia. Radiology 1970;95: 341–5.

Water-Soluble Contrast Media

Bowring AC, Jones RFC, Kern IB. The use of solvents in the intestinal manifestations of mucoviscidosis. J Pediatr Surg 1970;5:338–43.

Gastrointestinal problems in cystic fibrosis. Cystic Fibrosis Foundation Consensus Conference; 1991 June 9–13; Washington, D.C.

Campbell JB, Dunbar JS. Contrast in intussusception, controversy II. Presented at the 29th Annual Meeting of the Society for Pediatric Radiology; 1986 April 9–13; Washington, D.C.

Chiu CL, Gambach RR. Hypaque pulmonary oedema—a case report. Radiology 1974;111:91–2.

Cleghorn GJ, Stringer DA, Forstner GG, et al. Treatment of distal intestinal obstruction syndrome in cystic fibrosis with a balanced intestinal lavage solution. Lancet 1986; 1(8470):8–11.

Cohen MD, Smith JA, Slabaugh RD, Rust RJ. Neonatal necrotizing enterocolitis shown by oral metrizamide (Amipaque). AJR 1982;138:1019–23.

Cohen MD, Weber T. Metrizamide in neonatal and childhood small bowel obstruction. AJR 1982;139:689–92.

Franken EA. Meconium ileus: results of enema reduction. Symposium—gastrointestinal imaging: 1993 and beyond, a look at therapy and intervention. Society of Pediatric Radiology, 36th Annual Meeting; 1993 May 12; Seattle.

Ginai AZ. Experimental evaluation of various available contrast agents for use in the gastrointestinal tract in case of suspected leakage. Effects on peritoneum. Br J Radiol 1985;58:969–78.

Grantmyre EB, Butler GJ, Gillis DA. Necrotizing enterocolitis after renografin-76 treatment of meconium ileus. AJR 1981;136:990–1.

Harris PD, Neuhauser EBD, Gerth R. The osmotic effect of water soluble contrast media on circulating plasma volume. AJR 1964:694–8.

Hay M, Cant PJ. Case report: renal excretion of enteral gastrografin in the absence of free intestinal perforation. Clin Radiol 1990;41:137–8.

Leonides JC, Burry VF, Fellows RA, et al. Possible adverse effect of methylglucamine diatrizoate compounds on the bowel of newborn infants with meconium ileus. Radiology 1976;121:693–6.

Lutzger LG, Factor SM. Effects of some water-soluble contrast media on the colonic mucosa. Radiology 1976; 118:545–8.

Noblett HR. Treatment of uncomplicated meconium ileus by gastrografin enema: a preliminary report. J Pediatr Surg 1969;4:190–7.

Poole CA, Rowe MI. Clinical evidence of intestinal absorption of gastrografin. Radiology 1976a;118:151–3.

Poole CA, Rowe MI. Distal neonatal intestinal obstruction: the choice of contrast material. J Pediatr Surg 1976b;11:1011–22.

Ratcliffe JF. The use of Ioxaglate in the pediatric gastrointestinal tract: a report of 25 cases. Clin Radiol 1983;34:579–83.

Ratcliffe JF. Low osmolality water soluble (LOWS) contrast media and the pediatric gastrointestinal tract. Radiol Now 1985;8:8–11.

Reich SB. Production of pulmonary edema by aspiration of water soluble non-absorbable contrast media. Radiology 1969;92:367–70.

Sauvegrain J. The technique of upper gastro-intestinal investigation in infants and children. In: Karger S, editor. Progress in pediatric radiology. New York: Basel; 1969. p. 26–51.

Seltzer SE, Jones B. Cecal perforation associated with gastrografin cncma. AJR 1978;130.997–8.

Shaw A. Safety of N-acetylcysteine in treatment of meconium obstruction of the newborn. J Pediatr Surg 1969;4:119–25.

Wood BP, Katzberg RW, Ryan DH, et al. Diatrizoate enemas: facts and fallacies of colon toxicity. Radiology 1978;126:441–4.

Barium Examinations of the Upper Gastrointestinal Tract and Small Bowel

Barloon TJ, Franken EA. Plasma electrolyte status after small bowel enteroclysis. AJR 1986;146:323–5.

Becker MH, Genieser NB. A new device for feeding infants during fluoroscopy. J Pediatr 1972;80:291–2.

Bilbao MK, Frische LH, Dotter CT, et al. Hypotonic duodenography. Radiology 1967;89:438–43.

Ekberg O. Crohn disease of the small bowel examined by double contrast technique: a comparison with oral technique. Gastrointest Radiol 1977a;1:355–9.

Ekberg O. Double contrast examination of the small bowel. Gastrointest Radiol 1977b;1:349–53.

Eklof O, Erasmie U. The small bowel enema: an improved method of examination and its indications in childhood. Ann Radiol (Paris) 1978;21:143–8.

Heitzman ER, Berne AS. Roentgen examination of the cecum and proximal ascending colon with ingested barium. Radiology 1961;76:415–21.

Herlinger H. Small bowel. In: Laufer I, editor. Double contrast gastrointestinal radiology with endoscopic correlation. Philadelphia: WB Saunders; 1979. p. 423–94.

Herlinger H. The small bowel enema and the diagnosis of Crohn disease. Radiol Clin North Am 1982;20:721–42.

Hyde I, Danby B. An aid to barium meal examinations in infants. Br J Radiol 1980;53:997–8.

Hyslop JS, Mitchelmore AE, Cox RR, et al. Double contrast barium meal examination: a comparison of two high density barium preparations, E2HD and X-Opaque. Clin Radiol 1982;33:83–5.

Kellett MJ, Zboralske FF, Margulis AR. Peroral pneumocolon examination of the ileocecal region. Gastrointest Radiol 1977;1:361–5.

Kelvin FM, Gedgaudas RK, Thompson WM, et al. The peroral pneumocolon: its role in evaluating the terminal ileum. AJR 1982;139:115–21.

Kressel HY, Evers KA, Glick SN, et al. The per oral pneumocolon examination. Radiology 1982;144:414–6.

Laufer I. Upper gastrointestinal tract: technical aspects. In: Laufer I, editor. Double contrast gastrointestinal radiology with endoscopic correlation. Philadelphia: WB Saunders; 1979. p. 59–77.

Maglinte DDT, Lappas JC, Chernish SM, et al. Intubation routes for enteroclysis. Radiology 1986;158:553–4.

Pesquera GS. Method for direct visualization of lesions in small intestines. Clin Radiol 1929;22:254–7.

Pochaczevsky R. Oral examination of the colon: "the colonic cocktail." AJR 1974;121:318–25.

Poznanski A. A simple device for administering barium to infants. Radiology 1969;93:1106.

Ratcliffe JF. The small bowel enema in children: a description of a technique. Clin Radiol 1983;34:287–9.

Sanders DE, Ho CS. The small bowel enema: experience with 150 examinations. AJR 1976;127:743–51.

Sartoris DJ, Harell GS, Anderson MF, et al. Small bowel lymphoma and regional enteritis: radiographic similarities. Radiology 1984;152:291–6.

Sellink JL. Radiologic examination of the small intestine by duodenal intubation. Acta Radiol Diagn Stockholm 1974;15:318–32.

Stringer DA, Ein SH. Recurrent tracheoesophageal fistula: a protocol for investigation. Radiology 1984;151:637–41.

Stringer DA, Cloutier S, Daneman A, et al. The value of the small bowel enema in children. J Can Assoc Radiol 1986;37:13–6.

Stringer DA, Sherman PM, Liu P, et al. The value of the oral pneumocolon in pediatrics. AJR 1986;146:763–6.

Thomas PS, Chrispin AR. Congenital tracheoesopahgeal fistula without esophageal atresia. Clin Radiol 1969;20: 371–4.

Vallance R. An evaluation of the small bowel enema based on an analysis of 350 consecutive examinations. Clin Radiol 1980;31:227–32.

Vallance R, Smith RM. An analysis of 200 patients with negative small bowel enemas. Clin Radiol 1981;32:183–5.

Barium Examinations of the Large Bowel

Bigard M-A, Gaucher P, Lassalle C. Fatal colonic explosion during colonoscopic polypectomy. Gastroenterology 1979;77:1307.

Bo-Linn GW, Endrell V, Lee DD, et al. An evaluation of the significance of microscopic colitis in patients with chronic diarrhoea. J Clin Invest 1985;75:1559–69.

Burdelski M. Endoscopy in pediatric gastroenterology. Eur J Pediatr 1978;128:33–9.

Cadranel S, Rodesch P, Peeters JP, et al. Fiberendoscopy of the gastrointestinal tract in children: a series of 100 examinations. Am J Dis Child 1977;131:41–5.

Chong SKF, Bartram C, Campbell CA, et al. Chronic inflammatory bowel disease in childhood. BMJ 1982; 284:101–3.

Coblentz CL, Frost RA, Molinaro V, et al. Pain after barium enema: effect of CO_2 and air on double-contrast study. Radiology 1985;157:35–6.

Connolly BL, Alton DJ, Ein SH, et al. Partially reduced intussusception: when are repeated delayed reduction attempts appropriate? Pediatr Radiol 1995;25:104–7

Daneman A, Alton DJ, Ein SH, et al. Perforation during attempted intussuception reduction in children—comparison with barium and air. Pediatr Radiol 1995;25:81–8

Daneman A, Alton DJ. Intussusception: issues and controversies related to diagnosis and reduction. Radiol Clin North Am 1996;34:743–52

Ekberg O, Nylander G, Fork FT. Defecography. Radiology 1985;155:45–8.

Franken EA. Examination techniques and gastrointestinal symptoms in infants and children. In: Franken EA, editor. Gastrointestinal imaging in pediatrics. 2nd ed. Philadelphia: Harper and Row; 1982. p. 1–18.

Gans SL, Ament M, Christie DL, et al. Pediatric endoscopy with flexible fiberscopes. J Pediatr Surg 1975; 10:375–80.

Geenen JE, Schmitt MG, Wu WC, et al. Major complications of colonoscopy: bleeding and perforation. Am J Dig Dis 1975;20:231–5.

Grant DS, Bartram CI, Heron CW. A preliminary study of the possible benefits of using carbon dioxide insufflation during double contrast barium enema. Br J Radiol 1986; 59:190–1.

Gu L, Alton DJ, Daneman A, et al. Intussusception reduction in children by rectal insufflation of air. AJR 1988;150: 1345–8.

Habr-Gama A, Alves PRA, Gama-Rodrigues JJ, et al. Pediatric colonoscopy. Dis Colon Rectum 1979;22:530–5.

Harned RK, Consigny PM, Cooper NB, et al. Barium enema examination following biopsy of the rectum or colon. Radiology 1982;145:11–6.

Harned RK, Williams SM, Maglinte DDT, et al. Clinical application of in vitro studies for barium enema examination following colorectal biopsies. Radiology 1985;154: 319–21.

Kozarek RA, Earnest DL, Silverstein ME, et al. Air-pressure induced colon injury during diagnostic colonoscopy. Gastroenterology 1980;78:7–14.

Lappas JC, Miller RE, Lehman GA, et al. Post endoscopy barium enema examinations. Radiology 1983;149:655–8.

Laufer I, Mullens JE, Hamilton J. Correlation of endoscopy and double contrast radiography in the early stages of ulcerative and granulomatous colitis. Radiology 1976;118:1–5.

Laufer I, Smith NCW, Mullens JE. The radiological demonstration of colorectal polyps undetected by endoscopy. Gastroenterology 1976;70:167–70.

Laufer I. Double contrast enema: technical aspects. In: Laufer I, editor. Double contrast gastrointestinal radiology with endoscopic correlation. Philadelphia: WB Saunders; 1979. p. 495–515.

Maglinte DDT, Strong RC, Strate RW, et al. Barium

enema after colorectal biopsies: experimental data. AJR 1982;139:693–7.

Mahieu P, Pringot J, Bodart P. Defecography: 1. description of a new procedure and results in normal patients. Gastrointest Radiol 1984;9:247–51.

Miller M, Stringer DA, Chui-Mei T, et al. Lymphoid follicular pattern in the colon: an indicator of barium coating. J Can Assoc Radiol 1987;38:256–8.

Nussle D, Genton N, Bozic C. Functional radiological findings in Hirschsprung disease and in other causes of dyschezia. Ann Radiol (Paris) 1976;19:111–2.

Oh KS, Dorst JP, White JJ, et al. Positive contrast peritoneography and herniography. Radiology 1973;108:647–54.

Shiels WE II, Bisset GS III, Kirks DR. Simple device for air reduction of intussusception. Pediatr Radiol 1990; 20:472.

Shiels WE II, Maves CK, Hedlund GL, Kirks DR. Air enema for diagnosis and reduction of intussusception: clinical experience and pressure correlates. Radiology 1991;181:169.

Shiels WE II, Kirks DR, Keller GL, et al. Colonic perforation by air and liquid enemas: comparison study in young pigs. AJR 1993;160:931.

Shiels WE II. Intracolonic pressure and enemas in children: form follows function. Radiology 1995;196:19.

Simpkins KC, Stevenson GW. The modified Malmo double contrast enema in colitis: an assessment of its accuracy in reflecting sigmoidoscopic findings. Br J Radiol 1972; 45:486–92.

Stringer DA, Sherman PM, Jakowenko N. Correlation of double-contrast high density barium enema, colonoscopy and histology in children with special attention to disparities. Pediatr Radiol 1986;16:298–301.

Tedesco FJ, Waye JD, Raskin JB, et al. Colonoscopic evaluation of rectal bleeding: a study of 304 patients. Ann Intern Med 1978;89:907–9.

Thoeni RF, Menuck L. Comparison of barium enema and colonoscopy in the detection of small colonic polyps. Radiology 1977;124:631–5.

Williams CB, Hunt RH, Loose H, et al. Colonoscopy in the management of colon polyps. Br J Surg 1974;61:673–82.

Williams CB, Laage NJ, Campbell CA, et al. Total colonoscopy in children. Arch Dis Child 1982;52:49–53.

Winthrop JD, Balfe DM, Shackleford GD, et al. Ulcerative and granulomatous colitis in children. Comparison of double- and single-contrast studies. Radiology 1985;154: 657–60.

MISCELLANEOUS TECHNIQUES

Intestinal Tube Placement

Boros SJ, Reynolds JW. Duodenal perforation: a complication of neonatal nasojejunal feeding. J Pediatr 1974;85: 107–8.

Cheek JA, Staub GF. Nasojejunal alimentation for premature and full-term newborn infants. J Pediatr 1973;82: 955–62.

Chen JW, Wong PWK. Intestinal complications of nasojejunal feeding in low-birth-weight infants. J Pediatr 1974;85:109–10.

Ho CS. Percutaneous gastrostomy for jejunal feeding. Radiology 1983;149:595–6.

Ho CS, Gray RR, Goldfinger M, et al. Percutaneous gastrostomy for enteral feeding. Radiology 1985;156:349–51.

McAlister WH, Siegel MJ, Shackleford GD, et al. Intestinal perforations by tube feedings in small infants: clinical and experimental studies. AJR 1985;145:687–91.

McLean GK, Rombean JL, Caldwell MD, et al. Transgastrostomy jejunal intubation for enteric alimentation. AJR 1982;139:1129–33.

Merten DF, Mumford L, Filston HC, et al. Radiological observations during transpyloric tube feeding in infants of low birth weight. Radiology 1980;136:67–75.

Perez-Rodrigues J, Quero J, Frias EG, et al. Duodenorenal perforation in a neonate by a tube of silicone rubber during transpyloric feeding. J Pediatr 1978;92:113–6.

Rhea JW, Ahmad MS, Mange MS. Nasojejunal (transpyloric) feeding: a commentary. J Pediatr 1975;86:451–2.

Siegle RL, Rabinowitz JG, Sarasohn C. Intestinal perforation secondary to nasojejunal feeding tubes. AJR 1976;126:1229–32.

Strife JL, Rabinowitz JG, Sarasohn C. Jejunal intubation via gastrostomy catheters in pediatric patients. Radiology 1985;154:249.

Sun SC, Sanuels S, Lee J, et al. Duodenal perforation: a rare complication of neonatal nasojejunal tube feeding. Pediatrics 1975;55:371–5.

Video Velopharyngeal Examination

Croft CB, Sphrintzen RJ, Rakoff SJ. Patterns of velopharyngeal valving in normal and cleft palate subjects: a multiview videofluoroscopy and nasoendoscopic study. Laryngoscope 1981;91:265–71.

Glaser ER, Skolnick ML, McWilliams BJ, et al. The dynamics of Passavant's ridge in subjects with and without velopharyngeal insufficiency—a multiview videofluoroscopic study. Cleft Palate J 1979;16:24–33.

Kelsey CA, Ewanowski SJ, Crummy AB, et al. Lateral pharyngeal wall motion as a predictor of surgical success in velopharyngeal insufficiency. N Engl J Med 1982;287:64–8.

La Rossa D, Brown A, Cohen H, et al. Video-radiography of the velopharyngeal portal using the Towne's view. J Maxillofac Surg 1980;8:203–5.

McWilliams BJ, Musgrave RH, Crozier PA. The influence of head position upon velopharyngeal closure. Cleft Palate J 1968;5:117–24.

Quattromani FL, Benton C, Cotton RT. The Towne projection for evaluation of the velopharyngeal sphincter. Radiology 1977;125:540–2.

Sinclair SW, Davies DM, Bracka A. Comparative reliability of nasal pharyngoscopy and videofluoroscopy in the assessment of velopharyngeal incompetence. Br J Plast Surg 1982;35:113–7.

Skolnick ML. Video velopharyngography in patients with nasal speech, with emphasis on lateral pharyngeal motion in velopharyngeal closure. Radiology 1969;93:747–55.

Skolnick ML. Videofluoroscopic examination of the velopharyngeal portal during phonation in lateral and base projections—a new technique for studying the mechanics of closure. Cleft Palate J 1970;7:803–16.

Skolnick ML. A plea of an interdisciplinary approach to the radiological study of the velopharyngeal portal. Cleft Palate J 1977;14:329–30.

Skolnick ML, Zagzebski JA, Watkin KL. Two dimensional ultrasonic demonstration of lateral pharyngeal wall movement in real time—a preliminary report. Cleft Palate J 1985;12:299–303.

Sphrintzen RJ, Lencione RM, McCall GN, et al. A three dimensional cinefluoroscopic analysis of velopharyngeal closure during speech and nonspeech activities in normals. Cleft Palate J 1974;2:412–28.

Stringer DA, Witzel MA. The Waters projection for evaluation of lateral pharyngeal wall movement in speech disorders. AJR 1985;145:409–10.

Stringer DA, Witzel MA. Velopharyngeal insufficiency on multiview videofluoroscopy: a comparison of projections. AJR 1986;146:15–9.

Stringer DA, Witzel MA. Comparison of multiview videofluoroscopy and nasopharyngoscopy in the assessment of velopharyngeal insufficiency. Cleft Palate Craniofac J 1988. [In press]

Sialography

Evers K, Zito JL, Fine J, et al. CT sialography: utilising acinar filling. Br J Radiol 1985;58:839–43.

Manashil GB. A new catheter for sialography. AJR 1977; 128:518.

McGahan JP, Walter JP, Bernstein L. Evaluation of the parotid gland. Radiology 1984;152:453–8.

Rabinov KR, Joffe N. A blunt-tip side-injecting cannula for sialography. Radiology 1969;92:1438.

Rubin P, Holt JF. Secretary sialography in diseases of major salivary glands. AJR 1957;77:575–98.

Stacey-Clear A, Evans R, Kissini MW, et al. Sialography does not alter the management of parotid space-occupying lesions. Clin Radiol 1985;36:389–90.

Yune HY, Klatte EC. Current status of sialography. AJR 1972;115:420–8.

Rectal Manometry

Mahboubi S, Schnaufer L. The barium enema examination and rectal manometry in Hirschsprung disease. Radiology 1979;130:643–7.

COMPUTED TOMOGRAPHY

Afshani E. Computer tomography in abdominal abscesses in children. Radiol Clin North Am 1981;19:515–26.

Daneman A. Pediatric body CT. 1st ed. London: Springer-Verlag; 1986.

Kirks DR, Korobkin M. Computed tomography of the chest in infants and children: techniques and mediastinal evaluation. Radiol Clin North Am 1981;19:409–19.

Kirks DR, Merton DF, Grossman H, et al. Diagnostic imaging of pediatric abdominal masses: an overview. Radiol Clin North Am 1981;19:527–45.

Kirks DR, Fitz CR, Harwood-Nash DC, et al. Practical techniques for pediatric computed tomography. Pediatr Radiol 1983;13:148–55.

Kuhn JP, Berger PE. Computed tomography in the evaluation of blunt abdominal trauma in children. Radiol Clin North Am 1981;19:503–13.

Kuhns LR. Computed tomography of the retroperitoneum in children. Radiol Clin North Am 1981;19: 495–501.

MAGNETIC RESONANCE IMAGING

Boechat MI, Kangarloo H, Ortega J, et al. Primary liver tumours in children: comparison of CT and MR imaging. Radiology 1988;169:727–32.

Brant-Zawadski M, Badami JP, Mills CM, et al. Primary intracranial tumor imaging: a comparison of magnetic resonance and CT. Radiology 1984;150:435–40.

Brasch RC, Wesbey GE, Gooding CA, et al. Magnetic resonance imaging of transfusional hemosiderosis complicating thalassaemia major. Radiology 1984;150: 767–71.

Buonocore E, Borkowski GP, Pavlicek W, et al. NMR imaging of the abdomen: technical considerations. AJR 1983;141:1171–8.

Bydder GM, Steiner RE, Young IR, et al. Clinical NMR imaging of the brain: 140 cases. AJR 1982;139:215–36.

Cohen MD, Carr BE, Smith JA, et al. The visualization of major blood vessels by magnetic resonance in children with malignant tumours. Radiographics 1985;5:441–5.

Cohen MD. Advantages and disadvantages of magnetic resonance imaging. In: Cohen MD, editor. Pediatric magnetic resonance imaging. 1st ed. Philadelphia: WB Saunders; 1986a. p. 151–4.

Cohen MD. Contrast agents. In: Cohen MD, editor. Pediatric magnetic resonance imaging. 1st ed. Philadelphia: WB Saunders; 1986b. p. 142–5.

Cohen MD. Magnetic resonance imaging techniques in children. In: Cohen MD, editor. Pediatric magnetic resonance imaging. 1st ed. Philadelphia: WB Saunders; 1986c. p. 15–7.

Cohen MD. Body imaging: gastrointestinal system. In: Cohen MD, Edwards MK, editors. Magnetic resonance imaging of children. 1st ed. Philadelphia: BC Decker; 1990. p. 611–78.

Davis PL, Moss AA, Goldberg HI, et al. Nuclear magnetic resonance imaging of the liver and pancreas. Radiographics 1984;4:159–69.

Glaser GM, Aisen AM, Francis IR, et al. Hepatic cavernous hemangioma: magnetic resonance imaging. Work in progress. Radiology 1985;155:417–20.

Hahn PF, Starck DD, Vici L-G, et al. Duodenal hematoma: the ring sign in MR imaging. Radiology 1986;159:379–82.

Hope PL, Reynolds EOR. Investigation of cerebral energy metabolism in newborn infants by phosphorus nuclear magnetic resonance spectroscopy. Clin Perinatol 1985; 12:261–75.

Itai Y, Ohtomo K, Furui S, et al. Non-invasive diagnosis of small cavernous hemangioma of the liver: advantage of MR. AJR 1985;145:1195–9.

Johnston DL, Liu P, Wismer G, et al. Magnetic resonance imaging: present and future applications. Can Med Assoc J 1985:132:765–77.

Li KC, Glazer GM, Quint LE, et al. Distinction of hepatic cavernous hemangioma from hepatic metastases with MR imaging. Radiology 1988;169:409–15.

Ohtomo K, Ital Y, Furui S, et al. Hepatic tumours: differentiation by transverse relaxation time (T[2]) of magnetic resonance imaging. Radiology 1982;148:753–6.

Rhee RS, Ray CG, Kravetz MH, et al. Cervical esophageal duplication cyst: MR imaging. J Comput Assist Tomogr 1988;12:693–5.

Ros PR, Lubbers PR, Olmsted WW, Morillo GT. Hemangioma of the liver: heterogenous appearance on T2-weighted images. AJR 1987;147:1167–70.

Roth JL, Nugent M, Gray JE, et al. Patient monitoring during magnetic resonance imaging. Anaesthesiology 1985;62:80–3.

Simeone JF, Edelman RR, Starck DD, et al. Surface coil MR imaging of abdominal viscera. Part III. The pancreas. Radiology 1985;157:437–41.

Wall SD, Fisher MR, Amparo EG, et al. Magnetic resonance imaging in the evaluation of abscesses. AJR 1985; 144:1217–21.

Weinreb JC, Lowe T, Cohen JM, et al. Human fetal anatomy: MR imaging. Radiology 1985;157:715–20.

ANGIOGRAPHY

Buonocore E, Collman IR, Kerley HE. Massive upper gastrointestinal hemorrhage in children. AJR 1972;115: 289–96.

Franken EA. Gastrointestinal imaging in pediatrics. 2nd ed. Philadelphia: Harper & Row; 1982. p. 480–1.

Moore AV, Kirks DR, Mills SR, et al. Pediatric abdominal angiography: panacea or passe? AJR 1982;138:433–43.

Whitley NO, Hunt TM. Angiography in the diagnosis and management of gastrointestinal bleeding. Appl Radiol 1979;8(6):63–73.

NUCLEAR MEDICINE

Alavi A, Dann RW, Baum S, et al. Scintigraphic detection of acute gastrointestinal bleeding. Radiology 1977;124:753–6.

Alavi A, Ring EJ. Localization of gastrointestinal bleeding: superiority of 99mTc sulfur colloid compared with angiography. AJR 1981;137:741–8.

Arasu T, Fitzgerald J, Siddiqui A, et al. Gastroesophageal reflux in infants and children—comparative accuracy of diagnostic methods. J Pediatr 1980;96:798–803.

Armas RR. Clinical studies with spleen-specific radiolabeled agents. Semin Nucl Med 1985;15:260–75.

Berger RB, Zeman RK, Gotttschalk A. The technetium-99m-sulfur colloid angiogram in suspected gastrointestinal bleeding. Radiology 1983;147:555–8.

Camponovo E, Buck JL, et al. Scintigraphic features of choledochal cyst. J Nucl Med 1989;30(5):622–8.

Charron, M. Inflammatory bowel disease in pediatric patients. QJM 1998;41:309–20.

Chaudhuri TK, Polak JJ. Autoradiographic studies of distribution in the stomach of 99mTc-pertechnetate. Radiology 1977;123:223–4.

Cleveland R. Question and answer. AJR 1995;1548.

Cornwell EE, Rodriguez A, et al. Acute acalculous cholecystitis in critically injured patients. Preoperative diagnostic imaging. Ann Surg 1989;210(1):52–5.

Coughlin JR, Mann DA. Detection of acute cholecystitis in children. Can Assoc Radiol J 1990;41(4):213–6.

Dogan AS, Conway JJ, et al. Hepatobiliary scintigraphy in children with cystic fibrosis and liver disease. J Nucl Med 1994;35(3):432–5.

Erhlich CP, Papanicolaou N, Treves S, et al. Splenic scintigraphy using TC-99m-labeled heat-denatured red blood cells in paediatric patients: concise communication. J Nucl Med 1982;23:209–13.

Gaskin KJ, Waters DL, et al. Liver disease and common-bile-duct stenosis in cystic fibrosis. N Engl J Med 1988; 318(6):340–6.

Gelfand MJ, Smith HS, et al. Hepatobiliary scintigraphy in pediatric liver transplant recipients. Clin Nucl Med 1992;17(7):542–9.

Gerhold JP, Klingensmith WC, Kuni CC, et al. Diagnosis of biliary atresia with radionuclide hepatobiliary imaging. Radiology 1983;146:499–504.

Guillet J, Basse-Cathalinat B, Christopher E, et al. Routine studies of swallowed radionuclide transit in pediatrics: experience with 400 patients. Eur J Nucl Med 1984;9:86–90.

Heyman S. Pediatric nuclear gastroenterology: evaluation of gastroesophageal reflux and gastrointestinal bleeding. In: Freeman LM, Weissman HS, editors. Nuclear medicine annual. New York: Raven Press; 1985. p. 133–69.

Heyman S. The radionuclide salivagram for detecting the pulmonary aspiration of saliva in an infant. Pediatr Radiol 1989;208–9.

Heyman S. Pediatric gastrointestinal motility studies. Semin Nucl Med 1995;15:339–47.

Heyman S. Gastric emptying in children. J Nucl Med 1998;39:865–9.

Jewell FM, Davies A, et al. Technetium-99m-HMPAO labelled leukocytes in the detection and monitoring of inflammatory bowel disease in children. Br J Radiol 1996; 69:508–14.

Jobling JC, Lindley KJ, Yousef Y, et al. Investigating inflammatory bowel disease-white cell scanning, radiology, and colonoscopy. Arch Child Dis 1996;74:22–6.

Kennan N, Hayward M. Tc-HMPAO-labeled white cell scintigraphy in Crohn's disease of the small bowel. Clin Radiol 1992:45:331–4.

Kim CK, Heyman S. Scintigraphic evaluation of liver transplants. In: Murray IPC, Ell PJ, editors. Nuclear medicine in clinical diagnosis and treatment. New York: Churchill Livingstone; 1994. p. 69–75.

Klein H, Wald A. Computer analysis of radionuclide esophageal transit studies. J Nucl Med 1984;25:957–64.

Lette J, Morin M, et al. Standing views to differentiate gallbladder or bile leak from duodenal activity on cholescintigrams. Clin Nucl Med 1990;15(4):231–6.

Majd M, Reba RC, Altman RP. Effect of phenobarbital in 99mTc-IDA scintigraphy in the evaluation of neonatal jaundice. Semin Nucl Med 1981;11:194–204.

Malleson P, Petty RE, Nadel HR, Dimmick JE. Functional asplenia in childhood onset systemic lupus erythematosus. J Rheumatol 1988;15:1648–52.

Malmud LS, Fisher RS, Knight LC, et al. Scintigraphic evaluation of gastric emptying. Semin Nucl Med 1982; 12:116–25.

Mansfirel JC, Giaffer MH, Tindale WB, et al. Quantitative assessment of overall inflammatory bowel disease activity using labelled leukocytes: a direct comparison between indium-111 and technetium HMPAO methods. Gut 1995;37:679–83.

Miller JH, Gelfand MJ. Pediatric nuclear imaging. Philadelphia: WB Saunders; 1994.

Mirvis SE, Vainright JR, et al. The diagnosis of acute acalculous cholecystitis: a comparison of sonography, scintigraphy, and CT. AJR 1986;147(6):1171–5.

Nadel H. Where are we with nuclear medicine in pediatrics? Eur J Nucl Med 1995;22:1433–51.

Nadel H. Hepatobiliary scintigraphy in children. Semin Nucl Med 1996;26:25–42.

Nagel RA, Westaby D, et al. Liver disease and bile duct abnormalities in adults with cystic fibrosis. Lancet 1989; 2(8677):1422–5.

Nora PF, Davis RP, et al. Chronic acalculous gallbladder disease: a clinical enigma. World J Surg 1984;8(1):106–12.

Notghi A, Harding LK. The clinical challenge of nuclear medicine in gastroenterology. Br J Hosp Med 1995;54:80–6.

O'Brien S, Keogan M, et al. Biliary complications of cystic fibrosis. Gut 1992;33(3):387–91.

Oates E, Austin J, Becker J. Technetium-99m-sulfur colloid SPECT imaging in infants with suspected heterotaxy syndrome. J Nucl Med 1997;36:1368–71.

Oberg K. Neuroendocrine gastrointestinal tumours. Ann Oncol 1996;7:453–63.

Ota T, Tei M, Yoshioka A, et al. Intrapancreatic accessory spleen diagnosed by technetium-99m heat-damaged red blood cell SPECT. J Nucl Med 1997;38:494–5.

Oyens WJG, Corstens FHM. Scintigraphic techniques for delineation of infection and inflammation. Br J Hosp Med 1995;54:75–8.

Papos M, Varkonyi A, Buga K, et al. HM-PAO-labeled leukocytes in pediatric patients with inflammatory bowel disease. J Pediatr Gastroenterol Nutr 1996:23:547–52.

Paret G, Gilad E, et al. Acute acalculous cholecystitis in an infant after cardiac surgery. J Pediatr Surg 1994;29(12): 1580–1.

Pintelon H, Jonckheer MH, et al. Paediatric nuclear medicine procedures: routine sedation or management of anxiety? Nucl Med Commun 1994;15(8):664–6.

Savelli G, Spinelli A, et al. Bone lesions in a patient with transplanted liver for a metastatic carcinoid. The role of somatostatin receptor scintigraphy. Tumori 1998;84:82–4.

Schatzlein M, Ballantine T, Thirunavukkarasu S, et al. Gastroesophageal reflux in infants and children. Arch Surg 1979;114:505–10.

Seregni E, Chiti A, Bombardieri E. Radionuclide imaging of neuroendocrine tumours: biological basis and diagnostic results. Eur J Nucl Med 1998;25:639–58.

Sfakianakis GN, Conway JJ. Detection of ectopic gastric mucosa in Meckel's diverticulum and in other aberrations by scintigraphy: 1. Pathophysiology and 10-year old clinical experience. J Nucl Med 1981;22:647–54.

Shah AN, Dodson F, et al. Role of nuclear medicine in liver transplantation. Semin Nucl Med 1995;25(1):36–48.

Shah DB, Cosgrove M, Rees JIS, Jenkins HR. The technetium white cell scan as an initial imaging investigation for evaluating suspected childhood inflammatory bowel disease. J Pediatr Gastroenterol Nutr 1997;25:524–8.

Shi W, Johnson CF, et al. Localization of neuroendocrine tumours with [111In]DTPA-octreotide scintigraphy (Octreoscan): a comparative study with CT and MR imaging. QJM 1998;91:295–301.

Sty JR, Conway JJ. The spleen: development and functional evaluation. Semin Nucl Med 1985;15(3):276–98.

Ternberg JL, Keating JP. Acute acalculous cholecystitis. Complication of other illnesses in childhood. Arch Surg 1975;110(5):543–7.

Treves ST. Pediatric nuclear medicine. New York: Springer-Verlag; 1995.

Urbain JC, Charkes DC. Recent advances in gastric emptying scintigraphy. Semin Nucl Med 1995;15:318–37.

Waldman JD, Rosenthal A, et al. Sepsis and congenital asplenia. J Pediatr 1977;90: 555–9.

Weiss S. Sedation of pediatric patients for nuclear medicine procedures [review]. Semin Nucl Med 1993;23(3):190–8.

Weissmann HS, Badia J, et al. Spectrum of 99m-Tc-IDA cholescintigraphic patterns in acute cholecystitis. Radiology 1981;138(1):167–75.

Westra SJ, Zaninovic AC, et al. Imaging in pediatric liver transplantation. Radiographics 1993;13(5):1081–99.

Williams JG. Pertechnetate and the stomach—a continuing controversy. J Nucl Med 1983;24:633–6.

Yeker D, Buyukunal C, Benli M, et al. Radionuclide imaging of Meckel's diverticulum: cimetidine versus pentagastrin plus glucagon. Eur J Nucl Med 1984;9:316–9.

4

UPPER AND LOWER GASTROINTESTINAL ENDOSCOPY

Margaret A. Marcon, MD, FRCPC

The use of endoscopic equipment in the management of pediatric patients has changed dramatically over the past several decades. Beginning in the early 1970s, small-diameter fiberoptic bronchoscopes were used for gastrointestinal (GI) endoscopy in children (Freeman, 1973). Since that time, the development of video endoscopy as well as equipment in a range of sizes has expanded the use of GI endoscopy in pediatrics. Modern equipment allows the experienced endoscopist to perform diagnostic and therapeutic interventions even in very small infants.

Advances in the use of conscious sedation and cardiovascular monitoring allow a well-trained pediatric endoscopist to perform these procedures safely. Endoscopic evaluation of the upper and lower GI tract for diagnostic evaluation has become commonplace. It is important that one know the relative indications for these procedures in children, thus avoiding unnecessary investigation(s). There may be alternative or complementary procedures that may yield the same or additional information. The use of endoscopy for therapeutic intervention in children is also becoming common although the ability to perform this type of endoscopy is more limited. These procedures often require significant added expertise. For example, biliary endoscopy requires a coordinated effort with an experienced colleague in adult gastroenterology. Other procedures require a multidisciplinary approach involving staff from various areas such as surgery or radiology.

This chapter will discuss the specific uses for GI endoscopy as an investigative and therapeutic tool in the pediatric patient. The requirements for training to ensure competence to perform GI endoscopy in children have been developed (Hassall, 1997). The procedures must be performed in a setting with personnel trained in managing sedation in children. Reviews that address specific technique and set-up of equipment are available (Cotton, 1992; Fox, 1996). Guidelines for the use of sedation have been outlined by the American Academy of Pediatrics (1993). Endocarditis prophylaxis is recommended in those children at risk for serious infection from transient bacteremia. Recommendations have been developed and recently updated by the American Heart Association (Dajani et al., 1997; Gewitz, 1997).

UPPER GASTROINTESTINAL ENDOSCOPY

Two different types of flexible endoscopes are used. There are standard fiberoptic flexible scopes that transmit light through glass fibers bundled within a sheath. With the videoscopes, the transmitted signal is converted to a video or digital signal that can be transferred to a monitor. The endoscopes with an outside diameter of 8.7 mm or more can directly incorporate the digital technology. Although the small diameter of some endoscopes currently prohibits the incorporation of the video technology, video converters can be attached and thus allow capture of the digital image. Some degree of resolution is lost with the video converter but the images are still adequate.

There are flexible instruments with an external diameter down to 5 mm that have been developed for GI endoscopy. These smaller scopes allow endoscopy in very small infants (weighing less than 2 kg) but also are widely used in adults with esophageal strictures or cancer. The tips of the various scopes have a deflection range of 180° to 210° upward and 90° to 120° downward. The tip will move 100° to 120°, right to left. The diameter of the instrument or working channel will vary depending on the outside diameter of the endoscope. The size of the working channel may limit the availability to perform some procedures while using the smaller-diameter endoscopes. This is particularly true for therapeutic procedures. The choice of the endoscope used depends on the patient's size as well as what instruments may be used during the procedure. Larger-diameter scopes in smaller children may cause tracheal compression. If a larger endoscope is required or the child has airway problems such as tracheal stenosis, a general anesthetic is preferred over conscious sedation to ensure a patent airway.

An array of instruments is available for use through the instrument channel. A variety of biopsy forceps are also available. The "bite" size varies, with larger forceps giving a bigger sample by covering more surface area. Basically, these are pinch biopsies, done under direct vision, that include the mucosa and submucosa and occasionally part of the muscularis propria. If deeper biopsies are needed, a full-thickness surgical biopsy is necessary. There are other accessories such as grasping forceps and baskets for removing foreign bodies, wire snares for polypectomies, needles for injection, and probes for thermal coagulation (Figure 4–1). The smaller-diameter scopes will not allow passage of all the instruments available.

ESOPHAGOGASTRODUODENOSCOPY

The major indications for esophagogastroduodenoscopy (EGD) are listed in Table 4–1. For many diseases, endoscopy not only allows for gross visualization of the involved part of the GI tract but also allows for tissue sampling and sometimes even therapeutic intervention. The endoscopist must weigh the use of this tool compared with others that are available. There may be radiologic procedures that offer similar diagnostic yields. Cost and risk to the patient must be considered in the decision on which procedure(s) to perform.

There are few absolute contraindications for this procedure. If the patient has cardiovascular instability, the procedure is not warranted unless some therapeutic intervention such as endoscopic homeostasis is going to be performed. One must carefully weigh the risks and benefits in the patient with deteriorating neurologic or pulmonary status. If information gained from the procedure will significantly change the management, one must consider the most appropriate mode of sedation, including general anesthesia. Suspected cervical spine injuries must be stabilized prior to the procedure. Endoscopy should not be performed when there is suspected intestinal perforation. Bleeding diathesis in patients should be corrected before obtaining biopsies.

Complications

Although complications will occur, the incidence of serious complications is low (Rothbaum, 1996).

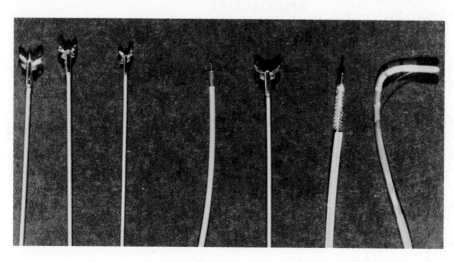

FIGURE 4–1. Various instruments that can be passed through the working channel in the endoscope. Left to right: biopsy forceps (three sizes); injection needle; grasping forceps; cytology brush; and papillitome for endoscopic retrograde cholangiopancreatography.

Complications can be divided into those associated with sedation and those directly related to the procedure. In a prospective study of 2046 upper endoscopies in pediatric patients, the overall complication rate was 1.7% (Ament, 1981). Most were related to sedation. The rate is higher with therapeutic endoscopy than in diagnostic endoscopy. The endoscopist must identify the high-risk patient and ensure that appropriate sedation and location for the procedure are chosen. Another pediatric center quotes their complication rate as less than 0.5% (Benaroch and Rudolph, 1994).

Complications directly related to the procedure include retropharyngeal hematoma, sore throat, loose or broken teeth, laryngeal trauma, and perforation. Insufflation may cause significant abdominal distention, which may cause respiratory compromise during the procedure. The endoscopist should remember to suck out the excess air as the endoscope is being withdrawn; this will decrease the incidence of vomiting and discomfort post procedure. There are added risks of complications during therapeutic endoscopy, and these are discussed in each section.

Indications

Esophageal Disease

Dysphagia and Odynophagia. Dysphagia and odynophagia can occur for a variety of reasons. One of the most common reasons for dysphagia in childhood is gastroesophageal reflux (GER) and esophagitis. A secondary peptic stricture may develop and cause obstruction (Plates 1 and 2). A stricture need not be present for children to complain of food sticking during swallowing; esophagitis alone may cause this sensation (Catto-Smith et al., 1991). Mucosal biopsies are necessary because gross visualization cannot exclude esophagitis (Biller et al., 1983). Motor disorders of the esophagus may be the etiology of the dysphagia but endoscopy is necessary to look for mucosal disease. In a study by Ament, (Ament and Christie, 1977) 12 of 39 children who underwent EGD for nausea, vomiting, dysphagia, odynophagia, or retrosternal pain had esophagitis. All 12 children had a barium swallow. Esophagitis was only diagnosed on the barium study in 1 of these 12 children. Barium studies are much better at delineating structural

TABLE 4–1. Indications for Esophagogastroduodenoscopy

Dysphagia or odynophagia
Unexplained chest or abdominal pain
Unexplained recurrent vomiting
Chronic infections or inflammatory diseases of the GI tract
Intestinal malabsorption or iron deficiency anemia
Upper GI bleeding
Caustic ingestion
Foreign body ingestion
Cancer surveillance
Treatment and follow-up surveillance for esophageal varices
Removal of polyps and follow-up surveillance
Surveillance for rejection in intestinal transplantation
Placement of percutaneous feeding tubes
Stricture dilation

problems such as a stricture or motor dysfunction than mucosal disease.

A recent study looked at the interpretation of endoscopic findings between experienced endoscopists and found it was acceptable (Armstrong et al., 1996). Several grading scales have been developed based on the endoscopic appearance of the esophagus (Hetzel et al., 1988; Savary and Miller, 1978) (Table 4–2). Use of these scales allows comparison between procedures as well as between endoscopists.

Severe esophagitis, sometimes with stricture, can occur in children undergoing treatment for malignancies or after bone marrow or solid organ transplantation. This may present as dysphagia or retrosternal or epigastric pain. The etiology of the esophagitis can range from simple peptic esophagitis to viral infections like herpes simplex or cytomegalovirus (CMV) infection or graft-versus-host disease. Again, mucosal biopsies and brushings are often necessary to determine the etiology and direct appropriate therapy. One needs to assess the hematological status of the child to ensure biopsies can safely be obtained.

Solid food dysphagia may be the only GI symptom in eosinophilic esophagitis (Attwood et al., 1993). Patients can even have food impaction that requires endoscopic removal. Despite the fact that one may find a narrowed area in the esophagus, particularly the more proximal esophagus, barium

TABLE 4–2.   Scoring of Esophagitis

Grade	Hetzel and Dent*	Savary and Miller[†]
Grade 0 =	Normal esophageal mucosa, no abnormalities noted	
Grade 1 =	No macroscopic erosions visible. Erythemia, hyperemia and/or friable esophageal mucosa	One or more longitudinal nonconfluent mucosal lesions with erythema, often covered with exudate above or extending from the gastroesophageal junction
Grade 2 =	Superficial erosions or ulceration involving less than 10% of the mucosal surface of the last 5 cm of the esophageal squamous mucosa	Confluent erosive and exudative mucosal lesions that do not cover the entire circumference of the esophagus
Grade 3 =	Superficial erosions or ulcerations involving 10–50% of the mucosal surface of the last 5 cm of the esophageal squamous mucosa	Circumferential mucosal lesions covering the whole esophageal mucous membrane
Grade 4 =	Deep ulceration anywhere in the esophagus or confluent erosion or ulceration of more than 50% of the mucosal surface of the last 5 cm of the esophageal squamous mucosa	Chronic mucosal lesions, such as ulceration with or without stricture formation

*Hetzel et al., 1988; [†]Savary and Miller, 1978.

swallows are usually reported as normal. In our experience, close attention to the proximal esophagus during barium swallow has shown tertiary contractions. Biopsies demonstrate diffuse eosinophilic infiltrate in the esophagus.

Achalasia can present during childhood. At endoscopy, the esophagus will be dilated and generally demonstrate no real peristalsis. As one passes the endoscope through the lower esophageal sphincter, a "pop" can be felt. Although patients may transiently have some symptom relief, more definitive intervention is necessary. Balloon dilation of the lower esophageal sphincter can result in significant improvement in symptoms that may last for many years (Boyle et al., 1981; Nakayama et al., 1987). The balloon can be passed over a guidewire placed endoscopically, or the balloon can be placed fluoroscopically. Botulinum toxin injection directly into the lower esophageal sphincter has also been used (Pasricha et al., 1996; Walton and Tougas, 1997). Some groups have begun using endoscopic ultrasonography of the lower esophageal sphincter to try and better direct the injections of the toxin (Hoffman et al., 1997).

Esophageal Stricture. A peptic stricture may develop in infants and children with severe reflux esophagitis (see Plate 2). Children who have undergone surgery for esophageal atresia typically develop strictures at the anastomotic site. Esophageal strictures can occur in children undergoing therapy for malignancy, such as chest radiation or aggressive chemotherapy in association with secondary mucositis. Stricture formation can occur following caustic injury, particularly ingestion of strong alkali. There are also congenital strictures or stenosis of the esophagus. Biopsies are often taken above and below the strictured area to look for inflammation and for Barrett's metaplasia.

The stricture may be dilated at the time of the endoscopy. The stenotic area is visualized and the appropriate size dilator or balloon chosen. A guidewire is placed through the working channel of the endoscope and then passed through the stenotic area. Hollow bougie dilators or small balloons are then passed over the guidewire. Balloon placement can be checked with the use of fluoroscopy. Strictures are often dilated over several sessions with progressively larger dilators or balloons. Refractory strictures may be treated by intralesional steroid injection (Bereson, 1994). Very thin membranous strictures can be excised with electrocautery or with laser therapy (Fox, 1996). Stents (plastic and metal) have been endoscopically placed in the esophagus to treat both benign and malignant strictures (Ell and May, 1997; Murphy, 1995; Nostrant, 1995). Although the vast experience with esophageal stents is in adults with malignant strictures, they have been used in children, especially those with caustic strictures (Berkovits et al., 1996).

Abdominal Pain, Vomiting, and Malabsorption

Esophagogastroduodenoscopy is warranted in children with unexplained vomiting. One looks for peptic ulcer disease associated with *Helicobacter pylori* gastritis or inflammatory diseases such as Crohn's disease or eosinophilic gastroenteritis (Plates 5 to 8). Mucosal lesions can be examined and biopsies obtained. This often leads to the precise diagnosis and thus guides therapy. Barium studies are not sensitive in picking up mucosal injury in the stomach. If a mass lesion is seen, biopsies again will be helpful. Polypoid lesions such as those associated with the familial polyposis syndromes may be removed from the stomach or duodenum. Antral or duodenal webs may be cut with electrocautery (Goenka et al., 1993) or laser (Ziegler et al., 1992). Balloon dilation has been used to treat strictures in the duodenum in peptic disease (Chan and Saing, 1994) as well as Crohn's disease (Murphy, 1991).

The role of endoscopy in evaluating abdominal pain is highly case dependent. The yield of positive findings depends on the patient selection. If history and physical examination suggest organic etiology, then endoscopy may be helpful and the yield would be higher. There are several studies looking at the role of endoscopy in children referred with abdominal pain but the patient groups are mixed and there are no controls. In one large study, 200 children underwent endoscopy for abdominal pain, of whom 47% had chronic recurrent pain. The endoscopy was normal in 82%. In those children with acute abdominal pain alone, the 67% had normal endoscopies (Quak et al., 1990). In the presence of added symptoms such as weight loss, vomiting or hematemesis, the endoscopy is more likely to be abnormal.

The role of endoscopy in the evaluation of malabsorption and chronic inflammatory disorders is more clear cut. A diagnosis of celiac disease may be made with a biopsy of the small intestine. Endoscopic biopsies have been shown to be histologically similar to suction-capsule biopsies (Granot et al., 1993). Endoscopic changes in celiac disease have also been described, such as notching or scalloping of the circular folds of the duodenum (Corazza et al., 1993). Although one may look for various serum antibodies to suggest celiac disease, a biopsy of the small intestine to confirm the diagnosis is still recommended (Chan et al., 1994). With intestinal lymphangiectasia, white plaques may be visualized, and biopsies from that area may confirm the diagnosis (Asakura et al., 1981). Furthermore, the ability to obtain biopsies of focal lesions as well as multiple areas of the mucosa contribute to the diagnosis of allergic, ischemic, or autoimmune disease, gastroduodenal Crohn's disease, or malignancy (Miller et al., 1997; Schmidt-Sommerfeld et al., 1990; Walker-Smith, 1993).

Upper Gastrointestinal Hemorrhage

Endoscopy has a major role in both the diagnosis and management of upper gastrointestinal (UGI) bleeding. Early studies demonstrated clear superiority over radiographic studies in determining the site of bleeding (Cox and Ament, 1979). The source of UGI bleeding can be identified in 85 to 90% of cases (Cadranel et al., 1977). As well as identifying the source of bleeding, endoscopic features have been described that predict the risk of rebleeding (Table 4–3). Depending on the etiology, therapeutic intervention may be undertaken at the time of endoscopy.

Careful history and physical examination will often suggest the etiology of the bleeding. It is important to examine the nasopharynx to ensure this is not the source of bleeding and thus avoid unnecessary GI endoscopy. The patient should be stabilized prior to endoscopy. The appropriate team should be assembled depending on the possible etiology and need for specific intervention. Fortunately, in children, most nonvariceal bleeding stops spontaneously. This does not negate the need for the procedure but makes it easier to visualize the lesion. Even in patients with

TABLE 4–3. Stigmata of Hemorrhage and the Role of Endoscopic Intervention*

Observation	Rebleeding Risk	Endoscopic Intervention
Spurting blood	High	Yes
Oozing blood	Moderate	Yes
Adherent clot, inactive	Moderate	Uncertain
Visible vessel	High	Yes
Clean ulcer base	Low	No

*Cadranel et al., 1977

variceal bleeding, often the bleeding has slowed or stopped by the time of endoscopy. This is not the case in adult patients, in whom significant bleeding may not cease until some type of therapeutic intervention is undertaken. One should be prepared for possible therapeutic intervention at the time the endoscopy is performed. Blood products should be on hand and the surgical or interventional radiology teams should be notified, if appropriate.

Nonvariceal Bleeding. Nonvariceal bleeding may be due to erosive esophagitis or gastritis, Mallory-Weiss tear, peptic ulcer with or without a visible vessel, medication-induced ulcers or gastritis, polyps, or vascular malformations. The possible etiology depends on the patient population. Peptic ulcers and Mallory-Weiss tears are the most common etiologies in otherwise well children. Erosive esophagitis and candidial infection may be the cause in a child on chemotherapy or after bone marrow transplantation. Biopsies for routine histopathology can be taken at the time of endoscopy. Additional procedures, such as brushing or biopsies for culture, depend on the patient population (Wara, 1985).

Various treatment modalities are available, depending on the lesions and the equipment available to the endoscopist. Injection of sclerosing or vasoconstrictive agents, thermal coagulation using monopolar and multipolar probes, heater probe and laser, (Stiegmann et al., 1992) all have all been used (Chung et al., 1991; Dorais and Haber, 1997; Laine, 1991, 1992; Lin et al., 1990). Ligation during endoscopy for bleeding from a postpolypectomy stump or some vascular lesions has been reported but experience is limited to case reports (Murray et al., 1996; Slivka et al., 1994). Studies evaluating these applications have been in adults, and use in children remains anecdotal. There are no large studies in children looking at the incidence and cost-effectiveness of endoscopic therapeutic intervention for nonvariceal bleeding.

Variceal Bleeding. Acute variceal bleeding due to either intrahepatic or extrahepatic portal hypertension can be managed by sclerotherapy or elastic band ligation. Both techniques have been used successfully in children (Fox et al., 1995; Hassall et al., 1989). Adult studies achieve control of active bleeding in at least 90% of patients. Similar success in the management of acute variceal bleeding has

been reported in children although spontaneous cessation of bleeding may partly account for this (Hassall, 1994; Maksoud et al., 1991; Thapa and Mehta, 1990). Children, more often than not, stop bleeding before the endoscopy. Various sclerosing agents have been used, including ethanolamine oleate, polidocanol, and sodium morrhuate alone or mixed with ethanol. Varices in the distal 3 to 5 cm of the esophagus are injected. Both intravariceal or paravariceal injection techniques have been used. Depending on the size of the patient, 0.5 to several milliliters of sclerosant are injected, with a maximum total volume between 6 and 30 mL. A series of procedures are done over many weeks until all the lesions are sclerosed. Surveillance endoscopy is then performed, and lesions are dealt with when they develop. Traditional esophageal variceal therapy is not useful for gastric varices but injection of tissue adhesives (glue) has been used successfully (Plates 3 and 4) (Ramond et al., 1989).

Several adult studies have shown fewer treatment-related complications and better survival with variceal ligation than with injection sclerotherapy (Laine et al., 1993; Stiegmann et al., 1992). A small tubular device with rubber bands on the outer surface is placed on the end of the scope. The trigger wire is passed through the instrument channel. The varix is suctioned into the device and a rubber band is released over the vessel. Newer devices allow the banding of multiple variceal lesions without having to reload the endoscope. Prior to this, the endoscope had to be withdrawn, loaded, and reintroduced for each varix that was ligated. Variceal ligation can easily be performed in children (Fox et al., 1995; Hall et al., 1988). Currently available equipment will fit down to an 8.6-mm diameter endoscope, thus limiting its use in very young children and infants.

Foreign Body Ingestion

Foreign bodies lodged in the esophagus should be removed promptly. Swallowed coins are the most common foreign body to cause problems although possibilities seem endless; bits of toys, pins, toothpicks and watch batteries have all been retrieved. Initially, a plain-film radiograph is taken to locate and define the object. One must look for more than one object, regardless of the history. Most lodge at the cricopharyngeal muscle, the area of the aortic arch, or the gastroesophageal junction.

The objects should be removed within 24 hours; the more proximal the object, the more urgent is retrieval. Although not universally accepted, one should consider airway protection during the procedure to avoid aspiration of the object into the airway during retrieval. Various instruments are available to use with the endoscope. The type of foreign body and the endoscopist's experience will direct the choice. These include polyp snares, helical baskets, alligator forceps, rat tooth forceps, and hooded sheaths (see Figure 4–1). Some tools have been developed for specific foreign bodies, such as the Clerf-Arrowsmith safety pin closer and the pin-bending forceps (Henderson et al., 1987; Holinger, 1990). If an underlying esophageal disorder may have predisposed to the problem, muscosal biopsies may also be helpful.

Caustic Ingestion

Children with a history of possible caustic ingestion should undergo endoscopy within 24 to 48 hours. Lack of oral or hypopharyngeal lesions does not negate the necessity for endoscopy (Gaudreault et al., 1983). There may be significant esophageal or gastric damage with few or no oropharyngeal lesions. Grading of the lesions by visual inspection on a scale of 1 to 3 helps with both prognosis and choice of treatment. In one large study, early complications and mortality only occurred in grade 3 burns (Zargar et al., 1991). The authors report no complications directly related to endoscopy. Circumferential ulceration at the time of the initial endoscopy suggests increased risk for stricture formation. Barium studies are not reliable in determining the extent of acute injury or in predicting stricture formation but may be useful several weeks later to assess for stricture formation.

Cancer Surveillance

Primary GI tumors are exceedingly rare in childhood. There are a handful of syndromes where surveillance is recommended. Endoscopic surveillance is suggested for several of the polyposis syndromes, including familial adenomatous polyposis, hereditary flat adenoma syndrome, and Gardner's syndrome (Burke and van Stolk, 1996; Flageole et al., 1994; Lynch et al., 1993; Noda et al., 1992). One can not only look for polyps but also remove them at the time of endoscopy.

Endoscopic surveillance is also part of the management of Barrett's esophagus. Histologic changes in Barrett's esophagus are considered premalignant. In a recent study, endoscopic photoablation laser treatment was performed using argon laser for the ablation of Barrett's epithelium (Berenson et al., 1993). This, along with acid suppression, facilitated regrowth of normal squamous epithelium. Although this study is in adults, this endoscopic therapy is theoretically applicable to children. Endoscopic laser therapy can also be used to activate tissue-sensitizing agents that then lead to tissue destruction (Lightdale et al., 1995; Nishioka, 1994). Photodynamic therapy is useful in adults with esophageal cancer but has not yet found a pediatric application.

PLACEMENT OF ENTERAL FEEDING CATHETERS

Feeding catheters have been placed percutaneously since 1980 (Gauderer et al., 1980). The percutaneous gastrostomy, or PEG, is the most common endoscopic intervention performed by a pediatric gastroenterologist. The two most common indications for PEG are providing fluid and nutrition in children and adults who cannot safely swallow or in whom for other reasons oral caloric intake is inadequate. Percutaneous gastrostomies are now placed in children with a variety of underlying disorders, from severe cerebral palsy to cancer. The decision to replace nasogastric nutritional supplement with a PEG must be made individually.

The technique itself is relatively simple. The PEG placement does not in itself require a general anesthesia. The choice of type of sedation (conscious or general anesthetic) is based on the endoscopist's experience with traditional UGI tract endoscopy in patients of similar age and disease. Perioperative antibiotics are used to decrease the risk of wound infection.

The endoscope is passed into the stomach, and the stomach and pylorus are surveyed. Endoscopy of the duodenum should be avoided, thus preventing unnecessary distention of the bowel. Bowel distention may cause interposition of the transverse colon between the abdominal wall and the stomach, increasing the risk of passing the tube through the bowel wall. A combination of gastric inflation, transillumination and indentation of the abdominal wall help in choice of the site of placement. One wants to place the PEG in the body of the stomach, rather than in the antrum. If the tube is too close to the antrum, the bolus feed may end up being delivered very rapidly into the duodenum, leading to dumping syndrome. If there is poor indentation of the abdominal wall, one should be concerned about the large bowel interposed between the stomach and abdominal wall. In this case, an open, surgically placed gastrostomy would be safer.

There are few absolute contraindications to PEG. These include previous abdominal surgery or abnormal abdominal anatomy, which may prevent adequate approximation of the stomach wall to the abdominal wall, and high-grade esophageal stricture. One must exercise caution in patients who have had previous abdominal surgery or ventriculoperitoneal shunt or are a poor anesthetic risk. One must also consider the risk of local infection or underlying disease complications directly related to the skin site. Despite these concerns, gastrostomy has been used successfully in patients with severe congenital and acquired immunodeficiencies, those with Crohn's disease or other inflammatory diseases, and children on high-dose immunosuppressive therapy (Mahajan et al., 1997; Mathew et al.,1996). Previous gastrostomy is not a relative contraindication. In fact, the new tube can be placed through the old, healed site.

Complications following PEG include cellulitis, gastrocolic fistula, peritonitis and anesthesia-related complications. Gauderer reported a 10-year follow-up experience in children (Gauderer, 1991). In his study, all the procedures were done in the operating room, and 50% received a general anesthetic. There were two deaths in 220 children; both children had severe heart disease, and the deaths were related to anesthesia. Of the 220, 2.3% developed a gastrocolic fistula, and 1.8% developed minor wound infections. Two patients were found at later surgery to have the catheter passing through the left lobe of the liver.

Some physicians suggest that children with severe neurologic impairment who require gastrostomy should not have a PEG because of the high incidence of GER in these patients. They feel that these children should have a combined antireflux operation and surgically placed gastrostomy tube. Several studies look at using preoperative evaluation to determine who actually needs an antireflux operation (Gauderer, 1991 Langer et al., 1988). The follow-up in these studies suggests that a significant number of children who have had a PEG without an antireflux operation do not need further surgery.

The type of infusion used to deliver nutrients may also affect the incidence of gastroesophageal reflux post gastrostomy (Coben et al., 1994). Bolus infusion is more likely to provoke reflux than a slower continuous infusion. The placement of a gastrojejunal tube may also be used in children with GER. During placement, once the tube is passed through the pylorus, it can be forwarded under fluoroscopic guidance. Nasojejunal tubes for feeding and for manometric studies can also be placed using endoscopy (Bosco et al., 1994). An endoscopically placed guidewire can be passed and the feeding tube or manometry catheter passed over it.

A wide variety of gastrostomy and gastrojejunostomy tubes are available. For both convenience and cosmetic reasons, many patients will prefer a skin-level tube. A button tube that lies flush with the skin has been used successfully and is now one of the most common devices (Gauderer et al., 1988; Treem et al., 1993). Choice of tube needs to be on an individual basis. All tube configurations allow for infusion of formula. If one plans to use the tube to vent or decompress the stomach and drain the gastric contents, some designs perform these functions better.

ENDOSCOPIC RETROGRADE CHOLANGIOPANCREATOGRAPHY

Endoscopic retrograde cholangiopancreatography (ERCP) has both a diagnostic and therapeutic role in the management of biliary and pancreatic disease in childhood (Brown et al., 1993; Buckley and Connon, 1990; Putnam et al., 1991; Werlin, 1994). The use of ERCP in childhood has expanded, particularly over the last decade. Currently available equipment allows for examination of children from infancy onward. The rate of successful cannulation of the biliary and pancreatic ducts depends on the level of skill of the endoscopist but successful cannulation rates of up to 95% can be obtained. One should also be prepared to perform therapeutic intervention, if necessary, during the procedure. Despite the increase in the use of this modality, the numbers performed at even a large pediatric center are far too few for the endoscopist to maintain his or her skills to perform these procedures independently. Close collaboration with adult colleagues with expertise in performing both diagnostic and therapeutic ERCP is mandatory (Plates 9 and 10).

The standard adult side-viewing endoscope can be used in most children past infancy. There is a smaller pediatric version of the side-viewing endoscope available but a smaller instrument channel limits the use of accessories available for the larger scope. Thus, the ability to perform therapeutic interventions may be significantly limited.

Endoscopic retrograde cholangiopancreatography is useful in managing the child with choledocholithiasis (both stone retrieval and sphincterotomy have been performed in children (Brown et al., 1993; Brown and Goldschmiedt, 1994). Although there are no studies looking at consequences of sphincterotomy in children, it has also become part of the routine preoperative evaluation for laparoscopic cholecystectomy in adult patients (Coppola et al., 1996). This has now carried over to pediatric patients (Al-Salem and Nourallah, 1997; Newman et al., 1997). Although there are studies in adults trying to establish which patients benefit from preoperative ERCP, no such studies in children exist (Coppola et al., 1996; Voyles et al., 1994).

The procedure is also useful in the diagnosis of congenital abnormalities of the biliary or pancreatic ducts, including choledochal cysts (Figure 4–2) and Caroli's disease. The diagnosis of primary sclerosing cholangitis is made at ERCP (Figure 4–3). It is now commonly used to look for the etiology of recurrent pancreatitis in childhood (Figure 4–4). In Guelrud's (Guelrud et al., 1994) review of 51 children with pancreatitis, 68% had findings on ERCP suggestive of a possible cause for the recurrent pancreatitis. Of these, 49% had some type of endoscopic therapeutic intervention performed. The authors felt that the intervention was helpful in 83%.

Children who present with evidence of obstruction of the common bile duct should undergo cholangiography. At the time of ERCP, stents may be placed to relieve biliary obstruction, whether due to stricture of the duct or compression from the head of the pancreas (Brown et al., 1993; Marcon et al., 1997) (Figure 4–5). Chronic pancreatic pseudocysts may be drained endoscopically. Endoscopic retrograde cholangiopancreatography is useful in the management of traumatic injury to the pancreatic or biliary ducts. It also allows for non-operative management of bile leaks in children who have undergone liver transplantation or other types of hepatobiliary surgery (Osorio et al., 1993).

The use of ERCP in the evaluation of neonatal cholestasis is less clear. Some groups have advocated it in the evaluation of such infants, particularly

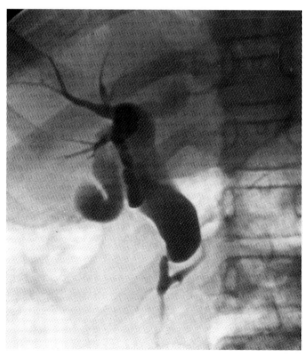

FIGURE 4–2. Choledochal cyst. An ERCP in a child with a choledochal cyst.

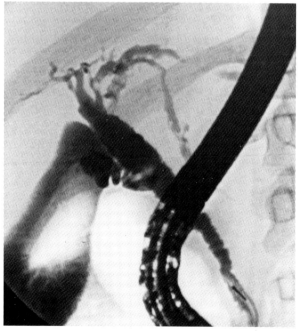

FIGURE 4–3. Sclerosing cholangitis. An ERCP in a 7-year-old girl with Crohn's colitis and primary sclerosing cholangitis.

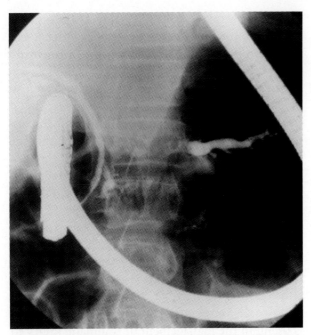

FIGURE 4–4. Chronic pancreatitis. An ERCP performed in a child with recurrent pancreatitis. The pancreatic duct is enlarged and irregular, consistent with chronic pancreatitis.

when one suspects extrahepatic biliary atresia (Derkx et al., 1994; Guelrud et al., 1991; Putnam et al., 1991; Wilkinson et al., 1991). Many others feel that the use of biliary scintigraphy and liver histology, along with a duodenal aspirate, will preclude most infants who do not have extrahepatic biliary atresia from laparotomy for intraoperative cholangiography (Brown et al., 1993). It is possible that, in a selected group of infants where supporting evidence for extrahepatic biliary atresia is less clear, ERCP would obviate laparotomy. Clinical protocols evaluating this group would be useful, rather than recommending ERCP for all cholestatic infants.

Complications include all those mentioned for standard EGD as well as some additional ones related specifically to ERCP. In adults, complications include cholangitis (5% in patients with obstructive jaundice) and pancreatitis (2 to 3%) (Chen et al., 1995; Sherman and Lehman, 1991; Werlin, 1994). The pancreatitis is usually chemically induced and short lived. However, deaths due to severe pancreatitis have been reported in adults. Other complications include bleeding, bowel perforation, or biliary tract leak. Most childhood series are small. The largest reviewed 121 children, and the incidence of post-ERCP pancreatitis was 3.3% (Brown et al.,

1993). A second group reported 17% incidence of post-ERCP pancreatitis in children undergoing ERCP for recurrent pancreatitis but this report only includes 18 children (Guelrud et al., 1994). Again, the risk of these complications also depends on the skill and experience of the endoscopist.

ENDOSONOGRAPHY

Endosonography or endoscopic ultrasound has become an important imaging tool in adult gastroenterology. Endoscopes can be equipped with a mechanical rotating sector scanner. These scopes have either a side or oblique view with a conical-shaped nose containing the scanner. With the newest equipment both high-resolution video and ultrasound images can be viewed simultaneously. Some include color Doppler signal detection as well. Biopsy forceps or an aspiration needle can be passed through the instrument channel. There are also ultrasonic probes that can be passed through the instrument channel on the larger endoscopes (working channel 2.8 mm).

The combination of endoscopy and ultrasound is now widely used in the staging of esophageal cancer. Studies show endoscopic ultrasound is superior to CT scanning for staging of both esophageal and gastric tumors (Tytgat and Fockens, 1996; Van Dam, 1997). The aspiration needle can be used to biopsy esophageal or gastric tumors, as well as into pancreatic lesions or abdominal or mediastinal lymph nodes (Chang and Wiersema, 1997). This technology is also useful in evaluating the biliary tract (Palazzo, 1997). An ultrasonic colonoscope is also available. What role ultrasonography combined with video endoscopy may play in pediatrics is unclear.

ENTEROSCOPY

Enteroscopy, or examination of the bowel beyond the third part of the duodenum, can be performed using several different techniques. This can be useful in occult GI bleeding. Esophagogastroduodenoscopy and colonoscopy should be performed first, and if no source is found enteroscopy may be helpful for diagnosis. Endoscopic intervention is also possible by passing a heater probe or laser through the instrument channel. Biopsies can also be obtained. Small intestinal polyps, such as those in familial adenomatous coli or Peutz-Jeghers syndrome, can be removed. Enteroscopy allows examination of the Roux-en-Y limb in patients with previous biliary tract surgery (Gostout and Bender, 1988). Percutaneous jejunostomies (JEPS) can also be placed with the enteroscope (Mellert et al., 1994).

The most common approach for enteroscopy is the push technique (Wilmer, 1998). A pediatric colonoscope was generally used although specialized enteroscopes are now available. The enteroscope is introduced under direct vision, just as for an EGD. An overtube may be used to prevent curling in the stomach. Fluoroscopy can aid in advancing the tube. With enteroscopes over two meters in length the entire jejunum can be examined. There is an instrument channel, so biopsies can be obtained and therapeutic intervention is possible.

Sonde enteroscopy depends on peristalsis to drag the slender instrument through the small bowel (Gostout, 1998). All enteroscopes of this type have a balloon on the end. The scope is passed nasally or orally and under direct visualization the tip-placed through the pylorus. The balloon is expanded and pulled down through the small intestine by peristalsis. The position of the enteroscope is checked with fluoroscopy. It takes 4 to 6 hours to complete, reaching the terminal ileum in 70 to 80% of patients. Inspection of the bowel is done while slowly withdrawing the scope. There is no instrument channel; thus, it is not possible to obtain biopsies. This procedure may be performed if the push enteroscopy did not allow viewing of enough of the small bowel to aid in diagnosis.

Interoperative enteroscopy is also reported. The enteroscope is introduced orally, just as for EGD. Then, at laporatomy, the surgeon can manually thread the bowel over the scope. This usually allows viewing of the entire small bowel, but is rather invasive.

Almost all reports of enteroscopy are in adults. Its role in children is unknown. The indications for use in childhood are really no different than adults (Benaroch and Rudolph, 1994). The current size of endoscope used for push enteroscopy limits the size of patient in which it can be used. The diameter of some sonde enteroscopy scopes is much smaller but the procedure is very time- and labor-intensive, and likely would not be well tolerated in most children. Enteroscopy combined with laporatomy has been done over the years in very select pediatric patients.

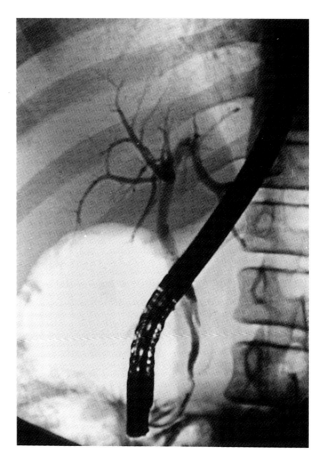

FIGURE 4–5 Fibrosing pancreatitis. An ERCP in a 14-year-old male who presented with jaundice, an enlarged pancreas (primarily the head of the pancreas) and distal common bile duct obstruction. A stent was placed into the common bile duct at the time of the procedure. He had fibrosing pancreatitis.

COLONOSCOPY

Full colonoscopy for both diagnostic and therapeutic use is now common in pediatrics. Equipment is available to examine the colon in even the smallest infant. Smaller endoscopes that were developed for the UGI tract can also be used. The stiffness of these scopes tends to be less than the marketed colonoscope. The UGI endoscopes are all shorter than the colonoscopes; so, one may not have enough length to reach the cecum. Successful completion of endoscopy of the entire colon with or without examination of the terminal ileum is possible but often technically challenging. Two additional problems that can hinder completion of a full colonoscopy are poor compliance with bowel preparation and inadequate sedation to complete the procedure.

Colonoscopes are available as both fiberoptic and video endoscopes, similar to the UGI tract endoscopes discussed in the previous section. Deflection range of the tip is from 180° upward and 160° right and left. Channel diameters are generally larger than those of the upper endoscopes to prevent clogging with fecal matter. This larger channel also allows for an array of instruments to be used for therapeutic procedures. Sigmoidoscopes are shorter (600 mm) than colonoscopes which are 1300 mm or longer.

The indications for colonoscopy in young patients are listed in Table 4–4. Chronic abdominal pain alone is not an indication for colonoscopy in a child. The yield of finding pathology without other findings is very low. Although at times only an examination of the rectosigmoid area may be necessary (sigmoidoscopy), one needs to determine prior to the procedure if a full colonoscopy is warranted. Colonic preparation and type of sedation can then be geared to the required procedure. Barium is hard to cleanse from the colon; so, timing of UGI tract studies should allow the patient to fully clear the barium before the bowel preparation for the colonoscopy. In most children, when one is interested in the bowel mucosa, a barium enema is unnecessary and usually adds no further information if a colonoscopy is to be performed. If suspicious lesions are found at the time of initial colonoscopy, the area may be marked or tattooed by submucosal injection of India ink (Salomon et al., 1993). The issues surrounding patient preparation and anesthetic risk, choice of sedation method and patient monitoring are similar to those for upper endoscopy. Respiratory compromise from the colonoscopy itself is usually

significantly less than that in upper endoscopy. Respiratory compromise during colonoscopy is related to oversedation alone. Although limited proctosigmoidoscopy may be performed with little or no sedation, there can be significant discomfort during a full colonoscopy. Pain may be intense while the bowel lumen is stretched or torsion is applied to the mesentery. Guidelines for administration and monitoring of pediatric patients as well as choice of anesthetic agents are reported elsewhere (Committee on Drugs of the American Academy of Pediatrics: Guidelines for monitoring and management of pediatric patients during and after sedation for diagnostic and therapeutic procedures, 1993; Ament and Brill, 1995; Balsells et al., 1997; Cote, 1994). A detailed description of the basic technique for colonoscopy is in the cited review (Fox, 1996). Endocarditis prophylaxis is recommended in the appropriate patients, as discussed at the beginning of this chapter.

Contraindications for colonoscopy included many of those for UGI tract endoscopy. Cardiovascular, respiratory, or neurological instability may preclude safe colonoscopy. At times, the procedure may be done but for patient safety it should be done with a general anesthetic and a protected airway. Coagulopathy or thrombocytopenia should be corrected before the procedure, especially if either pinch biopsies or therapeutic maneuvers are going to be performed. Neutropenia, suspected bowel ischemia or toxic megacolon are relative contraindications because of the increased risk of bowel perforation and sepsis. Adequate bowel preparation is necessary. One needs to be able to see the lumen to safely advance the colonoscope. If a full colonoscopy is really necessary and bowel preparation inadequate, the patient should be brought back again but prepared differently. Electrocautery in a poorly prepared colon also carries the risk of igniting volatile gases (Monahan et al., 1992).

Complications

As with UGI tract endoscopy, complications fall into two categories: those relating to sedation, and those relating to the procedure. Respiratory compromise results from oversedation alone. The endoscopist must be able to provide adequate pain relief with sedation to successfully complete the procedure. Thus, it is imperative that a member of the endoscopy team be experienced in administering

---

TABLE 4–4. Indications for Colonoscopy in Pediatric Patients

1. GI hemorrhage
2. Chronic diarrhea
3. Acute or chronic colitis
4. Suspected inflammatory bowel disease
5. Suspected polyposis syndrome
6. Cancer surveillance
7. Polyp removal
8. Foreign body removal
9. Dilation of a stricture
10. Decompression of an obstructed colon
11. Treatment of a bleeding lesion

sedation and monitoring the patient (Committee on Drugs of the American Academy of Pediatrics: Guidelines for monitoring and management of pediatric patients during and after sedation for diagnostic and therapeutic procedures, 1993; Ament and Brill, 1995; Balsells et al., 1997; Cote, 1994).

Based on literature on adults undergoing colonoscopy, the incidence of bacteremia during the procedure is likely quite low (Low et al., 1987). Endocarditis prophylaxis is still recommended for those at risk. More serious complications are bowel perforation and/or hemorrhage. Factors that may increase the risk of complications include excessive force, severe active colitis, polypectomy, injection or thermal cautery, stricture or adhesions, or any underlying condition that may weaken the bowel wall (Hunt, 1983; Rothbaum, 1996). The risk of perforation during diagnostic colonoscopy is less than 1% while during therapeutic colonoscopy, it may be as high as 3% (Damore et al., 1996). In one pediatric report of 234 children undergoing colonoscopy for rectal bleeding, there were no major complications (perforation, hemorrhage, septicemia) (Cynamon et al., 1989). Overall, colonoscopy in childhood is a safe and useful procedure when performed by an endoscopist with pediatric experience.

Indications

Gastrointestinal Hemorrhage

Colonoscopy is quite useful in determining the etiology of lower GI hemorrhage. Often therapeutic maneuvers can be performed during the same colonoscopy. The most common reason for blood per rectum is an anal fissure. This can be seen on simple inspection and does not require endoscopy. Most other lower GI tract bleeding in children is due to either colitis or benign juvenile polyps. Colitis may be due to infection, ischemia, allergy, or neoplastic or inflammatory bowel disease (largely ulcerative colitis or Crohn's disease). Often, these entities will look endoscopically different, and biopsies may add diagnostic information. The extent of disease can also be delineated.

Less common causes of lower GI bleeding in children include vascular malformations, including hemangiomas and telangiectasias. Bleeding vascular malformations in children have been described in association with Turner's syndrome, Rendu-Osler-Weber, blue rubber bleb nevus syndrome and diffuse

neonatal hemangiomatosis. Bleeding internal hemorrhoids are an unusual cause of bleeding in childhood. Although common in adults, in conjunction with constipation, these should raise suspicion of elevated portal hypertension in children (Heaton et al., 1992). All endoscopic techniques for hemostasis in the UGI tract have been used in the colon (Gallo and McClave, 1992; Noronha and Leist, 1988).

Polyps and Polypectomy

Juvenile polyps are by far the most common intestinal polyps seen in childhood. These benign lesions often present as painless rectal bleeding not associated with anemia, then undergo autoamputation, and do not recur. Less often, there may be more significant bleeding associated with chronic anemia, massive hemorrhage, or intermittent acute hemorrhage. Colonoscopy with polypectomy is then indicated. Coexistent adenomatous changes have been reported and, although it is exceedingly rare, support polypectomy (Cynamon et al., 1989; Tolia and Chang, 1990). The polyps may be seen on barium enema but very low lesions in the rectum may be missed. In one review, 18 children had a single-contrast barium enema before colonoscopy, and the polyps were not seen in 7 (39%) (Cynamon et al., 1989). Although these polyps are generally singular and in the rectosigmoid, there may be multiple polyps scattered throughout the colon. Colonoscopy also allows for removal of the polyp at the time of the procedure (Plate 13) (Jalihal et al., 1992). Other polyp syndromes may occur in childhood. The distribution, number, and histopathology of the polyps are important. Several syndromes carry a risk of malignancy, and surveillance is thus required.

The endoscopist should be prepared to perform a polypectomy at the time of endoscopy if a polyp is suspected. Bowel preparation must be adequate for visualization of the polyp(s). Poor preparation makes it difficult to see and snare or retrieve the polyp(s). Electrocautery is often used during the polypectomy and carries the risk of igniting volatile gases in the poorly prepared colon (Monahan et al., 1992). Adequate sedation is also necessary; movement may hinder snaring the polyp, cause premature garroting of the polyp before cautery is applied, and increase the risk of perforation and thermal injury during electrocautery.

Diminutive polyps (<5 mm) may be removed with biopsy forceps. Polyps larger than 5 mm are usually removed with a snare. Pedunculated polyps are ensnared around the stalk. Electrocautery may be applied while tightening the snare, helping prevent hemorrhage post polypectomy. Electrocautery may also be used during the removal of small polyps with forceps. There are both monopolar and bipolar hot forceps available. Thermal injury and perforation can occur with electrocautery; so, one must hold the polyp away from the bowel wall with the snare. Segmental resection of very large pedunculated polyps may be necessary. Saline injection around the base of a sessile polyp may facilitate its removal with the snare.

Very small polyps may be retrieved by aspiration through the scope channel. Larger polyps may be retrieved by withdrawal of the scope with strong suction applied to the polyp, using a basket or grasping forceps. Polyps may also be suctioned into a hood attached to the tip of the scope and carried out. Unfortunately, retrieval of larger polyps often requires repeated insertion and withdrawal of the scope. If one fails to retrieve the polyps, the initial bowel movements can be screened for the tissue. Post procedure, one must watch for delayed hemorrhage, and families should be prepared to quickly access medical care.

Colitis

Colonoscopy is useful in patients with suspected colitis. At the time of colonoscopy, the extent of involvement as well as the macroscopic pattern can be determined and biopsies can be sent for histology. This may lead to a diagnosis and also direct the medical or surgical management. Inspection of the terminal ileum may be helpful, especially when one is entertaining the diagnosis of Crohn's disease. In ulcerative colitis, the endoscopic abnormalities are usually contiguous, distally to the most proximal extent of the disease (Schmidt-Sommerfeld et al., 1990). Deep ulceration, cobblestoning and normal skip areas with some aphthous ulceration suggest Crohn's disease. Biopsies taken may also contain granulomata, again supportive of Crohn's disease. In cases where either the endoscopic appearance of the colitis or the biopsies are not able to differentiate the type of colitis, it is labeled indeterminate colitis (Plates 11 and 12).

Anyone presenting with acute colitis should have stool screening for infection prior to colonoscopy. Colonoscopy may be unnecessary in those with documented infection. Endoscopic features of infectious colitis are nonspecific and may not add anything to the diagnostic acumen. The exception is in *Clostridium difficile* associated pseudomembranous colitis, where endoscopically one sees sharply demarcated plaques of yellowish exudate, which vary from pinpoint size to large confluent areas. The endoscopic appearance of tuberculosis and *Yersinia* enterocolitis may mimic Crohn's disease. *Cytomegalovirus* colitis may have discrete ulceration. Biopsies taken during the endoscopy are very useful in making the correct diagnosis. Amebiasis can also be detected on colonic biopsy.

Allergic colitis, most commonly seen in infants, is usually due to either cow's milk or soy protein allergy (Jenkins et al., 1984). Endoscopic features are nonspecific. Biopsies show acute inflammation with a predominance of eosinophils. Eosinophilic colitis has been reported in older children but is significantly less common. In the infant group, the diagnosis is usually made clinically, and dietary manipulation solves the problem. Thus, colonoscopy usually is unnecessary. In cases where there is not rapid resolution of symptoms with dietary changes, colonoscopy may be helpful.

Colonoscopy is usually contraindicated in ischemic colitis and toxic megacolon. In patients with suspected graft-versus-host disease, there is often evidence of disease elsewhere, and colonoscopy may not add anything. The exception is where one is concerned about infectious complications such as colitis secondary to *CMV* infection.

Chronic Diarrhea

Colonoscopy is generally not indicated in the work-up of chronic diarrhea except where history suggests either chronic colitis or ileitis as the possible etiology (Schmidt-Sommerfeld et al., 1990). If one suspects Crohn's disease, the terminal ileum may be inspected and biopsied at the time of endoscopy. Occasional aphthous ulceration in the colon is also suggestive of Crohn's disease.

Cancer Surveillance

Although colon cancer is rare in childhood, there are several conditions where surveillance is recommended. The two major indications in childhood are the polyposis syndromes and longstanding ulcerative colitis. Children with a family history of familial adenomatous polyposis (FAP) need to begin screening in childhood. Careful biopsies of the early nodular changes will show adenomatous changes. Once it is determined that the child has FAP, he or she will ultimately require a colectomy. Other polyposis syndromes in which the polyps have a malignant potential require surveillance once the diagnosis is made (Cynamon et al., 1989; Jalihal et al., 1992; Tithecott et al., 1989; Tolia and Chang, 1990). Initiation of cancer surveillance is recommended after 7 to 8 years of ulcerative colitis (Griffiths and Sherman, 1997; Woolrich et al., 1992). Multiple biopsies are taken, to look for signs of dysplasia, which is considered a preneoplastic condition (Dajani et al., 1997; Gewitz, 1997).

REFERENCES

Committee on Drugs of the American Academy of Pediatrics. Guidelines for monitoring and management of pediatric patients during and after sedation for diagnostic and therapeutic procedures. Pediatrics 1993;89:1110–5.

Cotton P, Williams C. Practical Gastrointestinal Endoscopy. Oxford: Blackwell Scientific: 1992.

Dajani AS, Taubert KA, Wilson W, et al. Prevention of bacterial endocarditis: recommendaitons by the American Heart Association. Circulation 1997;96:358–66.

Fox VL. Endoscopy. In: Walker WA, et al., editors. Pediatric gastrointestinal disease. St. Louis: Mosby; 1996. p. 1533–41.

Freeman N. Clinical evaluation of the fiberoptic bronchoscope (Olympus BF 5b) for pediatric endoscopy. J Pediatr Surg 1973;8:213–20.

Gewitz MH. Prevention of bacterial endocarditis. Curr Opin Pediatr 1997;9:518–22.

Hassall E. Requirements for training to ensure competence of endoscopists performing invasive procedures in children. Training and Education Committee of the North American Society for Pediatric Gastroenterology and Nutrition (NASPGN), the Ad Hoc Pediatric Committee of American Society for Gastrointestinal Endoscopy (ASGE), and the Executive Council of NASPGN. J Pediatr Gastroenterol Nutr 1997;24:345–7.

UPPER GASTROINTESTINAL ENDOSCOPY

Al-Salem AH, Nourallah H. Sequential endoscopic/laparoscopic management of cholelithiasis and the choledocholithiasis in children who have sickle cell disease. J Pediatr Surg 1997;32:1432–5.

Albanese CT, Towbin RB, Ulman I, et al. Percutaneous gastrojejunostomy versus Nissen fundoplication for enteral feeding of the neurologically impaired child with gastroesophageal reflux. J Pediatr 1993;123:371–5.

Ament ME. Prospective study of risks of complications in 6424 procedures in pediatric gastroenterology. Pediatr Res 1981;15:524.

Ament ME, Christie DL. Upper gastrointestinal fiberoptic endoscopy in pediatric patients. Gastroenterology 1977;72:1244–8.

Armstrong D, Bennett JR, Blum AL, et al. The endoscopic assessment of esophagitis: a progress report on observer agreement. Gastroenterology 1996;111:85–92.

Asakura H, Miura S, Morishita T, et al. Endoscopic and histopathological study on primary and secondary intestinal lymphangiectasia. Dig Dis Sci 1981;26:312–20.

Attwood EA, Smyrk TC, DeMeester TR, et al. Esophageal eosinophilia with dysphagia: a distinct clinicopathologic syndrome. Dig Dis Sci 1993;38:109–16.

Benaroch LM, Rudolph CD. Pediatric endoscopy. Semin Gastrointest Dis 1994;5:32–46.

Berenson MM, Johnson TD, Markowitz NR, et al. Restoration of squamous mucosa after ablation of Barrett's esophageal epithelium. Gastroenterology 1993;104:1686–91.

Bereson GA. Intralesional steroids in the treatment of refractory esophageal strictures. J Pediatr Gastroenterol Nutr 1994;18:250–2.

Berkovits RN, Bos CE, Wijburg FA, et al. Caustic injury of the oesophagus. Sixteen years' experience, and introduction of a new model oesophageal stent. J Laryngol Otol 1996;110:1041–5.

Biller JA, Winter HS, Grand RJ, et al. Are endoscopic changes predictive of histologic esophagitis in children? J Pediatr 1983;103:215–8.

Bosco JJ, Gordon F, Zelig MP, et al. A reliable method for the endoscopic placement of a nasoenteric feeding tube. Gastrointest Endosc 1994;40:740–3.

Boyle JT, Cohen S, Watkins JB. Successful treatment of achalasia in childhood by pneumatic dilatation. J Pediatr 1981;99:35–40.

Brown CW, Werlin SL, Geenen JE, et al. The diagnostic and therapeutic role of endoscopic retrograde cholangiopancreatography in children. J Pediatr Gastroenterol Nutr 1993;17:19–23.

Brown KO, Goldschmiedt M. Endoscopic therapy of biliary and pancreatic disorders in children. Endoscopy 1994;26:719–23.

Buckley A, Connon JJ. The role of ERCP in children and adolescents. Gastrointest Endosc 1990;36:369–72.

Burke CA, van Stolk SR. Diagnosis and management of gastroduodenal polyps. Surg Oncol Clin N Am 1996;5:589–607.

Cadranel S, Rodesch P, Peeters JP, et al. Fiberendoscopy of the gastrointestinal tract in children. A series of 100 examinations. Am J Dis Child 1977;131:41–5.

Catto-Smith AG, Machida H, Butzner JD, et al. The role of gastroesophageal reflux in pediatric dysphagia. J Pediatr Gastroenterol Nutr 1991;12:159–65.

Chan KL, Saing H. Balloon dilation of peptic pyloric stenosis in children. J Pediatr Gastroenterol Nutr 1994;18:465–8.

Chan KN, Phillips AD, Mirakian R, et al. Endomysial antibody screening in children. J Pediatr Gastroenterol Nutr 1994;18:316–20.

Chen YK, Abdulian JD, Escalante-Glorsky S, et al. Clinical outcome of post-ERCP pancreatitis: relationship to history of previous pancreatitis. Am J Gastroenterol 1995;90:2120–3.

Chung SC, Leung JW, Sung JY, et al. Injection or heat probe for bleeding ulcer. Gastroenterology 1991;100:33–7.

Coben RM, Weintraub A, DiMarino AJ Jr, et al. Gastroesophageal reflux during gastrostomy feeding. Gastroenterology 1994;106:13–8.

Coppola R, D'Ugo D, Ciletti S, et al. ERCP in the era of laparoscopic biliary surgery. Experience with 407 patients. Surg Endosc 1996;10:403–6.

Corazza G, et al. Scalloped duodenal folds in childhood celiac disease. Gastrointest Endosc 1993;39:543–5.

Cox K, Ament ME. Upper gastrointestinal bleeding in children and adolescents. Pediatrics 1979;63:408–13.

Derkx HH, Huibregtse K, Taminiau JA. The role of endoscopic retrograde cholangiopancreatography in cholestatic infants. Endoscopy 1994;26:724–8.

Dorais J, Haber GB. Future of endoscopy in nonvariceal upper gastrointestinal bleeding. Gastrointest Endosc Clin N Am 1997;7:717–31.

Ell C, May A. Self-expanding metal stents for palliation of stenosing tumors of the esophagus and cardia: a critical review. Endoscopy 1997;29:392–8.

Flageole H, Raptis S, Trudel JL, et al. Progression toward malignancy of hamartomas in a patient with Peutz-Jeghers syndrome: case report and literature review. Can J Surg 1994;37:231–6.

Fox VL. Endoscopy. In: Walker WA, et al., editors. Pediatric gastrointestinal disease St. Louis: Mosby;1996. p. 1513–41.

Fox VL, Carr-Locke DL, Connors PJ, et al. Endoscopic ligation of esophageal varices in children. J Pediatr Gastroenterol Nutr 1995;20:202–8.

Gauderer MW. Percutaneous endoscopic gastrostomy: a 10-year experience with 220 children. J Pediatr Surg 1991;26:288–92.

Gauderer MW, Olsen MM, Stellato TA, et al. Feeding gastrostomy button: experience and recommendations. J Pediatr Surg 1988;23:1–8.

Gauderer MW, Ponsky JL, Izant RJJ. Gastrostomy without laparotomy: a percutaneous endoscopic technique. J Pediatr Surg 1980;15:872–5.

Gaudreault P, Parent M, McGuigan MA, et al. Predictability of esophageal injury from signs and symptoms: a study of caustic ingestion in 378 children. Pediatrics 1983;71:767–70.

Goenka AS, Dasilva MS, Cleghorn GJ, et al. Therapeutic upper gastrointestinal endoscopy in children: an audit of 443 procedures and literature review. J Gastroenterol Hepatol 1993;8:44–51.

Granot E, et al. Histologic comparison of suction capsule and endoscopic small intestinal biopsies in children. J Pediatr Gastroentol Nutr 1993;16:347–52.

Guelrud M, Jaen D, Mendoza S, et al. ERCP in the diagnosis of extrahepatic biliary atresia. Gastrointest Endosc 1991;37:522–6.

Guelrud M, Mujica C, Jaen D, et al. The role of ERCP in the diagnosis and treatment of idiopathic recurrent pancreatitis in children and adolescents. Gastrointest Endosc 1994;40:428–36.

Hall RJ, Lilly JR, Stiegmann GV. Endoscopic esophageal varix ligation: technique and preliminary results in children. J Pediatr Surg 1988;23:1222–3.

Hassall E. Nonsurgical treatment for portal hypertension in children. Gastrointest Endosc Clin North Am 1994; 4:223–58.

Hassall E, Berquist WE, Ament ME, et al. Sclerotherapy for extrahepatic portal hypertension in childhood. J Pediatr 1989;115:69–74.

Henderson CT, Engel J, Schlesinger P. Foreign body ingestion: review and suggested guidelines for management. Endoscopy 1987;19:68–71.

Hetzel DJ, Dent J, Reed WD, et al. Healing and relapse of severe peptic esophagitis after treatment with omeprazole. Gastroenterology 1988;95:903–12.

Hoffman BJ, Knapple WL, Bhutani MS, et al. Treatment of achalasia by injection of botulinum toxin under endoscopic ultrasound guidance. Gastrointest Endosc 1997;45:77–9.

Holinger LD. Management of sharp and penetrating foreign bodies of the upper aerodigestive tract. Ann Otol Rhinol Laryngol 1990;99:684–8.

Laine L. Determination of the optimal technique for bipolar electrocoagulation treatment. An experimental evaluation of the BICAP and Gold probes. Gastroenterology 1991;100:107–12.

Laine L. Endoscopic therapy for bleeding ulcers: which thermal method is best? Gastroenterology 1992;102:1083–4.

Laine L, El-Newihi HM, Igikovsky B, et al. Endoscopic ligation compared with sclerotherapy for treatment of bleeding esophageal varices. Ann Intern Med 1993; 119:1–7.

Langer JC, Wesson DE, Elin SH, et al. Feeding gastrostomy in neurology impaired children: is an antireflux procedure necessary? J Pediatr Gastroenterol Nutr 1988;7:837–41.

Lewis D, Khoshoo V, Pencharz PB, et al. Impact of nutritional rehabilitation on gastroesophageal reflux in neurologically impaired children. J Pediatr Surg 1994;29:167–9.

Lightdale CJ, Heier SK, Marcon NE, et al. Photodynamic therapy with porfirmer sodium versus thermal ablation therapy with Nd: YAG laser for palliation of esophageal cancer: a multicenter randomized trial. Gastrointest Endosc 1995;42:507–12.

Lin HJ, Lee FY, Kang WM, et al. Heat probe thermocoagulation and pure alcohol injection in massive peptic ulcer haemorrhage: a prospective, ransomised controlled trial. Gut 1990;31:753–7.

Lynch HT, Smyrk TC, Lanspa SJ, et al. Upper gastrointestinal manifestations in families with hereditary flat adenoma syndrome. Cancer 1993;71:2709–14.

Mahajan L, Olica L, Wyllie R, et al. The safety of gastrostomy in patients with Crohn's disease. Am J Gastroenterol 1997;92:985–8.

Maksoud JG, Goncalves ME, Porta G, et al. The endoscopic and surgical management of portal hypertension in children: analysis of 123 cases. J Pediatr Surg 1991; 26:178-181.

Marcon MA, Sylvester FA, Shuckett B, et al. Natural history of fibrosing pancreatitis in children. J Pediatr Gastroentol Nutr 1997;25:459A.

Mathew P, Bowman L, Williams R, et al. Complications and effectiveness of gastrostomy feedings in pediatric cancer patients. J Pediatr Hematol Oncol 1996;18:81–5.

Miller TL, McQuinn LB, Orav FJ. Endoscopy of the upper gastrointestinal tract as a diagnostic tool for children with human immunodeficieny virus infection. J Pediatr 1997;130:766–73.

Murphy GJ. Stents in the oesophagus. Postgrad Med J 1995;71:453–6.

Murphy VK. Repeated hydrostatic balloon dilation in obstructive gastroduodenal Crohn's disease. Gastrointest Endosc 1991;37:484–5.

Murray KF, Jennings RW, Fox VL. Endoscopic band ligation of a Dieulafoy lesion in the small intestine of a child. Gastrointest Endosc 1996;44:336–9.

Nakayama DK, Shorter NA, Boyle JT, et al. Pneumatic dilation and operative treatment of achalasia in children. J Pediatr Surg 1987;22:619–22.

Newman KD, Powell DM, Holcomb GW. The management of choledocholithiasis in children in the era of laparoscopic cholecystectomy. J Pediatr Surg 1997;32:1116–9.

Nishioka NS. Laser-induced fluorescence spectroscopy. Gastrointest Endosc Clin N Am 1994;4:313–26.

Noda Y, Watanabe H, Iida M, et al. Histologic follow-up of ampullary adenomas in patients with familial adenomatosis coil. Cancer 1992;70:1847–56.

Nostrant TT. Esophageal dilation. Dig Dis 1995;13:337–55.

Osorio RW, Freise CE, Stock PG, et al. Nonoperative management of biliary leaks after orthotopic liver transplantation. Transplantation 1993;55:1074–7.

Pasricha PJ, Rai R, Ravich WJ, et al. Botulinum toxin for achalasia: long-term outcome as predictors of response. Gastroenterology 1996;110:1410–5.

Putnam PE, Kocoshis Sa, Orenstein SR, et al. Pediatric endoscopic retrograde cholangiopancreatography. Am J Gastroenterol 1991;86:824–30.

Quak SH, Lam SK, Low PS. Upper gastrointestinal endoscopy in children. Singapore Med J 1990;31:123–6.

Ramond MJ, Valla D, Mosnier JF, et al. Successful endoscopic obturation of gastric varices with butyl cyanoacrylate. Hepatology 1989;10:488–93.

Rothbaum RJ. Complications of pediatric endoscopy. Gastrointest Endosc Clin N Am. 1996;6:445–59.

Savary M, Miller G. The esophagus. Handbook and atlas of endoscopy. Switzerland: Gassman Verlag AG; 1978.

Schmidt-Sommerfeld E, Kirschner BS, Stephens JK. Endoscopic and histologic findings in the upper gastrointestinal tract of children with Crohn's disease. J Pediatr Gastroenterol Nutr 1990;11:448–54.

Sherman S, Lehman GA. ERCP and endoscopic sphincterotomy-induced pancreatitis. Pancreas 1991;6:350–67.

Slivka A, Parsons WG, Carp-Locke DL. Endoscopic band ligation for treatment of post-polypectomy hemorrhage. Gastrointest Endosc 1994;40:230–2.

Stiegmann G, Goff JS, Michaletz-Onody PA, et al. Endoscopic sclerotherapy as compared with endoscopic ligation for bleeding esophageal varices. N Eng J Med 1992;326:1527-32.

Thapa BR, Mehta S. Endoscopic sclerotherapy of esophageal varices in infants and children. J Pediatr Gastroenterol Nutr 1990;10:430–4.

Treem WR, Etienne NL, Hyams JS. Percutaneous endoscopic placement of the "button": gastrostomy tube as the initial procedure in infants and children. J Pediatr Gastroenterol Nutr 1993;17:382–6.

Voyles CR, Sanders DL, Hogan R. Common bile duct evaluation in the era of laparoscopic cholecystectomy. 1050 cases later. Ann Surg 1994;219:744–50.

Walker-Smith JA. Fibre-optic techniques for investigation of gastrointestinal diseases in children. Pediatr Allergy Immunol 1993;4(Suppl 3):40–3.

Walton JM, Tougas G. Botulinum toxin use in pediatric esophageal achalasia: a case report. J Pediatr Surg 1997; 32:916–7.

Wara P. Endoscopic prediction of major rebleeding—a prospective study of stigmata of hemorrhage in bleeding ulcer. Gastroenterology 1985;88:1209–14.

Werlin SL. Endoscopic retrograde cholangiopancreatography in children. Gastrointest Endosc Clin Am 1994; 4:161–78.

Wilkinson ML, Mieli-Vergani G, Ball C, et al. Endoscopic retrograde cholangiopancreatography in infantile cholestasis. Arch Dis Child 1991;66:121–3.

Zargar SA, Kochhar R, Mehta S, et al. The role of fiberoptic endoscopy in the management of corrosive ingestion and modified endoscopic classification of burns. Gastrointest Endosc 1991;37:165–9.

Ziegler K, Schier F, Waldschmidt J. Endoscopic laser resection of a duodenal membrane. J Pediatr Surg 1992; 27:1582–3.

Endosonography

Chang KJ, Wiersema MJ. Endoscopic ultrasound-guided fine-needle aspiration biopsy and interventional endoscopic ultrasongraphy. Emerging technologies. Gastrointest Endosc Clin N Am 1997;7:221–35.

Palazzo L. Which test for common bile duct stones? Endoscopic and intraductal ultrasongraphy. Endoscopy 1997;29:655–65.

Tygat GN, Fockens P. Exploring the role of endosonography. Scand J Gastroenterol Supply 1996;220:71–4.

Van Dam J. Endosongraphic evaluation of the patient wih esophageal cancer. Chest 1997;112 (Suppl 4):1845–1905.

Enteroscopy

Benaroch LM, Rudolph CD. Pediatric endoscopy. Semin Gastrointest Dis 1994;5:32-46.

Gostout CJ. Sonde enteroscopy. Gastrointest Endosc Clin N Am 1998;6:777–92.

Gostout CJ, Bender CE. Cholangiopancreatography, sphincterotomy, and common duct stone removal via Roux-en-Y limb enteroscopy. Gastroenterology 1988;95: 156–63.

Mellert J, Naruhn MB, Grund KE, et al. Direct endoscopic percutaneous jejunostomy (EPJ). Clinical results. Surg Endoc 1994;8:867–9.

Wilmer A. Push enteroscopy. Gastrointest Endosc Clin N Am 1998;6:759–76.

Colonoscopy

Ament ME, Brill JE. Pediatric endoscopy, deep sedation, conscious sedation, and general anesthesia—what is best? Gastrointest Endosc 1995;41:173–5.

Balshells F, Wyllie R, Kay M, et al. Use of conscious sedation for lower and upper gastrointestinal endoscopic examination in children, adolescents, and young adults: a twelve-year review. Gastrointest Endosc 1997;45:375–80.

Committee on Drugs of the American Academy of Pediatrics: Guidelines for monitoring and managment of pediatric patients during and after sedation for diagnostic and therapeutic procedures. Pediatrics 1993;89:1110–5.

Cote CJ. Sedation for the pediatric patient. A review. Pediatr Clin in North Am 1994;41:31–58.

Cynamon HA, Milov DE, Andres JM. Diagnosis and management of colonic polyps in children. J Pediatr 1989;114:593–6.

Dajani AS, Taubert KA, Wilson W, et al. Prevention of bacterial endocarditis. Recommendations by the American Heart Association. Circulation 1997;96:358–66.

Damore LJ, Rantis PC, Varnava AM, et al. Colonoscopic perforations. Etiology, diagnosis, and management Dis Colon Rectum 1996;39:1308–14.

Fox VL. Colonoscopy. In: Walker WA, et al., eds. gastrointestinal disease 2 ed. St. Louis: Mosby 1996. p. 1533–41.

Gallo SH, McClave SA. Blue rubber bleb nevus syndrome: gastrointestinal involvement and its endoscopic presentation. Gastrointest Endosc 1992;38:72–6.

Gewitz MH. Prevention of bacterial endocarditis. Curr Opin Pediatr 1997;9:518–22.

Griffiths AM, Sherman PM. Colonoscopic surveillance for cancer in ulcerative colitisi: a crtical review. J Pediatr Gastroenterol Nutr 1997;24:202–10.

Heaton ND, Davenport M, Howard ER. Symptomatic hemmorrhoids and anorectal varices in children with portal hypertension. J Pediatr Surg 1992;27:833–5.

Hunt RH. Towards safer colonoscopy. Gut 1983;24:371–5.

Jalihal A, Misra SP, Arvind AS, et al. Colonoscopic polypectomy in children. J Pediatr Surg 1992;27:1220–2.

Jenkins HR, Pincott JR, Soothill JF, et al. Food allergy: the major cause of infantile colitis. Arch Dis Child 1984;59:326–9.

Low DE, Shoenut JP, Kennedy JK, et al. Prospective assessment of risk of bacteremia with colonscopy and polypectomy. Dig Dis Sci 1987;32:1239–43.

Monahan DW, Peluso FE, Goldner F. Combustible colonic gas levels during flexible sigmoidoscopy and colonscopy. Gastrointest Endosc 1992;38:40–43.

Noronha PA, Leist MH. Endoscopic laser therapy for gastrointestinal bleeding from congenital vascular lesions. J Pediatr Gastroenterol Nutr 1988;7:375–8.

Rothbaum RJ. Complications of pediatric endoscopy. Gastroinlest Endosc Clin N Am 1996;6:445–59.

Schmidt-Sommerfeld E, Kirschner BS, Stephens JK. Endoscopic and histologic findings in the upper gastrointestinal tract of children with Crohn's disease. J Pediatr Gastroenterol Nutr 1990;11:448–54.

Tithecott GA, Filler R, Sherman PM. Turcot's symdrome: a diagnostic consideration in a child with primary adenocarcinoma of the colon. J Pediatr Surg 1989;24:1189–91.

Tolia V, Chang CH. Adenomatons polyp in a four-year-old child. J Pediatr Gastroenterol Nutr 1990;10:262–4.

Woolrich AJ, DaSilva MD, Korelitz BI. Surveillance in the routine management of ulcerative colitis: the predictive value of a low-grade dysplasia. Gastroenterology 1992;103:431–8.

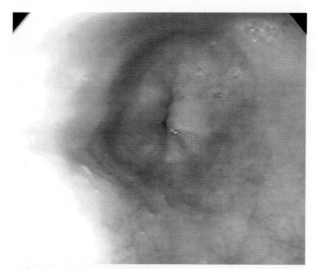

PLATE 1. Normal esophagus.

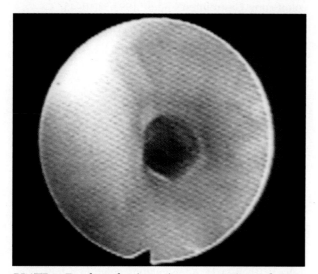

PLATE 2. Esophageal stricture in severe peptic esophagitis.

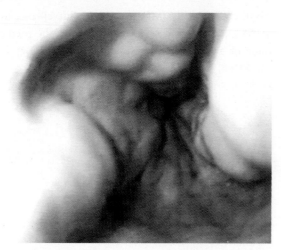

PLATE 3. Esophageal varices: the varices are the long ser-piginous lesions down the wall of the esophagus.

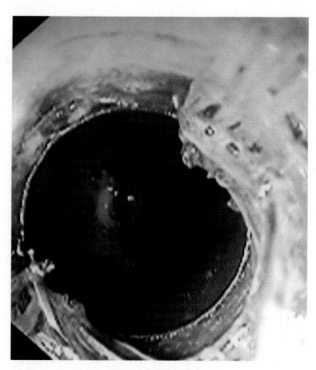

PLATE 4. Esophageal variceal banding: the view shows the banding apparatus on the tip of the endoscope and a ligat-ed varix (blue band). Notice that once banded, the varix collapses and the long serpiginous lesion is gone.

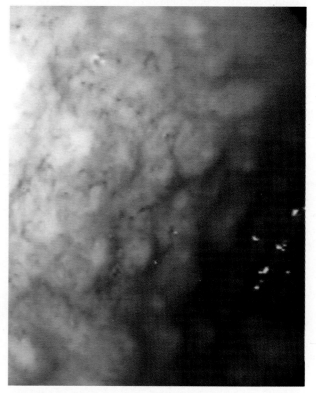

PLATE 5. Nodularity of the gastric antrum in a child with gastritis associated with *Helicobacter pylori*.

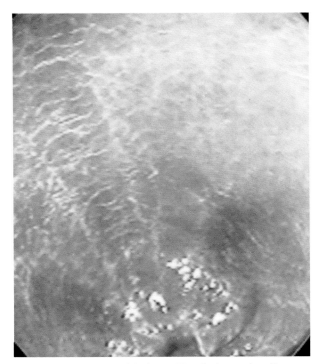

PLATE 6. Severe gastritis (non–*H. pylori*-associated).

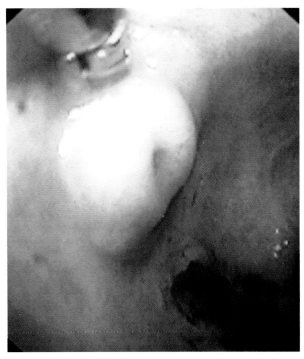

PLATE 8. Etopic pancreas. The raised umbilicated lesion is located in the gastric antrum.

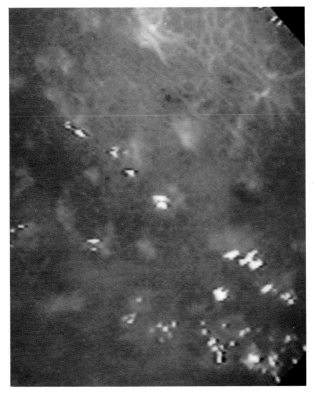

PLATE 7. Multiple aphthous ulcers seen in the body of the stomach in Crohn's disease.

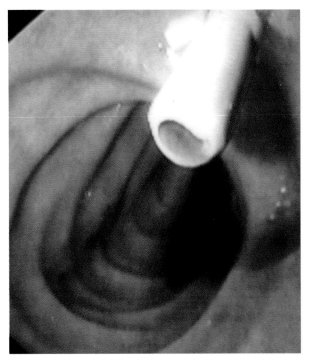

PLATE 9. A stent in the common bile duct placed during ERCP to relieve obstruction due to a stricture.

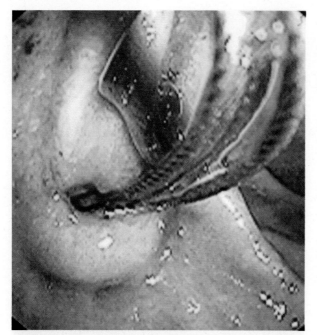

PLATE 10. The paplitome that is in the ampulae of Vater will be used to perform a sphincterotomy during the ERCP.

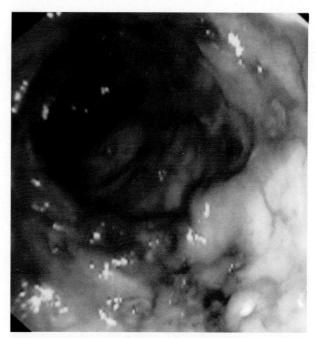

PLATE 12. Crohn's disease.

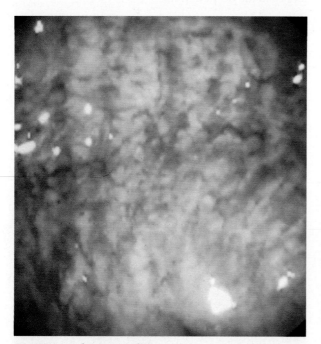

PLATE 11. Ulcerative colitis.

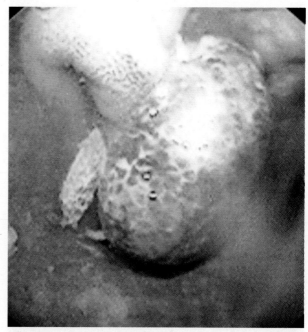

PLATE 13. A juvenile polyp.

5

PEDIATRIC GASTROINTESTINAL INTERVENTIONS

Peter Chait, MB, ChB, Kevin M. Baskin, MD,
Michael Temple, MD, and Bairbre Connolly, MB, ChB

INTERVENTIONAL RADIOLOGY SERVICES

Image-Guided Therapy

With the emergence of trained pediatric interventional radiologists, the provision of pediatric interventional radiology services has now become an essential feature of major children's hospitals. Interventional radiologists play an increasingly important role in clinical care, interacting directly with patients and their families, providing primary services for such needs as enterostomy access and vascular access as well as consultative services and procedures in collaboration with other specialists. Increased accessibility and accountability are important components of this emerging environment. In addition to performing procedures, the image-guided therapy (IGT) service must take responsibility for pre- and postprocedure care as well as for monitoring outcomes and treating complications (Ring and Kerlan, 1985; Goldberg, Mueller, et al., 1991).

The number and variety of pediatric interventional procedures performed with image guidance has grown as a direct result of improvements in imaging technology, particularly ultrasonography (US), fluoroscopy, and computed tomography (CT) (Diament, Boechat, et al., 1985; Hoffer, Fellows, et al., 1985; vanSonnenberg, Wittich, et al., 1987; Towbin and Ball, 1988; Towbin, 1989a; 1989b, 1991; Hubbard and Fellows, 1993; Chait, 1997). Rapid advances in biotechnology, with the development of different catheters, wires, balloons, and other devices, also contribute substantially to sustaining this growth. At the Centre for Image Guided Therapy at the Hospital for Sick Children in Toronto, over 3000 interventional cases are performed each year.

This has risen steadily over the last 7 years, largely due to close collaboration with referring physicians and other disciplines. The largest proportion of these procedures relates to the gastrointestinal system and includes enterostomy access, biopsies, and drainages.

The Image-Guided Therapy Team and Multidisciplinary Collaboration

A dedicated multidisciplinary team approach is fundamental to a successful interventional service (Ring and Kerlan, 1985; White, Rizer, et al. 1988; Katzen, Kaplan, et al., 1989; Goldberg, Mueller, et al., 1991). This approach includes 24-hour availability of trained pediatric interventional radiologists to patients and referring health care providers. Nurses and technologists specifically trained in an interventional radiology environment may act as first assistants and should understand the principles of minimally invasive procedures to anticipate and support the interventionists' efforts during critical points. They also help manage work flow and inventory control to assure a safe and efficient work environment. Close monitoring of patients throughout the procedure is required. In conjunction with the interventionist, interventional nurses triage patients for suitable pain control and sedation and work closely with pediatric anesthesiologists in preparing the patient for and administering general anesthetic agents when appropriate. Radiology technologists are trained in radiation safety and in the use of the various imaging modalities common to the interventional suite, including US, CT, fluoroscopy, and digital subtraction angiography (DSA). We maintain a prospective database of patient and procedure-related information, linked to other health information and imaging databases. In a larger service, nurse clinicians and pediatricians may assist with patient preparation and follow-up. The whole team must be familiar with patients' underlying diagnoses and must understand why each procedure is being performed.

Our team approach includes daily meetings and discussions about prioritization of patients, scheduling procedures, safe transport of patients, and appropriate periprocedural care of the patients' families. The team has a responsibility for effective communication with involved health care professionals, including referring physicians, anesthesiologists, clinical pathologists, and such allied health professionals as occupational therapists, social workers, discharge planners, and palliative care providers. This contributes to good continuity of care as well as to the satisfaction of patients, families, and colleagues. Such communication is especially important when interdisciplinary cooperation allows the performance of multiple procedures under the same anesthetic or the collaboration of multiple services in the same procedure.

Enterostomy Access Service

Procedures related to enterostomy catheters of all types (including gastrostomy, gastrojejunostomy, cecostomy, jejunostomy, and nasojejunal tubes) account for one-third of the pediatric interventional procedures performed at our institution. Because of the volume of patients we care for, we have developed an enterostomy access service (EAS). The EAS covers all aspects of enterostomy access from identification, referral, and education of patients through performance of the access procedure to postprocedure care and teaching. Our EAS team includes gastroenterologists, interventional radiologists, and nurse clinicians with special competency in the care of the enterostomy patient. The team works closely with admission and discharge planners, dietitians, and occupational therapists. Knowledgeable representatives of this team are available to patients and referring providers 24 hours a day (Borkowski, 1998). The team offers a single point of contact for referral, assessment, and prioritization of patients who are candidates for enterostomy access (Thorne and Radford, 1998). Usually, the enterostomy nurses, in coordination with the gastroenterologists, evaluate each patient's medical history and long-term nutritional requirements (this includes an

assessment for reflux, gastric outlet obstruction, motility disturbances, and swallowing disorders) and determine an appropriate feeding strategy. In consultation with the interventional radiologist, the procedure is scheduled, and patients and parents are scheduled for teaching. We run a weekly teaching session where information about catheters and catheter care is addressed and questions are answered. In this manner, there is adequate opportunity for patients and parents to understand the procedure and its implications, expected outcomes, and potential complications; the appropriate use and care of the enterostomy tube; discharge and follow up instructions; and contact information.

Consent and Assent

The required elements of an informed consent transaction differ from one jurisdiction to another. It is important to know what the standard of care is in your community (Rose, 1980; Reuter, 1986, 1987; Potchen, Potchen, et al., 1995). At a minimum, patients and parents must understand the procedure, its indications and contraindications, risks and benefits, surgical and medical alternatives, and expected outcomes prior to beginning any procedure. It is helpful to provide unbiased, up-to-date information in a format accessible to the patient (and family, where appropriate), targeted to a developmental level that matches the patient's (and parents') abilities. Assent refers to an informed agreement by minor children to planned procedures; it is obtained in addition to the informed consent of the patient's parents or guardian (Leikin, 1983; Bartholome, 1989; AAP, 1995). The knowledgeable and willing participation of the patient in the process increases comfort and cooperation and is well worth the effort. While informative pamphlets or digitized information may be helpful, it is ultimately the responsibility of the interventionist performing the procedure to verify informed consent through a one-on-one interaction with the patient and the parent. The acceptance of unavoidable complications by well-informed patients and parents cannot be overstressed.

PROCEDURE PLANNING

Pre-procedure Care

The referring physician must relate the reason for referral (the specific question to be answered or problem to be addressed), the patient's pertinent history and physical findings, and the diagnostic workup that led to the referral. In turn, the interventional radiologist must clarify the planned diagnostic or therapeutic approach. If a change of plan becomes necessary, the referring physician should be notified. While it may be unusual for diagnostic radiologists to question the appropriateness of a requested examination, interventional radiologists must recognize the different practice environment that an interventional procedure demands. On the other hand, where other procedure-based disciplines have a long-standing tradition, the recent emergence of pediatric interventional radiology may be less readily accepted by referring physicians and patients (Levin, Flanders, et al., 1995; Levin, Rao, et al., 1999; Schnyder, Capasso, et al., 1999). Close communication, attention to the development of outcomes-based information, and thorough involvement in pre-procedure workup and postprocedure care will lessen opposition and improve recognition of pediatric interventional radiology as a fully functional clinical specialty.

Immediately prior to the procedure, the patient's medical chart and imaging should be reviewed, and further imaging should be ordered if necessary. A specific search for any history of drug or environmental allergies is essential (e.g., latex allergy in spina bifida) (Moneret-Vautrin, Beaudouin, et al.,

1993; Cantani, 1999). Previous sedation and anesthetia records should also be specifically sought and reviewed.

Laboratory studies most frequently include a coagulation profile, platelet count, and hemoglobin level (Table 5–1). These should be obtained in close proximity to the procedure to reflect the patient's current condition. The coagulation profile generally includes the partial thromboplastin time (PTT) which measures thrombin generation in the intrinsic pathway and is a function of all coagulation factors except factor VII, and prothrombin time (PT), which measures thrombin generation in the extrinsic pathway and is a function of factors II, V, VII, and X as well as the fibrinogen level. Additional screening tests that may be considered are those for bleeding time (a measure of platelet-vessel interaction) and thrombin time (TT) which estimates the amount and function of fibrinogen. Alterations in common screening tests in neonates may be quite marked, and the tests are especially sensitive to contamination by heparin (for TT, PTT, and PT, in decreasing order of effect). Despite prolonged coagulation times in this population, neonates actually tend to be hypercoagulable. Procedures in this group should be approached with due caution.

There is generally a poor correlation between abnormalities in the coagulation profile or platelet counts and procedure-related bleeding complications.

TABLE 5–1. Reference Values for Coagulation*

Reference Group	Age	PT Mean (Boundary)	INR Mean (Boundary)	PTT Mean (Boundary)	Fibrinogen Mean (Boundary)
Healthy Fetuses[†]	Day 1	—	—	—	1.0 (0.57–1.43)
Premature Infants at Birth[‡]	Day 1	15.4 (14.6–16.9)	—	108 (80.0–168)	2.56 (1.60–5.50)
Healthy Premature Infants[§]	Day 1	13.0 (10.6–16.2)	1.3 (.09–1.6)	53.6 (27.5–79.4)	2.43 (1.50–3.73)
	Day 90	12.3 (10.0–14.6)	—	39.5 (28.3–50.7)	2.46 (1.50–3.52)
	Day 180	12.5 (10.0–15.0)	—	37.5 (27.1–53.3)	2.28 (1.50–3.60)
	Adult	12.4 (10.8–13.9)	1.00 (0.9–1.1)	33.5 (26.6–40.3)	2.78 (1.56–4.00)
Healthy Full-Term Infants	Day 1	13.0 (10.1–15.9)	1.00 (0.53–1.62)	42.9 (31.3–54.5)	2.83 (1.67–3.99)
	Day 90	11.9 (10.0–14.2)	1.00 (0.9–1.1)	37.1 (29.0–50.1)	2.43 (1.50–3.79)
	Day 180	12.3 (10.7–13.9)	1.00 (0.9–1.1)	35.5 (28.1–42.9)	2.51 (1.50–3.87)
	Adult	12.4 (10.8–13.9)	1.00 (0.9–1.1)	33.5 (26.6–40.3)	2.78 (1.56–4.00)

* Values are dependent upon the reagents used. Check with laboratory to determine normal values appropriate to each institution.
[†]19–27 weeks' gestational age
[‡]28–31 weeks' gestational age
[§]30–36 weeks' gestational age
INR, international normalized ratio; PT, prothrombin time; PTT, partial thromboplastin time

Especially in children, there is little documentation in the literature to support a hard-and-fast approach to the interpretation or application of these tests in pre-procedure planning. No matter what the numbers, a sick child with a history of bleeding problems should be treated with great caution.

With these cautions in mind, a generalized strategy for correcting bleeding abnormalities is offered in Table 5–2. Platelet dysfunction can be congenital or acquired, qualitative or quantitative. Acquired conditions such as renal failure (uremia), liver disease, and aspirin administration cause a qualitative defect whereas a consumptive coagulopathy results in a quantitative defect. Extrinsic pathway abnormalities, signaled by a prolonged PT or an elevated international normalized ratio (INR), are seen most often with warfarin administration, nutritional (vitamin K) deficiency, and disseminated intravascular coagulopathy. Intrinsic pathway abnormalities, with prolonged PTT, most often result from treatment with heparin or enoxaparin (low-molecular-weight heparin). Specific circumstances may require factor replacement or other specialized interventions beyond those outlined above to correct the defect underlying the abnormal value. Close consultation with a hematologist in such situations is essential. Aspirin, a nonreversible inhibitor of platelet function, should be withheld for 7 to 10 days prior to high-risk elective procedures. Nonsteroidal anti-inflammatory agents, as reversible platelet inhibitors, may need to be withheld for only 24 hours. Warfarin may need to be withheld for one to several days prior to the planned procedure, depending upon the specific regimen. Enoxaparin should be withheld for 24 hours, but heparin needs to be withheld only for 2 to 4 hours prior to the planned procedure. Finally, agents such as platelets and fresh frozen plasma that achieve peak blood levels at the time they are infused should be administered as close to the time of the procedure as possible for maximum effect.

Patients fasting for a procedure (see Sedation, Analgesia, and Anesthesia, below) should not become dehydrated, and orders for maintenance intravenous fluids (Table 5–3) should be part of routine pre-procedure orders. This is especially important for patients who will be receiving intravascular contrast during the procedure. Special considerations may be required for patients with borderline renal function and for those with cardiopulmonary compromise. Close consultation with the referring service (and in the latter case, with the cardiology service) will help avoid preventable complications. The insulin dose in diabetic patients may be cut in half on the morning of a procedure for the fasting patient although again, appropriate consultation will provide more specific guidance (Meyers, Alberts, et al., 1986; Kroenke, Gooby-Toedt, et al., 1998).

When either sedation or general anesthesia is planned, patients' intake must be restricted from solids for 8 hours prior to the procedure and clear fluids for 2 hours prior to the procedure (Schreiner, Triebwasser, et al., 1990; Splinter and Schaefer, 1990; Phillips, Daborn, et al., 1994; Soreide, Holst-Larsen, et al., 1995; Pandit and Pandit, 1997). All patients who require sedation or anesthesia must have adequate intravenous access. Emergency cases may require deviations from these guidelines and must be considered on a case-by-case basis. If proper fasting cannot be assured, use of the lightest sedation possible and maneuvers targeted to protecting the

TABLE 5–2. Guidelines for Pre-Procedure Correction of Bleeding Abnormalities

Defect	Parameter	Treatment
Qualitative platelet dysfunction	Bleeding time (normal < 8–9 min)	Desmopressin (DDAVP), 0.3 g/kg over 30 min, or transfuse 1 unit platelets/5–10 kg (for increase of 40–70 K), or cryoprecipitate, 1 unit/10 kg
	Platelet count	Transfuse 1 unit platelets/5–10 kg (for an increase of 40,000–70,000)
Extrinsic pathway	PT, INR	Hold warfarin (replace with heparin)
		Vitamin K1, 2 mg (infants), 5–10 mg (children), IM or SQ
		Fresh frozen plasma, 10–15 mL/kg
Intrinsic pathway	PTT	Hold heparin
		Fresh frozen plasma, 10–15 mL/kg

INR, international normalized ratio; PT, prothrombin time; PTT, partial thromboplastin time; IM, intramuscular; SQ, subcutaneous

airway from aspiration, reducing gastric contents, and increasing gastric pH may help reduce risk (Gombar, Dureja, et al., 1997).

In contrast to usual practice in adult patients, intravenous antibiotics are prescribed prophylactically in many pediatric gastrointestinal interventional procedures. Those involving the upper gastrointestinal system usually receive a first-generation cephalosporin (cefazolin 40 mg per kg) as a single dose prior to the procedure. Patients whose procedures involve the colon or rectum or in whom biliary manipulation is contemplated are given a combination of gentamicin (2.5 mg per kg), ampicillin (50 mg/kg) and metronidazole (10 mg/kg) as a single pre-procedure dose, and the same dosages are continued three times per day for several days following the procedure. In children who require prophylaxis due to cardiac conditions, a combination of ampicillin (50 mg per kg) and gentamicin (2.5 mg per kg) is administered within 30 minutes before starting the procedure. These patients receive a repeat dose of intravenous ampicillin (25 mg per kg) 6 hours following the procedure. Patients who are allergic to penicillin and cephalosporins receive vancomycin (20 mg per kg over an hour) and gentamicin (2.5 mg per kg).

Periprocedure Care

Access to the procedure room and movement of machines and instruments in and out of the room should be limited and should not compromise sterile technique. Thoughtful planning should be applied to properly positioning the patient before the start of a procedure. An effective position and judicious use of a tilting table facilitates successful completion of the procedure and promotes desirable movements of air, contrast agents, and fluids. For instance, a partial left decubitus position improves inflation of the cecum prior to cecostomy tube insertion while a fetal position (left-side-down decubitus) allows simultaneous imaging with US and fluoroscopy and improves access to the rectum during image-guided transrectal abscess drainage. Well-planned positioning will also improve visualization of monitors and the operative field and will decrease operator fatigue. We favor sitting on a rolling stool whenever possible to decrease low back and neck strain. The prospective position and movements of objects and personnel in the room (such as the fluoroscopic C-arm, the US machine, IV poles, monitors, the anesthetist, nurses, other clinicians, etc.) should be planned prior to

TABLE 5–3. Recommended Infusion Rates for Intravenous Maintenance Fluid Administration

Weight	Infusion Rate
<10 kg	4 mL/kg/hr
10 kg–20 kg	40 mL/hr plus 2 mL/kg/hr
>20 kg	60 mL/hr plus 1 mL/kg/hr

starting the case so as to provide a safe and effective work environment for all concerned. If oblique and lateral screening of the abdomen will likely be required, the patient's arms should be positioned above the head. A variety of restraining devices is available and should be employed strategically to maintain the patient in a safe, stable, and comfortable position throughout the procedure. In babies, monitored use of a warming device can help maintain body temperature (Table 5–4).

Sedation, Analgesia, and Anesthesia

Pediatric patients preparing for, undergoing, and recovering from interventional procedures should remain safe, comfortable, and free from anxiety. A discussion of the risks and benefits of sedation or anesthesia should be included under the umbrella of informed consent. Indications for sedation, analgesia, and general anesthesia are based on the physical status of the patient, the nature of the procedure, and in some cases, the needs of the physician. Arbitrarily dividing the continuum of comfort and control into five levels, from anxiety alleviation to gen-

TABLE 5–4. Warming Strategies for Procedures in Small Children*

Conservation
    Increase room temperature
    Warm blankets
    Plastic (cling) wrap
Convection
    Radiant heat from warming lamp
    Warm air flow (Bair Hugger)
Conduction
    Warm saline bags
    Chemical warming blanket (TransWarmer, Prism, Texas)

*Specific procedures should be in place to monitor and maintain body temperature during procedures in infants and small children

eral anesthesia can help guide an appropriate medical response (Table 5–5).

The specific goals for analgesia and anesthesia should be defined for each case, and an appropriate target level of sedation should be planned, understanding that patient responses may be unpredictable and that a change in plan may be required at any time. In general, most pediatric procedures that are painful or that require the child to be completely immobilized will require deep sedation or general anesthesia. General anesthesia may also be indicated for lengthy procedures and for procedures where the area of interest is close to a vital structure. On the other hand, some neonates and patients with oropharyngeal abnormalities may be poor candidates for endotracheal intubation. In these patients (and in older children undergoing less painful procedures), local anesthesia or light sedation may be all that is required.

The patient's physical status is categorized according to the American Society of Anesthesiologists (ASA) classification (Dripps and Lamont, 1961; Keats, 1978), slightly modified here (Table 5–6). This classification helps determine an appropriate selection of candidates for nurse-administered sedation under the direction of the interventional radiologist. In general, all ASA class I and II patients can be safely managed by registered nurses whose training includes specific competency in pediatric sedation, monitoring, and resuscitation. Class IV and V patients should be managed by pediatric anesthesiologists familiar with image-guided procedures. Class III patients should be managed only by experienced nursing personnel after appropriate consultation with the supervising anesthesiologist.

A wide variety of medications are available for analgesia and sedation (AAP, 1985; Strain, Harvey, et al., 1986; Strain, Campbell, et al., 1988; Sievers, Yee, et al., 1991; Ronchera, Marti-Bonmati, et al., 1992; AAP, 1993; Lefever, Potter, et al., 1993; Sectish, 1997; Riavis, Laux-End, et al., 1998). It is advisable to gain thorough familiarity with a limited selec-

TABLE 5–5. Levels of Comfort and Control in Intervention Procedures*

Level	Description	Examples	Sample Response
Anxiety alleviation	Decreased apprehension without a change in awareness	Gastrostomy tube change	Parental comfort Midazolam 0.3 mg/kg PO
Analgesia	Relief of pain without intentional sedation (may include some alteration in mental status)	Paracentesis	EMLA topical patch 2 hours prior to procedure Lidocaine 1% by local infiltration
Conscious sedation	A medically-controlled state of depressed consciousness that maintains — protective reflexes — a patent airway — patient responsiveness to stimulation or verbal commands	Percutaneous liver biopsy Cecostomy tube insertion	EMLA topical patch 2 hours prior to procedure Lidocaine 1% by local infiltration Diazepam 0.1 mg/kg IV Meperidine 1 mg/kg IV
Deep sedation	A medically controlled state of depressed consciousness or unconsciousness from which the patient is not easily aroused	Transrectal abscess drainage Esophageal dilatation and stent placement	Propofol 3 mg/kg IV induction, followed by 180 µg/kg/min IV for maintenance, titrated for effect by anesthesiology
General anesthesia	A medically controlled state of unconsciousness with — loss of protective reflexes — inability to independently maintain a patent airway — inability to respond purposefully to stimulation or verbal commands	Transjugular liver biopsy Percutaneous transcholecystic cholangiography	Endotracheal anesthesia, paralysis, and controlled respirations by anesthesiology

*The level of sedation, analgesia, and anesthesia should be directly targeted to the specific needs of the patient and the nature of the intended procedure.
IV, intravenously; PO, per os

TABLE 5–6. Classification of Patient Physical Status

ASA Class	Description
I	Healthy, no underlying organic disease
II	Mild or moderate systemic disease that does not interfere with daily routines (e.g., well-controlled asthma, essential hypertension)
III	Organic disease with definite functional impairment (e.g., severe steroid-dependent asthma, insulin-dependent diabetes, uncorrected congenital heart disease
IV	Severe disease that is life threatening (e.g., head trauma with increased intracranial pressure)
V	Moribund patient, not expected to survive
E	Physical status classification appended with an "E" connotes a procedure undertaken as an emergency (e.g., an otherwise healthy patient presenting for fracture reduction is classified as ASA physical status I E)

ASA, American Society of Anesthesiologists

tion. Monitoring of sedated patients includes cuff blood pressure each 5 to 10 minutes, continuous electrocardiography, and continuous pulse oximetry. Visual monitoring by physicians, nurses, and technologists (AAP, 1992; Lowrie, Weiss, et al., 1998) is by far the most important means of assuring safety and avoiding complications. Regardless of what level of sedation is chosen, full resuscitation and anesthetic equipment with suction should be immediately available.

The medications we prefer for analgesia and sedation in pediatric patients are summarized in Table 5–7. Infants weighing less than 5 kg may be given an oral dose of chloral hydrate followed with either intravenous morphine or oral diphenhydramine. In young children (5 to 20 kg), we prefer intravenous pentobarbital followed by intravenous meperidine, repeating as necessary. In older children and adolescents, sedation would include intravenous diazemuls followed by intravenous meperidine, repeated as necessary. Sedation for patients undergoing short procedures is usually accomplished with oral midazolam.

Liberal use of local anesthetics, even in sedated or anesthetized patients, improves postprocedure recovery and decreases pain experienced at the operative site. Local anesthetics may often be administered through a 27-Gauge needle with minimal discomfort. Patient acceptance is improved if the site has been prepared with topically applied EMLA cream (lidocaine 2.5% and prilocaine 2.5%, AstraZeneca) (Russell and Doyle, 1997) or Ametop gel (tetracaine 4%, Smith & Nephew). Raising the

TABLE 5–7. Approaches to Sedation and Analgesia for Interventional Procedures

Indication	Medication	Route	Dose	Maximum Dose	Comments
Patients < 5 kg	Chloral hydrate	PO	80 mg/kg	1 g/dose	May repeat in 30 min at half the dose
	and morphine or	IV	0.05 mg/kg	Individualized	
	diphenhydramine	PO	1 mg/kg	50 mg/dose	Naloxone and resuscitation equipment available
Patients 5–20 kg	Pentobarbital	IV	2–6 mg/kg	100 mg/dose	—
	Meperidine	IV	1 mg/kg	Individualized	Repeat each hour as needed
Patients > 20 kg	Diazepam	IV	0.1 mg/kg	0.6 mg/kg/8 h	Do not exceed 5mg/min
	Meperidine	IV	1 mg/kg	Individualized	
Oral sedation of older children	Midazolam	PO	0.3–0.5 mg/kg	Individualized	—
Local anesthesia	EMLA	Top	2.5 g/dose	—	Apply 2 hours prior
	Ametop	Top	1.5 g/dose	—	Apply 40 min prior
	Lidocaine 1%	Loc	—	0.5 cc/kg	Epinephrine (1:200,000) may be added for vasoconstriction
	Bupivacaine 0.25%	Loc	—	1 cc/kg	

IV, intravenously; PO, per os; Top, topical,; Loc, local

pH of the solution with a 1:9 mixture of injectable sodium bicarbonate to local anesthetic (Christoph, Buchanan, et al., 1988) decreases pain and improves distribution. If a longer duration of analgesia is desired, we use bupivacaine instead of lidocaine. In either case, mixture with epinephrine (1:200,000) will increase vasoconstriction and retention of the anesthetic at the site and will often significantly decrease bleeding at the site during the procedure.

POSTPROCEDURE MANAGEMENT

Immediately upon completion of the procedure, timed and dated medication and patient monitoring records are signed by the interventional radiologist. A brief note is written in the patient's chart outlining the procedure and its outcome, deviations from standard practice, complications, and recommendations for observation or further intervention. The interventional radiologist sits down with the parent or guardian, reviews the outcome of the procedure and any complications and unusual events, and gives specific instructions regarding care and followup. At our institution, if patients are awake enough, they are sent directly to the ward and do not need to go to the postanesthesia care unit (PACU). Patients who are still sedated or who have received endotracheal or intravenous general anesthesia are taken to the PACU, where they are monitored until they are awake enough to be transferred back to the ward or discharged to home. Patients are discharged from the PACU when their cardiovascular and airway stability are assured and they are awake, alert, and (if applicable) able to walk without help.

IMAGE GUIDANCE SYSTEMS

The scope of minimally invasive image-guided procedures is expanding with improvements in existing systems such as US, fluoroscopy, and CT. Recently, CT fluoroscopy (Silverman et al, 1999) and interventional magnetic resonance imaging [MR] are becoming more widely available. Although their role has yet to be defined, they will almost certainly find increasing use in the near future. By using a multimodality approach to patient problems and by combining procedures in a multidisciplinary format, we try to reduce the patient's exposure to ionizing radiation and anesthesia while maximizing the efficient use of resources. This "one-stop shop" environment is illustrated in Figures 5–1 and 5–2. Relative advantages and disadvantages of common imaging modalities are summarized in Table 5–8.

Ultrasonography

Ultrasonography guidance is ideal for the pediatric population due to the limited amount of subcutaneous and intraperitoneal fat. Furthermore, US uses no ionizing radiation and is a real-time modality. As technology has advanced, the quality of images obtained by high-frequency linear and curvilinear probes has improved dramatically, allowing most of our percutaneous biopsies to be performed under US control alone. At this point in time, we use US guidance for approximately 60% of the pediatric gastrointestinal procedures we perform, either alone or (more often) in combination with another modality. However, there are a number of situations in which US is not an ideal modality. For example, deep lesions or those obscured by intervening gas or bony structures are not well visualized on US. However, bone lesions that disrupt the cortex or have a soft-tissue element are ideally suited to US-guided sampling.

Fluoroscopy

Fluoroscopy is generally used for guidance where there is a differential density between structures. For example, the gas-tissue interface of the distended gastric lumen creates an easily visualized target for retrograde percutaneous gastrostomy. Dilatation, stenting, and vascular procedures are also performed primarily under fluoroscopic control. In such procedures as abscess drainage and biliary stenting or drainage, the initial needle access is obtained under US guidance, and the procedure is completed using fluoroscopic control.

Computed Tomography

In our practice, CT is primarily used as a diagnostic tool and for planning an approach prior to beginning a procedure. However, CT guidance may be indispensable in situations where lesions are deep and adjacent to vital structures or are obscured by bony structures.

Contrast Media

Water-soluble nonionic contrast media are used for most interventional and diagnostic procedures performed under fluoroscopic control, either primarily or after access under US or CT guidance. We use nonionic low-osmolar contrast media exclusively,

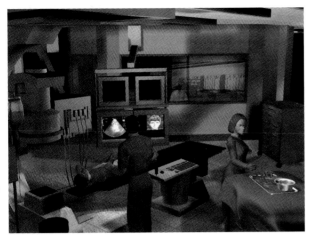

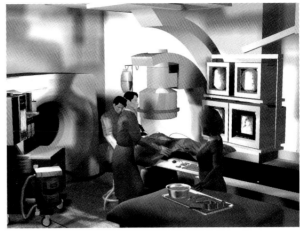

FIGURE 5–1. Simulated paediatric interventional radiology suite I. A high-resolution ceiling-mounted US unit is used for periprocedure screening. Controls are on the tableside rail. Medical imaging, video from wall-mounted cameras and audio are transmitted to a nearby conference. Two-way communication allows the interventional radiologist to discuss the procedure with a conference participant (monitor inset), or advise the technologist in the control room which images to database for later incorporation into the medical record and section teaching files. Illustration courtesy of Clive Bilewitz © 1999 3D-BioFX.

FIGURE 5–2. Simulated paediatric interventional radiology suite II. The simulated procedure continues (from Fig. 1) as the radiologist prepares to advance the catheter into the cecum under fluoroscopic guidance. Had a malpositioned cecum indicated the need for laparoscopic assistance from a surgical colleague, construction of the room to OR standards facilitates combined procedures. An interventional CT with fluoroscopic capability is currently parked against the left wall, but can be brought to the patient on rails as needed. Illustration courtesy of Clive Bilewitz © 1999 3D-BioFX.

and contrast reactions have been rare under this policy, as suggested by numerous reports (Bush and Swanson, 1991; Rubin and Cohan, 1991; Cohen and Smith, 1994). Although barium suspensions are helpful in outlining the colon prior to enterostomy tube insertion, they otherwise have limited use in pediatric interventions and are specifically avoided if there is any risk of peritoneal spill, extravasation

TABLE 5–8. Comparative Evaluation of Image Guidance Systems

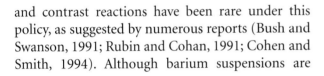

	Fluoroscopy	
	Advantages	*Disadvantages*
Fluoroscopy	Availability Rapid localization Needle tip easily visualized Real time	Poor tissue differentiation Ionizing radiation Not portable No quantitative depth measurement
Ultrasonography	Rapid localization Rapid multiplanar imaging No ionizing radiation Portable Real time	Needle difficult to visualize Limited anatomic information Obscured by gas or bone More technically demanding
Computed Tomography	Needle tip easily seen Fine anatomic detail No interference from overlying viscus or gas CT fluoroscopy allows real-time imaging	Expensive Ionizing radiation Not portable Longer procedure time

into soft tissues, or tracheal aspiration (Dodds, Stewart, et al., 1982; Foley, Ghahremani, et al., 1982; Cohen 1987, 1990). We frequently use air as a contrast medium in viscus organs. Many new contrast agents have recently been introduced, such as Levovist microbubbles (Berlex) in contrast-enhanced harmonic US, dysprosium and catheter-mounted coils in MR tracking and profiling, and carbon dioxide in fluoroscopic imaging. By and large, these have not yet come into common use for guidance of pediatric procedures.

ENTEROSTOMY ACCESS

Gastrostomy Catheter Insertion

Many specialists, including surgeons, gastroenterologists, and interventional radiologists, insert gastrostomy catheters. There are four basic approaches to gastrostomy tube insertion: (1) open surgical placement (Cunha, 1946), (2) laparoscopic guidance (Edelman, Unger, et al., 1991; Lee, Chao, et al., 1993; Raaf, Manney, et al., 1993; Sangster and Swanstrom, 1993), (3) percutaneous placement by endoscopic guidance (PEG) (Gauderer, Ponsky, et al., 1980), and (4) retrograde (King, Chait, et al., 1993; Chait, Weinberg, et al., 1996) or antegrade (Keller, Lai, et al., 1986; Towbin, Ball, et al., 1988) percutaneous placement under fluoroscopic guidance (Towbin, Ball, et al., 1988; Sanchez, vanSonnenberg, et al., 1992; Chait, Weinberg, et al., 1996; Bleck, Reiss, et al., 1998). The choice of technique depends on the availability of expertise and on the referral pattern. Open surgical gastrostomy is performed in our institution only when a patient is undergoing a simultaneous surgical procedure. For example, a patient undergoing tracheoesophageal fistula (TEF) repair might have an open gastrostomy done at the same time. Even in these cases, percutaneous gastrostomy is often performed by an interventional radiologist under image guidance in the operating room at the same time or just before the TEF is repaired.

Gastroenterologists oversee enterostomy services in many institutions and often elect PEG placement, a procedure first described by Gauderer and Ponsky in 1980 (Gauderer, Ponsky, et al., 1980). The procedure involves percutaneously puncturing the gastric and anterior abdominal walls with a needle guided by the light of an endoscope that has been advanced transorally into the stomach. A wire is snared, and a tapered gastrostomy tube is advanced through the mouth over the wire and out through the gastric and anterior abdominal walls.

The retrograde technique, described in detail below, can be performed on patients with esophageal stricture, tracheoesophageal fistula, or esophageal atresia, as well as on patients with oropharyngeal abnormalities and on very small patients. This technique is more versatile, allowing easier catheter exchange, removal, or conversion to gastrojejunostomy (Table 5–9). A similar antegrade percutaneous gastrostomy was described as an image-guided technique (Towbin, Ball, et al., 1988). In this approach, a needle is introduced percutaneously under fluoroscopic guidance after inflation of the stomach with air through a nasogastric tube. The wire is captured with a "gooseneck" snare introduced transorally in a manner similar to the PEG technique. Compared to the retrograde insertion technique, antegrade catheter placement offers the advantage of primary placement of a larger-bore catheter with a substantially lower rate of accidental dislodgment (Towbin, Ball, et al., 1988; Galat, Gerig, et al., 1990). This is achieved at the cost of substantially greater difficulty removing the catheter and its associated fixation device or bumper, which frequently must be removed either endoscopically or with a snare or basket (Coventry, Karatassas, et al., 1994; Mollitt, Dokler, et al., 1998). A variant of this technique has recently been described (Szymski, Albazzaz, et al., 1997; Clark, Pugash, et al., 1999). After percutaneous puncture under fluoroscopic guidance, a catheter and wire are guided up the esophagus and exteriorized through the mouth. The procedure is completed as in the PEG procedure previously described.

In the pediatric setting, the most common indication for gastrostomy tube insertion is failure to thrive (Table 5–10). This may result from a number of conditions, with cerebral palsy and neurologic impairment being the most common (Towbin, Ball, et al., 1988; Stuart, Tiley, et al., 1993; CPS, 1994; Steinkamp and von der Hardt, 1994; Chait, Weinberg, et al., 1996). With increasing complexity and acuity of care and with improved rates of survival of severe metabolic and generalized illnesses as well as liver, kidney, and bone marrow transplantation, there is an everincreasing number of patients who require long-term nutritional supplementation (Sant, Gilvarry, et al., 1993; 1994; Boyd and Beeken, 1994; Ganga, Ryan, et al., 1994; Steinkamp and von der Hardt, 1994; Israel and Hassall, 1995). Occasionally, gastrostomies are

TABLE 5–9. Relative Merits of Antegrade and Retrograde Gastrostomy Techniques

	Antegrade	*Retrograde*
Advantages	Primary insertion of large-bore catheter Low risk of accidental dislodgment	Possible in patients with esophageal atresia or stricture Can be removed or exchanged easily on an outpatient basis
Disadvantages	Risk of upper airway or esophageal trauma during insertion Increased risk of procedure-related pneumonia and exit-site infection Increased risk of injury to colon or liver (PEG technique)	Increased risk of dislodgment Requires multiple procedures to achieve large-bore catheter

PEG, percutaneous endoscopic guidance

used for gastric decompression or drainage (Stellato and Gauderer, 1987; Pricolo, Vittimberga, et al., 1989).

There are few contraindications to gastrostomy tube insertion. Abdominal masses, loops of intervening bowel, hepatomegaly, splenomegaly, or severe scoliosis may not allow a safe route of access to the stomach (Bell, Carmody, et al., 1995). If maneuvers designed to overcome the obstacles (see Method, under Gastrostomy Tube Insertion, below) are unsuccessful, the procedure can be deferred until a later date, allowing the dilated loop of bowel to collapse. Coagulopathies and bleeding abnormalities should be corrected before gastrostomy placement. Cardiorespiratory abnormalities may represent a contraindication to elective deep sedation or general anesthesia but the procedure can usually be safely completed with local anesthesia assisted by minimal intravenous sedation or judicious use of inhalational agents through a mask. Esophageal

TABLE 5–10. Common Indications for Enteral Tube Feeding

Failure to thrive

Anorexia associated with chronic illness (e.g., cystic fibrosis)

Chewing and swallowing disorders

Coma

Metabolic stress (e.g., trauma, burns, storage diseases)

Inflammatory bowel disease (e.g., Crohn's disease)

Neurodevelopmental handicaps (e.g., cerebral palsy)

Prematurity

Short gut

abnormalities, including stricture, stenosis, or the rare malignancy, should not be considered contraindications to gastrostomy placement as the stomach can be distended by air delivered through a needle placed percutaneously under US guidance (Figure 5–3). We do not regard the presence of a ventriculoperitoneal (VP) shunt a contraindication to the placement of any enterostomy tube since a site away from the VP shunt may usually be selected for access. In our experience, the rate of shunt infection in this population is not affected by gastrostomy tube placement (Sane, Towbin, et al., 1998). Patients with ascites (Lee, Saini, et al., 1991; McFarland, Lee, et al., 1995; Ryan, Hahn, et al., 1998), those receiving peritoneal dialysis (Geary and Chait, 1996), and patients with Crohn's disease (Cosgrove and Jenkins, 1997; Mahajan, Oliva, et al., 1997) may also safely receive enterostomy catheters. However, dialysate or ascitic fluid should be drained prior to the procedure.

The size of the catheter selected for primary gastrostomy insertion is usually based on the patient's weight. In children up to 10 kg, an 8.5 French catheter is used. In children from 10 to 30 kg, a 10 French catheter is used, and for patients over approximately 30 kg, a 12 French catheter is chosen. We currently use a 15-cm Dawson Mueller Mac-lock ultrathane catheter.

Materials required for the procedure include the following (Figure 5–4):

• A sharps container and needle counter
• EMLA topical anesthetic patch (AstraZeneca)
• Chlorhexidine gluconate 0.5% solution with 70%

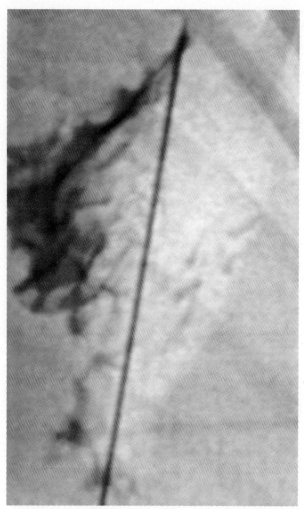

FIGURE 5–3. Transabdominal Gastric Insufflation. Using fluoroscopic guidance, a thin needle was introduced to inflate the stomach of this patient with esophageal atresia.

- Lubricating jelly (bacteriostatic Muko® [Ingram and Bell])
- Methylmethacrylate glue
- Gauze bandage (2 x 2)
- Antibiotic ointment (Polyderm [bacitracin zinc + polymyxin B sulfate] [Taro]
- Nasogastric tube (at least 10 French)
- Drainage bags (Holister U bag)
- Mefix adhesive bandage (Hypafix Dressing Retention Sheet [Smith and Nephew])
- K-lock adhesive catheter retention device

Outpatients are admitted the day of the procedure. An appropriate level of sedation or anesthesia is planned at the time the procedure is scheduled or in the pre-procedure teaching clinic. Most patients are sedated for this procedure according to protocol (see Sedation, Analgesia, and Anesthesia, above). Informed consent and assent are obtained by the interventional radiologist for the procedure and by the registered nurse or anesthesiologist providing sedation. Intravenous access is assured, and the patient is well hydrated, beginning the previous night for inpatients and on arrival for outpatients. An EMLA patch is placed on the skin over the left margin of the rectus abdominus muscle, centered approximately 2 cm below the costal margin, at least 2 hours prior to the planned procedure. Cefazolin (40 mg per kg) is given intravenously as a single dose just prior to the procedure.

Percutaneous Retrograde

InsertionRetrograde gastrostomy tube insertion is performed with the patient supine, preferably on a

isopropyl alcohol (Soluprep [tinted], Solumed, Inc.)
- Local anesthetic (1% lidocaine)
- #11 scalpel blade
- Syringes and needles, including a 27-Gauge 1.5-inch needle for administration of local anesthetic
- 18-Gauge single-wall puncture needle
- Slip ring extension set
- Low-osmolar contrast (Omnipaque (iohexol) 300 mg per mL [Nycomed])
- Pediatric gastrointestinal suture anchor set
- 70-cm non-Teflon-coated 0.035-inch guidewire (Reimer, Farres, et al., 1996)
- Dawson Mueller Mac-lock ultrathane catheter (15 cm, 8.5 to 12 French) (Cook, Inc.)
- Coons dilator (8, 10, or 12 French as appropriate)

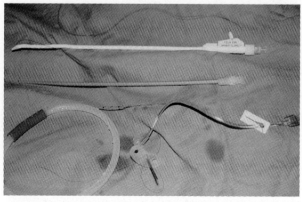

FIGURE 5–4. Equipment for percutaneous gastrostomy includes a single wall puncture needle, retention sutures, wire, dilator and Dawson Mueller catheter.

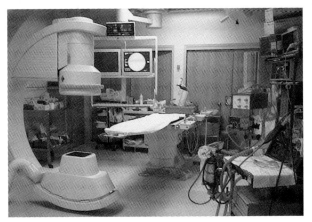

FIGURE 5–5. The interventional suite includes a digital fluoroscopic C-tube and on site anaesthesia equipment.

tilting procedure table, with a digital fluoroscopic C-arm (Figure 5–5). The costal margin is palpated, and the limits of the liver and spleen as well as any masses, pathology, or unusual anatomy that might interfere with safe completion of the procedure are identified and marked under US (Figure 5–6). Fluoroscopy is used to identify the transverse colon. A barium enema is performed with dilute barium if necessary (Figure 5–7). A nasogastric tube, at least 10 French if possible, is positioned under fluoroscopic control with the tip in the gastric lumen.

The skin of the epigastrium is prepared and draped in a sterile fashion, using Soluprep solution

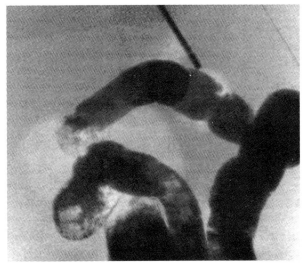

FIGURE 5–7. The transverse colon is filled with dilute barium and an NG tube is placed.

or a similar preparation (Figure 5–8). The preferred entry point for percutaneous gastric puncture is usually just lateral to the left margin of the rectus abdominus muscle, approximately 2 cm inferior to the costal margin. Development of a tract closer to the costal margin or through the body of the rectus muscle often leads to impingement and pain, especially for the ambulatory patient. Additionally, a margin of at least 2 cm should be left between the primary gastrostomy tube tract and any other trans-

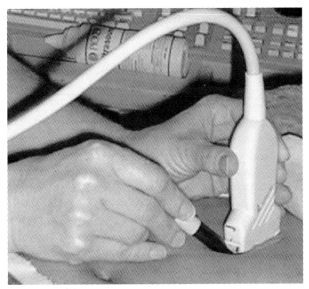

FIGURE 5–6. The edges of liver and spleen are marked using US guidance. This helps avoid inadvertent puncture during gastrostomy.

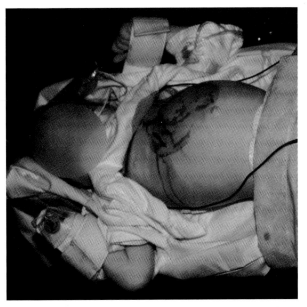

FIGURE 5–8. Patient in position with papoose and leg binder. The abdomen has been prepared with SoluPrep.

gastric catheters or percutaneous tubes (such as a pre-existing gastrojejunostomy tube) to avoid skin breakdown. The prospective entry site and needle tract are evaluated under fluoroscopic control with the tip of a forceps to assure that the tract will safely avoid transverse colon as well as the previously marked margins of liver and spleen. Glucagon is then administered intravenously (0.3 to 0.5 mg) to relax the stomach and small bowel and to keep the pyloric sphincter effectively closed to the passage of air.

The stomach is inflated via the nasogastric tube with boluses of air from a 60-cc syringe under fluoroscopic guidance until it appears full and tense (Figure 5–9). The final position for percutaneous puncture is selected with the tip of a sterile forceps. Frequently, the optimum window for development of a gastrostomy tube tract is quite narrow, between the costal, hepatic, splenic, and colonic margins previously described. Angling the C-arm and (as a last resort) tilting the table may be required to improve the window to a satisfactory level of safety. Even more complex angles may be needed to avoid vital structures in patients with severe scoliosis. If dilated colonic or small bowel loops intervene between the stomach and abdominal wall, they may be decompressed through a thin (27-Gauge) needle introduced percutaneously under fluoroscopic guidance (see Percutaneous Decompression of Intervening Bowel, below). Simultaneous endoscopic control has been helpful in a case of a patient with large gastric varices.

The skin at the puncture site is anesthetized by local infiltration of 1% lidocaine solution (to a maxi-

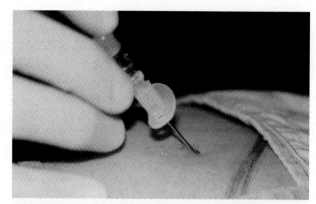

FIGURE 5–10. Needle in position ready for gastric puncture. This is performed with a sharp jabbing motion avoiding the posterior wall. Note the insertion site is well away from the marked costal margin.

mum of 0.5 cc per kg) through a 27-Gauge needle. Observation under fluoroscopy can help confirm a safe route of access to the stomach. A small skin nick is made with a #11 scalpel blade at the site for puncture. An 18-Gauge single-wall needle is preloaded with a pediatric retention suture. This is connected to a non-Luer-Lok T-connector attached to a 5-cc syringe filled with contrast.

Under fluoroscopic guidance, the stomach is punctured with a single thrusting motion (Figure 5–10). Care should be taken to avoid traversing the posterior wall. Contrast is injected to confirm the position of the needle (Figure 5–11). If there is any question whether the needle tip is within the lumen of the stomach, additional imaging should be per-

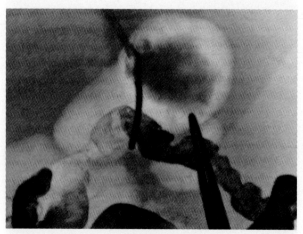

FIGURE 5–9. The stomach is distended with air and the prospective insertion site checked to assure safe access to the stomach.

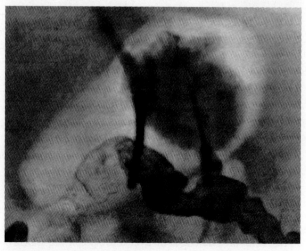

FIGURE 5–11. Intragastric location of the needle is confirmed with contrast injection.

formed in the lateral or oblique planes. The T-connector is removed without dislodging the retention suture, and a 0.035-inch straight guide wire is passed through the needle into the gastric lumen (Dewald, Hiette, et al., 1999, Moote, 1991). As the wire passes through the needle tip, it deploys the retention suture, which is visualized entering the stomach under fluoroscopy. The needle is then removed over the wire, and the retention suture is gently pulled up to the anterior abdominal wall and clamped with a forceps.

Maintaining gentle tension on the retention suture, a single dilatation is performed with the appropriately sized Coons dilator. The tips of the dilator and catheter should be lubricated with sterile jelly prior to insertion. To avoid pulling the retention suture through the gastric wall or losing the newly developed tract, dilatation is accomplished by rotating the tip of the dilator and pushing on the dilator rather than pulling on the retention suture. The dilator is exchanged over the wire for the appropriately sized gastrostomy catheter, which is passed into the stomach using the same "push-rather-than-pull" technique. The loop on the Mac-lock catheter is closed, and the locking device is fixed with a drop of methylmethacrylate glue (Figure 5–12). The retention suture is wrapped around a small piece of gauze and pulled up gently to appose the gastric and abdominal walls. A 2 x 2 gauze with antibiotic ointment is used to dress the catheter exit site (Figure 5–13), and this is all covered with a Mefix dressing. A K-lock device is used to secure the catheter to the skin. A feeding adapter is attached to the catheter,

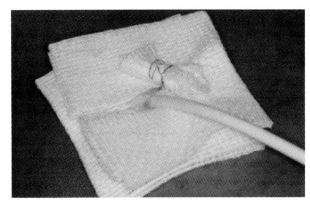

FIGURE 5–13. Bandages and antibiotic ointment are placed around the G tube. The retention suture is fastened around a gauze roll.

which is then left open to drain into a drainage bag (Figure 5–14).

Postprocedure Care

(See Postprocedure Management, above.) Postgastrostomy orders should specify that the nasogastric tube and gastrostomy tube be left open to drainage for 12 hours if active bowel sounds have resumed. Analgesia is provided in the form of intravenous morphine sulfate (0.05 mg per kg each 4 hours for 24 hours), followed by oral acetaminophen (15 mg per kg every 3 to 4 hours as needed). The patient should be observed on a regular basis for evidence of pain, infection, ileus, or obstruction. Enteral nutrition is usually started at least 12 hours following the procedure, after bowel sounds have resumed. We begin

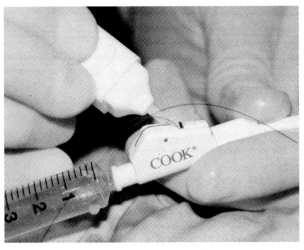

FIGURE 5–12. The locking string of the catheter is glued in place for additional protection.

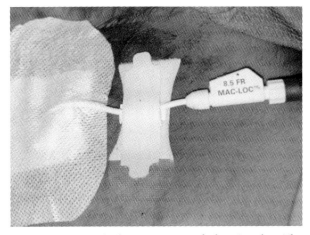

FIGURE 5–14. Final appearance of the G tube. The insertion site is covered with Mefix and further anchoring is provided by a K-lock.

with small amounts (5 cc) of clear fluids, advancing to half-strength then full-strength enteral solutions as tolerated. The patient is usually discharged 2 days after the procedure. The patient and parents are given a troubleshooting guide with recommended solutions to common problems explained in simple language. Round-the-clock contact information for routine and urgent calls is provided. For any tube-related problem, patients and parents are explicitly instructed to contact interventional radiology directly rather than the emergency department. For questions related to feeding or feeding solutions, they are directed to the enterostomy service nursing personnel, the clinical nutrition physicians, or the gastroenterologists, as appropriate.

Two weeks following the procedure, the retention suture is cut at the skin surface by the parents or primary caregiver at home. In our experience, no complications have resulted from either passage of the anchor suture or retention of the anchor suture in the gastric wall (Ho and Margulies, 1999). At this point, the dressings may be removed although some parents find a small dressing helps prevent the catheter from being accidentally caught and dislodged. We usually see these children as outpatients 6 weeks following the primary insertion procedure. If they are over 1 year of age, we exchange the catheter for a balloon-type G-tube. This allows sub-

sequent catheter changes to be performed at the patient's home or by a caregiver.

Results and Complications

Since 1991, we have performed over 1300 primary G-tube insertions on patients weighing from 800 g (27 weeks' gestation) to 80 kg. Postprocedure complications related to insertion of the gastrostomy catheter are uncommon and usually mild although severe complications may rarely be seen (Halkier, Ho, et al., 1989; Ciaccia, Quigley, et al., 1994; Chait, Weinberg, et al., 1996; Pien, Hume, et al., 1996; Ramage and Balfe, 1998; Ramage, Harvey, et al., 1999). The infection rate (Towbin, Ball, et al., 1988; Chait, Weinberg, et al., 1996; Pien, Hume, et al., 1996; Sane, Towbin, et al., 1998) after initial placement is extremely low, with local peritonism seen in several patients. In one patient with a VP shunt, a shunt-related infection developed 1 month after placement of the tube. There is a low incidence of skin surface infection, ranging from redness and irritation to local abscess formation. One neonate had significant postprocedure bleeding (Rose, Wolman, et al., 1986; Weiss, Fradkin, et al., 1999) due to gastritis that resolved with supportive care. Another patient developed peritonitis while being fed through a G-tube positioned outside the stomach (Figure 5–15) [Gray, 1987]. A patient whose bowel has been transfixed

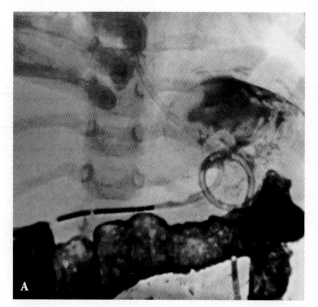 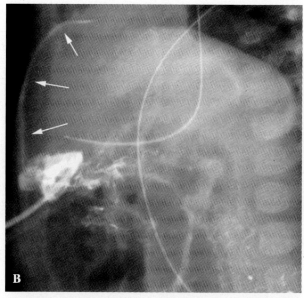

FIGURE 5–15. Extragastric G tube. *A,* AP image demonstrates the G tube overlying the stomach with contrast apparently pooling in the gastric fundus. A lateral view would have demonstrated the extragastric location of the tube and contrast. *B,* Lateral film from a subsequent tube study shows contrast outlining bowel loops and liver (*arrows*).

during placement of the enterostomy catheter may remain asymptomatic or may have discomfort, bilious vomiting, or other evidence of obstruction. In one such patient whose small bowel was traversed during the procedure (confirmed with CT), surgical intervention was needed to reposition the tube and close the hole in the small bowel. Erosions or ulcerations from the catheter itself are occasionally seen. One patient experienced erosion of the catheter with migration into the adjacent colon; the catheter required removal and re-insertion at a new site. Another child, whose Cope loop catheter migrated into the duodenum, developed perforation and subsequent peritonitis; such events are rare. The tissues may be extremely fragile in the neonatal patient, and care should be taken to avoid tearing of tissues. Pneumoperitoneum is frequently seen postoperatively with little clinical significance (Wojtowycz, Arata, et al., 1988). However, one patient with tracheoesophageal fistula developed tension pneumoperitoneum due to positive pressure ventilation. This was successfully aspirated percutaneously (Figure 5–16). Bilious vomiting and discomfort commonly accompany migration of the catheter into the duodenum (Hopens and Schwesinger, 1983; Huff, Rosenblum, et al., 1988; Ciaccia, Quigley, et al., 1994) and are relieved with repositioning or replacement of the catheter. We demonstrate to patients and parents at the conclusion of the procedure the length of catheter that should be seen externally, and we advise them to contact us if the catheter appears malpositioned or if the patient becomes symptomatic.

Continuing Care

As most of these patients require long-term enteral supplementation, they represent a cumulative population that requires long-term follow-up. Many of these patients progress to a low-profile type of catheter such as the Bard button or the MICC key devices (Figure 5–17) (Faller and Lawrence, 1993; Haas-Beckert and Heyman, 1993; Borge, Vesely, et al., 1995). These are placed electively as an outpatient procedure. At times, patients have gastrostomy tubes placed on a trial basis to determine whether they can tolerate bolus gastric feeding. Patients who aspirate into the tracheobronchial tree and have significant reflux may need to be converted to a gastrojejunostomy tube (McHugh, 1997). This is also performed as an outpatient elective procedure, after the gastrocutaneous tract has matured.

The G-tube is occasionally exchanged for a tube of larger diameter or is replaced because it leaks, becomes obstructed, or otherwise malfunctions (Lipscomb, Brown, et al., 1994; Vautier and Scott, 1994). The Mac-lock gastrostomy catheter is simply cut several centimeters from the skin surface to release the locking suture and exchanged over a 70-cm 0.035-inch guide wire. It is always preferable

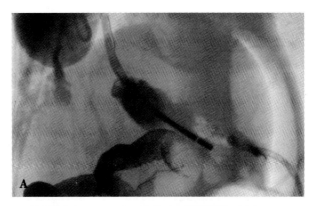
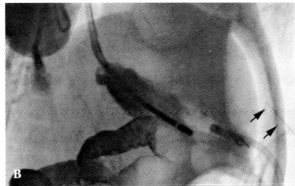
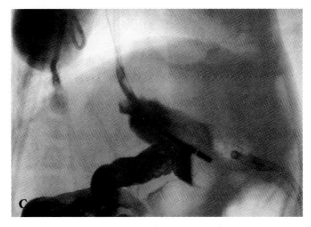

FIGURE 5–16. Pneumoperitoneum Aspiration. *A,* Lateral film shows a large pneumoperitoneum after G tube insertion. *B,* Air aspirated through needle (*arrows*) introduced into the peritoneum under fluoroscopic guidance. *C,* Appearance after successful aspiration.

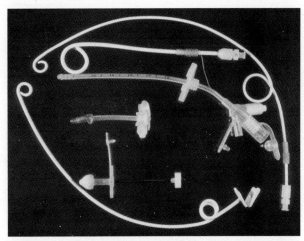

FIGURE 5–17. Numerous G and GJ tubes are available.

to change this catheter over a wire under fluoroscopic control to assure that access to the stomach is not lost. In the event the tube is completely obstructed, the wire may be introduced through the tract by gently probing alongside the catheter. Similarly, if the G-tube is accidentally dislodged, gentle probing with the soft tip of the wire may allow reaccess to the gastric lumen. In such cases, the position of the catheter within the stomach must be confirmed in at least two planes with a small amount of contrast as there is a substantial risk with intraperitoneal malposition of the tube.

Gastrojejunostomy Tube Insertion

As part of the pre-procedure evaluation for enterostomy insertion, patients are assessed for gastroesophageal reflux, tracheal aspiration, and gastric emptying. Children identified with significant abnormalities that contraindicate gastric feeding may be candidates for primary gastrojejunostomy (GJ) tube placement (Ho, 1983; Ho and Yeung, 1992). Since the introduction of this procedure, fundoplication procedures have no longer often been performed at our institution.

Materials

The size of catheter for primary gastrojejunostomy insertion is usually based on the patient's weight. In children weighing up to 10 kg, an 8.5 French gastrojejunostomy catheter is used. The same tube can be used in larger children, or for children 10 to 30 kg, a 10 French catheter can be used. For patients over approximately 30 kg, a 12 French catheter may be chosen. We use a 45-cm pediatric gastrojejunostomy

ultrathane catheter. However, for infants under 2 to 3 kg, we have found the pediatric or neonatal Carey-Alzate gastrojejunostomy tube most effective (Figure 5–18). Additional materials for this procedure are identical to those required for gastrostomy tube insertion, with the following exception: a longer 0.035-inch Benston wire (145 cm) is used to advance a 4 or 5 French catheter (JB-1 [Meditech]) past the ligament of Treitz.

Method

Primary gastrojejunostomy tube insertion is very similar to the retrograde insertion of a gastrostomy tube, described above. Intravenous glucagon administration can be deferred in most cases as peristalsis may ease initial placement of the catheter. However, if air is observed to traverse the pylorus during insufflation of the stomach prior to puncture, further attempts at inflation should be delayed, and glucagon should be administered. Percutaneous puncture is performed with an 18-Gauge single-wall needle loaded with a retention suture. After the initial puncture, the guide wire is advanced into the gastric lumen through the needle. The needle is exchanged over the wire for the catheter. Gentle tension is maintained on the retention suture held by a small mosquito clamp. The pylorus can usually be found posterosuperiorly, superior to the antrum and to the right of the spine. A small amount of contrast instilled through the catheter in this region will often outline the pylorus and proximal duodenum. Using fluoroscopy with contrast injection and

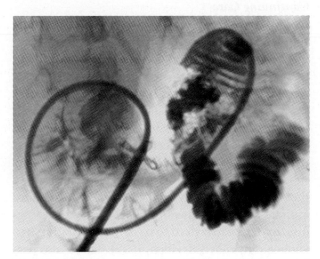

FIGURE 5–18. Carey-Alzate tubes are used in small neonates.

manipulation, the guide wire leads the catheter through the pylorus, around the duodenal loop, and into the jejunum. Leaving the wire in this position, the catheter is exchanged first for a Coons dilator, then for an 8, 10, or 12 French GJ tube. The stiffener tip should be parked in the pylorus, and the tube should be pushed off the stiffener until the catheter tip is well across the ligament of Treitz. The stiffener should then be redirected toward the fundus, and the proximal portion of the catheter, containing the Cope loop, is advanced into the stomach. The stiffener is removed, the intragastric Cope loop formed and locked, and the appropriate position and function is confirmed with a small amount of contrast in at least two imaging planes (Figure 5–19).

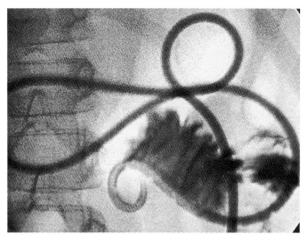

FIGURE 5–19. Chait GJ tube in normal positon. No contrast should leak into the stomach from the gastric loop.

Postprocedure Care

The postprocedure orders for these patients are similar except that the GJ tube is capped at the time of placement and is not left to drainage. A nasogastric tube is left to decompress the stomach until bowel sounds return. Unlike gastric feeding, nutrition through the GJ tube must be delivered as a constant infusion rather than periodic boluses. Under the direction of the nutrition team, tube feeding is slowly increased until an appropriate amount of calories is delivered.

Results

Gastrojejunostomy placement is more difficult than a simple gastrostomy. There are occasions in which placement of a gastrojejunostomy is not possible. Prior to the procedure, we explain to the patients and parents that a G-tube may be placed temporarily until a gastrojejunostomy tube can be safely and successfully navigated into position. This exchange is usually performed at approximately 3 to 5 days following the primary placement. At this time, the retention suture is still in place, and the tract has not yet matured, so due care must be taken to avoid losing the newly formed tract. This exchange is performed under sedation if necessary.

Complications

In addition to the complications mentioned in regard to gastrostomy insertion, long-term gastrojejunostomy catheter complications arise mainly from the fact that a longer catheter is used to feed the patient, and catheter blockages, breakages and replacements are more frequent. The introduction

of crushed tablets into catheters often results in clogging and requires a change of catheters. Leaking of feeding solutions through the intragastric Cope loop is seen and is usually due to the suture cutting through the catheter wall, as can occur following partial dislodgment. We have seen intermittent intussusception of the small bowel around the distal coil of the catheter in 12% of gastrojejunostomy recipients (Connolly, Chait, et al., 1998; Hughes, 1999), primarily in younger children (Figure 5–20). We have also seen several cases where "telescoping" small bowel gathers over the catheter (Figure 5–21). Both groups of children often present with bilious

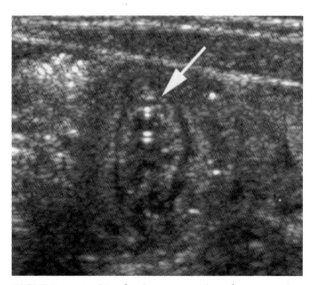

FIGURE 5–20. GJ tube intussusception demonstrating target appearance on ultrasound. Note the echogenic tube centrally (*arrow*).

vomiting and discomfort and may require replacement of the GJ catheter with a shortened GJ catheter from which the distal coil has been removed (see Figure 5–21). Just as with gastrostomy catheters, serious complications are possible but rare.

Continuing Care

GJ tubes are not changed at specific intervals. Patients are informed that if blockage occurs, they should attempt to unblock the catheter with forceful injection of soda water. If there are continued nonemergent problems, the patients or caregivers are directed to telephone the representative of the enterostomy access service (EAS) on call and are seen at the earliest available time. Vomiting of formula suggests an intragastric leak at the Cope loop, and vomiting of bile suggests intermittent intussusception; both require exchange of the catheter as described above.

Percutaneous Cecostomy Insertion

The number of young and old people with fecal soiling or loss of bowel control is quite large (Bishop

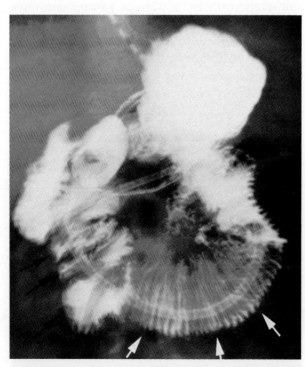

FIGURE 5–21. GJ tube intussusception demonstrating coiled spring appearance (*white arrows*). The gathered appearance of the bowel (*black arrows*) has been described as "telescoping." The coil has been removed fromr the distal end of the catheter.

and Nowicki, 1999). Spina bifida, the most common underlying disorder in children with fecal incontinence, occurs in about 1 out of 1000 births. Patients with other underlying diagnoses such as imperforate anus, cloacal abnormalities, sacral agenesis, paraplegia, and cerebral palsy may also be at risk for fecal soiling (Tagart, 1966; Langemeijer and Molenaar, 1991; Miglioli, 1991; Madoff, Williams, et al., 1992; Paidas, 1997; Bishop and Nowicki, 1999). There may be as many as 3 million people with poor bowel control in North America.

Bowel control depends on a normal internal sphincter, a normal external sphincter, sensation, peristalsis, a normal anorectal angle, psychosocial factors, and the absence of scarring. Normally, stool enters the rectum and results in relaxation of the internal anal sphincter. This is independent of the central nervous system. Voluntary contraction of the external sphincter is needed to contain flatus or feces. When any component of this system fails or is not normally developed, the result may be "fecal incontinence," or the inability to control bowel function. Treatment of fecal incontinence may include spontaneous defecation, dietary modification, laxatives, manual expression, disimpaction, bowel training, biofeedback, suppositories, electrostimulation, and large-volume enemas delivered via a special rectal balloon catheter (Bartolo, 1991; Younoszai, 1992; Keck, Staniunas, et al., 1994; Berquist, 1995; Lestar, Kiss, et al. 1998).

Antegrade colonic enemas (Sheldon, Minevich, et al., 1997) have been described as a surgical procedure where the appendix is used to form a cutaneous cecostomy for fluid irrigation (Malone, Antegrade Colonic Enema [MACE]) (Malone, Ransley, et al., 1990; Ellsworth, Webb, et al., 1996; Malone, Curry, et al., 1998; Wilcox and Kiely, 1998). Transcolonoscopic extraperitoneal cecostomies have also been described (Ganc, Netto, et al., 1988). A percutaneous approach to the placement of a cecostomy catheter was described for colonic decompression in adults (Casola, Withers, et al., 1986) and was adapted for the introduction of antegrade enemas in pediatric fecal incontinence by Chait and Shandling (Ramamurthy, 1996; Shandling, Chait, et al., 1996; Chait, Shandling, et al., 1997b; Towbin, 1997). We have had experience with 128 patients between June 1994 and August 1999.

Placement of the cecostomy tube involves two different procedures that take place about 6 weeks apart. In the first, a temporary cecostomy catheter (C-tube) is inserted into the patient's colon through the skin, usually in the lower right part of the abdomen. Approximately 6 weeks later, a more permanent tube is exchanged over the wire in a brief outpatient procedure. The C-tube insertion procedure is designed to allow a small-volume enema to be given through the tube to periodically clean out the colon. In this way, potentially embarrassing accidents are avoided, and the patient often gains freedom to pursue activities previously prevented by fear of incontinent episodes. The C-tube remains in the colon and provides a comfortable and convenient way to fully cleanse the bowel with an enema. Emptying the colon in this regular predictable way can prevent unexpected leakage. After their C-tube insertion, some patients are able to give themselves their own enemas for the first time. All of our patients have described almost complete resolution of their fecal incontinence, with few unexpected accidents.

Indications and Contraindications

A potential candidate for C-tube insertion may experience fecal incontinence with troublesome soiling or may not respond well to rectal enemas or may wear diapers (Chait, Shandling, et al., 1997b). Patients may not be candidates for C-tube insertion if they have had previous surgical procedures, coagulopathies, or known medical problems that unduly increase risk during the procedure or sedation. Although many of our patients are older, feedback from patients and parents indicates that the optimal time for primary placement is before the patient first attends school (age 4 to 6 years) (Temple, Chait, et al., 1999).

Materials

We normally place a 15-cm, 8.5 French Dawson Mueller Mac-lock catheter for primary C-tube insertion. We prepare a latex-free tray for patients predisposed to latex allergy (e.g., spina bifida) as well as for those with known latex sensitivity (Moneret-Vautrin, Beaudouin, et al., 1993; Cantani, 1999). Additional materials (Figure 5–22) required for the procedure include the following:

- *Nonlatex* gloves
- EMLA topical anesthetic patch (AstraZeneca)
- Chlorhexidine gluconate 0.5% solution with 70% isopropyl alcohol (Soluprep [tinted], Solumed, Inc.)

- A sharps container and needle counter
- #11 scalpel blade
- Local anesthetic (1% lidocaine)
- Syringes
- 18-Gauge, 1.5-inch needle to draw local anesthetic
- 27-Gauge, 1.25-inch needle for local anesthetic infiltration
- Glucagon
- Low-osmolar contrast (Omnipaque [iohexol] 300 mg I per mL [Nycomed])
- 22 French silicone (Nonlatex) Foley catheter
- 60-cc Luer-lok syringe (for inflation of the Foley catheter)
- Insufflation bulb
- 18-Gauge single-wall puncture needle
- Pediatric gastrointestinal suture anchor set
- Slip ring extension set, attached to a syringe filled with contrast.
- 125-cm Teflon-coated 0.035-inch Amplatz guide wire
- Small mosquito clamp
- Lubricating jelly (bacteriostatic Muko(r) [Ingram and Bell])
- 8 French Coons dilator
- 15-cm, 8.5 French Dawson Mueller Mac-lock (Nonlatex) catheter
- Antibiotic ointment (Polyderm [bacitracin zinc + polymyxin B sulfate]) [Taro])
- Gauze bandage (2 x 2)
- Mefix adhesive bandage (Hypafix Dressing Retention Sheet [Smith and Nephew])
- Drainage bag (Holister U bag)
- Methylmethacrylate glue
- K-lock adhesive catheter retention device

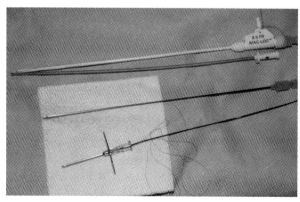

FIGURE 5–22. Cecostomy equipment includes a single wall puncture needle, wire, dilator and Dawson-Mueller catheter.

Preoperative Laboratory Studies and Pre-procedure Management

Most patients who have a C-tube placed are in good health except for their fecal incontinence. For this reason, we do not routinely order preoperative laboratory studies on this patient population. In select cases, in which the medical history is unknown or raises a suspicion of a bleeding diathesis, a coagulation profile, platelet count, and hemoglobin level are obtained. Because C-tube insertion is an elective procedure, an uncorrectable coagulopathy is an absolute contraindication.

Candidates for C-tube placement are maintained on a strict clear fluid diet for 2 days prior to the procedure to help assure a clean bowel preparation. Up to 45 mL of sodium phosphate oral solution (patient 4 to 6 years old, 10 mL; 7 to 9 years old, 20 mL; 10 years and older, 45 mL) is administered the night before the procedure (or per nasogastric [NG] tube for patients who cannot tolerate oral administration). The patient is admitted to the hospital on the morning of the procedure with a repeat dose of sodium phosphate as needed according to the results of pre-procedure abdominal radiography. Patients fasting for a procedure (see Sedation, Analgesia, and Anesthesia, above) should not become dehydrated, and orders for maintenance intravenous fluids should be part of the pre-procedure order regimen.

Two hours prior to the procedure, EMLA cream is applied topically to the prospective tube insertion site. A rectal dose of acetaminophen (15 mg per kg) is given 1 hour prior to the procedure. Patients are given a combination of gentamicin (2.5 mg per kg), ampicillin (50 mg per kg) and metronidazole (10 mg per kg) as a single pre-procedure dose. The same dosages are continued three times per day for several days following the procedure.

Technique and Alternatives

The cecostomy tube insertion procedure is performed on a tilting C-arm fluoroscopic interventional table. After US is performed to identify the liver, gallbladder, and urinary bladder, a 22 French silicone catheter is introduced into the rectum and the retention balloon is filled with a air from a 50-cc Luer-lok syringe. The abdomen is prepared and draped in sterile fashion using Soluprep solution. The sterile equipment and local anesthetic is prepared and is readily available prior to administra-

tion of glucagon. Up to 1 mg is given intravenously, and the colon is inflated with air via the rectal catheter. The position of the cecum is assessed, and the prospective tract site is determined.

Up to 0.5 cc per kg of 1% lidocaine should be infiltrated under fluoroscopic control into the skin and soft tissues down to the cecal wall, using a transperitoneal approach. One should see evidence of tenting of the cecal mucosa by the needle tip, and often a small bulge can be seen from deposition of anesthetic into the wall itself (Figure 5–23). After sufficient local anesthetic has been given, a small skin incision is made with a #11 scalpel. An 18-Gauge single-wall puncture needle, preloaded with two pediatric retention sutures is connected to a T-connector and a syringe filled with sterile water-soluble contrast. The needle is advanced through the skin and soft tissues until tenting of the cecal wall is again observed. Air should be insufflated as needed to maintain distention of the cecum. Under fluoroscopic guidance, the needle is rapidly advanced into the cecum with a single thrust. Contrast is then injected to confirm the position of the needle within the colon (Figure 5–24).

Under fluoroscopic control, a stiff 0.035-inch guide wire is advanced through the needle to deploy the retention sutures (Figure 5–25). The wire should

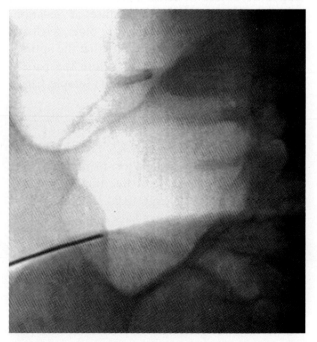

FIGURE 5–23. Bulging of the cecal wall is often seen with proper local anaesthetic administration.

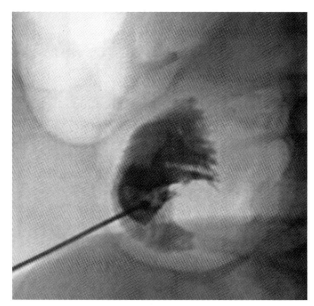

FIGURE 5–24. An intraluminal location of the needle is assured with contrast injection.

be advanced until the stiff portion is well within the lumen. The needle is then removed, and the two sutures are clamped with a mosquito forceps. Gentle tension on the sutures will appose the cecum against the anterior abdominal wall. An 8 French Coons dilator is introduced over the wire, maintain-

ing gentle tension on the retention sutures. This is followed by introduction of an 8.5 French Dawson Mueller Mac-lock 15-cm catheter. The catheter is locked, and its position within the cecum is confirmed in two planes with a small amount of contrast (Figure 5–26).

The locked "pigtail" of the catheter is pulled up against the anterior wall of the cecum, and the retention sutures are anchored to a small roll of gauze and fixed to the skin with adhesive tape. The skin at the tube exit site is dressed with a 2 x 2 gauze dressing and Polysporin antibiotic ointment and is covered with a Mefix dressing. The catheter is then left to drain to a drainage bag.

Postprocedure Care

Analgesia is provided in the form of intravenous morphine sulfate (0.05 mg per kg each 4 hours for 24 hours), followed by oral acetaminophen (15 mg/kg every 3–4 hours as needed). The patient is allowed to ambulate as tolerated. Clear fluids are initially given until the patient has normal bowel movements and bowel sounds. Gentamicin, ampicillin, and metronidazole are continued with the same dosages 3 times a day for 48 hours, and the metronidazole is then changed to an oral dose and given for a further 5 days.

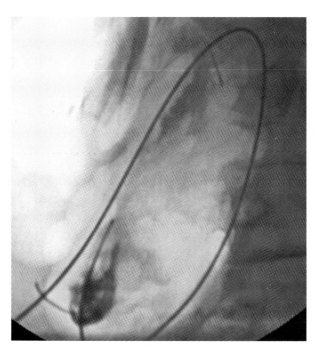

FIGURE 5–25. An Amplatz wire is introduced, displacing the retention sutures into the cecum.

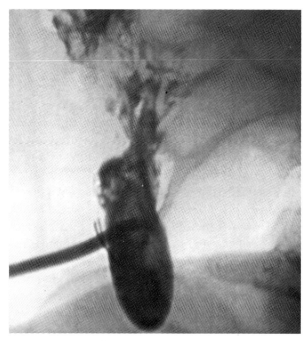

FIGURE 5–26. The cecostomy catheter loop is formed and the position reconfirmed with contrast injection.

The patient is usually discharged at 2 days post procedure, with orders to flush the catheter twice daily with 10 mL of saline. The pre-procedural rectal enema regime is continued for 9 days post procedure, at which time the antegrade enemas are begun. The retention sutures are cut at the skin by the parents 2 weeks following the procedure. The patients are provided with a contact list of physicians and nursing staff who will do any troubleshooting.

Variations

Occasionally, air introduced into the rectum does not fill the cecum. Placing the patient in the left-side-down or lateral decubitus position usually allows good filling of the cecum. Rotation of the C-arm may be necessary to separate loops of bowel that overlie the cecum. We have had one patient whose procedure was delayed because of very distended sigmoid overlying the cecum. The procedure was repeated, the cecum was clearly separated from the sigmoid, and a successful procedure was performed. Ventriculoperitoneal shunts are avoided if possible although evidence indicates that the procedure is safe even in this patient group. Occasionally, the cecum is high and just below the ribs, and a more lateral and superior approach is used. It is important to examine the borders of the liver, spleen, and gallbladder with US if this situation is found. If the retention sutures break during the procedure, the suture is replaced prior to further dilatation. Safe access obstructed by dilated loops of bowel may be improved by percutaneous needle decompression.

Results

Fecal incontinence is a difficult problem to treat. Most treatments have been unsatisfactory, unsuccessful, esthetically unappealing, or difficult for the child to administer without assistance. Administration of small-volume antegrade enemas via a percutaneously placed cecostomy is a safe and effective alternative for the treatment of fecal incontinence, with excellent patient response and acceptance and minimal complication, resulting in increased independence and mobility. In addition to the social benefits of alleviating incontinence, patients have reported decreased constipation, improved urinary bladder capacitance (with decompression of the colon and rectum), and decreased halitosis following insertion of their cecostomy tube.

Complications

We have successfully placed 128 cecostomy tubes since 1994. In the initial period, learning to use the tube effectively can be quite stressful for the patient and family. Two patients had their catheters removed due to emotional complications. The failure of antegrade enemas to alleviate incontinence in another patient was likely due to Hirschsprung's disease, and in retrospect, the procedure should not have been performed. Early complications include some pain at the site, which is successfully treated with oral analgesics. Several patients developed local tenderness and required intravenous antibiotics for a total of 5 days. We have seen no incidence of cellulitis (Maginot and Cascade, 1993) but have treated one patient for deep soft-tissue abscess by percutaneous drainage. Late complications seen in two patients were directly related to the volume of the phosphate enema; the dose was reduced, and the vomiting ceased. Following trauma to the exit site, one of our patients had a bleeding episode that resolved without any treatment. Several patients pulled the catheters out inadvertently. Temporary Foley catheters were placed by the parents at home. Later, the catheters were electively replaced with permanent catheters in the radiology suite. One patient was re-admitted for constipation; a high-fiber diet and stool softeners solved this problem. Granulation tissue has been seen fairly commonly; this is treated with a progression of saline soaks, hydrogen peroxide soaks, topical calcium carbonate, silver nitrate cauterization, and finally, surgical excision as indicated.

Continuing Care

At approximately 6 weeks post primary tube insertion, the tract has healed, and the catheter is exchanged for a Chait Trapdoor™ catheter (Figure 5–27) (Chait, Shandling, et al., 1997). This is an outpatient procedure that seldom needs sedation. No antibiotic coverage is given for this exchange. The position of the existing tube is checked, and once the new tube has been placed over a wire, the position of the trapdoor is confirmed with contrast. This device provides a low-profile catheter that is easily hidden under clothing or a small dressing, allowing the patient to lead a normal life (Figure 5–28). These catheters have been left in place for up to 3 years between changes but may become concreted and more difficult to remove over time. Our current technique for exchanging the trapdoor device is to clamp the catheter with forceps, cut off the trap-door, and introduce a wire into the catheter. The new catheter is then advanced over the wire, pushing the old catheter fragment into the cecum, where it passes in a few days.

Percutaneous Jejunostomy Insertion

Percutaneous jejunostomy has been performed occasionally as a primary procedure, as an alternative to gastrojejunostomy (Rosenblum, Taylor, et al. 1990; Hallisey and Pollard, 1994; Cope, Davis, et al., 1998). Indications for this procedure may include proximal stricture or obstruction of the duodenum (e.g., superior mesenteric artery syndrome) or other contraindications to permanent transgastric access. The difficulty in performing this procedure is reliably identifying and successfully puncturing a proximal loop of jejunum. This is, however, easier in a patient with a dilated segment of proximal jejunum. Placement of a nasojejunal catheter assists with identification of a jejunal loop. However, there is no functional sphincter that allows selective dilatation of the jejunum without decompression into the bowel distally.

Percutaneous Decompression of Intervening Bowel

If a distended loop of bowel is interposed anterior to the intended placement of an enterostomy catheter, air can be aspirated from the loop with a small (27-Gauge) needle. A small amount of contrast can then be injected into the offending loop to confirm that it has in fact deflated. This will allow for a clear route of access to the stomach, jejunum, or cecum.

Nasoduodenal and Nasojejunal Intubation

Nasoduodenal and nasojejunal catheters are primarily used for duodenal feeding, manometry, and pancreatic function tests. They may often be passed blindly on the ward, with position confirmed on the next chest radiograph. Difficult placements can be performed under image guidance. If a G-tube is present, it can be used to pass a gastroduodenal catheter more easily than the transnasal route. Initially, a directional catheter is placed over a wire to get into the proximal jejunum. The manometry catheter has multiple ports with a very small lumen, requiring either a 0.018- or 0.025-inch wire over which to introduce the catheter.

For nasojejunal catheter placement, a blind-

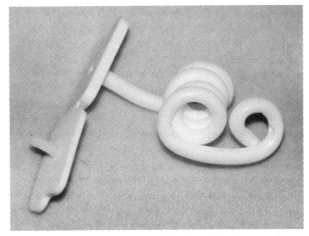

FIGURE 5–27. The low- profile Chait Trapdoor catheter forms a pigtail for internal retention.

ended silicone catheter with a stiffening wire may be advanced, sometimes with some difficulty, into the duodenum. Occasionally, one has to use a directional catheter with an exchange wire to traverse the duodenum and progress into the jejunum. This is then replaced with a cut nasojejunal tube such as a Frederick Miller feeding tube or even one of the silicone-type nasojejunal tubes.

PERCUTANEOUS BIOPSY

Image-guided percutaneous biopsy techniques (Sawhney, Berry, et al., 1987; Reading, Charboneau, et al., 1988; Gazelle and Haaga, 1989; Jaeger, MacFie, et al., 1990; Reddy, Gattuso, et al., 1991; Yeung 1992; Somers, Lomas, et al., 1993) have matured sufficiently to become the method of choice for obtaining diagnostic tissue specimens for pathologic

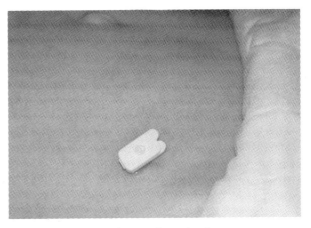

FIGURE 5–28. Trapdoor catheter in place.

analysis. At this time, biopsy procedures account for approximately 10% of all pediatric interventional procedures performed at our institution. These techniques have been especially useful in the abdomen and pelvis, improving tissue yield while decreasing morbidity and mortality. Increases in safety and effectiveness relate to improvements in three areas: image guidance modalities, biopsy needle technology, and pathologic technique.

Image Guidance

The following recommendations are useful in choosing the appropriate modality for a given biopsy procedure:

- Assure a safe window of access to the target lesion that avoids transgressing important vascular structures or organs where possible.
- Choose a route of access that avoids transgression (and possible contamination) of more than one anatomic compartment when malignancy or infection is suspected.
- Maximize visualization of the target lesion with respect to surrounding tissues, organs, and structures.
- Minimize exposure to radiation and contrast agents
- Obtain reliable documentation that the biopsy specimen was acquired from the target lesion.

The final choice of imaging modality will depend upon a variety of additional factors, including the size and location of the lesion and the experience and preference of the interventionist. The complementary use of multiple imaging modalities in the same procedure has already been helpful in the select cases described in this chapter. Multiple modalities will be of increasing use as development of interactive integrated multimodality systems continues, as illustrated by intraoperative probe tracking and dynamic image mapping onto preoperative volumetric imaging in image-guided neurosurgical procedures (Peters, Henri, et al., 1994; Comeau, Fenster, et al., 1998; St-Jean, Sadikot, et al., 1998).

Fluoroscopy generally has little use in percutaneous abdominopelvic biopsies, due to poor tissue differentiation. Although fluoroscopy is occasionally helpful in targeting obstructive biliary or urinary masses after ductal opacification, cross-sectional modalities (US, CT, MR) are preferred, both for preprocedure planning and for the performance of image-guided biopsies.

With the development of high-resolution image processing and real-time linear, curvilinear, and phased-array transducers with small footprints, US equipment has evolved to the point that lesions 3 to 4 mm in diameter can be sampled with a high yield even when implanted deeply within solid organs (Jaeger, MacFie, et al., 1990; Somers, Lomas, et al., 1993; Don, Kopecky, et al., 1994; Lencioni, Caramella, et al., 1995). Increased yields also relate to improved US visualization permitted by the small size of pediatric patients and by the decreased amount of subcutaneous and intraperitoneal fat in these patients. (Sawhney, Berry, et al., 1987; Reading, Charboneau, et al., 1988). Color Doppler imaging allows safer routes of access that avoid large vascular structures (Lencioni, Caramella, et al., 1995). The development of volumetric imaging techniques and improved contrast resolution with phased harmonic imaging may allow better definition of tissues and anatomic relationships than have been possible with conventional US systems. Mechanical needle guide systems are available to assist in obtaining an optimal relationship between the biopsy needle and the transducer. Most experienced interventionists prefer a "freehand" technique, especially where lesions are small or deeply situated, where the needle and US probe are distant from each other, or where the ultrasonographic window is very small. It is essential in either technique to maintain a perpendicular relationship between the needle and transducer (to increase reverberation artifact and therefore improve visualization of the needle, as shown in Figures 5–30, 5–34, 5–44, 5–45) and to keep both target lesion and needle in the imaging plane of the transducer. The movement of the needle is thus observed throughout its course. This is more easily accomplished if the target lesion is eccentrically located within the scanning field so that most of the field of view is available for observing the motion of the needle. Finally, it is a helpful rule of thumb to never move the needle and the transducer at the same time.

Computed tomography offers good tissue differentiation in the abdomen and pelvis and is usually used for biopsy planning. Helical CT techniques permit rapid scanning of small volumes with high resolution. Computed tomographic guidance may be especially advantageous in small, deeply situated lesions in larger patients; where the target lesion is adjacent to vital structures; or where the target lesion is obscured by overlying echogenic structures (e.g., lung, bowel gas, bone) (Reddy, Gattuso, et al., 1991; Wimmer and Wenz, 1991). During CT-guided approaches for biopsy, it is helpful to orient the needle perpendicular to the skin within the imaging plane, as compound angulation is difficult to perform. Angulation of the gantry is occasionally useful for lesions that are otherwise difficult to reach. Computed tomographic fluoroscopy (Katada, Anno, et al., 1994; Katada, Kato, et al., 1996; White, Templeton, et al., 1997) allows real-time navigation in anatomic regions not safely accessible or easily visualized with other modalities. Volumetric imaging on helical or MR scanners allows procedure planning and better definition of the anatomic relationships of nodules and masses but has added little to safety or efficacy so far. Positron emission tomography (PET), single photon emission computed tomography (SPECT), and MR systems differentiate pathophysiologic tissue characteristics and may yield improvements in specificity. As more tissue-specific contrast agents become available, these modalities may provide rich new areas for both tissue diagnosis and therapeutic intervention (Weissleder, 1999).

Biopsy Needles

Safe acquisition of sufficient tissue for a specific diagnosis without undue artifact or sampling error remains the central objective of all biopsy techniques. Fine-needle aspiration (FNA) may maximize safety (Smith, 1991; Smith, Katz, et al., 1993; Somers, Lomas, et al., 1993). If a pathologist skilled in cytopathology is available for preliminary diagnosis in the procedure room, sufficient yields for specific diagnoses may rival alternative techniques, especially for documentation of metastases or tumor recurrence in patients with known primary malignancies. Sampling error and a low negative predictive value (given a high false-negative rate and the high prevalence of malignancy in tertiary centers) continue to be limiting features of the FNA technique (Lerma, Musulen, et al., 1996). Thin-walled, small-gauge core biopsy needles with a variety of tips facilitate the collection of larger tissue specimens necessary for specific diagnosis of certain tumors such as sarcomas or the small round blue cell tumors that are more prevalent in the pediatric population (Sabbah, Ghandour, et al., 1981; Quinn, Sheley, et al., 1995; Tsang, Greenebaum, et al., 1995). A coaxial system using a larger needle (for control of

the target lesion and through which a thinner needle is passed for sampling), may improve both safety and yield in select cases (Moulton and Moore, 1993)

A variety of needles may be used for tissue acquisition. In general, they may be divided between noncutting and cutting needles, and between manual and automated devices. Noncutting (manual aspiration) needles (Chiba, spinal with a beveled edge of 25° and 45°, respectively) allow for sampling of cells and fluids for cytopathologic and microbiologic analysis. Manual cutting needles include end-cutting (Menghini, Turner, Jamshidi, Sure-cut, Madayag, Greene, Franseen) and side-cutting needles (Tru-cut, Westcott, Stylet-Gap). These bear various tip configurations, from smoothly beveled to serrated, each of which offers a particular advantage in specific situations. For example, a serrated tip may assist tissue acquisition in a firm resilient lesion while minimizing crush artifact. Automated systems include end-cutting (Angiomed Autovac) and side-cutting devices (Biopty, Monopty) (Figure 5–29). They allow a variable distance between the "cocked" and "fired" positions so that the length of the specimen can be adapted to the specific patient problem. Unless aspiration cytology is needed, automated cutting needles are our needles of choice. We use the Angiomed Autovac needle (18 to 21 Gauge), primarily for solid masses and organs. The automated side-cutting needles are used where gelatinous, resilient, or mobile

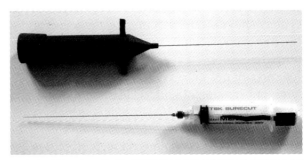

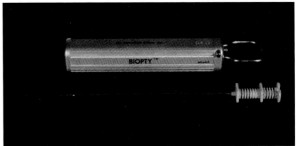

FIGURE 5–29. Biopsy devices. *A*, End cutting Tru-cut and Angiomed devices. *B*,. Side-cutting Biopty device.

tissue does not allow acquisition of good end-cutting core samples. Needles also vary by gauge. Thin needles (20 to 25 Gauge) are more often used for obtaining aspiration cytology and microbiology specimens or for core specimens in locations where there is a risk of entering vital structures, bowel loops, or blood vessels. Middle-gauge needles (18 to 20 Gauge) are used to obtain core (histologic) material and thicker fluid samples for microbiology. Larger needles less than 18 Gauge are available but are rarely used in the pediatric population except for bone biopsy procedures. Ultimately, the experience and preference of the operator and the nature of the target lesion determine needle selection. Special needles are manufactured for specific applications, including needles designed for easy visualization within the ultrasonographic beam, nonferrous needles for MR-guided procedures, kits for the performance of transjugular biopsies, and long flexible needles in holders designed to keep the operator's hands out of the CT fluoroscopy gantry. Although expensive, these needles are quite helpful for their dedicated purposes.

Pathologic Considerations

There are strengths and weaknesses to both cytologic and histologic examinations, depending upon the pathologist's experience as well as on the suitability of samples as representative of the target lesion. For the interpretation of cellular changes in the cytoplasm, nuclei, nucleoli, and chromatin, FNA may suffice; but FNA requires specific expertise in cytopathology on the part of the pathologist, and it benefits from the presence of the pathologist in the procedure room. Expertise in classic histologic interpretation is more readily available but depends upon preservation of both cellular morphology and architectural organization (including the intercellular matrix and supporting stroma) in the sample for proper diagnosis. Sampling the desired lesion has become more reliable as imaging modalities, especially US, have improved. However, nonrepresentative sampling from the target tissue may occur due to the presence of central necrosis, intense inflammatory reaction, or hemorrhage. Stains that characterize subcellular architecture and cellular biochemical products, immunocytochemical subclassification of mesenchymal malignancies (such as lymphomas), and ultrastructural analysis by electron microscopy all improve the diagnostic accuracy of core biopsies but may require a greater mass of sampled tissue and will certainly add to the overall cost of the procedure. However, with core biopsy techniques, the improved accuracy in analysis of mesenchymal malignancies and the improved ability to make a specific benign diagnosis increase the negative predictive value to nearly 100%. Since this may eliminate the need for repeat biopsies or open surgery in follow-up of negative results in these patients, the relative value of histologic material from core biopsy specimens in the pediatric population should not be underestimated.

Patient Preparation

Prior to the procedure, the patient's imaging studies should be reviewed with the referring physicians and surgeons to determine a likely clinicoradiologic diagnosis and to discuss the potential risks and benefits of the percutaneous approach. Close consultation with the pathologist is important to determine the need for histologic specimens, the amount of tissue required for specific diagnosis, and the desired transport medium and handling procedures for the biopsy material (Dabbs and Wang, 1998; Zardawi, 1998). Patient preparation is otherwise similar to that of other interventional procedures (see Preprocedure Care and Periprocedure Care sections, above). When sampling small lesions or lesions adjacent to vital structures, general anesthesia with control of respiration in end-expiration can be of considerable benefit in minimizing motion artifact and respiratory misregistration.

Indications and Contraindications

The primary indication for percutaneous biopsy is the nonsurgical diagnosis of malignancy (either primary or metastatic). Additional indications include

- confirmation of a benign diagnosis,
- investigation of nonmalignant pathology (e.g., transplant organ rejection, graft-versus-host disease, biliary atresia, neonatal hepatitis, sclerosing cholangitis), and
- acquisition of fluid or tissue for culture or other laboratory studies.

There are no absolute contraindications to percutaneous biopsy. The decision to obtain a biopsy should be made with consideration for the risks and benefits in each patient. However, percutaneous biopsy should not be employed when the result will not influence management or when surgical excision is planned regardless of the percutaneous result. Relative contraindications include the following:

- Coagulation abnormalities that might increase the risk of postprocedure bleeding. (Alternative methods, such as transjugular biopsy, may be used in patients with an uncorrectable bleeding diathesis.)
- Absence of a safe pathway from skin to target site.
- Intervening bowel. (Transgression of hollow viscus and nontarget solid organs is generally avoided if alternative pathways are available. However, thin-needle aspiration cytology is considered a safe procedure under almost any condition.)

Regional Considerations

Percutaneous Liver Biopsy

Liver biopsy is performed to diagnose suspected malignancy or to characterize diffuse hepatocellular disease. Blind (non image-guided) liver biopsies are still performed regularly (Esposito, Garipoli, et al., 1997). However, with a percutaneous intercostal approach, there is a significant risk of bleeding or other vascular trauma (pseudoaneurysm or arteriovenous fistula), bowel or gallbladder perforation, or pneumo- or hemothorax (Lachaux, Le Gall, et al., 1995). Since 1991, we have performed over 600 image-guided percutaneous liver biopsies without significant complications. Patients occasionally experience local pain or discomfort, which is relieved by analgesics. None have yet required hospitalization for biopsy-related complications.

For patients without focal pathology or bleeding diathesis, we use a subcostal midline approach with US guidance under sedation, using an 18-Gauge automated end-cutting needle (Figure 5–30). Two to three core specimens are obtained, depending on the pathologic quantities needed. Focal liver lesions as small as 3 to 4 mm are sampled with the same needle, using US control. It is helpful to choose an approach that interposes a rim of normal liver tissue between the liver capsule and the lesion to minimize bleeding from hypervascular lesions. Prior imaging studies are often helpful in localizing the lesion. Occasionally, CT guidance is required for lesions that are not well visualized with US.

Transjugular Liver Biopsy

Since 1992, we have performed 55 transjugular liver biopsies (Gamble, Colapinto, et al., 1985; Mewissen,

Lipchik, et al., 1988; Corr, Beningfield, et al., 1992; Furuya, Burrows, et al., 1992; Little, Zajko, et al., 1996), predominantly in children with uncorrectable coagulopathies or in children suspected of having portal hypertension, with a 12% rate of minor complication and one death due to a ventricular arrhythmia following the procedure. This procedure is facilitated by respiratory control under general anesthesia with the patient in the supine Trendelenburg position. Access is obtained under US guidance via the right internal jugular vein. Occasionally, where this vein is thrombosed, a left-sided jugular venous approach is used. The Quick-

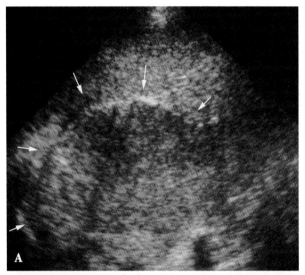

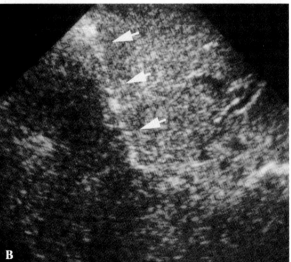

FIGURE 5–30 A, Transverse image of hepatic adenoma (*arrows*). B, Ultrasound guidance is required to constantly monitor the position of the biopsy needle (*arrows*) and assure adequate lesion sampling.

core transjugular set (Labs 100, Cook, Inc.) is our system of choice for all patients larger than 4 kg.

The catheter system is introduced through the sheath, and a directional catheter is advanced over a hydrophilic wire. Pressure recordings are taken in the inferior vena cava (IVC) and hepatic vein (free hepatic venous pressure). After selective access of the right hepatic vein, the portal pressure is measured indirectly by wedging an end-hole catheter into the peripheral portion of the hepatic vein. The corrected wedge pressure (portosystemic gradient) is calculated as the difference between the IVC pressure and the portal pressure. The normal portosystemic gradient is 2 to 4 mm Hg (Compra, 1988). A gradient greater than or equal to 6-mm Hg is evidence of portal hypertension, and a gradient greater than 15 mm Hg constitutes severe portal hypertension. A normal free hepatic venogram confirms patency of the main hepatic vein (useful in evaluation of Budd-Chiari syndrome) and should show fifth-order branching beyond the zero-order branch injected (the hepatic vein) (Figure 5–31). Hepatic fibrosis is indicated by loss of branching (mild: loss of fifth-order branching and beyond; moderate: loss of third- and fourth-order branching; severe: loss of first- and second-order branching). Retrograde portal venous filling during wedged hepatic venography indicates reversal of portal flow and suggests portal hypertension (Figure 5–32).

The biopsy needle is introduced through an 8 French cannula that has an internal stiffener. The needle tip is advanced to the tip of the catheter. We use US guidance to examine the liver with the nee-

dle and catheter in position so as to avoid any vital structures (including the gallbladder, major vessels, and bile ducts) and to make sure the needle throw will not extend outside the capsule of the liver (Figure 5–33). Combined US control also enables us to biopsy safely from the middle or left hepatic veins when necessary. Postbiopsy venography is performed to identify any evidence of bleeding. If significant hemorrhage is identified, it may be embolized via the indwelling catheter.

Percutaneous Splenic Biopsy

Splenomegaly and the development of focal splenic lesions may occur in immunosuppressed or immunodeficient patients and in those with a history of malignancy at risk for metastatic disease or relapse. The nature of splenic lesions is of primary diagnostic importance and defines the course of treatment in these patients. In the past, FNA biopsy was the procedure of choice in these patients (Zeppa, Vetrani, et al., 1994). Many of these patients eventually required

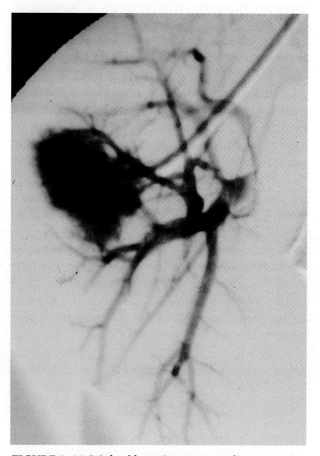

FIGURE 5–32 Wedged hepatic venogram demonstrating parenchymal blush and portal venous filling.

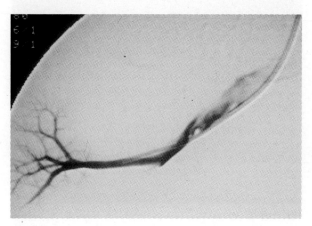

FIGURE 5–31. Free hepatic venogram demonstrates normal filling of up to fifth-order right hepatic venous branches.

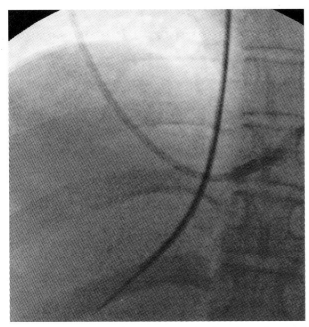

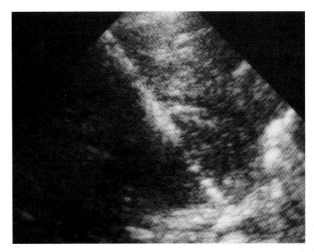

FIGURE 5–34 Transhepatic ultrasound guided biopsy of pancreatic head mass showing needle in place.

FIGURE 5–33. Fluoroscopic image showing sheathed transjugular needle after deployment. Ultrasound is used prior to deployment to help avoid vital structures.

splenectomy, with the pathologic diagnosis made by sampling tissue from the excised spleen. Ultrasonography-guided percutaneous core biopsy (UCB) of the spleen is a relatively new procedure used to obtain core tissue samples in patients with abnormal spleens (Quinn, vanSonnenberg, et al., 1986). Since 1991, we have performed 30 splenic UCBs. All were performed under US guidance, usually using a 7-MHz vector probe with an intercostal approach. General anesthesia is often used where the lesions are small and control of respiration is important. We have used 18- to 21-Gauge end-cutting automated biopsy devices for most of these procedures without significant complications. Adequate tissue is most often obtained with the 18-Gauge needle, which is now our device of choice for this procedure.

Percutaneous Pancreatic Biopsy

Primary pancreatic tumors are relatively rare in the pediatric population (Synn, Mulvihill, et al., 1988; Vane, Grosfeld, et al., 1989; Jaksic, Yaman, et al., 1992; Yagi, Shiraiwa, et al., 1994; Murakami, Ueki, et al. 1996; Willnow, Willberg, et al., 1996; Schwartz, 1997). Principles obtained for biopsies are similar to those for any other solid masses. The decision to perform percutaneous biopsy depends on the extent of the primary lesion and the presence of secondary pathology and the surgical alternatives. Visualization with US (Figure 5–34) or CT (Figure 5–35) is usually required to allow accurate placement of needles for small pancreatic lesions. Pancreatitis, bleeding, and seeding of the biopsy tract are the primary risks of this procedure. A window should be sought that allows biopsy without traversing bowel. If no such window is available, a transbowel route of access may usually be safely employed with a 21-Gauge needle.

Nodules and Masses

The results obtained from percutaneous lymph nodes are generally not as rewarding as those from biopsies of other organs. Often, several core biopsies are needed in several locations within a node to get an accurate diagnostic result. Excisional biopsy of suspicious superficial nodes is preferred to other

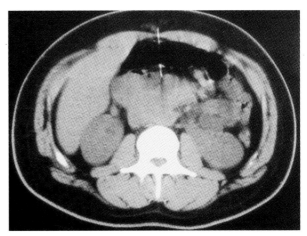

FIGURE 5–35. CT guided biopsy of pancreatic tumour.

approaches when possible. Otherwise, percutaneous biopsy of abdominal lymph nodes may be performed with fluoroscopic guidance following pedal lymphangiography. In the case of suspected lymphoma, percutaneous lymph node biopsy is usually performed with US or CT guidance.

PERCUTANEOUS ASPIRATION AND DRAINAGE

Description, Indications, and Contraindications

Percutaneous aspiration and drainage has been performed for many years, but it is with the advent of cross-sectional imaging techniques (predominantly CT and US) that this procedure has replaced surgical incision and drainage as the treatment of choice for the evacuation of most abdominopelvic fluid collections (Gerzof, 1981; Clark and Towbin, 1983; Mandel, Boyd, et al., 1983; vanSonnenberg, Mueller, et al., 1984; Gaisie, Jaques, et al., 1987; Gazelle, Haaga, et al., 1991; Hemming, Davis, et al., 1991; Lambiase, Deyoe, et al., 1992; Goletti, Lippolis, et al., 1993; Yeung and Ho, 1993; Gazelle and Mueller, 1994; Pereira, Chait, et al., 1996; Jamieson, Chait, et al., 1997; Kang, Gupta, et al., 1998; Okoye, Rampersad, et al., 1998; Yamini, Vargas, et al., 1998). Since 1991, we have performed more than 1000 primary drainage procedures. Procedures related to aspiration and drainage account for approximately 6% of all the pediatric interventional procedures we perform.

Absolute contraindications to abscess drainage include an uncorrectable bleeding diathesis and an unsafe route for drainage. In select cases, fluid collections in these patients may be safely aspirated through a thin needle.

Suspected fungal abscess, which can be quite invasive, may be considered a relative contraindication to percutaneous drainage unless local adjuvant therapy with direct injection of antifungal agents is anticipated. Interloop abscesses are also difficult to treat percutaneously, and aspiration with a small 22-Gauge needle may be all that is possible (Kuligowska, Keller, et al., 1995; Saluja, Fields, et al., 1998).

Image Guidance

Preprocedure Imaging

If a patient presents with clinical signs and symptoms of an abscess or fluid collection, cross-sectional imaging is usually requested. Clinical history and prior imaging are reviewed in close consultation with referring physicians to determine the likely source and nature of abnormal collections, and additional pre-procedure studies are obtained as required. Clinicoradiologic differential considerations should include abscess, sterile fluid collection (hematoma, seroma, biloma, urinoma), lymphocele, malignant fluid collection, pancreatic pseudocyst, and fluid-filled loops of bowel. Typically, CT is performed to confirm the presence and number of fluid collections, to distinguish a mature abscess from phlegmonous inflammatory tissue, to assess for the presence of an associated tumor, and to determine the availability of a safe access route. It is important to distinguish inflammatory tissue or cellulitis from a mature abscess, as drainage of inflammatory tissue without fluid is usually difficult. A combination of contrast-enhanced CT and US may be needed to differentiate these entities. For example, color flow by Doppler imaging or contrast enhancement by CT in the center of a mass suggests a phlegmonous mass rather than a fluid collection.

Fluid collections that appear smaller than the loop of a drainage catheter are usually aspirated. Collections may be drained through a single catheter if interconnected or through multiple catheters if discrete. Injection of radiographic contrast or dynamic ultrasonographic evaluation of fluid flow patterns can usually demonstrate whether each collection is accessible for aspiration or drainage. Multiseptate collections may be drained percutaneously if the septa can be disrupted with a guide-wire under ultrasonographic guidance. Again, noncommunicating cavities must be drained separately. All collections should be either drained or aspirated, and separate samples should be sent from each to improve antibiotic coverage (Heneghan, Everts, and Nelson, 1999). If any discrete collections cannot be safely accessed, surgical incision and drainage may be indicated.

Ultrasonography

Treatment of abdominopelvic fluid collections may be regarded as a two-stage procedure. The first stage, confirming the diagnosis, requires analysis of a fluid sample obtained from the abnormal area identified on pre-procedure imaging. In the case of small or poorly accessible collections, this may be accomplished with a thin needle under US guidance. Larger sterile collections (excepting lymphoceles and pancreatic pseudocysts) may be evacuated through a 16-Gauge angiocatheter or an 18-Gauge single-wall puncture or trocar needle under US guidance. Periprocedural imaging is usually performed directly on the C-arm fluoroscopic table. As soon as a safe route of access is determined, the site is identified with a surgical marker, and the patient is prepared and draped in sterile fashion as described elsewhere. A sterile cover is placed over the US probe (Civco) for intraprocedural guidance. The technique of needle insertion under US control is similar to that described under Percutaneous Biopsy, above. The most common US transducers useful for image guidance are 8-, 7-, or 5-MHz vector or small curvilinear probes. There is no substitute for a high-quality machine in image-guided applications. Larger, symptomatic, or infected collections will usually require progression to the second stage, catheter drainage, after using the same access needle to pass a guide wire. While the second stage is usually completed under fluoroscopic control, continued access to ultrasonographic imaging can assist disruption of septa within complex collections, confirm optimum positioning of the guide wire and catheter and document evacuation of the collection at the conclusion of the procedure (Jeffrey, Wing, et al., 1985).

Fluoroscopy
Having secured needle access to the fluid collection under US guidance, a wire is passed into the collection, and the catheter insertion is completed under fluoroscopic control as described under Percutaneous Technique, below. Initial access under fluoroscopic guidance is possible in gas-containing collections but is rarely the procedure of choice with abdominopelvic collections.

Computed Tomography and
Computed Tomographic Fluoroscopy
Guidance by CT is indicated to access fluid collections for which no adequate ultrasonographic window can be identified. In children, this is more often related to collections obscured by overlying gas or bone than simply to deeply situated lesions. Computed tomographic fluoroscopy permits maneuvering in real time around viscus organs and vital structures, but with a significant learning curve. The technique of needle insertion under CT control is similar to that described under Percutaneous Biopsy, above. As multiple imaging modalities are inte-

grated into unified interventional suites, image guidance will more likely be selected by task, based on safety and efficacy rather than convenience and availability. For example, diagnosis and initial access for select collections may be performed under CT or CT fluoroscopic guidance, the catheter placed under fluoroscopic guidance, and evacuation of the cavity confirmed with US, all as a continuous procedure without moving the patient.

Other Modalities
Fine anatomic and pathophysiologic detail; cross-sectional, multiplanar, and volumetric image rendering; and near real-time capability would make interventional MR an ideal modality for image-guided procedures were it not for the issues of cost and availability. Similarly, radionuclide scanning using gallium or agents labeled with white blood cells offers high sensitivity for the detection of infectious and inflammatory processes but limited anatomic detail. Intraoperative multimodality image registration and fusion will overcome some of these limitations. As economic concerns are addressed and when the technology can be integrated into a unified interventional suite, one would expect some more difficult procedures to be shifted to this environment.

Materials and Method
The following materials are required for percutaneous aspiration and drainage:

- Chlorhexidine gluconate (0.5%) with 70% isopropyl alcohol solution (Soluprep [tinted], Solumed, Inc.)
- Sterile US cover
- Angiocatheter, 16 Gauge
- Yueh 4 and 5 French sheathed needles with side holes
- Chiba needle, 22 Gauge (5, 10, and 15cm)
- Seldinger needle, 19 Gauge
- Single-wall puncture needle, 18 and 19 Gauge
- Trocar needle, 18 Gauge (11 and 20 cm)
- Neff introducer system (Cook, Inc.)
- Accustik introducer system (Meditech)
- All-purpose drains, 6 to 14 French (Meditech)
- Thalquick drainage catheter, 12 to 24 French (Cook, Inc.)
- Duan drainage catheter, 5 French (Cook, Inc.)
- Coons dilator, 5 to 22 French
- Abscess drainage bag

- Mefix adhesive bandage (Hypafix Dressing Retention Sheet [Smith and Nephew])
- K-lock adhesive catheter retention device

Percutaneous Technique

The procedure is performed under sterile technique. Most procedures are performed on a C-arm fluoroscopic table. The patient is sedated as described in Sedation, Analgesia, and Anesthesia, above. The position of the abscess and the site of percutaneous entry are marked with a surgical marker. When planning percutaneous drainage of an upper abdominal collection, care should be taken to avoid the pleura. Accordingly, the access site should be below the 8th rib anteriorly and the 12th rib posteriorly. A posterior approach often requires cranial angulation of the access needle. In these situations, transabdominal US allows visualization of the access needle entering posteriorly with the patient in the decubitus position. Having planned and marked a safe route of access, the patient is prepared with Soluprep, and sterile drapes are placed around the planned access site. Buffered lidocaine 1% solution (up to 0.5 cc per kg) is infiltrated into the subcutaneous tissues and along the prospective tract with a 27-Gauge needle.

Access

The size and type of needle depends upon the size, location, and viscosity of the collection. In large collections that are easily accessible, a 16-Gauge angiocatheter, a 5 French Yueh, or a single-wall 19-Gauge needle is used under US guidance. After sampling the contents of the collection, a 0.035-inch wire can be passed through these needles. For deeper collections, a 22-Gauge Chiba needle is advanced, using US guidance to avoid loops of bowel or vital structures and to enter the collection safely. Aspiration of the fluid confirms its character and informs further management decisions. If drainage is required, a 0.018-inch mandril wire placed through the thin needle may be exchanged for a Neff or Accustik introducer system. The inner dilator and wire can then be replaced with a larger Amplatz wire, over which a suitable drainage catheter may be inserted. Direct access with a trocar catheter system is less precise and is seldom used in the drainage of intra-abdominal abscesses unless they are very large and superficial. After obtaining samples for microbiologic or pathologic analysis, contrast is introduced through the needle or the sheath to outline the walls of the collection. This allows the introduction of a 0.035-inch wire into the fluid cavity without perforating the cavity walls.

Specimen Handling

Fluid samples obtained at initial access should be placed in a sterile container and transferred immediately to the microbiology laboratory for distribution, special stains, and preparation for culture. If no fluid is obtained, a small amount of nonbacteriostatic saline may be infiltrated through the needle to lavage the suspected site of infection. Any fluid then aspirated should be sent to the laboratory in the syringe in a sealed sterile container. Additionally, biopsy specimens from the region of the "dry" tap should be obtained for pathologic analysis. Not all dry taps are undrainable, and a large-bore catheter combined with a lytic adjuvant (such as urokinase) may assist drainage of symptomatic viscous fluid collections, including thick pus and maturing hematoma.

Drainage and Fixation

Once access to the collection is secured with a guide wire, the tract is enlarged with an appropriate series of fascial dilators. Lubricant may be used to assist passage of the dilator. After successful dilatation, a drainage catheter appropriate to the size, viscosity, and location of the collection is inserted under fluoroscopic guidance with a stiffener. Catheters range in size from as small as 4 French up to 22 French. For simple nonviscous fluid drainage, an 8, 10, or 12 French locking pigtail catheter with side holes (such as the Meditech All Purpose Drain) is usually used. For a larger or more viscous collection, a sump or Thalquick drain can be used. The stiffener is released from the catheter as it enters the collection, and the catheter is advanced to lie within the collection. Most catheters used for this purpose have an internal locking mechanism that is secured, and the catheter is connected to an abscess drainage system. This closed system has a one-way valve that allows aspiration of fluid using a Luer-Lok syringe. This decreases the odor and spillage of infected materials. Complete evacuation of the collection should be documented by US or CT. The one-way valve is then removed and the drainage catheter connected to gravity drainage. The catheter is fixed in position by suturing it to the skin or to an adhesive disk using a nonresorbing suture. Alternatively, a Mefix dressing at the exit site may be used with an adhesive K-lock catheter fixation device to avoid the discomfort of an external suture.

Regional Considerations

Deep Pelvic Collections

Pelvic abscesses are usually deep and obscured by overlying bowel, vessels, urinary bladder, and bony pelvis. If they are superficial and easily visualized with US or CT, they are easy to drain using the transabdominal approach described above. A transrectal approach has been our preferred technique in 67 cases where fluid collections have been located deeply within the pelvis. The patient is positioned in the left-side-down decubitus position. A digital rectal examination is performed while scanning through the anterior abdominal wall with US. The examining digit is visualized within the rectum, and the relationship between the rectal wall and the fluid collection is defined (Figure 5–36). For lesions higher up in the pelvis, an enema catheter is used to protect the mucosa from the sharp tip during introduction of the needle. Under US control, a long 18-Gauge trocar needle is advanced, either along the index finger or protected within the enema tip. The needle tip is positioned adjacent to the abscess collection and then advanced into the abscess under real-time imaging. The collection is aspirated, and the fluid is sent for laboratory assessment. Pus from a ruptured appendiceal abscess, a common indication for transrectal drainage, has a characteristically foul odor. A small amount of contrast is instilled to define the limits of the abscess cavity, and a 0.035-inch Amplatz guide wire is advanced through the needle into the collection. The tract is dilated, and an appropriately sized drain is inserted over the wire (Figure 5–37). Similar techniques may be used for transvaginal or transperineal access to pelvic fluid collections, but these are seldom employed in the pediatric population. A transgluteal route is used by some centers, but this approach is associated with a higher incidence of pain, bleeding, nerve damage, and other complications (Gazelle, Haaga, et al., 1991; Longo, Bilbao, et al., 1993; Yeung and Ho, 1993).

Periappendiceal and Interloop Abscesses

Following acute appendicitis or ruptured appendiceal abscess, the high risk of recurrent abscesses and postoperative adhesions is a relative contraindication to immediate appendicectomy (Finne, 1980;

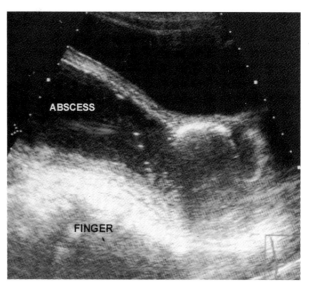

FIGURE 5–36. Transabdominal sonography is used to determine the relation of the abscess to the rectum. Here the abscess is indented posteriorly by the radiologist's finger during the rectal exam.

Kuligowska, Keller, et al., 1995; Jamieson, Chait, et al., 1997; Mazziotti, Marley, et al., 1997; Saluja, Fields, et al., 1998; Yamini, Vargas, et al., 1998). In our institution, US-guided percutaneous drainage is the preferred treatment of localized collections pre-

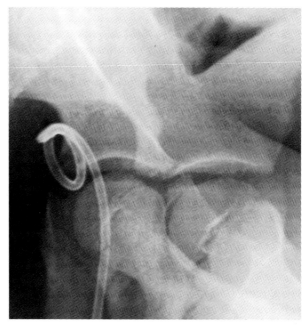

FIGURE 5–37. Lateral image of transrectal drain in place. Appropriately sized catheters are placed over a wire after tract dilation.

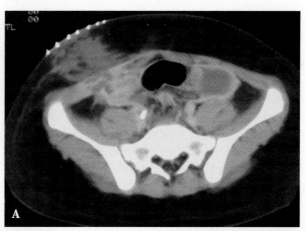

FIGURE 5–38. Appendiceal abscess drainage. *A*, CT demonstrated bilateral abscesses in the postoperative patient. *B*, Multiple drainage catheters may be required to treat multiple collections.

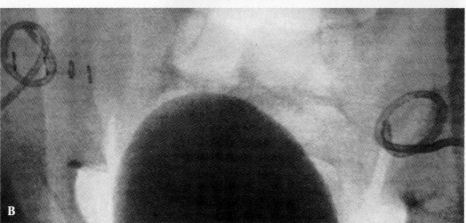

sumed to be due to a ruptured appendix (Figure 5–38). By their nature, interloop abscesses are surrounded by bowel and are often difficult to access or drain completely. Children with these may require several drains, repeated procedures, and a good deal of patience to achieve success. Aspiration with a 20- or 22-Gauge Chiba needle is an accepted treatment for collections that cannot be safely drained.

Lesser Sac Collections

Fluid in the lesser sac is often associated with pancreatitis and is typically drained transgastrically, in a manner similar to pancreatic pseudocysts (as below) (Amundson, Towbin, et al., 1990). If there is a clear window to the fluid collection under US, direct drainage or aspiration may be performed.

Subphrenic Collections

Subphrenic abscesses are usually seen as postoperative complications or in patients with ruptured appendix. They are often difficult to access and may require a transhepatic subcostal approach or an inter-

costal approach. Combined US and CT guidance may be necessary to access these collections, using fluoroscopy for final tube placement (van Gansbeke, Matos, et al., 1989; Eisenberg, Lee, et al., 1994)

Liver Abscesses

Primary hepatic abscesses are uncommon in the pediatric population (Wang, Chen, et al., 1989; Kong and Lin, 1994). Pyogenic abscesses are most commonly seen following abdominal trauma and in immunocompromised patients and patients with chronic granulomatous disease. Occasionally, pyogenic abscesses complicate appendicitis (septic emboli), portal vein thrombosis, or liver infarction (as in sickle cell disease or tumor necrosis) (Figure 5–39). Depending upon their size, pyogenic abscesses are aspirated or drained (Montoya, Alam, et al., 1983; Moore, Millar, et al., 1994; Ni, Chang, et al., 1995; Rajak, Gupta, et al., 1998) Small lesions are aspirated with a Chiba needle with US guidance. For larger collections, the standard drainage technique is used with access under US guidance, followed by contrast, wire placement, tract dilatation, and drainage catheter insertion under fluoroscopy. Just as for liver biopsy, a choice of access route that interposes normal liver tissue between the capsule and the collection will help prevent hemorrhage and, in this case, intraperitoneal contamination.

Percutaneous drainage plays an important role in the management of children with infected collections occurring after liver transplantation (Hoffer, Teele, et al., 1988; Letourneau, Hunter, et al., 1989). Retransplantation has been avoided in some children after successful drainage of infected bilomas secondary to hepatic arterial thrombosis. In the immunocompromised patient, focal microabscesses are often seen as a consequence of fungal infection. These are usually too small to allow for drainage but are often aspirated for diagnostic purposes.

The multiloculated cysts with satellite cysts characteristically seen on CT with *Echinococcus granulosa* infection are preferentially treated with antibiotics (albendazole) alone. Persistence of symptoms for more than 2 weeks while the patient is on appropriate medical therapy is an indication for percutaneous management. Standard access technique is used to catheterize the cysts, and portions of the cyst fluid are exchanged with equal volumes of hypertonic saline until the entire cyst volume has been replaced. This replacement technique avoids intraperitoneal spillage of infected fluid during the procedure. At this point, the cyst is completely evacuated and left to gravity drainage. If the cyst is intact (without connection to the biliary tree) and greater than 5 cm in diameter, it may be helpful to sclerose the cyst lining with absolute alcohol or silver nitrate solution (Men, Hekimoglu, et al., 1999). Antibiotic therapy is continued for 8 weeks or until the catheter is removed (Dilsiz, Acikgozoglu, et al., 1997; Khuroo, Wani, et al., 1997).

Patients who have immigrated from or traveled in underdeveloped areas, particularly Africa, South America, and Asia, are at increased risk for amebic liver abscesses. Such abscesses present as single or lobulated masses, usually in the right lobe, and are most often treated conservatively. Percutaneous drainage is indicated for failed antibiotic therapy or imminent rupture.

Cholecystic and Pericholecystic Collections

Drainage of pyogenic cholecystitis and infected pericholecystic collections is occasionally per-

formed in the pediatric population, using the transabdominal technique described above.

Splenic Abscesses

The optimum approach to splenic abscesses is controversial. There are concerns about the safety of trans-splenic percutaneous intervention. However, experience in both adult and pediatric patients suggests that percutaneous drainage of splenic abscesses can be performed safely and effectively (Quinn, vanSonnenberg, et al., 1986; Tikkakoski, Siniluoto, et al., 1992). Percutaneous drainage offers the advantage of preserving splenic function, important for host immune response. Percutaneous aspiration is indicated in any size of collection in the spleen. Drainage with a catheter should be considered in a significantly sized lesion that is not complex and is not close to any large vascular structures.

Pancreatic Collections

Percutaneous drainage of pancreatic fluid collections is indicated in the case of infected, symptomatic, or persistent pseudocysts (vanSonnenberg, Wittich, et al., 1985; Jaffe, Arata, et al., 1989; Amundson, Towbin, et al., 1990; Burnweit, Wesson, et al., 1990; Corbally, Blake, et al., 1992). Pancreatic phlegmon, peripancreatic necrosis, or pseudoaneurysms or varices are relative contraindications to percutaneous management.

Pancreatic abscesses are rare but have been seen in particularly immunocompromised children (Figure 5–40). Depending on their size and position,

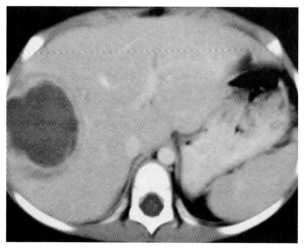

FIGURE 5–39. Hepatic abscesses can occur in infarcted liver in patients with sickle cell disease.

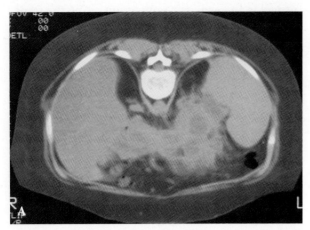
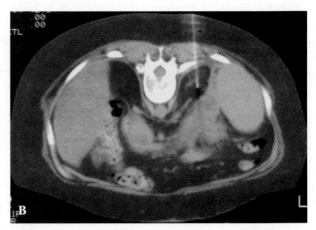

FIGURE 5–40. CT guidance was used to aspirate this *Pseudomonas* pancreatic abscess

they may be aspirated with a thin needle or drained. Because of the deep position of the pancreas, aspiration is usually performed as the initial procedure.

Pseudocysts usually develop as a result of acute pancreatitis from whatever cause. They may present as an upper abdominal mass, which appears hypoechoic on US, with or without debris. Computed tomography confirms the appearance of a low-density collection, which usually arises close to the pancreas in the region of the lesser sac. Clinically, most of these pseudocysts will resolve with bowel rest and parenteral nutrition. However, persistent symptomatic collections require treatment, preferably by transgastric drainage. After the extent of the cyst is defined on pre-procedure CT, drainage is usually performed under combined US and fluoroscopic control (Figure 5–41).

With the stomach deflated, the margins of the cyst are identified with US and marked on the skin.

Next, the stomach is inflated and accessed (as in the percutaneous retrograde gastrostomy procedure previous described), and a retention suture and safety wire are placed in the stomach. The stomach is now deflated, and a second needle is advanced through both walls of the stomach and into the pseudocyst itself. A sample of fluid is aspirated, and some contrast is introduced to outline the extent of the cavity. After dilatation of the tract, a drainage catheter is inserted and left to gravity drainage. Tubography is performed once drainage ceases or symptoms resolve to redefine the extent of the pseudocyst and to search for the presence of a fistula to the pancreatic duct. Normally, the catheter is left in position for at least 6 weeks to allow the tract between the stomach and the cyst to mature. This decreases the risk of enterocutaneous fistula formation by allowing the cyst to continue draining into the stomach until it resolves.

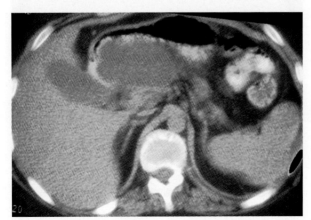
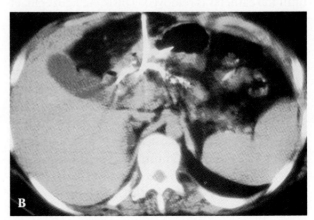

FIGURE 5–41. *A*, Lesser sac pseudocyst. *B*, Transgastric drainage was successful.

Special Considerations

Lymphoceles and Sclerotherapy

Lymphoceles are most commonly seen in renal transplantation patients and may result in impaired graft function or infection (Curry, Cochran, et al., 1984). Many asymptomatic lymphoceles resolve without intervention. Of the 28 lymphoceles we have treated since 1991, 13 required percutaneous aspiration or drainage and 7 were treated with transcatheter sclerosis with tetracycline, ethanol, povidone-iodine, or a combination of these. Although such patients often require treatment over a period of months to years, they are usually able to avoid surgery (Baskin, Chait, et al., 1999b). Frequent instillation of sclerosants (2 to 3 times per week) may help obliterate the cavity more quickly. Lymphoceles adjacent to or enclosing vital structures may not be candidates for sclerosis. After a trial of percutaneous drainage, they may be best served by open surgical or laparoscopic marsupialization (Figure 5–42). Other than pain, no complications were associated with percutaneous treatment in our experience.

Abscess Drainage in Neonates

Hepatic abscess is a known but rarely reported complication associated with umbilical venous catheter (UVC) placement (Montoya, Alam, et al., 1983). Umbilical venous catheters are used almost routinely in very low birth-weight (under 1000 g) infants. Percutaneous treatment of hepatic abscesses in very low birth-weight infants can be performed safely, with gentle technique and small (5 or 6 French) catheters, and may represent a desirable alternative to conservative treatment (Figure 5–43).

Infected Tumors and Hematomas

Successful percutaneous management of fluid associated with a hematoma or necrotic tumor, especially if infected, is usually not achievable. Instillation of a thrombolytic agent (such as urokinase or tissue plasminogen activator) as adjuvant therapy in the management of an uninfected hematoma may increase the likelihood of success.

Inflammatory Bowel Disease

Percutaneous and transrectal management of abdominopelvic fluid collections may be performed safely in children with inflammatory bowel disease (IBD) (Ayuk, Williams, et al., 1996). Such treatment may alleviate the need for open surgery during the

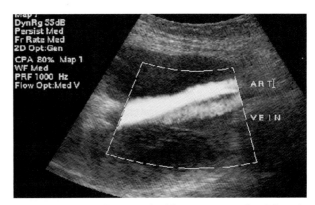

FIGURE 5–42. Ultrasound with power Doppler. Sclerosis of this 4-cm post-renal transplant lymphocele was contraindicated by the risk to encased vessels. The patient is now asymptomatic after percutaneous drainage, laparoscopic marsupialization, and finally surgical drainage.

active phase of disease and may reduce the morbidity of subsequent surgical intervention (Baskin, Chait, et al., 1999a). No enterocutaneous fistulae developed following percutaneous or transrectal drainage in 17 adolescents with IBD treated at our institution since 1992. One pre-existing fistula did not resolve with percutaneous intervention alone.

Ventriculoperitoneal Shunts and Foreign Bodies

The presence of a foreign body within a collection may result in recurrent abscess formation. Nevertheless, percutaneous drainage should be regarded as first-line therapy, in close consultation with the referring neurosurgeon. Infected collections associated with VP shunts may be aspirated percutaneously or drained surgically. The VP shunt is then surgically resited.

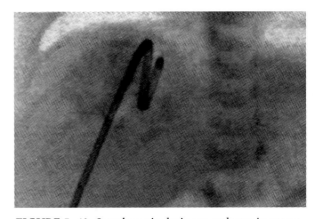

FIGURE 5–43. Intrahepatic drainage catheter in neonatal liver abscess.

Postprocedure Care

Analgesia is provided in the form of intravenous morphine sulfate (0.05 mg per kg every 4 hours for 24 hours) followed by oral acetaminophen (15 mg per kg every 3 to 4 hours as needed). The patient is allowed to ambulate as tolerated. Clear fluids are initially given until the patient has normal bowel movements and bowel sounds. The drainage catheter is left to gravity drainage. A three-way valve is usually placed on the catheter system. Saline lavage of the cavity (5 to 10 cc, 3 to 4 times per day) is followed by gentle irrigation (5 cc of normal saline flushed through the tube after aspiration of the lavaged fluid, 2 to 3 times a day). The volume of output from the tube, less irrigant, is recorded each shift.

Monitoring and Postprocedure Imaging

In children without an impairment of healing, symptoms should resolve substantially within 3 to 5 days following catheter placement. If symptoms persist or worsen, if the collection continues to drain, or if a contrast study reveals a fistula, further investigation is needed. Specifically, a search should be conducted for evidence of undiagnosed or undrained collections, foreign bodies, distal obstruction, or undiagnosed tumor that could account for continued symptoms or drainage. If imaging studies cannot document clear resolution, the catheter may be clamped for one to several days to evaluate for reaccumulation prior to removal.

Removal of Catheter

Progress is usually assessed at 48 to 72 hours with US. If the patient is asymptomatic, laboratory parameters (e.g., white cell counts) are returning to normal, negligible outputs are recorded from the catheter, and imaging (usually US) shows resolution of the collection, no further examinations are required, and the catheter can be removed. Most drainage failures are mechanical, attributed to undrained collections, catheter blockage, poor catheter position, or early removal of the catheter. Specific orders should be left not to remove the catheter without consulting the interventional service.

Results and Complications

Complications of percutaneous drainage are infrequent and usually minor. Fever shortly after initial drainage may represent bacteremia as a result of manipulation or lavage of an abscess cavity. Severe hemorrhage occurs infrequently and is related to unsuspected coagulopathy, laceration of a vessel, or pseudoaneurysm related to pancreatic inflammation. Disruption of the pleura during percutaneous drainage of subphrenic, hepatic, or splenic collections may result in pneumothorax, hemothorax, or pyothorax/empyema. It is possible to contaminate other spaces by traversing them during drainage (such as the subphrenic and subhepatic spaces during drainage of a hepatic abscess). Similarly, generalized peritonitis may develop due to perforation of an abscess cavity. Rarely, bowel perforation may occur at the time of initial puncture or due to catheter erosion. Overall, morbidity associated with image-guided percutaneous drainage is significantly lower than that associated with operative drainages, predominately related to the advantages of real-time US control. Mortality is rare in children treated by percutaneous aspiration or drainage and is more often related to underlying pathology and the clinical status of the patient than to the drainage procedure itself.

BILIARY INTERVENTIONS

General Considerations

Percutaneous transhepatic cholangiography (PTC), percutaneous transhepatic transcholecystic cholangiography (PTTC), percutaneous biliary drainage, dilatation of biliary strictures, and stone removal are all well-established techniques in the treatment of biliary disease (Ring and Kerlan, 1984; Burhenne, 1990; Coons, 1990; Gordon and Ring, 1990; Burke, 1991; Venbrux, 1992; Huard and Do-Xuan-Hop, 1937; Remolar, et al., 1956). The necessity for these procedures has increased substantially with the increasing number of liver transplantations performed in the pediatric population (Hoffer, Teele, et al., 1988; Letourneau, Hunter, et al., 1989; Morrison, Lee, et al., 1990; Klein, Savader, et al., 1991; Peclet, Ryckman, et al., 1994; Bhatnagar, Dhawan, et al., 1995; Chardot, Candinas, et al., 1995). With the increasing availability of transendoscopic management and the advent of magnetic resonance cholangiography, there are fewer applications for transhepatic image-guided biliary diagnosis. However, the percutaneous approach is still indicated prior to percutaneous therapeutic procedures and for patients in whom an endoscopic approach is not appropriate.

Hepatobiliary Structure and Function

Understanding the basic processes involved in normal liver and biliary function helps one gain a greater understanding of the manifestations and complications associated with cholestasis. The liver accounts for up to 5% of body mass in infants and young children. Through its dual blood supply (hepatic and portal), it receives 25% of cardiac output, filtering all splanchnic blood before its return to the heart. With its many specialized functions, including synthesis, storage, detoxification, phagocytosis, and excretion, the liver plays a major role in health and disease from birth through adulthood. The biliary system originates with the excretion of bile from hepatocytes into bile canaliculi. Terminal ductules carry bile from the canaliculi to interlobular ducts, then progressively through segmental ducts and the right and left intrahepatic ducts to leave the liver at the porta hepatis (parallel to the portal vein and hepatic artery) through the common hepatic duct (CHD). The CHD joins the cystic duct to form the common bile duct, draining finally at the ampulla of Vater (with the pancreatic duct in 85 to 90% of patients) or separately (10 to 15% of patients) into the duodenum.

Portal venous blood flow, supplying approximately 75% of afferent blood to the liver, is principally regulated by vascular resistance in extrahepatic vessels, namely, the intestinal, pancreatic, and splanchnic vascular beds. Hepatic arterial flow, which accounts for the remaining 25% of afferent supply, is regulated by sympathetic nerves, blood-borne factors (such as hormones and endotoxins), and the hepatic arterial buffer response (the inverse response of the hepatic artery to changes in portal vein flow) (Lautt, 1977, 1983, 1996; Gundersen, Corso, et al., 1998)

Enterohepatic Circulation

The gallbladder empties 70% of stored concentrated bile acids into the duodenum in a response to meals that is regulated by vagal stimulation and cholecystokinin. These bile acids emulsify dietary fats and facilitate the absorption of triglycerides and fat-soluble vitamins. The majority of bile acids are absorbed in the distal third of the terminal ileum by a specific active transport mechanism (Hofmann, Schteingart, et al., 1991). After deconjugation and dehydroxylation by colonic bacteria, most of the remaining bile acids are resorbed in the colon, with 3 to 5% of the bile salt pool lost through fecal excretion. The remaining bile acids complete the cycle of enterohepatic circulation by returning through the portal circulation for re-excretion into the hepatic sinusoids. The components of enterohepatic circulation pathways may not reach maturity until the end of the first year of life (Balistreri, Heubi, et al., 1983) and may produce cholestasis in the early neonatal period or more importantly, may increase the severity of symptoms related to liver disease in early infancy.

Jaundice in Infancy and Childhood

Infants who are icteric past the first week of life with an elevated conjugated (direct) bilirubin should be promptly evaluated for biliary atresia or other conditions known to cause cholestasis. Compared to physiologic and benign causes of jaundice in a child, the causes of childhood jaundice listed in Table 11–1 (Chapter 11) are quite rare, albeit disproportionately severe in their impact. The issue from an interventional standpoint often is the distinction between treatable and nontreatable causes of jaundice. Interventional radiologists may play a role in either diagnosis or treatment of many of the causes underlying jaundice in the newborn as well as in children after liver or bone marrow transplantation. These causes include intrahepatic disorders such as anatomic abnormalities (e.g., Caroli's disease, congenital hepatic fibrosis, and infantile polycystic disease), infectious, toxic, and metabolic disorders, and extrahepatic disorders such as biliary atresia, bile duct stricture or perforation, choledochal cyst, neoplasia

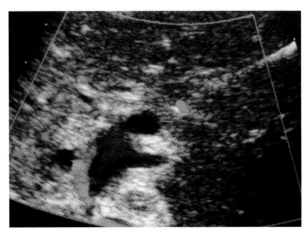

FIGURE 5–44. Percutaneous transhepatic biliary access obtained using ultrasound to avoid vascular structures.

and calculi. Absence of a normal gallbladder and presence of the ultrasonographic "triangular cord" sign support the diagnosis of biliary atresia (Choi, Park, et al., 1998). Other signs of liver injury or failure may not manifest until after the time period (birth to 2 months of age) when surgical treatment is most likely to be successful.

Percutaneous Transhepatic Biliary Access

All percutaneous biliary procedures begin with thin-needle access to the biliary tree under image guidance. These procedures are performed using strict sterile technique. Because these may be some of the more painful interventional procedures and because associated risks increase substantially in the uncooperative patient, we prefer to perform all biliary access procedures under general anesthesia. Patients are intubated, and suspended respiration is used as necessary. Just prior to the procedure, fluoroscopy is performed to identify the position of the diaphragm. Prior imaging is reviewed, and the procedure is performed according to the position of the ducts. Depressed immune function (Vane, Redlich, et al., 1988) and bacterial colonization with enteric organisms (Gallagher, 1990) are common in biliary obstruction, especially associated with liver transplantation (Saint-Vil, Luks, et al., 1991) and bile duct reconstruction (Liu, Li, et al., 1997; Chuang, Chen, et al., 1998). Biliary sepsis from manipulation of infected ducts is the most common cause of serious complications related to these procedures. Therefore, a low threshold should be maintained for the use of pre-procedure antibiotics. It is our practice to administer intravenous gentamicin (2.5 mg per kg), ampicillin (50 mg per kg), and metronidazole (10 mg per kg) as a single dose within 30 minutes prior to beginning the procedure. If there is no suspected cholangitis, pre-procedure cefazolin (40 mg per kg) is given.

Guidance by US is essential to identify dilated ducts or (when ducts are not dilated) the expected position of the ducts. Color Doppler interrogation is often helpful to distinguish ducts from vessels, but the more rapid refresh rate and resolution of gray-scale imaging maximize visualization while advancing the needle (Figure 5–44). The technique for US guidance during access has been discussed in percutaneous biopsy, image guidance, above. A subcostal approach is usually used for access to either right or left ducts. A left-sided subxiphoid approach avoids

the pleura, is more comfortable, and offers more favorable angles for advancement of wires and catheters through the ducts into the common bile duct and to the duodenum. When a right hepatic approach is necessary, the intercostal puncture should be as low as possible in the midaxillary line (below the 10th rib when possible) to decrease the risks of crossing the parietal pleura (e.g., bilo- or pneumothorax, empyema). Wide sterile preparation of the abdomen should be performed to accommodate any necessary change in approach. A 22-Gauge Chiba Hiliter, with a beveled stylet that locks to the needle, has been the most convenient access device for this procedure in our experience (Sukigara, Taguchi, et al., 1994). Upon access, the stylet is replaced by a slip ring (not Luer lock) extension set connected to a syringe. This allows the operator's hands to move out of the fluoroscopic field, and reduces movement of the needle. The selected biliary radicle is gently aspirated for culture, cytology, or other studies, then is slowly injected with contrast under fluoroscopy to outline the biliary tree. Injecting air should be diligently avoided because of potential confusion with the appearance of intraductal calculi. If certain access cannot be obtained under US guidance with the needle tip through the expected location of a bile duct, small amounts of 60% contrast are gently delivered through a small (3- to 5-cc) syringe under fluoroscopy. If persistent filling of a tubular structure is noted, an additional amount of contrast is injected to confirm access. If contrast fills a tubular structure but washes away, a vascular structure has been transgressed, and the needle should continue to be withdrawn. At the time of initial access, transcatheter opening and resting biliary pressures may be measured (McGlynn et al., 1978) using a manometric technique similar to the Whitaker test in the urinary collecting system (Whitaker and Johnston, 1966; vanSonnenberg et al., 1983). However, this is not routinely performed.

Percutaneous Transhepatic Cholangiography

The investigation of injury or obstruction in the biliary tree following liver transplant surgery is the most common indication for cholangiography at our institution. Other important indications include cholestasis and jaundice from primary biliary duct pathology or obstruction such as biliary atresia and choledochal cysts, infections (e.g., neonatal hepatitis) inflammatory conditions such as sclerosing cholangitis or ascending cholangitis, and other treatable causes of cholestasis such as calculi (Chen, 1985; Kim, Chung, et al., 1995). This study also can demonstrate the integrity of a surgical anastomosis and define communications between bilomas or intrahepatic abscesses and the biliary tree. In the evaluation of infantile cholestasis it is most important to distinguish these abnormalities for which surgical or interventional procedures may be vital (e.g., extrahepatic biliary aresia or chole-dochal cyst), and parenchymal infectious, inflammatory or metabolic disorders where such surgical interventions may be contraindicated.

Contraindications

Uncorrectable bleeding diathesis, a history of severe contrast reaction, vascular hepatic tumors, vascular malformations and ascites are regarded as relative contraindications to PTC.

Findings

During cholangiography, abnormal ducts may either be dilated or abnormally small, or may show filling defects or evidence of contrast extravasation (Table 5–11).

Dilated ducts are most often indicative of downstream obstruction or stricture, or following liver transplantation may represent denervation (with elevated resistance at the sphincter of Oddi,) or late-phase ischemic injury. It is not uncommon for ductal narrowing to occur due to accidental injury during surgical or interventional procedures. About 25% of patients with traumatic strictures develop calculi above the stricture. Chronic pancreatitis is another common cause of bile duct narrowing secondary to extrahepatic, extraductal fibrosis. Other causes of biliary ductal narrowing include sclerosing cholangitis and chronic ascending cholangitis. Both display diffuse intra- and extra-hepatic ductal thickening. Associated systemic inflammatory disorders (e.g., Crohn's disease, Riedel's thyroiditis) favor the diagnosis of sclerosing cholangitis while the identification of numerous pericholangitic abscesses favors the diagnosis of chronic ascending cholangitis. Biliary atresia remains the most common cause of cholestasis and liver-related death in neonates. Filling defects, especially following biliary manipulation or surgery, may often represent air bubbles. Positional changes may help distinguish these from

other filling defects. Spasm of Oddi's sphincter, hematomas, benign polypoid ductal tumors, and parasites can also present as filling defects. Biliary calculi are discussed in more detail below. Extravasation of contrast from the biliary tree may represent evidence of elevated intraluminal pressure related to hepatic abscesses, suppurative cholangitis, or other

TABLE 5–11. Abnormal Findings at Cholangiography

Findings	Common Causes
Dilated ducts	Obstruction: e.g.,
	• Extrahepatic biliary atresia
	• Post-surgical stricture
	• Intrahepatic biliary hypoplasia
	• Biliary calculi
	Choledochal cysts
	• Fusiform extrahepatic (Type I)
	• Saccular extrahepatic (Type II)
	• Choledochocele (Type III)
	• Multiple (Type IV)
	• Caroli's disease (Type V)
	Bacterial cholangitis
	Late phase ischemic injury
	Denervation
	Overfilling
Narrow or occluded ducts	Postinflammatory
	Postsurgical
	Biliary atresia
	Fibrosis
	Extrinsic compression (e.g., duodenal duplication)
	Sclerosing cholangitis
	Ascending cholangitis
	AIDS-related cholangitis
	Underfilling
Filling defects	Biliary calculi
	Thrombus
	Debris
	Parasites
	Tumor
	Air bubbles
Contrast extravasation	Obstruction
	Injury
	• Iatrogenic
	• Traumatic
	• Ischemic
	• Radiation
	Anastomotic dehiscence

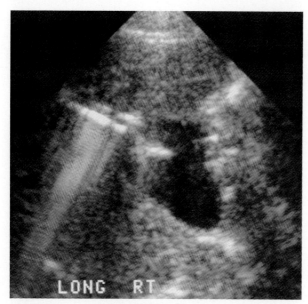

FIGURE 5–45. Ultrasound is used to access gallbladder for percutaneous transhepatic transcholecystic cholangiography. Note that reverberation artifact assists needle tracking.

causes of stricture or obstruction discussed above. It may also represent an intrinsic defect of the ductal wall itself, either through direct injury (e.g., penetrating trauma, surgical or interventional procedures), indirect injury (e.g., hepatic artery thrombosis, ischemia, irradiation) or adjacent inflammation

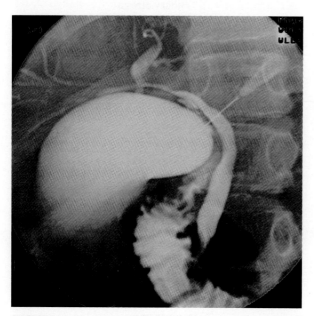

FIGURE 5–46. Contrast injected during a percutaneous transhepatic transcholecystic cholangiogram shows normal biliary anatomy.

(e.g., abscesses, bilomas, ascites, pancreatitis). Biliary leaks may fistulize to bowel, skin or wounds.

Percutaneous Transhepatic Transcholecystic Cholangiography and Transluminal Biopsy

When the bile ducts are undilated and repeated attempts at ERCP or transhepatic access to the intrahepatic ducts are unsuccessful, a transcholecystic approach may provide a route of access for cholangiography (Garel, Belli, et al., 1987; Giorgio, Amoroso, et al., 1988). This procedure is performed with antibiotic coverage. Controlled respiration is important. The needle of choice in this case is a 25-Gauge spinal needle, which has a sharp bevel that allows easier access to the gallbladder. Transhepatic access with US guidance (Figure 5–45) is performed as previously described. If possible, the gallbladder should be entred, where the wall is adherent to the liver, with a short jabbing motion. The free edge of the gallbladder should be avoided to reduce the risk of bile leak and peritonitis. Once the gallbladder has been accessed, bile is aspirated and sent to the laboratory. This is followed by the introduction of dilute contrast. The contrast is injected slowly to fill the biliary tree and identify the structures (Figure 5–46). If necessary, a Trendelenburg position is obtained to fill the intrahepatic ducts. If necessary, morphine can be given during the procedure to paralyze Oddi's sphincter and encourage intrahepatic filling.

Bile leakage is the main risk of the percutaneous transcholecystic approach. If the procedure is performed with diligence and the bile is evacuated from the gallbladder at the end of the procedure, the risk of bowel peritonitis is extremely small. Complete clearance of all bile and contrast is time consuming but necessary.

If a periductal obstructing mass is identified by imaging or suspected in relationship to a biliary stricture, the thin access needle may be exchanged for a suitable sheath. FNA biopsy may be performed through the sheath for cytopathologic analysis (Cozzi et al., 1999). If this is non-diagnostic, a biopsy forceps (Duber et al., 1991) or a transvascular needle, such as the flexible transjugular liver biopsy needle (described in Percutaneous Biopsy, above) (Valji, 1999), may be used to obtain histologic tissue specimens. In smaller children, a periductal tissue sample may be obtained through a second biopsy needle targeted at the region of obstruction under combined US and fluoroscopic guidance.

Biliary Drainage

Indications for biliary drainage include malignant obstruction associated with cholangitis and pleuritis, bile leakage post surgery or due to trauma and strictures related to either surgery or sclerosing cholangitis. The pediatric patients who most commonly need biliary drainage are transplant patients with ischemic strictures following hepatic artery thrombosis (Hoffer, Teele, et al., 1988; Chardot, Candinas, et al., 1995). Percutaneous transhepatic drainage is particularly well-suited to patients with large post-operative biliary defects or with bile leaks associated with severe acute necrotizing pancreatitis (Ernst et al., 1999). Percutaneous drainage may avoid the need for surgical re-exploration, surgical or endoscopic sphincterectomy, or even hepatic lobectomy. Although endoscopic drainage is an alternative, it is usually not possible in the presence of a hepaticojejunal anastomosis.

Initially, diagnostic cholangiography is performed, and a biliary duct is chosen for entry of the percutaneous drain. If the first duct to which access is obtained is not suitable for passage of a wire and drain to the duodenum, the needle is left in place for cholangiography. Using the "roadmap" provided by this cholangiogram, a second 22-Gauge Chiba Hiliter needle is placed in a more appropriate biliary radicle under US and fluoroscopic guidance. A small amount of bile is aspirated, and placement is confirmed with a gentle injection of contrast. This is followed by introduction of a 0.018-inch mandril wire or, if there is some concern about maintaining access, a hydrophilic wire. The tract is then dilated with an introducer system to allow access for a larger wire and catheter. Once access is obtained with a catheter and wire, the system is then further delineated and the area of abnormality or stricture identified (Figure 5–47). The catheter and wire are advanced to the area of abnormality and attempts are made to pass the wire (followed by the catheter) down past the stricture. If there is evidence of suppurative cholangitis, or if persistent attempts to pass a wire beyond the area of abnormality are unsuccessful, completion of the procedure is deferred. An external catheter is left in position for drainage and the patient is scheduled for completion of the procedure at a later date. Usually, following a day or two of decompression and antibiotics, infection or inflammation will subside and the area of abnormality may be more easily traversed.

After access to the abnormal area has been obtained, a stiff 0.035-inch Amplatz wire may be used to give better leverage. Balloon dilatation of the stricture can be performed at this time (Figure 5–48). An external/internal Cope loop drainage catheter is positioned with the loop fixed in the duodenum (Figure 5–49), and side holes added above and below the area of abnormality to divert bile flow from the defect and improve healing. The catheter is fixed in position with a suture through the skin or through a stoma device.

Patients are usually returned to the ward with the catheter initially left to gravity drainage. The catheter is flushed twice daily with 5- to 10-cc of sterile saline to keep the catheter and side-holes clear of thrombus or debris. To avoid protein and calorie malnutrition, fluid and electrolyte depletion, and to assist uptake of drugs (e.g., cyclosporine) that depend on enterohepatic circulation, early internalization of biliary drainage is desirable. Once the draining bile clears, a trial of internal drainage is attempted by capping the external drain. If this is successful and long-term drainage is anticipated, conversion to a completely internal drain or stent may be considered. If internalization is not feasible, clear bile drainage may be given to the patient transgastrically.

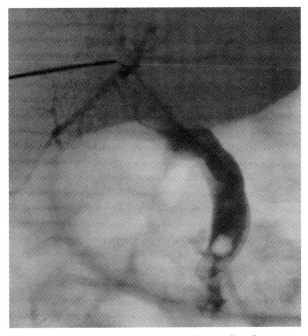

FIGURE 5–47. 22-Gauge needle and 0.018" Teflon-coated wire with contrast in dilated common bile duct with calculus.

Biliary Dilatation and Stenting

Dilatation of biliary strictures is usually performed with balloon catheters over a wire (Hancock, Wiseman, et al., 1989; Morrison, Lee, et al., 1990; Ward, Kiely, et al., 1990; Zajko, Sheng, et al., 1995). The size of the balloon used for dilatation should be gauged according to the diameter of the duct proximal and distal to the area of stricture. Often, several dilatations are performed, each lasting no more than 15 seconds. After dilatation, a biliary drain is usually left in position, with side holes made above and below this area of stricture. Internal biliary drains are seldom used in the pediatric population. Occasionally, expandable Palmaz stents have been used for anastamotic strictures in liver transplant patients.

T-tube cholangiography is performed in patients who have a T tube placed during surgical removal of the gallbladder or following liver transplant with hepatojejunal anastomosis. Retained stones or debris can be removed via this tract. The tract is usually allowed to mature for approximately 6 weeks. Then, either the tract may be safely dilated, removing residual stones using a sheath and basket, or the ampulla may be dilated with a balloon.

Transhepatic Removal of Biliary Calculi

Calculi within the biliary tree can be removed percutaneously through a mature biliary drain tract, using a basket and a sheath to remove the sludge, stones, and debris (Park, Choi, et al., 1987; Chiang, Shan, et al., 1994).

PORTAL VENOUS INTERVENTIONS

Access and Technique

The portal venous (PV) system can be accessed percutaneously via the transhepatic route easily and safely under US guidance. The technique is similar to percutaneous transhepatic biliary access, using a 22-Gauge Chiba needle. This is followed by placement of a 0.018-inch wire, then an introducer system. This allows for dilatation of strictures post transplantation (Figure 5–50), embolization of varices, and direct measurement of PV pressure when the PV and hepatic sinusoidal systems are discontinuous (e.g., extrahepatic PV obstruction, splenic vein obstruction, or presinusoidal portal hypertension (Egawa, Tanaka, et al., 1993; Funaki, Rosenblum, et al., 1995; Funaki, Rosenblum, et al., 1997). Embolization of PV-to-hepatic venous malformations is possible in patients with hepatic hemangiomas (Pereyra, Andrassy, et al., 1982; Burrows, Rosenberg, et al., 1985; Becker and Heitler, 1989). Recent reports have also raised the possibili-

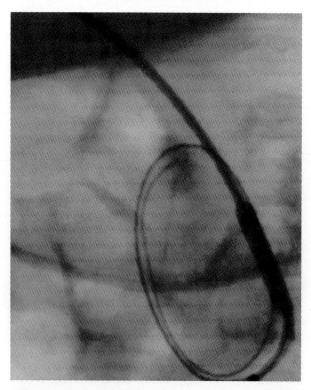

FIGURE 5–48. Common bile duct stricure is dilated using a balloon catheter.

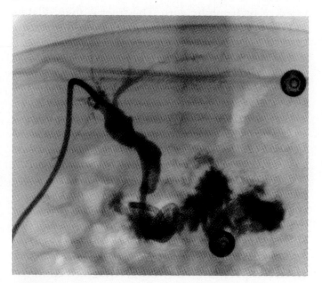

FIGURE 5–49. A catheter is placed after dilation for drainage and access.

ty of embolizing PV branches to induce hepatocyte replication for gene therapy (Duncan et al., 1999).

Transjugular Intrahepatic Portosystemic Shunt

The transjugular intrahepatic portosystemic shunt (TIPS) procedure involves the creation of a parenchymal tract between the hepatic and portal veins with a metallic stent (LaBerge, Ring, et al., 1993; Johnson, Leyendecker, et al., 1996; Cao, Monge, et al., 1997; Heyman, LaBerge, et al., 1997; Hackworth, Leef, et al., 1998; Boyvat, Cekirge, et al., 1999). Indications (Table 5–12) include treatment of GI bleeding, varices, or intractable ascites due to portal hypertension. Other indications for this procedure include relief of hepatic outflow obstruction (i.e., Budd-

Chiari syndrome) (Ganger et al., 1999) and reduction of intraoperative morbidity during liver transplantation surgery (Ochs, Sellinger, et al., 1993; McCormick, Dick, et al., 1994; Strunk, Textor, et al., 1997; Ganger, Klapman, et al., 1999; Ryu, Durham, et al., 1999; Sanyal, 1999; Yamada, Nakamura, et al., 1999). Candidates for TIPS should be evaluated with fiberoptic endoscopy to confirm the presence of varices and exclude other sources of hemorrhage for which alternative therapies would be more appropriate. Color and spectral Doppler US should be used to evaluate the size and patency of the portal and hepatic veins and to ascertain the presence of hepatic or abdominal masses or ascites (Feldstein, 1998). Contraindications include heart failure, polycystic liver disease, infection, severe hepatic encephalopathy, and severe liver failure. TIPS is described as a safe and effective procedure for the reduction of PV pressure in children as young as 3 years of age, with a short-term success rate of 75–90% (Johnson et al., 1996; Heymann et al., 1997). Long-term complications arise due to intimal hyperplasia, stricture, and thrombus within the shunt lumen (Freedman et al., 1993).

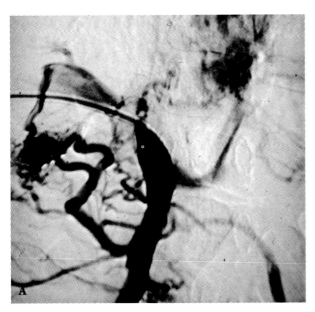

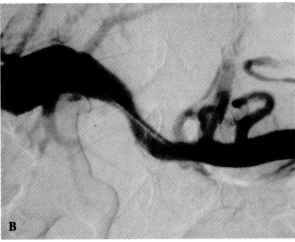

FIGURE 5–50. A, Portal venous stricture B, Portal vein dilation

TABLE 5–12. Indications and Contraindications for TIPS*

Accepted indications
  Acute variceal bleeding unresponsive to medical
    therapy (including sclerotherapy)
  Recurrent variceal bleeding unresponsive to medical
    therapy (including repeated sclerotherapy)
  Intractable ascites
Debated indications
  Portal hypertension from hepatic outflow
    obstruction (i.e., Budd-Chiari syndrome)
  Bridge to liver transplantation
  Initial therapy to treat or prevent variceal
    hemorrhage
Absolute contraindications
  Polycystic liver disease
  Severe hepatic failure
  Severe right-sided heart failure
Relative contraindications
  Severe hepatic encephalopathy
  Hypervascular liver tumor
  Portal vein thrombosis
  Severe active infection

*From Valji, 1999, with permission.

Minor procedural complications have occurred in approximately 10% of cases. Hepatic encephalopathy occurs in 5–35% of patients following TIPS (Sawhney et al., 1998). Other severe life-threatening complications are reported in less than 5% of patients, and include hemoperitoneum, hemobilia and biliary fistula, acute hepatic ischemia, pulmonary hypertension, and pulmonary edema. Chronic complications include PV thrombosis, hemolysis, and shunt stenosis. Typed and crossed blood should be available for emergent transfusion, and a PICU bed should be available for close monitoring, should the need arise.

The procedure is approached via a right internal jugular puncture under US guidance in the Trendelenberg position. A wire and catheter are introduced into the right hepatic vein selectively (although the middle or left hepatic veins may be used in the event the right is occluded). IVC pressure, free-, and wedge-hepatic pressures are measured and free- and wedge-hepatic venograms are performed (as described under Transjugular Liver Biopsy, above). The wedge hepatic venogram, (which may be performed with iodinated contrast or CO_2) usually demonstrates PV structures and direction of flow. A sheath and a Colapinto or Rosch-Uchida transjugular needle then replace the catheter. The needle is advanced through the sheath, either under US guidance (Longo et al., 1992) or by "road mapping" from the previous wedge venogram, until it enters the PV system. The PV entry point should be several centimeters away from the junction of the right and left PV to avoid massive hemorrhage, as this junction is extrahepatic in a large proportion of patients.

When blood is obtained, contrast is injected to confirm the position within a PV branch. A wire is then introduced securely into the splenic or superior mesenteric vein and the tract is dilated. The extent of dilatation depends on the size of the patient but usually ranges up to 8 mm. The balloon is deflated, and the transjugular catheter and a 9 French sheath are advanced into the vein. The transjugular catheter is then removed, and the sheath is left in position. A flexible wall stent (Schneider USA, Minneapolis) is then introduced on a balloon and positioned centrally within the hepatoportal tract. The balloon is inflated to distend the stent. PV pressures are recorded, and venography is performed to confirm patency. Additional stents are placed as needed to bridge the tract from the PV to the hepatic vein. Subsequent liver transplantation is less complicated if the stent does not extend into the IVC or deeply into the main PV.

Following the procedure, there is usually hepatopetal flow to the IVC, with collapse of varices. Rarely, the varices persist despite a well-functioning shunt, in which case embolization is performed. If the shunt is felt to be open but the pressure remains above 12 mm Hg, the stent is usually dilated up to 10 mm (Casado et al., 1998). If the pressure remains elevated, a second parallel stent can be placed (Haskal, Ring, et al., 1992). If the TIPS procedure was performed for uncontrolled variceal hemorrhage, gastric varices of splenic or coronary venous origin are often embolized with coils at the conclusion of the TIPS procedure.

Within 24 hours the TIPS procedure is followed up with Doppler US to confirm shunt patency and establish baseline flow measurements. If some stenosis or occlusion occurs or is suspected, the patient is restudied, and the stricture is dilated with an angioplasty catheter.

DILATATION OF HOLLOW VISCERA

Esophageal Dilatation

Balloon dilatation is probably the most common procedure performed in the esophagus (Cox, Winter, et al., 1994). Esophageal dilatation is often needed as a result of strictures caused by tracheoesophageal fistula, lye ingestion, reflux stricture, postoperative stricture, and achalasia. Complications following dilatation include pain, tracheal aspiration and perforation with mediastinitis or hemorrhage (Kim et al., 1993). The incidence of mediastinal infection is low and we have not experienced such a problem using the interventional techniques described below. We have successfully treated postoperative paraesophageal leakage and fluid collections with percutaneous drainage.

Technique

We usually perform oesophageal dilatations under general anesthesia. The esophagus is cannulated with a JB1 5 French catheter over a Benston 0.035-inch wire either transnasally or transorally. A small amount of contrast is instilled to outline the usual pre-stricture pouch and to delineate the length and character of the stricture itself (Figure 5–51). The wire is advanced past the stricture and coiled in the stomach. The directional catheter is exchanged for a balloon catheter. In postsurgical or lye strictures, dilatation is performed with an angioplasty balloon of a diameter similar to or smaller than the diameter of the esophagus above and below the stricture. We start with an undersized balloon and serially increase the diameter depending upon the tightness of the stricture and the acuteness of the "waist" seen during inflation (Figure 5–51). The balloon is inflated with iodinated contrast (Omnipaque 300) diluted in a 1:1 ratio with normal saline. Longer strictures are progressively dilated from the distal to the proximal extent. The balloon is ordinarily not inflated for more than 30 seconds at a time. Although pressure gauges are available, we usually inflate by hand. At the conclusion of the procedure the wire is removed and a contrast esophagram performed in two planes during withdrawal of the balloon catheter. It is not unusual for the stricture to appear unchanged immediately following dilatation due to mucosal edema. This appearance does not correlate with the clinical efficacy of the procedure. After deflation of the balloon, residual contrast in the pre-

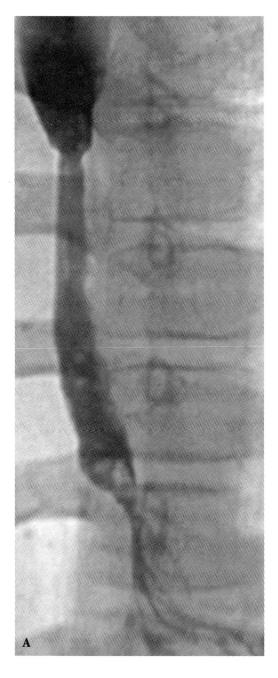

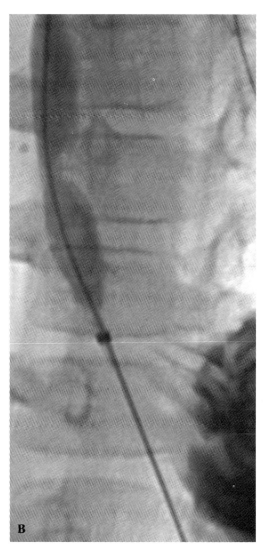

FIGURE 5–51. Post-reflux esophageal stricture and dilation

stricture pouch is aspirated through the balloon catheter as completely as possible, to reduce the risk of post-procedure tracheal aspiration. The child is observed in the PACU for several hours, and may be discharged if stable. Oral intake is restricted to clear fluids for the first 24 hours, after which normal feeding may be resumed.

Placement of an esophageal stent has been performed in children with persistent strictures (Chait et al., 1999), using either a nitinol coil-type stent or a solid silicone (Novathane) stent. The nitinol stent is easily placed but is frequently complicated by mucosal overgrowth.

Colonic Dilatation

Transcatheter balloon dilatation of strictures related to necrotizing enterocolitis (Figure 5–52) or other

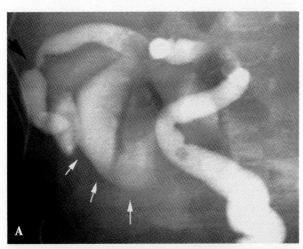

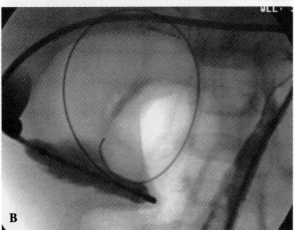

FIGURE 5–52. *A*, Colonic stricture (*black arrow*) related to necrotizing enterocolitis. Note prestenotic bowel dilation (*white arrows*). *B*, Balloon dilation of the stricure was performed.

causes is performed on occasion with variable results (Ball et al., 1985; Renfrew et al., 1986; Johnson and Lang, 1993). Antibiotic coverage is provided as previously outlined. Persistence of the stricture post dilatation may necessitate surgical resection.

GASTROINTESTINAL VASCULAR INTERVENTIONS

Management of Gastrointestinal Bleeding

Gastrointestinal (GI) bleeding in the pediatric population usually presents as a self-limited process and seldom requires angiographic intervention. Emergent surgical intervention for acute GI bleeding carries a high mortality. Prompt efforts

---

TABLE 5–13. Causes of Significant Gastrointestinal Bleeding in Children

---

Acute bleeding
    Varices (especially related to portal hypertension)
    Peptic ulcer disease (PUD)
    Meckel's diverticulum (with ectopic functional
      gastric mucosa)
    Intussusception
    Mallory-Weiss tear
    Intestinal infarction
    Hemobilia
    Anastomotic erosion or dehiscence
    Vascular malformation
Chronic recurrent bleeding
    Gastritis
    Inflammatory bowel disease
    Hemangioma
    Typhlitis
    Angiodysplasia
    Polyps
Gastrointestinal bleeding in the infant
    PUD
    Esophagitis
    Gastritis
    Meckel's diverticulum
    Nasopharyngeal bleeding
    Intussusception
    Necrotizing enterocolitis
    Vascular malformation
    GI duplication
    Tube erosion or perforation

---

to stop or slow massive bleeding by a transcatheter route may convert an emergent surgical procedure into a less-urgent or elective procedure and may significantly improve the final outcome. Even in those cases where transcatheter therapy has a lower success rate, such as angiodysplasia and arteriovenous malformations, coils placed pre-operatively may assist the surgeon in locating the site of bleeding, and methylene blue delivered through a catheter intraoperatively may help localize a vascular malformation, thus avoiding a blind laparotomy (Fishman et al., 1998). In general, transcatheter therapy is reserved for the approximately 25% of patients who do not respond to conservative therapy and who are poor surgical candidates. When GI bleeding manifests as a life-threatening condition (Table 5–13) it may represent a significant diagnostic and therapeutic problem. An initial hematocrit less than 20% or hemoglobin less than 7 g/100 ml, transfusions prior to intervention equal to or greater than 85 ml/kg, inability to identify the site of bleeding, presence of an associated coagulation abnormality and coexistence of another life-threatening disease are all predictive of a poor outcome (Cox and Ament, 1979). Stabilizing and supporting the patient are the first priorities. More than one large-bore IV, a nasogastric tube, transfusion, correction of coagulopathy, and gastric ice water lavage should be implemented before further measures are initiated. If one has not been placed, consideration should be given to insertion of a large-bore central venous line at the time of initial angiographic examination. Initial studies in these patients are directed toward locating the level and volume of blood loss.

Fiberoptic endoscopy is often beneficial in the diagnosis and treatment of bleeding above the ligament of Treitz and, to a lesser degree, in the lower intestinal tract. However, presence of a large volume of intraluminal blood will severely limit its value. US with Doppler, or CT- and MR-scans with contrast, may show evidence of a site of active bleeding or the compartment containing the resulting hematoma, but are otherwise not first-line studies for the evaluation of GI bleeding. For active bleeding of 0.05 to 0.4 ml/min, ^{99m}Tc-sulfur colloid scintigraphic scans (Alavi, 1982) with continuous dynamic imaging (Maurer, 1996) may be the most sensitive means of detecting the location of bleeding. A ^{99m}Tc-labeled red blood cell scan (Shah et al., 1979) does not require active bleeding at the time of injection and may help predict which patients require urgent angiographic intervention (Ng et al., 1997). If extravasated agent is not detected within the first 15 minutes, the patient may be periodically re-scanned over the following 24 hours (Winzelberg et al., 1982).

For active bleeding greater than 0.4 ml/min, or when there is persistent passage of large volumes of blood, or transfusion requirements for more than 12- to 20-ml packed-red-blood-cells/kg/24-hr, angiography should be promptly employed. If an upper GI bleed is suspected, the initial angiographic examination should include selective injection of the celiac axis and superior mesenteric artery (SMA), including visualization of the left gastric, gastroduodenal, pancreaticoduodenal and splenic arteries. A suspected lower GI bleed should lead to examination of the SMA then the inferior mesenteric artery (IMA). Repeat injections in multiple planes may be required to evaluate the complete distribution of each vessel. Injection of the aorta should be reserved for a last-resort search for alternative bleeding sites (e.g., inferior phrenic or lumbar arteries). Subselective injections should be used as needed to precisely identify the feeding vessels. The "pseudovein" sign from extravasation of contrast into an intraluminal thrombus, or a persistent blush in end-organ tissues may be helpful correlating signs of bleeding. False negative exams may relate to a lack of active bleeding at the time of injection, or to incomplete examination of the feeding vessels. False positive exams are reported from parenchymal blush, such as from the adrenal gland or hyperemic gastric mucosa. Active extravasation of contrast into a persistent "puddle" should be demonstrated to confirm the diagnosis and location of active bleeding.

Once the site of GI hemorrhage has been identified the angiographer must select the most appropriate therapeutic intervention, generally either induced vasoconstriction or embolization (Figure 5–53). Balloon tamponade, sclerotherapy, TIPS, electro- and thermal-coagulation, and laser photocoagulation also have been used under select circumstances.

Intra-arterial Vasopressin Infusion

Vasopressin is the most commonly used vasoconstricting agent. It causes a significant and prolonged reduction in splanchnic blood flow and PV pressure. The effect can be titrated by adjusting the rate of

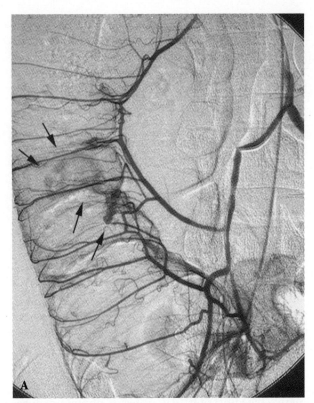 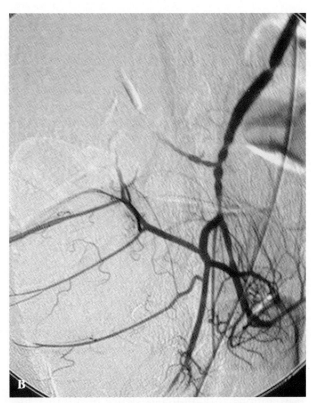

FIGURE 5–53. Selective superior mesenteric artery, right colic branch injection demonstrating active bleeding (*black arrows*) into the ascending colon which has been distended with air. *B*, Contrast injection after Gelfoam embolization demonstrates resolution of bleeding.

infusion, thereby posing little danger of significant end-organ ischemia in the GI tract. Vasopressin is particularly successful in the control of gastric mucosal bleeding. For bleeding in the large or small bowel, subselective catheterization may not be required, as SMA or IMA injection is often sufficient. Vasopressin is contraindicated in patients with dysrythmias or severe hypertension. It is not the therapy of choice for bleeding directly from a large artery, or for bleeding at sites with a dual blood supply (e.g., pyloroduodenal hemorrhage) (Waltman et al., 1979).

As yet, no vasopressin administration regimen has been specifically developed for use in the paediatric population. Most reports have relied upon adult dosages (Eckstein et al., 1984; Meyerovitz and Fellows, 1984; Afshani and Berger, 1986), although a dose of 0.1- to 0.4-U/min/1.73 m^2 body surface area has been recommended (Roy et al., 1981). Vasopressin is initially infused at a rate of 0.1- to 0.2-U/min/1.73 m^2 body surface area (0.1- to 0.2-U/min in adults) for 20- to 30-min through the selectively placed intra-arterial catheter. If repeat arteriography

demonstrates continued bleeding, the rate of administration may be doubled for an additional 20- to 30-min. If repeat arteriography at this point shows continued bleeding, further dosage increases are unlikely to be helpful, and embolization should be considered. One report (Tuggle et al., 1988) suggests that the highest rate of complications is associated with infusion rates greater than 0.01-U/kg/min., without improved control of bleeding. The infusion rate that corresponds to cessation of bleeding may be continued for 6- to 72-hours. If bleeding has stopped completely, the rate of infusion should be halved every 6- to 12-hours to a minimum rate of 0.1-U/min/1.73 m^2 body surface area. Heparinized D$_5$W (at approximately 25% of the weight-appropriate maintenance rate recommended in Table 5–3) should then be infused for an additional 4- to 6-hours. If there is no further bleeding, the catheter may be removed. Patients often report mild abdominal discomfort at the start of vasopressin infusion, which generally subsides in the first 10- to 15-min and should not recur. If pain persists it may herald more severe bowel ischemia. After assuring by repeat arteriography that the catheter tip position has not changed (Kadir and Athanq-soulis, 1978), the rate should be decreased until symptoms resolve. Urinary output and electrolytes must be monitored due to vasopressin's known antidiuretic effect. Abnormal changes should be treated with diuretics and electrolyte infusions, not by altering the rate of vasopressin administration.

Transcatheter Embolization

Embolotherapy has the potential for immediate and permanent cessation of bleeding without the risks associated with vasopressin and prolonged catheterization. The major risks of embolization include end-organ infarction and reflux of embolic material to unwanted sites. The extensive collateral circulation of the upper GI tract decreases the risk of infarction in this distribution. Embolization is indicated for patients who either fail or do not tolerate a trial of vasopressin infusion; to treat sites of greatest expected efficacy (e.g., duodenal or marginal ulcers; gastric, duodenal or pancreatic artery pseudoaneurysm complicating an adjacent inflammatory process such as pancreatitis or PUD); as a temporizing measure prior to surgical intervention; and as empiric therapy in the case of a massive unlocalized GI bleed.

Approximately 80% of massive upper GI hemorrhages are in the territory supplied by the left gastric artery. Empiric embolization of this vessel should be considered when all angiographic and endoscopic attempts at localization have failed, and the patient faces imminent multi-organ failure (Lang et al., 1992; Lang, pers. comm.). Embolotherapy should be avoided in the face of previous gastric or bowel surgery or radiation therapy or under other circumstances when adequate collateral circulation is impaired or in doubt. "Sandwiching" a site of persistent hemorrhage with a dual blood supply by placing embolic agents on either side of the site of bleeding may resolve the hemorrhage but increases the risk of end-organ infarction (Ring et al., 1977). A small area of infarction, which may be heralded by peritoneal signs, is well tolerated in most patients. A larger area of infarction will likely require surgery.

Macro- or microcoils are the preferred embolic devices for most GI bleeding applications, as they may be placed with the greatest precision of any permanent agent. Alternative agents for specific applications include Gelfoam "torpedoes" or slurries, polyvinyl alcohol particles (Ivalon), autologous blood clot (with or without co-treatment with aminocaproic acid), thrombin, isobutyl 2-cyanoacrylate (bucrylate) and detachable balloons. Coils should be deposited as distally in the arterial arcade as possible, but proximal to the bleeding vasa recta, to minimize the length of bowel at risk for ischemia (Valji, 1999).

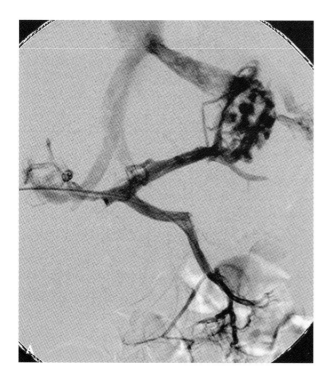

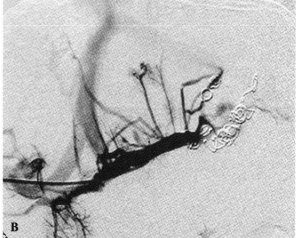

FIGURE 5–54. *A*, Selective portal venogram shows hemangioendotheliomas and hepatic venous (HV) shunting. *B*, After coil embolization HV shunting is improved. Following embolization there was stabilization of the patient's high output cardiac failure.

Embolization of tumors (usually pre-operatively), focal aneurysms (Kadir et al., 1980; Janik et al., 1981; Gow et al., 1996; Sawlani et al., 1996; Sidhu et al., 1999) and vascular malformations is occasionally performed using similar techniques. Embolization therapy for liver hemangoendotheliomas (Figure 5–54) is performed in patients who have failed conservative medical treatment with steroids and interferon (Pereyra et al., 1982; Burrows et al., 1985; Becker and Heitler, 1989). Angiography should be performed to confirm the hepatic arterial supply to the mass and to identify any supply from PV structures. The presence of hepatic arterial to hepatic venous shunts must also be identified prior to embolization, as they carry an increased risk of lung embolization.

REFERENCES

AAP. Guidelines for the elective use of conscious sedation, deep sedation, and general anesthesia in pediatric patients. Committee on Drugs. Section on anesthesiology. Pediatrics 1985;76(2):317–21.

AAP. American Academy of Pediatrics Committee on Drugs: guidelines for monitoring and management of pediatric patients during and after sedation for diagnostic and therapeutic procedures. Pediatrics 1992;89(6 Pt 1):1110–5.

AAP. American Academy of Pediatrics Committee on Drugs and Committee on Environmental Health: Use of chloral hydrate for sedation in children. Pediatrics 1993;92(3):471–3.

AAP. Informed consent, parental permission, and assent in pediatric practice. Committee on Bioethics, American Academy of Pediatrics. Pediatrics 1995;95(2):314–7.

Afshani E, Berger PE. Gastrointestinal tract angiography in infants and children. J Pediatr Gastroenterol Nutr 1986;5(2):173–86.

Alavi A. Detection of gastrointestinal bleeding with 99mTc-sulfur colloid. Semin Nucl Med 1982;12(2):126–38.

Amundson GM, Towbin RB, et al. Percutaneous transgastric drainage of the lesser sac in children. Pediatr Radiol 1990;20(8):590–3.

Ayuk P, Williams N, et al. Management of intra-abdominal abscesses in Crohn's disease. Ann R Coll Surg Engl 1996;78(1):5–10.

Ball WS Jr, Kosloske AM, et al. Balloon catheter dilatation of focal intestinal strictures following necrotizing enterocolitis. J Pediatr Surg 1985;20(6):637–9.

Bartholome WG. A new understanding of consent in pediatric practice: consent, parental permission, and child assent. Pediatr Ann 1989;18(4):262–5.

Bartolo DC. Gastroenterological options in faecal incontinence. Ann Chir 1991;45(7):590–8.

Baskin KM, Chait PG, et al. Percutaneous drainage of pelvic abscesses in children with inflammatory bowel disease. Canadian Association of Radiologists Journal 1999 [abstract];50(Suppl.): S67.

Baskin KM, Chait PG, et al. Minimally invasive management of lymphocoeles in pediatric renal transplant patients. Canadian Association of Radiologists Journal 1999 [abstract];50(Suppl.): S32.

Becker JM, Heitler MS. Hepatic hemangioendotheliomas in infancy. Surg Gynecol Obstet 1989;168(2):189–200.

Bell SD, Carmody EA, et al. Percutaneous gastrostomy and gastrojejunostomy: additional experience in 519 procedures. Radiology 1995;194(3):817–20.

Berquist WE. Biofeedback therapy for anorectal disorders in children. Semin Pediatr Surg 1995;4(1):48–53.

Bhatnagar V, Dhawan A, et al. The incidence and management of biliary complications following liver transplantation in children. Transpl Int 1995;8(5):388–91.

Bishop PR, Nowicki MJ. Defecation disorders in the neurologically impaired child. Pediatr Ann 1999;28(5):322–9.

Bleck JS, Reiss B, et al. Percutaneous sonographic gastrostomy: method, indications, and problems. Am J Gastroenterol 1998;93(6):941–5.

Borge MA, Vesely TM, Picus D. Gastrostomy button placement through percutaneous gastrostomy tracts created with fluoroscopic guidance: experience in 27 children. J Vasc Interv Radiol 1995;6(2):179–83.

Borkowski S. Pediatric stomas, tubes, and appliances. Pediatr Clin North Am 1998;45(6):1419–35.

Boyd KJ, Beeken L. Tube feeding in palliative care: benefits and problems. Palliat Med 1994;8(2):156–8.

Boyvat F, Cekirge S, et al. Treatment of a TIPS-biliary fistula by stent-graft in a 9–year-old boy. Cardiovasc Intervent Radiol 1999;22(1):67–8.

Burhenne HJ. The history of interventional radiology of the biliary tract. Radiol Clin North Am 1990;28(6):1139–44.

Burke DR. Biliary and other gastrointestinal interventions. Curr Opin Radiol 1991;3(2):151–9.

Burnweit C, Wesson D, et al. Percutaneous drainage of traumatic pancreatic pseudocysts in children. J Trauma 1990;30(10):1273–7.

Burrows PE, Rosenberg HC, Chuang HS. Diffuse hepatic hemangiomas: percutaneous transcatheter embolization with detachable silicone balloons. Radiology 1985;156(1): 85–8.

Bush WH, Swanson DP. Acute reactions to intravascular contrast media: types, risk factors, recognition, and specific treatment. AJR Am J Roentgenol 1991;157(6):1153–61.

Campra J, Reynolds T. The hepatic circulation. In: The liver: biology and pathobiology. New York: Raven Press 1988:911–930.

Cantani A. Latex allergy in children. J Investig Allergol Clin Immunol 1999;9(1):14–20.

Cao S, Monge H, et al. Emergency transjugular intrahepatic portosystemic shunt (TIPS) in an infant: a case report. J Pediatr Surg 1997;32(1):125–7.

Casado M, Bosch J, et al. Clinical events after transjugular intrahepatic portosystemic shunt: correlation with hemodynamic findings. Gastroenterology 1998;114(6): 1296–303.

Casola G, Withers C, et al. Percutaneous cecostomy for decompression of the massively distended cecum. Radiology 1986;158(3):793–4.

Chait P. Future directions in interventional pediatric radiology. Pediatr Clin North Am 1997;44(3):763–82.

Chait P, Temple M, et al. Use of esophageal stents in children with tracheosophageal fistula. European Society for Pediatric Radiology Meeting Syllabus 1999 [abstract]; Jerusalem, June 1999.

Chait PG, Baskin KM, et al. Access to the gastric lumen during percutaneous gastrostomy in paediatric patients with intervening gas-filled bowel. European Society of Pediatric Radiology Meeting Syllabus 1999 [abstract].

Chait PG, Shandling B, et al. Fecal incontinence in children: treatment with percutaneous cecostomy tube placement—a prospective study. Radiology 1997;203(3):621–4.

Chait PG, Weinberg J, et al. Retrograde percutaneous gastrostomy and gastrojejunostomy in 505 children: a 4 1/2–year experience. Radiology 1996;201(3):691–5.

Chardot C, Candinas D, et al. Biliary complications after paediatric liver transplantation: Birmingham's experience. Transpl Int 1995;8(2):133–40.

Chen LY. [Percutaneous transhepatic cholangiography in the diagnosis of congenital choledochal cyst in infants and children]. Chung Hua Fang She Hsueh Tsa Chih 1985;19(2):93–5.

Chiang HJ, Shan TY, Chen CJ. Percutaneous biliary stone removal under fluoroscopy. Chung Hua I Hsueh Tsa Chih (Taipei) 1994;54(5):343–8.

Christoph RA, Buchanan L, et al. Pain reduction in local anesthetic administration through pH buffering. Ann Emerg Med 1988;17(2):117–20.

Chuang JH, Chen WJ, et al. Prompt colonization of the hepaticojejunostomy and translocation of bacteria to liver after bile duct reconstruction. J Pediatr Surg 1998; 33(8):1215–8.

Ciaccia D, Quigley RL, et al. A case of retrograde jejunoduodenal intussusception caused by a feeding gastrostomy tube. Nutr Clin Pract 1994;9(1):18–21.

Clark JA, Pugash RA, Pantalone RR. Radiologic peroral gastrostomy. J Vasc Interv Radiol 1999;10(7):927–32.

Clark RA, Towbin R. Abscess drainage with CT and ultrasound guidance. Radiol Clin North Am 1983;21(3): 445–59.

Cohen MD. Choosing contrast media for the evaluation of the gastrointestinal tract of neonates and infants. Radiology 1987;162(2):447–56.

Cohen MD. Choosing contrast media for pediatric gastrointestinal examinations. Crit Rev Diagn Imaging 1990;30(4):317–40.

Cohen MD, Smith JA. Intravenous use of ionic and nonionic contrast agents in children. Radiology 1994;191(3): 793–4.

Comeau RM, Fenster A, Peters TM. Intraoperative US in interactive image-guided neurosurgery. Radiographics 1998;18(4):1019–27.

Connolly BL, Chait PG, et al. Recognition of intussusception around gastrojejunostomy tubes in children. AJR Am J Roentgenol 1998;170(2):467–70.

Coons H. Biliary intervention—technique and devices: a commentary. Cardiovasc Intervent Radiol 1990;13(4): 211–6.

Cope C, Davis AG, et al. Direct percutaneous jejunostomy: techniques and applications—ten years experience. Radiology 1998;209(3):747–54.

Corbally MT, Blake NS, Guiney EJ. Management of pancreatic pseudocyst in childhood: an increasing role for percutaneous external drainage. J R Coll Surg Edinb 1992;37(3):169–71.

Corr P, Beningfield SJ, Davey N. Transjugular liver biopsy: a review of 200 biopsies. Clin Radiol 1992;45(4):238–9.

Cosgrove M, Jenkins HR. Experience of percutaneous endoscopic gastrostomy in children with Crohn's disease. Arch Dis Child 1997;76(2):141–3.

Coventry BJ, Karatassas A, et al. Intestinal passage of the PEG end-piece: is it safe? J Gastroenterol Hepatol 1994; 9(3):311–3.

Cox JG, Winter RK, et al. Balloon or bougie for dilatation of benign esophageal stricture? Dig Dis Sci 1994; 39(4): 776–81.

Cox K, Ament ME. Upper gastrointestinal bleeding in children and adolescents. Pediatrics 1979;63(3):408–13.

Cozzi G, Alasio L, et al. Percutaneous intraductal sampling for cyto-histologic diagnosis of biliary duct strictures. Tumori 1999;85(3):153–6.

CPS. Undernutrition in children with a neurodevelopmental disability. Nutrition Committee, Canadian Paediatric Society. Cmaj 1994;151(6):753–9.

Cunha F. Gastrostomy: its inception and evaluation. Am J Surg 1946;72:610–634.

Curry NS, Cochran S, et al. Interventional radiologic procedures in the renal transplant. Radiology 1984;152 (3):647–53.

Dabbs DJ, Wang X. Immunocytochemistry on cytologic specimens of limited quantity. Diagn Cytopathol 1998;18(2):166–9.

Dewald CL, Hiette PO, et al. Percutaneous gastrostomy and gastrojejunostomy with gastropexy: experience in 701 procedures. Radiology 1999;211(3):651–6.

Diament MJ, Boechat MI, Kangarloo H. Interventional radiology in infants and children: clinical and technical aspects. Radiology 1985;154(2):359–61.

Dilsiz A, Acikgozoglu S, et al. Ultrasound-guided percutaneous drainage in the treatment of children with hepatic hydatid disease. Pediatr Radiol 1997;27(3):230–3.

Dodds WJ, Stewart ET, Vlymen WJ. Appropriate contrast media for evaluation of esophageal disruption. Radiology 1982;144(2):439–41.

Don S, Kopecky KK, et al. Ultrasound-guided pediatric liver transplant biopsy using a spring- propelled cutting needle (biopsy gun). Pediatr Radiol 1994;24(1):21–4.

Dripps R, Lamont A. ASA Classification. JAMA 1961; 178:261–266.

Duber C, Klose KJ, et al. [Obstructive jaundice: its histological diagnosis by percutaneous endoluminal bile duct biopsy]. Rofo Fortschr Geb Rontgenstr Neuen Bildgeb Verfahr 1991;155(3):246– 50.

Duncan JR, Hicks ME, et al. Embolization of portal vein branches induces hepatocyte replication in swine: a potential step in hepatic gene therapy. Radiology 1999; 210(2):467–77.

Eckstein MR, Kelemouridis V, et al. Gastric bleeding: therapy with intraarterial vasopressin and transcatheter embolization. Radiology 1984;152(3):643–6.

Edelman DS, Unger SW, Russin DR. Laparoscopic gastrostomy. Surg Laparosc Endosc 1991;1(4):251–3.

Egawa H, Tanaka K, et al. Relief of hepatic vein stenosis by balloon angioplasty after living- related donor liver transplantation. Clin Transplant 1993;7(4):306–11.

Eisenberg PJ, Lee MJ, et al. Percutaneous drainage of a subphrenic abscess with gastric fistula [clinical conference]. AJR Am J Roentgenol 1994;162(5):1233–7.

Ellsworth PI, Webb HW, et al. The Malone antegrade colonic enema enhances the quality of life in children undergoing urological incontinence procedures. J Urol 1996;155(4):1416–8.

Ernst O, Sergent G, et al. Biliary leaks: treatment by means of percutaneous transhepatic biliary drainage. Radiology 1999;211(2):345–8.

Esposito C, Garipoli V, et al. Percutaneous blind needle biopsy versus combined laparoscopic excisional and guided needle biopsy in the diagnosis of liver disorders in pediatric patients. Ital J Gastroenterol Hepatol 1997; 29(2):179–81.

Faller N, Lawrence KG. Comparing low-profile gastrostomy tubes. Nursing 1993;23(12):46–8.

Feldstein V, JM L. Sonography before, during, and after TIPS. Techniques in Vascular and Interventional Radiology 1998;1(2):86–93.

Finne CO. Transrectal drainage of pelvic abscesses. Dis Colon Rectum 1980;23(5):293–7.

Fishman SJ, Burrows PE, et al. Gastrointestinal manifestations of vascular anomalies in childhood: varied etiologies require multiple therapeutic modalities. J Pediatr Surg 1998;33(7):1163–7.

Foley MJ, Ghahremani GG, Rogers LF. Reappraisal of contrast media used to detect upper gastrointestinal perforations: comparison of ionic water-soluble media with barium sulfate. Radiology 1982;144(2):231–7.

Freedman AM, Sanyal AJ, et al. Complications of transjugular intrahepatic portosystemic shunt: a comprehensive review. Radiographics 1993;13(6):1185–210.

Fulcher AS, Turner MA. Orthotopic liver transplantation: evaluation with MR cholangiography. Radiology 1999;211(3):715–22.

Funaki B, Rosenblum JD, et al. Angioplasty treatment of portal vein stenosis in children with segmental liver transplants: mid-term results. AJR Am J Roentgenol 1997;169(2):551–4.

Funaki B, Rosenblum JD, et al. Portal vein stenosis in children with segmental liver transplants: treatment with percutaneous transhepatic venoplasty. AJR Am J Roentgenol 1995;165(1):161–5

Furuya KN, Burrows PE, et al. Transjugular liver biopsy in children. Hepatology 1992;15(6):1036–42.

Gaisie G, Jaques PF, Mauro MA. Radiologic management of fluid collections in children. Pediatr Radiol 1987;17(2): 143–6.

Galat SA, Gerig KD, et al. Management of premature removal of the percutaneous gastrostomy. Am Surg 1990; 56(11):733–6.

Gallagher PG. Enterobacter bacteremia in pediatric patients. Rev Infect Dis 1990;12(5):808–12.

Gamble P, Colapinto RF, et al. Transjugular liver biopsy: a review of 461 biopsies. Radiology 1985;157(3):589–93.

Ganc AJ, Netto AJ, et al. Transcolonoscopic extraperitoneal cecostomy. A new therapeutic and technical proposal. Endoscopy 1988;20(6):309–12.

Ganga UR, Ryan JJ, Schafer LW. Indications, complications, and long-term results of percutaneous endoscopic gastrostomy: a retrospective study. S D J Med 1994;47(5): 149–52.

Ganger DR, Klapman JB, et al. Transjugular intrahepatic portosystemic shunt (TIPS) for Budd-Chiari syndrome or portal vein thrombosis: review of indications and problems. Am J Gastroenterol 1999;94(3):603–8.

Garel LA, Belli D, et al. Percutaneous cholecystography in children. Radiology 1987;165(3):639–41.

Gauderer MW, Ponsky JL, Izant RJ Jr. Gastrostomy without laparotomy: a percutaneous endoscopic technique. J Pediatr Surg 1980;15(6):872–5.

Gazelle GS, Haaga JR. Guided percutaneous biopsy of intraabdominal lesions. AJR Am J Roentgenol 1989;153 (5):929–35.

Gazelle GS, Haaga JR, et al. Pelvic abscesses: CT-guided transrectal drainage. Radiology 1991;181(1):49–51.

Gazelle GS, Mueller PR. Abdominal abscess. Imaging and intervention. Radiol Clin North Am 1994;32(5):913–32.

Geary DF, Chait PG. Tube feeding in infants on peritoneal dialysis. Perit Dial Int 1996;16(Suppl 1): S517–20.

Gerzof SG. Percutaneous drainage of renal and perinephric abscess. Urol Radiol 1981;2(3):171–9.

Giorgio A, Amoroso P, et al. Ultrasonically-guided percutaneous transcholecystic cholangiography—an alternative approach in cases of biliary obstruction and failure of percutaneous transhepatic cholangiography. Hepatogastroenterology 1988;35(6):268–70.

Goldberg MA, Mueller PR, et al. Importance of daily rounds by the radiologist after interventional procedures of the abdomen and chest. Radiology 1991;180(3):767–70.

Goletti O, Lippolis PV, et al. Percutaneous ultrasound-guided drainage of intra-abdominal abscesses. Br J Surg 1993;80(3):336–9.

Gombar S, Dureja J, et al. The effect of pre-operative intake of oral water and ranitidine on gastric fluid volume and pH in children undergoing elective surgery. J Indian Med Assoc 1997;95(6):166–8.

Gordon RL, Ring EJ. Combined radiologic and retrograde endoscopic and biliary interventions. Radiol Clin North Am 1990;28(6):1289–95.

Gow KW, Murphy JJ 3rd, et al. Splanchnic artery pseudoaneurysms secondary to blunt abdominal trauma in children. J Pediatr Surg 1996;31(6):812–5.

Guibaud L, Lachaud A, et al. MR cholangiography in neonates and infants: feasibility and preliminary applications. AJR Am J Roentgenol 1998;170(1):27–31.

Haas-Beckert B, Heyman MB. Comparison of two skin-level gastrostomy feeding tubes for infants and children. Pediatr Nurs 1993;19(4):351–4, 364.

Hackworth CA, Leef JA, et al. Transjugular intrahepatic portosystemic shunt creation in children: initial clinical experience. Radiology 1998;206(1):109–14.

Halkier BK, Ho CS, Yee AC. Percutaneous feeding gastrostomy with the Seldinger technique: review of 252 patients. Radiology 1989;171(2):359–62.

Hallisey MJ, Pollard JC. Direct percutaneous jejunostomy. J Vasc Interv Radiol 1994;5(4):625–32.

Hancock BJ, Wiseman NE, Rusnak BW. Bile duct stricture in an infant with gastroschisis treated by percutaneous transhepatic drainage, biliary stenting, and balloon dilation. J Pediatr Surg 1989;24(10):1071–3.

Haskal ZJ, Ring EJ, et al. Role of parallel transjugular intrahepatic portosystemic shunts in patients with persistent portal hypertension. Radiology 1992;185(3):813–7.

Hemming A, Davis NL, Robins RE. Surgical versus percutaneous drainage of intra-abdominal abscesses. Am J Surg 1991;161(5):593–5.

Heneghan J, RJ E, RC N. Multiple fluid collections: CT- or US-guided aspiration—evaluation of microbiologic results and implications for clinical practice. Radiology 1999;212:669–72.

Heyman MB, LaBerge JM, et al. Transjugular intrahepatic portosystemic shunts (TIPS) in children. J Pediatr 1997; 131(6):914–9.

Ho CS. Percutaneous gastrostomy for jejunal feeding. Radiology 1983;149(2):595–6.

Ho CS, Yeung EY. Percutaneous gastrostomy and transgastric jejunostomy. AJR Am J Roentgenol 1992;158(2):251–7.

Ho T, Margulies D. Pneumoperitoneum from an eroded T-fastener. Surg Endosc 1999;13(3):285–6.

Hoffer FA, Fellows KE, et al. Therapeutic catheter procedures in pediatrics. Pediatr Clin North Am 1985;32(6): 1461–76.

Hoffer FA, Teele RL, et al. Infected bilomas and hepatic artery thrombosis in infant recipients of liver transplants. Interventional radiology and medical therapy as an alternative to retransplantation. Radiology 1988;169(2):435–8.

Hopens T, Schwesinger WH. Complications of tube gastrostomy: radiologic manifestations. South Med J 1983; 76(1):9–11.

Hovsepian DM, Steele JR, et al. Transrectal versus transvaginal abscess drainage: survey of patient tolerance and effect on activities of daily living. Radiology 1999;212 (1):159–63.

Huard P, Do-Xuan-Hop. La ponction transhepatique des canaux bilares. Bull Soc Med Chir Indochine 1937;15: 1090.

Hubbard AM, Fellows KE. Pediatric interventional radiology: current practice and innovations. Cardiovasc Intervent Radiol 1993;16(5):267–74.

Huff JP, Rosenblum J, Camara DS. Complications of gastrostomy. South Med J 1988;81(8):1050–2.

Hughes U, Connolly B, et al. Further report of small-bowel intussusceptions related to gastrojejunostomy tubes. Society for Pediatric Radiology Meeting Syllabus;1999 May;Vancouver, BC. [Abstract] p.104.

Israel DM, Hassall E. Prolonged use of gastrostomy for enteral hyperalimentation in children with Crohn's disease. Am J Gastroenterol 1995;90(7):1084–8.

Jaeger HJ, MacFie J, et al. Diagnosis of abdominal masses with percutaneous biopsy guided by ultrasound. BMJ 1990;301(6762):1188–91.

Jaffe RB, Arata JA Jr, Matlak ME. Percutaneous drainage of traumatic pancreatic pseudocysts in children. AJR Am J Roentgenol 1989;152(3):591–5.

Jaksic T, Yaman M, et al. A 20–year review of pediatric pancreatic tumors. J Pediatr Surg 1992;27(10):1315–7.

Jamieson DH, Chait PG, Filler R. Interventional drainage of appendiceal abscesses in children. AJR Am J Roentgenol 1997;169(6):1619–22.

Janik JS, Culham JA, et al. Balloon embolization of a bleeding gastroduodenal artery in a 1–year- old child. Pediatrics 1981;67(5):671–4.

Jeffrey RB Jr, Wing VW, Laing FC. Real-time sonographic monitoring of percutaneous abscess drainage. AJR Am J Roentgenol 1985;144(3):469–70.

Johnson DL, Lang E. Technical aspects of nonoperative dilation of a complex colon anastomotic stricture. Dig Dis Sci 1993;38(10):1929–32.

Johnson SP, Leyendecker JR, et al. Transjugular portosystemic shunts in pediatric patients awaiting liver transplantation. Transplantation 1996;62(8):1178–81.

Kadir S, Athanasoulis CA. Catheter dislodgement: a cause of failure of intraarterial vasopressin infusions to control gastrointestinal bleeding. Cardiovasc Radiol 1978;1(3):187–91.

Kadir S, Athanasoulis CA, et al. Transcatheter embolization of intrahepatic arterial aneurysms. Radiology 1980;134(2):335–9.

Kang M, Gupta S, et al. Ilio-psoas abscess in the paediatric population: treatment by US-guided percutaneous drainage. Pediatr Radiol 1998;28(6):478–81.

Katada K, Anno H, et al. [Development of real-time CT fluoroscopy]. Nippon Igaku Hoshasen Gakkai Zasshi 1994;54(12):1172–4.

Katada K, Kato R, et al. Guidance with real-time CT fluoroscopy: early clinical experience. Radiology 1996; 200(3):851–6.

Katzen BT, Kaplan JO, Dake MD. Developing an interventional radiology practice in a community hospital: the interventional radiologist as an equal partner in patient care. Radiology 1989;170(3 Pt 2):955–8.

Keats AS. The ASA classification of physical status—a recapitulation. Anesthesiology 1978;49(4):233–6.

Keck JO, Staniunas RJ, et al. Biofeedback training is useful in fecal incontinence but disappointing in constipation. Dis Colon Rectum 1994;37(12):1271–6.

Keller MS, Lai S, Wagner DK. Percutaneous gastrostomy in a child. Radiology 1986;160(1):261–2.

Khuroo MS, Wani NA, et al. Percutaneous drainage compared with surgery for hepatic hydatid cysts. N Engl J Med 1997;337(13):881–7.

Kim IO, Yeon KM, et al. Perforation complicating balloon dilation of esophageal strictures in infants and children. Radiology 1993;189(3):741–4.

Kim OH, Chung HJ, Choi BG. Imaging of the choledochal cyst. Radiographics 1995;15(1):69–88.

King SJ, Chait PG, et al. Retrograde percutaneous gastrostomy: a prospective study in 57 children. Pediatr Radiol 1993;23(1):23–5.

Klein AS, Savader S, et al. Reduction of morbidity and mortality from biliary complications after liver transplantation. Hepatology 1991;14(5):818–23.

Kong MS, Lin JN. Pyogenic liver abscess in children. J Formos Med Assoc 1994;93(1):45–50.

Kroenke K, Gooby-Toedt D, Jackson JL. Chronic medications in the perioperative period. South Med J 1998; 91(4):358–64.

Kuligowska E, Keller E, Ferrucci JT. Treatment of pelvic abscesses: value of one-step sonographically guided transrectal needle aspiration and lavage. AJR Am J Roentgenol 1995;164(1):201–6.

LaBerge JM, Ring EJ, et al. Creation of transjugular intrahepatic portosystemic shunts with the wallstent endoprosthesis: results in 100 patients. Radiology 1993; 187(2):413–20.

Lachaux A, Le Gall C, et al. Complications of percutaneous liver biopsy in infants and children. Eur J Pediatr 1995;154(8):621–3.

Lambiase RE, Deyoe L, et al. Percutaneous drainage of 335 consecutive abscesses: results of primary drainage with 1–year follow-up. Radiology 1992;184(1):167–79.

Lang EV, Picus D, et al. Massive upper gastrointestinal hemorrhage with normal findings on arteriography: value of prophylactic embolization of the left gastric artery. AJR Am J Roentgenol 1992;158(3):547–9.

Langemeijer RA, Molenaar JC. Defaecation problems in children: anatomy, physiology and pathophysiology of the defaecation mechanism. Neth J Surg 1991;43(6): 208–12.

Lee MJ, Saini S, et al. Malignant small bowel obstruction and ascites: not a contraindication to percutaneous gastrostomy. Clin Radiol 1991;44(5):332–4.

Lee WJ, Chao SH, et al. Laparoscopic-guided gastrostomy. J Formos Med Assoc 1993;92(10):911–3.

Lefever EB, Potter PS, Seeley NR. Propofol sedation for pediatric MRI [letter]. Anesth Analg 1993;76(4):919–20.

Leikin SL. Minors' assent or dissent to medical treatment. J Pediatr 1983;102(2):169–76.

Lencioni R, Caramella D, Bartolozzi C. Percutaneous biopsy of liver tumors with color Doppler US guidance. Abdom Imaging 1995;20(3):206–8.

Lerma E, Musulen E, et al. Fine needle aspiration cytology in pancreatic pathology. Acta Cytol 1996;40(4):683–6.

Lestar B, Kiss J, et al. Clinical significance and application of anorectal physiology. Scand J Gastroenterol 1998;228 (Suppl):68–72.

Letourneau JG, Hunter DW, et al. Biliary complications after liver transplantation in children. Radiology 1989; 170(3 Pt 2):1095–9.

Levin DC, Flanders SJ, et al. Participation by radiologists and other specialists in percutaneous vascular and nonvascular interventions: findings from a seven-state database. Radiology 1995;196(1):51–4.

Levin DC, Rao VM, et al. Turf battles in radiology: how the radiology community can collectively respond to the challenge. Radiology 1999;211(2):301–5.

Lipscomb GR, Brown CM, et al. Blocked gastrostomy tubes [letter]. Lancet 1994;343(8900):801–2.

Little AF, Zajko AB, Orons PD. Transjugular liver biopsy: a prospective study in 43 patients with the Quick-Core biopsy needle. J Vasc Interv Radiol 1996;7(1):127–31.

Liu J, Li G, Lai B. A study on cholangitis after hepatic portoenterostomy for biliary atresia. Chin Med J (Engl) 1997;110(5):335–7.

Longo JM, Bilbao JI, et al. CT-guided paracoccygeal drainage of pelvic abscesses. J Comput Assist Tomogr 1993;17(6):909–14.

Longo JM, Bilbao JI, et al. Color Doppler-US guidance in transjugular placement of intrahepatic portosystemic shunts. Radiology 1992;184(1):281–4.

Lowrie L, Weiss AH, Lacombe C. The pediatric sedation unit: a mechanism for pediatric sedation. Pediatrics 1998;102(3): E30.

Madoff RD, Williams JG, Caushaj, PF. Fecal incontinence. N Engl J Med 1992;326(15):1002–7.

Maginot TJ, Cascade PN. Abdominal wall cellulitis and sepsis secondary to percutaneous cecostomy. Cardiovasc Intervent Radiol 1993;16(5):328–31.

Mahajan L, Oliva L, et al. The safety of gastrostomy in patients with Crohn's disease. Am J Gastroenterol 1997; 92(6):985–8.

Male C, Johnston M, et al. The influence of developmental haemostasis on the laboratory diagnosis and management of haemostatic disorders during infancy and childhood. Clin Lab Med 1999;19(1):39–69.

Malone PS, Curry JI, Osborne A. The antegrade continence enema procedure why, when and how? World J Urol 1998;16(4):274–8.

Malone PS, Ransley PG, Kiely EM. Preliminary report: the antegrade continence enema. Lancet 1990;336(8725): 1217–8.

Mandel SR, Boyd D, et al. Drainage of hepatic, intraabdominal, and mediastinal abscesses guided by computerized axial tomography. Successful alternative to open drainage. Am J Surg 1983;145(1):120–5.

Maurer AH. Gastrointestinal bleeding and cine-scintigraphy. Semin Nucl Med 1996;26(1):43–50.

Mazziotti MV, Marley EF, et al. Histopathologic analysis of interval appendectomy specimens: support for the role of interval appendectomy. J Pediatr Surg 1997;32(6):806–9.

McCormick PA, Dick R, Burroughs AK. Review article: the transjugular intrahepatic portosystemic shunt (TIPS) in the treatment of portal hypertension. Aliment Pharmacol Ther 1994;8(3):273–82.

McFarland EG, Lee MJ, et al. Gastropexy breakdown and peritonitis after percutaneous gastrojejunostomy in a patient with ascites [clinical conference]. AJR Am J Roentgenol 1995;164(1):189–93.

McGlynn M, Jefferies S, et al. The experimental assessment of techniques of measuring biliary pressure. Aust N Z J Surg 1978;48(5):581–5.

McHugh K. Conversion of gastrostomy to transgastric jejunostomy in children. Clin Radiol 1997;52(7):550–1.

Men S, Hekimoglu B, et al. Percutaneous treatment of hepatic hydatid cysts: an alternative to surgery. AJR Am J Roentgenol 1999;172(1):83–9.

Mewissen MW, Lipchik EO, et al. Liver biopsy through the femoral vein. Radiology 1988;169(3):842–3.

Meyerovitz MF, Fellows KE. Angiography in gastrointestinal bleeding in children. AJR Am J Roentgenol 1984;143(4):837–40.

Meyers EF, Alberts D, Gordon MO. Perioperative control of blood glucose in diabetic patients: a two-step protocol. Diabetes Care 1986;9(1):40–5.

Miglioli M. Constipation: physiopathology and classification. Ital J Gastroenterol 1991;23(8 Suppl 1):10–2.

Miyazaki T, Yamashita Y, et al. Single-shot MR cholangiopancreatography of neonates, infants, and young children. AJR Am J Roentgenol 1998;170(1):33–7.

Mollitt DL, Dokler ML, et al. Complications of retained internal bolster after pediatric percutaneous endoscopic gastrostomy. J Pediatr Surg 1998;33(2):271–3.

Moneret-Vautrin DA, Beaudouin E, et al. Prospective study of risk factors in natural rubber latex hypersensitivity. J Allergy Clin Immunol 1993;92(5):668–77.

Montoya F, Alam MM, et al. [Liver abscess in a newborn infant. Cure following percutaneous puncture under echographic control]. Pediatrie 1983;38(8):547–51.

Moore SW, Millar AJ, Cywes S. Conservative initial treatment for liver abscesses in children. Br J Surg 1994;81(6): 872–4.

Morrison MC, Lee MJ, et al. Percutaneous balloon dilatation of benign biliary strictures. Radiol Clin North Am 1990;28(6):1191–201.

Moulton JS, Moore PT. Coaxial percutaneous biopsy technique with automated biopsy devices: value in improving accuracy and negative predictive value. Radiology 1993;186(2):515–22.

Murakami T, Ueki K, et al. Pancreatoblastoma: case report and review of treatment in the literature. Med Pediatr Oncol 1996;27(3):193–7.

Ng DA, Opelka FG, et al. Predictive value of technetium Tc 99m-labeled red blood cell scintigraphy for positive angiogram in massive lower gastrointestinal hemorrhage. Dis Colon Rectum 1997;40(4):471–7.

Ni YH, Chang MH, et al. Ultrasound-guided percutaneous drainage of liver abscess in children. Chung Hua Min Kuo Hsiao Erh Ko I Hsueh Hui Tsa Chih 1995; 36(5):336–41.

Ochs A, Sellinger M, et al. Transjugular intrahepatic portosystemic stent-shunt (TIPS) in the treatment of Budd-Chiari syndrome. J Hepatol 1993;18(2):217–25.

Okoye BO, Rampersad B, et al. Abscess after appendicectomy in children: the role of conservative management. Br J Surg 1998;85(8):1111–3.

Paidas CN. Fecal incontinence in children with anorectal malformations. Semin Pediatr Surg 1997;6(4):228–34.

Pandit UA, Pandit SK. Fasting before and after ambulatory surgery. J Perianesth Nurs 1997;12(3):181–7.

Park JH, Choi BI, et al. Percutaneous removal of residual intrahepatic stones. Radiology 1987;163(3):619–23.

Peclet MH, Ryckman FC, et al. The spectrum of bile duct complications in pediatric liver transplantation. J Pediatr Surg 1994;29(2):214–9;discussion 219–20.

Pereira JK, Chait PG, Miller SF. Deep pelvic abscesses in children: transrectal drainage under radiologic guidance. Radiology 1996;198(2):393–6.

Pereyra R, Andrassy RJ, Mahour GH. Management of massive hepatic hemangiomas in infants and children: a review of 13 cases. Pediatrics 1982;70(2):254–8.

Peters TM, Henri CJ, et al. Integration of stereoscopic DSA and 3D MRI for image-guided neurosurgery. Comput Med Imaging Graph 1994;18(4):289–99.

Phillips S, Daborn AK, Hatch DJ. Preoperative fasting for paediatric anaesthesia. Br J Anaesth 1994;73(4):529–36.

Pien EC, Hume KE, Pien FD. Gastrostomy tube infections in a community hospital. Am J Infect Control 1996; 24(5):353–8.

Pitt HA, Doty JE, et al. The role of altered extrahepatic biliary function in the pathogenesis of gallstones after vagotomy. Surgery 1981;90(2):418–25.

Potchen EJ, Potchen JE, et al. Medical-legal issues in radiology: prevention and control. Curr Probl Diagn Radiol 1995;24(4):141–75.

Pricolo VE, Vittimberga GM, et al. Decompression after gastric surgery. Gastrostomy versus nasogastric tube. Am Surg 1989;55(7):413–6.

Quinn SF, Sheley RC, et al. The role of percutaneous needle biopsies in the original diagnosis of lymphoma: a prospective evaluation. J Vasc Interv Radiol 1995;6(6): 947–52.

Quinn SF, vanSonnenberg E, et al. Interventional radiology in the spleen. Radiology 1986;161(2):289–91.

Raaf JH, Manney M, et al. Laparoscopic placement of a percutaneous endoscopic gastrostomy (PEG) feeding tube. J Laparoendosc Surg 1993;3(4):411–4.

Rajak CL, Gupta S, et al. Percutaneous treatment of liver abscesses: needle aspiration versus catheter drainage. AJR Am J Roentgenol 1998;170(4):1035–9.

Ramage IJ, Balfe JW. Risks of gastrostomy tubes in children on peritoneal dialysis [letter]. Perit Dial Int 1998; 18(1):84–5.

Ramage IJ, Harvey E, et al. Complications of gastrostomy feeding in children receiving peritoneal dialysis. Pediatr Nephrol 1999;13(3):249–52.

Ramamurthy H. Percutaneous Cecostomy: a new technique in the management of fecal incontinence. J Pediatr Surg 1996;31(12):1737.

Reading CC, Charboneau JW, et al. Sonographically guided percutaneous biopsy of small (3 cm or less) masses. AJR Am J Roentgenol 1988;151(1):189–92.

Reddy VB, Gattuso P, et al. Computed tomography-guided fine needle aspiration biopsy of deep-seated lesions. A four-year experience. Acta Cytol 1991;35(6):753–6.

Reimer W, Farres MT, Lammer J. Gastric wall dissection as a complication of percutaneous gastrostomy. Cardiovasc Intervent Radiol 1996;19(4):288–90.

Remolar J, S K, et al. Percutaneous transhepatic cholangiography. Gastroenterology 1956;31:39.

Renfrew DL, Smith WL, Pringle KC. Per anal balloon dilatation of a post-necrotizing enterocolitis stricture of the sigmoid colon. Pediatr Radiol 1986;16(4):320–1.

Reuter SR. Some legal aspects of angiography and interventative radiology. Leg Med 1986;124–33.

Reuter SR. An overview of informed consent for radiologists. AJR Am J Roentgenol 1987;148(1):219–27.

Riavis M, Laux-End R, et al. Sedation with intravenous benzodiazepine and ketamine for renal biopsies. Pediatr Nephrol 1998;12(2):147–8.

Ring EJ, Kerlan RK Jr. Interventional biliary radiology. AJR Am J Roentgenol 1984;142(1):31–4.

Ring EJ, Kerlan RK Jr. Inpatient management: a new role for interventional radiologists. Radiology 1985;154(2):543.

Ring EJ, Oleaga JA, et al. Pitfalls in the angiographic management of hemorrhage: hemodynamic considerations. AJR Am J Roentgenol 1977;129(6):1007–13.

Ronchera CL, Marti-Bonmati L, et al. Administration of oral chloral hydrate to paediatric patients undergoing magnetic resonance imaging. Pharm Weekbl Sci 1992; 14(6):349–52.

Rose C. The radiologist, the patient and Canadian law. J Can Assoc Radiol 1980;31(3):198–201.

Rose DB, Wolman SL, Ho CS. Gastric hemorrhage complicating percutaneous transgastric jejunostomy. Radiology 1986;161(3):835–6.

Rosenblum J, Taylor FC, et al. A new technique for direct percutaneous jejunostomy tube placement. Am J Gastroenterol 1990;85(9):1165–7.

Roy CC, Morin CL, Weber AM. Gastrointestinal emergency problems in paediatric practice. Clin Gastroenterol 1981;10(1):225–54.

Rubin JD, Cohan RH. Iodinated radiographic contrast media: comparison of low-osmolar with conventional ionic agents [corrected] [published erratum appears in Curr Opin Radiol 1991 Dec;3(6):975]. Curr Opin Radiol 1991;3(5):637–45.

Russell SC, Doyle E. A risk-benefit assessment of topical percutaneous local anaesthetics in children. Drug Saf 1997;16(4):279–87.

Ryan JM, Hahn PF, Mueller PR. Performing radiologic gastrostomy or gastrojejunostomy in patients with malignant ascites. AJR Am J Roentgenol 1998;171(4):1003–6.

Ryu RK, Durham JD, et al. Role of TIPS as a bridge to hepatic transplantation in Budd-Chiari syndrome. J Vasc Interv Radiol 1999;10(6):799–805.

Sabbah R, Ghandour M, et al. Tru-cut needle biopsy of abdominal tumors in children: a safe and diagnostic procedure. Cancer 1981;47(10):2533–5.

Saint-Vil D, Luks FI, et al. Infectious complications of pediatric liver transplantation. J Pediatr Surg 1991; 26(8):908–13.

Saluja S, Fields JM, et al. Percutaneous needle aspiration of small interloop abscesses in children. Pediatr Surg Int 1998;13(7):528–30.

Sanchez RB, vanSonnenberg E, et al. CT guidance for percutaneous gastrostomy and gastroenterostomy. Radiology 1992;184(1):201–5.

Sane SS, Towbin A, et al. Percutaneous gastrostomy tube placement in patients with ventriculoperitoneal shunts. Pediatr Radiol 1998;28(7):521–3.

Sangster W, Swanstrom L. Laparoscopic-guided feeding jejunostomy. Surg Endosc 1993;7(4):308–10.

Sant SM, Gilvarry J, et al. Percutaneous endoscopic gastrostomy—its application in patients with neurological disease. Ir J Med Sci 1993;162(11):450–1.

Sanyal AJ. Budd-Chiari syndrome: is TIPS tops? Am J Gastroenterol 1999;94(3):559–61.

Sawhney R, SA W. TIPS complications. Techniques in Vascular and Interventional Radiology 1998;1(2):80–5.

Sawhney S, Berry M, Bhargava S. Percutaneous real-time ultrasonic guided biopsy in the diagnosis of deep-seated, non-palpable intra-abdominal masses (initial experience). Australas Radiol 1987;31(3):295–9.

Sawlani V, Phadke RV, et al. Arterial complications of pancreatitis and their radiological management. Australas Radiol 1996;40(4):381–6.

Schnyder P, Capasso P, Meuwly JY. Turf battles in radiology: how to avoid/how to fight/how to win. Eur Radiol 1999;9(4):741–8.

Schreiner MS, Triebwasser A, Keon TP. Ingestion of liquids compared with preoperative fasting in pediatric outpatients. Anesthesiology 1990;72(4):593–7.

Schwartz MZ. Unusual peptide-secreting tumors in adolescents and children. Semin Pediatr Surg 1997;6(3):141–6.

Sectish TC. Use of sedation and local anesthesia to prepare children for procedures. Am Fam Physician 1997; 55(3):909–16.

Shah GK, Stoler BB, Rovere J. Demonstration of bleeding site by 99mTc-labeled red cells. Radiology 1979;132(1): 169–70.

Shandling B, Chait PG, Richards HF. Percutaneous cecostomy: a new technique in the management of fecal incontinence. J Pediatr Surg 1996;31(4):534–7.

Sheldon CA, Minevich E, et al. Role of the antegrade continence enema in the management of the most debilitating childhood recto-urogenital anomalies. J Urol 1997; 158(3 Pt 2):1277–9;discussion 1279–80.

Sidhu MK, Shaw DWW, et al. Post-traumatic hepatic pseudoaneurysms in children. Pediatr Radiol 1999;29(1): 46–52.

Sievers TD, Yee JD, et al. Midazolam for conscious sedation during pediatric oncology procedures: safety and recovery parameters. Pediatrics 1991;88(6):1172–9.

Silverman S, K T, et al. CT fluoroscopy-guided abdominal interventions: techniques, results, and radiation exposure. Radiology 1999;212:673–81.

Silverman SG, Deuson TE, et al. Percutaneous abdominal biopsy: cost-identification analysis. Radiology 1998;206 (2):429–35.

Smith EH. Complications of percutaneous abdominal fine-needle biopsy. Review. Radiology 1991;178(1):253–8.

Smith MB, Katz R, et al. A rational approach to the use of fine-needle aspiration biopsy in the evaluation of primary and recurrent neoplasms in children. J Pediatr Surg 1993;28(10):1245–7.

Somers JM, Lomas DJ, et al. Radiologically-guided cutting needle biopsy for suspected malignancy in childhood. Clin Radiol 1993;48(4):236–40.

Soreide E, Holst-Larsen H, et al. The effects of chewing gum on gastric content prior to induction of general anesthesia. Anesth Analg 1995;80(5):985–9.

Sperling DC, Needleman L, et al. Deep pelvic abscesses: transperineal US-guided drainage. Radiology 1998; 208(1):111–5.

Splinter WM, Schaefer JD. Unlimited clear fluid ingestion two hours before surgery in children does not affect volume or pH of stomach contents. Anaesth Intensive Care 1990;18(4):522–6.

Steinkamp G, von der Hardt H. Improvement of nutritional status and lung function after long-term nocturnal gastrostomy feedings in cystic fibrosis. J Pediatr 1994; 124(2):244–9.

Stellato TA, Gauderer MW. Percutaneous endoscopic gastrostomy for gastrointestinal decompression. Ann Surg 1987;205(2):119–22.

Strain JD, Campbell JB, et al. IV Nembutal: safe sedation for children undergoing CT. AJR Am J Roentgenol 1988;151(5):975–9.

Strain JD, Harvey LA, et al. Intravenously administered pentobarbital sodium for sedation in pediatric CT. Radiology 1986;161(1):105–8.

Strunk HM, Textor J, et al. Acute Budd-Chiari syndrome: treatment with transjugular intrahepatic portosystemic shunt. Cardiovasc Intervent Radiol 1997;20(4):311–3.

Stuart SP, Tiley EHD, Boland JP. Feeding gastrostomy: a critical review of its indications and mortality rate. South Med J 1993;86(2):169–72.

Sukigara M, Taguchi Y, et al. Percutaneous transhepatic biliary drainage guided by color Doppler echography. Abdom Imaging 1994;19(2):147–9.

Synn AY, Mulvihill SJ, Fonkalsrud EW. Surgical disorders of the pancreas in infancy and childhood. Am J Surg 1988;156(3 Pt 1):201–5.

Szymski GX, Albazzaz AN, et al. Radiologically guided placement of pull-type gastrostomy tubes. Radiology 1997;205(3):669–73.

Tagart RE. The anal canal and rectum: their varying relationship and its effect on anal continence. Dis Colon Rectum 1966;9(6):449–52.

Temple M, Chait P, et al. Transrectal abscess drainage in children. Canadian Association of Radiologists Journal 1999;50(Suppl.): S32.

Temple M, Chait P, et al. Long term followup of cecostomy patients. Canadian Association of Radiologists Journal 1999;50(Suppl.): S35 [abstract].

Temple M, Chait P, et al. Risk of Infection with percutaneous gastrostomy tube placement in children with ventriculoperitoneal shunts. Society for Pediatric Radiology Meeting Syllabus;1999 May;Vancouver, BC. [Abstract] p. 105.

Thorne SE, Radford MJ. A comparative longitudinal study of gastrostomy devices in children. West J Nurs Res 1998;20(2):145–59, discussion 159–65.

Tikkakoski T, Siniluoto T, et al. Splenic abscess. Imaging and intervention. Acta Radiol 1992;33(6):561–5.

Towbin RB. Current advances in pediatric interventional radiology. Curr Opin Radiol 1989;1(4):572–6.

Towbin RB. Pediatric interventional procedures in the 1980s: a period of development, growth, and acceptance. Radiology 1989;170(3 Pt 2):1081–90.

Towbin RB. Pediatric interventional radiology. Curr Opin Radiol 1991;3(6):931–5.

Towbin RB. Percutaneous cecostomy. Radiology 1997; 203(3):604.

Towbin RB, Ball WS Jr. Pediatric interventional radiology. Radiol Clin North Am 1988;26(2):419–40.

Towbin RB, Ball WS Jr, Bissett GSD. Percutaneous gastrostomy and percutaneous gastrojejunostomy in children: antegrade approach. Radiology 1988;168(2):473–6.

Tsang P, Greenebaum E, et al. Image-directed percutaneous biopsy with large-core needles. Comparison of cytologic and histologic findings. Acta Cytol 1995; 39(4):753–8.

Tuggle DW, Bennett KG, et al. Intravenous vasopressin and gastrointestinal hemorrhage in children. J Pediatr Surg 1988;23(7):627–9.

Valji K. Vascular and interventional radiology. Philadelphia: W. B. Saunders Company, 1999.

van Gansbeke D, Matos C, et al. Percutaneous drainage of subphrenic abscesses. Br J Radiol 1989;62(734):127–33.

Vane DW, Grosfeld JL, et al. Pancreatic disorders in infancy and childhood: experience with 92 cases. J Pediatr Surg 1989;24(8):771–6.

Vane DW, Redlich P, et al. Impaired immune function in obstructive jaundice. J Surg Res 1988;45(3):287–93.

vanSonnenberg E, Ferrucci JT Jr, et al. Biliary pressure: manometric and perfusion studies at percutaneous transhepatic cholangiography and percutaneous biliary drainage. Radiology 1983;148(1):41–50.

vanSonnenberg E, Mueller PR, Ferrucci JT Jr. Percutaneous drainage of 250 abdominal abscesses and fluid collections. Part I: Results, failures, and complications. Radiology 1984;151(2):337–41.

vanSonnenberg E., Wittich GR, et al. Complicated pancreatic inflammatory disease: diagnostic and therapeutic role of interventional radiology. Radiology 1985;155(2):335–40.

vanSonnenberg E, Wittich GR, et al. Percutaneous diagnostic and therapeutic interventional radiologic procedures in children: experience in 100 patients. Radiology 1987;162(3):601–5.

Vautier G, Scott BB. Blocked gastrostomy tubes. Lancet 1994;343(8905):1105.

Venbrux AC. Interventional radiology in the biliary tract. Curr Opin Radiol 1992;4(3):83–92.

Waltman AC, Greenfield AJ, et al. Pyloroduodenal bleeding and intraarterial vasopressin: clinical results. AJR Am J Roentgenol 1979;133(4):643–6.

Wang DS, Chen DS, et al. Bacterial liver abscess in children. J Singapore Paediatr Soc 1989;31(1–2):75–8.

Ward EM, Kiely MJ, et al. Hilar biliary strictures after liver transplantation: cholangiography and percutaneous treatment. Radiology 1990;177(1):259–63.

Weiss B, Fradkin A, et al. Upper gastrointestinal bleeding due to gastric ulcers in children with gastrostomy tubes. J Clin Gastroenterol 1999;29(1):48–50.

Weissleder R. Molecular imaging: exploring the next frontier. Radiology 1999;212:609–14.

Whitaker J, Johnston GS. Estimation of urinary outflow resistance in children: simultaneous measurement of bladder pressure, flow rate, and exit pressure. Invest Urol 1966;3(4):379–89.

White CS, Templeton PA, Hasday JD. CT-assisted transbronchial needle aspiration: usefulness of CT fluoroscopy. AJR Am J Roentgenol 1997;169(2):393–4.

White RI Jr, Rizer DM, et al. Streamlining operation of an admitting service for interventional radiology. Radiology 1988;168(1):127–30.

Wilcox DT, Kiely EM. The Malone (antegrade colonic enema) procedure: early experience. J Pediatr Surg 1998;33(2):204–6.

Willnow U, Willberg B, et al. Pancreatoblastoma in children. Case report and review of the literature. Eur J Pediatr Surg 1996;6(6):369–72.

Wimmer B, Wenz W. CT-guided interventions. Present and future aspects. Acta Radiol Suppl 1991;377:46–9.

Winzelberg GG, McKusick KA, et al. Detection of gastrointestinal bleeding with 99mTc-labeled red blood cells. Semin Nucl Med 1982;12(2):139–46.

Wojtowycz MM, Arata JA Jr, et al. CT findings after uncomplicated percutaneous gastrostomy. AJR Am J Roentgenol 1988;151(2):307–9.

Yagi M, Shiraiwa K, et al. A solid and cystic tumor of the pancreas in a 10–year-old girl: report of a case and review of the literature. Surg Today 1994;24(9):826–8.

Yamada K, Nakamura K, et al. A case of Budd-Chiari syndrome successfully treated by transcatheter recanalization of the right hepatic vein and transjugular intrahepatic portosystemic shunt. Radiat Med 1999;17(1):85–9.

Yamini D, Vargas H, et al. Perforated appendicitis: is it truly a surgical urgency? Am Surg 1998;64(10):970–5.

Yeung EY. Percutaneous abdominal biopsy. Baillieres Clin Gastroenterol 1992;6(2):219–44.

Yeung EY, Ho CS. Percutaneous radiologic drainage of pelvic abscesses. Ann Acad Med Singapore 1993;22(5):663–9.

Younoszai MK. Stooling problems in patients with myelomeningocele. South Med J 1992;85(7):718–24.

Zajko AB, Sheng R, et al. Transhepatic balloon dilation of biliary strictures in liver transplant patients: a 10–year experience. J Vasc Interv Radiol 1995;6(1):79–83.

Zardawi IM. Fine needle aspiration cytology in a rural setting. Acta Cytol 1998;42(4):899–906.

Zeppa P, Vetrani A, et al. Fine needle aspiration biopsy of the spleen. A useful procedure in the diagnosis of splenomegaly. Acta Cytol 1994;38(3):299–309.

6

PHARYNX AND ESOPHAGUS

Sambasiva R. Kottamasu, MD, and
David A. Stringer, BSc, MBBS, FRCR, FRCPC

ANATOMY OF THE PHARYNX AND ESOPHAGUS

The pharynx is divided into three parts: the nasopharynx, oropharynx, and hypopharynx. It is surrounded by the superior, middle, and inferior constrictor muscles, which insert posteriorly into a median raphe, with the exception of the transverse and oblique inferior fibers of the inferior constrictor that constitute cricopharyngeus. On a barium swallow examination, cricopharyngeus is normally seen as a posterior impression on the upper esophagus (Figure 6–1) (see also Chapter 3).

The nasopharynx communicates with the oropharynx through the velopharyngeal portal, which is closed during normal swallowing and phonation by a complex interaction of constrictor and palatine muscles. A prominent muscle band, the pharyngeal (Passavant's) ridge, may be seen during closure of the velopharyngeal portal in patients with cleft palate and in some normal patients. The ridge may help compensate for any abnormality (Swischuk et al., 1974) although it is often inconsistent in action and may lie below the palate. The oropharynx lies between the tonsillar pillars and the larynx. The hypopharynx surrounds the larynx and ends at the cricopharyngeus.

There are a number of important anatomic differences between the adult pharynx and the child pharynx. In the newborn, adenoid, a midline lymphoid tissue in the nasopharynx, is not radiologically visible. Recognizable adenoid is seen in all infants over 6 months of age but in only half of infants under this age (Capitanio and Kirkpatrick, 1970). Adenoid becomes prominent in early childhood and disappears in early adulthood. It varies widely in size, although it should never be large enough to cause nasal speech or difficulty in nasal breathing. Adenoid helps close the velopharyngeal portal during swallowing and speech. Methods of measuring adenoid (Hibbert and Whitehouse, 1978; Jeans et al., 1981) are cumbersome and are not routinely used. Hypertrophy of the lingual tonsils may be associated with dysphagia (Fitzgerald and O'Connell, 1987).

The pharynx develops and reaches adult form during the first 6 years of life. The trachea is initially long, with the hyoid located at a level between the second and third cervical vertebrae. By the age of 6 years, the hyoid has reached the fourth cervical vertebra, where it remains.

The variation in the size and shape of the retropharyngeal space relates to the position of the head, the degree of flexion or extension of the cervical spine, and the phase and vigor of respiration (Ardran and Kemp, 1968; 1969). In the infant, the retropharyngeal space is wide during quiet breathing with the head in the neutral position. When the infant cries, prominence of the soft tissues is seen in the posterior pharyngeal space on plain films (Figure 6–2). This results in the trachea having a characteristic buckle on plain films, which varies in size and disappears during some phases of respiration. The buckle can be quickly demonstrated with a few seconds of fluoroscopy if doubt about normality arises; fluoroscopy may involve less radiation and is often easier than repeated attempts to obtain plain films. Extrinsic pressure on the trachea may be used to eliminate normal tracheal buckling (Berger et al., 1974). This normal appearance should not be confused with the more elongated and permanent widening of the posterior pharyngeal space seen when there is a retropharyngeal abscess or a neoplasm.

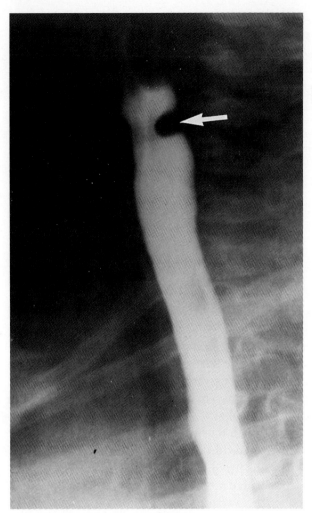

FIGURE 6–1. Normal cricopharyngeus. The cricopharyngeus (*arrow*) is intermittently seen and causes no obstruction.

The esophagus in infants and children is similar to the adult esophagus but with a few important radiologic differences. Air is more often seen in the esophagus in children, especially neonates. If persistent or unusually marked, respiratory disease (Keats and Smith, 1974) or tracheoesophageal fistula should be suspected (Smith et al., 1976). The normal impressions of aorta, left main stem bronchus, and left atrium may be seen on the esophagogram but are frequently less prominent than in adults. In infants, the entire esophagus is often filled on rapid swallowing of liquids, and all or part of the esophagus may transitorily dilate relative to the size of the chest (see Chapter 3, Figures 3–6B and 3–10B). The normal esophagus may be deviated by extrinsic structures such as the heart (Figure 6–3).

DEGLUTITION

The mechanism of deglutition involves sucking (with bolus formation due to mandibular and tongue movements) and swallowing (due to pharyngeal movements).

Normal Sucking and Bolus Formation

Sucking and swallowing of amniotic fluid by 26- to 36-week-old fetuses has been observed on real-time ultrasonography (US). One to two mandibular movements per minute occur in 20% of fetuses. Distinct pharyngeal and tongue movements are harder to assess and are less commonly seen. Apparent vomiting as suggested by mouth opening, extension of the neck, and protrusion of the tongue has been noted in esophageal atresia and tracheoesophageal fistula (Bowie and Clair, 1982).

Sucking and swallowing are easier to study after delivery. In immature preterm infants, there may be only apposition of the jaws, with an occasional suck. As the infant matures, sucking becomes more normal. In normal-term infants, for the first 2

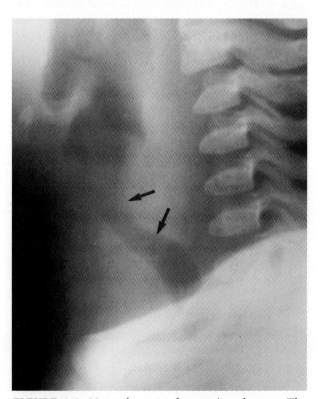

FIGURE 6–2. Normal neonatal posterior pharynx. The apparent soft tissue mass buckles the trachea (*arrows*) when the infant cries. The mass is not present during quiet respiration.

days of life there are bursts of 4 to 6 sucks followed by a short rest. After this time, the suck-swallow mechanism matures, with bursts of 10 to 30 sucks followed by short rests. The longer bursts of sucking are accompanied by cessation of esophageal peristalsis, and the entire esophagus fills with liquid.

When the tongue moves posteriorly during sucking, negative pressure traps air in the mouth. This generally means that some air precedes or accompanies fluid in passage to the stomach; hence, all babies need to be burped at the end of feeds.

Sucking is to some extent a learned response. Neonates fed for long periods via a gastrostomy because of esophageal atresia often have difficulty feeding if denied oral feeding for prolonged periods. After esophageal atresia repair, those infants with a cervical esophagostomy, who are provided with opportunities to swallow, have less difficulty feeding (Ardran and Kemp, 1970).

Normal Swallowing

The normal sequence (Ardran and Kemp, 1969) is as follows:

1. The tongue moves to the roof of the mouth, squeezing the bolus posteriorly in the mouth to the oropharynx.
2. The soft palate elevates and, due to the combined sphincter action of the constrictors and palatine muscles, takes a more horizontal position with closure of the velopharyngeal portal.
3. The bolus of food in the oropharynx passes inferiorly by a combination of gravity and contraction of the constrictor muscles. This pharyngeal contraction occurs craniocaudally, driving the bolus inferiorly. When liquids are swallowed in the erect position, this contraction is less important, as gravity causes the liquid to descend from the oropharynx to the hypopharynx.
4. As the pharyngeal contraction reaches the level of the larynx, the larynx rises, respiration ceases, and the epiglottis depresses (Figure 6–4).
5. The bolus is mainly diverted laterally over the lateral pharyngoepiglottic folds down the lateral food channels (the piriform sinuses). A small portion of the bolus may enter the laryngeal vestibule and subsequently be squeezed out by the further descent of the epiglottis (Ekberg and Nylander, 1982a). (There is some controversy regarding the normality of this finding: Ekberg and Nylander, 1982b.)

6. The cricopharyngeus opens, and the bolus reaches the proximal esophagus where a peristaltic wave carries it toward the stomach.

Imaging of Sucking and Swallowing

The mechanism of sucking and swallowing is complex and rapid. It takes less than a second for a mouthful of fluid to reach the upper esophagus. Hence, the radiologic evaluation has to be in real time, and static images are rarely helpful.

Sucking and swallowing have been observed prenatally on US but with no clinical significance. The sucking mechanism has been assessed using cineradiography during bottle-feeding and breast-feeding (Ardran et al., 1958) but this technique has a relatively high radiation dosage. More recently, real-time US (Smith et al., 1985) and scintigraphy have been used (Llamas-Elviras et al., 1986) but US has not been fully evaluated and the value of scintig-

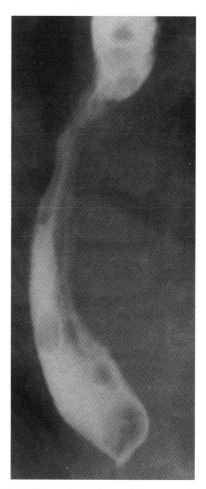

FIGURE 6–3. Normal esophagus. The normal esophagus is deviated to the right by an enlarged heart.

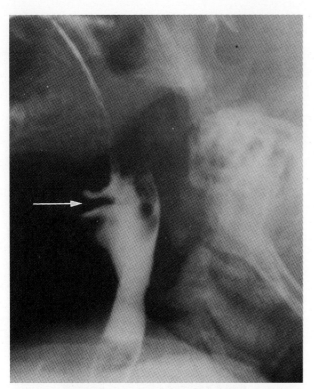

FIGURE 6–4. Normal swallow. As the pharyngeal contraction reaches the level of the larynx, the larynx rises, respiration ceases, and the epiglottis (*arrow*) depresses.

raphy is disputed (Gilchrist et al., 1987). Videofluoroscopy is currently the most available method of studying the swallowing mechanism because it involves less radiation than cineradiography (Ott and Pikna, 1993). However with videofluoroscopy, the speed of successive images can be controlled only with expensive video equipment since freeze-frame images made with standard video equipment are usually of poor quality. Excellent freeze-frame (single frame) images can be obtained with cine loop digital fluoroscopy.

The indications for barium study to assess swallowing are in clinical situations concerned with bolus formation, nasal escape, or aspiration. Every videofluoroscopic barium study should answer three questions (Chen et al., 1990; Ott and Pikna, 1993): Is the bolus formation normal? Does nasal escape occur? Is aspiration present?

Bolus Formation
By understanding the normal sucking mechanisms it is possible to detect subtle abnormalities, the most common being inadequate movement of the tongue, resulting in a lack of bolus formation.

Chapter 3 describes an effective method of studying this abnormality.

Nasal Escape
Nasal escape may be seen in the first few days of life in a normal term infant but is more common in those with swallowing disorders and is always abnormal after the first few days of life (Figure 6–5). In older children with nasal escape, speech is usually hypernasal due to velopharyngeal incompetence (Skolnick et al., 1980), which can be assessed by velopharyngeal videofluoroscopic function studies in lateral and Towne's projections (usually done to assess speech) (Stringer and Witzel, 1986).

Aspiration
Aspiration is the most serious finding associated with swallowing disorders. Intermittent slight aspi-

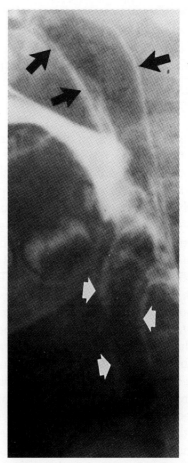

FIGURE 6–5. Nasal escape and aspiration. Swallowing produces nasal aspiration (*black arrows*) shown on barium swallow. This cerebral palsy patient also aspirated contrast into the trachea (*white arrows*).

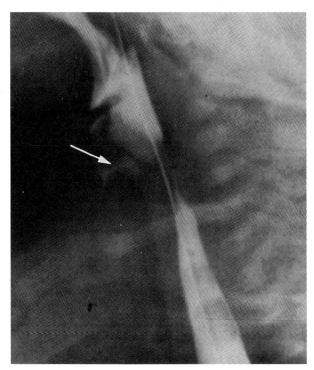

FIGURE 6–6. Tracheal aspiration. Intermittent aspiration of contrast media into the proximal part of the trachea (*arrow*).

ration may occur in crying or struggling infants and children, probably related to their uncooperativeness. This slight aspiration is usually accompanied by coughing and prompt clearing of barium. If no cough follows aspiration, the child is more likely to have aspiration-related respiratory problems. Fatigue aspiration accompanied by a decreased cough reflux toward the end of feeding is associated with recurrent pneumonia (Cumming and Reilly, 1972). Its cause is uncertain.

The contrast examination for suspected aspiration should concentrate on the upper esophagus and be recorded on video as otherwise intermittent aspiration may be missed, especially if the aspiration occurs only into the uppermost portion of the trachea (Figure 6–6).

Repeated spontaneous aspiration from the beginning of the procedure is highly significant, and caution should be used in continuing the examination (Figure 6–7). A change in the position of a patient's head or body may eliminate aspiration of liquid barium during videofluoroscopic swallowing studies in patients with oropharyngeal dysphagia. In patients with substantial language or cognitive

defects or restricted head movement, postural changes were less beneficial in preventing aspiration (Rasley et al., 1993). If further information is required following significant aspiration, such as a check for gastroesophageal reflux, the stomach can be filled via a nasogastric tube. Care should be taken to ensure that reflux does not result in aspiration during this part of the procedure. The lights should be kept fully on during the examination of patients at risk, especially if infants, and an experienced assistant should constantly monitor the color and status of the child. At the end of the examination, the barium should be removed from the stomach via the nasogastric tube.

If aspiration occurs, the child is at risk of acute lung collapse and consolidation, which in infants classically affects the right upper lobe (Figure 6–8). In older children and some infants, other lobes can be affected to a variable extent, and intermittent lung changes may be seen if the aspiration is chronic (Figure 6–9).

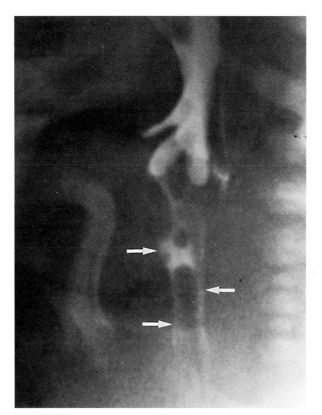

FIGURE 6–7. Gross tracheal aspiration. Contrast media preferentially entered the proximal part of the trachea (*arrows*), with no contrast media entering the esophagus. The examination was stopped at this point.

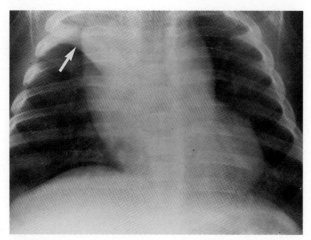

FIGURE 6–8. Acute aspiration. There is right upper lobe collapse and consolidation (*arrow*) due to acute aspiration of a feed in an 8-month-old infant.

Abnormal Sucking and Swallowing

Abnormalities of sucking and swallowing can be classed as anatomic, neuromuscular, or a combination of both. Anatomic abnormalities in the neonate such as cleft palate, macroglossia, or micrognathia are usually obvious on clinical examination. Macroglossia and micrognathia are associated with many conditions (Table 6–1) (Taybi, 1982). In older children, pharyngitis may be found. Radiology may help in

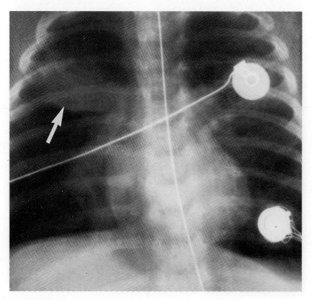

FIGURE 6–9. Chronic aspiration: Riley-Day syndrome (familial dysautonomia). Patchy consolidation occurred intermittently, affecting many areas of the lung, on this occasion primarily in the right upper lobe (*arrow*).

diagnosing foreign bodies, tumors, and diverticula. If reconstructive surgery is considered in children over 5 years of age, velopharyngeal evaluation can aid in assessing speech, which may be altered by the surgery.

Many neuromuscular disorders may affect swallowing (Table 6–2). Myelomeningocele can result in poor bolus formation, nasal escape, and aspiration, possibly related to the Arnold Chiari malformation (Fernbach and McLone, 1985). Cerebral palsy, cricopharyngeal dysfunction, Riley-Day syndrome, collagen disorders, and achalasia are considered in more detail, below.

Cerebral Palsy

Cerebral palsy is the most common cause of disordered swallowing in infancy when no anatomic abnormality is present. In cerebral palsy, swallowing worsens with age whereas functional defects associated with prematurity improve. Any part of the swallowing mechanism can be disturbed, and there may be other clinical manifestations of cerebral palsy.

In older children with cerebral palsy and feeding problems, occupational therapists can work closely with the parents and child to find the most effective method of feeding. When difficulty is encountered, a feeding study under fluoroscopy can be helpful. The child is placed in the position in which he or she is usually fed. Then the parent, with the occupational therapist present, can feed fluid or semi-solid or solid food mixed with barium to assess how effective normal feeding is for that child (Figure 6–10). The child with cerebral palsy often has the most difficulty forming an adequate bolus due to tongue dysfunction (Chen et al., 1990). The feeding technique can be modified during the procedure to find the most effective method, which may incorporate various nipples, a spoon of different size, shape, or position, or a tube placed over the tongue. If aspiration is detected, gastrostomy is considered. Prior to any gastrostomy the competence of the gastroesophageal junction is assessed, as reflux is common in children with cerebral palsy. If needed, an antireflux procedure can be performed at the time of gastrostomy tube placement.

Cricopharyngeal Dysfunction

While the normal anatomy and physiology of the cricopharyngeus muscles are imperfectly known, their dysfunction is understood even less (Palmer, 1976). In normal infants and children, it is common to see intermittent posterior indentation of the cricopha-

TABLE 6–1. Some Causes of Macroglossia and Micrognathia.

Macroglossia
- Debré-Sémélaigne syndrome
- EMG syndrome
- Glycogen storage disease type II
- Hypothyroidism
- Mucopolysaccharidosis I H
- Robinow's syndrome

Micrognathia
- Cockayne's syndrome
- Cri du chat syndrome
- de Lange's syndrome
- First arch syndrome
- Klippel-Feil syndrome
- Mandibulofacial dysostosis (Treacher Collins syndrome)
- Noonan's syndrome
- Oculoauriculovertebral dysplasia (Goldenhar's syndrome)
- Pyknodysostosis
- Trisomy 13, 18, and 22
- Turner's syndrome

ryngeus that does not impede the passage of solids or fluids (see Figure 6–1). Cricopharyngeal achalasia is the failure of effective relaxation of the cricopharyngeus, especially in infancy (Macauley, 1951). Some feel that this condition is relatively common (Caffey, 1978) but most believe it to be rare (Franken and Smith, 1982). Prematurity and maternal diabetes have been associated with this abnormality. One infant with dysphagia from birth, a nonopening cricopharyngeus shown on barium study, and an obstructing ring on endoscopy was found to have fibroblastic replacement of cricopharyngeal muscle fibers on biopsy (Cumming et al., 1986). In adults, a cricopharyngeal defect may be associated histologically with muscle hypertrophy (Torres et al., 1984) but the clinical significance of these histologic findings is still uncertain (Curtis et al., 1984). Myotomy is considered by some to be useful in treating cricopharyngeal achalasia (Bishop, 1974).

Riley-Day Syndrome

Riley-Day syndrome (familial dysautonomia) is a recessively inherited autosomal condition that affects mainly Ashkenazi Jews. It often presents in infancy with gagging, vomiting, and aspiration of food (Figure 6–11). Autonomic dysfunction is indicated by increased sweating, decreased lacrimation, labile hypertension, and orthostatic hypotension.

Cricopharyngeal dysfunction may be associated with the Riley-Day syndrome (Margulies et al., 1968; Gyepes and Linde, 1968). When aspiration occurs, as it often does, coughing may be absent due to a depressed cough reflex (Harris, 1969) (see Figure 6–11). Patients with associated megaesophagus have been successfully treated by the Heller operation (Santel, 1971). Riley-Day syndrome is also associated with a high incidence of scoliosis and fractures (Yoslow et al., 1971).

Scleroderma

Scleroderma (progressive systemic sclerosis) is a well-established cause of disordered esophageal motility in adults. It is rare in children, and findings are similar to those in esophagography and esophageal motility studies in adults. The major signs are distal esophageal dysmotility and reflux, often with esophagitis (Tatelman and Keech, 1966).

Secondary to esophagitis, columnar metaplasia (Barrett's esophagus) may develop, with an asso-

TABLE 6–2. Neuromuscular Causes of Swallowing Disorders.

Bulbar and pseudobulbar palsies
Cerebral palsy—common
Cranial nerve palsies—V, VII, IX, X, XI, XII
Cricopharyngeal dysfunction
Dermatomyositis
Familial dysautonomia (Riley-Day syndrome)
Infections
- Acute infectious polyneuritis
- Diphtheria
- Poliomyelitis
- Tetanus
Myelomeningocele
Muscular dystrophy
Myasthenia gravis
Myotonia dystrophica
Scleroderma
Syndromes
- de Lange's
- Möbius'
- Prader-Willi

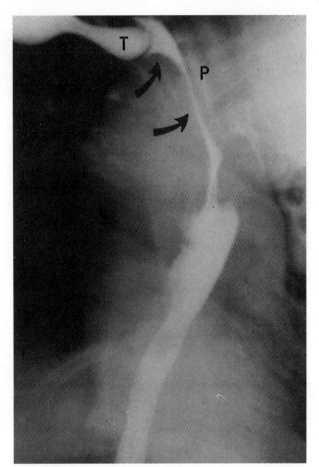

FIGURE 6–10. Normal swallowing study with good bolus formation with neck extended. The tongue is elevated (*arrows*) against the teat (*T*) and palate (*P*), pushing a bolus of barium into the oropharynx.

ciated increased risk of adenocarcinoma (Halpert et al., 1983). Even though rare in children, due to their longer life expectancy, this condition should be followed carefully. Squamous cell carcinoma has also been reported as a rare associated disorder.

Plain films or barium studies will show dilatation due to both atrophy and fibrous replacement of the smooth muscle. A similar process can result in small-bowel dilatation and decreased motility and in the large bowel can result in pseudosacculation, loss of haustration, and occasional dilatation (Olmsted and Madewell, 1976; Martel et al., 1976), although less often in children than adults. Hand contractures and erosive arthropathy are also less common in children than adults (Shanks et al., 1983). Systemic lupus erythematosus rarely may be evident in conjunction with the scleroderma, producing esophageal dysmotility (Dabich et al., 1974).

Dermatomyositis

The most common and earliest finding on esophagography in patients with dermatomyositis is nasal escape of barium due to reduced hypopharyngeal muscle tone. The valleculae and piriform sinuses broaden and the upper esophagus dilates (Grunebaum and Salinge, 1971). The vasculitis affecting the bowel may rarely cause ulceration or even perforation (Figure 6–12). Peristalsis of the small bowel may be reduced and its mucosa thickened (Steiner et al., 1974).

Other manifestations of dermatomyositis include chronic pulmonary parenchymal disease, acro-osteolysis, and soft tissue calcification. Soft tissue calcification is present in at least 40% of patients and is one of four distinct patterns, of which the two most common are deep linear and deep calcaneal deposits. Superficial calcaneal and lacy, reticular, subcutaneous calcification are less common, and the

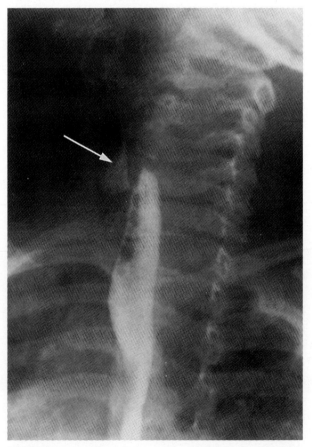

FIGURE 6–11. Chronic aspiration: Riley-Day syndrome (familial dysautonomia). There is intermittent aspiration into the trachea (*arrow*). Due to a depressed cough reflex, there was no coughing.

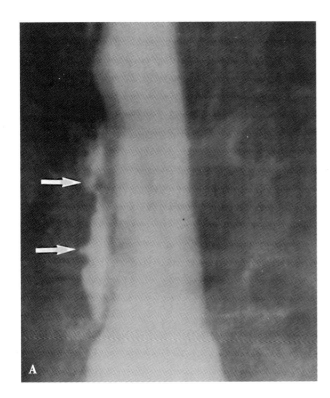

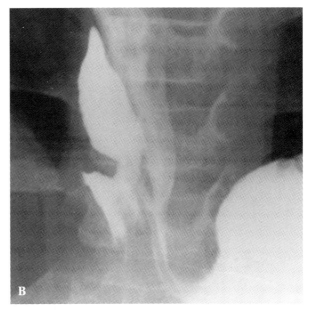

FIGURE 6–12. Dermatomyositis. *A*, Esophageal ulceration (*arrows*) and *B*, perforation arise secondary to the vasculitis.

latter is associated with a severe clinical course of the disease (Blane et al., 1984).

Achalasia

Esophageal achalasia is a neuromuscular disorder of the esophagus with abnormal motility and failure of relaxation of the distal esophagus. It is usually due to absence of the myenteric plexuses in the lower esophagus although rarely it can result from damage to the vagus nerve.

Achalasia is encountered usually in adults between the third and fifth decade inclusive. Less

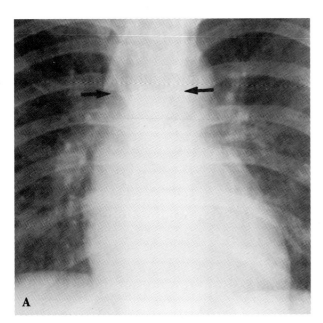

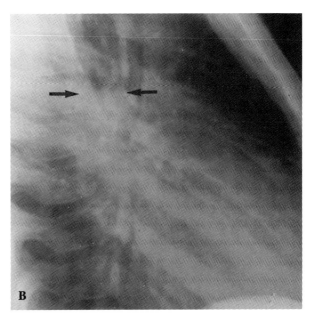

FIGURE 6–13. Achalasia. The stomach gas bubble is absent. A gas-fluid level (*arrows*) in the esophagus is shown on frontal (*A*) and lateral (*B*) chest films.

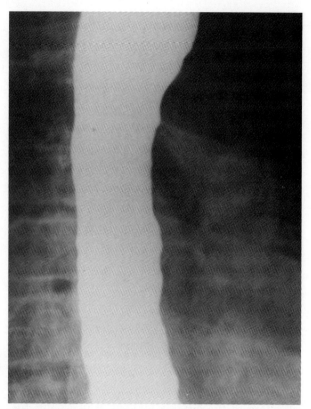

FIGURE 6–14. Achalasia. The esophagogram shows disordered motility with irregular peristaltic contractions giving an irregular outline to the esophagus.

Chest radiography may show evidence of pulmonary disease with parenchymal changes due to aspiration seen as early as infancy (Vaughan and Williams, 1973). There may be an air-filled dilated esophagus (House and Griffiths, 1977) with or without a gas-fluid level, and the stomach gas bubble may be absent in approximately one-third of patients (Figure 6–13) (Muralidharan et al., 1978). In initial achalasia, the esophagogram shows disordered motility (Figure 6–14); in long-standing achalasia, the esophagus is dilated and the obstruction obvious (Figure 6–15). The esophagogram is usually sufficient for diagnosis.

Transabdominal ultrasonography at the level of the gastroesophageal junction may show a large residual in a markedly dilated esophagus (Spence and Fitzgerald, 1996).

In children, manometry may be useful for early diagnosis of achalasia. They demonstrate that the obstruction in achalasia is not due to spasm of the esophagus and cardia (Willich, 1973). Transesophageal US shows promise in evaluating achalasia, demonstrating thickening of the circular and longitudinal muscle layers at the lower esophageal sphincter (Ziegler et al., 1990). Although amyl nitrite has been used during a barium swallow to

than 5% of cases involve children under the age of 14 years (Moersch, 1929; Olsen et al., 1953) and most are older children. However, children of any age can be affected, and there are occasional reports of achalasia in infants (Asch et al., 1974; Magilner and Isard, 1971; Moazam and Rogers, 1976; Starinsky et al., 1984). Although there is seldom a family history, achalasia may be inherited as an autosomal recessive condition (Westley et al., 1975).

The most common symptom of achalasia is dysphagia (Muralidharan et al., 1978) which is usually worse with solid foods; regurgitated food on the child's pillow is a characteristic sign (Sorsdahl and Gay, 1965). Up to one-third of children with achalasia have pulmonary complications (Sorsdahl and Gay, 1965) which are usually secondary to aspiration and may be accompanied by a nocturnal cough and stridor (Tasker, 1995). A rare syndrome of combined esophageal achalasia, alacrima (decreased tear production), and ACTH insensitivity has been reported (Ambrosino et al., 1986; Tuck et al., 1991) and is referred to as triple-A syndrome.

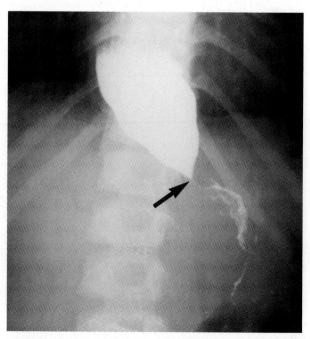

FIGURE 6–15. Achalasia. The dilated barium-filled esophagus shows characteristic tapering and obstruction at the gastroesophageal junction (*arrow*).

distinguish achalasia from pseudoachalasia (Dodds et al., 1986), its value in children is uncertain.

Achalasia is associated with a risk of esophageal carcinoma, usually occurring in the middle third of the esophagus, corresponding to the top level of a column of retained food and probably a result of chronic irritation (Carter and Brewer, 1975). In children (with their long life expectancy), a myotomy is generally the preferred treatment. However, balloon dilatation, used in adults to treat achalasia (Agha and Lee, 1986), may be useful in children (Figure 6–16). This technique is not without complications, and perforations occur in 4 to 6% of cases (Zegel et al., 1979; Stewart et al., 1979; Ott et al., 1984). Post-dilatation contrast swallows are useful in demonstrating perforations but are poor predictors of patient response (Ott et al., 1984).

Chronic Granulomatous Disease

Chronic granulomatous disease, a dysfunction of the leukocytes which predisposes to chronic granulomatous reactions to infections, has been reported to markedly affect esophageal motility. This can result in aperistalsis or irregular peristalsis with an associated tight gastroesophageal sphincter, requiring gastrostomy feeding for nutrition (Markowitz et al., 1982).

CONGENITAL AND DEVELOPMENTAL ANOMALIES OF THE PHARYNX AND ESOPHAGUS

Branchial Arch and Pouch Remnants

Embryogenesis of Branchial Arch and Pouch Remnants

Vertebral (somatic) differentiation and development of body structures occurs at all levels except for the neck and some of its surrounding structures. Here development is due to a complex rearrangement of relationships between branchial clefts and pharyngeal pouches.

In the fifth week of gestation, five branchial arches form (Figure 6–17). Each consists of a cartilaginous bar, muscle and artery derived from mesoderm, and nerve tissue derived from neural crest cells. The arches are separated by branchial clefts, which lie on the external surface of the fetus. In the primitive foregut, there are a similar number of pharyngeal pouches, which do not quite meet the branchial clefts. (In the lower vertebrates, pouches and clefts communicate to form gills.)

The branchial arches, which form in the fifth week, virtually disappear by the seventh week, coinciding with the descent of the thyroid gland. Thus,

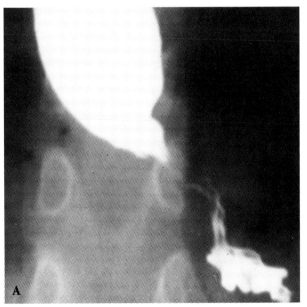
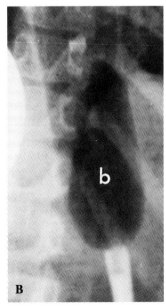

FIGURE 6–16. Achalasia. (*A*) The barium swallow shows a markedly dilated barium-filled esophagus with characteristic tapering and obstruction. (*B*) A balloon catheter (b) is positioned and dilated within the narrowing.

TABLE 6–3. Derivatives of Branchial Arches and Pouches.*

First arch and pouch
    Meckel's cartilage (forms the mandible)
    Body and tongue
Second arch and pouch
    Palatine tonsil and supratonsillar fossa
    Part of tongue
    Foramen cecum
    Hyoid (lesser horn and part of body)
Third arch and pouch
    Part of epiglottis
    Thymus
    Hyoid (greater horn and part of body)
Fourth arch and pouch
    Part of right subclavian artery
    Arch of aorta
    Part of epiglottis
    Cuneiform cartilage
    Thyroid
    Superior parathyroid (thymus—inconsistent)
Fifth arch and pouch
    Ultimobranchial body (becomes lost in the
        developing thyroid)
Sixth arch and pouch
    Pulmonary artery
    Ductus arteriosus
    Cricoid, arytenoid, and corniculate cartilages

*Related to the gastrointestinal tract, thyroid, and parathyroid.

in this short period the arches have undergone the complex changes necessary to form their ultimate structures (Table 6–3).

The second branchial arch overgrows the third and fourth arches and reaches approximately to the fifth arch, making the second branchial cleft larger than the others (Figure 6–17). Of branchial cleft abnormalities, 75 to 95% arise from the second branchial arch (Maran and Buchanan, 1978; Neal and Pemberton, 1945). Most of the remainder arise from the first branchial cleft, and a few arise from the third branchial cleft. Abnormalities from the fourth branchial cleft are exceptionally rare.

Presentation and Investigation

Branchial cleft abnormality can present as a sinus, cyst, or fistula. If there is communication between the branchial cleft and the corresponding pharyn-

geal pouch, a fistula develops (see Figure 6–18); with no communication, a sinus forms to the skin. If the branchial cleft remains patent without a communication to the pharyngeal pouch and to the skin, then a cyst develops. Only rarely may a cyst communicate through a sinus to the pharynx.

Sinus and fistula tracts are usually discovered in infancy or early childhood. They may present with mucoid drainage and are less likely than cysts to become infected. Cysts often present as mass lesions in later childhood or even in adulthood.

Investigation of sinus or fistula consists of injecting water-soluble contrast media via a fine catheter such as a sialogram catheter (see Figure 6–18). Contrast injection of the tract may be combined with a computed tomography (CT) evaluation, which can definitively diagnose 80% of patients, based on characteristic morphology, location, and displacement of surrounding structures (Harnsberger et al., 1984). Computed tomography is very useful in the evaluation of branchial fistula (Herman et al., 1992) and in the demonstration of a branchial cleft cyst in an unusual location such as posterior and medial to the sternocleidomastoid muscle, displacing

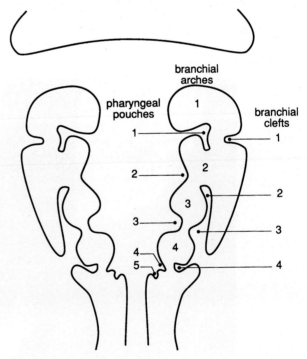

FIGURE 6–17. Coronal section through a 5- to 6-week-old fetus. The second arch grows inferiorly to lie over the third and fourth arches. This predisposes to the formation of branchial cleft anomalies.

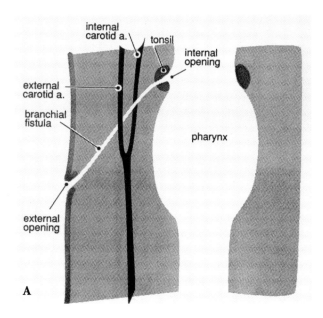

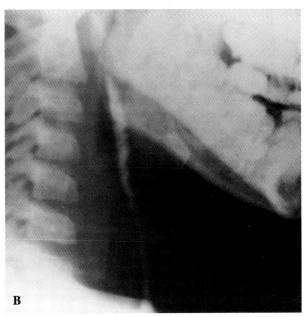

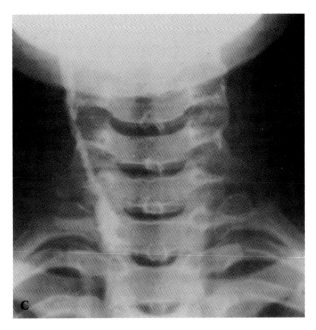

FIGURE 6–18. Second branchial cleft fistula. *A,* Line drawing demonstrates how the second branchial cleft fistula passes between the external and internal carotid arteries. The fistulograph shows the superior end of the fistula in the region of the tonsils and the inferior end of the lower neck on lateral (*B*) and frontal (*C*) views.

the carotid artery and internal jugular vein anteromedially or extending between the external and internal carotid arteries (Salazar et al., 1985). Cysts can be seen well on US of the neck (Figure 6–19). Esophagography is usually not indicated but may occasionally demonstrate a persistent isolated pharyngeal pouch.

Types of Anomalies

First Arch and Cleft Anomalies. Anomalies of the first arch and cleft usually involve the ear, producing auricular pits or a cervicoaural fistula, sinus, or cyst. Auricular pits alone are not a branchial cleft anom-

aly, since they were found in 1% of British military personnel and may well be familial (Fourman and Fourman, 1955). A cyst can occur at any point along the potential course. The fistula, from the skin in the submandibular triangle superolateral to the hyoid bone, passes through the region of the parotid gland and facial nerve to reach the bony/cartilagenous junction of the external auditory canal. It is unusual for radiologic examinations to diagnose a cervicoaural fistula, sinus, or cyst, but US, sinography, or CT may be helpful. In cysts involving the parotid, US and CT cannot clearly distinguish branchial

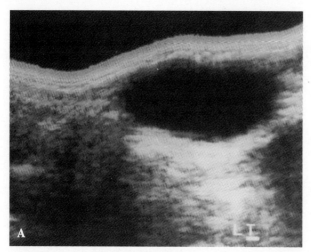 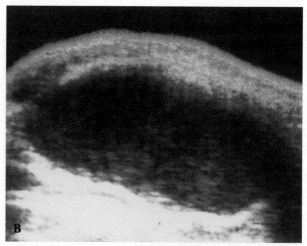

FIGURE 6–19. Second branchial cleft cyst. Longitudinal ultrasonography of the neck can demonstrate either an echo-free cyst (*A*) or an echogenic mass (*B*). The increased through transmission of sound in both examples indicates the fluid nature of the mass and aids differentiation from a solid lesion.

cysts from inflammatory cysts of the parotid but in practice, most anomalies do not involve the parotid gland (Harnsberger et al., 1984).

Second Arch and Cleft Anomalies. These are the most common branchial anomalies and consist of a fistula, cyst, or sinus. A complete fistula passes from the region of the tonsillar bed to the anterior border of the sternocleidomastoid, typically in the lower third of the neck (see Figure 6–18). It passes between the internal and external carotid arteries. A fistulograph is the study of choice in patients with this anomaly (Harnsberger et al., 1984).

A cyst can occur anywhere along this tract but is usually superficial in the neck and lined with stratified squamous epithelium. Cysts show well on US and can contain a variable internal echogenicity (see Figure 6–19). A cyst is typically echo free but may be echogenic if it is infected or contains desquamated cells. The presence of through transmission helps distinguish it from a solid lesion (see Figure 6–19 A and B).

Cysts at the mandibular angle usually have a characteristic appearance on CT. The cyst is usually fluid-filled, displacing the sternocleidomastoid posteriorly or posterolaterally, the carotid artery and jugular vein medially or posteromedially, and the submandibular gland anteriorly (Harnsberger et al., 1984). Occasionally there are other patterns, especially when a cyst is located posterior and medial to the sternocleidomastoid muscle; in this position there is displacement of the carotid artery and internal jugu-

lar vein anteromedially. The extension of the cyst between external and internal carotid arteries may be helpful in these cases (Salazar et al., 1985). Deeper cysts are rarely seen and are probably pharyngeal pouch remnants and contain ciliated epithelium.

Sinuses to the skin are uncommon, and many are secondary to previous drainage of an infected cyst. Sinuses to the pharynx are rare.

Third Branchial Cleft and Pharyngeal Pouch Anomalies. These rare cystic anomalies usually lie deep to the internal carotid artery, intimately related to the vagus nerve. Infected cysts may infrequently extend into the retropharynx or chest, causing diagnostic difficulty in differentiation with other retropharyngeal abscesses and chest pathology. The distinction is important because the surgical treatment is different (Hewel et al., 1995; Murdoch et al., 1995). Internal sinuses are also rare (Fowler, 1962).

Fourth Branchial Cleft and Pharyngeal Pouch Anomalies. Many doubt the existence of fourth arch or cleft anomalies. The single-case report of Tucker and Skolnick (1973) differs in some respects from the projected descriptions proposed from the embryology of the fourth arch (Gray and Skandalakis, 1972).

Esophageal Atresia and Tracheoesophageal Fistula

Esophageal atresia and tracheoesophageal fistula are the most common anomalies affecting the esophagus and trachea. Their etiology and normal embryogenesis are discussed below.

Embryogenesis of the Esophagus and Trachea

The esophagus begins just distal to the level of the fifth pharyngeal pouch. A laryngotracheal groove develops at this level during the fourth week of gestation, growing caudally and forming lateral lung buds at its caudal end (Figure 6–20). The normal development and separation of the trachea and esophagus depends on three events occurring during the fourth and fifth weeks of gestation: differentiation of the primitive foregut endoderm into the trachea anteriorly and into the esophagus posteriorly, the appearance of lateral ridges which grow into a separate trachea and esophagus, and the elongation of the trachea and esophagus craniocaudally.

Failure of any of these events can result in atresia or fistula of the esophagus or trachea although the exact mechanism is poorly understood. It is thought to be a failure not of recanalization but of probably either malfunction of lateral ridge fusion or rapid elongation that outstrips the capacity for separate tracheal and esophageal formation.

Clinical Features and Presentation

There are four important types of esophageal atresia and tracheoesophageal fistula (Figure 6–21): esophageal atresia without fistula (5 to 10% of

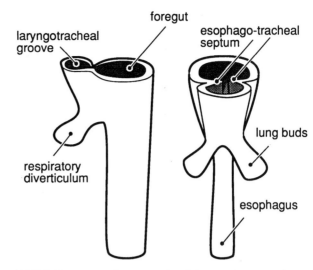

FIGURE 6–20. Embryogenesis of the esophagus and trachea. A laryngotracheal groove develops during the fourth week of gestation, growing caudally and forming lateral lung buds at its caudal end.

cases), esophageal atresia with distal fistula with or without proximal fistula (85 to 94%), esophageal atresia with proximal fistula only (this type is rare), and H-type tracheoesophageal fistula without atresia (1 to 5%).

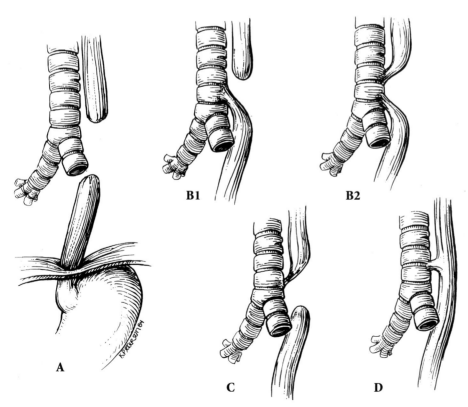

FIGURE 6–21. Types and frequency of occurrence of tracheoesophageal fistula. *A,* Esophageal atresia without tracheoesophageal fistula, 5–10%. *B1,* Esophageal atresia with distal tracheoesophageal fistula, 85–94%. *B2,* Esophageal atresia with proximal and distal tracheoesophageal fistula, rare. *C,* Esophageal atresia with proximal tracheoesophageal fistula, rare. *D,* H-type tracheoesophageal fistula without atresia, 1–5%.

The reported incidence of esophageal atresia with tracheoesophageal fistula varies between 1 in 2000 (Shapiro et al., 1958) and 1 in 5083 live births (Ingalls and Prindle, 1949). Familial tracheoesophageal atresia has occurred in siblings, identical twins (Blank et al., 1967; Ohkuma, 1978), in 2 children with different mothers but the same father (Mackenzie, 1980), and in a mother and her children (Engel et al., 1970). Other anomalies of tracheal and esophageal separation occur but are rare (Figure 6–22).

Esophageal atresia presents on the first day of life with coughing and choking, which may be associated with cyanosis. Excessive salivation may occur, especially in esophageal atresia without fistula. Esophageal atresia should be considered if maternal polyhydramnios was present, if there is excessive salivation, if a catheter could not be passed into the stomach after delivery, or if coughing, choking, or cyanosis occur during the infant's first feeding. The abdomen is often distended since the fistula opens in expiration and closes in inspiration, allowing air to enter the stomach. This distention, if severe, may interfere with respiration. A scaphoid abdomen is associated with the rare forms of atresia that have no distal fistula.

The H-type fistula usually presents later in childhood and may even be found in adulthood. It usually presents with chronic or intermittent respiratory symptoms and can be difficult to diagnose if small (see Chapter 3).

Imaging of Esophageal Atresia and Tracheoesophageal Fistula

The association of polyhydramnios with esophageal atresia and tracheoesophageal fistula is well known and can occur as early as 24 weeks. In one-third of patients, antenatal ultrasonographic diagnosis is possible as little amniotic fluid passes the fistula, resulting in polyhydramnios and absent stomach fluid. However, antenatal US fails to detect two-thirds of cases, presumably because the tracheoesophageal fistula is large enough to allow the passage of amniotic fluid (Pretorius et al., 1987). In the rare cases with no distal fistula, antenatal diagnosis is more reliable and is based on absent gastric fluid and polyhydramnios (Farrant, 1980; Pretorius et al., 1987). Antenatal US can also show associated anomalies such as the VATER association (Claiborne et al., 1986) (see Associations, below). Amniography (used to diagnose bowel obstruction) may fail to show an esophageal atresia if there is a distal fistula (Rao, 1978). Hence, diagnosis in the majority of cases is made after birth.

Following delivery, plain-film radiography is usually sufficient to diagnose the more common atresias. After attempted placement of a nasogastric tube, frontal and lateral radiographs of the chest and upper abdomen will show the extent of the proximal pouch and the presence of a distal fistula (Figure 6–23). If there is no gas in a scaphoid abdomen, there is no distal fistula (Figure 6–24). Frontal and

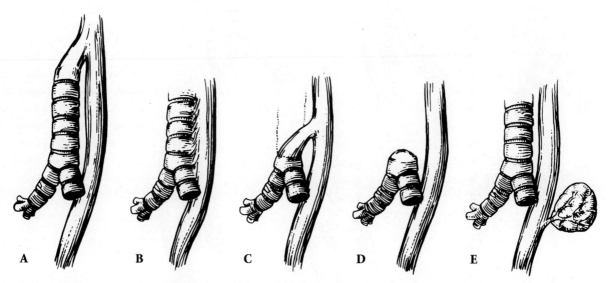

FIGURE 6–22. Rare anomalies of tracheal and esophageal separation. *A,* Laryngotracheoesophageal cleft. *B,* Esophagotrachea. *C,* Tracheal agenesis with fistula. *D,* Tracheal agenesis. *E,* Esophageal bronchus.

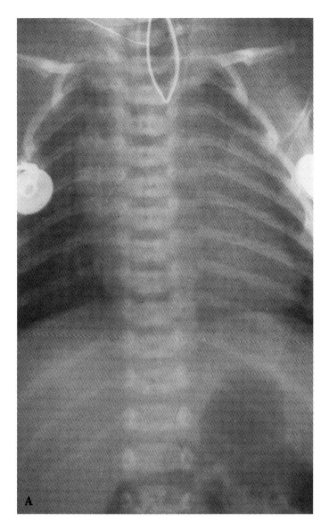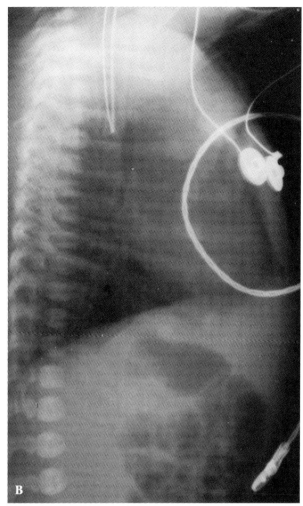

FIGURE 6–23. Esophageal atresia and tracheoesophageal fistula in the newborn infant. The nasogastric tube is doubled up in the proximal esophageal pouch on frontal (*A*) and lateral (*B*) projections. Gas in the abdomen demonstrates the presence of a tracheoesophageal fistula.

lateral chest radiographs can be used to delineate the size of the pouch after injecting air into the proximal pouch. This procedure must be carried out with heart rate monitoring, as profound bradycardia and respiratory problems can occur secondary to esophageal distension.

Contrast medium may be injected into the proximal pouch by nasoesophageal tube to exclude a proximal fistula (a pouchogram); occasionally more than one proximal fistula is present (Goodwin et al., 1978). However, we do not find this necessary preoperatively at our hospital. The rare proximal fistula in the chest will be found intraoperatively, and the rare proximal fistula in the neck is more approachable from the neck at a separate operation after the first esophageal oper-

ation has healed. If a pouchogram is performed, less than 0.5 mL of a solution of unflavored barium and water (Figure 6–25) or (preferably) one of the newer non-ionic low-osmolar contrast media should be used. The contrast media should be instilled under fluoroscopic control while monitoring the pulse rate; fluoroscopy is necessary to prevent aspiration of barium (Figure 6–26). Water-soluble bronchographic media may also be used (Thomas and Chrispin, 1969) but barium or the newer non-ionic low-osmolar contrast media are preferable. Videotape or cine loop recording of the procedure will avoid needless repetition of the examination. After filling the pouch, the barium should be removed through the nasoesophageal tube by prompt suction with a syringe.

Management

The common atresias with distal fistula are usually repaired by primary anastomosis with division of the fistula. The anastomosis can be end-to-end or end-to-side (a Duhamel procedure). The apparent increased incidence of recurrent fistula (Ein et al., 1983) and other complications (Ein and Theman, 1973) with the end-to-side anastomoses is not universally found (Beardmore, 1973). Rarely the atresia may be due to an esophageal web proximal to the tracheoesophageal fistula (Fox, 1978; Jona and Belin, 1977) which simplifies surgery.

Atresia without distal tracheoesophageal fistula is usually treated by initially performing a gastrostomy, as primary closure is rarely possible. A cervical esophagostomy may be created to enable sham feeding, which allows the swallow reflex to be learned prior to a definitive repair and helps to drain secretions.

A considerable gap usually exists between the proximal pouch and the distal pouch, except when there is a proximal fistula (Berdon and Baker, 1975). To assess whether primary repair is feasible, the length of the gap can be found by passing a tube through the gastrostomy into the distal esophageal pouch, while another tube lies in the proximal pouch (Figure 6–27) (Ein and Friedberg, 1981). To demonstrate the smallest gap, gentle pressure is exerted on the tubes to approximate the ends of the pouches (see Figure 6–27). Barium can be used to show the distal pouch (Figure 6–28) but it does not demonstrate the smallest gap.

A ruler can be used to measure the gap, provided allowance is made for magnification and dif-

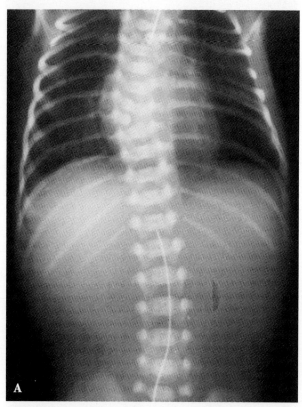

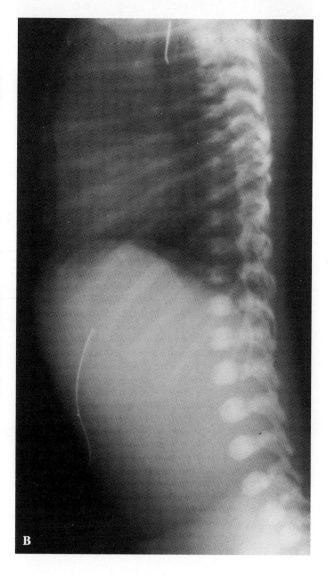

FIGURE 6–24. Esophageal atresia without a tracheoesophageal fistula in a newborn infant. A nasogastric tube is present in the proximal esophagus pouch on frontal (*A*) and lateral (*B*) projections. The lack of air in a scaphoid abdomen demonstrates that tracheoesophageal fistula is not present. The multiple rib and vertebral anomalies with scoliosis indicate the VATER association. An umbilical venous catheter is present.

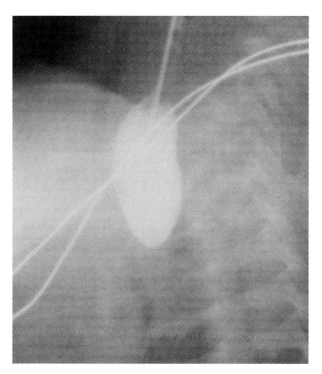

FIGURE 6–25. Esophageal atresia. Barium instilled into the proximal pouch excludes a proximal pouch fistula. The air-filled trachea is deviated anteriorly by the distended proximal pouch.

ferences in projection. When comparing films, the gap and ruler should be compared to the height of the same midthoracic vertebral body. If the esophageal deficit is within a few centimeters, then further waiting is advised to see if growth of the pouches helps bridge the gap (Ein and Friedberg, 1981). Manual bouginage of the upper esophageal pouch can be performed to stimulate growth (Howard and Meyers, 1965) but is rarely used today. An alternative stretching procedure involves elongation of the proximal pouch using mercury-filled bags and stretching the distal pouch by bouginage. However, spontaneous growth of the esophageal segments may occur without any stretching or bouginage (Puri et al., 1981), and no stretching is performed at our hospitals. A circular esophageal myotomy may aid primary anastomosis and give good long-term results. It will be seen as a somewhat dilated proximal esophagus on barium swallow (see Figure 6–36) (Vizas et al., 1978; Janik et al., 1980).

If a primary repair cannot be undertaken, a colonic interposition can be performed (Figures 6–29 and 6–30) or a gastric tube can be fashioned

(Figures 6–31 and 6–32). Early complications of colonic interposition include anastomotic leaks, aspiration, and ischemic necrosis of the colon. These complications also can arise later along with gastrocolic reflux and reflux into the residual esophagus (Christensen and Shapir, 1986). In addition, a colonic interposition becomes increasingly tortuous as colon growth exceeds growth of the thorax, leading to stasis, inflammation, obstruction, and aspiration (see Figure 6–30) (Ein and Friedberg, 1981). However, many surgeons prefer colonic interposition (Azar et al., 1971).

Complications also occur with gastric tubes, as the small diameter of their lumen makes the anastomosis in the neck more difficult (Ein and Friedberg, 1981). The gastric tube is created from the greater curvature of the stomach and can be fashioned retrosternally (see Figure 6–32) (Ein et al., 1973). Anastomosis between the gastric tube and the esophagostomy takes place 2 to 4 weeks later, following

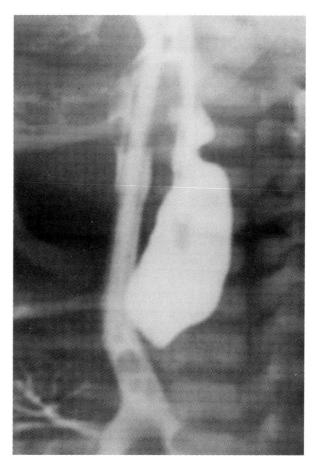

FIGURE 6–26. Esophageal atresia. Overfilling of the proximal pouch has caused severe aspiration.

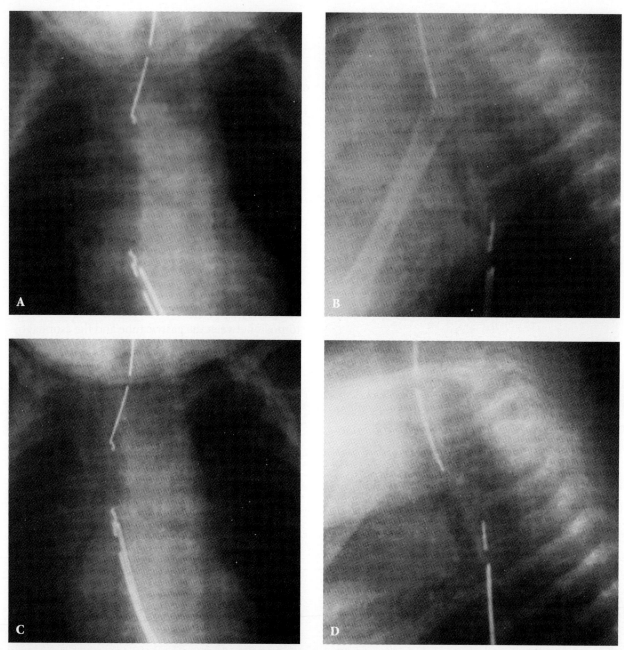

FIGURE 6–27. Esophageal atresia without tracheoesophageal fistula. Tubes are positioned in proximal and distal esophageal pouches, the latter via a gastrostomy shown on frontal (*A*) and lateral (*B*) spot films. Pressing the tubes gently toward each other will demonstrate the smallest distance between the pouches as shown on frontal (*C*) and lateral (*D*) spot films.

satisfactory contrast studies through the neck gastric tube stoma and gastrostomy (see Figure 6–32). Examination with water-soluble contrast material should precede barium study to assure postoperative integrity prior to anastomosis of the cervical esophagostomy and the gastric tube. Meanwhile, until healing is complete, feeding continues either by gastrostomy, by gastrostomy jejunal tube, or by hyperalimentation. The cervical anastomosis leaks in 63% of cases regardless of whether antral or parietal cell mass is brought up to the esophagus; the leak usually heals spontaneously but almost half (43%) develop a stricture (Ein et al., 1978). Occasionally there is a proximal pouch fistula in associa-

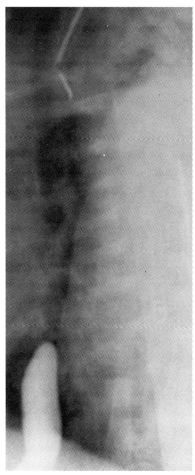

FIGURE 6–28. Esophageal atresia without tracheoesophageal fistula. A tube is in the proximal esophageal pouch. Barium instilled via a gastrostomy has refluxed into the lower esophageal pouch. This does *not* demonstrate the smallest gap between pouches.

tion with atresia and no distal fistula. In these cases, the distal pouch is generally large, facilitating surgery (Berdon, 1975).

Associations

The VATER Association. Most of the associations with esophageal atresia and tracheoesophageal fistula are covered by the acronym VATER, which represents Vertebral anomalies, Anal atresia, Tracheoesophageal fistula with Esophageal atresia, and Radial dysplasia (Quan and Smith, 1972; 1973). However, pulmonary, vascular and renal anomalies have also been observed (Barnes and Smith, 1978). Various types of tracheoesophageal fistula are associated (Barry and Auldist, 1974) but distal tracheoesophageal fistula is the most common (Barnes and Smith, 1978).

Vertebral anomalies can occur anywhere in the spine and may consist of aplasia or hypoplasia of pedicles or vertebral bodies (Figure 6–33). Scoliosis may develop as the child grows, and rib deformities are often seen when a vertebral anomaly affects the dorsal spine (see Figure 6–25).

Vascular abnormalities include cardiac lesions and a single umbilical artery. A ventricular septal defect is the most common cardiac lesion, either as a solitary finding or combined with other cardiac anomalies. Other defects include patent ductus arteriosus, tetralogy of Fallot, single ventricle, and transposition of the great vessels.

Approximately 5% of infants with VATER association have a right aortic arch which may cause surgical problems if the usual right thoracotomy is performed and hence, some surgeons prefer this information preoperatively (Harrison et al., 1977). If this information is required and is not apparent from the plain films, CT can accurately localize the aorta (Day, 1985). (At our hospitals, the surgeons do not require this information preoperatively.)

The anorectal anomaly is often a high rectal atresia with a bladder fistula (Barnes, 1978).

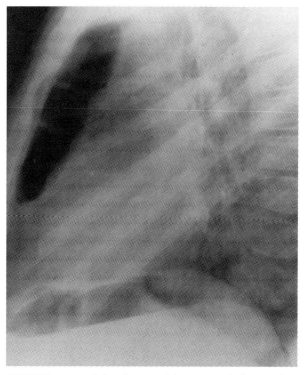

FIGURE 6–29. Colon interposition. Lateral chest radiograph shows the retrosternal location of the colon interposition.

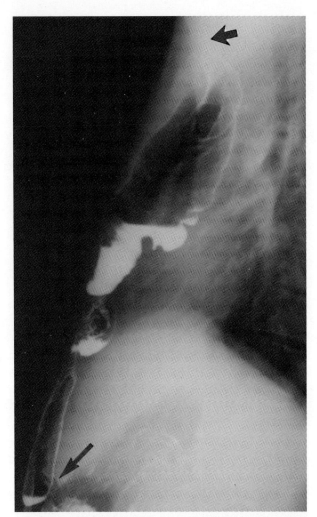

FIGURE 6–30. Colon interposition for esophageal atresia without tracheoesophageal fistula. Lateral view after barium swallow shows the interposed colon in the left anterior mediastinum. The proximal anastomosis (*short arrow*) is to the esophagus; the distal anastomosis (*long arrow*) is to the gastric corpus.

The kidneys can be dysplastic, hypoplastic, or ectopic. Other associated genitourinary or muscular anomalies include caliceal diverticulum, hydronephrosis, persistent urachus, and deficient abdominal musculature (Taybi, 1982).

The radius may be hypoplastic (Figure 6–34) or aplastic, and polydactyly and triphalangeal thumb may be present.

Other Associations. In the absence of a vertebral abnormality, 13 pairs of ribs have been seen (Hodson and Shaw, 1973) as well as duodenal atresia (McCook and Felman, 1978). A variety of bronchopulmonary anomalies may be associated, such as

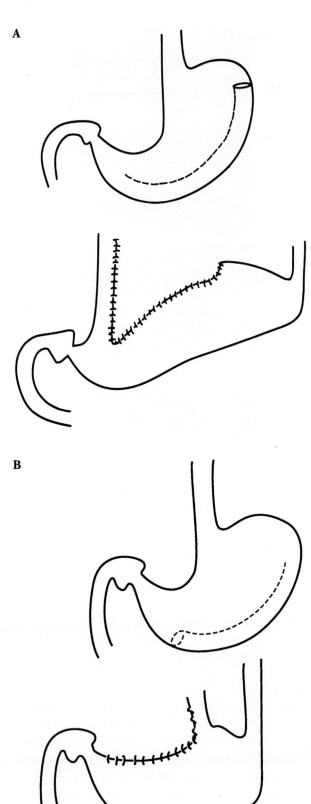

FIGURE 6–31. Gastric tube. The gastric tube is created from the greater curvature of the stomach and can be fashioned as a peristaltic (*A*) or antiperistaltic tube (*B*).

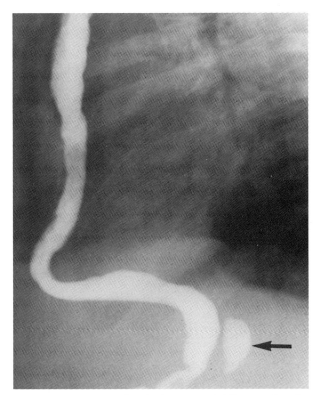

FIGURE 6–32. Gastric tube loopogram. The gastric tube is in the anterior mediastinum. Reflux into the distal esophageal remnant has occurred (*arrow*).

a single pleural cavity (Marshall et al., 1986), and a spectrum of lobar or pulmonary hypoplasia or agenesis (Black and Welch, 1986; Benson et al., 1985).

Segmental esophageal stenosis distal to an esophageal atresia may rarely be found at the junction of the middle and lower thirds of the esophagus. Most of these patients have a distal tracheoesophageal fistula, and the stenosis is probably fibromuscular thickening although tracheobronchial remnants could also give this appearance (Thomason and Gay, 1987) and gastroesophageal reflux could result in a similar stricture. All should be amenable to esophageal dilatation using Gruentzig angioplasty balloon catheters (see Figure 6–34) (Stringer et al., 1985).

Duodenal atresia is an association most often found in Down syndrome children with esophageal atresia. The plain-film findings are characteristic if a tracheoesophageal fistula is present, with a double bubble appearance due to gaseous distension of the stomach and duodenum (Figure 6–35).

A surprising association reported by Ahmed (1970), and which we have also encountered in our hospital, is infantile hypertrophic pyloric stenosis. Although acquired esophageal strictures are a well-known association of epidermolysis bullosa dystroficans, congenital esophageal atresia has been described with this condition (Doi et al., 1986). It is uncertain whether there is a true association.

Complications

The three early complications that may follow operative treatment of esophageal atresia are leak, recurrent fistula, and stricture. Long-term problems that may present early or late and can be interrelated include stricture with or without impaction of food, problems related to esophageal dysmotility, respiratory complications, and progressive scoliosis.

Respiratory Symptoms and Complications. Coughing, choking, gagging, apnea, dying spells,

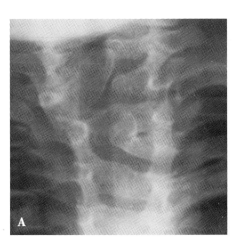
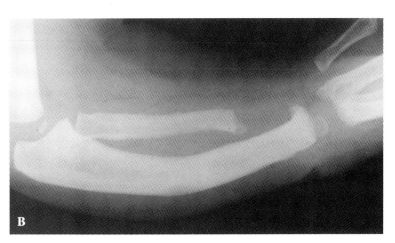

FIGURE 6–33. VATER association. A 6-year-old boy has anomalies of the vertebral bodies and laminae (*A*) in association with ulnar bowing and a hypoplastic radius (*B*).

cyanosis, wheezing, and recurrent chest infections from aspiration can all occur secondary to anastomotic stricture, gastroesophageal reflux, esophageal dyskinesia, or recurrent tracheoesophageal fistula. An abnormal tracheal nerve plexus innervation is present, which may be related to some of the tracheal dysfunction and respiratory symptoms (Nakazato and Landing et al., 1986; Nakazato and Wells et al., 1986).

Tracheomalacia can produce stridor (Daum, 1971) with life-threatening anoxic spells; it may require surgery (Filler et al., 1976). On fluoroscopy during barium examination, the trachea will be seen to collapse on expiration in tracheomalacia (Figure 6–36). Other respiratory complications that are less common include tracheal stenosis (Daum, 1971) and hemorrhagic right upper lobe infarction (Lindham et al., 1979).

Anastomotic Leak. Anastomotic leak is serious and can be fatal (Daum, 1971). A leak usually presents early, often with an associated pneumothorax, and can be confirmed by an esophagogram with a non-ionic low-osmolar water-soluble contrast

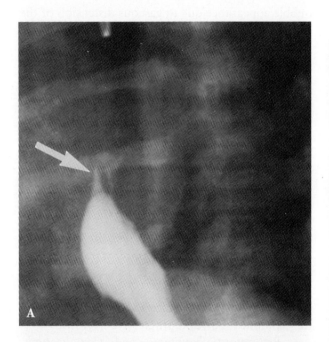

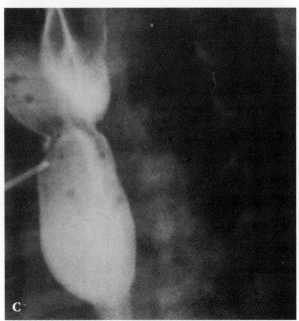

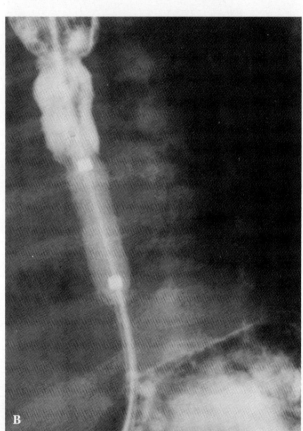

FIGURE 6–34. Esophageal dilatation. *A,* Barium instilled via a gastrostomy showed a tight lower esophageal stricture (*arrow*) in an infant. *B,* Dilatation of the stricture can be performed using Gruentzig angioplasty balloon catheters. *C,* A follow-up study showed a marked improvement.

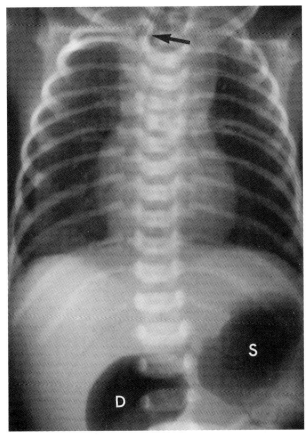

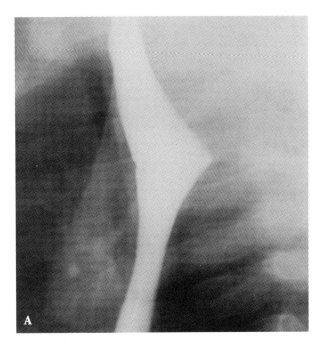

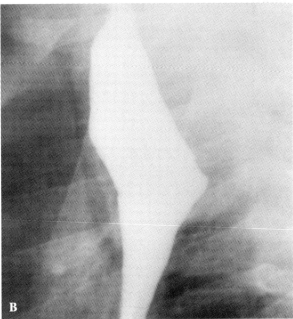

FIGURE 6–35. Esophageal atresia, tracheoesophageal fistula, and duodenal atresia. The plain films show the high location of the nasogastric tube in the proximal esophageal pouch (*arrow*) and a characteristic double bubble appearance due to gaseous distension of the stomach (*S*) and duodenum (*D*).

FIGURE 6–36. Tracheomalacia. The trachea is of normal caliber during inspiration (*A*) but collapses during each expiration (*B*) independent of the presence of barium. A myotomy has resulted in a dilated proximal esophagus.

medium. (If barium is used, it may enter the pleura or mediastinum, remaining there for years.) To exclude a leak and other complications, postoperative esophagogram is performed before oral feeding. Barium can be used if a leak is not suspected. However, for the first postoperative swallow, the relatively new non-ionic low-osmolar water-soluble contrast media are preferred although water-soluble bronchographic contrast media also can be used.

Recurrent Fistula. Approximately 10% of tracheoesophageal fistula recur (Kafrouni et al., 1970; Stanford et al., 1973) although higher and lower incidences have been reported (Ein and Theman, 1973; Daum, 1971). Diagnosis is difficult (Kafrouni et al., 1970; Filston et al., 1982) and may be delayed for some years (Kiser et al., 1972; Slim and Tabry, 1974; Falletta, 1964). The fistula may be asymptomatic although many are associated with respiratory symptoms. It is generally agreed that the number of symptoms is directly related to the size of the fistula (Daum, 1971).

Plain films of the chest and abdomen may show a dilated, air-filled esophagus and an abdomen

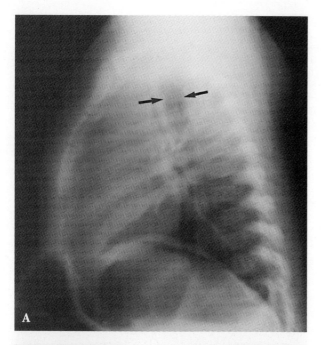

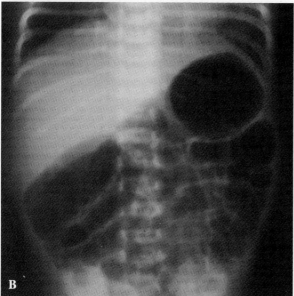

FIGURE 6–37. Recurrent tracheoesophageal fistula. Plain films show (*A*) a dilated, air-filled esophagus (*arrows*) in the chest and an abdomen (*B*) distended with bowel gas.

distended with bowel gas (Figure 6–37) (Stringer, 1984). A chest radiograph shows evidence of chronic lung disease secondary to the repeated aspiration of esophageal contents.

Many techniques advocated for investigating recurrent fistula are similar to those used in H-type fistula examinations. Routine esophagography may show recurrent fistula (Figure 6–38) or unusual

anterior beaking of the esophagus in the region of the anastomosis, which indicates the possible presence of a recurrent fistula even in the absence of symptoms (Figure 6–39) (Stringer, 1983). A tube esophagogram using videotape or cine loop recording should be performed, ideally in the prone position (Stringer, 1983) (Figure 6–40). This may have to be repeated at different times to demonstrate the fistula. Though usually not necessary, selective catheterization of the fistula has been advocated to confirm the diagnosis, demonstrate the position and course of the fistula, and assist the surgeon (Filston et al., 1982; Kirks and Briley, 1979).

Other methods of investigation include injecting methylene blue into the esophagus during bronchoscopy or instilling it into the trachea during esophagoscopy. Alternatively, bubbles may be seen during esophagoscopy if saline is instilled into the esophagus and positive pressure is applied to the airway (Kafrouni et al., 1970; Stanford et al., 1973).

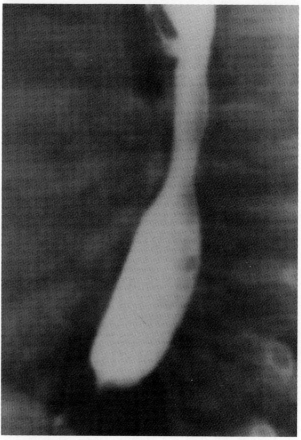

FIGURE 6–38. Recurrent tracheoesophageal fistula. The fistula extends from the esophagus inferiorly to the trachea superiorly.

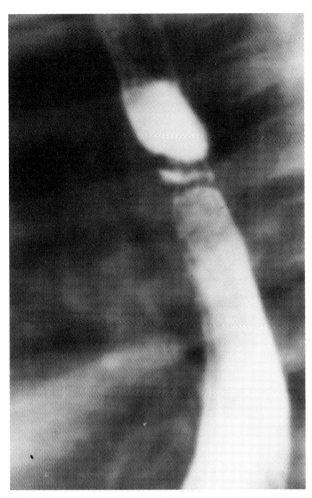

FIGURE 6–39. Recurrent tracheoesophageal fistula. Tube esophagogram using video recording shows beaking of the anterior esophagus, which suggests a recurrent fistula despite the absence of symptoms.

A missed proximal pouch fistula may mimic a recurrent tracheoesophageal fistula. However, a missed fistula tends to be some distance proximal to the anastomosis, or it would have been found at surgery (Daum, 1971, Hays et al., 1966).

Stricture and Esophageal Dysmotility. Between 35 to 50% of patients develop strictures (Laks et al., 1972) that may be secondary to the anastomotic repair or to esophageal dysmotility and reflux esophagitis. If due to a tight anastomosis, the initial follow-up barium esophagograph will demonstrate the abnormality, and the stricture can be dilated.

Late strictures tend to be secondary to reflux esophagitis. The gastroesophageal junction is sometimes patulous following repair of an atresia, and this probably predisposes it to reflux (Figure 6–41). In addition, the esophagus below the anastomosis is invariably dyskinetic with disordered and ineffectual peristalsis. The cause of this dysmotility is uncertain but there is an abnormality of the myenteric plexus of the esophagus and stomach (Nakazato, 1986; Landing et al., 1986). The dysmotility is often associated with reflux, which in the absence of normal esophageal peristalsis leads to esophagitis (Figure 6–42) and stricture (Figure 6–43), a situation that is exacerbated by the recumbent position usually favored for babies. The stricture is usually seen at the level of the anastomosis but is sometimes at a lower level. Multiple strictures may be infrequently encountered (see Figure 6–43). Plain films may show air-fluid levels if the strictures are severe (Figure 6–44), and complete

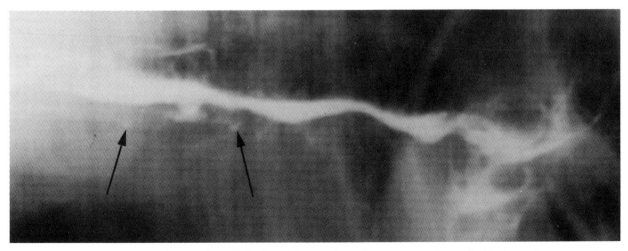

FIGURE 6–40. Recurrent tracheoesophageal fistula. Videotaped esophagogram performed with the patient prone shows a recurrent fistula that could not be demonstrated by other techniques. Faint traces of barium are in the trachea (*arrows*).

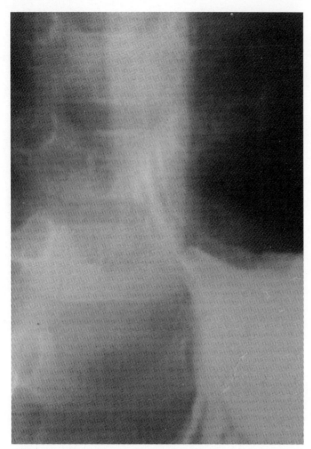

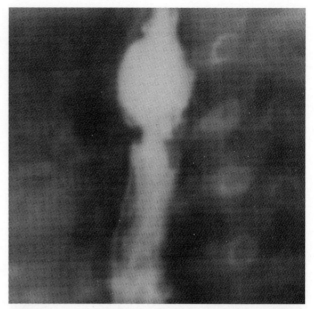

FIGURE 6–42. Reflux esophagitis following esophageal atresia repair. The mucosa of the esophagus below the anastomosis is irregular on this single-contrast barium esophagram performed by injecting the barium through a nasoesophageal tube.

FIGURE 6–41. Patulous gastroesophageal junction. A barium study shows a sliding hiatus hernia with patulous gastroesophageal junction following repair of an esophageal atresia that probably predisposes to reflux.

obstruction may be seen on a contrast study (Figure 6–45).

Aspiration pneumonia and dysphagia can occur without a stricture, probably secondary to esophageal dyskinesia (Chrispin et al., 1966).

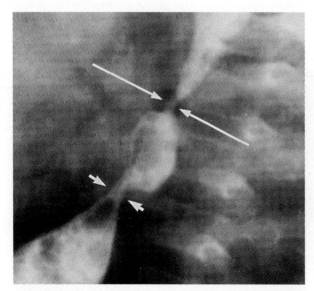

FIGURE 6–43. Esophageal strictures following esophageal atresia repair. Two strictures are present, near (*long arrows*) and below (*short arrows*) the site of the anastomosis.

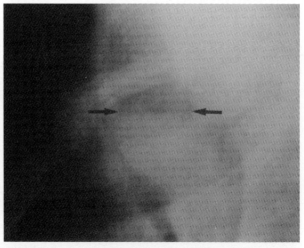

FIGURE 6–44. Esophageal stricture following esophageal atresia repair. Complete obstruction is indicated by the air-fluid level (*arrows*) in the upper esophagus on this lateral chest radiograph. The upper esophagus is compressing the trachea anteriorly.

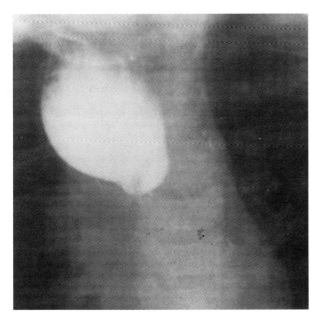

FIGURE 6–45. Esophageal stricture following esophageal atresia repair. There is complete obstruction to passage of barium at the site of the anastomosis and dilatation of the upper esophagus.

Reflux may be reduced by the use of smaller, more frequent feeds and by placing the baby in a semirecumbent position. Surgical antireflux procedures such as Nissen fundoplication may occasionally be required if reflux is gross. However, since there is an increased risk of esophageal obstruction associated with the dysmotility, fundoplication should be performed only when absolutely necessary.

A food bolus or swallowed foreign body may impact at the site of the anastomosis in later childhood (Figure 6–46).

Progressive Scoliosis. Progressive scoliosis concave to the side of the thoracotomy may develop years after the surgery if there has been severe mediastinitis and empyema secondary to dehiscence of the esophageal anastomosis. This inflammation can heal with marked scarring and rib fusion and the scoliosis can develop and progress rapidly at the time of the adolescent growth spurt (Gilsanz et al., 1983).

H-Type Tracheoesophageal Fistula

Although H-type tracheoesophageal fistula may be acquired, it is usually congenital. It is occasionally present at multiple levels (Eckstein, 1966) but is more commonly single, with 62% of the fistula at or above the level of the second thoracic vertebrae;

hence, repair can be accomplished by a cervical approach, a safer surgical technique than a thoracotomy (Schneider and Becker, 1962).

Acquired nonmalignant esophagorespiratory fistulae are rare complications of trauma, infection (Wychulis et al., 1966), foreign body (Rahbar and Farhar, 1978), esophageal diverticula, and necrotizing vasculitis (Wesselhoeft and Keshishian, 1968). Fistulous communications following lye ingestion are rare but may occur early as a direct result of the caustic or later, after dilatation of a resulting stricture (Amoury et al., 1975; Wychulis et al., 1966). The H-type fistulae without atresia present later than those with atresia (Eckstein et al., 1970), with symptoms that include choking, coughing, attacks of cyanosis, and recurrent pneumonias (Sundar et al., 1975). Also, the abdomen may be distended.

Plain films may show gaseous abdominal distension (Helmsworth and Pryles, 1951) and pneumoesophagus (Smith et al., 1976), especially after endotracheal intubation and positive pressure ventilation. The fistula may easily show on an esophagogram (Figure 6–47) or it may be difficult and require a number of examinations. The prone esophagograph with videotape recording is the best method of demonstrating an H-type fistula (Thomas and Chrispin, 1969). To prevent filling of

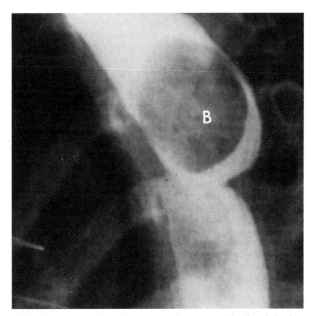

FIGURE 6–46. Esophageal stricture with food bolus impaction. Two years after repair of esophageal atresia, a food bolus (*B*) is impacted at a stricture in the upper esophagus.

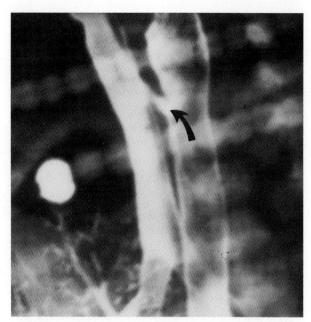

FIGURE 6–47. H-type tracheoesophageal fistula. The fistula passes obliquely and superiorly from the esophagus to the trachea. More of the tracheobronchial tree is filled with barium than is desirable.

the tracheobronchial tree, the examination should be stopped as soon as barium enters the trachea.

Although other studies are rarely indicated, CT can show an H-type fistula as a single chamber coalescence of the esophagus and trachea (Johnson et al., 1985). Bronchoscopy occasionally may be helpful in a few patients when there are still diagnostic problems and the contrast study has not shown the fistula (Winslow et al., 1966).

Gastric tubes, usually successfully inserted, may occasionally fail and result in a fistula (Ein et al., 1973; Stringer and Pablot, 1985).

Rare Anomalies of Tracheal and Esophageal Separation

There is a spectrum of rare anomalies of tracheal and esophageal separation (see Figure 6–22).

Laryngotracheoesophageal Cleft

Laryngotracheoesophageal cleft is a rare anomaly with a persistent communication via a cleft through the larynx, cricoid cartilages, and part of the trachea. The cleft is variable in size with a defect in the posterior part of the cricoid cartilage and a large H-type fistula representing one end of the spectrum of laryngotracheoesophageal cleft (Figure 6–48).

A cleft usually presents early with choking on feeding, excessive oral mucus, and cyanosis. Stridor may occasionally be present, and polyhydramnios and prematurity are often part of the clinical picture (Blumberg et al., 1965). Other anomalies may be associated, especially esophageal atresia and tracheoesophageal fistula (Burroughs and Leape, 1974). The prognosis is good if the defect is small.

The diagnosis is best made by laryngoscopy and endotracheal intubation (Felman and Talbert, 1972). The radiologist may be the first to discover an unsuspected lesion during a barium examination. Because of the risk of aspiration, great care must be taken during a barium examination when there is the possibility of any type of fistula. When small, clefts may be difficult to demonstrate. Like H-type fistulae, they are best seen radiologically using a videoesophagogram (Morgan et al., 1979).

Esophagotrachea

The most severe form of laryngotracheoesophageal cleft is the esophagotrachea with no division between the trachea and the esophagus (Griscom, 1966).

Tracheal Agenesis with and without Fistula

Tracheal agenesis is extremely rare. Typically, there is

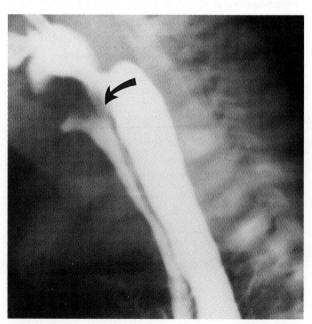

FIGURE 6–48. Laryngotracheoesophageal cleft. A defect in the posterior part of the cricoid cartilage with a large H-type fistula (*arrow*) represents one end of the spectrum of laryngotracheoesophageal cleft.

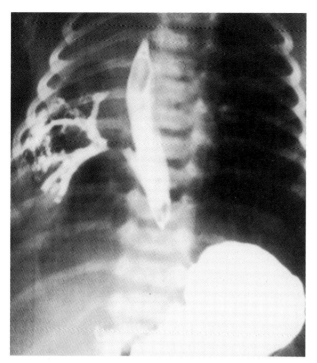

FIGURE 6–49. Esophageal bronchus. The esophageal bronchus fills with barium.

a connection between the carina and anterior esophagus; less often, there may be a short section of trachea. In the rarest form, no fistula occurs.

The baby will have respiratory difficulties at birth with cyanosis. Associated cardiovascular, gastrointestinal, or genitourinary anomalies are usually present. The condition is invariably fatal.

Plain films may show a marked pneumoesophagus with anterior displacement of tracheal tube, and contrast studies will outline the anatomy (Morgan et al., 1979).

Esophageal Bronchus

Esophageal bronchus is a rare anomaly in which the bronchus arises directly from the esophagus; it may be a main stem bronchus supplying an entire lung or it may be a lobular bronchus (Figure 6–49). Rarely, other anomalies such as an anomalous pulmonary artery (Graves et al., 1975) or esophageal atresia and tracheoesophageal fistula may be present (Leithiser et al., 1986). The blood supply may occasionally arise from the systemic ciculation (Stanley et al., 1985). The child presents with respiratory difficulty or recurrent infections and may have abnormal chest radiology findings such as a hypoplastic lung (Reilly et al., 1973).

Esophagogram usually demonstrates an abnormal bronchus (see Figure 6–49) although repeat examinations or esophagogram with barium injected through a nasoesophageal tube may be necessary. Bronchography is not usually required as there is no communication with the sequestered lung. Preoperative angiography or magnetic resonance angiography (MRA), if available, is often required to show the arterial supply and venous drainage (Reilly et al., 1973; Graves et al., 1975; Stanley et al., 1985).

Cysts and Duplications of the Foregut

Foregut malformations are complex and varied. Despite overlap in some individual cases, they can be divided into 3 broad categories: bronchogenic cysts, enteric (including neurenteric) cysts, and tubular esophageal duplications. The origin of a duplication cannot be determined from its type of epithelium; for example, respiratory pseudostratified ciliated epithelium is found in the prenatal esophagus as well as in the respiratory tract. All primitive foregut epithelium appears to have this potential for development (Amendola et al., 1982).

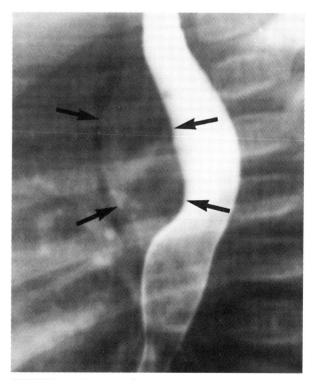

FIGURE 6–50. Bronchogenic cyst. Rarely, a bronchogenic cyst appears as a mass (*arrows*) between the esophagus and the trachea, mimicking an aberrant left main pulmonary artery.

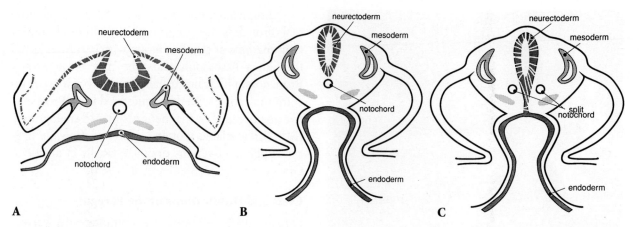

FIGURE 6–51. Embryogenesis of a neurenteric cyst. *A,* In early gestation the notochord normally separates the endoderm and neurectoderm. *B,* In the first trimester, part of the neurectoderm has separated from the rest of the ectoderm to form the spinal cord. It normally remains separated from the endoderm by the notochord. In a neurenteric cyst *C,* there is imperfect separation, and the notochord is split by a connection between endoderm and neurectoderm.

Bronchogenic Cysts

Bronchogenic cysts are formed from groups of epithelial cells that have separated from the tracheobronchial tree. They are derivatives of the trachea and lung buds of the anterior part of the primitive foregut and usually present with respiratory symptoms such as wheezing, dyspnea, and coughing secondary to compression of adjacent structures. The cysts usually occur in the middle mediastinum (Amendola et al., 1982).

Plain films demonstrate the mass lesion and any tracheal deviation and an esophagogram may show a deviated but otherwise normal esophagus. The radiologic appearance is often similar to that of an enteric cyst. Rarely, a bronchogenic cyst may lie between the esophagus and the trachea, mimicking an aberrant left main pulmonary artery (Figure 6–50). It may occasionally communicate with the esophagus via a fistula, usually secondary to infection (Mindelyun and Long, 1978). Bronchoscopy can show the tracheal compression but is not usually indicated. Computed tomography or MR demonstrates the anatomy, and CT with intravenous contrast or MR is used preoperatively to show the relationship of a cyst to the vascular structures. Some investigators advocate CT with transbronchial or transesophageal needle aspiration as an alternative to surgery in evaluating congenital mediastinal cysts (Kuhlman et al., 1988). However, re-accumulation of fluid after needle aspiration has been reported (van Beers, 1989).

Enteric and Neurenteric Cysts

Enteric cysts tend to be more posterior in position than bronchogenic cysts. They are derived from the posterior part of the primitive foregut (Gray and Skandalakis, 1972) and commonly contain gastric or intestinal mucosa and neural tissue. Respiratory pseudostratified epithelium is occasionally present. Cysts containing neural tissue are termed neurenteric cysts.

Enteric cysts usually present early in life and are sometimes associated with other foregut anomalies such as esophageal atresia (Kirks and Filston, 1981). Secretions from the lining epithelium increase the size of the cyst and cause pressure symptoms, usually respiratory. The thoracic cysts may traverse the diaphragm and communicate with gut or even pancreatic ducts (Filler et al., 1979). Enteric cysts can reach a great size and cause respiratory embarrassment.

The embryologic development of neurenteric cysts is complex and imperfectly understood. As the notochord grows cranially from a primitive knot of cells, it normally separates and lies between the endoderm and ectoderm, accompanying the ectoderm in its faster cranial growth. If separation is imperfect, endodermal tissue is dragged cranially, interfering with the notochord's normal development and preventing the lateral mesoderm from growing in to separate the ectoderm and endoderm growth (Figure 6–51) (Beardmore and Wiglesworth, 1958). The resulting malformation is a neurenteric cyst, usually in the posterior mediastinum.

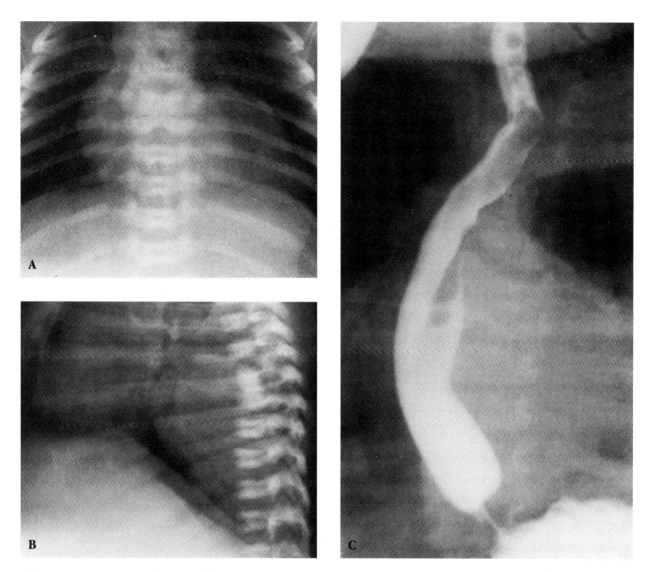

FIGURE 6–52. Neurenteric cyst. A large posterior mediastinal mass and associated midthoracic vertebral anomaly can be seen on the frontal (*A*) and lateral (*B*) chest radiographs. (*C*) The mass deviates the esophagus to the right but does not communicate with its lumen.

The cyst is in contact with the spinal canal either through a fibrous tract or a fistula, which may even extend to the skin surface. This intraspinal extension may cause serious problems such as cord compression and paraplegia (Piramoon and Abbassioun, 1974). However, the patient may be neurologically normal (Superina et al., 1984). The resulting vertebral anomalies, always superior to the neurenteric cyst, include butterfly vertebrae with anterior spina bifida, hemivertebrae, and scoliosis (Figure 6–52). The distance from cyst to spinal anomaly depends on how early in utero the adhesion of notochord to endoderm occurred. An enteric cyst of the duodenum may communicate via a fistulous tract to the cervical spinal cord and present with intermittent meningitis and a normal radiographic chest examination (Boivin et al., 1964).

Complications and Unusual Features of Enteric Cysts. Acid secretion by the cyst can cause ulceration with fatal hemorrhage. Depending on where the ulcer erodes, it may present with hematemesis or hemoptysis (Chang et al., 1976). There may be a direct association between feeding and the onset of hemorrhage.

A partial pericardial defect may be present on the same side as an enteric cyst (Kassner et al., 1975). Enteric cysts may rarely present as a mass lesion in the

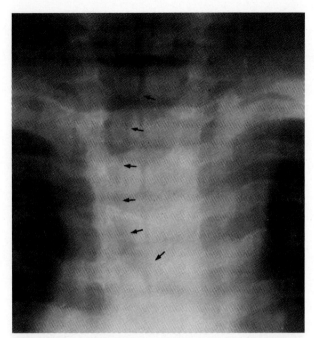

FIGURE 6–53. Enteric cyst. A soft tissue mass narrows and displaces the trachea (*arrows*) to the right.

neck, causing diagnostic problems; they may be asymptomatic or cause respiratory distress (Gans et al., 1968). Enteric cysts have been found in the thorax communicating with the small bowel (Gross et al., 1950) and are associated with small-bowel cysts. Many other uncommon associations may exist (Ware and Conrad, 1953). A communicating esophageal duplication cyst containing a foreign body has been reported (Stringel et al., 1985) but usually a perforating foreign body would form its own cavity. Esophageal duplication cyst and aberrant right subclavian artery mimicking a symptomatic vascular ring has been described (Helund and Bisset, 1989). Spontaneous resolution of some mediastinal cysts has been documented (Martin et al., 1988), and a case of bilateral gastric bronchopulmonary-foregut malformation arising from the stomach has been reported (Pan et al., 1989).

Imaging of Enteric Cysts. Initially, plain films will show the position of the cyst and any vertebral anomalies (see Figure 6–52), possibly showing the cyst as a soft tissue mass displacing the trachea (Figures 6–52 and 6–53).

Ultrasonography may delineate enteric cysts well and is particularly useful if anomalies are suspected in the neck or abdomen and occasionally in the thorax in infants. The cysts lie adjacent to the esophagus but do not usually communicate with it,

though the esophagus may be displaced by the mass (Figure 6–54).

If an associated vertebral anomaly is identified, MR may be used to delineate any fistula or anterior spina bifida. Intraspinal anomalies can coexist with these mediastinal masses in almost 25% of patients who are often initially asymptomatic. Hence, MR, myelography, or CT with simultaneous contrast myelography (depending on availability) should be performed in all patients with associated vertebral anomalies (Superina et al., 1984). All these give excellent delineation of the mass (Figure 6–55) and may give extra information on the intraspinal anomalies (Figure 6–56). Computed tomography is helpful to demonstrate the relations of a cyst preoperatively and can be diagnostically reliable (Fitch et al., 1986), although often such information preoperatively is not required. Which modalities to use depends on their availability and the exact clinical problem.

A (technetium) Tc 99m sodium pertechnetate scan (Meckel scan) can image duplications if they

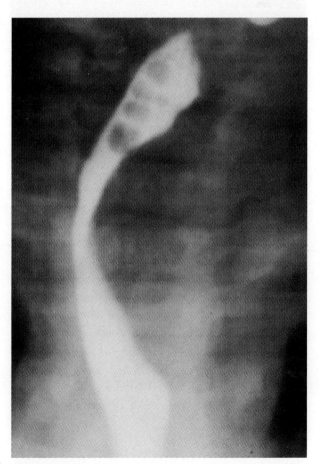

FIGURE 6–54. Enteric cyst. The soft tissue mass displaces but does not communicate with the esophagus.

contain ectopic gastric mucosa and thus confirm the diagnosis (see small bowel duplications, Chapter 9). Rarely, an esophageal duplication cyst may present in adult life and may be diagnosed and managed by CT with transesophageal needle aspiration (Kuhlman et al., 1985).

Neurogenic tumors may cause problems in differential diagnosis. These tumors frequently affect the posterior ribs and may involve the spinal canal.

Tubular Esophageal Duplications

Tubular esophageal duplications are rare and may communicate with the normal esophagus or stomach (Figure 6–57) (Moir, 1970). The embryogenesis is probably different from other foregut malformations and may be due to faulty recanalization of the esophageal lumen (Amendola et al., 1982). These anomalies can present with dysphagia or can be completely asymptomatic. Esophageal carcinoma in a duplication has been found in an adult (Boivin et al., 1964).

Vascular Anomalies

Vascular anomalies of the aortic arch system may be associated with formation of a vascular ring. These abnormalities may be symptomatic and become

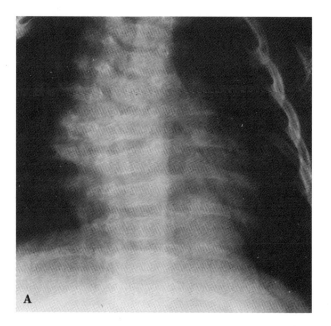

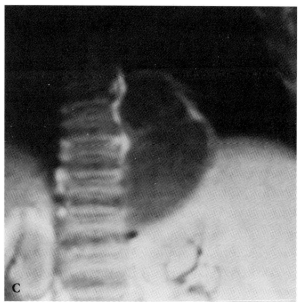

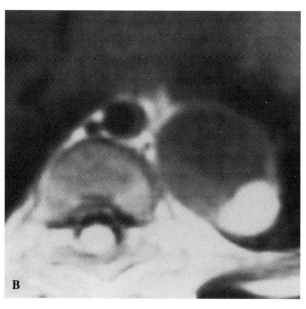

FIGURE 6–55. Neurenteric cyst. A large posterior mediastinal mass and associated midthoracic vertebral anomaly can be seen on the frontal chest radiograph (*A*). Axial (*B*) and coronal (*C*) MR clearly shows the position of the mass adjacent to the thoracic vertebrae.

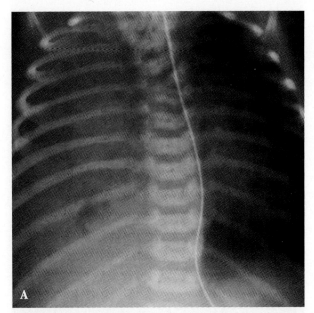
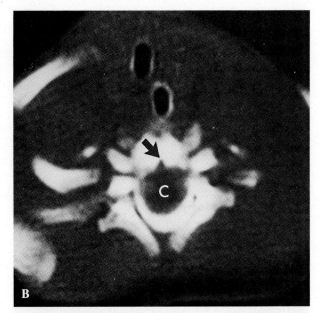

FIGURE 6–56. Neurenteric cyst. *A,* A large mass opacifies the right hemithorax. The nasogastric tube is deviated to the left, and there is an associated upper thoracic vertebral anomaly. *B,* Postoperative CT myelography shows the deformed vertebrae with an expanded cord (*C*) and an anterior projection arising from the cord at the site of a fibrous connection (*arrow*).

apparent in the neonatal period, present in later life, or remain asymptomatic. Early symptoms are usually respiratory in nature, such as dyspnea, stridor, and cyanotic spells especially during feeding. The infant may also become limp and apneic due to reflex apnea, a sometimes fatal condition that is poorly understood (Fearon and Shortreed, 1963).

Embryogenesis
Within each of the six paired branchial arches, there is a vascular or aortic arch from which the pulmonary, carotid, and subclavian vessels develop (Figure 6–58). The fourth arch forms the true aortic arch, and the sixth arch gives rise to both of the pulmonary arteries and the ductus arteriosus. Maldevelopment can lead to a wide range of vascular anomalies. The variations in vascular anomalies are legion (Klinkhamer, 1969). The relevant embryogenesis will be discussed separately under each anomaly section.

Imaging of Vascular Anomalies
Plain chest radiography is the first examination usually performed, assessing the position of the trachea and aorta. In normal individuals with a left aortic arch, the trachea is slightly deviated to the

right or can be buckled to the right due to head flexion. An aortic arch anomaly should be suspected if the trachea is midline or deviated to the left (Strife et al., 1989) or if there is increased soft tissue density in the right paratracheal region. Tracheal indentation, either on the right as seen on the anteroposterior view or posteriorly as seen on the lateral view, is abnormal. A high Kv radiograph using a copper/tin/aluminum filter (Fearon and Shortreed, 1963) helps show mediastinal detail as well as aortic position (Wolf et al., 1978), tracheal impressions (Deanfield and Chrispin, 1981), bronchial situs (Deanfield et al., 1980), and the proximal airway (Dunbar, 1970).

An esophagogram is helpful, and there are four patterns that cover most tracheal and esophageal abnormalities (Figure 6–59).

Contrast-enhanced CT is used to demonstrate aberrant left pulmonary artery sling and may help investigate other anomalies.

Angiography is the definitive diagnostic step. While not considered necessary by most pediatric surgeons, some surgeons find angiography of assistance in determining the exact vascular anatomy prior to operation. Digital subtraction angiography has not yet been widely used for assessing vascular

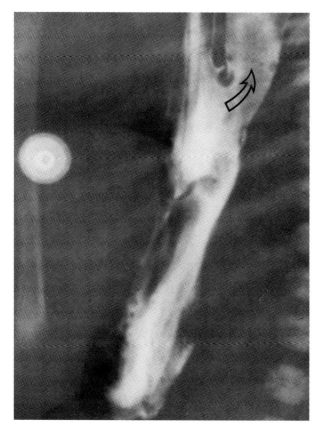

FIGURE 6–57. Tubular esophageal duplication. A communicating tubular duplication extends superiorly from the lower esophagus and retrogradely fills with barium (*arrow*) instilled via a nasoesophageal tube.

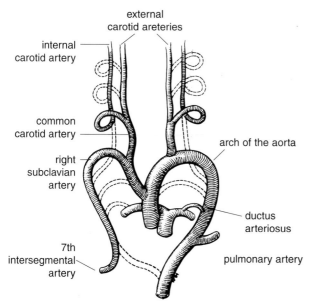

FIGURE 6–58. Formation of aortic arch and major vessels. Originally, six paired vascular arches are present. Some components become obliterated (*dotted lines*) with time.

rings but could be a useful alternative to arteriography (Tonkin et al., 1984). Magnetic resonance angiography, increasingly the diagnostic modality of choice, is noninvasive and helpful in preoperative evaluation of selected children with complicated vascular anomalies.

Bronchoscopy, suggested by some physicians, is not generally helpful and may actually be detrimental.

Vascular Anomalies on Lateral Barium Swallow

Posterior Esophageal Impression and Normal Trachea. This is the most common abnormal appearance, caused by either an aberrant right subclavian artery with a left aortic arch or less commonly by an aberrant left subclavian artery with a right aortic arch. It is due to the disappearance of the fourth arch between the origin of the common carotid artery and subclavian artery. This anomaly has been seen in 0.5% of autopsies (Beaubout et al., 1964) but does not generally cause symptoms in childhood. Rarely, an associated anterior tracheal narrowing occurs when the innominate and common carotid arteries arise from a common trunk. A vascular ring may occasionally occur if there is a left-sided ductus with

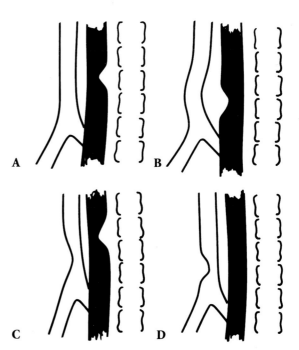

FIGURE 6–59. The four lateral esophagograph patterns. *A,* Posterior esophageal impression and normal trachea. *B,* Anterior esophageal and posterior tracheal impression. *C,* Posterior esophageal and anterior tracheal impression. *D,* Anterior tracheal impression and normal esophagus.

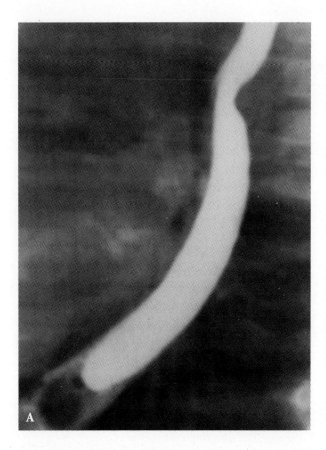

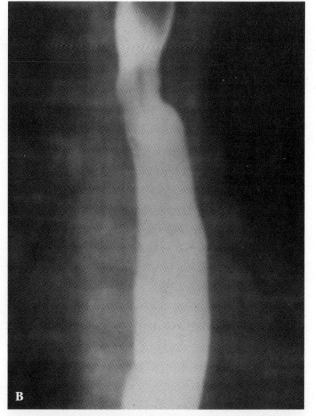

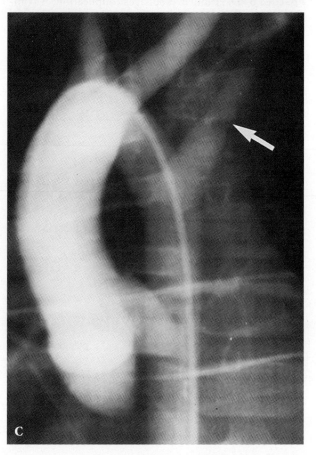

FIGURE 6–60. Aberrant left subclavian artery with right-sided aortic arch. Esophagogram shows a posterior indentation on the lateral view (*A*) and a slightly oblique indentation on the frontal view (*B*). Arch aortograph (*C*) demonstrates the right-sided aortic arch and the aberrant left subclavian artery (*arrow*).

a right aortic arch and aberrant left subclavian artery. This will result in symptoms only if the ductus is sufficiently close to the trachea to cause compression. More rarely, a left or right aberrant subclavian artery may cause pulmonary collapse (Montgomery and Partridge, 1981). An aneurysm of the aberrant subclavian artery has been reported in adults. In the absence of respiratory symptoms or signs, treatment of aberrant subclavian artery is not indicated.

On plain films, no abnormality is seen unless a right sided aorta is present. Esophagography shows a posterior indentation on the esophagus on the lateral view and an oblique or transverse defect on the frontal view (Figure 6–60). The indentation of the esophagus on the lateral view is often longer and smoother from an aberrant right subclavian than from an aberrant left subclavian because the former artery takes a more oblique course as it crosses the esophagus (Figure 6–61). An aberrant left subclavian artery tends to run more horizontally as it is usually tethered by a left ductus arteriosus. In some patients with a right aortic arch with aberrant left subclavian artery (ALSA), a left-sided esophageal indentation is noted, which may be related to an aortic diverticulum extending to the left of the esophagus or ALSA or to the ligamentum arteriosum (Kleinman et al., 1994). Angiography is usually not indicated but will show the aberrant vessels if a vascular ring is suspected (see Figure 6–60). Magnetic resonance angiography is an excellent alternative to angiography in patients with vascular rings when further anatomic delineation of the abnormality is required (Bisset et al., 1987).

Although aberrant subclavian arteries that pass between the trachea and esophagus have apparently been reported, such an occurrence now seems doubtful (Beaubout et al., 1964).

Anterior Esophageal and Posterior Tracheal Impression. There has been a case report of this deformity being caused by a collateral systemic artery to the lung (Castenada-Zuniga et al., 1978) but otherwise the only vascular cause is a pulmonary sling where the left pulmonary artery arises from the right pulmonary artery and then loops posteriorly around the trachea before passing to the left. The embryogenesis is complex. This pulmonary artery branch of the left sixth arch either fails to develop or becomes obliterated at an early stage. However, the distal portion of the left sixth arch develops normally, as shown by a normally situated

ductus arteriosus. The developing lung bud has an area of relative ischemia, and a collateral branch from the pulmonary portion of the right sixth arch develops. As the lung divides, the left lung takes this collateral with it, forming a left pulmonary artery which hence arises on the right.

An aberrant left pulmonary artery often presents at birth with severe respiratory difficulty. Milder cases have been reported, however, including a 79-year-old man with dysphagia only during the last few months of life (Gray and Skandalakis, 1972).

On plain films, there may be evidence of air trapping or collapse secondary to tracheobronchial obstruction, complications that are unusual in other vascular anomalies (Berdon and Baker, 1972). Rarely, the aberrant left pulmonary artery may be seen as a soft tissue mass indenting the posterior aspect of the trachea (Figure 6–62).

If a tracheal bronchus to the right upper lobe lies superior to the pulmonary sling, there may be compensatory emphysema in this lobe together with collapse of the middle and lower lobes of the right lung (Capitanio et al., 1971).

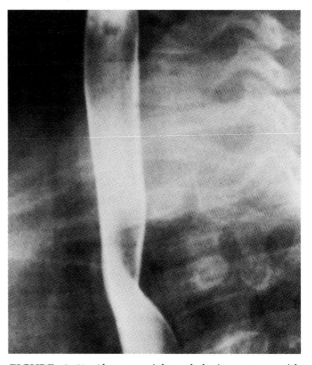

FIGURE 6–61. Aberrant right subclavian artery with left-sided aortic arch. Esophagogram shows a posterior indentation on the lateral view slightly more triangular than the indentation caused by an aberrant left subclavian artery due to the more oblique course of the vessel.

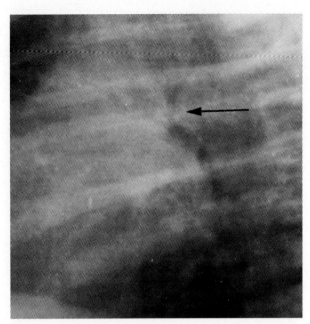

FIGURE 6–62. Aberrant left pulmonary artery. A faint soft tissue mass (*arrow*) posteriorly indents the inferior part of the trachea.

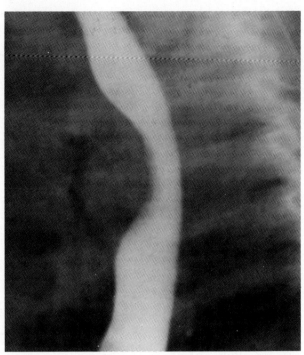

FIGURE 6–63. Aberrant left pulmonary artery. A constant indentation is present on the anterior aspect of the esophagus.

The aberrant left pulmonary artery is usually seen as an oval mass between the trachea and esophagus (Figure 6–63). It is essential to view the carinal area, checking with the ribs and vertebrae to ensure a true lateral projection. Videofluoroscopy helps reduce screening time. Computed tomography during the intravenous injection of contrast material or angiography may confirm the diagnosis. Preoperative diagnosis is important because intraoperative identification of the vessels can be difficult and the aberrant vessel may be missed or mistakenly ligated for a ductus arteriosus (Berdon and Baker, 1972). Rarely, a complete cartilage ring tracheal stenosis may also be present and require surgical treatment as well (Berdon et al., 1984; Han et al., 1980). Failure to recognize this ring-sling complex may result in death due to continuing respiratory embarrassment.

The appearance of an anterior esophageal and posterior tracheal impression in the appropriate clinical context is diagnostic of an anomalous left pulmonary artery sling. Bronchogenic cysts and lymph node enlargement which could be considered in the differential are usually more lateral in location rather than being localized between the esophagus and trachea. However, exceptions do occur (see Figure 6–50).

Posterior Esophageal and Anterior Tracheal Impression. The combination of a posterior eso-phageal and anterior tracheal impression is usually caused by a vascular ring such as a double aortic arch (Figure 6–64). A right aortic arch combined with an aberrant left subclavian artery and a left ductus arteriosus has a similar appearance when the ring is tight (Neuhauser, 1946; 1949). An indentation on both sides of the esophagus can be seen on the frontal projection, with the right indentation usually being higher and larger than the left (Figure 6–65). Very rarely, a left ductus may compress the left main bronchus rather than the trachea, resulting in unilateral obstructive pulmonary hyperinflation (Pirtle and Clarke, 1983).

Double aortic arch develops due to the bilateral persistence of aortic arches. The arches are usually of unequal size; the smaller can be divided along with the ductus arteriosus to relieve the tracheal compression. Angiography or MRA, if required preoperatively, will show the double aortic arch (Figure 6–66).

A right aortic arch with an aberrant left subclavian artery is a relatively common anomaly. However, if the ductus arteriosus arises sufficiently close to the origin of the aberrant artery to cause tracheal compression, a deformity identical to a double aortic arch will be produced.

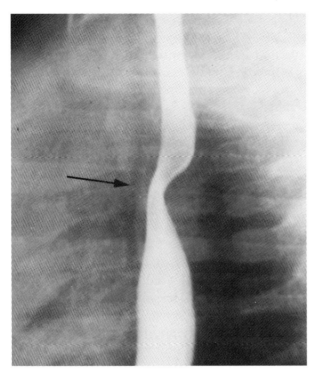

FIGURE 6–64. Double aortic arch. The double arch indents the posterior aspect of the esophagus and narrows the trachea anteriorly (*arrow*).

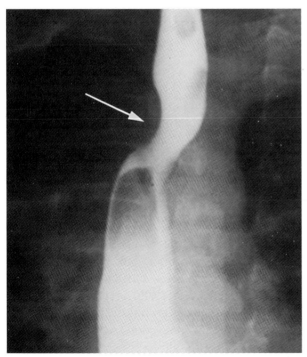

FIGURE 6–65. Double aortic arch. The right side of the esophagus is indented from a high right-sided arch (*arrow*). Just inferiorly, the esophagus deviates around a left-sided arch.

Surgical treatment of the two anomalies is similar, so preoperative differentiation may not be required. However, in cases of double aortic arch, knowledge of the vascular arrangement helps the surgeon decide which is the smaller arch to divide.

Anterior Tracheal Impression and Normal Esophagus. The innominate artery may produce anterior tracheal indentation (Gross and Neuhauser, 1948) but its reported frequency and perceived importance varies (Berdon and Baker, 1972; Moes et al., 1975). Although it does not affect the esophagus, anterior tracheal indentation on plain lateral chest radiograph is seen in this condition. When indentation is not found on a barium swallow, the trachea should be carefully examined fluoroscopically. An anterior constant curvilinear indentation of the trachea midway between the carina and sternal notch may be seen in this condition. Even when this can be demonstrated, surgery may neither be indicated nor curative (Moes et al., 1975; Berdon et al., 1969).

Rare Vascular Impressions on the Esophagus

An oblique posterior-to-anterior extrinsic vascular impression on the distal esophagus may be demonstrated in total anomalous pulmonary venous return below the diaphragm caused by a common pulmonary vein (Ablin et al., 1989).

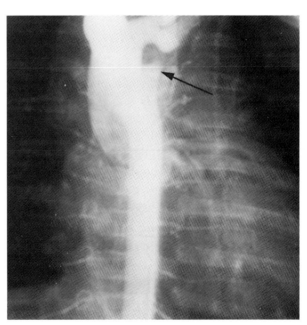

FIGURE 6–66. Double aortic arch. Arch aortograph shows a large right-sided aortic arch and a smaller left-sided arch (*arrow*).

Congenital Stenosis of the Esophagus

Although most childhood stenoses are associated with trauma, reflux esophagitis, or ingestion of toxic substances, a few stenoses are truly congenital and may be more common than is generally accepted (Dominguez et al., 1985). They have been seen in association with a cartilaginous ring (Anderson et al., 1973) and secondary to the lack of submucosa (Takayanagi et al., 1975).

Congenital stenoses have been associated with tracheoesophageal fistula (Jewsbury, 1971) and are similar to upper esophageal webs. Congenital stenosis of the lower esophagus has been found in a neonate when introduction of solid food produced dysphagia. The infant had undergone repair of a more proximal esophageal atresia but a congenital etiology is supported since stenosis appeared on the first day of life (Mortensson, 1975). Congenital strictures are most often between the middle (Gross, 1964) and the junction of the middle and lower third of the esophagus (Dominguez et al., 1985).

Any child with dysphagia following esophageal atresia repair may have a secondary stricture from reflux esophagitis, which is especially likely due to disordered motility in the lower esophagus. Dilatation of the stricture may be possible using Gruentzig angioplasty balloons (Stringer et al., 1985).

Congenital Tracheomalacia

Tracheomalacia is usually secondary to intubation or esophageal atresia. Occasionally a neonate presents with stridor from birth with uncertain etiology. This can be considered a case of congenital tracheomalacia, a rare anomaly with a grave prognosis. What is important from a gastrointestinal point of view is the appearance on a barium swallow. The trachea may be almost obliterated on expiration (Figure 6–67), and care should be taken during the examination to maintain respiratory function.

ACQUIRED DISEASES OF THE PHARYNX AND ESOPHAGUS

Inflammation of the Pharynx and Esophagus

Retropharyngeal Abscess

Retropharyngeal abscesses occur most commonly in the first few years of life which may be related to the presence of an increased number of peripharyngeal lymph nodes which occur in this age group (Harner, 1975). Such abscesses are usually secondary to infection in the regions drained by these nodes, namely, the middle ear, pharynx, and nose. The usual cause of a retropharyngeal abscess in older children is trauma.

The child looks ill and will not swallow, drools, and spits out all saliva. A lateral neck radiograph is necessary to exclude a foreign body or airway obstruction. On radiographic examination, a soft tissue mass is visible (Figure 6–68), which must be distinguished from the apparent soft tissue mass due to tracheal buckling, which is a normal appearance (see Figure 6–2).

Retropharyngeal soft tissue masses may be secondary to hypothyroidism in young infants (Grunebaum and Moskowitz, 1970), and an increase in such tissue may be secondary to other pathology such as tumor, bleeding, (especially in trauma [Andrew, 1978] or hemophilia [Markowitz, 1981]). The clinical status and history of the patient should allow ready differentiation.

Treatment usually entails incising the abscess to permit drainage and prevent serious complications which include periesophageal abscess from extension into the mediastinum and empyema from extension into the pleural space (Ramilo et al., 1978).

Esophagitis

Esophagitis usually results from gastroesophageal reflux (see Chapter 7) but other causes include ingestion of caustic substances, infections, and non-infectious inflammatory disorders as discussed below. Many radiologic features, such as aperistalsis (Simeone et al., 1977), are common to all these etiologies, and in the evaluation of any patient, clinical details must be known.

Caustic Esophagitis: Clinical Features. Ingestion of caustics by children is nearly always accidental. The most commonly swallowed substances are household cleaning products, including ammonium chloride, alkaline caustics, and acids.

The diagnosis is usually obvious from the history. Examination of the mouth may show burns but their absence does not exclude esophageal lesions and these should be sought if caustic ingestion is suspected. The diagnosis must be made quickly so that steroids, antibiotics, and supportive measures can be instituted. Treatment is aimed at preventing the main complications of caustic inges-

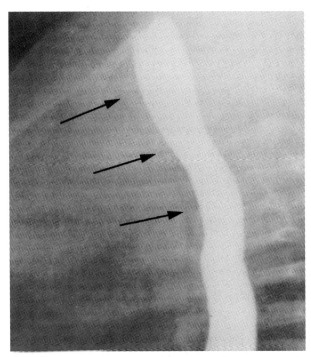

FIGURE 6–67. Congenital tracheomalacia. There is almost complete obliteration of the trachea (*arrows*) on expiration in this neonate who had stridor from birth.

tion, namely mediastinitis, esophageal perforation, and long-term stricture formation.

Caustic Esophagitis: Imaging. In the acute phase of severe cases, plain chest films may show a dilated, air-filled, atonic esophagus with either mediastinal widening due to mediastinitis or widening of the left lateral paraspinal pleural reflection due to esophageal wall thickening.

Esophagoscopy can be used to grade the severity and extent of esophageal involvement (Alford and Harris, 1959). In view of the danger of perforation, however, it may not be wise to pass the endoscope beyond the first evidence of esophagitis; its use should be only to confirm that the esophagus is involved (Daly, 1968).

The extent of the esophagitis can be more safely demonstrated with esophagography (Middlekamp et al., 1969) although it may underestimate the damage (Franken, 1973). An iso-osmolar water-soluble contrast medium esophagograph is advisable as perforation is a common and serious complication. If a tracheoesophageal fistula is also suspected, the new iso-osmolar water-soluble contrast medium is preferred to bronchographic medium. The esophagogram may show a rigid, narrow esophagus (Figure

6–69) with a variable degree of ulceration (Figure 6–70), or there may be a variety of appearances including a dilated, atonic esophagus or an irritable esophagus with tertiary waves (Levine, 1991). Aspiration due to swallowing incoordination may also be present (Franken and Smith, 1982). In less severely affected children, a double-contrast esophagograph may show transverse folds that are contractions of the muscularis mucosae, often followed by stricture formation at the same site at a later date (Reeder, 1985).

Complications of Caustic Esophagitis. Perforation and mediastinitis may occur as acute complications, especially following esophagoscopy. Perforation which occurs some time after the initial trauma is usually associated with surgical dilatation of a stricture. Frequent dilatations may produce a low-grade mediastinitis.

Strictures occur in up to 30% of cases, and the incidence of reflux is increased regardless of whether

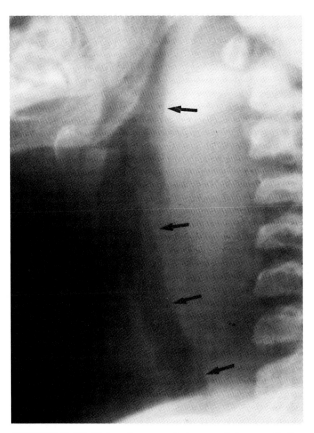

FIGURE 6–68. Retropharyngeal abscess. A large soft-tissue retropharyngeal mass of smooth outline extends along the entire cervical spine (*arrows*). In comparison with the buckling seen with crying (see Figure 6–2), this mass produces less abrupt bulging.

a hiatus hernia is present or not (Franken, 1973). They occur at any level of the esophagus and can involve all or part of the circumference, together with a variable length of the esophagus (Karasick and Lev-Toaff, 1995). Radiologically, strictures in the chronic phase generally appear tapered with smooth mucosa (see Figure 6–70) although strictures may be irregular or shouldered, mimicking carcinoma (Figure 6–71). Sporadic cases of carcinoma arise in caustic strictures many years after the initial injury (Franken and Smith, 1982). Rarely, the grave complications of a tracheoesophageal or esophagoaortic fistula may ensue (Amoury et al., 1975). Strictures can be dilated with Gruentzig angioplasty balloon catheters as described in Chapters 3 and 5.

Infective Esophagitis: Clinical Features. Infective esophagitis is most commonly caused by *Candida albicans* in patients who are immunosuppressed or receiving cytoxic chemotherapy but it also occurs in association with achalasia and occasionally in

previously healthy patients (Guyer and Rooke, 1971). Pain and dysphagia are the usual presenting symptoms; oral candidiasis is not necessarily pre-

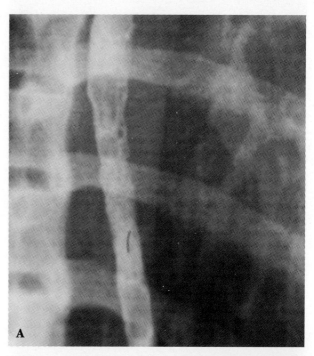

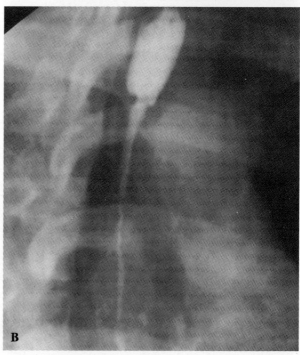

FIGURE 6–70. Chronic esophageal stricture due to lye ingestion. (*A*) Irregularity and rigidity indicate esophageal ulceration and edema 2 weeks after ingestion of lye. (*B*) A tight esophageal stricture developed over the next 6 months.

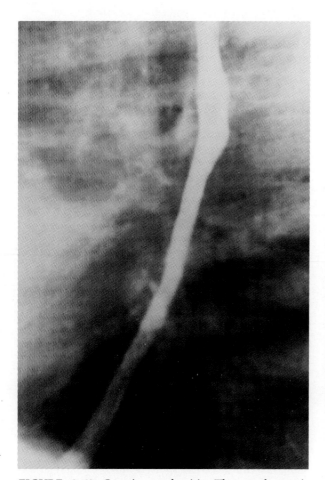

FIGURE 6–69. Caustic esophagitis. The esophagus is rigid and narrow following ingestion of sulfuric acid.

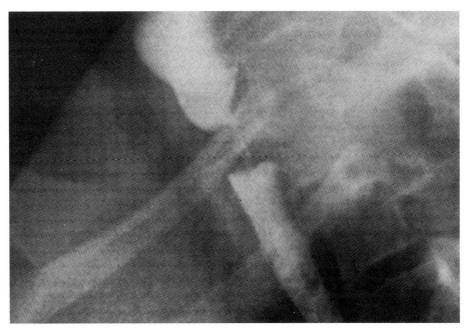

FIGURE 6–71. Chronic esophageal stricture due to lye ingestion. A chronic stricture due to lye ingestion shows shouldering.

sent. Herpes virus or cytomegalovirus infections are less common but have similar symptoms and radiologic appearances. Cytomegalovirus has also been found to cause esophagitis and gastritis in acquired immune deficiency syndrome (AIDS) patients (Balthazar et al., 1985). Herpes virus is often found along with *Candida* and may be the cause of persistent esophagitis despite adequate antifungal therapy. Herpes virus occasionally causes esophagitis in an otherwise healthy patient (DeGaeta et al., 1985; Shortsleeve and Levine, 1992).

Infective Esophagitis: Imaging. Double-contrast esophagography is more accurate than single-contrast study and has an 88% sensitivity (Levine et al., 1985). The lower two thirds of the esophagus are particularly affected on esophagography. Initially, decreased motility or spasm (Rohrman and Kidd, 1978) is a nonspecific finding (Simeone et al., 1977). The mucosa of the esophagus then becomes irregular with raised nodules (Figure 6–72) that are initially probably due to edema although plaques of fungi can give a similar appearance and develop later (Figure 6–73), along with fine mucosal ulceration. The wall of the esophagus may appear thick. The diagnosis is difficult initially but can later be demonstrated well by double-contrast esophagogram (Levine et al., 1985) (see Figure 6–73).

Plaque-like lesions in the esophagus can occur with herpes or candidiasis (Figure 6–74). Discrete ulcers on an otherwise normal mucosa suggests herpes esophagitis (Levine et al., 1981). Many children with esophagitis will not tolerate gas tablets or granules; with these patients, a single-contrast examination has to be performed even though it is much less sensitive than a double-contrast examination (Levine et al., 1985). In cases of herpes or candidal esophagitis, barium may adhere to the esophageal mucosa for several hours (Guyer and Rooke, 1971), which may aid diagnosis.

In one unusual instance, an immunosuppressed patient receiving cytoxic chemotherapy presented with hematemesis, with the esophagus full of coagulated blood secondary to severe csophagitis and thrombocytopenia (Figure 6–75). Esophageal histoplasmosis has been reported in a child with immunodeficiency with hyper-IgM (Tu et al., 1991).

Severe infective esophagitis may progress to formation of strictures (see Figure 6–74), which can be dilated using Gruentzig angioplasty balloon catheters as described in Chapters 3 and 5.

A differential radiologic diagnosis should include peptic (reflux) esophagitis, intramural diverticulosis, and the rare types of noninfective esophagitis. Rarely, the radiologic appearance mim-

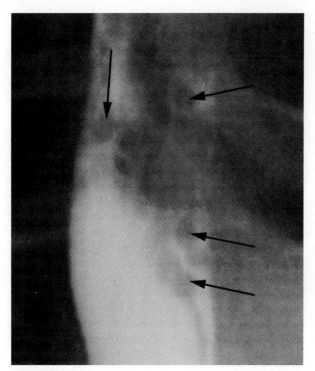

FIGURE 6–72. Early monilial esophagitis. Raised nodules, outlined with barium (*arrows*), represent localized edema in the early phase.

ics varices (Figure 6–76) but the clinical history should make diagnosis easy. An uncertain diagnosis can be confirmed by esophagoscopy but as this often requires a general anesthetic, the barium study is usually relied upon. The endoscopic examination has the advantage of enabling bioptic diagnosis of the etiologic organism.

Tuberculous Esophagitis. Fortunately, tuberculous esophagitis is rare and usually is a manifestation of advanced or disseminated tuberculous disease in an adult patient. However, occasionally the condition may be seen in children (Hamilton et al., 1977). Patients may present with signs of disseminated tuberculosis or occasionally just with dysphagia (Hamilton et al., 1977). If there is dysphagia, a barium study as an early examination can show a number of features including irregular mucosa often eccentric in position, extrinsic compressions from adjacent nodes, large discrete ulcers, sinus or fistulous tracks, or a raised irregular ulcerated mass.

Rare types of Noninfective Esophagitis. Epidermolysis bullosa. Epidermolysis bullosa is the most common of the rare types of esophagitis. It is a congenital hereditary disorder of the skin and mucosa,

with a blistered appearance related to mild trauma. There are two types of the disease, simple and dystrophic. The simple form does not scar; lesions appear after slight trauma but then heal. The dystrophic form can be mutilating and potentially lethal; it is inherited either as a dominant (two types) or recessive condition, the recessive being the most severe. Scarring occurs after the vesicles have ruptured, leading to progressive contractures of the extremities. The hands develop a characteristic mitten deformity due to soft tissue syndactyly, and long bones become slender and overconstricted. The esophagus and mucous membranes are affected, often leading to dysphagia due to strictures (Tischler et al., 1983). Bullae can form in the mucous membranes of the esophagus, pharynx, tongue, buccal membranes, trachea, conjunctiva, and even the vulva and vagina (Burkhart and Ruppert, 1981;

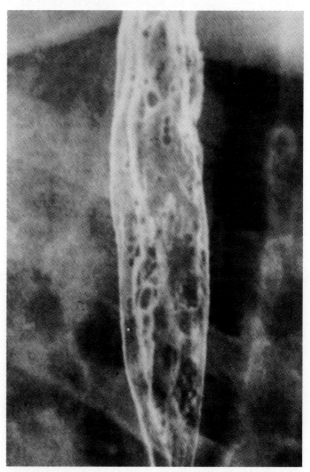

FIGURE 6–73. Early and later monilial esophagitis. As the infection develops, the raised nodules representing monilial plaques become more defined.

Thiers, 1981; DuPree et al., 1969; Shackelford et al., 1982; Johnston et al., 1981; Katz et al., 1967; Becker and Swinyard, 1968; Hillemeir et al., 1981; Thompson et al., 1980; Schuman and Arciniegas, 1972).

The esophageal bullae occur at the carina or at the very proximal or distal esophagus—the sites of most trauma. The bullae may heal without permanent damage but can also ulcerate, bleed, and

progress to strictures or (rarely) webs. The upper half of the esophagus often shows a smooth, short stricture, which may be present even when the skin is relatively clear (Figure 6–77) (Becker and Swinyard, 1968; Hillemeier et al., 1981; Kabakian and Dahmash, 1978).

Although the radiologic appearance is similar to other causes of esophagitis, the presence of the

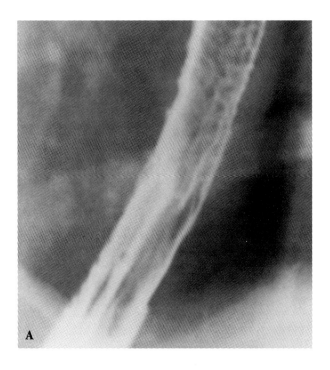

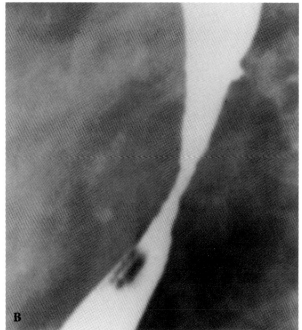

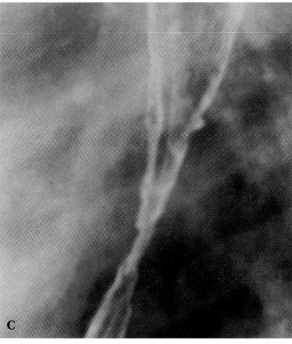

FIGURE 6–74. *Candida albicans* and herpes virus esophagitis. *A,* Double-contrast esophagograph shows the mucosa to be irregular, ulcerated, and nodular due to combined fungal and viral infections in an immunosuppressed leukemic child. Stricture rapidly developed as seen on subsequent single- (*B*) and double-contrast (*C*) examinations.

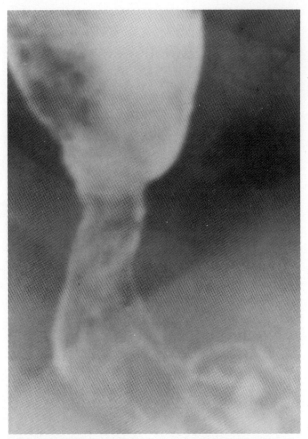

FIGURE 6–75. Monilial esophagitis and thrombocytopenia resulting in hemorrhage. A cast of blood was outlined by barium and was present throughout the esophagus.

associated skin abnormality is diagnostic. Esophagoscopy and stricture dilatations should only be performed if absolutely necessary because of the risk of rupturing the very fragile esophagus or causing hemorrhage or more bulla formation (Tischler et al., 1983).

Eosinophilic gastroenteritis. Eosinophilic gastroenteritis is an uncommon condition of unknown etiology characterized by peripheral eosinophilia and infiltration of the gastrointestinal tract with eosinophils. The stomach and small bowel are the most commonly affected areas and are discussed in Chapters 8 and 9. Colonic involvement, which is rare, is discussed in Chapter 10.

Eosinophilic infiltration of the esophagus is rare but can produce strictures (Figure 6–78). Eosinophilic esophagitis presents with dysphagia, which may be superimposed on symptoms caused by involvement of other parts of the gastrointestional tract (Matzinger and Daneman, 1983; Feczko et al., 1985).

On barium examination, the findings vary from a normal swallow with abnormal manometry and biopsy to irregular mucosa and stricture formation (Dobbins et al., 1977; Landres et al., 1978; Picus and Frank, 1981; Matzinger and Daneman, 1983).

The clinical course is generally self-limiting. Steroids are used for more severe cases and surgery is reserved for persistent obstructive symptoms (Matzinger and Daneman, 1983).

Crohn's disease. Crohn's disease rarely affects the esophagus in children and gives a radiologic appearance similar to that in adults, particularly mucosal ulceration and stricture formation (Tischler and Helman, 1984). Filiform postinflammatory polyps in the esophagus reported in adults have not yet been seen in children (Cockey et al., 1985).

Graft-versus-host disease. Chronic graft-versus-host disease is an immunologic disorder which can occur following bone marrow transplantation for severe aplastic anemia, immunodeficiency disorders, and certain malignancies. The donor lymphocytes damage host tissues, particularly the skin, liver, and intestinal mucosa. The effects on the small

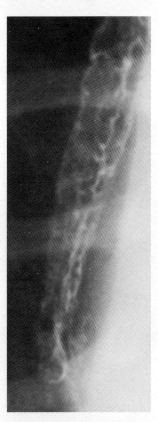

FIGURE 6–76. Monilial esophagitis. The marked serpiginous filling defects in the esophagram mimic varices.

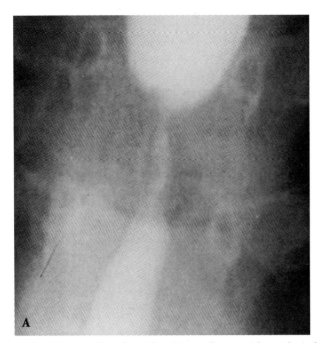 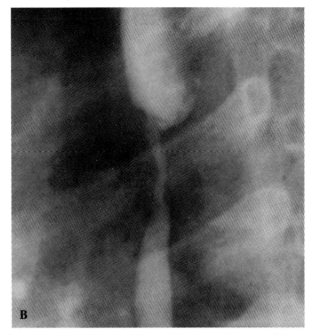

FIGURE 6–77. Esophageal stricture from epidermolysis bullosa. Frontal (*A*) and oblique (*B*) views show an abrupt, narrow stricture.

bowel are discussed in Chapter 9. The esophagus can also be affected with resulting dysphagia, chest pain, painful swallowing, regurgitation, and weight loss (McDonald et al., 1984).

Webs, ring-like narrowing, and tapering strictures in the mid and upper esophagus may all be seen radiologically (McDonald et al., 1984). Less apparent is the characteristic desquamation best detected on esophagoscopy.

Rare Miscellaneous Causes of Esophagitis. Radiologic appearances identical to those found in candidal esophagitis have been seen in adults with acanthosis nigricans (Itai et al., 1976), which is associated with visceral malignancies and characterized clinically by pigmentation, hyperkeratosis, and papillomatous hyperplasia.

Pemphigoid (Al-Katoubi and Eliot, 1984), Behçet syndrome (Vlymen and Muskowitz, 1981), and lipoid proteinosis (Francis, 1975) are other rare causes of esophagitis. Pemphigoid more commonly affects the oral and conjunctival mucosa but occasional smooth esophageal strictures or webs have been seen in adults (Al-Katoubi and Eliot, 1984).

Iatrogenic esophagitis may result from radiation (Lepke and Libshitz, 1983) or medication (Creteur et al., 1983; Daunt et al., 1985). Its radiologic features include abnormal motility with and without mucosal edema, stricture formation, ulceration, and pseudodiverticulum or fistula formation (Lepke and Libshitz, 1983). The abnormal motility occurs less than 4 months after radiotherapy and the strictures occur more than 4 months after radiotherapy; the other abnormalities occur at no specific time. Radiation-induced injury occurs more frequently and rapidly if there is adjuvant chemotherapy.

Many medications have been implicated in esophagitis, including Vibramycin (doxycycline), tetracycline, and quinidine. The diagnosis has often been made endoscopically, with evidence of redness and friability of the esophageal mucosa, erosions, ulcers, and strictures. The erosions, variable-sized ulcers, and strictures can all be seen on double-contrast barium examinations (Daunt et al., 1985; Creteur et al., 1983), which are preferable to endoscopy in small children. This esophagitis is relatively benign and generally improves following cessation of medication and symptomatic therapy.

In contrast, toxic epidermal necrolysis is a generalized disease usually of high mortality which also has been linked to many antibiotics and medications which can result in esophagitis. Usually there is evidence of acute esophagitis but stricture formation has been reported recently (Herman et al., 1984). Treatment is similar to that for burns.

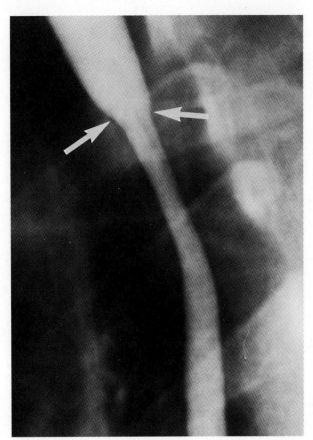

FIGURE 6–78. Esophageal stricture from eosinophilic gastroenteritis. A long stricture with a tapered upper end (*arrows*) is present in the mid esophagus.

Neoplasms of the Esophagus

Benign Tumors of the Esophagus

Esophageal tumors, both benign and malignant, are very rare in children. Of the benign tumors, leiomyomas (Schmidt and Lockwood, 1967; Levine et al., 1996), hemangiomas (Govoni, 1982; Wesenberg, 1982), hamartomas (Dieter, Riker, et al., 1970), and angiofibromatous polyps (Dieter, Holinger, et al., 1970; Styles et al., 1985) have all been reported in children. The most common symptoms are dysphagia, regurgitation, and vomiting, although respiratory difficulties can predominate.

Esophagography is the preferred initial examination by which to demonstrate esophageal tumors although both it and esophagoscopy may yield false-negative results. If esophagography reveals a smooth or crenated filling defect, CT with oral and intravenous contrast or endoscopy or MR should be used to determine the nature of the lesion.

Malignant Tumors of the Esophagus

Esophageal carcinoma is exceptionally rare in children; it sometimes follows lye ingestion (Kinnman et al., 1968) or it may arise spontaneously (Moore, 1958). The radiologic features are similar to those seen in adults with mucosal irregularity with or without a mass lesion, which may be ulcerated and cause obstruction (Figure 6–79). More common in childhood are lymphomas which may affect the esophagus by extrinsic pressure and compromise the tracheobronchial tree (Mandell et al., 1982). Malignant tumors in children are similar in appearance to the irregular destructive mass lesions or strictures seen in adults.

Trauma to the Esophagus

Swallowed Foreign Body

Clinical Features. Although no age is exempt, swallowed foreign bodies are common in pediatric prac-

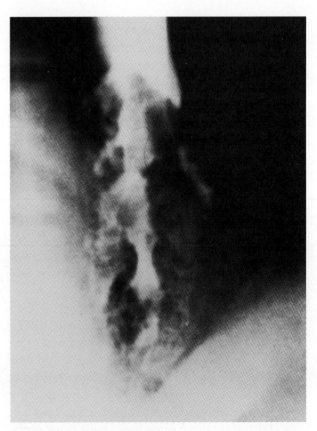

FIGURE 6–79. Esophageal carcinoma. A barium swallow shows mucosal irregularity with a mass lesion in the lower esophagus. This was seen to cause obstruction on fluoroscopy.

tice due to the childhood propensity to put things into the mouth (Figure 6–80). Coins are generally the most commonly swallowed foreign bodies found in children (Franken and Smith, 1982) but geographic variations exist, such as in Hong Kong, where fish bones are the most common swallowed foreign body (Nandi and Ong, 1978). An endotracheal tube has been reportedly swallowed in the first week of life (Bowen and Dominquez, 1981). In adults, the main culprit is a bolus of meat (Baraka and Bikhazi, 1975).

Most swallowed foreign objects pass through the bowel without complication. Of foreign bodies which impact, 80% do so at the level of the thoracic inlet below the cricopharyngeus (Nandi and Ong, 1978). A few foreign bodies impact at the level of the left main bronchus, and fewer impact just above the gastroesophageal sphincter. If impaction occurs at any other level as seen on plain film, an underlying anomaly should be assumed unless proven otherwise by examination. Thus, a barium study would be indicated if endoscopy has not already been performed. The underlying anomaly is usually a stricture, such as may follow the repair of tracheoesophageal fistula and esophageal atresia (Figure 6–81). Other anomalies include congenital strictures (Jewsbury, 1971), webs, or extrinsic masses, and the more common acquired strictures from esophagitis.

Although many children give a history of foreign body ingestion, some cases may be unsuspected and present with gastrointestinal or, less commonly, respiratory symptoms. Gastrointestinal symptoms include dysphagia, drooling, gagging, vomiting, and poor feeding. Respiratory symptoms are more common in young children in whom an esophageal foreign body is more likely to impinge on the trachea, producing wheezing and stridor (Newman, 1978; Beer et al., 1982).

Diagnosis must be made quickly so that the object can be removed promptly (see Chapter 3). A coin will lodge in the esophagus so that its flat surfaces face anteriorly and posteriorly (Figure 6–82). A coin in the trachea tends to lie at right angles to this, with the flat surfaces facing sideways. A foreign body impacted in the esophagus is unlikely to pass spontaneously. The longer it remains impacted, the more difficult it is to remove and the greater the risk as edema from the attendant local trauma grips the object more firmly and manipulation becomes more difficult (Nandi and Ong, 1978; Towbin et al., 1989; Macpherson et al., 1996). Ensuing complications may include stenosis, ulceration, or perforation of the esophagus. The latter can result in local infection with abscess formation or mediastinitis; tracheoesophageal fistula, or esophagoaortic fistula (Nandi and Ong, 1978; Newman, 1978). Pneumopericardium has been reported from a bronchial foreign body (Tjhen et al., 1978).

The radiologic investigation of foreign body ingestion initially consists of plain films. All areas must be surveyed but usually a combination of

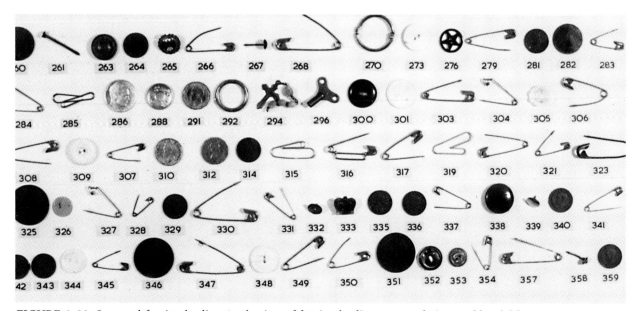

FIGURE 6–80. Ingested foreign bodies. A selection of foreign bodies commonly ingested by children.

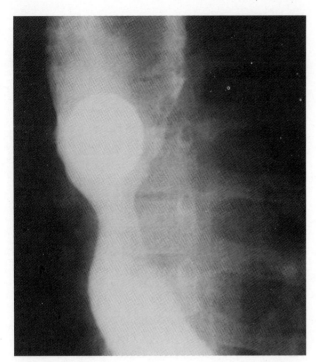

FIGURE 6–81. Coin proximal to esophageal stricture. Routine barium examination of a stricture, which developed after repair of esophageal atresia, serendipitously revealed a coin.

abdomen and chest radiographs (frontal and lateral) and lateral neck plain radiographs are sufficient to localize a radiopaque foreign body. However, not all foreign bodies are radiopaque (Newman, 1978), and they may be overlooked unless extra care is taken (Figure 6–83). The frontal view of the neck is not useful. Some types of fish bones are radiopaque and others are easily missed on plain radiographs (Campbell et al., 1968; Ell and Sprigg, 1991). Aluminum can tops are of surprisingly low radiodensity and may easily be overlooked, remaining unsuspected for some time and leading to complications (Burrington, 1976; Eggli et al., 1986; Levick and Spitz, 1977). Barium studies are useful in diagnosing radiolucent foreign bodies (Figures 6–83 and 6–84) (Newman, 1978) but barium itself may obscure small foreign objects (Campbell et al., 1968).

Prompt endoscopic removal is recommended for a sharp-edged foreign body because of its potential for wall penetration and perforation. Likewise, small disk batteries such as those used in electronic watches and calculators should be removed without delay to prevent caustic erosion and perforation (Shaffer et al., 1986). Blunt, smooth foreign bodies

(such as coins) present for less than 24 hours may be removed with a Foley catheter (Shackelford et al., 1972; Carlson, 1972) although this technique is controversial (see Chapter 3). A technique to remove blunt foreign bodies from the esophagus using a wire basket under fluoroscopic guidance has been described (Shaffer et al., 1986). To hasten passage of nontoxic foreign bodies with smooth surfaces, a number of noninvasive pharmacologic and mechanical measures have been advocated, such as glucagon

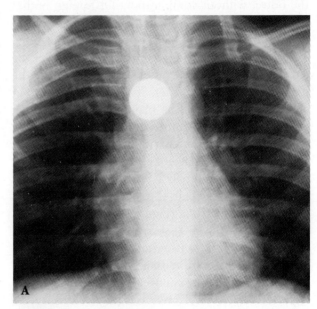

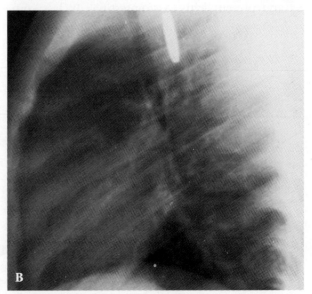

FIGURE 6–82. Coin in the esophagus. A coin lodged in the esophagus will appear face on in the frontal view (*A*) and on end in the lateral view (*B*). Coins in the trachea have the reverse appearance.

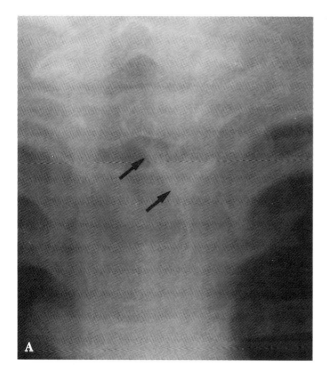 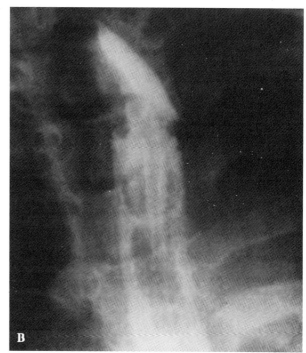

FIGURE 6–83. Foreign body in the esophagus. A faintly radiopaque suction cap (arrows) from a toy arrow is only faintly visible on plain film (*A*) and is more obvious on barium study (*B*).

to relieve lower esophageal sphincter spasm, and carbonated beverages to distend the esophagus and force impacted food or foreign bodies into the stomach (Mohammed and Hegedus, 1986; Robbins and Shortsleeve, 1994). Metallic foreign bodies may be removed from the upper gastrointestinal tract by means of a magnet inserted into the end of an orogastric tube (Volle et al., 1986; Towbin et al., 1990; Paulson and Jaffe, 1990).

If a foreign body is missed and becomes impacted in the esophagus, a perforation is likely to occur; the patient may be referred some time after the event with no history of foreign body ingestion. The radiologist may be the first to suggest the diagnosis as plain films may show localized air in the mediastinum (Figure 6–85), and contrast studies can outline the cavity arising from the esophagus (Figure 6–85).

Iatrogenic Perforation

Infants. It is increasingly recognized that in infants, and especially in newborn preterm infants, instrumentation with laryngoscope, endotracheal intubation, and feeding tube manipulation can all lead to submucosal or transmural perforation of the pharynx or esophagus (Tucker et al., 1975; Touloukian et

al., 1977; Lee and Kuhn, 1976; Eklof et al., 1969; Grunebaum et al., 1980; Faerber et al., 1980). Although such perforation was thought at one time

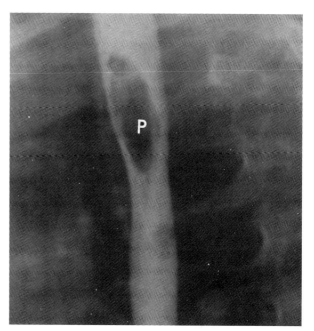

FIGURE 6–84. Foreign body in the esophagus. A nonradiopaque foreign body (plum pit) could not be seen on plain films but is easily visible (*P*) with barium.

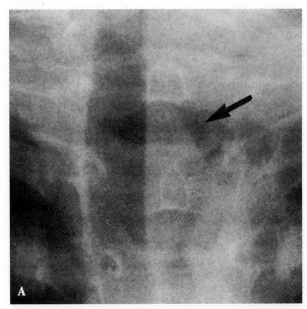

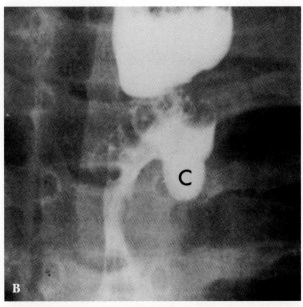

FIGURE 6–85. Foreign body perforation. Plain films show localized air (*arrow*) in the mediastinum (*A*). A barium swallow outlines the cavity (*C*) arising from the esophagus (*B*).

to be associated with a fulminating course and high mortality, if recognized and treated promptly by antibiotics and removal of any feeding tube, the out-

look is good and surprisingly free of sequelae. Occasionally it may even go unrecognized and be found to have occurred serendipitously at a later date

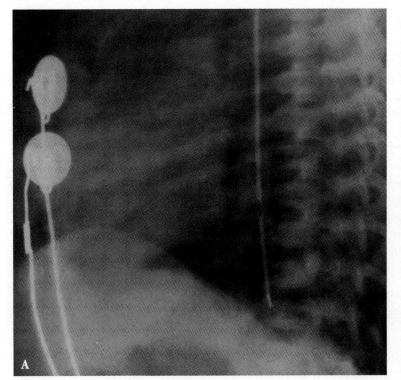

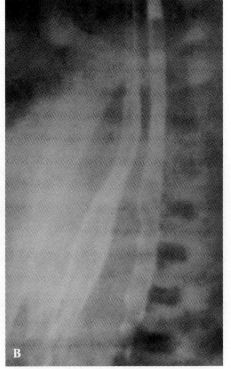

FIGURE 6–86. Pharyngoesophageal perforation. A feeding tube tracks an unusually straight and more posterior course than is usual for a nasoesophageal tube on the lateral chest radiograph (*A*). Low ionic water-soluble contrast swallow shows a large posterior track (*B*).

(Faerber et al., 1980). The perforation often occurs at or above the pharyngoesophageal level, and a feeding tube may track through the mediastinum and on into the abdomen (Figure 6–86). The clinical presentation may mimic an esophageal atresia with excessive salivation, choking, coughing, and failure to pass a nasogastric tube.

Diagnosis is made by careful examination of plain films, which can demonstrate subcutaneous emphysema in the neck or a pneumomediastinum (Amodio et al., 1986). The location of feeding tubes should always be carefully assessed. In esophageal atresia, the nasogastric tube occupies a characteristic position in the upper thorax, immediately behind the trachea and sometimes outlined by gas in the proximal esophageal pouch (see esophageal atresia). The nasogastric tube will have a different appearance in perforation often lying further posteriorly. An air-filled pouch has not been seen in these traumatic patients (Faerber et al., 1980). Instilling iso-osmolar water-soluble contrast media down the tube may be helpful in the few cases when diagnosis is difficult (see Figure 6–86).

An esophageal perforation has been reported secondary to gastrostomy tube replacement with a Foley catheter and balloon inflation in the esophagus (Kenigsberg and Levenbrown, 1986). Gastrostomy Foley catheters can migrate into the esophagus (Figure 6–87) or small bowel, and care should be taken if balloon inflation is to be performed.

Older Children. Iatrogenic perforation in older children is similar to that seen in adults (Parkin, 1973). It can occur following feeding tube placement, esophagoscopy, bougie dilatation, or sclerotherapy for varices. The perforation may be incomplete with hematoma formation (Bradley and Han, 1979) or there may be perforation of adjacent structures such as the pleura. Feeding tubes passed inadvertently into the trachea and bronchi are especially liable to transgress the pleura (Sheffner et al., 1985). Rarely, the abdominal segment of the esophagus may be perforated by instrumentation (Han and Tischler, 1984).

The appearance of the perforation will vary according to its size and location. Due to the arrangement of the pleura, adjacent to the midesophagus on the right and the lower esophagus on the left, the collection of fluid or air will be on the right or left if the perforation is in the mid or lower esophagus, respectively. Pneumomediastinum, pneumoperitoneum, or cervical emphysema (Han et al., 1985) may all occur depending on the site of perforation (Figure 6–88). Again, instilling iso-osmolar water-soluble contrast media down the tube may help in the few cases where diagnosis is difficult. Follow-up of these patients may

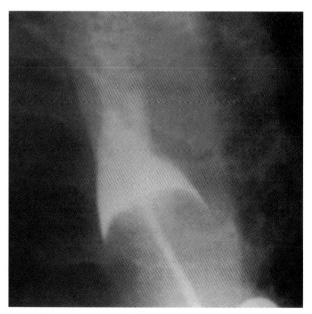

FIGURE 6–87. Foley catheter in the esophagus. There is a complete obstruction to flow of barium due to an inflated Foley gastrostomy catheter which has entered the lower esophagus.

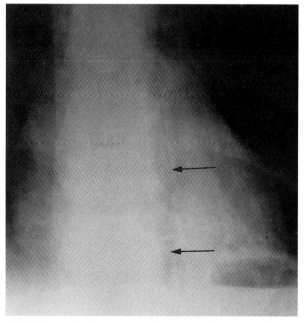

FIGURE 6–88. Pneumomediastinum from esophageal perforation. There is a faint pneumomediastinum (*arrows*) secondary to an endoscopic lower esophageal perforation.

show an almost complete disappearance of even large sinus tracks (Figure 6–89).

Ventriculoperitoneal shunt tips occasionally migrate to unusual locations. At our hospital we have seen the intra-abdominal portion perforate the rectum and appear from the anus. In another unusual instance, a patient presented complaining of a leaking tube coming out of the mouth. The patient was otherwise well despite the tube having perforated the stomach and refluxed up the esophagus to reach the mouth (Figure 6–90).

Mallory-Weiss Syndrome

Mallory-Weiss syndrome is rare but is occasionally reported in children. It consists of a lower esophageal mucosal tear, best seen endoscopically although it can occasionally be seen by esophagography. Where hemorrhage is severe and endoscopy not available, selective celiac angiography can be used to demonstrate the bleeding site. Radiologic and clinical findings are similar to those found in adults (Knauer, 1976).

Boerhaave's Syndrome

Boerhaave's syndrome—spontaneous esophageal rupture—occurs in children and infants but is more common in adults. The mechanism of rupture is uncertain, but the following factors have been implicated: increased pressure in the esophagus due to cricopharyngeal incoordination during swallowing; vomiting and increased pressure during delivery (Dubos et al., 1986); pre-existent esophagitis (Harell et al., 1970); and rarely, an obstructing lesion such as an esophageal web (Aaronson et al., 1975). The infant usually presents within 48 hours of birth. Clinically, progressive respiratory distress with dyspnea and cyanosis occur due to the formation of a tension hydropneumothorax. Occasionally blood regurgitates into the mouth.

The radiologic appearances are different in neonates from those in adults (Aaronson et al., 1975). Radiographic chest examination in infants typically shows a right-sided hydropneumothorax or occasionally a pneumothorax. In adults the hydropneumothorax tends to be left-sided. The difference may be due to the more right-sided position of the neonatal esophagus (Harell et al., 1970). Mediastinal gas is unusual; indeed, the presence of pneumomediastinum is nonspecific and may be found in gastrointestinal disease without gut perforation presumably from a ruptured alveolus as it is often self limiting (Woodruff et al., 1985). The diagnosis of gut perforation can be confirmed by a water-soluble contrast media esophagogram. An isotonic contrast medium should be used if there is any risk of medium entering the lungs and is the safest medium to use if there is any gut leak.

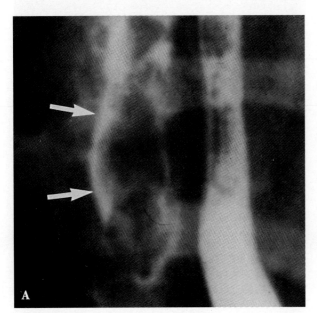 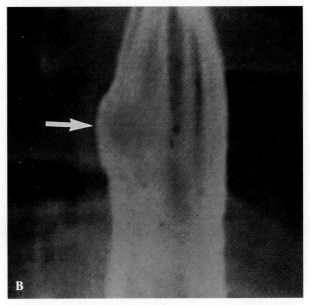

FIGURE 6–89. Esophageal perforation. A large sinus secondary to an endoscopic midesophageal perforation was demonstrated on a low-osmolar water-soluble contrast swallow (*A*). Follow-up of this sinus showed progressive reduction in sinus size with minimal esophageal outpouching (*arrow*) at 6 months (*B*).

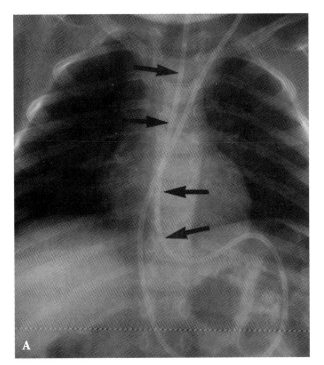
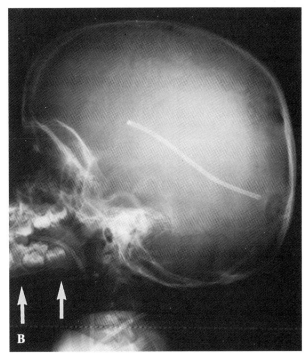

FIGURE 6–90. Ventriculoperitoneal shunt. A ventriculoperitoneal shunt perforated the stomach (*A*) and refluxed up the esophagus (*black arrows*) to reach the mouth and protrude through the lips (*B, white arrows*).

Needle aspiration of the chest to relieve respiratory embarrassment can be a necessary emergency measure but a definite surgical repair must quickly be undertaken to prevent death. Occasionally a stricture of the esophagus develops following the repair.

Miscellaneous Disorders of the Mouth, Pharynx, Esophagus, and Salivary Glands

Abnormalities of the Salivary Glands

Acute sialadenitis is not uncommon in children and usually does not require imaging. Organisms implicated include *Streptococcus viridans*, hemolytic streptococci, *Staphylococcus aureus* and *albus* and pneumococcus (Pearson, 1961). More chronic disease may indicate calculus formation secondary to infection and inflammation, or rarely, the presence of a tumor, for which imaging can be helpful.

Ultrasonography is the modality of choice if there is a mass such as hemangioma, mixed salivary tumor, or lymphadenopathy (Seibert and Seibert, 1986; Gritzmann, 1989). Ultrasonography can delineate the mass from the adjacent muscles and vascular structures and may show a calculus as a dense shadowing echogenic focus (Grunebaum et al., 1985).

Plain film radiography is useful for demonstrating radiopaque calculi (Figure 6–91). Submandibular calculi are more often radiopaque than parotid stones (Yune and Klatte, 1972).

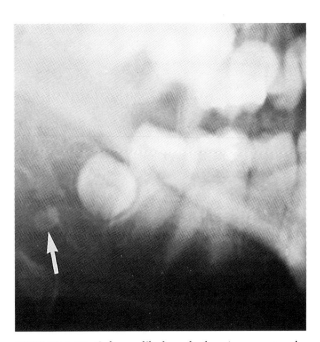

FIGURE 6–91. Submandibular calculus. An opaque submandibular calculus (*arrow*) is present.

Sialography is reserved for diagnostic problems usually related to recurrent pain or swelling in a salivary gland. The technique is discussed in Chapter 3. An improved technique for sialography in difficult cases involves passing a cannula into the salivary duct ostium over a thin, flexible, blunt guide wire (Aslam et al., 1991). Sialography is particularly useful in demonstrating lucent calculi, which appear as filling defects in contrast-filled duct systems (Figure 6–92) (Nicholson, 1990). Calculi may rarely produce obstruction of a ball valve type, best seen on postsialogogue films, and which, if suspected, is the only indication for these extra views. Infection proximal to an obstruction may result in alternating areas of dilatation and stricture that appear like a string of sausages. The punctate, globular, cavitary, and destructive sialographic changes found in parotitis (Figure 6–93) have been termed sialectasis or sialodochiectasis (Rubaltelli et al., 1987). The term pseudosialectasis has recently been introduced for these appearances in autoimmune disease, as they probably represent duct disruption rather than ectasia (Som et al., 1981). The stone is occasionally visible on clinical examination during sialography, perhaps brought to the duct orifice by the effect of the sialogogue. It can sometimes be gently removed by the radiologist after minimal duct dilatation.

Salivary gland scanning with Tc 99m pertechnetate is sensitive to minor disturbances of gland function. A mild abnormality will show normal perfusion but diminished early uptake at 1 minute; however, by 15 minutes uptake is usually normal. With more progressive involvement, there is increasingly less uptake in the parotid glands even at 15 minutes. In addition, the spontaneous accumulation of activity in the mouth which is usually seen by 15 minutes may be reduced or delayed. Following stimulation with lemon, however, the activity is discharged normally into the mouth. With severe dysfunction there is very little activity in the parotid glands, and the submandibular glands may also be involved.

Congenital absence of the major salivary glands is rare with only a few reported cases in the world literature. Following clinical exclusion of the more common causes of a dry mouth, salivary gland agenesis can be confirmed by a Tc-99m-pertechnetate scan or CT (Whyte and Hayward, 1989).

Many causes of salivary gland dysfunction will show a similar appearance and nuclear medicine scanning is relatively nonspecific. Benign mixed tumors may either be cold or have uptake equal to that of the surrounding gland. Blood flow and blood pool images are variable and may show hyperemia or hypoperfusion.

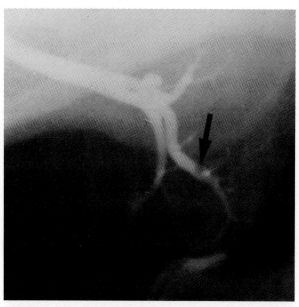

FIGURE 6–92. Submandibular calculus. A lucent calculus (*arrow*) appears as a defect in a duct during sialography. Air bubbles can also give this appearance if accidentally introduced.

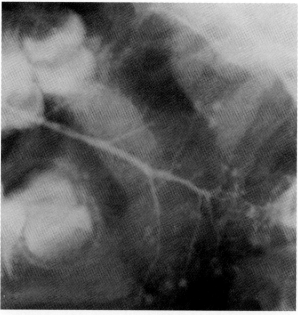

FIGURE 6–93. Sialectasis. Small pools of contrast in the parotid gland indicate sialectasis in a 6-year-old girl with parotitis.

Hemangiomas present a typical picture and are highly vascular on the flow phase and cold on the functional phase. Although uncommon, hemangiomas constitute a significant proportion of salivary gland tumors seen in childhood.

Warthin's tumor is unique in that it is able to concentrate the pertechnetate to a greater degree than the normal tissue and retains the concentrated secretions as there is no communication with the patent duct system. Thus, Warthin's tumor has a pathognomonic appearance on scintigraphy; it is hot on the early phase and remains hot on wash-out phase.

Malignant neoplasms show variable blood flow and are usually cold on delayed scans. Inflammatory lesions show hyperemia on blood flow images and decreased function on delayed scans. Obstruction shows decreased blood flow, dilated ducts proximal to obstruction, and decreased uptake in the parenchyma on delayed scans.

Gallium 67 citrate localizes in a variety of neoplastic and inflammatory lesions. It will demonstrate persistent increased uptake in lymphomatous and other malignant involvement of salivary glands. Gallium uptake in inflammatory and infectious conditions tends to peak early by 24 hours; however, in some patients the differentiation between neoplasm and sialadenitis is difficult. Because a great deal of gallium normally accumulates in the salivary glands, it is difficult to distinguish a mild increase from normal. Parotid glands may show an avid gallium accumulation after irradiation and this can complicate the differentiation of a lymphoma and postradiation adenitis. Gallium 67 citrate has been useful in showing salivary gland involvement by sarcoidosis.

Time activity curves may be generated over the parotid glands, and analysis of the time to maximum activity as well as time to half peak activity (T-1/2) may be helpful in distinguishing chronic from acute inflammation as well as obstructive disorders.

Computed tomography and MR have been helpful in assessing salivary glands in children (Bryan et al., 1982; Mandelblatt et al., 1987; Teresi et al., 1987; Bronstein et al., 1987). The technique of enhancing the salivary glands by sialography immediately followed by CT (CT sialography) is particularly useful in adults when space-occupying lesions are present (McGahon et al., 1984; Evers et al., 1985) and can be incorporated into an aspiration biopsy procedure. However, whether this affects patient management is controversial (Stacey-Clear et al.,

1985). Non-CT sialography is often unhelpful in space-occupying lesions but valuable in infective conditions (McGahon et al., 1984).

Esophageal Webs

Upper esophageal webs are uncommon in children except for the webs associated with atresia of the esophagus. Upper esophageal webs may be associated with the iron deficiency anemia common in adolescents (Crawford et al., 1965; Maclean and Houghton-Allen, 1975).

Upper esophageal webs associated with dysphagia have been found in a 5-year-old girl and a 6-year-old boy (Maclean and Houghton-Allen, 1975). The girl had consistently refused to eat solid food and lived on fluids alone; she was cured following esophageal dilatation. The boy developed dysphagia, which was cured by esophagoscopy. In our hospital, a teenage boy developed an upper esophageal web following extensive radiotherapy and cervical spine surgery. He had dysphagia until the web was disrupted by limited esophagoscopy (Figure 6–94). Other causes of pharyngeal and esophageal webs include pemphigus, epidermolysis bullosa, and dyskeratosis congenita (Franken and Smith, 1982). In adults, upper esophageal webs are often of doubtful clinical significance (Nosher et al., 1975).

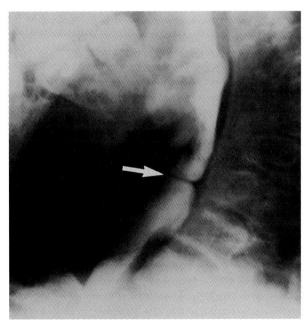

FIGURE 6–94. Esophageal web. The web appears as a linear lucency (*arrow*) on this esophagograph. The cervical vertebrae are surgically fused.

Lower esophageal webs, also rare in children, may be related to gastroesophageal reflux (Weaver et al., 1984).

Diverticula of the Pharynx and Esophagus

Congenital diverticula are extremely rare in the esophagus. Only 1 was found in 7000 autopsies (Guthrie, 1945) and this was a form of pulsion diverticulum at the cricopharyngeal level. Congenital posterior midline pharyngoesophageal diverticula have been found. They may be asymptomatic, found only when a foreign body impacts in them, or may simulate esophageal atresia (Nelson, 1957; Brintnall and Kridelbaugh, 1950; Theander, 1973; MacKellar and Kennedy, 1972).

Acquired diverticula can be secondary to trauma (Girdany et al., 1969) and usually occur in neonates (Eklof et al., 1969) when they are induced during nasogastric intubation although they have been found in older children (Osman and Girdany, 1973). Clinically, they mimic the rare congenital type and can produce symptoms of esophageal atresia (Eklof et al., 1969). Acquired diverticula may be more common than is currently appreciated as they may remain undetected for many years. A traumatic perforation usually occurs in the neck, and the tip of a perforating nasogastric tube has been seen as low as the third lumbar vertebra and may even enter the pericardial space (see Iatrogenic Perforation in this chapter) (Touloukian et al., 1977). It is important to check the position of a nasogastric tube in the early diagnosis of perforation (Grunebaum et al., 1980). Early recognition of traumatic perforation is essential as death can occur from sepsis (Lee and Kuhn, 1976).

Traction and pulsion diverticula (Zenker's diverticula) are uncommon in children but are occasionally seen in older children. They are similar to those seen in adults and consist of a posterolateral outpouching through Killian's dehiscence, a site of potential weakness in the lowermost part of the inferior constrictor muscle where the posterior raphe ends and the cricopharyngeus begins. An underlying anomaly such as cutis laxa may predispose to diverticulum formation (Figure 6–95).

Intramural Diverticulosis of the Esophagus

Intramural diverticulosis is a rare disorder associated with esophageal dysphagia and is usually seen in adults (Castillo et al., 1977). It is very rare in children, and only a few cases have been documented in children between 5 years of age (Peters et al., 1982; Braun et al., 1978) and adolescence (Weller, 1972; Cramer, 1972; Braun et al., 1978; Peters et al., 1982; Markle and Hanson, 1992). The "diverticula" are dilated esophageal glands obstructed by desquamated squamous cells and hence do not involve the entire wall of the esophagus and so are sometimes called pseudodiverticula (Castillo et al., 1977; Peters et al., 1982). The cause of the desquamated squamous cells is uncertain but may be related to chronic irritation (Wrightman and Wright, 1974), most likely due to gastroesophageal reflux (Peters et al., 1982).

The barium swallow appearance of the pseudodiverticula is similar to a flask or collar stud with a narrow neck and wider base, often seen in association with an adjacent stricture. Associated hiatus hernia, gastroesophageal reflux, and disordered motility may also be present.

Although CT is not the best modality for investigating the pediatric esophagus, it can show marked thickening of the esophageal wall with irregularity of the lumen and intramural gas collections (Pearlberg et al., 1983).

Varices of the Esophagus

In children, esophageal varices are usually secondary to portal hypertension. They are similar to the varices of adults in most respects, with vermiform vessels arising from below the diaphragm and passing through the esophagogastric junction. The rare solitary esophageal varix (Trenkner et al., 1983) has not been described in children.

Initial investigation can be ultrasonographic to evaluate the echotexture of the liver, presence of portal vein, and collaterals. A widening of the mesenteric base to 1.7 times the width of the aorta is compatible with esophageal varices. Duplex rangegated US has also been useful in evaluating portal and collateral flow (Stringer et al., 1985). (Ultrasonographic, CT, and MR findings are discussed further in Chapter 11).

Plain film radiography is generally not helpful although a few cases (less than 5%) may show evidence of varices with posterior mediastinal masses (Figure 6–96), lesions in the inferior pulmonary ligament, or obliteration of the descending aorta (Ishikawa et al., 1985).

Contrast investigation with barium swallow follows the adult approach (Waldram et al., 1977), except that antispasmodics are used less in children

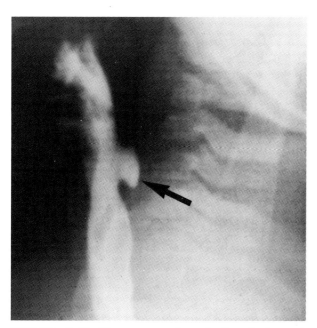

FIGURE 6–95. Pharyngoesophageal diverticulum, A posterolateral diverticulum (*arrow*) found in a 6-month-old girl with cutis laxa probably represents a pulsion or Zenker's diverticulum.

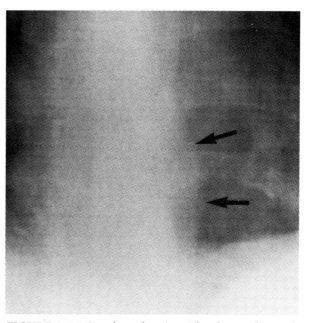

FIGURE 6–96. Esophageal varices. The chest radiograph shows a posterior mediastinal mass (*arrows*) but not obliteration of the descending aorta.

and Valsalva's and Müller's maneuvers may be difficult to perform, especially in the very young. The varices appear as vermiform filling defects in the lower esophagus (Figure 6–97). The increase in intrathoracic pressure during crying may mask small varices but they can be seen to fill during the gasp between cries when the child is horizontal. The esophagus should be examined with small mouthfuls of dense barium (liquid or paste) for good mucosal coating; occasionally a more diluted barium better demonstrates the varices. Persistence and patience may be needed, as radiologic diagnosis of varices can be difficult. The barium study should also include the stomach and duodenum to show other possible varices (Figure 6–98).

Varices may be demonstrated by CT. If CT is being performed for some other reason, it can be useful to include the gastroesophageal region during dynamic contrast enhancement to detect any varices (Balthazar et al., 1987). The varices show up as dense rounded and tubular structures. Other collaterals such as periadrenal and adrenal portosystemic shunts may also be demonstrated (Brady et al., 1985), and CT may demonstrate gastric varices (Balthazar, 1984) as well as evidence of hepatic cirrhosis and portal cavernoma (Stringer et al., 1985).

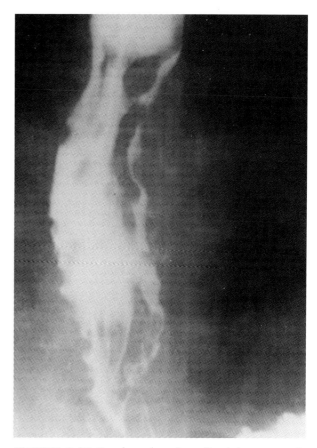

FIGURE 6–97. Esophageal varices. Serpiginous vermiform filling defects in the lower esophagus indicate varices.

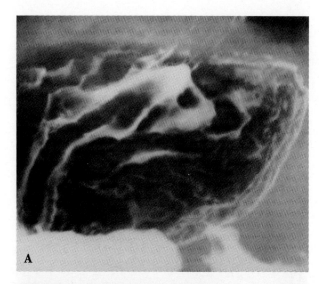

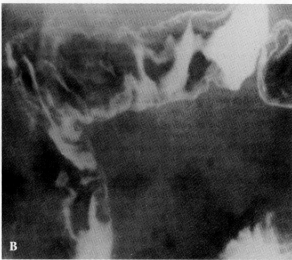

FIGURE 6–98. Gastric and duodenal varices. Serpiginous filling defects in the fundus of the stomach (*A*) and duodenum (*B*) were confirmed as varices on endoscopy.

By showing contrast between flowing blood and the surrounding soft tissue, MR can demonstrate varices but its true value in children is still to be fully determined (see Chapter 11).

Endoscopy is valuable in the assessment of varices but is difficult in children and may require a general anesthetic. In addition, there is a small but appreciable risk of hemorrhage. An advantage of esophagoscopy is that it allows sclerotherapy during the procedure. Radiologic appearance after sclerotherapy is discussed below.

Angiography or digital subtraction angiography can demonstrate varices in a number of ways, including delayed films on celiac and superior mesenteric arteriography, or immediate films on splenoportocavography, or percutaneous transhepatic portal or gastric coronary venography. Percutaneous transhepatic gastric coronary venography has a sensitivity of 78% and a specificity of 100% compared to endoscopy in adults (Takashi et al., 1985). Its advantage is that embolization of the varices is possible (Lunderquist et al., 1978).

Management of Varices. In our hospital, endoscopic sclerotherapy and/or occasionally the Siguira operation or (rarely) a shunt procedure are preferred to embolization, as in our experience recurrence is less common.

Sclerotherapy using a flexible endoscope is a well-accepted technique but it often requires repeated procedures, and complications—including perforation—do occur. Immediately after sclerotherapy, there is narrowing of the distal esophagus at the site of the injection (Tihansky et al., 1984; Van Steenbergen et al., 1984), and in the first 30 days there may be mucosal ulceration, intramural defects, sinuses, fistulae, esophageal dissection, and even perforation (Agha, 1984; DeMarino et al., 1988). After 60 days following sclerotherapy, esophageal dysmotility, strictures, and luminal obstruction along with irregular contour and mural defects can occur (Agha, 1984). Over 7 months later, double-contrast barium studies will show sharp-edged, longitudinal tramline filling defects and a patchy nodularity with loss of normal longitudinal folds. Healed ulcers, epithelial tags, and redundant epithelial folds cause these appearances (Rose et al., 1985).

The Siguira operation involves transection of the esophagus with re-anastomosis, splenectomy, and division of varices. Pyloroplasty and selective vagotomy may also be performed. This major operation appears to be relatively well tolerated and results are good. Follow-up barium examination can demonstrate irregularity at the site of re-anastomosis that may be associated with focal outpouchings (pseudodiverticula) (Greenspan et al., 1982).

Percutaneous transhepatic embolization of gastroesophageal varices is a safe and effective therapeutic procedure for the control of bleeding in patients with this disorder (L'Hermine et al., 1989).

Lingual Tonsils

Lingual tonsils may appear as an irregular space-occupying lesion in the hypopharynx, especially if there has been tonsillitis, and should be considered in the differentiation of malignant disease in this region

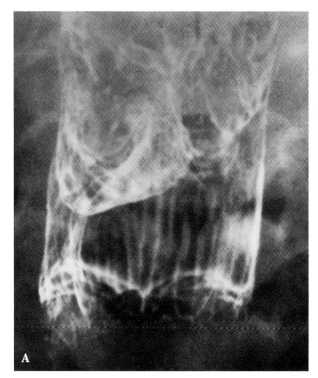
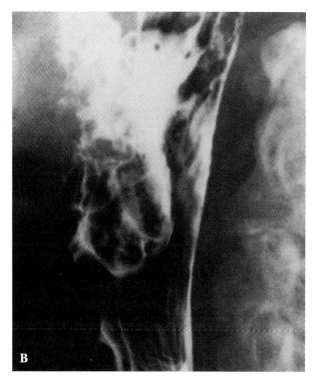

FIGURE 6–99. Lingual tonsils. A barium swallow showed an irregular space-occupying lesion in the hypopharynx extending inferiorly on the lateral view (*A*) and more on the right than the left on the frontal view (*B*). Enlarged inflamed lingual tonsils were found on endoscopy.

(Figure 6–99). Hypertrophy of the lingual tonsils may cause dysphagia (Fitzgerald and O'Connell, 1987).

REFERENCES

ANATOMY OF THE PHARYNX AND ESOPHAGUS

Ardran GM, Kemp FH. The mechanism of changes in form of the cervical airway in infancy. Med Radiol Photogr 1968;44:26–54.

Ardran GM, Kemp FH. Normal and disturbed swallowing. Prog Pediatr Radiol 1969;2:151–69.

Ardran GM, Kemp FH. Some important factors in the assessment of oropharyngeal function. Dev Med Child Neurol 1970;12:158–66.

Ardran GM, Kemp FH, Lind J. A cineradiographic study of bottle feeding. Br J Radiol 1958;31:11–22, 156–62.

Berger PE, Kuhns LR, Poznanski AK. A simple technique for eliminating tracheal buckling on lateral neck roentgenograms. Pediatr Radiol 1974;2:69–72.

Bishop HC. Cricopharyngeal achalasia in childhood. J Pediatr Surg 1974;9:775–8.

Blane CE, White ST, Braunstein EM, et al. Patterns of calcification in childhood dermatomyositis. AJR 1984;142:397–400.

Bowie JD, Clair MR. Fetal swallowing and regurgitation: observation of normal and abnormal activity. Radiology 1982;144:877–8.

Caffey J. Pediatric x-ray diagnosis. 7th ed. Chicago: Year Book; 1978. p. 1708.

Capitanio MA, Kirkpatrick JA. Nasopharyngeal lymphoid tissue. Radiology 1970;96:389–91.

Chen MYM, Ott AJ, Peele VN, Gelfand DW. Oropharynx in patients with cerebrovascular disease: evaluation with videofluoroscopy. Radiology 1990;176:641–3.

Cumming WA, Akhtar M, Ferentzi C, et al. Cricopharyngeal ring: a case report. Pediatr Radiol 1986;16:152–3.

Cumming WA, Reilly BJ. Fatigue aspiration. Radiology 1972;105:387–90.

Curtis DJ, Cruess DF, Berg T. The cricopharyngeal muscle: a video recording review. AJR 1984;142:497–500.

Dabich L, Sullivan DB, Cassidy JT. Scleroderma in the child. J Pediatr 1974;85:770–5.

Ekberg O, Nylander G. Cineradiography of the pharyngeal stage of deglutition in 150 individuals without dysphagia. Br J Radiol 1982a;55:253–7.

Ekberg O, Nylander G. Cineradiography of the pharyngeal stage of deglutition in 250 patients with dysphagia. Br J Radiol 1982b;55:258–62.

Fernbach SK, McLone DG. Derangement of swallowing in children with myelomeningocele. Pediatr Radiol 1985;15:311–4.

Fitzgerald P, O'Connell D. Massive hypertrophy of the lingual tonsils: an unusual cause of dysphagia. Br J Radiol 1987;60:505–6.

Franken EA Jr, Smith WL, editors. Gastrointestinal imaging in pediatrics. 2nd ed. Philadelphia: Harper & Row; 1982. p. 30.

Gilchrist AM, Laird JD, Ferguson WR. What is the significance of the abnormal oesophageal scintigram? Clin Radiol 1987;38:509–11.

Grunebaum M, Salinge H. Radiologic findings in polymyositis—dermatomyositis involving the pharynx and upper esophagus. Clin Radiol 1971;22:97–100.

Gyepes MT, Linde LM. Familial dysautonomia: the mechanism of aspiration. Radiology 1968;91:471–5.

Halpert RD, Laufer I, Thompson JJ, et al. Adenocarcinoma of the esophagus in patients with scleroderma. AJR 1983;140:927–30.

Harris GBC. A special form of disturbed swallowing: one aspect of familial dysautonomia. Prog Pediatr Radiol 1969;2: 184–9.

Hibbert J, Whitehouse GM. The assessment of adenoidal size by radiological means. Clin Otolaryngol 1978;3:43–7.

Jeans WD, Fernando DCJ, Maw AR. How should adenoidal enlargement be measured? A radiological study based on interobserver agreement. Clin Radiol 1981;32:337–40.

Keats TE, Smith TH. Air esophagram: a sign of poor respiratory excursion in the neonate. AJR 1974;120:300–4.

Llamas-Elviras JM, Martinez-Parades M, Sopena-Monforte R, et al. Value of radionuclide oesophageal transit studies of functional dysphagia. Br J Radiol 1986;59:1073–8.

Macauley JC. Neuromuscular incoordination of swallowing in the newborn. Lancet 1951;1:1208–12.

Margulies SI, Brunt PW, Donner MW, et al. Familial dysautonomia: a cineradiographic study of the swallowing mechanism. Radiology 1968;90:107–12.

Martel W, Chang SF, Abel MR. Loss of colonic haustration in progressive systemic sclerosis. AJR 1976;126:704–13.

Olmsted WW, Madewell JE. The esophageal and small-bowel manifestations of progressive systemic sclerosis. Gastrointest Radiol 1976;1:33–6.

Ott DJ, Pikna LA. Clinical and videofluoroscopic evaluation of swallowing disorders. AJR 1993;161:507–13.

Palmer ED. Disorders of the cricopharyngeus muscle: a review. Gastroenterology 1976;71:510–9.

Rasley A, Logemann JA, Kahrilas PJ, et al. Prevention of barium aspiration during videofluoroscopic swallowing studies: value of change in posture. AJR 1993;160:1005–9.

Santel L. Megaesophagus in two cases of familial dysautonomia. J Pediatr Surg 1971;6:501.

Shanks MJ, Blane CE, Adler DD, et al. Radiographic findings of scleroderma in childhood. AJR 1983;141:657–60.

Skolnick ML, Glaser ER, McWilliams BJ. The use and limitations of the barium pharyngogram in the detection of velopharyngeal insufficiency. Radiology 1980;135:301–4.

Smith WH, Erenberg A, Nowak A, et al. Physiology of sucking in the normal term infant using real-time US. Radiology 1985;156:379–81.

Smith WL, Franken EA Jr, Smith JA. Pneumoesophagus as a sign of H-type tracheoesophageal fistula. Pediatrics 1976;58:907–9.

Steiner RM, Glassman L, Schwartz MW, et al. The radiological findings in dermatomyositis of childhood. Radiology 1974;111:385–93.

Stringer DA, Witzel MA. Velopharyngeal insufficiency on videofluoroscopy: comparison of projections. AJR 1986;146:15–9.

Swischuk LE, Smith PC, Fagan CJ. Abnormalities of the pharynx and larynx in childhood. Semin Roentgenol 1974;9:283–300.

Tatelman M, Keech MK. Esophageal motility in systemic lupus erythematosus, rheumatoid arthritis and scleroderma. Radiology 1966;86:1041–6.

Taybi H. Radiology of syndromes and metabolic disorders. 2nd ed. Chicago: Year Book; 1982. p. 447–8.

Torres WE, Clements JL, Austin GE, et al. Cricopharyngeal muscle hypertrophy: radiologic anatomic correlation. AJR 1984;141:927–30.

Yoslow W, Becker MH, Bartels J, et al. Orthopedic defects in familial dysautonomia: a review of sixty-five cases. J Bone Joint Surg Am 1971;53:1541–50.

Achalasia

Agha FP, Lee HH. The esophagus after endoscopic pneumatic balloon dilatation for achalasia. AJR 1986;146:25–9.

Ambrosino MM, Genieser NB, Banguru BS, et al. The syndrome of achalasia of the esopahgus, ACTH insensitivity and alacrima. Pediatr Radiol 1986;16:328–9.

Asch MJ, Liebman W, Lachman RS, et al. Esophageal achalasia: diagnosis and cardiomyotomy in a newborn infant. J Pediatr Surg 1974;9:911–2.

Carter R, Brewer LA. Achalasia and esophageal carcinoma—studies in early diagnosis for improved surgical management. Am J Surg 1975;130:114–20.

Dodds WJ, Stewart ET, Kistik SM, et al. Radiologic amyl nitrite test for distinguishing pseudoachalasia from idiopathic achalasia. AJR 1986;146:21–3.

House AJS, Griffiths GJ. The significance of an air esophagram visualized on conventional chest radiographs. Clin Radiol 1977;28:301–5.

Magilner AD, Isard HJ. Achalasia of the esophagus in infancy. Radiology 1971;98:81–2.

Markowitz JF, Aronow E, Rausen AR, et al. Progressive esophageal dysfunction in chronic granulomatous disease. J Pediatr Gastroenterol Nutr 1982;1:145–9.

Moazam F, Rodgers BM. Infantile achalasia: brief clinical report. J Thorac Cardiovasc Surg 1976;72:809–12.

Moersch HJ. Cardiospasm in infancy and in childhood. Am J Dis Child 1929;38:294–8.

Muralidharan S, Jairaj PS, Periyanayagam WJ, et al. Achalasia cardia: a review of 100 cases. Aust N Z J Surg 1978;48:167–70.

Olsen AM, Holman CB, Anderson HA. Diagnosis of cardiospasm. Dis Chest 1953;23:447–97.

Ott DJ, Wu WC, Gelfand DW, et al. Radiographic evaluation of the achalasic esophagus immediately following pneumatic dilatation. Gastrointest Radiol 1984;9:185–91.

Sorsdahl OA, Gay BB. Achalasia of the esophagus in childhood. Am J Dis Child 1965;109:141–5.

Spence LD, Fitzgerald E. Case report: transabdominal ultrasound detection of achalasia. Clin Radiol 1996;51:297–8.

Starinsky R, Berlovitz I, Mares AJ, et al. Infantile achalasia. Pediatr Radiol 1984;14:113–5.

Stewart ET, Miller WN, Hogan WJ, et al. Desirability of roentgen esophageal examination immediately after pneumatic dilatation for achalasia. Radiology 1979;130:589–91.

Tasker AD. Achalasia: an unusual cause of stridor. Clin Radiol 1995;50:496–8.

Tuck JS, Bisset RAL, Doig CM. Achalasia of the cardia in childhood and the syndrome of achalasia alacrima and ACTH insensitivity. Clin Radiol 1991;44:260–4.

Vaughan WH, Williams JL. Familial achalasia with pulmonary complications in children. Radiology 1973;107:407–9.

Westley CR, Herbst JJ, Goldman S, et al. Infantile achalasia: inherited as an autosomal recessive disorder. J Pediatr 1975;87:243–6.

Willich E. Achalasia of the cardia in children: manometric, cinematographic and pharmacoradiographic studies. Pediatr Radiol 1973;1:229–36.

Zegel HG, Kressel HY, Levine GM, et al. Delayed esophageal perforation after pneumatic dilatation for the treatment of achalasia. Gastrointest Radiol 1979;4:219–21.

Ziegler K, Sanft C, Friedrich M, et al. Endosonographic appearances of the esophagus in achalasia. Endoscopy 1990;22:1–4.

Branchial Arch and Pouch Remnants

Fourman P, Fourman J. Hereditary deafness in a family with ear pits. Br J Med 1955;2:1354–6.

Fowler WG. Lateral pharyngeal diverticula. Ann Surg 1962;155:161–6.

Gray SW, Skandalakis JE. Embryology for surgeons: the embryological basis for the treatment of congenital defects. Philadelphia: WB Saunders; 1972. p. 39–40.

Harnsberger HR, Mancuso AA, Maraki AS, et al. Branchial cleft anomalies and their mimics: computed tomographic evaluation. Radiology 1984;152:739–48.

Herman TE, McAlister WH, Siegal MJ. Brachial fistula: CT manifestations. Pediatr Radiol 1992;22:152–3.

Hewel K, Kioumehr F, Wang M. Infected third branchial cleft cyst: retropharyngeal extension to the superior mediastinum. J Can Assoc Radiol 1995;47:111–3.

Maran AG, Buchanan PR. Branchial cysts, sinuses and fistulae. Clin Otolaryngol 1978;3:77–92.

Murdoch MJ, Culham JAG, Stringer DA. Pediatric case of the day: infected third branchial cleft cyst. Radiographics 1995;15:1027–30.

Neal HB, Pemberton J. Lateral cervical (branchial) cysts and fistulas; a clinical and pathological study. Surgery 1945;18:267–86.

Salazar JE, Duke RA, Ellis JV. Second branchial cleft cyst: unusual location and a new CT diagnostic sign. AJR 1985;145:965–6.

Tucker HM, Skolnick ML. Fourth branchial cleft (pharyngeal pouch) remnant. Trans Am Acad Opthalmol Otolaryngol 1973;77(1):368–71.

Esophageal Atresia and Tracheoesophageal Fistula

Ahmed S. Infantile pyloric stenosis associated with major anomalies of the alimentary tract. J Pediatr Surg 1970;5:660–6.

Amoury RA, Hrabovsky EE, Leonidas JD, et al. Tracheoesophageal fistula after lye ingestion. J Pediatr Surg 1975;10:273–6.

Azar H, Chrispin AR, Waterston DJ. Esophageal replacement with transverse colon (in) infants and children. J Pediatr Surg 1971;6:3–9.

Barnes JC, Smith WL. The VATER association. Radiology 1978;126:445–9.

Barry JE, Auldist AW. The Vater association: one end of a spectrum of anomalies. Am J Dis Child 1974;128:769–71.

Beardmore H, Touloukian R. [discussion]. J Pediatr Surg 1973;8:645.

Benson JE, Olsen MM, Fletcher BD. A spectrum of bronchopulmonary anomalies associated with tracheoesophageal malformations. Pediatr Radiol 1985;15:377–80.

Berdon WE, Baker DH. Radiographic findings in esophageal atresia with proximal pouch fistula (type B). Pediatr Radiol 1975;3:70–4.

Black PR, Welch KJ. Pulmonary agenesis (aplasia), esophageal atresia, and tracheoesophageal fistula: a different treatment strategy. J Pediatr Surg 1986;21:936–8.

Blank RH, Prillaman PR, Minor GR. Congenital esophageal atresia with tracheoesophageal fistula occurring in identical twins. J Thorac Cardiovasc Surg 1967;53:192–6.

Chrispin AR, Friedland GW, Waterston DJ. Aspiration pneumonia and dysphagia after technically successful repair of esophageal atresia. Thorax 1966;21:104–10.

Christensen LR, Shapir J. Radiology of colonic interposition and its associated complications. Gastrointest Radiol 1986;11:233–40.

Claiborne AK, Blocker SH, Martin CM, et al. Prenatal and postnatal sonographic delineation of gastrointestinal abnormalities in a case of the VATER syndrome. J Ultrasound Med 1986;5:45–7.

Daum R. Postoperative complications following operation for esophageal atresia and tracheoesophageal fistula. In: Rickman PP, Hecker WC, Prevot J, editors. Progress in pediatric surgery. Baltimore: University Park; 1971. p. 209–37.

Day DL. Aortic arch in neonates with esophageal atresia: preoperative assessment using CT. Radiology 1985;155:99–100.

Doi O, Aoyama K, Mori S, et al. A case of epidermolysis bullosa dystrophicans with congenital esophageal atresia. J Pediatr Surg 1986;21:943–5.

Eckstein HB, Aberdeen E, Chrispin A, et al. Tracheoesophageal fistula without esophageal atresia. Z Kinderchir 1970;9:43–9.

Eckstein HB, Somasundaram K. Multiple tracheoesophageal fistulas with atresia. J Pediatr Surg 1966;1:381–3.

Ein SH, Friedberg J. Esophageal atresia and tracheoesophageal fistula: review and update. Otolaryngol Clin North Am 1981;14:219–49.

Ein SH, Shandling B, Simpson JS, et al. A further look at the gastric tube as an esophageal replacement in infants and children. J Pediatr Surg 1973;8:859–67.

Ein SH, Shandling B, Simpson JS, et al. Fourteen years of gastric tubes. J Pediatr Surg 1978;13:638–42.

Ein SH, Stringer DA, Stephens CA, et al. Recurrent tracheoesophageal fistula—a 17 year review. J Pediatr Surg 1983;18:436–41.

Ein SH, Theman TE. A comparison of the results of primary repair of esophageal atresia with tracheoesophageal fistulas using end to side and end to end anastomoses. J Pediatr Surg 1973;8:641–4.

Engel PhMA, Vos LJM, de Vries JA, et al. Esophageal atresia with tracheoesophageal fistula in mother and child. J Pediatr Surg 1970;5:564–5.

Falletta GP. Recommunication on repair of congenital tracheoesophageal fistula. Arch Surg 1964;88:779–86.

Farrant P. The antenatal diagnosis of esophageal atresia by ultrasound. Br J Radiol 1980;53:1202–3.

Filler RM, Roselle PJ, Lebowitz RL. Life-threatening anoxic spells caused by tracheal compression after repair of esophageal atresia: correction by surgery. J Pediatr Surg 1976;11:739–48.

Filston HC, Rankin JS, Kirks DR. The diagnosis of primary and recurrent tracheoesophageal fistulas: value of selective catheterization. J Pediatr Surg 1982;17:144–8.

Fox PF. Unusual esophageal atresia with tracheoesophageal fistula. J Pediatr Surg 1978;13:373.

Gilsanz V, Boechat IM, Birnberg FA, et al. Scoliosis after thoracotomy for esophageal atresia. AJR 1983;141:457–60.

Goodwin CD, Ashcraft KW, Holder TM, et al. Esophageal atresia with double tracheoesophageal fistula. J Pediatr Surg 1978;13:269–73.

Harrison MR, Hanson BA, Mahour GH, et al. The significance of the right aortic arch in repair of esophageal atresia and tracheoesophageal fistula. J Pediatr Surg 1977;12: 861–9.

Hays DM, Wooller MM, Snyder WH. Esophageal atresia and tracheoesophageal fistula: management of the uncommon types. J Pediatr Surg 1966;1:240–5l.

Helmsworth JA, Pryles CV. Congenital tracheoesophageal fistula without esophageal atresia. J Pediatr 1951;38:610–7.

Hodson CJ, Shaw DG. Congenital atresia of the esophagus and thirteen pairs of ribs. Pediatr Radiol 1973;1:248–9.

Howard R, Myers NA. Esophageal atresia: a technique for elongating the upper pouch. Surgery 1965;58:725–7.

Ingalls TH, Prindle RA. Esophageal atresia with tracheoesophageal fistula. Epidemiologic and teratologic implications. N Engl J Med 1949;240:987–95.

Janik JS, Filler RM, Ein SH, et al. Long-term follow-up of circular myotomy for esophageal atresia. J Pediatr Surg 1980;15:835–41.

Johnson JF, Sneoka BL, Mulligan ME, et al. Tracheoesophageal fistula: diagnosis with CT. Pediatr Radiol 1985;15:134–5.

Jona JZ, Belin RP. Intramural tracheoesophageal fistula associated with esophageal web. J Pediatr Surg 1977;12: 227–32.

Kafrouni G, Baick CH, Woolley MM. Recurrent tracheoesophageal fistula: a diagnostic problem. Surgery 1970;68: 889–94.

Kirks DR, Briley CA, Currarino G. Selective catheterization of tracheoesophageal fistula. AJR 1979;133:763–4.

Kiser JC, Peterson TA, Johnson FE. Chronic recurrent tracheoesophageal fistula. Chest 1972;62:222–4.

Laks H, Wilkinson RH, Schuster SR. Long-term results following correction of esophageal atresia with tracheoesophageal fistula: a clinical and cinefluorographic study. J Pediatr Surg 1972;7:591–7.

Lindham S, Lohr G, Sylven M. Hemorrhagic right upper lobe infarction as a complication in primary end-to-end anastomosis of esophageal atresia. Pediatr Radiol 1979;8: 183–4.

Mackenzie M. Malformations of esophagus. Arch Laryngol 1980;1:301–15.

Marshall DG, Reid WD, Armstrong R. A case of single pleural cavity with esophageal atresia and tracheoesophageal fistula. J Pediatr Surg 1986;21:939–40.

McCook TA, Felman AH. Esophageal atresia, duodenal atresia, and gastric distension: report of two cases. AJR 1978;131:167–8.

Nakazato Y, Landing BH, Wells TR. Abnormal Auerbach plexus in the esophagus and stomach of patients with esopahgeal atresia and tracheoesophageal fistula. J Pediatr Surg 1986;21:831–7.

Nakazato Y, Wells TR, Landing BH. Abnormal tracheal innervation in patients wtih esophageal atresia and tracheoesopahgeal fistula: study of the intrinsic tracheal nerve plexuses by a microdissection technique. J Pediatr Surg 1986;21:838–44.

Ohkuma R. Congenital esophageal atresia with tracheoesophageal fistula in identical twins. J Pediatr Surg 1978; 13:361–2.

Pretorius DH, Drose JA, Dennis MA, et al. Tracheoesophageal fistula in utero: twenty-two cases. J Ultrasound Med 1987;6:509–13.

Puri P, Blake N, O'Donnell B, et al. Delayed primary anastomosis following spontaneous growth of esophageal segments in esophageal atresia. J Pediatr Surg 1981;16:180–3.

Quan L, Smith DW. The VATER association: vertebral defects, anal atresia, tracheoesophageal fistula with esophageal atresia, radial dysplasia. Birth Defects 1972;8:75–8.

Quan L, Smith DW. The VATER association: vertebral defects, anal atresia, tracheoesophageal fistula with esophageal atresia, radial and renal dysplasia: a spectrum of associated defects. J Pediatr 1973;82:104–7.

Rahbar A, Farha SJ. Acquired tracheoesophageal fistula. J Pediatr Surg 1978;13:375–6.

Rao SB, Slovis TL, Cradock TV, et al. Visualization of the intestinal tract by amniography in a fetus with esophageal atresia. Pediatr Radiol 1978;7:241–2.

Schneider KM, Becker JM. The "H type" tracheoesophageal fistula in infants and children. Surgery 1962;51:677–86.

Shapiro RN, Eddy W, Fitzgibbon J, et al. The incidence of congenital anomalies discovered in the neonatal period. Am J Surg 1958;96:396–400.

Slim MS, Tabry IF. Left extrapleural approach for the repair of recurrent tracheoesophageal fistula. J Thorac Cardiovasc Surg 1974;68:654–7.

Smith WL, Franken EA Jr, Smith JA. Pneumoesophagus as a sign of H-type tracheoesophageal fistula. Pediatrics 1976;58:907–9.

Stanford W, Armstrong RG, Cline RE, et al. Recurrent tracheoesophageal fistula. Ann Surg 1973;15:452–5.

Stringer DA, Ein SH. Recurrent tracheo-esophageal fistula: a protocol for investigation. Radiology 1984;151:637–41.

Stringer DA, Pablot SM. Bronchogastric tube fistulas as a complication of esophageal replacement. J Can Assoc Radiol 1985;36:61–2.

Stringer DA, Pablot SM, Mancer K. Gruentzig angioplasty dilatation of an esophageal stricture in an infant. Pediatr Radiol 1985;15:424–6.

Sundar B, Guiney EJ, O'Donnell B. Congenital H-type tracheoesophageal fistula. Arch Dis Child 1975;50:862–3.

Taybi H. Radiology of syndromes and metabolic disorders. 2nd ed. Chicago: Year Book; 1982. p. 405.

Thomas PS, Chrispin AR. Congenital tracheo-esophageal fistula without esophageal atresia. Clin Radiol 1969;20:371–4.

Thomason MA, Gay BB. Esophageal stenosis with esophageal atresia. Pediatr Radiol 1987;17:197–201.

Vizas D, Ein SH, Simpson JS. The value of circular myotomy for esophageal atresia. J Pediatr Surg 1978;13:357–9.

Wesselhoeft CW, Keshishian JH. Acquired non-malignant esophagotracheal and esophagobronchial fistulas. Ann Thorac Surg 1968;6:187–95.

Winslow PR, Bryant LR, Hasbrouck JD. Cystoscope endoscopy in the "H-type" tracheoesophageal fistula. Arch Surg 1966;93:520–2.

Wychulis AR, Ellis FH, Anderson HA. Acquired non-malignant esophagotracheobronchial fistula. Report of 36 cases. JAMA 1966;196:103–8.

Rare Anomalies of Tracheal and Esophageal Separation

Blumberg JB, Stevenson JK, Lemire RJ, et al. Laryngotracheoesophageal cleft, the embryological implications, review of literature. Surgery 1965;57:559–66.

Burroughs N, Leape LL. Laryngotracheoesophageal cleft: report of a case successfully treated and review of the literature. Pediatrics 1974;53:516–22.

Felman AH, Talbert JL. Laryngotracheoesophageal cleft. Radiology 1972;103:641–4.

Graves VB, Dahl DD, Power HW. Congenital bronchopulmonary foregut malformation with anomalous pulmonary artery. Radiology 1975;114:423–4.

Griscom NT. Persistent esophagotrachea: the most severe degree of laryngotracheo-esophageal cleft. AJR 1966;97:211–5.

Leithiser RE, Capitanio MA, MacPherson RI, et al. "Communicating" bronchopulmonary foregut malformations. AJR 1986;146:227–31.

Morgan CL, Grossman H, Leonidas J. Roentgenographic findings in a spectrum of uncommon tracheoesophageal anomalies. Clin Radiol 1979;30:353–8.

Reilly BJ, McDonald P, Cumming WA, et al. Three cases of congenital bronchopulmonary foregut malformation. Ann Radiol 1973;16:281–5.

Stanley P, Vachon L, Gilsanz V. Pulmonary sequestration with congenital gastroesophageal communication. Pediatr Radiol 1985;15:343–5.

Cysts and Duplications of the Foregut

Amendola MA, Shirazi KK, Brooks J, et al. Transdiaphragmatic bronchopulmonary foregut anomaly: "dumbbell" bronchogenic cyst. AJR 1982;138:1165–7.

Beardmore HE, Wiglesworth FW. Vertebral anomalies and alimentary duplications: clinical and embryological aspects. Pediatr Clin North Am 1958;5:457–74.

Boivin Y, Cholette JP, Lefebrve R. Accessory esophagus complicated by an adenocarcinoma. J Can Med Assoc 1964;90:1414–7.

Chang SH, Morrison L, Shaffner L, et al. Intrathoracic gastrogenic cysts and hemoptysis. J Pediatr 1976;88:594–6.

Fallon M, Gordon ARG, Lendrum AC. Mediastinal cysts of foregut origin associated with vertebral abnormalities. Br J Surg 1954;41:520–33.

Filler RM, Simpson JS, Ein SH. Mediastinal masses in infants and children. Pediatr Clin North Am 1979;26:677–90.

Fitch SJ, Tonkin ILD, Tonkin AK. Imaging of foregut duplication cysts. Radiographics 1986;6:189–201.

Gans SL, Lackey DA, Zuckerbraun L. Duplications of the cervical esophagus in infants and children. Surgery 1968;63:849–52.

Gray SW, Skandalakis JE. Embryology for surgeons: the embryological basis for the treatment of congenital defects. Philadelphia: WB Saunders; 1972. p. 80–5, 311–14.

Gross RE, Neuhauser EBD, Longino LA. Thoracic diverticula which originate from the intestine. Ann Surg 1950;131:363–75.

Helund GL, Bisset GS III. Esophageal duplication cyst and aberrant right subclavian artery mimicking a symptomatic vascular ring. Pediatr Radiol 1989;19:543–4.

Kassner EG, Rosen Y, Klotz DH. Mediastinal esophageal duplication cyst associated with a partial pericardial defect. Pediatr Radiol 1975;4:53–6.

Kirks DR, Filston HC. The association of esophageal duplication cyst with esophageal atresia. Pediatr Radiol 1981;11:214–6.

Kuhlman JE, Fishman EK, Wang K-P, et al. Esophageal duplication cyst: CT and transesophageal needle aspiration. AJR 1985;145:531–2.

Kuhlman JE, Fishman EK, Wang KP, et al. Mediastinal cysts: diagnosis by CT and needle aspiration. AJR 1988;150:75–8.

Martin KW, Siegel MJ, Chesna E. Spontaneous resolution of mediastinal cysts. AJR 1988;150: 1131–2.

Mindelyun R, Long P. Mediastinal bronchogenic cyst with esophageal communication. Radiology 1978;126:28.

Moir JD. Combined duplication of the esophagus and stomach. J Can Assoc Radiol 1970;21:257–62.

Pan G, Singleton E, Nihill M, Harberg F. A case of bilateral gastric bronchopulmonary-foregut malformation. Pediatr Radiol 1989;19:463–4.

Piramoon AM, Abbassioun K. Mediastinal enterogenic cyst with spinal cord compression. J Pediatr Surg 1974; 9:543–5.

Stringel G, Mercer S, Biggs V. Esophageal duplication cyst containing a foreign body. J Can Med Assoc 1985;132: 529–31.

Superina RA, Ein SH, Humphreys RP. Cystic duplications of the esophagus and neurenteric cysts. J Pediatr Surg 1984;19:527–30.

van Beers B, Trigaux J, Weynants P, et al. Foregut cyst of the mediastinum: fluid re-accumulation after transbronchial needle aspiration. Br J Radiol 1989;62:558–60.

Ware GW, Conrad HA. Thoracic duplication of alimentary tract. Am J Surg 1953;86:264–71.

Vascular Anomalies

Ablin DS, Newell JD, Davis M. Esophageal vascular impression in total anomalous pulmonary venous return below the diaphragm. Pediatr Radiol 1989;19:454–5.

Beaubout JW, Stewart JR, Kincaid OW. Aberrant right subclavian artery: dispute of commonly accepted concepts. AJR 1964;92:855–64.

Berdon WE, Baker DH. Vascular anomalies and the infant lung: rings, slings and other things. Semin Roentgenol 1972;7:39–64.

Berdon WE, Baker DH, Bordiuk J, et al. Innominate artery compression of the trachea in infants with stridor and apnea: method of roentgen diagnosis and criteria for surgical treatment. Radiology 1969;92:272–8.

Berdon WE, Baker DH, Wung J-T, et al. Complete cartilage—ring tracheal stenosis associated with anomalous left pulmonary artery: the ring-sling complex. Radiology 1984;152:57–64.

Bisset GS III, Strife JL, Kirks DR, Bailey WW. Vascular rings: MR imaging. AJR 1987;149:251–6.

Capitanio MA, Ramos R, Kirkpatrick JA. Pulmonary sling: roentgen observations. AJR 1971;112:28–34.

Castenada-Zuniga WR, Amplatz K, Edwards JE. Anterior vascular indentation of the oesophagus. Br J Radiol 1978; 51:633–5.

Deanfield JE, Chrispin AR. The investigation of chest disease in children by high kilovoltage filtered beam radiography. Br J Radiol 1981;54:856–60.

Deanfield JE, Leanage R, Stroobant J, et al. The use of high kilovoltage filtered beam radiographs for the detection of bronchial situs in infants and children. Br Heart J 1980;44:577–83.

Dunbar JS. Upper respiratory tract obstruction in infants and children. AJR 1970;109:227–46.

Fearon B, Shortreed R. Tracheobronchial compression by cardiovascular anomalies in children: syndrome of apnoea. Ann Otol Rhinol Laryngol 1963;72:949–69.

Gray SW, Skandalakis JE. Embryology for surgeons: the embryological basis for the treatment of congenital defects. Philadelphia: WB Saunders; 1972. p. 340–1.

Gross RE, Neuhauser EBD. Compression of the trachea by an anomalous innominate artery: an operation for its relief. Am J Dis Child 1948;75:570–4.

Han BK, Dunbar JS, Bove K, et al. Pulmonary vascular sling with tracheobronchial stenosis and hypoplasia of the right pulmonary artery. Pediatr Radiol 1980;9:113–5.

Kleinman PK, Spevak MR, Nimkin K. Left-sided esophageal indentation in right aortic arch with aberrant left subclavian artery. Radiology 1994;191:565–7.

Klinkhamer AC. Esophagography in anomalies of the aortic arch system. Baltimore: Williams & Wilkins; 1969. p. 1–126.

Moes CAF, Izukawa T, Trusler GA. Innominate artery compression of the trachea. Arch Otolaryngol 1975;101:733–8.

Montgomery DP, Partridge JB. Vascular rings causing pulmonary collapse. Clin Radiol 1981;32:277–80.

Neuhauser EBD. The roentgen diagnosis of double aortic arch and other anomalies of the great vessels. AJR 1946;56:1–12.

Neuhauser EBD. Tracheo-esophageal constriction produced by right aortic arch and left ligamentum arteriosum. AJR 1949;62:493–9.

Pirtle T, Clarke E. Vascular ring: unusual cause of unilateral obstructive pulmonary hyperinflation. AJR Am J Roentgenol 1983;140:1111–2.

Strife JL, Matsumoto J, Bisset GS III, Martin R. The position of the trachea in infants and children with right aortic arch. Pediatr Radiol 1989;19:226–9.

Tonkin ILD, Gold RE, Moser D, et al. Evaluation of vascular rings with digital subtraction angiography. AJR 1984;142:1287–91.

Wolf EL, Berdon WE, Baker DH. Improved plain film diagnosis of the right aortic arch and anomalies with high kilovoltage selective filtration magnification technique. Pediatr Radiol 1978;7:141–6.

Congenital Stenosis of the Esophagus

Anderson LS, Shackleford GD, Mancilla-Jimenez R, et al. Cartilaginous esophageal ring: a cause of esophageal stenosis in infants and children. Radiology 1973;108:665–6.

Dominguez R, Zarabi M, Oh KS, et al. Congenital oesophageal stenosis. Clin Radiol 1985;36:263–6.

Gross RE. Esophageal stenosis or stricture. The surgery of infancy and childhood. WB Saunders: Philadelphia; 1964. p. 103–13.

Jewsbury P. An unusual case of congenital esophageal stricture. Br J Surg 1971;58:475–6.

Mortensson W. Congenital esophageal stenosis distal to esophageal atresia. Pediatr Radiol 1975;3:149–51.

Stringer DA, Pablot SM, Mancer K. Gruentzig angioplasty dilatation of an esophageal stricture in an infant. Pediatr Radiol 1985;15:424–6.

Takayanagi K, Li K, Komi N. Congenital esophageal stenosis with lack of submucosa. J Pediatr Surg 1975;10: 425–6.

Retropharyngeal Abscess

Andrew WK. The soft tissue sign: a new parameter in the diagnosis of the fractures of the base of the skull. Clin Radiol 1978;29:442–3.

Grunebaum M, Moskowitz G. The retropharyngeal soft tissues in young infants with hypothyroidism. AJR 1970;108:543–5.

Harner SG. Peritonsillar, peripharyngeal and deep neck abscesses. Postgrad Med 1975;57:147–9.

Markowitz RI. Retropharyngeal bleeding in haemophilia. B J Radiol 1981;54:521–3.

Ramilo J, Harris VJ, White H. Empyema as a complication

of retropharyngeal and neck abscesses in children. Radiology 1978;126:743–6.

Esophagitis

Al-Katoubi MA, Eliot C. Oesophageal involvement in benign mucous membrane pemphigoid. Clin Radiol 1984;35:131–5.

Alford BR, Harris HH. Chemical burns of the mouth, pharynx and esophagus. Ann Otol Rhinol Laryngol 1959; 68:122–8.

Amoury RA, Hrabovsky EE, Leonidas JC, et al. Tracheo-esophageal fistula after lye ingestion. J Pediatr Surg 1975; 10:273–6.

Balthazar EJ, Mcgibow AJ, Hulnick DH. Cytomegalovirus esophagitis and gastritis in AIDS. AJR 1985;144:1201–4.

Becker MH, Swinyard LA. Epidermolysis bullosa dystrophica in children: radiologic manifestations. Radiology 1968;90:124–8.

Burkhart CG, Ruppert ES. Dystrophic epidermolysis bullosa. Clin Pediatr (Phila) 1981;20:493–6.

Cockey BM, Jones B, Bayless TM, et al. Filiform polyps of the esophagus with inflammatory bowel disease. AJR 1985;144:1207–8.

Creteur V, Laufer I, Kressel HY, et al. Drug induced esophagitis detected by double-contrast radiography. Radiology 1983;147:365–8.

Daly JF. Corrosive esophagitis. Otolaryngol Clin North Am 1968;1:119–31.

Daunt N, Brodribb TR, Dickey JD. Oesophageal ulceration due to doxycycline. Br J Radiol 1985;58:1209–11.

DeGaeta L, Levine MS, Guglielmi GE, et al. Herpes esophagitis in an otherwise healthy patient. AJR 1985;144:1205–6.

Dobbins JW, Sheaham DG, Behar J. Eosinophilic gastroenteritis with esophageal involvement. Gastroenterol 1977;72:1312–16.

DuPree E, Hodges F Jr, Simon JL. Epidermolysis bullosa of the esophagus. Am J Dis Child 1969;117:349–51.

Feczko PJ, Halpert RD, Zonca M. Radiographic abnormalities in eosinophilic esophagitis. Gastrointest Radiol 1985;10:321–4.

Francis RS. Lipoid proteinosis. Radiology 1975;117:301–2.

Franken EA Jr. Caustic damage of the gastrointestinal tract: roentgen features. AJR 1973;118:77–85.

Franken EA Jr, Smith WC, editors. Gastrointestinal imaging in pediatrics. 2nd ed. Philadelphia: Harper & Row; 1982. p. 68–9, 74–5.

Guyer PB, Rooke HWP. Candidiasis of the esophagus. Br J Radiol 1971;44:131–6.

Hamilton R, Mellow M, Braun NMT, et al. Esophageal tuberculosis presenting with dysphagia. J Pediatr 1977;91:678–9.

Herman TE, Kushner DC, Cleveland RH. Esophageal stricture secondary to drug-induced tonic epidermal necrolysis. Pediatr Radiol 1984;14:439–40.

Hillemcier C, Touloukian R, McCallum R, Grybowski J. Esophageal web: a previously unrecognized complication of epidermolysis bullosa dystrophica. Pediatrics 1981;67:678–82.

Itai Y, Kogure T, Okuyama Y. Radiological manifestations of esophageal involvement in acanthosis nigricans. Br J Radiol 1976;49:592–3.

Johnston DE, Koehler RE, Balfe DM. Clinical manifestations of epidermolysis bullosa dystrophica. Dig Dis Sci 1981;26:144–9.

Kabakian HA, Dahmash NS. Pharyngoesophageal manifestations of epidermolysis bullosa. Clin Radiol 1978;29:91–2.

Karasick S, Lev-Toaff AS. Esophageal strictures: findings on barium radiographs. Pictorial essay. AJR 1995:165:561–5.

Katz J, Gryboski JD, Rosenbaum HM, et al. Dysphagia in children with epidermolysis bullosa. Gastroenterology 1967;52:259–62.

Kinnman J, Shin HI, Wetteland P. Carcinoma of the oesophagus after lye corrosion in a 15-year old. Acta Chir Scand 1968;134:489–93.

Landres RT, Kuster GGR, Strum WB. Eosinophilic esophagitis in a patient with vigorous achalasia. Gastroenterology 1978;74:1298–1301.

Lepke RA, Libshitz HI. Radiation-induced injury of the esophagus. Radiology 1983;148:375–8.

Levine MS, Laufer I, Kressel HY, et al. Herpes esophagitis. AJR 1981;136:863–6.

Levine MS, Macones AJ, Laufer I. Candida esophagitis: accuracy of radiographic diagnosis. Radiology 1985;154: 581–7.

Levine MS. Radiology of esophagitis: a pattern approach. Radiology 1991:179:1–7.

Matzinger MA, Daneman A. Esophageal involvement in eosinophilic gastroenteritis. Pediatr Radiol 1983;13:35–8.

McDonald GB, Sullivan KM, Plumley TF. Radiographic features of esophageal involvement in chronic graft-vs-host disease. AJR 1984;142:501–6.

Middlekamp JN, Ferguson TB, Roper CL, et al. The management and problems of caustic burns in children. J Thorac Cardiovasc Surg 1969;57:341–7.

Nelson WE. Textbook of pediatrics. 12th ed. Philadelphia: WB Saunders; 1983. p. 897–9.

Picus D, Frank PH. Eosinophilic esophagitis. AJR 1981;136:1001–3.

Reeder JD. Transverse esophageal folds: association with corrosive injury. Radiology 1985;155:303–4.

Rohrman CA, Kidd R. Chronic mucocutaneous candidiasis: radiologic abnormalities in the esophagus. AJR 1978;130:473–6.

Schuman BM, Arciniegas E. The management of esophageal complications of epidermolysis bullosa. Dig Dis Sci 1972;17:875–80.

Shackleford GD, Bauer EA, Graviss ER, et al. Upper airway and external genital involvement in epidermolysis bullosa dystrophica. Radiology 1982;143:429–32.

Shortsleeve MJ, Levine MS. Herpes esophagitis in otherwise healthy patients: clinical and radiographic findings. Radiology 1992;182:859–61.

Simeone JF, Burrell M, Toffler R, et al. Aperistalsis and esophagitis. Radiology 1977;123:9–14.

Thiers BH. The mechanobullous disease. Hereditary epidermolysis bullosa and epidermolysis bullosa acquisita. J Am Acad Dermatol 1981;5:745–8.

Thompson JW, Ahmed AR, Dudley JP. Epidermolysis bullosa dystrophica of the larynx and trachea. Acute airway obstruction. Ann Otol Rhinol Laryngol 1980;89:428–9.

Tischler JM, Han SY, Helman CA. Esophageal involvement in epidermolysis bullosa dystrophica. AJR 1983;141:1283–6.

Tishler JMA, Helman CA. Crohn's disease of the esophagus. J Can Assoc Radiol 1984;35:28–30.

Tu RK, Peters ME, Gourley GR, Hong R. Esophageal histoplasmosis in a child with immunodeficiency with hyper-IgM. AJR 1991;157:381–2.

Vlymen WJ, Muskowitz PS. Roentgenographic manifestations of esophageal and intestinal involvement in Behçet's disease in children. Pediatr Radiol 1981;10:193–6.

Neoplasms of the Esophagus

Dieter RA, Holinger PH, Maurizi DG. Angiofibromatous polyp of the pharynx. Am J Dis Child 1970;119:91–3.

Dieter RA, Riker WL, Holinger PH. Pedunculated esophageal hamartoma in a child—a case report. J Thorac Cardiovasc Surg 1970;59:851–4.

Govoni AF. Hemangiomas of the esophagus. Gastrointest Radiol 1982;7;113–7.

Kinnman J, Shin HI, Wetteland P. Carcinoma of the esophagus after lye corrosion: report of a case in a 15-year-old Korean male. Acta Chir Scand 1968;134:489–93.

Levine MS, Buck JL, Pantongrag-Brown L, et al. Esophageal leiomyomatosis. Radiology 1996;199:533–6.

Mandell GA, Lantieri R, Goodman LR. Tracheobronchial compression in Hodgkin lymphoma in children. AJR 1982;139:1167–70.

Moore C. Visceral squamous cancer in children. Pediatrics 1958;21:573–81.

Schmidt A, Lockwood K. Benign neoplasms of the esophagus. Acta Chir Scand 1967;133:640–4.

Styles RA, Gibb SP, Tarshis A, et al. Esophagogastric polyps: radiographic and endoscopic findings. Radiology 1985;154:307–11.

Wesenberg RL. Evaluation of an esophageal infantile hemangioma using ultra-low-dose real-time fluoroscopy. General Electric X-Ray Clinical Symposium, Milwaukee, 1982(2):1.

Swallowed Foreign Body

Baraka A, Bikhazi G. Oesophageal foreign bodies. BMJ 1975;1:561–3.

Beer S, Avidan G, Viure E, et al. A foreign body in the esophagus as a cause of respiratory distress. Pediatr Radiol 1982;12:41–2.

Bowen A, Dominguez R. Swallowed neonatal endotracheal tube. Pediatr Radiol 1981;10:178–9.

Burrington JD. Aluminum "pop tops": a hazard to child health. JAMA 1976;235:2614–17.

Campbell DR, Brown B. St John, Manchester JS. An evaluation of the radiopacity of various ingested foreign bodies in the pharynx and esophagus. J Can Assoc Radiol 1968;19: 183–6.

Campbell JB, Condon VR. Catheter removal of blunt esophageal foreign bodies in children: survey of the Society for Pediatric Radiology. Presentation at the 28th Annual Meeting of the Society of Pediatric Radiology; 1985; Boston.

Campbell JB, Davis WS. Catheter technique for extraction of blunt esophageal foreign bodies. Radiology 1973;108:438–40.

Carlson DH. Removal of coins in the esophagus using a Foley catheter. Pediatrics 1972;50:475–6.

Eggli KD, Potter BM, Garcia V, et al. Delayed diagnosis of esophageal perforation by aluminum foreign bodies. Pediatr Radiol 1986;16:511–3.

Ell SR, Sprigg A. The radio-opacity of fishbones—species variation. Clin Radiol 1991;44:104–7.

Franken EA Jr, Smith WC, editors. Gastrointestinal imaging in pediatrics. 2nd ed. Philadelphia: Harper & Row; 1982. p. 69.

Jewsbury P. An unusual case of congenital oesophageal stricture. Br J Surg 1971;58:475–6.

Lederman H, Towbin R, Ball WS, et al. Esophageal edema as a predictor of unsuccessful balloon extraction of esophageal foreign bodies. Presentation at the 28th Annual Meeting of the Society for Pediatric Radiologists; 1985; Boston.

Levick RK, Spitz L. The "invisible" can top. Br J Radiol 1977;50:594–6.

Macpherson RI, Hill JG, Othersen HB, et al. Esophageal foreign bodies in children: diagnosis, treatment and complications. AJR 1996;166:919–24.

Mohammed SH, Hegedus V. Dislodgement of impacted oesophageal foreign bodies with carbonated beverages. Clin Radiol 1986;37:589–92.

Nandi P, Ong GB. Foreign body in the oesophagus: Review of 2394 cases. Br J Surg 1978;65:5–9.

Newman DE. The radiolucent esophageal foreign body: an often forgotten cause of respiratory symptoms. J Pediatr 1978;92:60–3.

Nixon GW. Foley catheter method of esophageal foreign body removal: extension of applications. AJR 1979; 132:441–2.

O'Connor JF, Layton RG, Feins NR. Peroral removal of a sewing needle and attached thread from the esophagus in an infant. Pediatr Radiol 1977;5:236–8.

Paulson EK, Jaffe RB. Metallic foreign bodies in the stom-ach: fluoroscopic removal with a magnetic orogastric tube. Radiology 1990;174:191–4.

Rice BT, Spiegel PK, Dombrowski PJ. Acute esophageal food impaction treated by gas-forming agents. Radiology 1983;146:299–301.

Robbins MI, Shortsleeve MJ. Treatment of acute esophageal food impaction with glucagon, an effervescent agent and water. AJR 1994;162:325–8.

Shackleford GD, McAlister WH, Robertson CL. The use of a Foley catheter for removal of blunt esophageal foreign bodies from children. Radiology 1972;105:455–6.

Shaffer HA Jr, Alford BA, de Lange EE, et al. Basket extraction of esophageal foreign bodies. AJR 1986; 147:1010–3.

Tjhen KY, Schmaltz AA, Ibrahim Z, et al. Pneumopericardium as a complication of foreign body aspiration. Pediatr Radiol 1978;7:121–3.

Towbin RB, Dunbar JS, Rice S. Magnet catheter for removal of magnetic foreign bodies. AJR 1989; 154;149–50.

Towbin R, Lederman HM, Dunbar JS, et al. Esophageal edema as a predictor of unsuccessful balloon extraction of esophageal foreign body. Pediatr Radiol 1989; 19:359–60.

Trenkner SW, Maglinte DDT, Lehman GA, et al. Esophageal food impaction: treatment with glucagon. Radiology 1983;149:401–3.

Volle E, Hanel D, Beyer P, Kaufmann H. Ingested foreign bodies: removal by magnet. Radiology 1986;160:407–9.

Iatrogenic Perforation

Amodio JB, Berdon WE, Abramson SJ, et al. Retrocardiac pneumomediastinum in association with tracheal and esophageal perforation. Pediatr Radiol 1986;16:380–3.

Bradley JL, Han SY. Intramural hematoma (incomplete perforation) of the esophagus associated with esophageal dilatation. Radiology 1979;130:59–62.

Eklof O, Lohr G, Okmian L. Submucosal perforation of the esophagus in the neonate. Acta Radiol (Diagn) 1969; 8:187–92.

Faerber EN, Schwartz AM, Pinch LW, et al. Unusual manifestations of neonatal pharyngeal perforation. Clin Radiol 1980;31:581–5.

Grunebaum M, Horodniceanu C, Wilunsky E, et al. Iatrogenic transmural perforation of the oesophagus in the preterm infant. Clin Radiol 1980;31:257–61.

Han SY, McElvein RB, Aldrete JS, et al. Perforation of the esophagus: correlation of site and cause with plain film findings. AJR 1985;145:537–40.

Han SY, Tishler JM. Perforation of the abdominal segment of the esophagus. AJR 1984;143:751–4.

Kenigsberg K, Levenbrown J. Esophageal perforation secondary to gastrostomy tube placement. J Pediatr Surg 1986;21:946–7.

Lee SB, Kuhn JP. Esophageal perforation in the neonate. A review of the literature. Am J Dis Child 1976;130:325–9.

Parkin GJS. The radiology of perforated oesophagus. Clin Radiol 1973;24:324–32.

Sheffner SE, Gross BH, Birnberg FA, et al. Iatrogenic bronchopleural fistula caused by feeding tube insertion. J Can Assoc Radiol 1985;36:52–5.

Tucker AS, Soine L, Izant RJ. Gastrointestinal perforations in infancy, anatomic and etiologic gamuts. AJR 1975;123:755–63.

Touloukian RJ, Beardsley GP, Ablow RC, et al. Traumatic perforation of the pharynx in the newborn. Pediatrics 1977;59:1019–22.

Mallory-Weiss and Boerhaave's Syndromes

Aaronson IA, Cywes S, Louw JH. Spontaneous esophageal rupture in the newborn. J Pediatr Surg 1975;10:459–66.

Dubos JP, Bouchez MC, Kacet N, et al. Spontaneous rupture of the esophagus in the newborn. Pediatr Radiol 1986;16:317–9.

Harell GS, Friedland GW, Daily WJ, et al. Neonatal Boerhaave's syndrome. Radiology 1970;95:665–8.

Knauer CM. Mallory-Weiss syndrome. Gastroenterology 1976;71:5–8.

Woodruff WW, Merton DF, Kirks DR. Pneumomediastinum: an unusual complication of acute gastrointestinal disease. Pediatr Radiol 1985;15:196–8.

Miscellaneous Disorders of the Mouth, Pharynx, Esophagus, and Salivary Glands

Agha FP. The esophagus after endoscopic injection sclerotherapy: acute and chronic changes. Radiology 1984;153:37–42.

Balthazar EJ. Computed tomographic recognition of gastric varices. AJR 1984;142:1121–5.

Balthazar EJ, Naidich DP, Megibow AJ, Lefleur RS. CT evaluation of esophageal varices. AJR 1987;148:131–5.

Brady TM, Gross BH, Glazer GM, et al. Adrenal pseudomasses due to varices: angiographic-CT-MRI-pathologic correlations. AJR 1985;145:301–4.

Braun P, Nussle D, Roy CC, et al. Intramural diverticulosis of the esophagus in an eight year old boy. Pediatr Radiol 1978;6:235–7.

Brintnall ES, Kridelbaugh WW. Congenital diverticulum of the posterior hypopharynx simulating atresia of the esophagus. Ann Surg 1950;131:564–74.

Castillo S, Aburashed A, Kimmelman J, et al. Diffuse intramural esophageal pseudodiverticulosis. New cases and review. Gastroenterology 1977;72:541–5.

Cramer KR. Intramural diverticulosis of the esophagus. Br J Radiol 1972;45:857–9.

Crawford MD'A, Jacobs A, Murphy B, et al. Paterson-Kelly syndrome in adolescence: a report of five cases. BMJ 1965:1:693–5.

DeMarino GB, Sumkin JH, Leventhal R, Van Thiel DH. Pneumatosis intestinalis and pneumoperitoneum after sclerotherapy. AJR 1988;151:953–4.

Eklof O, Lohr G, Okniran L. Submucosal perforation of the esophagus in the neonate. Acta Radiol 1969;8:187–92.

Fitzgerald P, O'Connell D. Massive hypertrophy of the lingual tonsils: an unusual cause of dysphagia. Br J Radiol 1987;60:505–6.

Franken EA Jr, Smith WC, editors. Gastrointestinal imaging in pediatrics. 2nd ed. Philadelphia: Harper & Row; 1982. p. 24.

Girdany BR, Sieber WK, Osman MZ. Traumatic pseudo-diverticulum of the pharynx in newborn infants. N Engl J Med 1969;280:237–40.

Greenspan R, Kressel HY, Laufer I, et al. Radiographic findings in the esophagus following the Sigiura procedure. Radiology 1982;144:245–7.

Grunebaum M, Horodniceanu C, Wilunsky E, et al. Iatrogenic transmural perforation of the esophagus in the preterm infant. Clin Radiol 1980;31:257–61.

Guthrie KS. Congenital malformations of the esophagus. J Pathol Bact 1945;57:363–73.

Ishikawa T, Saeki M, Tsukune Y, et al. Detection of para-esophageal varices by plain film. AJR 1985;144:701–4.

Lee SB, Kuhn JP. Esophageal perforation in the neonate. Am J Dis Child 1976;130:325–9.

L'Hermine C, Chastanet P, Delemazure O, et al. Percutaneous transhepatic embolization of gastroesophageal varices: results in 400 patients. AJR 1989;152:755–60.

Lunderquist A, Borjesson B, Owman T, et al. Isobutyl 2-cyanoacrylate (bucrylate) in obliteration of gastric coronary vein and esophageal varices. AJR 1978;130:1–6.

MacKellar A, Kennedy JC. Congenital diverticulum of the pharynx simulating esophageal atresia. J Pediatr Surg 1972;7:408–11.

Maclean AD, Houghton-Allen BW. Upper esophageal web in childhood. Pediatr Radiol 1975;3:240–1.

Manashil GB. Sialography—a simple procedure. Med Radiogr Photogr 1976;52:34–42.

Manashil GB. A new catheter for sialography. AJR 1977;128:518.

Markle BM, Hanson K. Esophageal pseudodiverticulosis: two new cases in children. Pediatr Radiol 1992;22:194–5.

Nelson AR. Congenital true esophageal diverticulum: report of a case unassociated with other esophagotracheal abnormality. Ann Surg 1957;145:258–64.

Nosher JL, Campbell WL, Seaman WB. The clinical significance of cervical, esophageal and hypopharyngeal webs. Radiology 1975;117:45–7.

Osman MZ, Girdany BR. Traumatic pseudodiverticulums of the pharynx in infants and children. Ann Radiol 1973;16:143–7.

Pearlberg JL, Sandler MA, Madrazo BL. Computed tomographic features of esophageal intramural pseudodiverticulosis. Radiology 1983;147:189–90.

Peters ME, Crummy AB, Wojtowycx MM, et al. Intramural esophageal pseudodiverticulosis. A report in a child with a sixteen-year follow-up. Pediatr Radiol 1982; 12:262–3.

Rabinov KR, Joffe N. A blunt-tip side-injecting cannula for sialography. Radiology 1969;92:1438.

Rose JD, Roberts GM, Smith PM. The radiological appearance of the esophagus after sclerotherapy for varices. Clin Radiol 1985;36:355–8.

Rubin P, Holt JF. Secretory sialography in diseases of major salivary glands. AJR 1957;77:575–98.

Stringer DA, Daneman A, St. Onge O. Doppler assessment of abdominal and peripheral vessels in children. Presented at the 71st meeting of the Radiological Society of North America; 1985 Nov 17–22; Chicago.

Takashi M, Igarashi M, Hino S, et al. Esophageal varices: correlation of left gastric venography and endoscopy in patients with portal hypertension. Radiology 1985; 155:327–31.

Theander G. Congenital posterior midline pharyngoesophageal diverticula. Pediatr Radiol 1973;1:153–5.

Tihansky DP, Reilly JJ, Schade RR, et al. The esophagus after injection sclerotherapy of varices: immediate postoperative changes. Radiology 1984;153:43–7.

Touloukian RJ, Beardsley GP, Ablow RC, et al. Traumatic perforation of the pharynx in the newborn. Pediatrics 1977;59:1019–22.

Trenkner SW, Levine MS, Laufcr I, ct al. Idiopathic esophageal varix. AJR 1983;141:43–4.

Van Steenbergen W, Fevery J, Broeckaert L, et al. Intramural hematoma of the esophagus: unusual complication of variceal sclerotherapy. Gastrointest Radiol 1984; 9:293–5.

Waldram R, Nunnerley H, Davis M, et al. Detection and grading of oesophageal varices by fiber-optic endoscopy and barium swallow with and without buscopan. Clin Radiol 1977;28:137–41.

Weaver JW, Kaude JV, Hamlin DJ. Webs of the lower esophagus: a complication of gastroesophageal reflux? AJR 1984;142:289–92.

Weller MH. Intramural diverticulosis of the esophagus: report of a case in a child. J Pediatr 1972;80:281–5.

Wrightman AJA, Wright EA. Intramural esophageal diverticulosis: a correlation of radiological and pathological findings. Br J Radiol 1974;47:496–8.

Abnormalities of the Salivary Glands

Aslam MO, Hussain S, Rizvi I, Bley W. Technical report: wire guided sialography. Clin Radiol 1991;44:350–1.

Bronstein AD, Nyberg DA, Schwartz AN, et al. Increased salivary gland density on contrast-enhanced CT after head and neck radiation. AJR 1987;149:1259–63.

Bryan RN, Miller RH, Ferreyo RI, et al. Computed tomography of the major salivary glands. AJR 1982;139:547–54.

Evers K, Zito JL, Fine J, et al. CT sialography: utilising acinar filling. Br J Radiol 1985;58:839–43.

Gritzmann N. Sonography of the salivary glands. AJR 1989;153:161–6.

Grunebaum M, Ziv N, Mankuta DJ. Submaxillary sialadenitis with a calculus in infancy diagnosed by ultrasonography. Pediatr Radiol 1985;15:191–2.

Mandelblatt SM, Braun IF, Davis PC, et al. Parotid masses: MR imaging. Radiology 1987;163:411–4.

McGahon JP, Walter JP, Bernstein L. Evaluation of the parotid gland. Radiology 1984;152:453–8.

Nicholson DA. Contrast media in sialography: a comparison of Lipiodol ultra fluid and Urografin 290. Clin Radiol 1990;42:423–6.

Pearson RSB. Recurrent swellings of the parotid gland. Gut 1961;2:210.

Rubaltelli L, Sponga T, Candiani F, et al. Infantile recurrent sialectatic parotitis: the role of sonography and sialography in diagnosis and follow up. Br J Radiol 1987;60:1211–4.

Seibert RW, Seibert JJ. High resolution ultrasonography of the parotid gland in children. Pediatr Radiol 1986;16:374–9.

Som PM, Shugar JMA, Train JS, et al. Manifestations of parotid gland enlargement: radiographic, pathologic, and clinical correlations: Part I. The autoimmune pseudosialectasias. Part II. The diseases of Mikulicz syndrome. Radiology 1981;141:415–9, 421–6.

Stacey-Clear A, Evans R, Kissini MW, et al. Sialography does not alter the management of parotid space-occupying lesions. Clin Radiol 1985;36:389–90.

Teresi LM, Lufkin RB, Wortham DG, et al. Parotid masses: MR imaging. Radiology 1987;163:405–9.

Yune HY, Klatte EC. Current status of sialography. AJR 1972;115:420–8.

Whyte AM, Hayward MWJ. Agenesis of the salivary glands: a report of two cases. Br J Radiol 1989;62:1023–6.

7

DIAPHRAGM AND ESOPHAGOGASTRIC JUNCTION

Sambasiva R. Kottamasu, MD, and
David A. Stringer, BSc, MBBS, FRCR, FRCPC

The diaphragm is a structure of complex developmental origin which can be affected by developmental or acquired abnormalities. This chapter considers first the embryology, then the developmental anomalies, which are primarily a variety of hernias, and finally acquired abnormalities such as hiatus hernia, gastroesophageal reflux, and diaphragm paralysis.

EMBRYOGENESIS

The ventral part of the diaphragm is formed from the septum transversum, a thick plate of mesodermal tissue occupying the space between the pericardial cavity and the stalk of the yolk sac (Figure 7–1) (Gray and Skandalakis, 1972). As this part develops, there are two relatively weak areas anteriorly at either side of the sternum through which the anterior hernia of Morgagni can develop. Defects elsewhere in the septum transversum may result in a peritoneopericardial hernia.

Posteriorly, the septum transversum is connected to the posterior aspect of the coelomic cavity by the mesoesophagus (the esophageal mesentery) that surrounds the inferior vena cava (see Figure 7–1). The pleuroperitoneal canals, which connect the thoracic and abdominal cavities, lie on either side of the mesoesophagus (Panicek et al., 1988). The pleuroperitoneal membrane, a double-layered membrane consisting of both pleura and peri-

toneum, grows in and closes off the canals. A defect in this membrane allows the herniation of abdominal viscera (Panicek et al., 1988). The exact defect may be only a part of the pleuroperitoneal canal or it may extend to the entire canal and even further. For convenience these are all called Bochdalek's hernias (Snyder and Greaney, 1965). Striated muscle normally develops between layers of the pleuroperitoneal membrane and forms the muscular diaphragm. If this muscle layer fails to form completely, in whole or in part of the hemidiaphragm, then the abdominal contents can bulge into the thorax; this is called eventration. The diaphragm is completed by peripheral muscular ingrowth from the body wall around the pleuropericardial canals. Defective development in any of the above can produce the hernias discussed below.

CONGENITAL AND DEVELOPMENTAL ANOMALIES

A diaphragmatic hernia in a child is almost always congenital in origin although it can result from trauma. Excluding hiatus hernia, there are five types of congenital diaphragmatic hernia: Bochdalek's (pleuroperitoneal) hernia, eventration of the diaphragm, Morgagni's (retrosternal) hernia, peritoneopericardial hernia, and miscellaneous hernial defects, e.g., a localized defect or complete absence

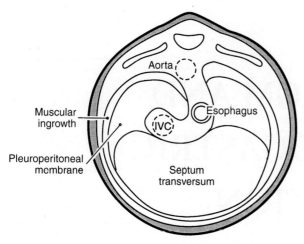

FIGURE 7–1. Embryology of the diaphragm. The diaphragm is formed by the septum transversum, the pleuroperitoneal membranes, and muscular ingrowth from the thoracoabdominal wall.

of the diaphragm. Hiatus hernias are discussed later in this chapter.

Bochdalek's (Pleuroperitoneal) Hernia

There is confusion over the definition of a Bochdalek defect, and the original description differs from that in general usage (Whittaker et al., 1968). Bochdalek originally described herniation through the costolumbar triangles, but in addition, herniation through a persistent pleuroperitoneal canal with an obvious posterior lip to the defect, and herniation through larger posterolateral defects with no posterior lip are now all grouped together as Bochdalek's hernias (Whittaker et al., 1968; Bonham-Carter et al., 1962; Harrington, 1942; Cerilli, 1964; Snyder and Greaney, 1965).

In 90% of cases, Bochdalek's hernia has no containing sac and the herniated bowel lies freely in the thoracic cavity. However, in 10% of cases, the hernia is contained in a hernial sac. If there is a major or complete diaphragmatic defect (unlike the partial posterior defect of a Bochdalek's hernia) and the sac contains a few muscular elements, then the condition is an eventration of the diaphragm rather than a true Bochdalek's hernia (Snyder and Greaney, 1965).

Eventrations and Bochdalek's hernias with a sac are less likely to allow the hemithorax to fill with bowel, and most eventrations are asymptomatic and found incidentally in later life as an asymptomatic chest mass on plain-film chest radiography. When

eventration presents acutely in the neonatal period with respiratory distress, distinguishing it from Bochdalek's hernia is often not possible preoperatively. Differentiation is unimportant since the true diagnosis will be discovered at the time of operation and the treatment of these symptomatic herniations is the same.

Clinical Features

Bochdalek's hernia is the commonest congenital diaphragmatic hernia, with an incidence of approximately 1 in 2200 and occurring between 2 and 9 times more commonly on the left side than on the right (Gale, 1985).

Bochdalek's hernias frequently present acutely at birth with severe respiratory distress, including cyanosis and dyspnea (Bonham-Carter et al., 1962), and can rapidly result in death if not quickly recognized and treated. Suction of bowel gas via a nasogastric tube may be life saving. Turning the infant on the affected side may facilitate spontaneous reduction of the hernia (Allen and Thomson, 1966). It follows that a chest radiograph examination is mandatory for any neonate in respiratory distress.

If presentation is not at birth, symptoms usually occur any time in the early neonatal period but occasionally a Bochdalek's hernia may present in later life (Day, 1972; Glasson et al., 1975; Berman et al., 1988). If so, it may present acutely although the symptoms and signs may be more gradual in onset and include dyspnea, respiratory infections, vomiting, and cyanosis (Bonham-Carter et al., 1962). Occasionally there may be severe abdominal colic, discomfort after eating, constipation, bowel obstruction, or even no symptoms as when the hernia is discovered serendipitously on a chest radiograph taken for other reasons (Berman et al., 1988).

Imaging

The diagnosis of diaphragmatic hernia has occasionally in the past been made antenatally by fetography (Bell and Ternbert, 1977). Antenatal ultrasonography (US) has replaced this technique; specific evidence of diaphragmatic hernia are now the findings of movement of abdominal contents into the chest on inspiration, peristalsis of chest contents, or malposition of the heart. Less specific signs are small abdominal circumference, absent intra-abdominal stomach, and a solid or cystic intrathoracic mass (Comstock, 1986; Guibaud et al., 1996). Antenatal

US is useful in alerting the clinician to a diaphragmatic hernia so that delivery can be performed at an institution which can take care of these cases.

A chest radiograph examination is mandatory for any neonate in respiratory distress or if a diaphragmatic hernia is suspected for other reasons. If air has been swallowed, the diagnosis of a left-sided diaphragmatic hernia is usually easy to make as the intra-abdominal gas pattern is abnormal (Figure 7–2).

Characteristically, there are multiple radiolucencies due to bowel gas in the thorax (see Figure 7–2), the heart and superior mediastinum are shifted to the opposite side, the esophagus is of normal length, and there is a relative absence of bowel gas in the abdomen. It is important to perform abdominal radiography (if the abdomen was not included in the chest radiography) because the bowel gas pattern can indicate that the chest shadows are not caused by pneumonia or by cystic adenomatoid

malformation. The radiologic size of the hernia does not reflect the true size of the diaphragmatic hernia (Reed and Lang, 1959). The spleen or the left lobe of the liver or kidney occasionally may be herniated on the left side (Figure 7–3), which can be demonstrated by US (Sumner et al., 1982).

If the infant presents at birth with severe respiratory distress, or if the child is too young or sick to have swallowed much air, the radiologic appearance may be that of a water-density mass obscuring the hemithorax and deviating the heart to the opposite side. Delayed films will show swallowed air entering the intrathoracic bowel (see Figure 7–2). The abdomen may appear scaphoid in outline due to absence of intra-abdominal contents. If the condition of the infant precludes waiting for delayed films, a small amount of air can be injected through a nasogastric tube to demonstrate the abnormal position of the bowel. Care is necessary

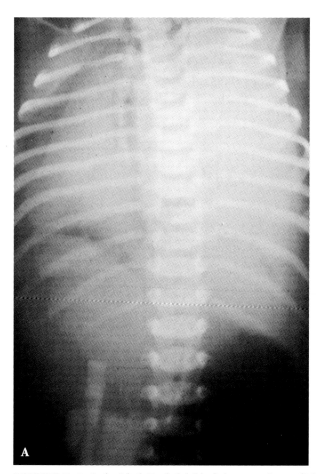
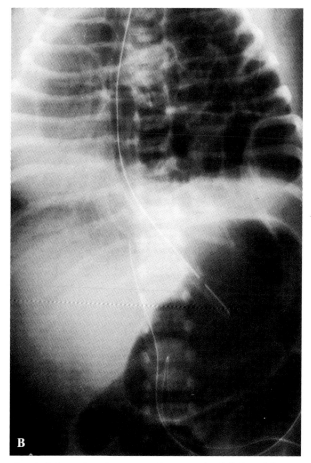

FIGURE 7–2. Left-sided Bochdalek's (pleuroperitoneal) hernia. *A,* Water-density mass obscures the left hemithorax and deviates the heart to the right. *B,* Delayed film shows gas entering the intrathoracic bowel. Unlike in this patient, the stomach often herniates into the thorax.

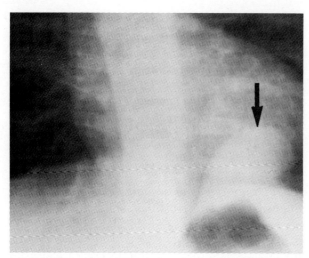

FIGURE 7–3. Left-sided Bochdalek's (pleuroperitoneal) hernia with renal herniation. A reniform soft-tissue density mass (*arrow*) is posterior to the heart. This 9-month-old girl also has tetralogy of Fallot with a right-sided aortic arch and an elevated cardiac apex, which produces an appearance resembling a sabot (coeur en sabot).

as too much gas in the intrathoracic stomach or small bowel can fatally exacerbate the respiratory distress. Similarly, in the acute situation, aspiration of gas via a nasogastric tube can be life saving (Fig-ure 7–4). If there is difficulty in passing the nasogastric tube (as can happen if the herniated stomach has undergone volvulus in the chest) or if the patient is in extreme distress, then a needle should be inserted straight through the chest wall to rapidly deflate the viscus.

A right-sided Bochdalek diaphragmatic hernia is relatively rare (Canino et al., 1964), probably because the right pleuroperitoneal canal closes earlier in gestation than the left (Figure 7–5). Occasionally, following streptococcal infection a right-sided hernia may appear (McCarten et al., 1981; Akierman and Mayock, 1983). Diagnosing a right-sided Bochdalek's hernia may be difficult. The liver may fill part of the thorax (Figure 7–6), and the intra-abdominal gas pattern may initially appear normal. Diagnosis can most often be made by judging the position of the liver from the changing gas pattern on a plain film and by US. The superior margin of the liver may be rounded; blunting of the costophrenic angle suggests pleural fluid (Canino et al., 1964).

A large hydrothorax may be present that may be associated with incarcerated peritoneal sacs. The hydrothorax can obscure the diaphragmatic hernia on plain-film radiography but US before or after delivery will show the nature of the chest opacification. An

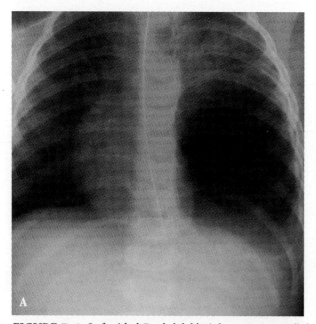
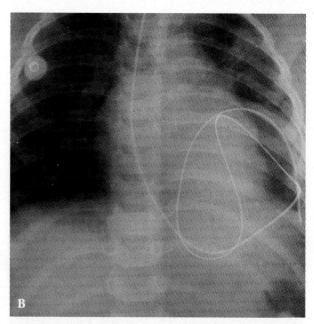

FIGURE 7–4. Left-sided Bochdalek's (pleuroperitoneal) hernia. *A,* Gas in the intrathoracic stomach is displacing the heart to the right, exacerbating the respiratory distress. The tip of the nasogastric tube lies at the esophagogastric junction. The stomach has twisted up into the chest. *B,* In the acute situation, aspiration of gas via a nasogastric tube can decompress the stomach and be life saving.

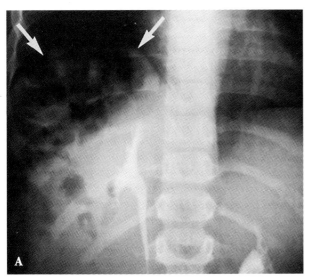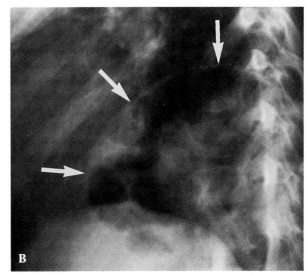

FIGURE 7–5. Right-sided Bochdalek's (pleuroperitoneal) hernia. The right kidney and bowel gas is shown in an abnormally high (*A*) and posterior (*B*) location due to herniation into a right-sided Bochdalek's (pleuroperitoneal) hernia (*arrows*). This hernia was discovered serendipitously in a 5-year-old boy during intravenous urography and was found at surgery to be a Bochdalek's (pleuroperitoneal) hernia lying within a sac.

unusual association is ascites, which may be due to obstruction of the hepatic veins similar to Budd-Chiari syndrome (Gilsanz et al., 1986).

Postnatal US is useful in diagnosing right-sided hernias and easily shows the intrathoracic position of the liver. Technetium Tc 99m sulfur colloid liver scans have been used to diagnose diaphragmatic hernia by identifying the position of the liver and spleen in difficult cases. Umbilical arteriography and venography have been used to diagnose Bochdalek's hernia (Miller et al., 1977; Sagel and Ablow, 1968) but such arteriography is no longer indicated because of the high risk of major complications (Baker and Berdon, 1977), which is unacceptable especially when careful perusal of plain films is sufficient.

An antegrade examination of the small bowel is more useful in doubtful cases of right-sided rather than left-sided diaphragmatic hernia but is not usually needed. A contrast enema will show the abnormal gut location but also is rarely indicated. There is a well-known association of malrotation/malfixation of the midgut with diaphragmatic hernia (Berman et al., 1988).

Computed tomography (CT) can diagnose Bochdalek's hernia but is rarely indicated. It is interesting that CT has detected many asymptomatic small hernias in later life; such hernias may be more common than previously thought (Gale, 1985).

Differential Diagnoses. The major differential diagnoses are congenital cystic adenomatoid malformation of the lung, streptococcal pneumonia, staphylococcal pneumonia with pneumatoceles or other inflammatory lung processes (Canino et al., 1964), and eventration. In practice, differentiation from eventration is not important since the identical surgery will be indicated when there is respiratory distress in a neonate due to lung compression. In streptococcal and staphylococcal pneumonia, there are usually other clinical indicators of the infection, which must be severe to mimic a hernia.

Though it is rare, cystic adenomatoid lung malformation is the main differential consideration (Craig et al., 1956; Davies et al., 1979). Antenatal US can detect this anomaly as either a cystic or solid mass which can be distinguished from a hernia by the finding of an intact diaphragm on the ipsilateral side of the mass (Claiborne et al., 1985). Cystic adenomatoid lung malformation can closely mimic the postnatal plain-film appearance of a hernia, initially being of soft-tissue density and later containing radiolucencies. The abdominal gas pattern, normal in cystic adenomatoid malformation and abnormal in diaphragmatic hernia, usually is a clue to the true diagnosis. Differentiation is important because a cystic adenomatoid malformation requires a thoracic operation whereas a hernia usually is corrected abdominally (Davies et al., 1979).

Associations and Complications

The major causes of death from congenital diaphragmatic hernia postoperatively are related to hypoplasia of the lungs, persistent fetal circulation, and major associated cardiovascular anomalies. In this regard, the initial uncorrected blood pH of a child appears to have prognostic significance with good survival above pH 7.0 and a poor survival below pH 7.0 (Mishalany et al., 1979). A major cause of death or severe morbidity in patients who present late is midgut malrotation with associated strangulation (Gaisie et al., 1983; Berman et al., 1988).

Lung Hypoplasia. The major association with Bochdalek's hernia is lung hypoplasia, which can range from unilateral and mild to bilateral and severe. When bilateral, the hypoplasia is more severe on the side of the hernia. The extent of the lung hypoplasia depends on the stage at which the developing lungs are compressed.

The diaphragm forms by the 9th intrauterine week, at which time a large portion of the small bowel is extra-abdominal. If a defect occurs in the diaphragm, bowel will tend to herniate into the thorax as the small bowel returns to the abdomen. Bronchioles develop mainly between the eighth and twelfth weeks of gestation (Berdon et al., 1968) but some development occurs up to the sixteenth week.

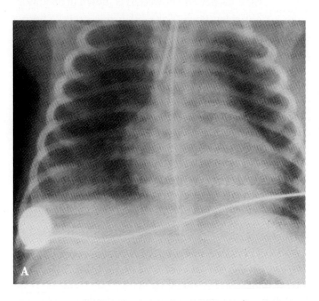

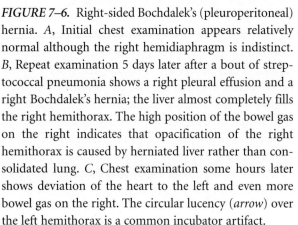

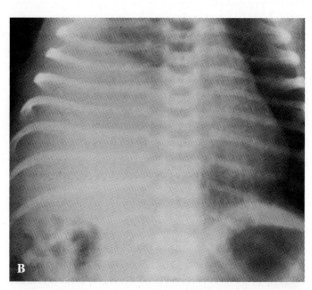

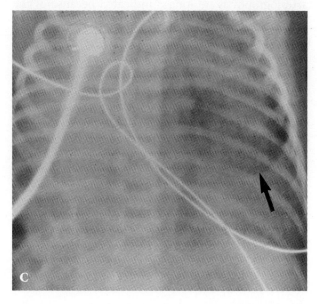

FIGURE 7–6. Right-sided Bochdalek's (pleuroperitoneal) hernia. *A,* Initial chest examination appears relatively normal although the right hemidiaphragm is indistinct. *B,* Repeat examination 5 days later after a bout of streptococcal pneumonia shows a right pleural effusion and a right Bochdalek's hernia; the liver almost completely fills the right hemithorax. The high position of the bowel gas on the right indicates that opacification of the right hemithorax is caused by herniated liver rather than consolidated lung. *C,* Chest examination some hours later shows deviation of the heart to the left and even more bowel gas on the right. The circular lucency (*arrow*) over the left hemithorax is a common incubator artifact.

If lung compression occurs early, the hypoplasia is usually bilateral and so severe that the infant dies before surgery can be performed. If lung compression occurs later, bronchiole development is more normal with a much improved prognosis.

Lung hypoplasia is the major cause of death, and the prognosis is determined by the degree of hypoplasia. The patients can be divided into three groups (Table 7–1) according to the extent of the lung hypoplasia, which may be apparent from the chest radiographs (Berdon et al., 1968).

In stage I with insignificant hypoplasia, the overall prognosis is excellent. In stage II, severe, bilateral hypoplasia is nearly always fatal. Stage III gives the greatest challenge to surgeons and intensive care personnel. Unilateral lung hypoplasia is seen as a small hypoplastic lung (Figure 7–7) in the immediate postoperative period. With survival, this will slowly re-expand to fill the hemithorax but will appear hyperlucent with decreased lung vessels secondary to the bronchiolar hypoplasia (Berdon et al., 1968). Because of the early development of the hypoplasia, active intervention in the third trimester has not been advocated in cases discovered on antenatal US.

Persistent Fetal Circulation. An associated complication is persistent fetal circulation (Levy et al., 1977), with the maintenance of high pulmonary artery pressure after birth related to the lung hypoplasia. This can cause respiratory distress, cyanosis, and right-to-left shunting. In a normal heart, the shunting occurs through a ductus arteriosus or foramen ovale. The chest radiograph shows normal lungs despite shunting. Vasodilator therapy may be helpful in infants with unilateral hypoplasia but with bilateral hypoplasia drug therapy is not helpful (Ein et al., 1980). The relationship of arterial pCO_2 and ventilation parameters may be valuable in predicting survival postoperatively in Bochdalek's hernia cases. The presence of carbon dioxide retention as measured 2 hours after surgery, despite hyperventilation with high pressure and high respiratory rate, has a mortality of 90%. However, in those in whom hyperventilation caused a good response with reversible ductal shunting, the favorable prognosis improves to 97% (Bohn et al., 1984).

Malrotation. Malrotation of the intestine is invariably associated with Bochdalek's hernia because normal fixation of the bowel is not possible due to its abnormal position. Therefore, the bowel is theoretically more likely to undergo volvulus. When operating for diaphragmatic hernia, some surgeons perform a Ladd procedure at the same time (Bonham-Carter et al., 1962).

Hernial Sac. In addition to recurrence of the hernia, a hernial sac may either be missed or incompletely removed at operation. A hernial sac will be present if herniation occurs after closure of the pleuro-peritoneal canals by the membrane. A hernia is more likely to reach the apex of the lung, as seen on chest radiograph examination, if a sac is not present than if one is; however, since this cannot be relied on, a search should always be made at surgery for the hernial sac (Karasick et al., 1978; Kenigsberg and Gwinn, 1965). With or without a sac, the hernia presents at a similar age (Bonham-Carter et al., 1962).

Hiatus hernia may follow Bochdalek's hernia repair and be associated with severe vomiting (Cohen and Beck, 1980).

Miscellaneous. Emphysema of the hypoplastic lungs, especially of the lower lobes, is a well recognized complication (Berdon et al., 1968) and is usually asymptomatic. However, occasionally there are symptoms, which may exceptionally require lobectomy (Omojola et al., 1981).

Other associations include cardiac anomalies, Meckel's diverticulum, chest wall deformities, Turner's syndrome, and pulmonary sequestrations, which may be multiple (Bonham-Carter et al., 1962; Allen and Thomson, 1966; Tovar and Benavent, 1979). A rare complication found at operation for Bochdalek's hernia is gut obstruction and gangrene. Occasionally, a kidney, spleen, or liver may herniate and present as an intrathoracic mass (Burke et al., 1967). Bilateral intrathoracic kidneys are even rarer but have been reported. This is usually asymptomatic, and the organ may occlude the diaphragmatic defect

TABLE 7–1.   Grading of Bochdalek Hernia*

Group	Extent of Hypoplasia	Prognosis
Stage I	Insignificant hypoplasia	Excellent
Stage II	Severe bilateral hypoplasia	Usually fatal
Stage III	Unilateral hypoplasia	Moderate

*According to lung hypoplasia.

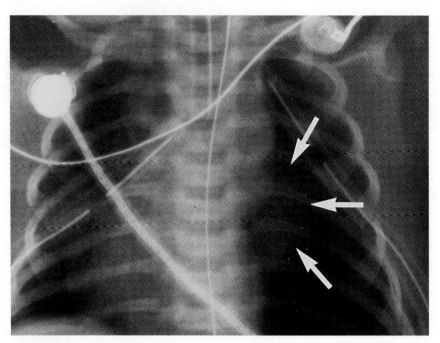

FIGURE 7–7. Hypoplastic left lung. Immediately following repair of a left-sided Bochdalek's hernia, the left hemidiaphragm is flat, and a small hypoplastic lung (*arrows*) is seen within the pneumothorax.

and thus prevent bowel herniation. The diagnosis of a herniated organ may be facilitated by US, which can differentiate normal intrathoracic kidneys (Sumner et al., 1982).

Late Presentation

Streptoccocal pneumonia. In infants, streptoccocal pneumonia may rarely be associated with the late appearance of a right-sided diaphragmatic hernia (Akierman and Maycock, 1983; McCarten et al., 1981). The mechanism is uncertain but is probably due to the changed lung compliance from the pneumonia, resulting in a change in transdiaphragmatic pressures such that the liver can no longer plug the right diaphragmatic defect.

The herniation may become apparent due to clinical deterioration after an initial improvement. A large pleural effusion and loss of visualization of the right hemidiaphragm with or without a mediastinal shift can also occur (Akierman and Maycock, 1983). The use of US in diagnosing these sick infants is possible at the incubator in the intensive care unit, and US was used in the patient illustrated in Figure 7–6. Diaphragmatic hernias presenting outside the neonatal period are frequently associated with mis-

leading clinical and radiologic assessments, resulting in diagnostic delay and inappropriate therapy (Berman et al., 1988). When a diagnostic dilemma continues, fluoroscopy, upright views, and plain-film radiographs after nasogastric intubation are occasionally helpful. Contrast study of the upper gastrointestinal tract or contrast study per rectum may aid delineation of the anomaly, with beaking corresponding to the constriction at the site of the diaphragmatic defect (Siegel et al., 1981).

Miscellaneous. Late presentation of diaphragmatic hernia occur more often on the right side than the left and may occasionally present late with no history of chest infection. Late presentation usually indicates a better prognosis (Wiseman and MacPherson, 1977) as there will be little or no problem with lung hypoplasia. Occasionally a previous chest radiograph performed for other reasons shows normal lungs although our experience is that in those patients who develop delayed left hernias the gastric air bubble may be further below the level of the left hemidiaphragm than usual on initial radiographs (Figure 7–8). However, a significant number will present acutely and may die secondary to strangulation or volvulus (Figure 7–9) (Gaisie et al., 1983). Hence, diagnosis and treatment should be prompt, an often difficult task due to the unusual modes of presentation associated with misleading clinical signs and radiologic assessments. This has occasionally resulted in both diagnostic delay and misguided therapeutic intervention such as insertion of chest drains into the stomach.

The cause of delayed presentation is uncertain. It has been proposed that in some patients, the viscera is initially confined to a sac and presents when the sac ruptures (Osebold and Soper, 1976). Another theory presumes the diaphragmatic defect to have been occluded by spleen, kidney, or liver and its presentation delayed until an insult such as trauma dislodges the occlusions. A diaphragmatic hernia may even occasionally present long after trauma.

Delayed presentation may also be due to the lack of initial symptoms, the abnormality only being discovered when symptoms occur. This is documented in one case in which a chance radiographic

finding of an asymptomatic Bochdalek's hernia presenting in 1912 eventually proved fatal from complications of strangulation 46 years later (Kirkland, 1959). This indicates that there is a group whose viscera may have herniated at an early stage but who present only when a complication such as volvulus or strangulation occurs.

As can be imagined from the above, the radiologic appearance, like the clinical presentation, can be protean. The appearance on plain-film may show gas-filled loops of bowel in the chest similar to those of neonates. However, the appearance may be less obvious, mimicking pneumonia with or without aeroceles, gastric volvulus, tension pneumothorax, or pleural effusion (see Figures 7–6, 7–8, and 7–9) (Siegel et al., 1981). Bowel obstruction can be superimposed, which may cause diagnostic difficulty. A pleural effusion may be present, which, if there is bowel necrosis or perforation, may be serosan-

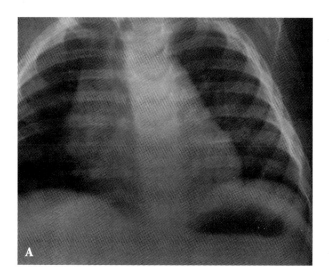

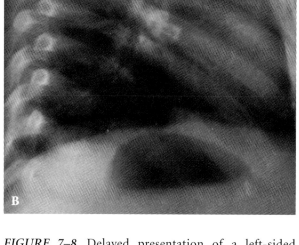

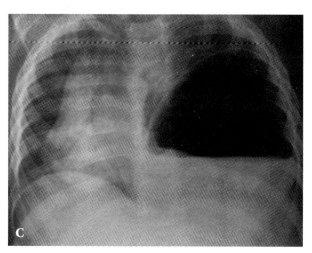

FIGURE 7–8. Delayed presentation of a left-sided Bochdalek's (pleuroperitoneal) hernia. A chest radiograph of a 6-month-old patient shows normal lungs in frontal (*A*) and lateral (*B*) projections. *C*, At 2 years of age and associated with acute respiratory embarrassment, there is a dilated stomach full of air and fluid in the thorax, displacing the heart and mediastinum to the right. A Bochdalek's hernia with sac was found at operation.

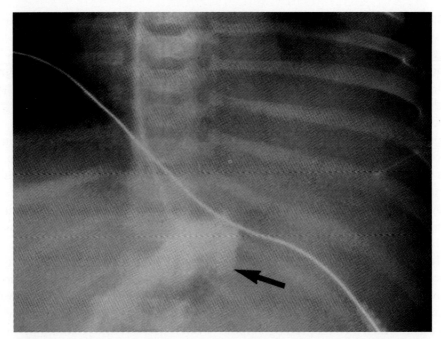

FIGURE 7–9. Delayed presentation of a left-sided Bochdalek's (pleuroperitoneal) hernia in a 4-month-old boy. A chest radiograph shows a large pleural effusion, an indistinct left hemidiaphragm, and a stomach (*arrow*) containing contrast material displaced inferomedially by necrotic bowel secondary to volvulus in a Bochdalek's hernia.

guinous, full of pus or even blood (see Figure 7–9) (Carter and Giuseffi, 1948; Bosher et al., 1960; Deaner et al., 1983). In our experience, the presence of an effusion or an abnormal bowel-gas pattern can be a serious sign of bowel necrosis possibly secondary to volvulus. Many patients with diaphragmatic hernia have malfixation of the midgut and hence are susceptible to volvulus.

Eventration

Failure of formation of the muscular component of the hemidiaphragm results in protrusion of the abdominal contents into the chest. Part or all of the hemidiaphragm may be affected, and occasionally both hemidiaphragms are involved (Lundstrom and Allen, 1966; Rodgers and Hawks, 1986). Bilateral eventrations have a high mortality but may occasionally respond to surgery (Rodgers and Hawks, 1986).

Eventration may present in infancy as respiratory distress and mimic a Bochdalek's hernia (Bonham-Carter et al., 1962). A prenatal diagnosis of eventration of the diaphragm has been reported but the findings may be indistinguishable from a diaphragmatic hernia (Jurcak-Zaleski et al., 1990). A membrane

containing little if any striated muscle is found at surgery. The prognosis in these infants is similar to that of a Bochdalek's hernia and depends mainly on the degree of associated pulmonary hypoplasia.

However, most eventrations are found incidentally in later life as an asymptomatic mass on plain chest radiographic examination (Figure 7–10). Ultrasonography can be useful in the diagnosis, especially on the right side (see Figure 7–10) and even when the eventration is quite small (Figure 7–11) (Moccia et al., 1981). Peritoneography will show the diaphragm to be intact but is rarely indicated (see Figure 7–10).

Eventration may show as a superiorly located stomach (Figure 7–12) with the antrum higher than the fundus. On the left it is associated with a high spleen or splenic flexure; when it is on the right, the liver appears high. US or a liver-spleen radionuclide scan can be used to confirm that a chest mass is an eventration containing portions of liver or spleen; it can also be combined with a chest radiography examination or a lung scan (Spencer et al., 1971).

Among the many anomalies associated with eventration are hypoplastic lungs or ribs, gastric volvulus, multiple hemivertebrae, cleft palate, coarctation of the aorta, and other congenital heart defects (Wayne et al., 1974).

Morgagni's (Retrosternal) Hernia

The original description of Morgagni's hernia has been expanded to include a series of retrosternal hernias (Bingham, 1959) including

- a defective attachment of the anterior portion of the diaphragm to the ribs and sternum
- true defects in the diaphragm posterior to the sternal and costal insertion
- combinations of the above

Morgagni's hernias represent 3% of diaphragmatic hernias (Comer and Clagett, 1966). They occur most often on the right, occasionally on both sides, and only rarely on the left. They are usually asymptomatic but may present with abdominal pain or discomfort, bloating, diarrhea or vomiting. Rarely, chest pain or even dyspnea may be present (Schneidau et al., 1982). The herniation and its symptoms may be intermittent. The presence of a sac is generally thought to be common (Bingham, 1959), and the omentum is the most common herniating tissue.

Morgagni's hernias are usually easily diagnosed radiologically although occasionally they may be mistaken for middle-lobe pathology. On plain films, herniating omentum can appear as a large right-sided cardiophrenic mass (Figure 7–13). If the hernia contains bowel, it is usually the transverse colon although the small bowel, stomach, or liver may be herniated (Baran et al., 1967). Supradiaphragmatic gas-containing bowel may be seen on plain films and may mimic a Bochdalek's hernia.

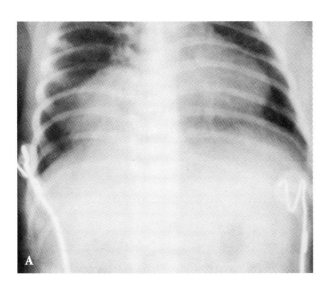

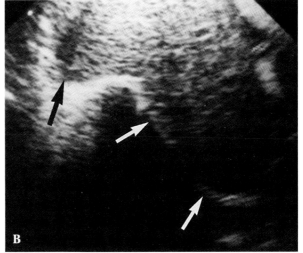

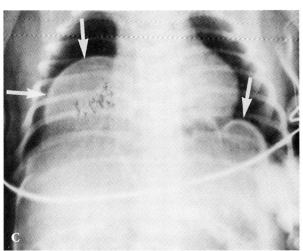

FIGURE 7–10. Eventration of the diaphragm. *A*, A mass contiguous with the right hemidiaphragm is shown on chest examination. *B*, Longitudinal ultrasonography demonstrates a normal hemidiaphragm posteriorly (*white arrows*) and bulging of the liver (*black arrow*) into the thorax anteriorly. *C*, Peritoneography shows the intact hemidiaphragm and multiple eventrations (*arrows*) but this technique is rarely indicated.

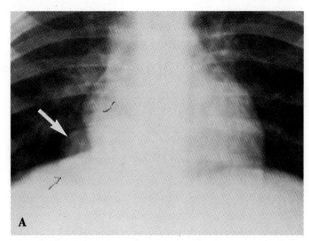
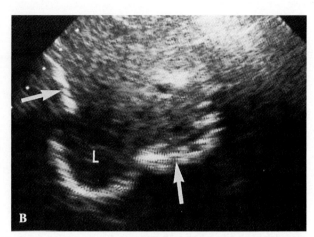

FIGURE 7–11. Eventration of the diaphragm. *A,* Chest radiograph shows a mass in the right cardiophrenic angle. *B,* Longitudinal US shows the mass to be a small portion of liver (*L*) bulging into the thorax with a normal hemidiaphragm adjacent (*arrows*).

Differentiation is easily made on the lateral view due to the retrosternal location of Morgagni's hernia (Forshall, 1966) (Figure 7–14). Barium examination may also discover herniated bowel, and a barium enema is the best contrast examination if the diagnosis is in doubt. The transverse colon is deviated upwards toward or through the hernial opening.

Morgagni's hernia is associated with an increased incidence of cardiac anomalies and Down syndrome. This hernia is best treated surgically to prevent complications (Baran et al., 1967; Forshall, 1966).

Peritoneopericardial Hernia

Peritoneopericardial hernia is a rare hernia caused by faulty development of the septum transversum (Wilson et al., 1947). It may be associated with anomalies of the anterior abdominal and thoracic walls (see Chapter 9). Bowel contents may occasionally protrude into the pericardial cavity. Rarely, this hernia may follow surgery.

Traumatic Diaphragmatic Hernia

Rupture of the diaphragm can result from blunt

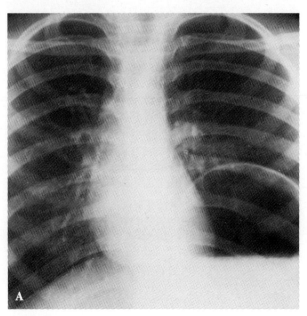
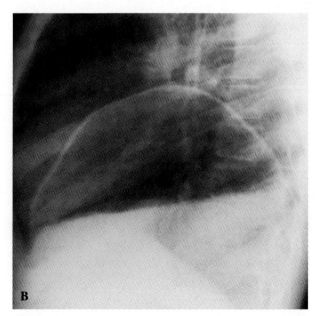

FIGURE 7–12. Eventration of the left hemidiaphragm. Eventration affects the complete left hemidiaphragm on frontal (*A*) and lateral (*B*) views. The stomach bulges into the left hemithorax.

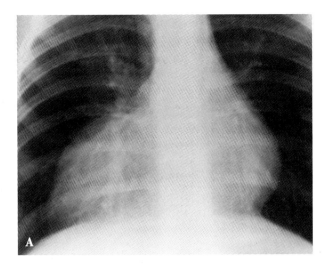

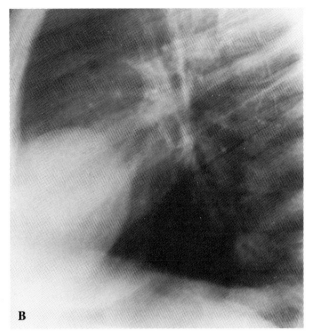

FIGURE 7–13. Morgagni's hernia. *A,* A large herniation of omentum fills the right cardiophrenic angle on the frontal view. *B,* Its anterior position is clearly shown on the lateral view.

trauma, and a high index of suspicion is required to make the correct diagnosis. It occurs more commonly on the left side than on the right. However, the right half of the diaphragm is more difficult to evaluate because of adjacent liver. Ultrasonography or a radionuclide liver/spleen scan are helpful when a right-sided diaphragmatic injury is suspected (Ball et al., 1982; Fung and Vickar, 1991). Findings on chest radiographs may be abnormal but aerated bowel may not be seen in the chest. The diaphragm can rupture without immediate visceral herniation. Chest radiographs obtained at admission and repeated soon after are valuable in suggesting the diagnosis of traumatic rupture of the diaphragm

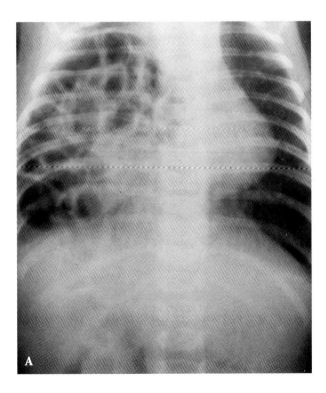

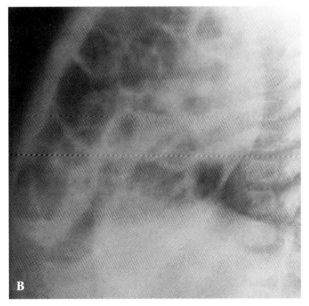

FIGURE 7–14. Morgagni's hernia. *A,* Loops of bowel fill the right hemithorax and mimic a Bochdalek's hernia. *B,* Lateral view shows the retrosternal location of the hernia.

(Gelman et al., 1991). Findings on CT scans may be subtle and include discontinuity of the diaphragm, herniation of abdominal viscera or omentum, and narrowing of the stomach or bowel with an hourglass configuration (Worthy et al., 1995). Delayed herniation through a trauma-induced defect in the diaphragm can cause bowel obstruction (Cruz and Minagi, 1994). Once a delayed presentation of traumatic diaphragmatic hernia is suspected, contrast studies of the gastrointestinal tract are useful confirmatory investigations (McHugh et al., 1991).

Miscellaneous Hernial Defects

Other congenital hernial defects such as total absence of the diaphragm are found only rarely. The prognosis depends on the degree of lung hypoplasia and the extent of other associated malformations.

DIAPHRAGM PARALYSIS

Etiology

Movement of the diaphragm may be abnormal due to a number of conditions. Central diseases such as intracerebral bleeding, upper motor neuron abnormality secondary to trauma or myelitis, abnormal diaphragm response due to myositis, dystrophy, eventration, or juxtadiaphragmatic pathology may all be causes seen in children. However, the most common cause of paralysis is a lower motor neuron (phrenic nerve) paralysis secondary to birth trauma or thoracic surgery (McCauley and Labib, 1984). Odita et al. reported four neonates with phrenic nerve paralysis complicating chest tube placement for pneumothorax. In all four, phrenic nerve paralysis developed on the side of chest tube placement and was associated with impingement of the chest tube on the mediastinum or spine; Odita and colleauges suggested that the medial end of the chest tube should be no less than 1 cm from the spine (Odita et al., 1992).

Imaging

There is a wide range of normal and abnormal movements of the hemidiaphragm and any radiologic assessment must be made in conjunction with a knowledge of the clinical status. Fluoroscopy has been the major imaging technique used to evaluate diaphragm movement but ultrasonographic assessment is now the initial modality of choice (Houston

et al., 1995). In our experience, there is a close correlation between ultrasonographic and clinical findings. In patients in whom fluoroscopy findings conflict with those of US, the anterior third (the dome) of the hemidiaphragm often moves incongruously with respect to the posterior third. Hence, apparent paradoxical movement on anteroposterior fluoroscopy may be relatively unimportant if there was a good normal excursion of the posterior part of the hemidiaphragm. Fast gradient-recalled-echo (GRE) magnetic resonance imaging (MR) can be used to assess diaphragmatic motion (Gierada et al., 1995). Each modality is discussed below.

Plain Films

Plain films can be useful in monitoring the position of a hemidiaphragm if chest radiographs are being taken regularly for other reasons, e.g., following thoracic surgery. However, the left hemidiaphragm may occasionally be higher than the right without any diaphragm paralysis, and plain films will not give any dynamic information.

Ultrasonography

Ultrasonography has the advantage that it can be performed at the bedside with minimal disturbance to the sick infant or child. Furthermore, US is safe in that no ionizing radiation is used, an important point when multiple serial examinations have to be performed. It is also of use in detecting the presence of intra-abdominal pathology adjacent to the hemidiaphragms such as subphrenic abscesses (Khan and Gould, 1984) or pleural pathology such as effusions with hemidiaphragm depression (Lowe et al., 1981). A relatively minor difficulty is encountered if the dome of the right hemidiaphragm is partially obscured by ribs or if the left hemidiaphragm is obscured by gas in the stomach or splenic flexure (Haber et al., 1975).

Recent ultrasonographic evaluation of normal adults has shown that there is greater movement of the middle and posterior thirds of the diaphragm than of the anterior third (Harris et al., 1983). Hence, the ultrasonographic assessment should evaluate all parts of the hemidiaphragms with the patient breathing spontaneously to assess overall movement. The hemidiaphragm can be viewed from a number of projections even if any surgical dressings are present.

When tachypnea is present, US can be difficult to evaluate. We have overcome this problem by having one observer call out the time of inspiration while a second observer looks at the television monitor. A possible refinement could be pneumotachography (Harris et al., 1983) or using the respiratory impedance for judging the phase of respiration.

Fluoroscopy

At our hospital, fluoroscopy is reserved for patients in whom US has been unsuccessful or has given results contrary to the clinical impression, such as when US is normal but the patient cannot be weaned from the ventilator.

So that the status of the patient can be closely watched, the lights in the fluoroscopic room should not be dimmed although this will degrade the image somewhat. The positioning of the ventilated infant with multiple intravenous lines under the fluoroscope can be difficult or even hazardous. As mentioned earlier, if there is tachypnea, it is helpful to have an assistant who calls out when inspiration occurs while a second observer watches the TV monitor.

The movement of the hemidiaphagms is complex (Alexander, 1966). The left hemidiaphragm may occasionally be higher than the right, and inequality of movement is common (Young and Simon, 1972). The anterior part (the dome) is the only part of the hemidiaphragm routinely visualized on frontal fluoroscopy (Alexander, 1966; Haber et al., 1975). The excursion seen radiographically in the anteroposterior projection in normal adults is unrelated to vital capacity, and small excursions of less than 3 cm still may mean an expiration of 5 L of air (Young and Simon, 1972). Lateral or oblique fluoroscopy is often useful but occasionally may be difficult to interpret (Alexander, 1966; Haber et al., 1975) and can be hazardous to a sick child.

Magnetic Resonance Imaging

Gierada et al. reported that it is feasible to assess diaphragmatic motion using fast gradient-recalled-echo MR and acquiring dynamic images during real-time breathing in healthy subjects (Gierada et al., 1995). The applications of dynamic MR in the evaluation of pathologic conditions affecting diaphragmatic motion need further investigation.

Phrenic Nerve Stimulation

Phrenic nerve stimulation, which has been suggested as an adjunct to ultrasonographic or fluoroscopic assessment, entails faradic stimulation of the phrenic nerve during US or fluoroscopy. The technique may aid the examination of patients who respire poorly when not ventilated, and it may distinguish neuropraxia from more severe disruption as neuropraxia may demonstrate only partial paralysis on faradic stimulation (McCauley and Labib, 1984); this is important in determining prognosis. Further studies are necessary to further elucidate this interesting technique.

ESOPHAGOGASTRIC JUNCTION AND LOWER ESOPHAGEAL SPHINCTER

General Considerations

The lower esophagus, containing the esophagogastric junction and lower esophageal sphincter, is a region of complex anatomy and function which passes through a series of stages of development during childhood. A knowledge of these changes is helpful in understanding the pathogenesis of both gastroesophageal reflux and hiatus hernia.

Anatomy and Physiology

Many anatomic terms such as cardia and phrenic ampulla used with respect to the esophagogastric junction and the lower esophageal sphincter are still confused and ill defined (Friedland, 1978). Hence, the terms are defined in the following discussion.

The Esophagogastric Junction

The esophagogastric junction is the point at the inferior end of the lower esophageal sphincter where sling fibers from the stomach and diaphragm loop around the base of the esophagus posterolaterally (Figure 7–15). Unfortunately, there are no radiologic landmarks to show the junction anteromedially. When the junction is closed, the adjacent gastric mucosa has a rosette appearance which can be appreciated on double-contrast study (Figure 7–16). These folds extending into the esophagus form the "mucosal choke" (Steiner, 1977).

The Lower Esophageal Sphincter

The normal lower esophageal sphincter is generally the area of the inferior end of the esophagus above the stomach between the phrenoesophageal membranes, approximately 4 cm long in adults and shorter in children. The length of the lower esophageal sphincter increases with age. The shorter lower esophageal sphincter is thought to be physiologically important and usually contains the junction of columnar and squamous epithelium, a macroscopically visible zigzag line (see Figure 7–15).

The lower esophageal sphincter is the functional junction of the esophagus and stomach and includes a zone of relatively high pressure about 15 to 30 mm Hg above gastric pressure (Steiner, 1977). This high pressure falls to gastric fundal pressure at the onset of swallowing (Wolf, 1970). Lower esophageal sphincter pressure in infants is well developed by 2 weeks of age, and until 1 year of age, this pressure is significantly higher than in older children.

The lower esophageal sphincter is controlled by the vagus nerve. This enables the sphincter to relax when the patient swallows, even if nothing passes down the esophagus. Higher intra-abdominal pressure is associated with an increase in the lower

esophageal sphincter pressure. Gastrin, cholinesterase inhibitors, and parasympathomimetics all increase the sphincter tone (Steiner, 1977).

Phrenoesophageal Membranes. The esophagus is attached to the diaphragm by phrenoesophageal membranes (Eliska, 1973). There are four types of attachment of the phrenoesophageal membrane depending on the age of the patient: fetal type, juvenile type, old-age type, and transitional type (Eliska, 1973; Friedland, 1978). Only the fetal and juvenile types are seen in children.

Fetal type. In the fetal type, there are two elastic phrenoesophageal membranes which arise from either side of the diaphragm, thoracic and abdominal, and are attached to each other and to the adventitia of the esophagus. The hiatus is narrowed, the margins are thick, and the infradiaphragmatic portion of the esophagus is short in comparison with

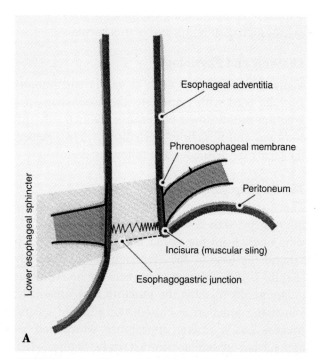
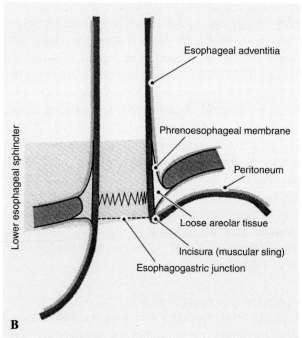

FIGURE 7–15. The esophagogastric junction. *A,* The fetal type of esophagogastric junction has elastic phrenoesophageal membranes which arise from either side of the diaphragm, thoracic and abdominal, and which are attached to each other and to the adventitia of the esophagus. The hiatus is narrowed, the margins are thick, and the infradiaphragmatic portion of the esophagus is short compared to that in adults. The result is a firm attachment between the esophagus and hiatus. *B,* In the juvenile type, the esophagogastric junction matures so that in infancy the margins of the hiatus are still thick but the hiatus is less narrow and is no longer always attached to the esophagus. This juvenile type, which is present until the third decade, has a thinned upper membrane and a double lower phrenoesophageal membrane. The two limbs of the lower membrane are separated by loose alveolar tissue, which allows for greater mobility of the esophagus through the hiatus than in the fetal type.

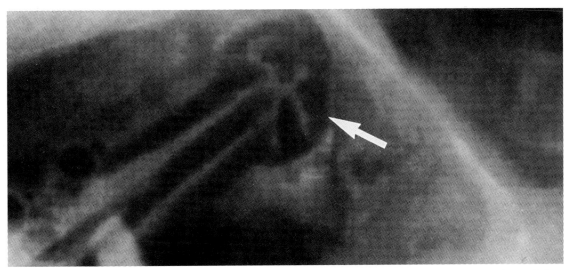

FIGURE 7–16. The esophagogastric junction. The gastric mucosa has a rosette appearance (*arrow*) best appreciated on double-contrast study.

that of adults. The result is a firm attachment between the esophagus and hiatus (Eliska, 1973; Friedland, 1978).

Juvenile type. In the juvenile type, the esophagogastric junction matures so that in infancy the margins of the hiatus are still thick but the hiatus is wider and no longer always attached to the esophagus (Eliska, 1973; Friedland, 1978). This type, which is present until the third decade, has a thinned upper membrane and a double lower phrenoesophageal membrane. The two limbs of the lower membrane are separated by loose alveolar tissue, which allows for greater mobility of the esophagus through the hiatus than in the fetal type (Eliska, 1973).

Old-age and transitional types. These two types are briefly described so that the spectrum of changes can be appreciated. After the third decade, the upper phrenoesophageal membrane atrophies, elastic tissue decreases, and the distance between the membranes increases so that mobility of the esophagus increases (Eliska, 1973; Friedland, 1978). The amount of fat between the phrenoesophageal membranes also increases, compounding this mobility (Eliska, 1973).

Other Factors of Physiologic Importance
Other factors thought physiologically important in maintaining competence of the esophagogastric junction are the length of the intra-abdominal esophagus and the acute angle between the esophagus and stomach. The portion of esophagus which is intra-

abdominal has been seen as part of the mechanism preventing gastroesophageal reflux but this portion is variable, decreasing on inspiration and swallowing (Friedland, 1978). The intra-abdominal esophagus is 3 cm long in adults but shorter in children. The angle between the esophagus and the stomach is acute in adults and is also called the incisura or angle of His. This angle is less acute in infancy.

Overall, the physiology of the normal gastroesophageal junction and the pathophysiology of gastroesophageal reflux and hiatus hernia are still poorly understood. They are probably closely related to the anatomy, however, particularly to the presence of a high-pressure area localized to the lower esophageal sphincter.

HIATUS HERNIA AND GASTROESOPHAGEAL REFLUX

General Considerations

Hiatus hernia occurs most often in infants and middle-aged patients. Its etiology is uncertain. Pressure differences between the thorax and abdomen are thought to be important but certainly not essential. In adults, raised intra-abdominal pressure may produce a hiatus hernia but there is little evidence for this in infancy.

The infantile esophagogastric junction differs from the juvenile in some respects. The hiatus is more of a narrow canal and the angle at which the esophagus enters the stomach is less acute in infants, with the squamocolumnar junction usually not seen (Steiner, 1977). In addition, infants have a more fetal type of lower esophageal sphincter with very elastic upper and lower phrenoesophageal membranes, which are attached to each other in the hiatus and weld the hiatal margin to the esophagus and its adventitia. These features may predispose to hiatus hernia and gastroesophageal reflux although the exact mechanism is unclear.

There is a well-recognized association between hiatus hernia and delayed gastric emptying, suggesting that raised intragastric pressure with active gastric peristalsis may be an important etiologic factor, and hypertrophic pyloric stenosis producing gastric outlet obstruction has been found in up to 10% of infants with hiatus hernia (Johnston, 1965; McCallum et al., 1981; Smellie, 1954). Other associated anomalies in children with gastroesophageal reflux include midgut malrotation and duodenal web (Humphreys et al., 1965; Thommesen et al., 1977). Therefore, the gastric outlet and the duodenum should be examined at the initial barium investigation whenever reflux is detected. A hiatus hernia associated with severe vomiting is occasionally a complication of Bochdalek's hernia repair in infants (Cohen and Beck, 1980).

Clinical Findings

General

Gastroesophageal reflux can produce problems starting at birth. In the first weeks of life, a minor degree of lower esophageal reflux is common and usually settles quickly as the infant matures and becomes capable of upright posture. In some infants, however, more pronounced reflux may occur, with esophagitis evidenced by repeated, often bloodstained vomiting. If reflux is still present at 18 months of age, it is less likely to resolve spontaneously and may require surgery.

The infant with hiatus hernia and/or gastroesophageal reflux may present with failure to thrive and is often below the tenth percentile (Cahill et al., 1969). Dysphagia is unusual and when present indicates esophagitis with or without stricture.

Secondary iron deficiency anemia can occur. Pulmonary complications such as aspiration pneumonia are related to the severity of the reflux (Darling et al., 1978). Delay in gastric emptying or hypertrophic pyloric stenosis may underlie hiatus hernia as

may chronic unremitting asthma (Friedland et al., 1973). The differential diagnosis for recurrent aspiration pneumonia includes H-type tracheoesophageal fistula and swallowing abnormalities with aspiration.

A large hiatus hernia may occasionally produce gastric obstruction and volvulus (Gerson and Lewicki, 1976; Daneman and Kozlowski, 1977). Total herniation of the stomach into the thorax occurs rarely (Harp et al., 1965) and may be accompanied by herniation of the duodenum. Reflux has been implicated in the production of apnea (Leape et al., 1977) and sudden infant death syndrome (Herbst et al., 1978) although this is not an invariable finding (Walsh et al., 1981). Hiatus hernia and reflux may rarely be familial (Steiner, 1977). Neurologic disorders can be associated with reflux, and mental retardation is the most frequent associated clinical finding in children with reflux esophagitis at our hospital. Rarely, a central nervous system tumor may cause reflux.

Sandifer's Syndrome

Sandifer's syndrome is the association of hiatus hernia and abnormal movements of the head and neck during or after eating (Sutcliffe, 1969). The gastrointestinal symptoms may be overlooked and the patient referred to a neurologist. Dramatic relief can be obtained with surgical repair of the hiatus hernia. Torticollis may be associated with gastroesophageal reflux without hiatus hernia (Taybi, 1982).

Cystic Fibrosis

Gastroesophageal reflux with and without hiatus hernia has been reported as an association of cystic fibrosis documented by barium esophagography, endoscopy, and 24-hour pH-probe monitoring (Bendig et al., 1982; Scott et al., 1985). Gastroesophageal reflux is also associated with a decrease in lung function tests (Stringer et al., 1988). The exact cause of gastroesophageal reflux in cystic fibrosis is uncertain but a combination of lung hyperinflation, increased coughing, and physiotherapy (Foster et al., 1982) or drug treatment (Bendig et al., 1982) may be implicated. Hyperinflation, which depresses the diaphragm, may alter the relationship of intrathoracic and intra-abdominal pressures, resulting in reflux (Bendig et al., 1982). An increase in episodes of gastroesophageal reflux is associated with postural chest physiotherapy in children with cystic fibrosis (Foster et al., 1982). Gastroesophageal reflux may also be preceded or exacerbated by coughing (Bendig et al., 1982; Pellegrini et al., 1979) but we have not noticed any correlation of gastroesophageal reflux with coughing during our barium meal studies.

In normal adults and children, reflux is often associated with a transient, inappropriate reduction in lower esophageal sphincter pressure (Dent et al., 1980; Werlin et al., 1980). In cystic fibrosis, medications such as β-adrenergic agonists or methylxanthine compounds can reduce lower esophageal sphincter pressure (Berquist et al., 1981). In addition, cholecystokinin, which is elevated in patients with pancreatic insufficiency, may decrease lower esophageal sphincter pressure (Harvey et al., 1973). However, initial investigations have not confirmed such a reduction in resting lower esophageal sphincter pressure in patients with cystic fibrosis and gastroesophageal reflux (Scott et al., 1985).

Although gastroesophageal reflux is associated with reduced pulmonary function in cystic fibrosis patients, gastroesophageal reflux does not necessarily cause reduced function. Children with severe disease may have greater lung hyperinflation and increased coughing, and they may require drugs or physiotherapy that predisposes to further reflux. Gastroesophageal reflux may in turn exacerbate the already reduced pulmonary function through recurrent aspiration of gastric contents. However, the association of cystic fibrosis, gastroesophageal reflux, and pulmonary aspiration is unproved.

Occasionally severe complications of gastroesophageal reflux occur (Bendig et al., 1982), such as esophagitis with stricture formation (Figure 7–17). These complications may be difficult to treat because of the severe lung disease. The hypersecretion of gastric acid in cystic fibrosis (Cox et al., 1982), if aspirated, could be related to the severity of the complications although no association has been proved. It is important to give symptomatic relief in addition to preventing the complications of gastroesophageal reflux because of the increased hazard of surgery in these already debilitated children.

Imaging and Other Investigations

Diagnosis of gastroesophageal reflux is best made clinically but when there is clinical concern over the diagnosis or if medical management fails, further investigation is warranted. In addition, structural abnormalities primary or secondary to the reflux can be excluded by imaging studies. However, just as the mechanism of hiatus hernia and gastro-

esophageal reflux is controversial, so are the methods of diagnosis.

Plain Film

Plain films are not usually advocated for diagnosing hiatus hernia or gastroesophageal reflux. They are of value for patients in whom a gastroesophageal abnormality is unsuspected and in whom the films suggest lung aspiration secondary to reflux or show a hiatus hernia, which appears as a retrocardiac lucency (Figure 7–18).

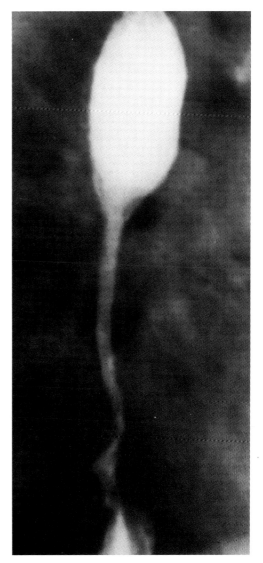

FIGURE 7–17. Reflux esophagitis stricture in a child with cystic fibrosis. A long stricture is present with gradual tapering at either end and some mucosal irregularity in a child with cystic fibrosis and gross gastroesophageal reflux despite previous Nissen fundoplication.

Ultrasonography

Ultrasonography can play an important role in the diagnosis of gastroesophageal reflux in children under the age of 5 years (Naik and Moore, 1984; Naik et al., 1985) as it is noninvasive and safe. The patient drinks water or, in the case of babies, dextrose water to fill the stomach with fluid. Ultrasonography is then performed with the patient supine. A sagittal section slightly to left of the midline on real time is obtained with the transducer in the epigastrium. The heart is seen to lie above and anterior to the aorta and above the crus of the diaphragm. It is in the triangle delineated by these structures that gastroesophageal reflux is looked for, and it is indicated by opening of the gastric cardia and bubbling fluid entering the space from below the diaphragm (Figure 7–19).

Initial results show reasonable correlation with a barium meal examination (Naik et al., 1985). The major disadvantages are that it may be time consuming and the region of interest may not be easily visualized.

Barium Studies

Previously, a lower incidence of hiatus hernia and reflux was found in the United States compared with

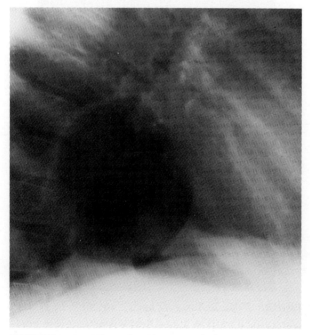

FIGURE 7–18. Hiatus hernia. Lateral chest examination shows a large hiatus hernia producing a retrocardiac lucency.

that in the U.K. and Canada. The disparity disappeared when spot films of the gastroesophageal junction, using a thick barium, were taken with patients in the prone, oblique, and supine positions. The prone position is least helpful because in this position, swallowed and refluxed air rather than barium collects adjacent to the gastroesophageal junction. A delayed film is often useful and may demonstrate gastroesophageal reflux during a small-bowel study (Friedland et al., 1974; Darling, 1975; Swyer, 1955; Darling et al., 1974).

Even using a standardized method of examination, however, the high sensitivity can result in low specificity (Leonidas, 1984; Cleveland et al., 1983). The barium study can be performed when conservative treatment of a refluxing child fails or there is concern over a possible anatomic abnormality such as stricture, gastric outlet or duodenal obstruction. The examination technique is described in Chapter 3. The examination can be used specifically to look for hiatus hernia or gastroesophageal reflux and also to exclude gastric outlet obstruction.

Barium meal findings of hiatus hernia. In contrast to the normal parallel esophageal mucosal folds, esophagography may show a small hiatus hernia with gastric folds converging above the hiatus. The earliest manifestation of this abnormality is tenting or beaking of the esophagogastric junction (Cleveland et al., 1983) (Figure 7–20). The areae gastricae traversing the esophageal hiatus have been used as a criterion for the presence of a hiatus hernia in adults (Gelfand and Ott, 1979). This has not been described in children, and the areae gastricae are more difficult to see in children than in adults. A moderate-sized hiatus hernia is more obvious (Figure 7–21). When a major portion of the stomach lies within the thorax, it is sometimes called a partial intrathoracic stomach (Figure 7–22). The diagnosis is usually obvious but may cause problems in infancy especially when a nasogastric tube has been inserted into an unusually located stomach (Figure 7–23). Gastric volvulus may also be associated with a partial intrathoracic stomach.

Barium meal findings of gastroesophageal reflux. There is no general agreement on the best method of testing for gastroesophageal reflux on barium swallow, and indeed, there is no general agreement on the usefulness of any radiologic observations. If spontaneous reflux is not seen, it may be elicited by gently rocking the supine infant or child

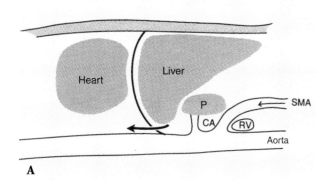

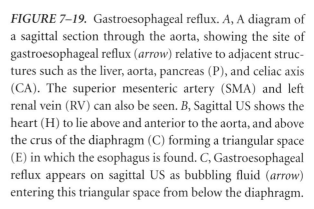

FIGURE 7–19. Gastroesophageal reflux. *A,* A diagram of a sagittal section through the aorta, showing the site of gastroesophageal reflux (*arrow*) relative to adjacent structures such as the liver, aorta, pancreas (P), and celiac axis (CA). The superior mesenteric artery (SMA) and left renal vein (RV) can also be seen. *B,* Sagittal US shows the heart (H) to lie above and anterior to the aorta, and above the crus of the diaphragm (C) forming a triangular space (E) in which the esophagus is found. *C,* Gastroesophageal reflux appears on sagittal US as bubbling fluid (*arrow*) entering this triangular space from below the diaphragm.

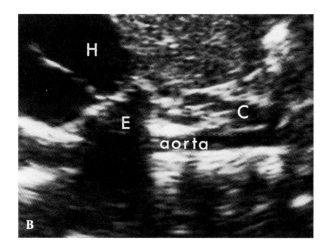

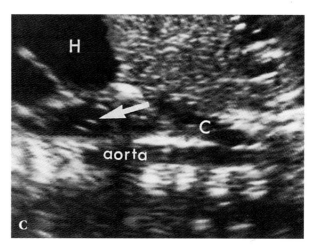

from left to right posterior oblique positions. Palpating the abdomen and placing the patient in a head-down position are nonphysiologic maneuvers; reflux elicited in this manner is of uncertain significance. Valsalva's maneuver in children is usually impractical (Blumhagen and Christie, 1979).

The presence of major or minor reflux is determined by the anatomic level reached by the reflux (McCauley et al., 1978). Reflux is most significant if it occurs spontaneously and repeatedly reaches a level above the clavicles in a quiet infant lying supine after having been burped. Major reflux, above the clavicles and into the cervical esophagus, has a higher incidence of pulmonary complications (Darling et al., 1978).

Water Siphon Test

The water siphon test as used in adults has a reasonable correlation with the symptoms of reflux (Crummy, 1966). Using pH-probe testing as the reference standard, the water siphon test detects 95% of cases of reflux in infants and children whereas only 38% of these patients will have spontaneous reflux of barium. Since the false-positive rate is high, the test is useful mainly for excluding, rather than making, the diagnosis of reflux (Blumhagen and Christie, 1979).

Twenty-Four-Hour pH-Probe Test

The 24-hour pH-probe test is a sensitive test for gastroesophageal reflux (Euler and Byrne, 1981) but a number of false-positive results occur (Tuttle and Grossman, 1958). The disadvantages of the pH-probe test are that it is technically demanding and relatively invasive.

Manometry

Various techniques for manometry of the lower esophageal sphincter zone have been devised. In adults with gastroesophageal reflux, the lower esophageal sphincter pressure is generally less than it is in adults without reflux; individual pressure readings are less helpful, however (Richter and Castell, 1982). The results in children are even less

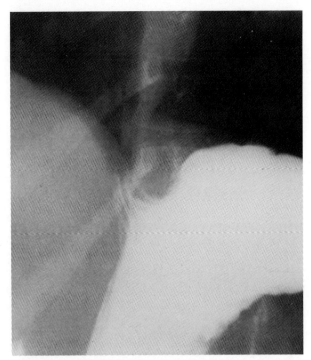

FIGURE 7–20. Small hiatus hernia. The esophagogastric junction is tented with converging gastric folds entering the hiatus, the earliest sign of hiatus hernia.

clear because less than half of those with reflux show the expected decrease in lower esophageal sphincter pressure (Moroz et al., 1976).

Nuclear Medicine Studies

Technetium Tc 99m sulfur colloid mixed with milk or the patient's normal feeding is given orally or by nasogastric tube which is removed after feeding or through a gastrostomy. The patient should be kept NPO for 4 hours and should not have any barium studies for at least 24 hours as contrast in the bowel attenuates photons and renders scintigraphic evaluation suboptimal. Serial posterior gamma camera images are obtained to evaluate gastroesophageal reflux or lung aspiration as shown by the presence of radionuclide in the esophagus or lungs, respectively (Figure 7–24) (Heyman et al., 1979; Heyman et al., 1982; Rudd and Christie, 1979; Fisher et al., 1976). The associated delay in gastric emptying is also routinely evaluated by milk formula labeled with technetium Tc 99m sulfur colloid (Hillemeier et al., 1981). When a child is given a meal via nastogastric tube or gastrostomy, dynamic scanning is performed at the time of tracer administration to ensure proper location of the tube. If delivery of food into antrum or duodenum occurs, the study should be terminated and rescheduled. The scintigraphic technique is relatively easy and sensitive and allows for quantification of gastroesophageal reflux and gastric emptying (Piepsz et al., 1981; Fisher et al., 1976). There is good correlation between the 24-hour esophageal pH-probe test and scintigraphic evaluation of gastroesophageal reflux in some institutions

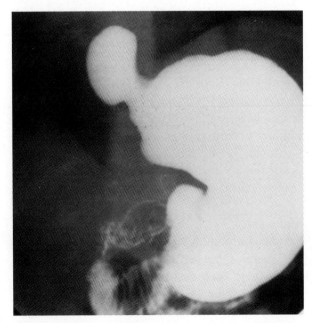

FIGURE 7–21. Moderate-sized hiatus hernia. A large part of the stomach has herniated superior to the diaphragm.

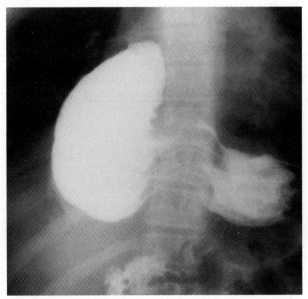

FIGURE 7–22. Partial intrathoracic stomach. Having herniated through the hiatus, a major portion of the stomach lies within the thorax.

(Siebert et al., 1983); we have found the latter not quite as sensitive but much less invasive. The technique is discussed in more detail in Chapter 3.

Radionuclide salivagram is a clinically valuable and safe test for evaluating aspiration of oral secretions in neurologically impaired children with dysphagia in whom a fluoroscopic barium swallow may be difficult to perform due to their inability to swallow. Technetium Tc 99m sulfur colloid in 1 mL of saline is placed in the patient's mouth, and dynamic images are obtained up to 30 minutes for evaluation of tracheobronchial and pulmonary aspiration. This is a simple and sensitive technique for detecting aspiration prior to attempting oral feeds in neurologically impaired children.

Endoscopy

Esophagoscopy is primarily used to detect esophagitis and assess the need for operative treatment if other studies have not been helpful. Biopsies can show infective esophagitis (see Chapter 6) or columnar-lined (Barrett's) esophagus (see Chapter 7). The presence of intraepithelial eosinophils may indicate prolonged reflux, and biopsies of the esophagus have been recommended since observation alone is less reliable (Winter et al., 1982).

Treatment of Uncomplicated Gastroesophageal Reflux

Many healthy infants have clinical or imaged evidence of reflux but only a few will require surgical attention. In most cases, it is best to treat infants conservatively, with no specific investigation (Leonidas, 1984). Conservative treatment consisting of small, frequent thickened feedings and appropriate positioning (Herbst, 1981) will yield curative results in most infants. Further study such as barium meal examination can be reserved for children over 1 year

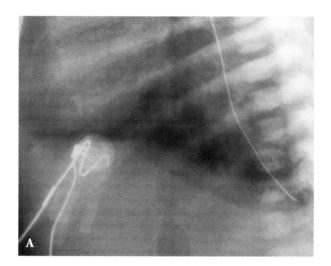

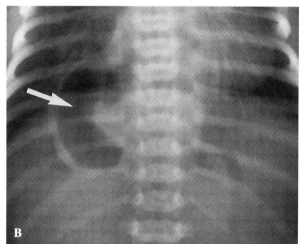

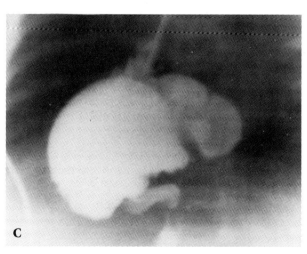

FIGURE 7–23. Intrathoracic stomach. *A,* Plain lateral film taken after nasogastric tube insertion shows a posterior location of the tube, suggesting perforation. *B,* Follow-up film shows a gas-filled structure resembling gut (*arrow*). *C,* Contrast study confirms the structure as an intrathoracic stomach.

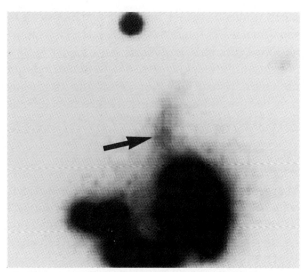

FIGURE 7–24. Gastroesophageal reflux. Activity of technetium Tc 99m sulfur colloid reappears in the esophagus (*arrows*) after a milk radionuclide feed.

of age who have continuing symptoms or signs as these more often require surgical management.

Complications of Gastroesophageal Reflux

Esophagitis and Strictures

Reflux esophagitis can occur without any predisposing abnormality but is more likely when there is defective esophageal peristalsis. This occurs after repair of esophageal atresia because peristalsis of the esophagus is normal above but abnormal below the site of the surgical repair (see Chapter 6). Swallowed food reaches the lower esophagus below the anastomosis in these conditions and tends to stagnate due to lack of peristalsis.

The lower esophageal sphincter usually opens in response to the normal peristaltic wave of the esophagus but in the absence of this wave, the sphincter can still open in response to deglutition. This still occurs after transection of the esophagus following primary anastomosis for esophageal atresia or following colon interposition in esophageal atresia without fistula (Chrispin and Friedland, 1966). After deglutition, the lower esophageal sphincter still relaxes and gastroesophageal reflux can occur. As a result of defective peristalsis, refluxed gastric contents remain in the esophagus with the swallowed food and produce inflammation.

Debilitated patients, such as those with severe neurologic problems who spend long periods of time supine, are also at risk of esophagitis as reflux drains less efficiently when a patient is recumbent.

One of the earliest radiologic signs of esophagitis is the presence of irregular contractions, which may be present when reflux occurs into the esophagus (Figure 7–25). Transverse striations (feline contractions or "shiver") are more common with gastroesophageal reflux (Williams et al., 1983). Irregularity of the esophageal wall develops later and is best seen on careful double-contrast views as a granular pattern or erosions (Creteur et al., 1983; Maglinte et al., 1983). Unfortunately, double-contrast views may not be possible in many younger children, and the assessment of early mucosal involvement becomes difficult especially since there is poor correlation of single-contrast examination and esophageal biopsy when there is mild esophagitis (Darling et al., 1982; Creteur et al., 1983).

Stricture formation secondary to reflux esophagitis may occur rapidly, and the appearance is easily demonstrated (Figure 7–26). A subtle early manifestation of stricture formation may be a stepladder appearance secondary to transverse folds from longitudinal scarring (Levine et al., 1984). These are not to be confused with the more transitory feline "shiver" of esophagitis. Rarely, pseudomembranes may be seen (Levine et al., 1986).

Barrett's Esophagus

Barrett's esophagus (columnar-lined esophagus) in children is secondary to gastroesophageal reflux, as in adults. This etiology is supported by evidence of Bremner et al. who stripped the squamous epithelium from the esophagi of dogs and noted its predominant replacement by columnar epithelium in those animals with induced gastroesophageal reflux and hypersecretion (Bremner et al., 1970). In addition, a number of conditions predisposing to lower esophageal incompetence and gastroesophageal reflux have also been associated with Barrett's esophagus, namely scleroderma, previous myotomy for achalasia, previous gastric surgery, and indwelling nasogastric tubes (Halpert et al., 1984).

The columnar mucosa histologically resembles stomach but the mucous glands are esophageal in type, parietal cells are lacking, and the mucosa may contain patches of squamous epithelium (Pierce and Creamer, 1963; Bremner et al., 1970; Robbins et al., 1978).

Radiologically, the appearance is of a stricture or ulceration that classically is in the proximal

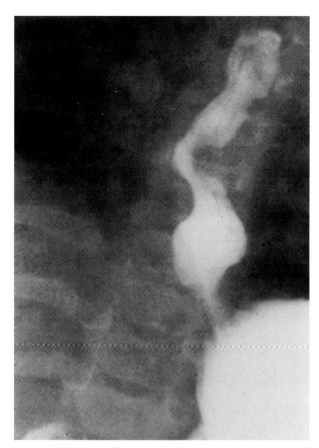

FIGURE 7–25. Reflux esophagitis. Irregular esophageal contractions giving a serpiginous outline to the esophagus, an early sign of esophagitis, accompany an episode of gastroesophageal reflux.

esophagus but can often be found more distally (Robbins et al., 1978; Halpert et al., 1984). In 13% of cases, however, neither a stricture nor radiologic evidence of ulceration is present (Robbins et al., 1978).

The presence of hiatus hernia, gastroesophageal reflux, and esophagitis with the strictures is common (Shapir et al., 1985; Halpert et al., 1984) but is not diagnostic of Barrett's esophagus (Levine et al., 1983; Halpert et al., 1984). Other signs reported on double-contrast examinations include distal esophageal widening; a granular, nodular, or reticular mucosal pattern; and intramural pseudodiverticula (Chen et al., 1985; Levine et al., 1983; Halpert et al., 1984; Shapir et al., 1985; Vincent et al., 1984). The reticular pattern is the most commonly noted distinctive feature. However, when the areas affected by this pattern are examined histologically, the mucosa may be normal or abnormal, squamous or columnar, and benign or malignant. Hence,

although a strong indicator of Barrett's esophagus, the reticular pattern is not specific for any type of mucosa (Vincent et al., 1984).

In addition, there is an increased incidence of adenocarcinoma of the esophagus (Levine et al., 1984; Agha, 1985) occurring in later life—a grave cause of concern as our children have a long life expectancy.

Although the radiographic features in children are similar to those in adults, there are some important differences. Hiatus hernia is much less common in children. Ulceration is usually detectable by double-contrast study but these are more difficult in children and may not be possible in younger children. Detection of ulceration with single-contrast studies is poor. Abnormal esophageal motility is present in approximately one-third of cases, often related to underlying disorders such as esophageal atresia. Strictures are present in approx-

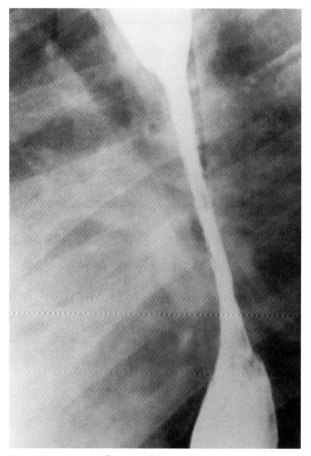

FIGURE 7–26. Reflux esophagitis stricture. A long stricture with gradual tapering at either end and some mucosal irregularity is present in a child with cerebral palsy and gross gastroesophageal reflux.

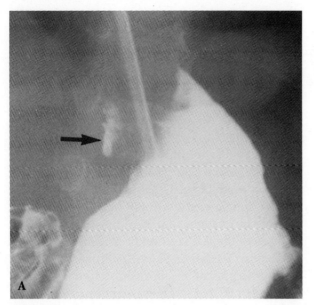
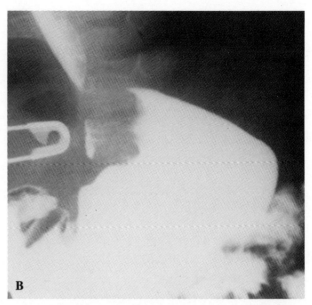

FIGURE 7–27. Nissen fundoplication. The fundus is wrapped around the lower esophagus in a Nissen fundoplication. *A,* A small amount of barium is present in the wrap (*arrow*); the nasogastric tube shows the position of the esophageal lumen. *B,* After removal of the tube, the supradiaphragmatic esophagus fills with barium.

imately 40%. The most common radiographic finding is gastroesophageal reflux but this is nonspecific (Yulish et al., 1987).

Technetium Tc 99m pertechnetate scintigraphy may demonstrate uptake in the ectopic gastric mucosa of Barrett's esophagus. Following an intravenous injection of Tc 99m pertechnetate, scanning

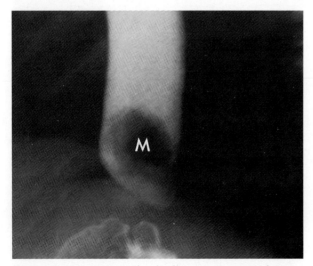

FIGURE 7–28. Nissen fundoplication causing obstruction. A bolus of meat appearing as a negative filling defect on barium swallow (M), has become impacted at the tight Nissen fundoplication.

is performed with the patient in a right lateral decubitus position to reduce the possibility of activity in the esophagus due to gastroesophageal reflux. Posterior, anterior, and left lateral planar images or three-dimensional single photon emission computed tomography (SPECT) images may be obtained. If activity is detected in the esophagus, the imaging is repeated (following ingestion of water) to distinguish persistent focal uptake in Barrett's esophagus from gastroesophageal reflux.

The definitive diagnostic modality in children and adults remains endoscopy and biopsy because of the nonspecific nature of imaging findings (Shapir et al., 1985).

Follow-Up

Treatment and Clinical Features

The majority of infants with vomiting and a small hiatus hernia resolve their symptoms spontaneously (Carre, 1959; Carre, 1960). This can be expedited by positional therapy (Carre and Astley, 1960; Carre, 1952), thickening of the feeds, and weaning to solid foods (Carre et al., 1952). Surgery should be reserved for patients who have serious complications or in whom medical management fails (Friedland et al., 1975). A 20-year follow-up has shown that over 90% of children treated nonoperatively

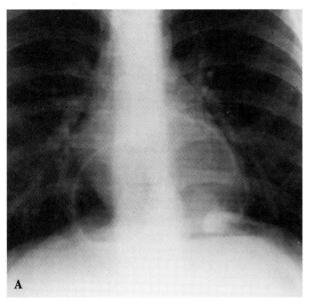 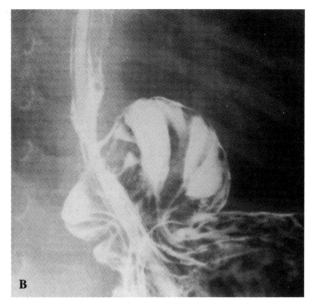

FIGURE 7–29. Herniation of Nissen fundoplication. *A*, The plication has herniated, producing a paraesophageal hernia shown on plain film as a relative lucency overlying the heart. *B*, The same, seen on barium study. The nasogastric tube helps show the position of the esophagus.

were asymptomatic whereas the majority of the more severe cases who required surgery or had strictures were still symptomatic (Astley et al., 1977). The indications for surgery are failure to thrive, persistent vomiting, and the development of complications including hematemesis, anemia, and stricture, and a large hiatus hernia or a partial thoracic stomach (Ein et al., 1979).

Postoperative Appearance
Fundoplication can appear as a soft-tissue mass in the gastric fundus on plain films. Barium examination demonstrates the fundal deformity (Figure 7–27). If the plication is tight, the passage of barium or food is delayed (Figure 7–28) or eructation is impeded (the "gas bloat" syndrome). This complication occurs less frequently if a partial wrap is used (Ein et al., 1979). Gastric stenosis with an hourglass configuration may result from Nissen fundoplication (Thoeni and Moss, 1979). Herniation of a plication may sometimes occur and can be clearly demonstrated on plain film as well as barium examination (Figure 7–29).

When severe esophageal complications develop, the esophagus can be replaced either by a gastric tube or an interposed colon (see section on tracheoesophageal fistula and esophageal atresia in Chapter 6).

REFERENCES

EMBRYOGENESIS

Gray SW, Skandalakis JE. Embryology for surgeons: the embryological basis for the treatment of congenital defects. Philadelphia: WB Saunders; 1972.

Panicek DM, Benson CB, Gottlieb RH, Heitzman ER. The diaphragm: anatomic, pathologic, and radiologic considerations. Radiographics 1988;8:385–425.

Snyder WH, Greaney EM. Congenital diaphragmatic hernia: 77 consecutive cases. Surgery 1965;57:576–88.

CONGENITAL AND DEVELOPMENTAL ANOMALIES

Bochdalek's (Pleuroperitoneal) Hernia

Akierman AR, Mayock DE. Group B streptococcal septicemia and delayed onset congenital right sided diaphragmatic hernia. Can Med Assoc J 1983;129:1289–90.

Allen MS, Thomson SA. Congenital diaphragmatic hernia in children under one year of age: a 24 year review. J Pediatr Surg 1966;1:157–61.

Baker DH, Berdon WE. Arteriography for diagnosis of congenital diaphragmatic hernia. J Pediatr 1977;90:1034.

Bell MJ, Ternbert JL. Antenatal diagnosis of diaphragmatic hernia. Pediatrics 1977;60:738–40.

Berdon WE, Baker DH, Amoury R. The role of pulmonary hypoplasia in the prognosis of newborn infants with diaphragmatic hernia and eventration. AJR 1968; 103:413–21.

Berman L, Stringer DA, Ein SH, Shandling B. Childhood diaphragmatic hernias presenting after the neonatal period. Clin Radiol 1988;39:237–44.

Bohn DJ, James I, Filler RM, et al. The relationship between PaCO2 and ventilation parameters in predicting survival in congenital diaphragmatic hernia. J Pediatr Surg 1984;19:666–71.

Bonham-Carter RE, Waterston DJ, Aberdeen E. Hernia and eventration of the diaphragm in childhood. Lancet 1962;1:656–9.

Bosher LH, Fishman L, Webb WR, et al. Strangulated diaphragmatic hernia with gangrene and perforation of the stomach. Dis Chest 1960;37:505–12.

Burke EC, Wenzl JE, Utz DC. The intrathoracic kidney. Am J Dis Child 1967;113:487–90.

Canino CW, Eichmann J, Rominger CJ, et al. Congenital right diaphragmatic hernia. Radiology 1964;82:249–52.

Carter BN, Giuseffi J. Strangulated diaphragmatic hernia. Ann Surg 1948;128:210–25.

Cerilli GJ. Foramen of Bochdalek's hernia. Ann Surg 1964;159:385–9.

Claiborne AK, Martin CM, McAlister WH, et al. Antenatal diagnosis of cystic adenomatoid malformation: effect on patient management. Pediatr Radiol 1985;15:337–9.

Cohen MD, Beck JM. Hiatus hernia: a complication of posterolateral diaphragmatic herniation (Bochdalek's hernia) in infants. Clin Radiol 1980;31:215–19.

Comstock CH. The antenatal diagnosis of diaphragmatic anomalies. J Ultrasound Med 1986;5:391–6.

Craig JM, Kirkpatrick J, Neuhauser EBD. Congenital cystic adenomatoid malformation of the lung in infants. AJR 1956;76:516–26.

Davies MRQ, Cywes S, Rode H. Cystic pulmonary hamartoma simulating posterolateral diaphragmatic hernia. S Afr Med J 1979;56:947–50.

Day B. Late appearance of Bochdalek's hernia. BMJ 1972; 1:786.

Deaner S, McMenemey WH, Smith SM. Hemothorax due to strangulated hernia. BMJ 1983;1:22.

Ein SH, Barker G, Olley P, et al. The pharmacologic treatment of newborn diaphragmatic hernia: a 2 year evaluation. J Pediatr Surg 1980;15:384–94.

Gaisie G, Young LW, Oh KS. Late onset Bochdalek's hernia with obstruction: radiographic spectrum of presentation. Clin Radiol 1983;34:267–70.

Gale ME. Bochdalek's hernia: prevalence and CT characteristics. Radiology 1985;156:449–52.

Gilsanz V, Emons D, Hansmann M, et al. Hydrothorax, ascites and right diaphragmatic hernia. Radiology 1986; 158:243–6.

Glasson MJ, Barter W, Cohen DH, et al. Congenital left posterolateral diaphragmatic hernia with previously normal chest x-ray. Pediatr Radiol 1975;3:201–5.

Guibaud L, Filiatrault D, Garel L, et al. Fetal congenital diaphragmatic hernia: accuracy of US in the diagnosis and prediction of the outcome after birth. AJR 1996;166: 1195–1202.

Harrington SW. Diaphragmatic hernia of children. Ann Surg 1942;115:705–15.

Karasick S, O'Hara B, Karasick D, et al. Supradiaphragmatic cyst following surgical repair of congenital diaphragmatic hernia. Radiology 1978;129:142.

Kenigsberg K, Gwinn JL. The retained sac in repair of posterolateral diaphragmatic hernia in the newborn. Surgery 1965;57:894–7.

Kirkland JA. Congenital posterolateral hernia in the adult. Br J Surg 1959;47:16–22.

Levy RJ, Rosenthal A, Freed MD, et al. Persistent pulmonary hypertension in a newborn with congenital diaphragmatic hernia: successful management with tolazoline. Pediatrics 1977;60:740–2.

McCarten KM, Rosenberg HK, Borden S, et al. Delayed appearance of right diaphragmatic hernia associated with group B streptococcal infection in newborns. Radiology 1981;139:385–9.

Miller FJ, Varano LA, Shocat SJ. Umbilical arteriography for the rapid diagnosis of congenital diaphragmatic hernia in the newborn infant. J Pediatr 1977;90:993–4.

Mishalany HG, Nakada K, Woolley MM. Congenital diaphragmatic hernias. Eleven years' experience. Arch Surg 1979;114:1118–23.

Omojola MF, Reilly BJ, Mancer K. Emphysema associated with pulmonary hypoplasia in congenital diaphragmatic hernia. AJR 1981;136:1007–9.

Osebold WR, Soper RT. Congenital posterolateral diaphragmatic hernia past infancy. Am J Surg 1976;131:748–54.

Reed JO, Lang EF. Diaphragmatic hernia in infancy. AJR 1959;82:437–49.

Sagel SS, Ablow RC. The use of umbilical venography for the diagnosis of congenital right-sided diaphragmatic hernia. Radiology 1968;91:797–8.

Siegel MJ, Shackleford GD, McAlister WH. Left-sided congenital diaphragmatic hernia: delayed presentation. AJR 1981;137:43–6.

Snyder WH, Greaney EM. Congenital diaphragmatic hernia: 77 consecutive cases. Surgery 1965;57:576–88.

Sumner TE, Volberg FM, Smolen PM. Intrathoracic kidney: diagnosis by ultrasound. Pediatr Radiol 1982;12:78–80.

Tovar J, Benavent MI. Diaphragmatic hernia associated with double pulmonary sequestration. J Pediatr Surg 1979;14:604–6.

Whittaker LD, Lynn HB, Dawson B, et al. Hernias of the foramen of Bochdalek in children. Mayo Clin Proc 1968;43:580–91.

Wiseman NE, MacPherson R. "Acquired" congenital diaphragmatic hernia. J Pediatr Surg 1977;12:657–65.

Eventration

Bonham-Carter RE, Waterston DJ, Aberdeen E. Hernia and eventration of the diaphragm in childhood. Lancet 1962;1:656–9.

Jurcak-Zaleski S, Comstock CH, Kirk JS. Eventration of the diaphragm: prenatal diagnosis. Case report. J Ultrasound Med 1990;9:351–4.

Lundstrom CH, Allen RP. Bilateral congenital eventration of the diaphragm. AJR 1966;97:216–7.

Moccia WA, Kaude JV, Felman AH. Congenital eventration of the diaphragm. Pediatr Radiol 1981;10:197–200.

Rodgers BM, Hawks P. Bilateral congenital eventrations of the diaphragms: successful surgical management. J Pediatr Surg 1986;21:858–64.

Spencer RP, Spackman TJ, Pearson HA. Diagnosis of right diaphragmatic eventration by means of liver scan. Radiology 1971;99:375–6.

Wayne ER, Campbell JB, Burrington JD, et al. Eventration of the diaphragm. J Pediatr Surg 1974;9:643–51.

Morgagni's (Retrosternal) Hernia

Baran EM, Houston HE, Lynn HB, et al. Foramen of Morgagni hernias in children. Surgery 1967;62:1076–81.

Bingham JAW. Hernia through congenital diaphragmatic defects. Br J Surg 1959;201:1–15.

Comer TP, Clagett OT. Surgical treatment of hernia of the foramen of Morgagni. J Thorac Cardiovasc Surg 1966;52:238–40.

Forshall I. Less common herniae through the diaphragm in infants and children. Proc R Soc Med 1966;59:212–4.

Schneidau A, Baron HJ, Rosin RD. Morgagni revisited: a case of intermittent chest pain. Br J Radiol 1982;55:238–40.

Peritoneopericardial Hernia

Wilson AK, Rumel WR, Ross OL. Peritoneopericardial diaphragmatic hernia. AJR 1947;57:42–9.

Traumatic Diaphragmatic Hernia

Ball T, McCrory R, Smith JO, et al. Traumatic diaphragmatic hernia: errors in diagnosis. AJR 1982;138:633–7.

Cruz CJ, Minagi H. Large bowel obstruction resulting from traumatic diaphragmatic hernia: imaging findings in four cases. AJR 1994;162:843–5.

Fung HMY, Vickar DB. Traumatic rupture of the right hemidiaphragm with hepatic herniation: real-time ultrasound demonstration. J Ultrasound Med 1991;10:295–8.

Gelman R, Mirvis SE, Gens D. Diaphramatic rupture due to blunt trauma: sensitivity of plain chest radiographs. AJR 1991;156:51–7.

McHugh K, Ogilvie BC, Brunton FJ. Delayed presentation of traumatic diaphragmatic hernia. Clin Radiol 1991;43:246–50.

Worthy SA, Kang EY, Hartman TE, et al. Diaphragmatic rupture: CT findings in 11 patients. Radiology 1995;194:885–8.

DIAPHRAGM PARALYSIS

Alexander C. Diaphragm movements and the diagnosis of diaphragmatic paralysis. Clin Radiol 1966;17:79–83.

Gierada DS, Curtin JJ, Erickson SJ, et al. Diaphramatic motion: fast gradient-recalled-echo MR imaging in healthy subjects. Radiology 1995;194:879–84.

Haber K, Asher WM, Freimanis AK. Echographic evaluation of diaphragmatic motion in intra-abdominal diseases. Radiology 1975;114:141–4.

Harris RS, Giovanetti M, Kim BK. Normal ventilatory movement of the right hemidiaphragm studied by US and pneumotachography. Radiology 1983;146:141–4.

Houston JG, Fleet M, Cowan MD, McMillan NC. Comparison of ultrasound with fluoroscopy in the assessment of suspected hemidiaphragmatic movement abnormality. Clin Radiol 1995;50:95–8.

Khan AN, Gould DA. The primary role of ultrasound in evaluating right-sided diaphragmatic humps and juxtadiaphragmatic masses: a review of 22 cases. Clin Radiol 1984;35:413–18.

Lowe SH, Cosgrove DO, Joseph AEA. Inversion of the right hemidiaphragm shown on ultrasound examination. Br J Radiol 1981;54:754–7.

McCauley RGK, Labib KB. Diaphragmatic paralysis evaluated by phrenic nerve stimulation during fluoroscopy or real-time ultrasound. Radiology 1984;153:33–6.

Odita JC, Khan ASSI, Dincsoy M, et al. Neonatal phrenic nerve paralysis resulting from intercostal drainage of pneumothorax. Pediatr Radiol 1992;22:379–81.

Young DA, Simon G. Certain movements measured on inspiration-expiration, chest radiographs correlated with pulmonary function studies. Clin Radiol 1972;23:37–41.

ESOPHAGOGASTRIC JUNCTION AND LOWER ESOPHAGEAL SPHINCTER; HIATUS HERNIA AND GASTROESOPHAGEAL REFLUX

Agha FP. Barrett carcinoma of the esophagus: clinical and radiographic analysis of 34 cases. AJR 1985;145:41–6.

Astley R, Carre IJ, Langmead-Smith R. A 20 year prospective follow-up of childhood hiatal hernia. Br J Radiol 1977;50:400–3.

Bendig DW, Seilheimer DK, Wagner ML, et al. Complications of gastroesophageal reflux in patients with cystic fibrosis. J Pediatr 1982;100:536–40.

Berquist WE, Rachelefsky GS, Kadden M, et al. Effect of theophylline on gastroesophageal reflux in normal adults. J Allergy Clin Immunol 1981;67:407–11.

Blumhagen JD, Christie DL. Gastroesophageal reflux in children. Evaluation of the water siphon test. Radiology 1979;131:345–9.

Bremner CG, Lynch VP, Ellis FH. Barrett's esophagus: congenital or acquired? An experimental study of esophageal mucosal regeneration in dogs. Surgery 1970;68:209–16.

Cahill JL, Aberdeen E, Waterston DJ. Results of surgical treatment of esophageal hiatus hernia in infancy and childhood. Surgery 1969;66:597–602.

Carre IJ. Scientific Communications: proceedings of the British Pediatric Association. Arch Dis Child 1952;27:300.

Carre IJ. The natural history of the partial thoracic stomach (hiatus hernia) in children. Arch Dis Child 1959;34:344–53.

Carre IJ. Postural treatment of children with a partial thoracic stomach (hiatus hernia). Arch Dis Child 1960;35:569–80.

Carre IJ, Astley R. The fate of the partial thoracic stomach (hiatus hernia) in children. Arch Dis Child 1960;35:484–6.

Carre IJ, Astley R, Smellie JM. Minor degrees of partial thoracic stomach in childhood. Lancet 1952;1:1150–3.

Chen YM, Gelfand DW, Ott DJ, et al. Barrett esophagus as an extension of severe esophagitis: an analysis of radiologic signs in 29 cases. AJR 1985;145:275–81.

Chrispin AR, Friedland GW. A radiological study of the neural control of oesophageal vestibular function. Thorax 1966;21:422–7.

Cleveland RH, Kushner DC, Schwartz AN. Gastroesophageal reflux in children: results of a standardized fluoroscopic approach. AJR 1983;141:53–6.

Cohen MD, Beck JM. Hiatus hernia: a complication of posterolateral diaphragmatic herniation (Bochdalek's hernia) in infants. Clin Radiol 1980;31:215–9.

Cox KL, Isenberg JN, Ament ME. Gastric acid hypersecretion in cystic fibrosis. J Pediatr Gastroenterol Nutr 1982;1:559–65.

Creteur V, Theoni RF, Federle MP, et al. Role of single and double contrast radiography in the diagnosis of reflux esophagitis. Radiology 1983;147:71–4.

Crummy AB. The water siphon test in the evaluation of gastroesophageal reflux. Its correlation with pyrosis. Radiology 1966;87:501–4.

Daneman A, Kozlowski K. Large hiatus hernia in infancy and childhood. Aust Radiol 1977;21:133–9.

Darling DB. Hiatal hernia and gastroesophageal reflux in infancy and childhood. AJR 1975;123: 724–36.

Darling DB, Fisher JH, Gellis SS. Hiatal hernia and gastroesophageal reflux in infants and children: analysis of the incidence in North American children. Pediatrics 1974;54:450–5.

Darling DB, McCauley RGK, Leonidas JC, et al. Gastroesophageal reflux in infants and children: correlation of radiological severity and pulmonary pathology. Radiology 1978;127:735–40.

Darling DB, McCauley RGK, Leape LL, et al. A child with peptic esophagitis: correlation of radiographic signs with esophageal pathology. Radiology 1982;145:673–7.

Dent J, Dodds WJ, Friedman RH, et al. Mechanism of gastroesophageal reflux in recumbent asymptomatic human subjects. J Clin Invest 1980;65:256–67.

Ein SH, Shandling B, Stephens CA, et al. Partial gastric wrap-around as an alternative procedure in the treatment of hiatal hernia. J Pediatr Surg 1979;14:343–6.

Eliska O. Phreno-oesophageal membrane and its role in the development of hiatal hernia. Acta Anat (Basel) 1973;86:137–50.

Euler AR, Byrne WJ. Twenty-four hour esophageal intraluminal pH probe testing: a comparative analysis. Gastroenterology 1981;80:957–61.

Fisher RS, Malmud LS, Roberts GS, et al. Gastroesophageal (GE) scintiscanning to detect and quantitate GE reflux. Gastroenterology 1976;70:301–8.

Foster AC, Voyles JB, Murray BL, et al. Twenty-four hour pH monitoring in children with cystic fibrosis: association of chest physical therapy to gastroesophageal reflux [abstract 609]. Pediatr Res 1983;17:188A.

Friedland GW. Historical review of the changing concept of lower esophageal anatomy: 430 B.C.–1977. AJR 1978;131:373–88.

Friedland GW, Dodds WJ, Sunshine P, et al. The apparent disparity in incidence of hiatal hernia in infants and children in Britain and the United States. AJR 1974;120:305–14.

Friedland GW, Sunshine P, Zboralske FF. Hiatal hernia in infants and young children: a 2- to 3-year follow-up study. J Pediatr 1975;87:71–4.

Friedland GW, Yamate M, Marinkovitch VA. Hiatal hernia and chronic unremitting asthma. Pediatr Radiol 1973; 1:156–60.

Gelfand DW, Ott DJ. Areae gastricae traversing the esophageal hiatus: a sign of hiatus hernia. Gastrointest Radiol 1979;4:127–9.

Gerson DE, Lewicki AM. Intrathoracic stomach: when does it obstruct? Radiology 1976;119:257–64.

Halpert RD, Feczko P, Chason DP. Barrett's esophagus: radiologic and clinical considerations. J Can Assoc Radiol 1984;35:120–3.

Harp RA, Gonzalez JL, Graham J. Total gastric hiatal herniation in an infant. Surgery 1965;57:302–4.

Harvey RF, Dowsett L, Hartog M, Read AE. A radioimmunoassay for cholecystokinin-pancreozymin. Lancet 1973;2:826–8.

Herbst JJ. Gastroesophageal reflux. J Pediatr 1981;98: 859–70.

Herbst JJ, Book LS, Bray PF. Gastroesophageal reflux in the "near miss" sudden infant death syndrome. J Pediatr 1978;92:73–5.

Heyman S. Esophageal scintigraphy (milk scan) in infants and children with gastroesophageal reflux. Radiology 1982;144:891–3.

Heyman S, Kirkpatrick JA, Winter HS, et al. An improved radionuclide method for the diagnosis of gastroesophageal reflux and aspiration in children (milk scan). Radiology 1979;131:479–82.

Hillemeier AC, Lange R, McCallum R, et al. Delayed gastric emptying in infants with gastroesophageal reflux. J Pediatr 1981;98:190–3.

Humphreys GH, Wiedel PH, Baker DH, et al. Esophageal hiatus hernia in infancy and childhood. Pediatrics 1965; 36:351–8.

Johnston JH. Hiatus hernia in childhood. Arch Dis Child 1965;35:61–5.

Leape LL, Holder TM, Franklin JD, et al. Respiratory arrest in infants secondary to gastroesophageal reflux. Pediatrics 1977;60:924–9.

Leonidas JC. Gastroesophageal reflux in infants: role of the upper gastrointestinal series. AJR 1984;143:1350–1.

Levine MS, Caroline D, Thompson JJ, et al. Adenocarcinoma of the esophagus: relationship to Barrett mucosa. Radiology 1984;150:305–9.

Levine MS, Kressel HY, Caroline DF, et al. Barrett esophagus: reticular pattern of the mucosa. Radiology 1983; 147:663–7.

Maglinte DDT, Schultheis TE, Krol KL, et al. Survey of the esophagus during the upper intestinal examination in 500 patients. Radiology 1983;147:65–7.

McCallum RW, Berkowitz DM, Lerner E. Gastric emptying in patients with gastroesophageal reflux. Gastroenterology 1981;80:285–91.

McCauley RGK, Darling DB, Leonidas JC, et al. Gastroesophageal reflux in infants and children: a useful classification and reliable physiological technique for its demonstration. AJR 1978;130:47–50.

Moroz SP, Espinoza J, Cumming WA, et al. Lower esophageal sphincter function in children with and without gastroesophageal reflux. Gastroenterology 1976;71:236–41.

Naik DR, Bolia A, Moore DJ. Comparison of barium swallow and ultrasound in diagnosis of gastroesophageal reflux in children. BMJ 1985;290:1943–5.

Naik DR, Moore DJ. Ultrasound diagnosis of gastroesophageal reflux. Arch Dis Child 1984;59:366–79.

Pellegrini CA, DeMeester TR, Johnson LF, et al. Gastroesophageal reflux and pulmonary aspiration: incidence, functional abnormality, and results of surgical therapy. Surgery 1979;86:110–9.

Piepsz A, Georges B, Perlmutter N, et al. Gastroesophageal scintiscanning in children. Pediatr Radiol 1981; 11:71–4.

Pierce JW, Creamer B. The diagnosis of the columnar lined esophagus. Clin Radiol 1963;14:64–9.

Richter JE, Castell DO. Gastroesophageal reflux: pathogenesis, diagnosis and therapy. Ann Intern Med 1982;97:93–103.

Robbins AH, Vincent ME, Saini M, et al. Revised radiologic concepts of the Barrett's esophagus. Gastrointest Radiol 1978;3:377–81.

Rudd TG, Christie DL. Demonstration of gastroesophageal reflux in children by radionuclide gastroesophagography. Radiology 1979;131:483–6.

Scott RB, O'Loughlin EV, Gall DG. Gastroesophageal reflux in patients with cystic fibrosis. J Pediatr 1985;106: 223–7.

Shapir J, DuGrow R, Frank P. Barrett's esophagus: analysis of 19 cases. Br J Radiol 1985;58:491–3.

Siebert JJ, Byrne WJ, Euler AR, et al. Gastroesophageal reflux—the acid test: scintigraphy or the pH probe. AJR 1983;140:1087–90.

Smellie JM. Discussion on hiatus hernia. Proc R Soc Med 1954;47:531–9.

Steiner GM. Review article: gastro-esophageal reflux, hiatus hernia and the radiologist, with special reference to children. Br J Radiol 1977;50:164–74.

Stringer DA, Sprigg A, Juodis E, et al. The association of cystic fibrosis, gastroesophageal reflux, and reduced pulmonary function. Can Assoc Radiol J 1988;39:100–2.

Sutcliffe J. Torsion spasms and abnormal postures in children with hiatus hernia: Sandifer's syndrome. Prog Pediatr Radiol 1969;2:190–7.

Swyer PR. Partial thoracic stomach and esophageal hiatus hernia in infancy and childhood. Am J Dis Child 1955; 90:421–51.

Taybi H. Radiology of syndromes and metabolic disorders. 2nd ed. Chicago: Year Book; 1982. p. 348–9.

Thoeni RF, Moss AA. The radiographic appearance of complications following Nissen fundoplication. Radiology 1979;131:17–21.

Thommesen P, Gravesan M, Garsdal L. The significance of abnormal duodenal loop on radiological and clinical care in infants with sliding hiatus hernia. Pediatr Radiol 1977;6:88–91.

Tuttle SG, Grossman MI. Detection of gastroesophageal reflux by simultaneous measurements of intraluminal pressure and pH. Proc Soc Exp Biol Med 1958;98:225–7.

Vincent ME, Robbins AH, Spechler SJ, et al. The reticular pattern as a radiographic sign of the Barrett esophagus: an assessment. Radiology 1984;153:333–5.

Walsh JK, Farrell MK, Keenan WJ, et al. Gastroesophageal reflux in infants: relation to apnea. J Pediatr 1981;99: 197–201.

Werlin SL, Dodds WJ, Hogan WJ, et al. Mechanisms of gastroesophageal reflux in children. J Pediatr 1980;97:244–9.

Williams SM, Harned RK, Kaplan P, et al. Work in progress: transverse striations of the esophagus: association with gastroesophageal reflux. Radiology 1983;146:25–7.

Winter HS, Madara JL, Stafford RJ, et al. Intraepithelial eosinophils: a new diagnostic criterion for reflux esophagitis. Gastroenterology 1982;83:818–23.

Wolf BS. The inferior esophageal sphincter—anatomic, roentgenologic and manometric correlation, contradictions, and terminology. AJR 1970;110: 260–77.

Yulish BS, Rothstein FC, Halpin TC. Radiographic findings in children and young adults with Barrett's esophagus. AJR 1987;148:353–7.

8

THE STOMACH

Sambasiva R. Kottamasu, MD, and
David A. Stringer, BSc, MBBS, FRCR, FRCPC

EMBRYOGENESIS

In the fifth week of development, the stomach appears as a fusiform dilatation of the foregut but soon rotates about the longitudinal and anteroposterior axes (Figure 8–1). The 90° rotation about the longitudinal axis brings the left margin of the stomach to the anterior position; hence, the left vagus lies anterior to the stomach and the right vagus lies posterior. The differential growth of the opposite sides of the stomach results in the relatively longer greater curvature. The stomach then rotates on its anteroposterior axis to assume its final position.

Gastric acid production probably begins at about 32 weeks of gestation. In the first 24 hours of life, there is a rapid rise in acid production, which then gradually decreases (Franken and Smith, 1982).

ANATOMY

The stomach is often more horizontal in infancy than in later life and may be filled with a large quantity of gas. The amount of gas is increased when air is swallowed during feeding or crying.

During a barium meal in infancy, the pylorus displays a wide range of emptying times. Initially, the appearance of the pylorus may mimic that of pyloric stenosis, but with time (and with radiation kept to a minimum) the pylorus will be seen to open normally, emptying gastric contents into the duodenum. Caution must be taken not to make a false diagnosis of hypertrophic pyloric stenosis (see Chapter 8).

In older children, the appearance approximates that of adults. Double-contrast examinations of an infant's stomach are rarely necessary unless gastric bleeding occurs or epigastric pain is present; when performed, excess mucus often prevents good mucosal coating. The areae gastricae can be seen on double-contrast examinations using very high-density barium in older and some younger children. The techniques of barium examination are discussed in detail in Chapter 3.

CONGENITAL AND DEVELOPMENTAL ANOMALIES

Abdominal Situs Inversus

Normally on the left, the stomach gas bubble demonstrates the position of the stomach. If the stomach lies on the right (i.e., situs inversus), then the apex of the heart and the lower hemidiaphragm are usually also on the right (dextrocardia). Situs inversus is occasionally associated with the cardiac apex on the left and a lower left hemidiaphragm (levocardia); this unusual form is commonly associated with cyanotic heart disease (Jefferson and Rees, 1980). Therefore, the position of the cardiac apex may point toward serious congenital heart disease although this in itself gives no indication of the internal arrangement of the cardiac chambers.

Situs Ambiguus

Situs ambiguus is associated with polysplenia or asplenia, and the stomach may be on the left or right. The right and left lobes of the liver may be symmetric in children with situs ambiguus.

Diverticulum

A gastric diverticulum is usually found in adults and is most often an asymptomatic radiologic curiosity. It is found in 0.1 to 2.6% of autopsies (Meeroff et al.,

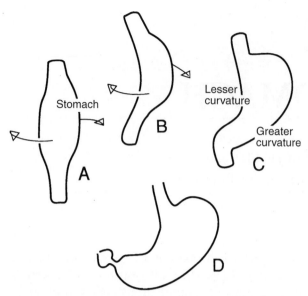

FIGURE 8–1. Embryogenesis of the stomach. The stomach appears as a fusiform dilatation of the foregut in the fifth week of development, (*A*). The stomach then rotates about the longitudinal and anteroposterior axes (*B*). The differential growth of the opposite sides of the stomach results in the relatively longer greater curvature (*C*). The stomach then rotates on its anteroposterior axis to assume its final position (*D*).

1967). It occurs most frequently in the posterior aspect of the fundus, just inferior to the esophagogastric junction (Figure 8–2) (Dodd and Sheft, 1969) but

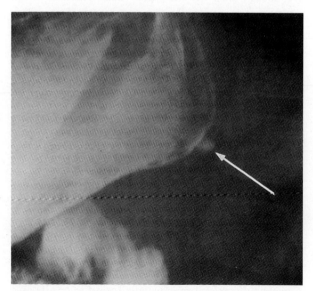

FIGURE 8–2. Gastric diverticulum. A small diverticulum (*arrow*) arises from the posterior aspect of the fundus, inferior to the esophagogastric junction.

may occur elsewhere and if large, may mimic a mass separate from the stomach on computed tomography (CT) examination (Schwartz et al., 1986).

Intramural diverticula can occur in adults but are rare. They arise from the greater curvature of the antrum and characteristically vary in size and shape with different phases of peristalsis, position of the patient, gastric distension, and extrinsic compression (Flachs et al., 1965; Cockrell et al., 1984). Although not reported in children as yet, they are important because they have a superficial resemblance to an antral ectopic pancreatic rest. It is important not to mistake barium artifact for a diverticulum or an ulcer, which may subject the child to unnecessary endoscopy or surgery (Shackelford, 1982).

Duplication

Duplication of the stomach accounts for only 3.8% of all gastrointestinal duplications (Thornhill et al., 1982). Gastric duplications most often occur along the greater curvature of the stomach, with the majority in the antrum (Wieczorek et al., 1984). They may or may not communicate with the gastric lumen. It is more prevalent in females and usually presents in infancy with pain, vomiting, fever, or anemia. The most frequent complication is partial or complete small-bowel obstruction but ulceration with bleeding, perforation, or fistula can occur. Rarely there may be multiple duplications affecting other areas in the bowel (Egelhoff et al., 1986).

Imaging of Gastric Duplication

Antenatal ultrasound (US) may detect a gastric duplication as a cystic upper abdominal mass in the fetus. However, the appearance is nonspecific as specific US signs have not been described antenatally (Bidwell and Nelson, 1986).

Postnatal US is diagnostic; it usually shows the wall of the cyst to be bowel having an echogenic line (mucosa) surrounded by a hypoechoic line (muscle) (Figure 8–3) (Moccia et al., 1981). These specific signs are not seen antenatally but are well seen in the baby soon after delivery (Bidwell and Nelson, 1986). In addition, US will show the size of the duplication, which is usually fluid filled. Occasionally there may be echogenic debris within the cyst representing hemorrhage or inspissated material (Kangarloo et al., 1979).

On barium meal examination, there is an indentation, usually on the greater curvature, due to the mass effect of the duplication (Kremer et al., 1970).

Lung sequestration is a rare association of gastric duplication, and CT can be helpful in diagnosis (Thornhill et al., 1982). Technetium Tc 99m pertechnetate will often be taken up by a duplication cyst with ectopic gastric mucosa but is rarely needed for a preoperative diagnosis.

Microgastria and Agastria

Microgastria (a small underdeveloped stomach) and agastria (absent stomach) are rare anomalies. Microgastria is frequently associated with other malformations such as malrotation (Hochberger and Swoboda, 1974), congenital heart disease, aganglionosis, and especially asplenia (Shackelford et al., 1973; Kessler and Smulewicz, 1973).

In microgastria the stomach is underdeveloped and has a tubular configuration with a small fundus. Stomach capacity is reduced, and associated gastroesophageal reflux is common but the histologic differentiation of gastric cell types is normal (Gorman and Shaw, 1984). Thus, the infant presents early with feeding difficulties and for many years may tolerate only pureed food. Despite these problems, if there is no associated malformation, the usual prognosis is healthy survival into adult life (Blank and Chisholm, 1973).

In agastria, the stomach is absent; this is the most extreme part of the microgastria-agastria spectrum and has earlier and more severe symptoms. Agastria can be associated with atresia, thus representing the most extreme form of gastric atresia (Figure 8–4).

Atresia or Web of the Stomach

Gastric atresia or web is a rare form of gastrointestinal atresia. It may be complete, may have a fibrous connection, or may be membranous, forming a web that is complete or incomplete (Figures 8–5 and 8–6). Gastric atresia is probably caused by gastric ischemia rather than failure of recanalization, as it may be associated with other bowel atresias of ischemic etiology. The rarity of the condition is probably related to the abundant vascular supply of the stomach. It can occasionally be familial with an autosomal recessive inheritance (Melhem et al., 1975), and it is associated (rarely) with epidermolysis bullosa (DeGroot et al., 1978; Orense et al., 1987).

Gastric atresia is associated with polyhydramnios during pregnancy and with patients who show an atresia or complete web soon after birth with abdominal distension and nonbilious vomiting. With an incomplete gastric web, presentation is similar to a complete atresia if, as is common, there is a small defect in the membrane. However, if the defect in the web is larger, presentation occurs later. The etiology of some cases which present in later life is uncertain but may be related to annular ulceration and scarring rather than congenital factors (Felson et al., 1969; Rhind, 1959; Farman et al., 1968).

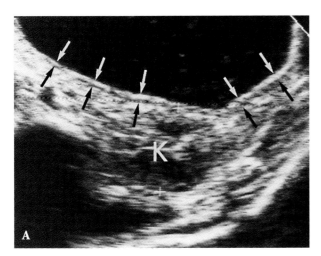
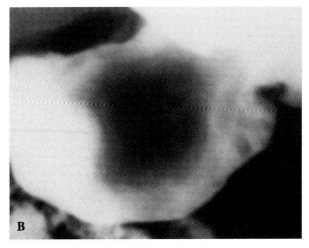

FIGURE 8–3. Gastric duplication. *A*, Transverse ultrasonography shows a large cyst lying anterior to the left kidney (K). The wall of the cyst is bowel as it has an echogenic line (the mucosa, *white arrows*) surrounded by a hypoechoic line (the muscle, *black arrows*). *B*, A barium meal examination in another patient shows a filling defect due to extrinsic compression from a duplication cyst.

Imaging of Atresia or Web

With a complete atresia or web, abdominal plain film shows a large distended gas-filled stomach and no small-bowel gas (Bronsther et al., 1971). A barium meal is usually unnecessary but if performed will confirm complete obstruction (see Figure 8–6). Differential diagnosis includes duodenal atresia, annular pancreas, and malrotation with high peritoneal bands (Ladd's bands).

With an incomplete web, the appearance is similar to a complete atresia but some gas is present in the small bowel (Cremin, 1969). A barium study will confirm the diagnosis (Figure 8–7). Care should be taken to ensure that any suspected web is constant, especially if the defect in the web is large; the appearance of a web can be mimicked in normal children, producing a pseudo-web pattern on barium examination (Fujioka et al., 1980).

Ectopic Pancreas

Ectopic pancreatic tissue can be found especially in the stomach and duodenum. The usual location is the antrum and pyloric region of the stomach. Very rarely, surrounding antral mucosa may be duodenal rather than gastric (Stringer et al., 1986).

The embryologic origin of an ectopic pancreas is unknown (Beseman et al., 1969).

Gastric ectopic pancreas is usually asymptomatic but an association with vague epigastric pain is reported (Rooney, 1959) and vomiting may be

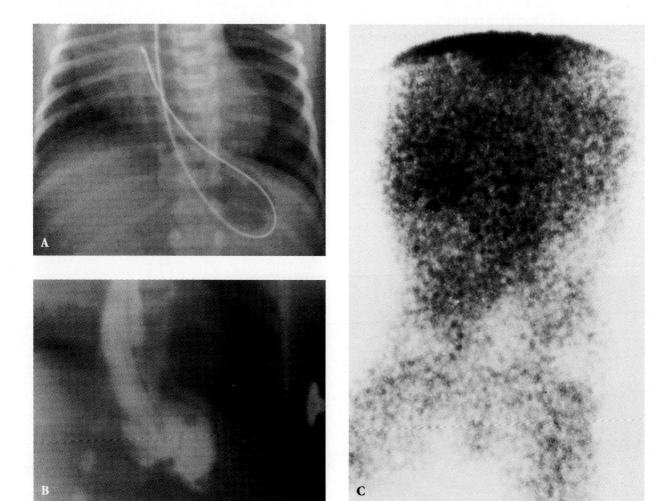

FIGURE 8–4. Agastria (absent stomach) with atresia. *A,* On plain film, a nasogastric tube curled back into the esophagus from below the hemidiaphragm. *B,* Injected barium confirmed the complete obstruction. *C,* A technetium Tc 99m scan showed no functioning gastric mucosa. No stomach was found at operation, and there was a dilated distal esophagus in which the nasogastric tube was curled. An example of the most extreme form of gastric atresia.

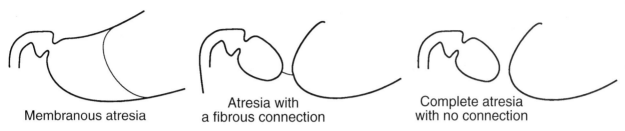

FIGURE 8–5. Types of gastric atresia. Gastric atresia may be membranous and form a web, may have a fibrous connection, or may be complete.

present (Eklof et al., 1973; Lucaya and Ochoa, 1976). If the ectopic tissue involves the pylorus, symptoms may develop early in life and mimic hypertrophic pyloric stenosis (Matsumoto et al., 1974).

Imaging of Ectopic Pancreas

Rarely, focal gastric antral thickening associated with the ectopic pancreas may be seen on US (Stringer et al., 1986), leading to the discovery of the

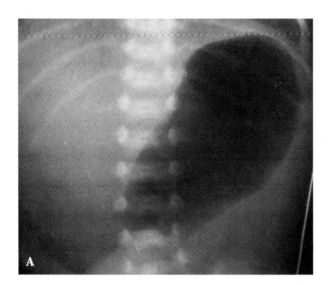

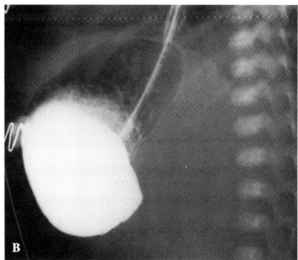

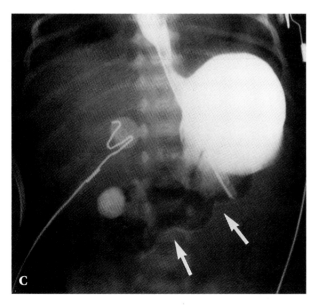

FIGURE 8–6. Gastric atresia. *A,* The plain film of a newborn girl with nonbilious vomiting shows a dilated air-filled stomach. *B,C,* The barium study confirmed a complete obstruction of the gastric antrum, and hyperperistalsis was present on fluoroscopy (*arrows*). The barium study was not necessary for diagnosis.

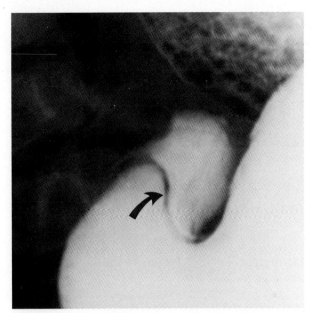

FIGURE 8–7. Gastric antral web. A constant linear defect (*arrow*) is present in the gastric antrum. This membranous web caused delayed emptying of the proximal stomach.

lesion. However, the diagnosis is usually made by barium meal examination.

Classically, a smooth, dome-shaped umbilicated mass projects into the lumen of the gastric antrum on the greater curvature (Figure 8–8). The central niche present in less than half of cases is part of a rudimentary duct system (Kilman and Berk, 1977); it may mimic an ulcer and project outside the gastric wall or into the gastric lumen (Stone et al.,

1971). Sometimes the central niche is difficult to discern and the mass appears more polypoid. However, location and careful examination will usually confirm the diagnosis (Figure 8–9).

Gastroscopic confirmation is usually unnecessary because an aberrant pancreas has a characteristic appearance on barium meal, similar to its appearance on gastroscopy (see Chapter 4) (Strobel et al., 1978).

ACQUIRED OUTLET OBSTRUCTION

The many causes of gastric outlet obstruction in infancy and early childhood can be divided into three groups, namely, decreased peristalsis, abnormal anatomy or function of the pylorus, and other anatomic causes such as atresia, webs, ulcers, annular pancreas, or extrinsic mass lesions (Table 8–1).

Decreased Peristalsis

Ileus

Generalized adynamic ileus affects the stomach as well as the rest of the gastrointestinal tract (Franken et al., 1980). In some girls it may have associated headache or migraine. In neonates, this ileus is often secondary to sepsis, anoxia, and neurologic disease. Plain films may show gross distension of the stomach with gas and fluid. Occasionally a barium meal examination may be indicated to exclude other anomalies. Gastroesophageal reflux and vomiting commonly occur with gastric hypotonia, and so care must be taken to prevent spontaneous aspi-

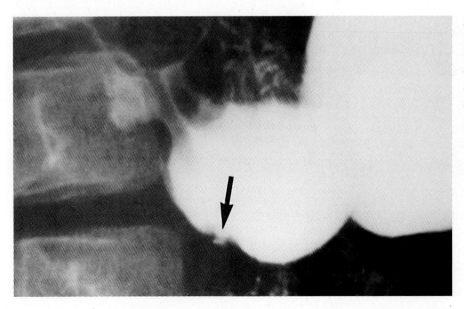

FIGURE 8–8. Ectopic pancreas. A smooth dome-shaped umbilicated mass projects into the lumen of the antrum on the greater curvature. The central niche (*arrow*) represents a rudimentary duct system.

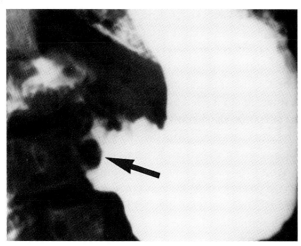

FIGURE 8–9. Ectopic pancreas. A central niche is difficult to appreciate in this polypoid mass (*arrow*) arising in the antrum. However, the location is characteristic.

ration of barium into the lungs. Barium should be withdrawn from the stomach at the end of the examination.

Antral Dysmotility

Antral dysmotility is a rare and controversial abnormality in infants who present with chronic vomiting (Bryne et al., 1981). On barium meal, the infants show a characteristic funnel-shaped antrum, absent antral peristalsis, delayed gastric emptying, and gastroesophageal reflux. The lower esophageal sphincter pressure is normal or increased, which suggests that the reflux is secondary to gastric outlet obstruction. Initial treatment is medical, with hourly feeds, upright positioning of the infant, and possibly cisapride; however, some children eventually require pyloroplasty. Further study is needed to fully evaluate this unusual condition.

Hypoperistalsis Syndromes

Hypoperistalsis may be idiopathic rather than caused by ileus. It can occur as an isolated finding or may form part of the megacystis-microcolon-intestinal hypoperistalsis syndrome or other forms of pseudo-obstruction. It can affect the stomach but more often involves the rest of the bowel (see Chapter 9).

Abnormal Pylorus

Pylorospasm

Pylorospasm—spasm of the pylorus delaying gastric emptying—is an ill-defined, controversial, self-limiting entity that does not require surgery. In the opinion of many radiologists and gastroenterologists, it represents a radiologic observation of normal delay in gastric emptying. Care must be taken to distinguish this condition from hypertrophic pyloric stenosis. The pylorus of normal infants may have a delayed opening of up to 15 to 20 minutes, especially at the beginning of a barium study, and may be accompanied by marked peristaltic activity. Thus, the initial appearance on US and barium study may suggest hypertrophic pyloric stenosis with narrowing of the pyloric canal; however, with time the pylorus will be seen to open (Figures 8–10 and 8–11). If the pyloric canal fails to open to its full extent, then the pylorospasm is more likely significant. Surgery is not indicated, however, as infants invariably stop vomiting and show rapid clinical improvement.

Hypertrophic Pyloric Stenosis

Clinical Findings. Hypertrophic pyloric stenosis (HPS) is a common cause of gastric outlet obstruction in infancy; its etiology is unknown. In the rare cases that run in families, hypertrophic pyloric stenosis may be a dominant polygenic trait with a lower threshold level for expression in boys than in girls (Bilodeau, 1971). The incidence is three times greater in boys than girls and varies geographically; as high as 1 in 250 male births in Sweden (Wallgren, 1946), to the low overall

---

Table 8–1. Causes of Gastric Outlet Obstruction in Infancy and Early Childhood

Decreased peristalsis
    Ileus
    Antral dysmotility
    Hypoperistalsis syndromes
Abnormal pylorus
    Pylorospasm
    Hypertrophic pyloric stenosis (HPS)
    Postoperative (burned-out) HPS
    Rare anomalies
Other anatomic causes
    Atresia / webs
    Ulcers
    Annular pancreas
    Extrinsic mass lesions

incidence of approximately 1 case for every 780 live births in North America. The condition is less common in black infants. Rarely, it may sequentially coexist with esophageal atresia (Magilner, 1986), an association which is difficult to explain but which we also have noticed in our hospital.

The patient with hypertrophic pyloric stenosis is usually a full-term infant who usually presents at 2 to 4 weeks of age. It is uncommon to present before 1 week or later than 3 months of age (Konvolinka and Wernuth, 1971). However, 20% of patients with classic hypertrophic pyloric stenosis have symptoms from birth (Andressy et al., 1977), and the few who present in the first week of life generally have less muscle hypertrophy than those presenting later, suggesting an early gradual onset in at least some (Geer et al., 1985). Curiously, premature infants are rarely affected. The patient presents with vomiting, which is often projectile. Diagnosis is best made clinically following a feed by palpating an olive-shaped pyloric tumor. Gastric hyperperistalsis may be visible in the upper abdomen, passing from left to right. In the classic case with an experienced clinician, no other diagnostic procedure is necessary, and the infant can undergo surgery as soon as any fluid and electrolyte disturbance such as hypochloremic alkalosis has been remedied. Some cases, however, pose a diagnostic dilemma, in which imaging can be of help (Table 8–2) (Shopfner et al., 1964).

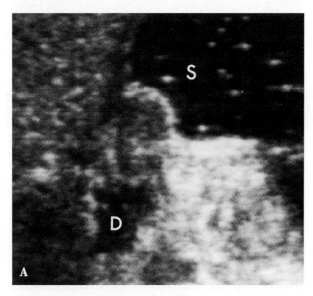

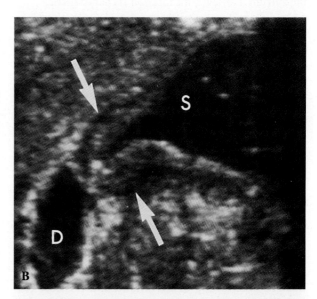

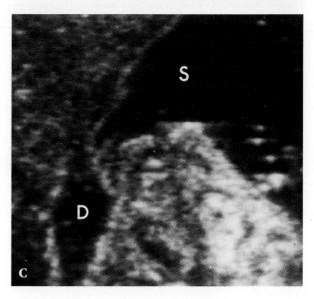

FIGURE 8–10. Pylorospasm. *A,* On ultrasonography the pylorus between the stomach (S) and duodenal cap (D) initially failed to open, mimicking hypertrophic pyloric stenosis. *B,* After 15 minutes, the pylorus starts to open but the pyloric muscle appears somewhat thick (*arrows*). *C,* By 20 minutes, the pylorus appears more normal.

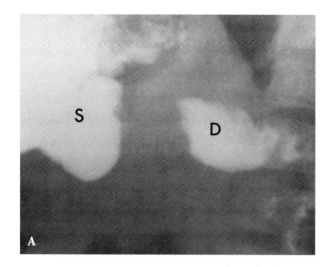

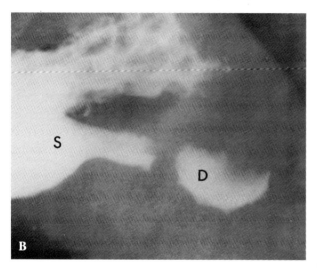

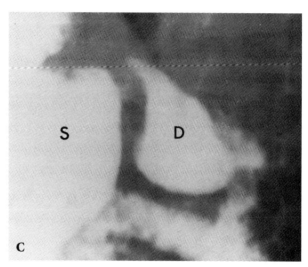

FIGURE 8–11. Pylorospasm. *A*, The pylorus between the stomach (S) and duodenal cap (D) was initially narrow on barium meal study, mimicking hypertrophic pyloric stenosis. *B*, After 15 minutes the pylorus starts to open. *C*, By 20 minutes the pylorus appears normal and there is good gastric emptying.

Ultrasonographic Imaging. Ultrasonography, due to its lack of radiation, is the imaging mode of choice (Teele and Smith, 1977; Blumhagen and Coombs, 1981; Pilling, 1983; Hayden et al., 1984; Ball et al., 1983; Sauerbrei and Paloschi, 1983; Graif et al., 1984; Stundar et al., 1986; Neilson and Hollman, 1994; Hernanz-Schulman et al., 1994).

However, an ultrasound examination for hypertrophic pyloric stenosis has to be performed properly (Blumhagen, 1986). If the infant's stomach is not full or if the contents are very echoic, it should be filled with a dextrose water solution either via a nasogastric tube or by bottle-feeding. A nasogastric tube is routinely used at our hospital so that air or other strongly echoic gastric contents can be aspirated; any fluid should be aspirated at the end of the examination. The examination is performed in real time, with the infant positioned so that the fluid is adjacent to the

pylorus. Viewing this area must be continuous to assess whether any "pyloric tumor" is constant and whether there is free drainage into the duodenum.

High-frequency transducers to visualize a field of view 3.5 cm deep are advisable (Blumhagen, 1986). Patience with a fractious baby is well rewarded, especially as gentle abdominal pressure with the transducer can give an excellent view. Timing changes in the angle of the transducer with respiration is also helpful and is soon perfected by practice.

The hypertrophied pyloric muscle on cross section appears as a thick, echolucent ring with central dense echoes which represent the convoluted compressed mucosa (Figure 8–12). The hypertrophied pyloric muscle may demonstrate nonuniform echogenicity related to the orientation of the ultrasound beam to the circular fibers of the pyloric muscle (Spevak et al., 1992). By performing oblique cuts

Table 8–2. Investigation of Infant Vomiting Caused by Suspected Hypertrophic Pyloric Stenosis

	Procedure	
Investigation Step	*Tumor Found*	*No Tumor Found*
(1) Abdominal palpation	Pyloromyotomy	US
(2) US	Pyloromyotomy	Barium meal examination
(3) Barium meal	Pyloromyotomy	HPS excluded; seek other causes of vomiting

US=ultrasonography; HPS=hypertrophic pyloric stenosis.

along the long axis of the pylorus, the continuity of the thickened muscle with the stomach wall can be seen, which helps to confirm the diagnosis as well as showing gastric hyperperistalsis and shouldering and beaking in the gastric antrum (Figure 8–13).

An experienced US technician seldom requires measurements to make a diagnosis but they may be helpful especially to those just learning the techniques (Blumhagen, 1986). Of the many criteria for diagnosing hypertrophic pyloric stenosis (Westra et al., 1989), an accurate one appears to be a thick pyloric muscle greater than 3 mm on one side of the lumen (O'Keeffe et al., 1991; Lamki et al., 1993). Antropyloric muscle thickness less than 2 mm should be con-

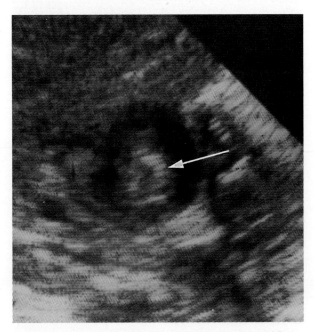

FIGURE 8–12. Hypertrophic pyloric stenosis. Oblique longitudinal US shows a cross section through the pylorus; the central dense echoes (*arrow*) from compressed mucosa are surrounded by echolucent hypertrophied muscle.

sidered normal (O'Keeffe et al., 1991). The pyloric canal in infants with HPS may be longer than 17 mm (Stundar et al., 1986; Haller and Cohen, 1986). According to Stundar et al. (1986) this is a most accurate and invariable measurement, with 14 mm as the upper limit of normal. However, we have had a severely premature infant who had hypertrophic pyloric stenosis at 2 weeks of age (30 weeks corrected) and whose pyloric canal measured only between 10 and 12 mm. For such a tiny neonate, these measurements were abnormally large (Bisset and Gupta, 1988) (Figure 8–14). Some normal and abnormal patients occasionally have a pylorus measuring between 14 and 17 mm. In some premature infants with surgically proven HPS, the thickness of pyloric muscle on transverse ultrasonographic scans may measure only between 2 and 3 mm (Bisset and Gupta, 1988; Lamki et al., 1993). Hence, these measurements should always be interpreted in conjunction with patient size and other radiologic and clinical findings.

Other diagnostic criteria include the demonstration, on longitudinal section, of continuity between the abnormal pyloric and normal antral muscle (Hayden et al., 1984). Sometimes the transition is gradual with an extension of the thickening into the pylorus (Ball et al., 1983). The fluid in the antrum may show the beak and shoulders of the tumor (see Figure 8–13). A curved echogenic structure in the middle of the hypertrophied muscle on longitudinal section represents the mucosa and may appear as a double track that has a similar characteristic appearance on barium study (see Figure 8–13) (Cohen et al., 1987). Prominent gastric peristalsis and lack of fluid drainage into the duodenum may also be seen. Gastroesophageal reflux, which often accompanies HPS, can be assessed with the stomach full of fluid (see Chapter 7).

Still, 8% of cases of hypertrophic pyloric stenosis can be missed by US (Blumhagen and Noble,

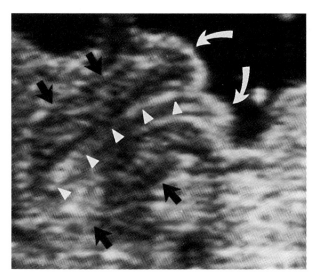

FIGURE 8–13. Hypertrophic pyloric stenosis. The continuity of the thickened muscle with the stomach wall can be seen on oblique ultrasonographic cuts on the long axis of the pylorus. The pyloric canal appears as an echogenic curved line (*white arrow heads*) in the middle of the hypertrophied muscle (*black arrows*). Other signs are shouldering and beaking in the gastric antrum (*white curved arrows*) and gastric hyperperistalsis.

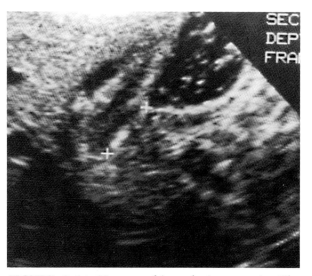

FIGURE 8–14. Hypertrophic pyloric stenosis. The pyloric tumor measured only between 10 and 12 mm but this was abnormally large for a severely premature infant who had hypertrophic pyloric stenosis at 2 weeks of age (30 weeks, corrected). Hence, measurements are only a rough indicator of muscle thickening.

1983). Hence, if no definite tumor is seen on US, a barium meal is advisable.

Plain-Film Imaging. Plain films prior to a barium meal are rarely required. Plain films may show either gaseous distension of the stomach with evidence of prominent peristaltic waves or thickening of the wall of the gastric antrum with decreased gas content in the rest of the bowel (Riggs and Long, 1971).

Barium Meal Imaging. If there is still clinical concern or if gastroesophageal reflux was the initial diagnosis, a barium study can be performed (although rarely if ever indicated in practice).

The barium meal appearance is characteristic. The pyloric canal shows a constant elongation (the string sign) (Meuwissen and Sloof, 1932), with a gentle curve that is concave superiorly (Figure 8–15). The pyloric canal often has a double track of barium due to folding of the compressed mucosa (Figure 8–16). This double track is said to be a reliable differentiating factor between pylorospasm and hypertrophic pyloric stenosis (Haran et al., 1966) but the constant nature of the deformity is more

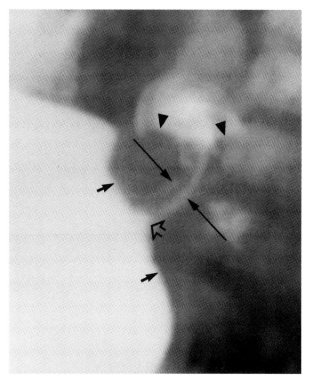

FIGURE 8–15. Hypertrophic pyloric stenosis. The distal antrum is shouldered (*short arrows*) and ends in a beak (*open arrow*). The narrowed pylorus produces a double track (*long arrows*). The base of the duodenal bulb is umbrella shaped (*arrowheads*).

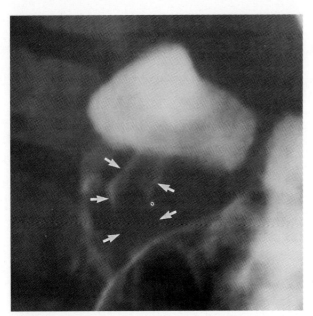

FIGURE 8–16. Hypertrophic pyloric stenosis. A characteristic double track (*arrows*) of barium connects the antrum to the duodenal cap.

important. The hypertrophied pyloric muscle bulges into the distal antrum and base of the duodenal cap, producing an appearance of a shoulder, a mushroom, or an umbrella (see Figure 8–15). A pyloric tit deformity may be seen on the lesser curve

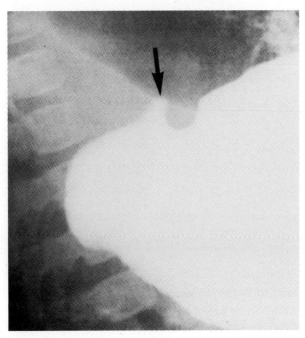

FIGURE 8–17. Hypertrophic pyloric stenosis. A pyloric tit deformity (*arrow*) lies adjacent to the pyloric mass.

adjacent to the pyloric mass (Figure 8–17), possibly the result of a persistent peristaltic wave blocked by the pyloric tumor (Shopfner, 1964).

Sometimes, barium passing into the pyloric canal is markedly delayed despite active peristalsis and may appear pinched off in a beak at the canal's entrance (Figure 8–18). Where the diagnosis is not obvious, spot compression films of the antrum may delineate the above signs more quickly and clearly (Currarino, 1964).

Gastroesophageal reflux with or without hiatus hernia is very commonly associated with infantile HPS and is probably secondary to gastric outlet obstruction. Other gastrointestinal associations include esophageal atresia (Franken and Saldino, 1969) and webs in the gastric antrum (Mandell, 1978). Rarely, peritoneal bands associated with midgut malrotation may cross the pyloric canal and resemble hypertrophic pyloric stenosis on imaging.

Postoperative or Burned-Out Hypertrophic Pyloric Stenosis

Hypertrophic pyloric stenosis is treated surgically in North America, the United Kingdom, and most of Europe. In Scandinavia, however, a medical approach is often taken because the natural history of the condition is such that over many months the gastric outlet obstruction disappears. After some years the radiologic appearance also returns to normal; this occurs more quickly in those patients treated by surgery (Steinicke and Roelsgaard, 1960).

In the immediate postoperative period, the pylorus remains deformed on barium meal. Radiologic assessment by barium meal of persistent hypertrophic pyloric stenosis due to an incomplete pyloromyotomy can be difficult. In this situation, continued symptoms combined with persistent hyperperistalsis and delayed gastric emptying (Figure 8–19) are more important in the diagnosis of incomplete pyloromyotomy than the observation of pyloric canal elongation since the latter may also be seen following clinically successful pyloromyotomy. Serial US is probably the most helpful investigation.

Serial US postoperatively shows changes in the pyloric muscle thickness and may be used in assessing the effectiveness of a pyloromyotomy. However, in the first postoperative week the muscle may appear thicker away from the operative site than it appeared in preoperative scans due to contraction with bunching-up of cut muscle. Careful examination will show that there is a depression and little muscle over the operative site. The next 3 weeks shows rapid involution of the muscle. A return to normal thickness by between 6 weeks and 6 months is then seen (Sauerbrei and Paloschi, 1983).

Persistent hypertrophic pyloric stenosis due to an incomplete pyloromyotomy appears as a persistent gastric outlet obstruction and muscle hypertrophy although it may have a tapered appearance (Jamroz et al., 1986).

Chronic Granulomatous Disease

Chronic granulomatous disease is a rare inherited disorder of phagocytes. Eighty percent of patients are boys with some evidence of an X-linked inheritance. Inheritance in the 20% who are girls is uncertain.

The patient's phagocytes can ingest but cannot kill microbes, hence, intracellular bacteria survive, infection persists, and granulomatous lesions result.

Although rarely affected by this disease, the stomach can be involved resulting in marked antral wall thickening with narrowing of the lumen (Mascatello et al., 1977; Kopen and McAlister, 1984; Griscom et al., 1974; Bowen and Gibson, 1980; Stringer et al., 1986). The antral thickening may be asymptomatic and discovered accidentally during US looking for lesions elsewhere (Figure 8–20) (Stringer et al., 1986) or may cause gastric outlet obstruction (Hartenberg and Kodroff, 1984). Ultrasonography is the initial modality of choice as it avoids radiation in these children, especially as they often require many examinations over the years. It is also valuable for monitoring the abnormality during treatment. Surprisingly, the condition may improve without antibiotics, suggesting that infection is not the cause (Kopen and McAlister, 1984). One theory suggests foreign antigens may trigger a hyperplastic granulomatous reaction from gastric macrophages.

Barium meal examination can be useful in initially evaluating gastric outlet obstruction and will demonstrate considerable antral narrowing and deformity which may mimic linitis plastica (see Figure 8–20) (Stringer et al., 1986). The body of the stomach may occasionally also be involved (Hartenberg and Kodroff, 1984).

Although not generally necessary, if being performed to assess some other pathology such as hepatic abscesses, CT can also show the marked antral thickening (see Figure 8–19) (Stringer et al., 1986).

Rare Disorders of the Pylorus

Gastric outlet obstruction may be produced by rare pyloric abnormalities such as congenital double pylorus (Sufian et al., 1977), extrinsic compression of the pylorus by falciform ligament (Dassonville et al., 1986), hypertrophy of the pyloric mucosa without muscle hypertrophy (Slim et al., 1964), and gastroduodenal intussusception (Apfelberg et al., 1971; Lichtman et al., 1986). Barium meal examination is usually the best way to demonstrate these rare anomalies.

Gastroduodenal intussusception can occur from rare tumors. It may present with chronic vomiting, and weight loss (Lichtman et al., 1986), and amylase elevation. The intussusception may be well seen on US as multiple hyperechoic and hypoechoic rings. The lead point may have a different echo pattern. In such a case, CT can be useful by showing that the stomach is incorporated into the mass and that there are no adjacent or retroperitoneal nodes involved (Figure 8–21) (Lichtman et al., 1986; Stringer et al., 1986).

A pyloroduodenal deformity due to a malpositioned liver has been reported in children following omphalocele repair (Oh et al., 1977).

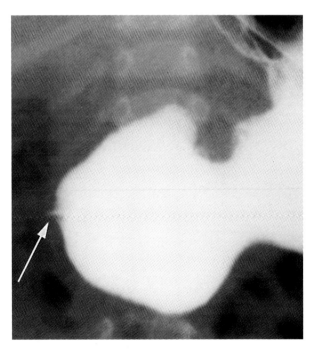

FIGURE 8–18. Hypertrophic pyloric stenosis. Despite hyperactive peristalsis as shown by marked indentations in the stomach, passage of barium is delayed. A beak of barium (*arrow*) is at the antral end of the narrow pylorus.

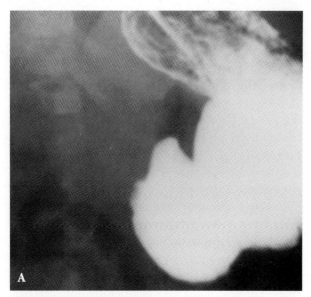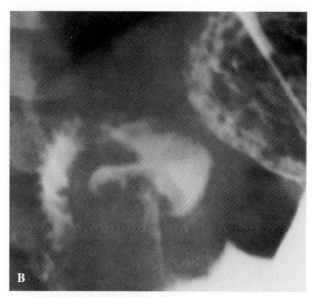

FIGURE 8–19. Hypertrophic pyloric stenosis. *A,* Persistent hyperperistalsis and delayed gastric emptying are important in diagnosing incomplete pyloromyotomy. *B,* The observation of pyloric canal elongation is less reliable as it may also be seen following a clinically successful pyloromyotomy.

ACQUIRED ABNORMALITIES

Gastritis

Gastritis, an inflammation of the stomach wall, can be of various types, classed by radiologic appearance or etiology. This book will use a radiologic classification of erosive, corrosive, emphysematous, and miscellaneous forms of gastritis.

Gastritis can have a primary or secondary etiology. Primary causes include Crohn's disease, eosinophilic gastritis, and varioliform gastritis (although the last may have an allergic basis) (Caporali and Luciano, 1986). Secondary causes include stress, local infection, and medications. Stress includes shock, burns, trauma, systemic infection, and postoperative effects. *Helicobacter pylori* is now

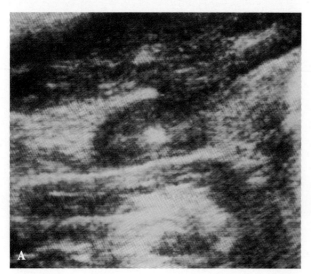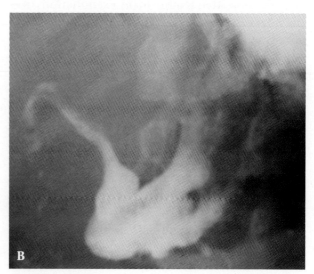

FIGURE 8–20. Chronic granulomatous disease. *A,* The marked antral muscle thickening on ultrasonography mimics hypertrophic pyloric stenosis (Reprinted with permission, Stringer et al., 1986). *B,* Barium study may show gastric outlet obstruction with a narrow deformed gastric antrum.

implicated as a cause of gastritis and peptic ulceration (McNulty and Wise, 1985; Marshall and Warren, 1984; Cello, 1995). Medications that have been implicated include steroids, aspirin, and other nonsteroidal anti-inflammatory drugs.

Erosive Gastritis

Clinical Findings. Erosive gastritis is more common in adults but may be seen in children, especially adolescents. Erosive gastritis in children usually presents with abdominal pain, nausea, and vomiting. Hematemesis may occur without preceding symptoms, in which case aspirin ingestion should be suspected. In some patients the diagnosis is clear and no radiologic or endoscopic examination is neccessary.

Imaging. Acute erosions may occur in childhood but radiologic demonstration is uncommon. Hence, the

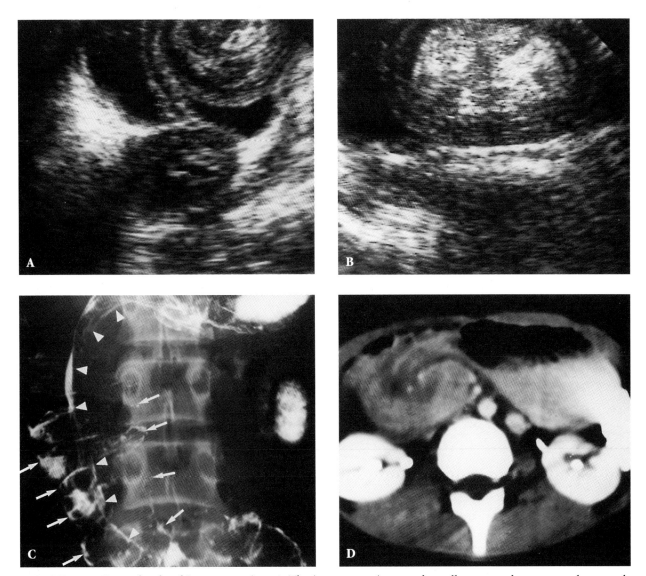

FIGURE 8–21 Gastroduodenal intussusception. *A,* The intussusception may be well seen on ultrasonography as multiple hyperechoic and hypoechoic rings and the lead point *B,* may have a different echo pattern. *C,* Barium study demonstrates the intussusception with barium passing through a narrow track in the intussusceptum (*arrow heads*), and refluxing back around the intussuscipiens (*arrows*). *D,* CT can also show the mass and provide further information excluding adjacent or retroperitoneal node involvement and showing contiguity with the stomach. A gastric hamartoma was removed at operation. (Reprinted with permission, Lichtman et al., 1986.)

definitive diagnosis of gastritis in children is by gastroscopy, with the added advantage of the ability to take biopsies. However, gastroscopy is an invasive procedure with some hazards and may require general anesthesia especially in younger children. Hence, it may be preferable to use radiologic study as a screening procedure and an aid in excluding other abnormalities.

Radiologic diagnosis is best made with a barium meal examination using graded compression (McLean et al., 1982). Double-contrast techniques are more effective at demonstrating erosions than single-contrast techniques (Theoni et al., 1983; Ott et al., 1982). Although both techniques have poor sensitivity (Ott et al., 1982), finding erosive gastritis on double-contrast barium meal is becoming more frequent, and there is an overall incidence of detection of between 0.5 and 20% in adults (Levine et al., 1986). The most common radiologic abnormality is "varioliform" erosion where a small punctate or slit-like collection of barium is surrounded by a relatively radiolucent halo due to edematous mucosa (Figure 8–22). This gives the appearance of smooth raised centrally umbilicated lesions 3 to 11 mm in diameter, most commonly seen in the antrum (Levine et al., 1986). Rarely, the elevated lesions may appear more polypoid (Figure 8–23). The relatively high detection rate of this specific abnormality on barium meal is partly due to its distinctiveness whereas other evidence of erosions has no radiolucent halo and is more subtle.

Other radiologic findings include mucosal irregularity (Turner et al., 1974) and erosions without edema. More controversial signs include a hypertrophied antral-pyloric fold (Glick et al., 1985) and serpiginous erosions (Levine et al., 1986). Coarse areae gastricae in the body and fundus of the stomach and prominent folds have both been reported as associated with gastric hypersecretion and possibly gastritis (Smith, 1984; Watanabe et al., 1983) but there is no histologic proof (Keto et al., 1983).

Other radiologic modalities are generally considered unsuitable for the detection of gastritis although we have followed up a patient with gastritis with US, noting a decrease in gastric wall thickness with reducing symptoms. The normal gastric wall in children measures 2 to 3 mm when the stomach is distended with fluid and is more than 5 mm when affected by gastritis. The normal echo pattern of the gastric wall may also be disturbed in gastritis, resulting in loss of differentiation of muscle and mucosa (Stringer et al., 1986). Thickened stomach may also be noted with gastric malignancy as well as congestive gastropathy secondary to dilated and tortuous veins in the submucosa in some patients with portal hypertension (Saverymuttu et al., 1990).

Technetium Tc 99m labelled white-blood-cell scintigraphy has also been used to detect gastritis (Wilton et al., 1984), but its usefulness is uncertain and hence rarely used.

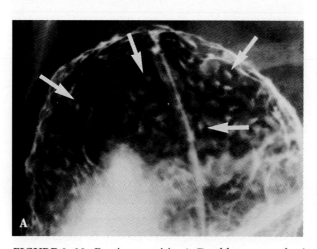 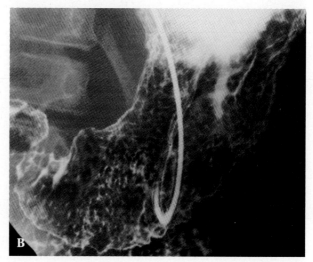

FIGURE 8–22. Erosive gastritis. *A,* Double-contrast barium meal examination shows "varioliform" erosions where a small punctate or slit like collection of barium is surrounded by a relatively radiolucent halo due to edematous mucosa (*arrows*), giving the appearance of smooth, raised, centrally umbilicated lesions 3 to 11 mm in diameter. *B,* The erosions were seen throughout the stomach.

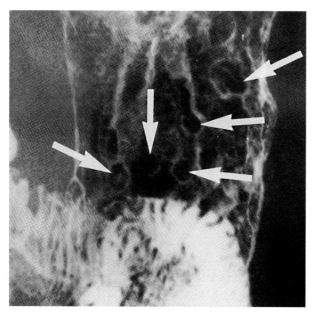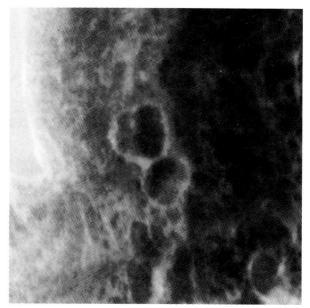

FIGURE 8–23. Erosive gastritis. *A*, Double-contrast barium meal shows elevated polypoid lesions in the body of the stomach (*arrows*). *B*, Spot film shows two lesions, one with an irregular outline and a central collection of barium.

Corrosive Gastritis

Acid ingestion characteristically causes narrowing of the gastric antrum, which is also seen in up to 20% of patients following alkali ingestion. Intense pylorospasm immediately following ingestion causes the antrum to act as a reservoir for the caustic material. The resulting inflammation and necrosis progress to fibrosis with aperistaltic narrowing, which may mimic carcinoma. Interstitial gas may be present, which can form bullae (Franken, 1973; Levitt et al., 1975).

Acute iron ingestion may be associated with a nonspecific ileus and radiopaque material in the stomach on plain-film radiographs and with diffuse thickening of the gastric wall and echogenic material within the gastric lumen on US (Newman et al., 1992).

Emphysematous Gastritis

In adults, emphysematous gastritis with gas in the stomach wall is a rare and severe form of phlegmonous gastritis caused by gas-forming organisms. This occurs only very rarely in infants, usually preceded by gastroenteritis. It occurs especially in the malnourished and may be amenable to treatment by hyperalimentation (Udassin et al., 1984).

In children, gas in the stomach wall is occasionally seen in pneumatosis intestinalis (Colquhoun, 1965) or secondary to bowel obstruction or following endoscopy (Figure 8–24) (Kay-Butler, 1962; Myhre and Wilson, 1948; Katz et al, 1972). These latter causes are more common in children than infectious emphysematous gastritis.

The radiologic appearance on plain film is of gas outlining the stomach. This may also be detected on CT when performed for some other purpose (Martin and Hartley, 1986).

Miscellaneous Causes of Gastritis

Crohn's Disease. Crohn's disease of the stomach can produce antral narrowing and mucosal irregularity on single- and double-contrast studies (Figure 8–25) but only high-quality double-contrast studies will show early disease as shown by subtle umbilicated aphthae, often misleadingly termed aphthous ulcers (see Chapter 9) (Figure 8–26). When Crohn's disease affects the stomach, it is often symptomatic and may be associated with a poor prognosis (Tootla et al., 1976). In our experience it affects the stomach in approximately 1% of patients with Crohn's disease and is nearly always associated with upper abdominal symptoms.

Eosinophilic Gastroenteritis. Eosinophilic gastroenteritis can produce a nodular pattern to the gastric

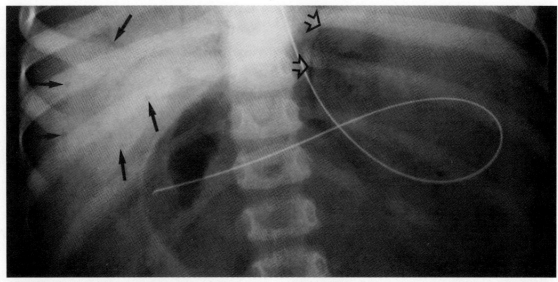

FIGURE 8–24. Emphysematous gastritis. Plain films show gas in the stomach wall (*open arrows*) and in the intrahepatic portal veins (*arrows*) secondary to gastric volvulus and gangrene in the stomach wall. Perforation rapidly occurred and emergency partial gastrectomy was successfully performed.

antrum, less marked than when present in the small bowel (see Chapter 9) (Teele et al., 1979).

Candidiasis. Unusual infections may affect the stomach in immunodepressed children. Invasive gastric candidiasis has been reported in an immunocompromised child with Crohn's disease and results in thick gastric folds, superficial erosions, and decreased distensibility of the stomach (Pugh and Fitch, 1986).

Toxoplasmosis. Toxoplasmosis has long been recognized as an opportunistic infection in immunocompromised patients caused by an intracellular protozoan parasite, *Toxoplasma gondii.* Over the past decade, and with the advent of the acquired immunodeficiency syndrome (AIDS) epidemic, there has been a marked increase in cases of toxoplasmosis, with primary affinity for the central nervous system. The mode of infection is by ingestion of cysts or by transplacental transmission of trophozoites. Toxoplasmosis has also been acquired by organ transplantion or blood transfusion. Individuals infected with *Toxoplasma gondii* may have no clinical symptoms or may present with lymphadenopathy, malaise, and fever. The brain, lung, myocardium, liver, skin, skeletal muscle, and stomach may be involved, with ocular involvement seen primarily with congenital infection. Gastric involvement with toxoplasmosis may manifest as antral narrowing (Smart et al., 1990). Other causes of stomach involvement in AIDS patients include infections such as cryptosporidiosis and cytomegalovirus and neoplasms such as lymphoma.

Ménétrier's Disease (Giant Hypertrophic Gastritis). Ménétrier's disease is rare in childhood (Sandberg, 1971) but can occur in patients as young as 3 years of age (Degnan, 1957; Henderson and Sprague, 1979). Abdominal pain or nausea and vomiting may be present. Affected children usually have protein-losing enteropathy with hypoproteinemia, which may result in peripheral edema, ascites, and effusions. Hemorrhage can occur, causing hematemesis, melena, or anemia (Baker et al., 1986), and peripheral eosinophilia is common (Baker et al., 1986; Marks et al., 1986). There are two forms of the disease, acute and chronic. The acute form is self-limiting and is of uncertain etiology (Sandberg, 1971). This acute form remits and is the usual form seen in childhood. An association with *Cytomegalovirus* has been found on culture and by intranuclear inclusions on biopsy in a number of patients, suggesting a possible causal relationship, especially as there is often a prodromal viral illness (Henderson and Sprague, 1979; Lachman et al., 1971; Leonidas et al., 1973; Marks et al., 1986; Coad, 1986). Recently, an association with *Campylobacter pylori* has also been reported.

The incidence of gastric carcinoma may be higher in Ménétrier's disease, (Scharschmidt, 1977) and prophylactic gastrectomy has been used in the treatment of its chronic form in adults. However, in children the disease appears more benign and transient than in adults, and malignancy has not been reported (Burns and Gay, 1968; Chouraqui et al., 1981).

Ultrasonography can demonstrate the hypertrophied folds (Derchi et al., 1982) but diagnosis is made primarily by barium meal examination (Figure 8–27) with confirmatory endoscopy and biopsy. The signs in children on barium meal of hypertrophic tortuous gastric folds, usually confined to the fundus and body of the stomach, are similar to those of adults (see Figure 8–27) (Burns and Gay, 1968). Gastroscopy will confirm large rugae when there is still clinical doubt, and biopsies may show eosinophilic infiltration in the gastric mucosa or cytomegalic inclusions in hyperplastic mucosa with marked hypertrophy and hyperplasia of the mucous glands (Leonidas et al., 1973; Chouraqui et al., 1981).

Chronic Granulomatous Disease. Antral narrowing has also been seen in chronic granulomatous disease (see Figure 8–20) (Bowen and Gibson, 1980; Griscom et al., 1974), pernicious anemia (O'Connell and Chrispin, 1976), and as a late complication of iron ingestion (Vuthibhagdee and Harris, 1972).

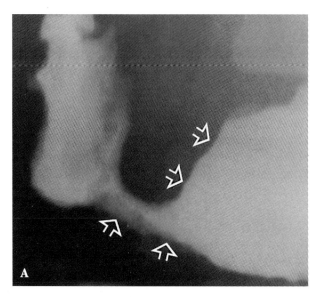

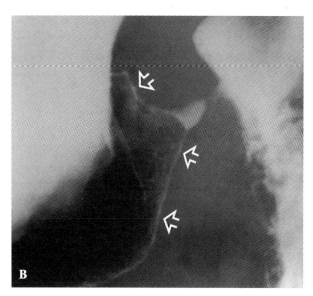

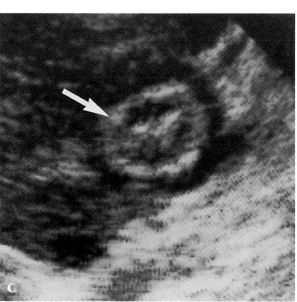

FIGURE 8–25. Crohn's disease. Single- and double-contrast barium meal studies, *A* and *B*, respectively, show antral narrowing and mucosal irregularity (*arrows*). *C*, Longitudinal US shows the central echogenic mucosa surrounded by hypoechoic muscle but also a further hyperechoic ring (*arrow*) that probably represents submucosal inflammation.

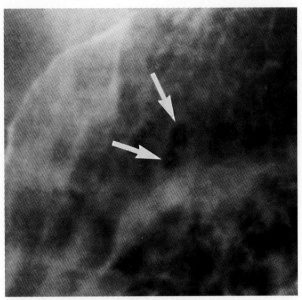

FIGURE 8–26. Crohn's disease. Double-contrast barium study of the gastric antrum shows subtle umbilicated apthae (*arrows*). (Reprinted with permission, Stringer DA. Imaging inflammatory bowel disease in the pediatric patient. Radiol Clin North Am 1987;25:93–113).

Gastric Ulcer

Acute gastric ulcers, erosions, and chronic gastric ulcers may all be seen in children, even in infants, but they occur only rarely (Block, 1963) and are less

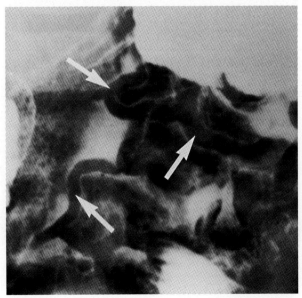

FIGURE 8–27. Ménétrier's disease. Double-contrast barium meal demonstrates hypertrophied gastric folds (*arrows*).

common than duodenal ulcers (Singleton and Faykus, 1964; Daryabeigi et al., 1977). The ulcer may be primary or secondary to stress (such as burns), cerebral disease (Daryabeigi et al., 1977), or medication (frequently aspirin) (Seagram et al., 1973). Primary gastric ulcers are unusual in children under 10 years of age (Drumm et al., 1988).

Helicobacter pylori has been implicated as a cause of gastritis and peptic ulceration (McNulty and Wise, 1985; Marshall and Warren, 1984; Cello, 1995). The name of the organism has changed from *Campylobacter*-like organisms to *Campylobacter pylori* and now to *Helicobacter pylori*. *Helicobacter pylori* is a motile spiral organism found within the gastric antrum of over 90% of patients with duodenal ulcers, 80% of patients with gastric ulcers, and virtually 100% of patients with chronic active gastritis (Cello, 1995). Its prevalence increases with the patient's age. About 10% of Americans under the age of 30 are infected with *Helicobacter pylori* whereas nearly 60% of Americans over the age of 60 are infected. Although its prevalence in the gastric mucosa of patients with the lesions mentioned above is higher than that in matched controls without peptic lesions, the majority of infected individuals remain asymptomatic. *Helicobacter pylori* has not been isolated from food, water, or stools, and the precise mode and vehicle of transmission are not documented. The mode of transmission is most likely person-to-person contact, probably from oropharyngeal secretions (Drumm et al., 1990). Health professionals caring for patients with gastrointestinal diseases are more than twice as likely to harbor the organism (Peterson, 1986). At our hospital we have found these organisms in patients with duodenal ulceration (Drumm et al., 1988). Diagnosis is by culture, silver stain, and urease test.

In all children with gastric ulcers, gastrointestinal bleeding is a major presenting symptom but pain is more evident in older children, perhaps because younger children are less able to verbalize their symptoms (Drumm et al., 1988). Perforation may occasionally occur. Young children with secondary ulcers more often require emergency surgery. Neonates have a particularly high perforation rate and a higher mortality rate compared to older children with primary ulcers, who require surgery only occasionally and have an excellent prognosis (Drumm et al., 1988).

Imaging

In a sick child, plain films may show free intraperitoneal air, indicating a perforation. A low-osmolar water-soluble contrast meal may show the leak (Figure 8–28).

Ultrasonography can detect thickening of the gastric antral wall in some gastric ulcers (Figure 8–29) (Stringer et al., 1986; Hayden et al., 1987) but should not be relied on to make the diagnosis. It may occasionally be useful for detecting unsuspected lesions or following up known disease (Stringer et al., 1986). In infants, gastric ulcers can give a thickened deformed antropyloric region on US, with elongation of the antropyloric canal and delay in gastric emptying (Hayden et al., 1987). Ulcers in older children can also appear as asymmetrical thickening of the wall. The normal distended gastric wall is usually 2 to 3 mm thick (Stringer et al., 1986). If the stomach is not distended, the gastric wall is contracted and will appear thicker than normal. Hence, the correct technique entails filling the stomach with fluid to ensure adequate distension.

If a contrast study is indicated, a double-contrast barium meal should be performed as single-contrast studies are poor at detecting gastric ulcers (Drumm et al., 1988; Ament and Christie, 1977; Ott et al., 1982; Laufer et al., 1975) although large lesser-curve ulcers may be detected (Figure 8–30). In young children, double-contrast barium examinations are more difficult to perform because lack of cooperation can limit the swallowing of gas

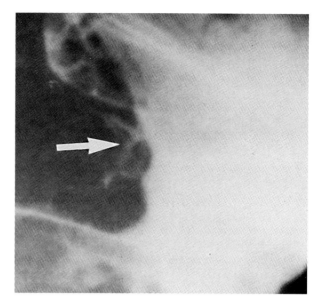

FIGURE 8–28. Gastric ulcer. An iso-osmolar water-soluble contrast (Hexabrix) meal shows a perforation with leak of contrast medium (*arrow*).

tablets, and the high-density barium preparations are relatively unpalatable. If necessary, barium with air can be instilled via a nasogastric tube (one is often already present in sick young children). To tailor the examination to the patient, close rapport with referring clinicians is essential regarding the patient's condition, as well as for consultation regarding the suitability for a nasogastric tube.

The radiologic appearance in children is similar to that in adults. On single-contrast study the ulcer is

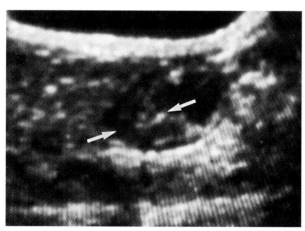

FIGURE 8–29. Gastric ulcer. Longitudinal US shows thickening of the gastric antral wall (*arrow*). A large gastric ulcer was found endoscopically. (Reprinted with permission, Stringer et al., 1986.)

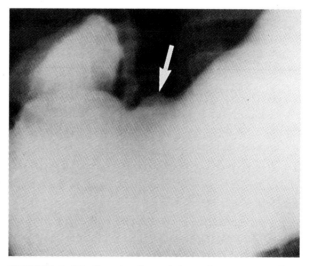

FIGURE 8–30. Gastric ulcer. A large lesser-curve ulcer niche (*arrow*) is seen on a single-contrast barium meal.

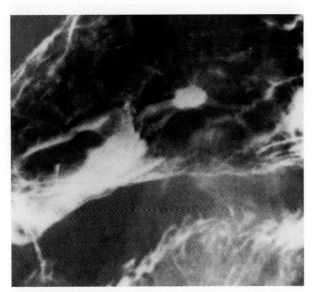

FIGURE 8–31. Gastric ulcer. A large posterior ulcer crater is filled with a pool of barium on double-contrast examination and shows radiating folds.

seen as an outpouching from the lesser curvature of the stomach (see Figure 8–30). Large ulcer craters may fill with a pool of barium on double-contrast examinations; more subtle findings include folds radiating

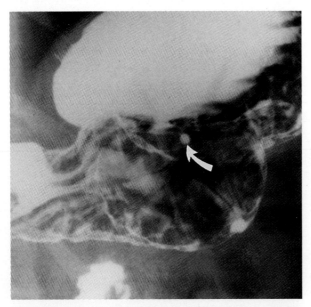

FIGURE 8–32. Stalactite phenomenon. A drip of barium is suspended from the anterior wall of the stomach (*arrow*), mimicking an ulcer niche on the posterior wall. This diagnosis was made because the barium changed shape and position whereas an ulcer crater should be constant.

from a central ulcer niche (Figure 8–31). This must not be confused with the stalactite phenomenon where a drip of barium is suspended from the anterior wall of the stomach, mimicking an ulcer niche on the posterior wall (Figure 8–32) (Gohel et al., 1978). A stalactite phenomenon will change shape and position whereas an ulcer crater should be constant.

Rarely, gastric ulcers may be multiple and cause considerable scarring (Figure 8–33). Shallow gastric ulcers may be better visualized with graded compression (Amaral, 1978).

Endoscopy

Endoscopy remains the gold standard in the detection of gastric ulcers, even when compared to the double-contrast technique (Dooley et al., 1984) (see Chapter 4). However, gastroscopy is an invasive technique with attendant risks, usually requiring a general anesthetic or heavy sedation in children under 10 years of age. Hence, a properly performed double-contrast barium meal examination should remain the screening procedure but if there is clinical concern, endoscopy should be used early to prevent the catastrophic complications of peptic ulcer disease in childhood (Drumm et al., 1988; Mougenot et al., 1976).

Neoplasms

Benign Tumors

Polyps in the stomach can be found in association with polyposis syndromes such as Gardner's syndrome, familial polyposis coli, and Peutz-Jeghers syndrome (see Chapters 9 and 10). In familial polyposis coli many gastric polyps are regenerative in type but adenomatous polyps also occur (Denzler et al., 1979). Single-contrast barium studies may show large polyps but double-contrast studies are more accurate for smaller polyps (Figure 8–34). Endoscopy is necessary to assess the histology as most polyps do not require surgery (Feczko et al., 1985). The polyps in this condition may be absent from the antrum but are found in the rest of the stomach. Occasionally, there may be a large number of adenomatous gastric polyps in Gardner's syndrome (Figure 8–35) or familial polyposis.

Benign lymphoid hyperplasia of the stomach in children is rare and is usually associated with immunoglobulin abnormality (Odes et al., 1981; Stringer et al., 1986). Ultrasonography may detect a mild antral thickening of approximately 5 mm but

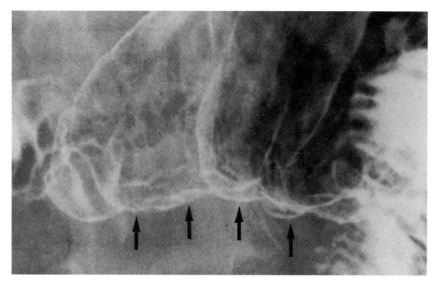

FIGURE 8–33. Gastric ulcers. Multiple gastric ulcers confirmed at endoscopy have caused greater curve deformity due to scarring (*arrows*).

this is a subtle finding and may easily be missed (Stringer et al., 1986). More obvious are the gastric nodules well seen on double-contrast barium meal (Figure 8–36) (Odes et al., 1981; Ou Tim et al., 1977; Stringer et al., 1986). Umbilication may be present (Batik et al., 1971); the term "état mammelonné" has been used to describe this appearance (Ou Tim et al., 1977).

Intramural gastric hematomas are rare and when they affect the pylorus as in hemophilia, the barium meal appearance may be identical to that seen in hypertrophic pyloric stenosis. However, ultrasonography may demonstrate the pyloric lumen and the surrounding hematoma, which rapidly resolves over several days (Bisset et al., 1988).

Other benign tumors in children are often mesenchymal. These rare benign tumors are usually found in adolescents and include leiomyoma, neurofibroma, fibroma, hemangioma, inflammatory fibroid polyp (Schroeder et al., 1987), carcinoid, lipoma (Herlinger, 1966), and teratoma. Multiple gastric leiomyomas (Figure 8–37), pulmonary hamartoma, and neuroblastoma, have been reported in a few children and is commonly referred to as Carnie's triad.

The rare gastric teratomas are benign and unlike teratomas in the rest of the gastrointestinal

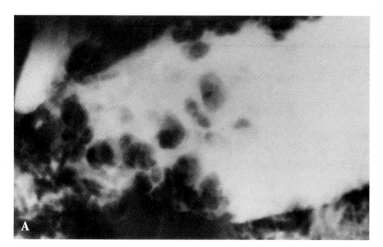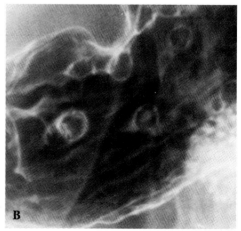

FIGURE 8–34. Gastric polyps. *A*, Single-contrast barium meal shows large polypoid filling defects in the stomach. *B*, Double-contrast studies, however, more accurately show smaller polyps.

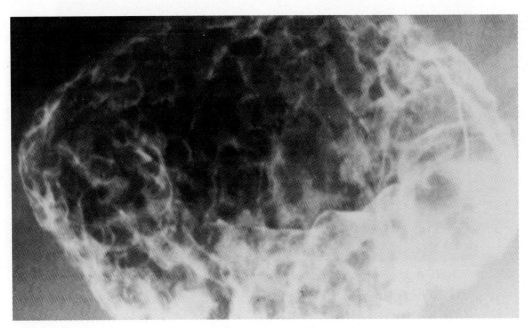

FIGURE 8–35. Gastric polyps in Gardner's syndrome. There are multiple polyps throughout the gastric fundus.

tract, have a strong male predominance (Haley et al., 1986). Clinically, they present in the first year of life, often in the first 2 weeks, with a palpable abdominal mass or abdominal distension. Respiratory distress, vomiting, constipation, a difficult delivery, and hemorrhage secondary to tumor ulceration may all occur (Siegel and Shackelford, 1978; Haley et al., 1986). Computed tomography and US may demonstrate a well-defined mass with cystic and solid components of varying proportions, frequently possessing areas of fat and calcification (Bowen et al., 1987). We have seen a benign gastric hamartoma present in a patient of 14 years with chronic anorexia and intermittent vomiting due to chronic intussusception (see Figure 8–21).

Imaging. A benign gastric teratoma may show on plain films as a soft tissue mass with calcification, and the left kidney may be depressed (Siegel and Shackelford, 1978). Preoperative diagnosis is difficult because exogastric neurogenic tumors are much more common than gastric teratomas and because renal or hepatic tumors and adrenal hemorrhage can all mimic the appearance of gastric teratomas.

Ultrasonography and occasionally CT may show the origin of the mass; a barium study will show the gastric abnormalities. Ultrasonography is the initial modality if there is an upper abdominal palpable mass. Both CT and US will clearly show the exogastric extent of these tumors, and CT may also demonstrate the size and extent of a gastric wall mass (Megibow et al., 1985). If the mass has intussuscepted into small bowel, the US and CT appearance may be characteristic (see Figure 8–21). Gastric teratomas are well marginated and have one or more cystic components of variable proportions, frequently possessing areas of calcification and fat clearly shown by CT and US (Bowen et al., 1987).

Barium studies are not usually performed unless the mass is not palpable or there is hematemesis or a suspected polyposis syndrome. Small benign gastric wall masses such as polyps are usually smooth in outline and are best seen by double-contrast examinations (see Figure 8–34), although mesenchymal tumors may have a large exogastric component which may cavitate and communicate with the stomach (Herlinger, 1966).

Malignant Tumors

Gastric carcinoma is rare in childhood but can occur in early life. *Helicobacter pylori* has been implicated as a cause of gastric and duodenal ulcers as well as gastric carcinoma (Levine et al., 1996). By

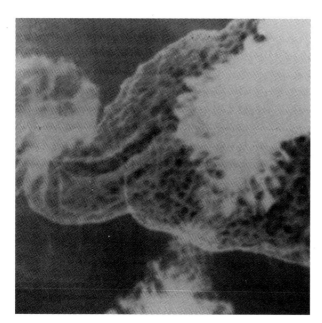

FIGURE 8–36. Benign lymphoid hyperplasia of the stomach. Numerous 2 to 3 mm gastric nodules are seen clearly on double-contrast barium meal. Umbilication of the nodules is not present. This patient has dysgamma-globulinemia and enteric giardiasis.

fied. Gastroscopy is performed and biopsies taken if a malignant mass is suspected.

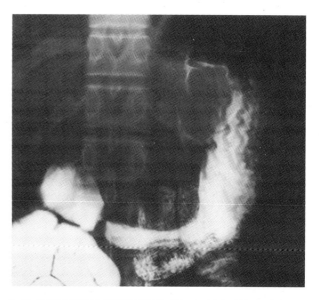

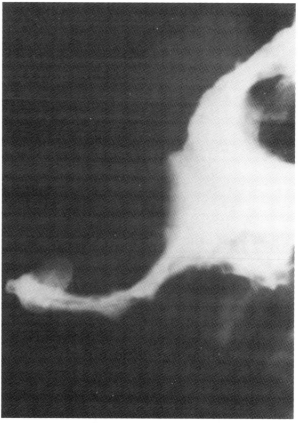

FIGURE 8–37. Multiple gastric leiomyomas. Single-contrast barium meal (*A* and *B*) shows multiple masses in the fundus, body, and antrum of the stomach in a 5-year-old child who presented with hematemesis.

the time of diagnosis, the lesion is often advanced and the prognosis is poor (Dixon and Fazzari, 1976). Gastric carcinoma also occurs in association with familial polyposis coli. It may present as a chronic gastric ulcer (Figure 8–38); because this is also a rare lesion, follow-up examinations are essential to ensure complete healing of any allegedly benign gastric ulcer. Endoscopy should be undertaken if healing does not progress.

Leiomyosarcoma and lymphoma of the stomach are more common in adults but may present in childhood (Wurlitzer et al., 1973) as can undifferentiated sarcoma. *Helicobacter pylori* may also play a role in the development of non-Hodgkin's gastric lymphoma (Levine et al., 1996). The radiologic appearance of malignant tumors in children is similar to that seen in adults, with thickening of the gastric wall, mucosal irregularity and ulceration, nodular mass lesions (Figure 8–39), and (possibly) obstruction. This is generally best shown on double-contrast barium meals although US or CT may help delineate the size and extent of spread of tumor. Mass lesions may be large, particularly in Burkitt's lymphoma. Additional disease in abdominal lymph nodes, omentum, liver, or spleen may also be identi-

MISCELLANEOUS DISORDERS

Bezoar

A bezoar is a concretion of various ingested substances in the stomach or intestines. In children there are four types: trichobezoar, phytobezoar, lactobezoar, and miscellaneous bezoars.

Trichobezoar

Trichobezoar, the most common type of bezoar in childhood, mainly affects females. It consists of hair, usually found in the stomach but also extending a variable distance into the bowel. The hair usually has been swallowed by an emotionally disturbed child. The bezoar is always dark in color and contains undigested, putrid fat mixed with the hair (DeBakey and

Ochsner, 1938). A trichobezoar produces a foul, nauseating smell, which can be noticeable on examination. The failure of swallowed hair to pass through bowel is an enigma; the occasional finding of hairballs in the stool indicates that passage can occur.

The symptoms of a trichobezoar are often vague and are present for a variable period of time. Anorexia, dyspepsia, loss of weight, weakness, and headaches may be followed by epigastric pain, nausea, and vomiting. Complications such as ulceration, perforation, intestinal obstruction, and hematemesis may occur. Besides the foul breath, examination may reveal alopecia, a furred tongue, and an abdominal mass (DeBakey and Ochsner, 1938). Protein-losing enteropathy has also been found (Valberg et al., 1966).

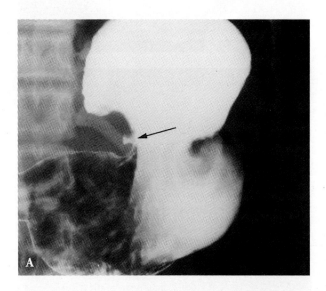

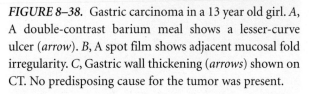

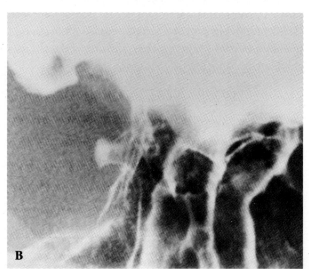

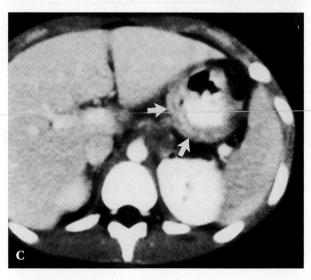

FIGURE 8–38. Gastric carcinoma in a 13 year old girl. *A,* A double-contrast barium meal shows a lesser-curve ulcer (*arrow*). *B,* A spot film shows adjacent mucosal fold irregularity. *C,* Gastric wall thickening (*arrows*) shown on CT. No predisposing cause for the tumor was present.

Phytobezoar

Phytobezoars are formed of vegetable material, in North America most often from persimmons although other foods such as coconut fiber, celery, and various roots have also been found (DeBakey and Ochsner, 1938). A food bezoar may be seen in myotonica dystrophia due to decreased gastric peristalsis (Kuiper, 1971). In the majority of patients, however, there is no underlying defect of peristalsis. A history of ingestion is easier to obtain than in cases of trichobezoar but otherwise the symptoms are similar.

Lactobezoar

Lactobezoars are the most common type of bezoar seen in infancy and are unusual in later childhood. Undiluted milk powder has been implicated as a cause (Wolf and Davis, 1963). Concentrated feeds are thought to precipitate diarrhea and vomiting, which can produce dehydration and thus initiate a vicious circle, allowing the formation of a lactobezoar (Cremin et al., 1974). Prematurity may predispose to lactobezoar, so special care is advised in feeding premature babies (Schreiner et al., 1979). Symptoms can be minimal but abdominal distension is common. Diarrhea may be present, and an abdominal mass is sometimes palpable. Gastric perforation is an occasional complication. (Cremin et al., 1974; Schreiner et al., 1979).

Treatment of lactobezoar consists of replacing all formula feeds with a dilute glucose solution given by mouth. This usually produces a prompt favorable response.

Miscellaneous Bezoars

Various concretions may produce bezoars of a more solid character. Shellac (in furniture polish), bismuth (e.g., following ingestion of bismuth for peptic ulceration), and various medicinal compounds have been implicated (DeBakey and Ochsner, 1938).

Imaging

The radiologic appearance of all bezoars is characteristic, and plain films are often sufficient to make the diagnosis. A bezoar produces a mottled gastric shadow that mimics food but it may characteristically be rimmed by gas (Figures 8–40 and 8–41). It is important to know when the child last ate in order to avoid mistaking a recent meal for a bezoar (though meals are not generally outlined by gas). A delayed fasting film may be helpful in case of doubt.

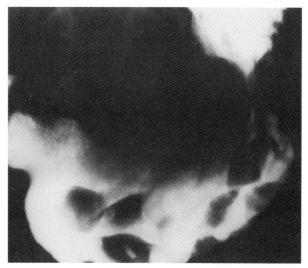

FIGURE 8–39. Burkitt's lymphoma of the stomach. A target lesion with central ulceration and several nodular masses scattered throughout the body and antrum of the stomach in a six-year-old child who presented with upper gastrointestinal bleeding.

If necessary, US will show the bezoar (see Figure 8–40). If it is a trichobezoar, US will demonstrate an echogenic rim due to the spongy nature of the bezoar at the periphery but generally will show a very echogenic edge as the first acoustic interface will reflect most of the sound (Ratcliffe, 1982; McCracken et al., 1986; Malpani et al., 1988; Tennenhouse and Wilson, 1990). A lactobezoar is also hyperechoic but does not have such a strong first interface reflection and so appears more as a hyperechoic mass of mixed echo texture (Naik et al., 1987).

If contrast studies are needed, either air passed through a nasogastric tube or orally administered barium will demonstrate the space-occupying mass. This is often best seen after barium has emptied from the stomach as some residual barium will coat the crevices in the bezoar (Figure 8–42). Extension into the small bowel may also be seen.

Except for lactobezoars, bezoars are best treated surgically.

Foreign Body Ingestion

A variety of ingested foreign bodies (Desrentes, 1990) can be visualized radiologically. Once a foreign body has reached the stomach it is unlikely to require any active treatment other than observation as it usually is passed per rectum in time.

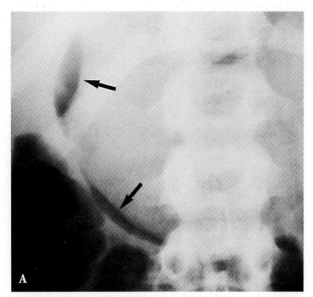 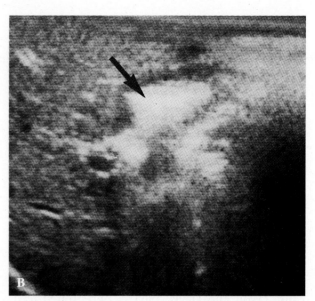

FIGURE 8–40. Trichobezoar. *A,* Plain film shows a curvilinear gas shadow (*arrows*) faintly surrounding part of a mottled intragastric mass. *B,* Ultrasonography shows highly echogenic antral contents (*arrow*) but, unusually, relatively little acoustic shadowing.

Spontaneous Rupture of the Stomach in Neonates

Spontaneous rupture of the stomach very occasionally occurs in neonates. This was first thought to be due to muscular defects in the stomach wall but rupture secondary to gastric distension in experimental animals has a similar histologic appearance to that of the spontaneous rupture seen in neonates

(Shaw et al., 1965). Selective circulatory ischemia (as part of the response to stress, hypoxia, or shock), peptic ulceration, and trauma following intubation have been implicated in the etiology (Lloyd, 1969). Perforation may also occur proximal to duodenal obstruction (Takebayaski et al., 1975).

Radiologically, pneumoperitoneum is the usual sign of intestinal perforation, and absence of

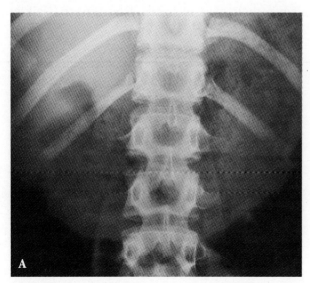 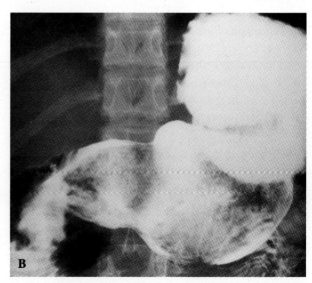

FIGURE 8–41. Trichobezoar. *A,* Plain film shows a curvilinear gas shadow (*arrow*) faintly surrounding part of a mottled intragastric mass. *B,* Barium outlines the bezoar.

gas in the stomach may suggest the site of perforation. The absence of a gas-fluid level in the stomach on erect films and a paucity of gas in the small and large bowel are suggestive but not definitive of gastric rupture (Figure 8–43). The presence of a gas-fluid level in the stomach in association with dilated gas-filled loops of small and large bowel suggests a perforation due to necrotizing enterocolitis of the bowel even in the absence of specific evidence for this diagnosis such as portal vein or intramural gas (Pochaczevsky and Bryk, 1972).

Massive subcutaneous emphysema can develop following gastric rupture secondary to duodenal obstruction (Takebayaski et al., 1975).

Gastric Rupture following Blunt Abdominal Trauma

A rare condition, especially in children, gastric perforation following blunt abdominal trauma requires prompt diagnosis and treatment; it leads to significant morbidity and mortality. Gastric perforation follows severe abrupt pressure applied to a distended stomach. (An empty stomach is more pliable and is protected behind the costal margin.) This injury is strongly associated with trauma to other organs, particularly the spleen and kidney.

Plain-film radiography and CT may show evidence of free subdiaphragmatic air and visualize the falciform ligament outlined by air. Computed tomography may also show the intraperitoneal location of the tip of a nasogastric tube as well as intraperitoneal layering of food and fluid (Tu et al., 1992).

Pneumatosis

Linear lucencies in the stomach wall indicate pneumatosis, which in infancy often signals serious underlying disease. Gastric pneumatosis may be seen in association with gastric outlet obstruction, usually secondary to hypertrophic pyloric stenosis (Leonidas, 1976) or necrotizing enterocolitis (Bell et al., 1971; Santulli et al., 1975) but also as an isolated finding (Figure 8–44) (Robinson et al., 1974; Holgerson et al., 1974). The cause of gastric pneumatosis is uncertain; in cases of gastric obstruction it may be caused by elevated intragastric pressure that forces gas through superficial mucosal tears (Holgerson et al., 1974). Pneumatosis in necrotizing enterocolitis may be due to invasion of the necrotic mucosa by gas-forming bacteria (Stone et al., 1968).

Gastric pneumatosis is rare in older children. Gastric outlet obstruction, usually volvulus, is often the underlying cause. Linear lucencies can be seen in the stomach wall on radiography, and the gastric gas pattern may indicate the underlying cause. (See also emphysematous gastritis and Figure 8–24.)

Acute gastric dilatation may be associated with pneumatosis and is a rare cause of portal venous gas and does not require surgical intervention (Radin et al., 1987). When branching lucencies are seen in the right upper quadrant on an abdominal radiograph, portal venous gas must be distinguished from pneumobilia. Although a central distribution of gas is more common with pneumobilia than with portal venous gas, it is not a reliable distinguishing feature. Gastric emphysema, a rapid resolution of the extra-intestinal gas, and absence of an enterobiliary fistula all help in distinguishing portal venous gas from pneumobilia.

Diffuse Neonatal Gastric Infarction

Diffuse neonatal gastric infarction can be a devastating complication of invasion of the gastric wall and

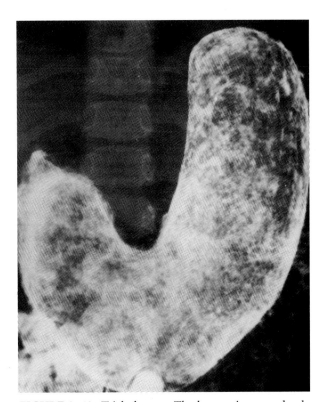

FIGURE 8–42. Trichobezoar. The bezoar is most clearly seen following a barium meal examination, when barium coats its crevices.

vessels by fungi colonizing the gastric mucosa. The predisposing factors for this hazard include broad-spectrum antibiotic therapy and the shunting of blood flow away from the stomach during an episode of asphyxia. Plain radiographs and positive contrast studies in neonates with diffuse gastric infarction prior to perforation may suggest an erroneous diagnosis of mechanical gastric outlet obstruction due to the devitalized stomach being aperistaltic, dilated, and fixed in position (Johnson et al., 1988). Gastric infarction should be included in the differential diagnosis of a dilated aperistaltic stomach that fails to propel air or contrast material distally.

Volvulus

Gastric volvulus is unusual in children because the stomach is usually tethered by the esophagus, the retroperitoneal duodenum, the gastrohepatic, gastrophrenic, gastrosplenic, and gastrocolic (the greater omentum) ligaments. These attachments must be abnormal or the ligaments stretched for the stomach to undergo volvulus (Ziprkowski and Teele, 1979). It is not surprising, therefore, that gastric volvulus is often associated with other congenital anomalies such as midgut malrotation, diaphragmatic hernia, and eventration.

Volvulus can be mesenteroaxial or organoaxial (Figure 8–45). Mesenteroaxial volvulus often has an axis through the esophagogastric junction as that is often the least mobile point of the stomach in children. The axis is more perpendicular to a line joining the esophagogastric junction and duodenal cap if the former is more mobile. With organoaxial volvulus, the twist occurs around an axis passing through the duodenal cap and esophagogastric junction.

Volvulus may be total or partial, the latter usually limited to the pylorus. It may be asymptomatic or range from acute abdominal crisis to more chronic symptoms (Cole and Dickinson, 1971; Yousef et al., 1983). Chronic intermittent abdominal pain, distension, and failure to thrive may all be due to a chronic gastric volvulus, frequently associated with a large hiatal hernia (Yousef et al., 1983).

Mesenteroaxial Volvulus

Mesenteroaxial volvulus is the most common form of volvulus in children and neonates (Ziprkowski and Teele, 1979; Campbell et al., 1972; Campbell, 1979). Though usually associated with midgut malrotation or diaphragmatic hernia (see Chapter 7), occasionally no predisposing cause is found (Kilcoyne et al., 1972).

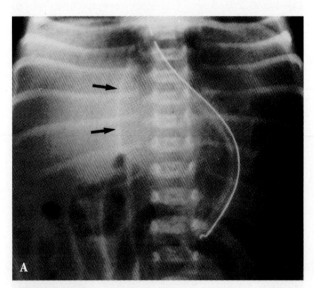

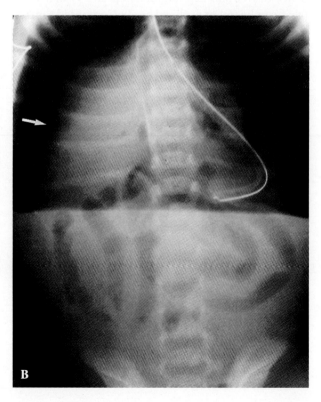

FIGURE 8–43. Neonatal gastric rupture. Massive hydropneumoperitoneum is present. *A,* The stomach is devoid of gas on the supine film. *B,* There is no gastric gas-fluid level on the erect film. The falciform ligament (*A, arrows*) and liver (*B, arrow*) are outlined by free intraperitoneal gas.

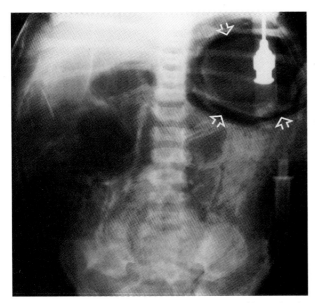

FIGURE 8–44. Gastric pneumatosis. Linear lucencies in the stomach wall (*arrows*) and in other loops of bowel indicate pneumatosis in this child with Hirschsprung's disease, causing obstruction.

It often presents acutely with pain and vomiting, but chronic symptoms such as poor growth, failure to thrive, and respiratory problems may be present.

The distended stomach appears spherical on supine plain radiographic examinations (Figure 8–46); on erect films a gas-fluid level may be present in the fundus inferiorly and in the antrum superiorly. Ultrasonography is rarely indicated but may show the grossly distended stomach (see Figure 8–46).

Obstruction may be found on a barium meal examination at the esophagogastric junction or more distally. If barium reaches the stomach, the orientation and inferior position of fundus relative to the antrum can be seen (Ziprkowski and Teele, 1979).

Organoaxial Volvulus

Organoaxial volvulus is uncommon in children (Ziprkowski and Teele, 1979; Cole and Dickinson, 1971). A distended stomach is easier to twist than an empty one (Dalgaard, 1952), and organoaxial volvulus is seen in retarded children with aerophagia (Ziprkowski and Teele, 1970). Transverse colonic distension along with gastric distension may predispose to organoaxial volvulus; this type of volvulus may also occur in association with a large hiatal hernia or (rarely) with Morgagni's hernia (Cybulsky and Himal, 1985).

The diagnosis of organoaxial volvulus on plain films may be difficult with a nonspecific dilated round stomach. On barium examination, the reversal of greater and lesser curvatures of a horizontally oriented stomach can be difficult to appreciate; the characteristic appearance is the inferior position of the duodenal cap relative to the antrum (Figure 8–47). Partial volvulus will give an intermediate appearance (Figure 8–48).

Displacement

A child's stomach may occasionally be displaced by an extrinsic mass. Gastrointestinal causes include pancreatic pseudocyst; hepatic, splenic, choledochal, or duplication cyst; hematoma secondary to bleeding diathesis or trauma; retroperitoneal tumor; left-sided gallbladder (Grossman and Redo, 1966); lymphangioma (Siegel et al., 1978); and liver malformation associated with omphalocele (Oh et al., 1977).

The symptoms and signs depend on the size and position of the mass. When the mass is adjacent to the pylorus, obstruction may result; in other locations, the mass may be a chance finding.

Ultrasonography should be the initial examination for suspected mass lesions. The results will deter-

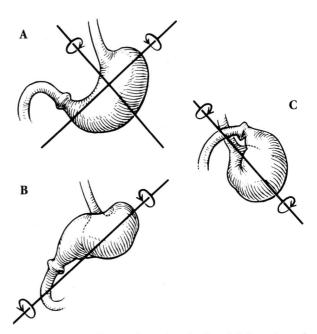

FIGURE 8–45. Types of gastric volvulus. (*A*) Rotation of the stomach can occur around two axes. (*B*) Rotation around axis X results in organoaxial volvulus. (*C*) Rotation around axis Y results in mesenteroaxial volvulus.

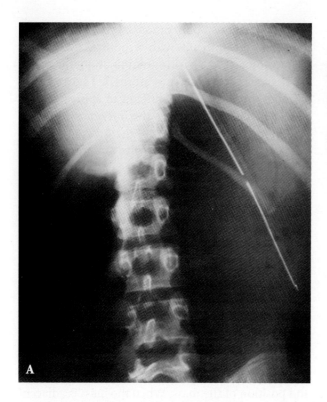

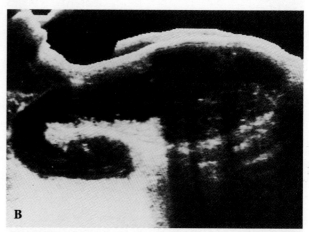

FIGURE 8–46. Mesenteroaxial volvulus. *A*, Supine plain film shows the grossly distended spherical stomach just after a nasogastric tube had been passed with some difficulty. *B*, Fluid within the distended stomach and duodenum shown on US. The study was performed after several liters of gas and fluid had been aspirated via the nasogastric tube.

mine the most appropriate subsequent examinations (such as barium study, radionuclide scan, or CT).

MISCELLANEOUS PROCEDURES

Percutaneous Gastrostomy

Enteral alimentation is a crucial component of care for the malnourished child who cannot eat. Until recently, long-term alimentation was delivered through nasogastric tubes or gastrostomy tubes placed at surgery but percutaneous gastrostomy (PG) is replacing these traditional methods. The advantages of PG over nasogastric tubes include improved comfort, increased mobility, greater social acceptance, increased ease of feedings, and decreased gastroesophageal reflux. This simple technique for jejunal feeding requires no general anesthesia or gastroscopy in adults (Ho, 1983; Ho et al., 1985; Van Sonnenberg et al., 1986; Wills and Oglesby, 1985; Tao and Gilles, 1983) and is now well accepted for both adults and children (Keller et al., 1986; Wollman et al., 1995).

There are many nonradiologic techniques for inserting a gastrostomy but some consider a fluoroscopic method preferable (see Chapter 5). A common radiologic technique entails insufflation of the stomach via a nasogastric tube, delineation of the liver with US (or CT) to ensure it is not lying anterior to the stomach, and fluoroscopically guided gastric percutaneous puncture with placement of gastrostomy or jejunostomy feeding tube by guidewire exchange (McLean et al., 1982; Cory et al., 1988; Towbin et al., 1988; Wills and Oglesby, 1988; Ho and Yeung, 1992; McLoughlin et al., 1996). (For further details, see Chapter 5.)

Gastrostomy Complications

Following gastrostomy by any method, a variety of complications can occur which require radiologic examination. A suspected malposition or migration of the catheter or a suspected leak can be investigated by injecting a small volume of iso-osmolar water-soluble contrast media under fluoroscopic control. This easily demonstrates the position of the catheter.

A correctly positioned PG tube lies in the body of the stomach anchored to the anterior abdominal wall. Correct initial placement does not protect against eventual migration beyond the gastric lumen. A gastrocutaneous track is formed 2 to 3 weeks after initial placement of a PG tube. After the track has matured, tube replacement is usually simple. However, because tube exchange creates an opportunity for misplacement, the position of the newly placed tube must be verified fluoroscopically after the injection of contrast material.

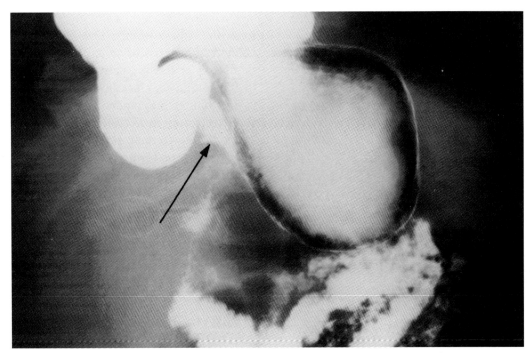

FIGURE 8–47. Organoaxial volvulus. A large esophageal hiatus allowed superior movement of the antrum into the chest with resultant organoaxial rotation. The duodenal cap (*arrow*) lies inferior to the antrum.

After PG, pneumoperitoneum and abdominal wall or gastric hematoma are commonly present. Presence of subcutaneous emphysema, free peri-toneal fluid, or a loculated abdominal fluid collection are signs of possible complication (Wojtowycz and Arata, 1988).

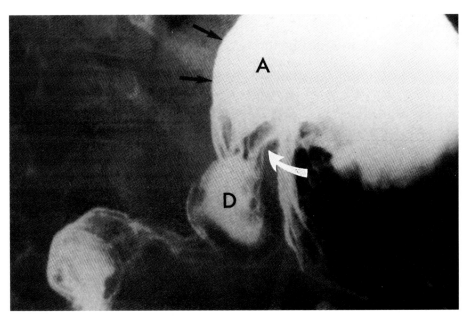

FIGURE 8–48. Partial organoaxial volvulus. The barium examination shows reversal of greater (*black arrows*) and lesser (*white arrow*) curvatures of the stomach, causing the duodenal cap (D) to lie inferior to the gastric antrum (A).

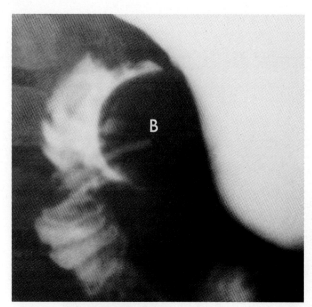

FIGURE 8–49. Duodenal obstruction from Foley gastrostomy. The inflated balloon (B) of a Foley balloon catheter has migrated into the duodenum, causing almost complete obstruction.

Percutaneous gastrostomy tubes with antral stomas subject the feeding tube to increased peristalsis, which predisposes the tube to dislodgment and antegrade propulsion. Tube migration is more common with Foley catheter-type feeding tubes than with newer tubes. They can migrate into the duodenum (Figure 8–49) or even the esophagus and cause obstruction. In addition to luminal occlusion, migrating tubes may rarely incite an intestinal obstruction by causing a retrograde jejunoduodenogastric intussusception (Weber and Nadel, 1991; Levine et al., 1995). Findings in this rare condition on CT include gastric distension associated with a soft tissue mass in the antrum and duodenum with an eccentrically placed fatty area of attenuation that represents the intussusception and intussuscepted mesentery, and a coiled-spring appearance resulting from coating of the intussusception by contrast material (Weber and Nadel, 1991).

Local infection may occur following PG tube placement. The infection is usually a local wound infection in the abdominal wall that responds well to antibiotics; rarely, a more serious necrotic fasciitis may occur. Ultrasonography may be requested if an underlying abscess is suspected. Findings include thickening of the rectus muscles, the abdominal wall, and the soft tissue encasing the PG tube.

Gastroesophageal reflux may be more evident following a gastrostomy. This is especially true in children at high risk of reflux such as those with cystic fibrosis or cerebral palsy and whose intake prior to gastrostomy may have been reduced. Ideally, a pre-gastrostomy scintigraphic gastroesophageal reflux study or barium meal examination will show who is at risk for this complication, and an anti-reflux procedure can be performed at the time of gastrostomy.

Less common complications include gastric ulcers, gastric perforation, penetration into the pancreas, separation of stomach from abdominal wall, and (rarely) gastric torsion and gastric pneumotosis (Vade et al., 1983). (For more details, see Chapter 5.)

REFERENCES

EMBRYOGENESIS; CONGENITAL AND DEVELOPMENTAL ANOMALIES

Beseman EF, Auerbach SH, Wolfe WW. The importance of roentgenologic diagnosis of aberrant pancreatic tissue in the gastrointestinal tract. AJR 1969;107:71–6.

Bidwell JK, Nelson A. Prenatal ultrasonic diagnosis of congenital duplication of the stomach. J Ultrasound Med 1986; 5:589–91.

Blank E, Chisholm AJ. Congenital microgastria, a case report with a 26 year follow-up. Pediatrics 1973;51:1037–41.

Bronsther B, Nadeau MR, Abrams MW. Congenital pyloric atresia: a report of three cases and review of the literature. Surgery 1971;69:130–6.

Cockrell CH, Cho SR, Messmer JM, et al. Intramural gastric diverticula: a report of three cases. Br J Radiol 1984; 57:288.

Cremin BJ. Congenital pyloric antral membranes in infancy. Radiology 1969;92:509–12.

De Groot WG, Postumu R, Hunter AGW. Familial pyloric atresia associated with epidermolysis bullosa. J Pediatr 1978;92:429–31.

Dodd GD, Sheft D. Diverticulum of the greater curvature of the stomach: a roentgenographic curiosity. AJR 1969;107:102–4.

Egelhoff JC, Bisset GS, Strife JL. Multiple enteric duplications in an infant. Pediatr Radiol 1986;16:160–1.

Eklof O, Lassrich A, Stanley P, et al. Ectopic pancreas. Pediatr Radiol 1973;1:24–7.

Farman J, Cywes S, Weberloff L. Pyloric mucosal diaphragms. Clin Radiol 1968;19:98–9.

Felson B, Berkman YM, Hoyumpa AM. Gastric mucosal diaphragm. Radiology 1969;92:513–7.

Flachs K, Stelman HH, Matsumoto PJH. Partial gastric diverticula. AJR 1965;94:339–42.

Franken EA Jr, Smith WL, editors. Gastrointestinal imaging in pediatrics. 2nd ed. Philadelphia: Harper & Row; 1982. p. 110.

Fujioka M, Fisher S, Young LW. Pseudoweb of the gastric antrum in infants. Pediatr Radiol 1980;9:73–5.

Gorman B, Shaw DG. Congenital microgastria. Br J Radiol 1984;57:260–2.

Hochberger O, Swoboda W. Congenital microgastria: a follow-up observation over six years. Pediatr Radiol 1974;2:207–8.

Jefferson K, Rees S. Clinical cardiac radiology. 2nd ed. London: Butterworths; 1980. p. 10.

Kangarloo H, Sample WF, Hansen G, et al. Ultrasonic evaluation of abdominal gastrointestinal tract duplication in children. Radiology 1979;131:191–4.

Kessler H, Smulewicz JJ. Microgastria associated with agenesis of the spleen. Radiology 1973;107:393–6.

Kilman WJ, Berk RN. The spectrum of radiographic features of aberrant pancreatic rests involving the stomach. Radiology 1977;123:291–6.

Kremer RM, Lepoff RB, Izant RJ, et al. Duplication of the stomach. J Pediatr Surg 1970;5:360–4.

Lucaya J, Ochoa JB. Ectopic pancreas in the stomach. J Pediatr Surg 1976;11:101–2.

Matsumoto Y, Kawai Y, Kimura K. Aberrant pancreas causing pyloric obstruction. Surgery 1974;76:827–9.

Meeroff M, Gollan JRM, Meeroff JC. Gastric diverticulum. Am J Gastroenterol 1967;47:189–203.

Melhem RE, Salem G, Mishalany H, et al. Pyloro-duodenal atresia: a report of three families with several similarly affected children. Pediatr Radiol 1975;3:1–5.

Moccia WA, Astacio K, Kande JV. Ultrasonography demonstration of gastric duplication in infancy. Pediatr Radiol 1981;11:52–4.

Orense M, Garcia Hernandez JB, Celorio C, et al. Pyloric atresia associated with epidermolysis bullosa. Pediatr Radiol 1987;17:435.

Rhind JA. Mucosal stenosis of the pylorus. Br J Surg 1959;46:534–40.

Rooney DR. Aberrant pancreatic tissue in stomach. Radiology 1959;73:241–4.

Schwartz AN, Goiney RC, Graney DO. Gastric diverticulum simulating an adrenal mass: CT appearance and embryogenesis. AJR 1986;146:553–4.

Shackelford G. Barium collections in the stomach mimicking intraluminal diverticula. AJR 1982;139:805–6.

Shackelford G, McAlister WH, Brodeur AE, et al. Congenital microgastria. AJR 1973;118:72–6.

Stone DD, Riddervold HO, Keats TE. An unusual case of aberrant pancreas in the stomach: a roentgenographic and gastrophotographic demonstration. AJR 1971;113:128.

Stringer DA, Daneman A, Brunelle F, et al. US of the normal and abnormal stomach (excluding hypertrophic pyloric stenosis) in children. J Ultrasound Med 1986;5:183–8.

Strobel CT, Smith LE, Fonkalsrud EW, et al. Ectopic pancreatic tissue in the gastric antrum. J Pediatr 1978;92:586–8.

Thornhill BA, Cho KC, Morehouse HT. Gastric duplication associated with pulmonary sequestration: CT manifestations. AJR 1982;138:1168–71.

Wieczorek RL, Seidman I, Ranson JH, et al. Congenital duplication of the stomach: case report and review of the literature. Am J Gastroenterol 1984;8:597–602

ACQUIRED OUTLET OBSTRUCTION

Andressy RJ, Haff RC, Larsen GL. Infantile hypertrophic pyloric stenosis during the first week of life. Clin Pediatr 1977;16:476–8.

Apfelberg DB, Glicklich M, Tang TT. Gastroduodenal intussusception in a child. Surgery 1971;69:736–40.

Ball TI, Atkinson GO, Gay BB. Ultrasound diagnosis of hypertrophic pyloric stenosis: real time application and demonstration of a new US sign. Radiology 1983;147:499–502.

Bilodeau RG. Inheritance of hypertrophic pyloric stenosis. AJR 1971;133:241–4.

Bisset RAL, Gupta SC. Hypertrophic pyloric stenosis, ultrasonic appearances in a small baby. Pediatr Radiol 1988;18:405.

Blumhagen JD. The role of ultrasonography in the evaluation of vomiting in infants. Pediatr Radiol 1986;16:267–70.

Blumhagen JD, Coombs JB. Ultrasound in the diagnosis of hypertrophic pyloric stenosis. J Clin Ultrasound 1981;9:289–92.

Blumhagen JD, Noble HGS. Muscle thickness in hypertrophic pyloric stenosis: US determination. AJR 1983;140:221–3.

Bowen A III, Gibson MD. Chronic granulomatous disease with gastric antral narrowing. Pediatr Radiol 1980;10:119–20.

Bryne WJ, Kangarloo H, Ament ME, et al. Antral dysmotility: an unrecognized cause of chronic vomiting during infancy. Ann Surg 1981;193:521–4.

Cohen HL, Schechter S, Mestel AL, et al. Ultrasonic "double tract" sign in hypertrophic pyloris stenosis. J Ultrasound Med 1987;6:139–43.

Currarino G. The value of double contrast examination of the stomach with pressure "spots" in the diagnosis of infantile hypertrophic pyloric stenosis. Radiology 1964;83:873–8.

Dassonville M, Verstreken L, De Laet M-H. Falciform ligament: a cause of extrinsic antral obstruction in the neonatal period. J Pediatr Surg 1986:21:977–8.

Franken EA Jr, Saldino RN. Hypertrophic pyloric stenosis complicating esophageal atresia with tracheoesophageal fistula. Am J Surg 1969;117:647–9.

Franken EA Jr, Smith WL, Smith JA. Paralysis of the small bowel resembling mechanical intestinal obstruction. Gastrointest Radiol 1980;5:161–7.

Geer LL, Gaisie G, Mandell VS, et al. Evolution of pyloric stenosis in the first week of life. Pediatr Radiol 1985;15:206–8.

Graif M, Itzchak Y, Argaid I, et al. The pylorus in infancy: overall US assessment. Pediatr Radiol 1984;14:14–7.

Griscom NT, Kirkpatrick JA, Girdany BR, et al. Gastric antral narrowing in chronic granulomatous disease of childhood. Pediatrics 1974;54:456–60.

Haller JO, Cohen HL. Hypertrophic pyloric stenosis: diagnosis using US. Radiology 1986;161:338–9.

Haran PJ, Darling DB, Sciammas F. The value of the double tract sign as a differentiating factor between pylorospasm and hypertrophic pyloric stenosis. Radiology 1966;86:723–5.

Hartenberg MA, Kodroff MB. Chronic granulomatous disease of childhood: probable diffuse gastric involvement. Pediatr Radiol 1984;14:57–8.

Hayden CK, Swischuk LE, Lobe TE, et al. Ultrasound: the definitive imaging modality in pyloric stenosis. Radiographics 1984;4:517–30.

Hernanz-Schulman M, Sells LL, Ambrosino MM, et al. Hypertrophic pyloric stenosis in the infant without a palpable olive: accuracy of US diagnosis. Radiology 1994;193:771–6.

Jamroz GA, Blocker SH, McAlister WH. Radiographic findings after incomplete pyloromyotomy. Gastrointest Radiol 1986;11:139–41.

Konvolinka CW, Wernuth CR. Hypertrophic pyloric stenosis in older infants. Am J Dis Child 1971;122:76–9.

Kopen PA, McAlister WH. Upper gastrointestinal and ultrasound examinations of gastric antral involvement in chronic granulomatous disease. Pediatr Radiol 1984;14:91–3.

Lamki N, Athey PA, Round ME, et al. Hypertrophic pyloric stenosis in the neonate—diagnostic criteria revisited. J Can Assoc Radiol 1993;44:21–4.

Lichtman S, Hayes G, Stringer DA, et al. Chronic intussusception due to antral myoepithelioma. J Pediatr Surg 1986;21:956–8.

Magilner AD. Esophageal atresia and hypertrophic pyloric stenosis: sequential coexistance of disease (case report). AJR 1986;147:329–30.

Mandell GA. Association of antral diaphragms and hypertrophic pyloric stenosis. AJR 1978;131:203–6.

Mascatello VJ, Carrera GF, Teele RL, et al. The ultrasonic demonstration of gastric lesions. J Clin Ultrasound 1977;5:383–7.

Meuwissen T, Sloof JP. Roentgenologic diagnosis of congenital hypertrophic pyloric stenosis. Acta Paediatr 1932;14:19–48.

Neilson D, Hollman AS. The ultrasonic diagnosis of infantile hypertrophic pyloric stenosis: technique and accuracy. Clin Radiol 1994;49:246–7.

Oh KS, Strife JL, Fischer KC, Teele R. Pyloroduodenal deformity due to liver malformation associated with omphalocele. AJR 1977;128:957–60.

O'Keeffe FN, Stansberry SD, Swischuk LE, Hayden CK Jr. Antropyloric muscle thickness at US in infants: what is normal? Radiology 1991;178:827–30.

Pilling DW. Infantile hypertrophic pyloric stenosis: a fresh approach to the diagnosis. Clin Radiol 1983;34:51–3.

Riggs W Jr, Long L. The value of the plain film roentgenogram in pyloric stenosis. AJR 1971;112:77–82.

Sauerbrei EE, Paloschi GGB. The ultrasonic features of hypertrophic pyloric stenosis, with emphasis on the postoperative appearance. Radiology 1983;147:503–6.

Shopfner CE. "Pyloric tit" in hypertrophic pyloric stenosis. AJR 1964;91:674–9.

Shopfner CE, Kalmon EH, Coin CG. The diagnosis of hypertrophic pyloric stenosis. AJR 1964;91:796–800.

Slim MS, Bitar JG, Idriss H. Hypertrophy of the pyloric mucosa: a rare cause of congenital pyloric obstruction. Am J Dis Child 1964;107:636–9.

Spevak MR, Ahmadjian JM, Kleinman PK, et al. US of hypertrophic pyloric stenosis: frequency and cause of nonuniform echogenicity of the thickened pyloric muscle. AJR 1992;158:129–32.

Steinicke O, Roelsgaard M. Radiographic follow-up in hypertrophic pyloric stenosis. Acta Paediatr 1960;49:4–16.

Stringer DA, Daneman A, Brunelle F, et al. US of the normal and abnormal stomach (excluding hypertrophic pyloric stenosis) in children. J Ultrasound Med 1986;5:183–8.

Stundar RJ, Le Quesne GW, Little KET. The improved ultrasound diagnosis of hypertrophic pyloric stenosis. Pediatr Radiol 1986;16:200–5.

Sufian S, Ominsky S, Matsumoto T. Congenital double pylorus: a case report and review of the literature. Gastroenterology 1977;73:154–7.

Teele RL, Smith EH. Ultrasound in the diagnosis of idiopathic hypertrophic pyloric stenosis. N Engl J Med 1977;296:1149–50.

Wallgren A. Preclinical stage of infantile hypertrophic pyloric stenosis. Am J Dis Child 1946;72:371–6.

Westra SJ, de Groot CJ, Smits NJ, Staalman CR. Hyper-trophic pyloric stenosis: use of the pyloric volume measurement in early US diagnosis. Radiology 1989;172:618–9.

Gastritis

Baker A, Volberg F, Sumner T, et al. Childhood Menetrier's disease: four new cases and discussion of the literature. Gastrointest Radiol 1986;11:131–4.

Bowen A, Gibson MD. Chronic granulomatous disease with gastric antral narrowing. Pediatr Radiol 1980;10:119–20.

Burns B, Gay BB. Menetrier's disease of the stomach in children. AJR 1968;103:300–6.

Caporali R, Luciano S. Diffuse varioliform gastritis. Arch Dis Child 1986;61:407–8.

Cello JP. *Helicobacter pylori* and peptic ulcer disease. AJR 1995;164:283–6.

Chouraqui JP, Roy CC, Brochu P, et al. Menetrier's disease in children: report of a patient and review of sixteen other cases. Gastroenterology 1981;80:1042–7.

Coad NAG, Shah KJ. Menetrier's disease in childhood associated with cytomegalovirus infection: a case report and review of the literature. Br J Radiol 1986;59:618–20.

Colquhoun J. Intramural gas in hollow viscera. Clin Radiol 1965;16:71–85.

Degnan TJ. Idiopathic hypoproteinemia. J Pediatr 1957;51:448–51.

Derchi LE, Biggi GARE, Cicio GR, et al. US findings of Menetrier's disease: a case report. Gastrointest Radiol 1982;7:323–5.

Franken EA Jr. Caustic damage of the gastrointestinal tract: roentgen features. AJR 1973;118:77–85.

Glick SN, Cavanaugh B, Teplick SK. The hypertrophied antral-pyloric fold. AJR 1985;145:547–9.

Griscom NT, Kirkpatrick JA, Girdany BR, et al. Gastric antral narrowing in chronic granulomatous disease of childhood. Pediatrics 1974;54:456–60.

Henderson SE, Sprague PL. A case of hypertrophic protein losing enteropathy. Pediatr Radiol 1979;8:261–2.

Johnson JF, Woisard KK, Cooper GL. Diffuse neonatal gastric infarction. Pediatr Radiol 1988;18:161–3.

Katz D, Gans R, Antonelle M. Benign air dissection of the

esophagus and stomach at fibroesophagoscopy. Gastrointest Endosc 1972;19:72–4.

Kay-Butler JJ. A case of interstitial gastric emphysema. Br J Surg 1962;50:99–107.

Keto P, Suoranta H, Myllarniemi H, et al. Areae gastricae in gastritis: lack of correlation between size and histology. AJR 1983;141:693–6.

Lachman RS, Martin DJ, Vawter GF. Thick gastric folds in childhood. AJR 1971;112:83–92.

Leonidas JC, Beatty EC, Wenner HA. Menetrier's disease and cytomegalovirus infection in childhood. Am J Dis Child 1973;126:806–8.

Levine MS, Verstandig A, Laufer I. Serpiginous gastric erosions caused by aspirin and other nonsteroidal anti-inflammatory drugs. AJR 1986;146:31–4.

Levitt R, Stanley RJ, Wise L. Gastric bullae. Radiology 1975;115:597–8.

Marks MP, Lanza MV, Kahlstrom EJ, et al. Pediatric hypertrophic gastropathy. AJR 1986;147:1031–4.

Marshall BJ, Warren JR. Unidentified curved bacilli in the stomach of patients with gastritis and peptic ulceration. Lancet 1984:1311–5.

Martin DF, Hartley G. Gastric emphysema demonstrated by computed tomography. Br J Radiol 1986;59:507–8.

McLean AM, Paul RE, Phillips E, et al. Chronic erosive gastritis—clinical and radiological features. J Can Assoc Radiol 1982;33:158–62.

McNulty CAM, Wise R. Gastric microflora. BMJ 1985; 291:366–7.

Myhre J, Wilson JA. A study on the occurrence of pneumoperitoneum after gastrostomy and the observance of interstitial emphysema of the stomach. Gastroenterology 1948;11:118–9.

Newman B, Bowen A, Meza MP, Towbin RB. Pediatric case of the day. Acute iron ingestion. Radiographics 1992; 12:606–8.

O'Connell DJ, Chrispin AR. Unusual gastrointestinal features in a child with pernicious anemia. Gastrointest Radiol 1976;1:263–5.

Ott DJ, Gelfand DW, Wu WC, et al. Sensitivity of single- vs. double-contrast radiology in erosive gastritis. AJR 1982;138:263–6.

Pugh TF, Fitch SJ. Invasive gastric candidiasis. Pediatr Radiol 1986;16:67–8.

Sandberg DH. Hypertrophic gastropathy (Ménétrier's disease) in childhood. J Pediatr 1971;78:866–8.

Saverymuttu AH, Corbishley CM, Maxwell JD, Joseph AEA. Thickened stomach—an ultrasound sign of portal hypertension. Clin Radiol 1990;41:17–8.

Scharschmidt BF. The natural history of hypertrophic gastropathy (Menetrier's disease). Am J Med 1977;63: 641–4.

Smart PE, Weinfeld A, Thompson NE, Defortuna AM. Toxoplasmosis of the stomach: a cause of antral narrowing. Radiology 1990;174:369–70.

Smith HJ. Radiographic response to cimetidine in patients with basal gastric acid hypersecretion. AJR 1984;142:118.

Stringer DA, Daneman A, Brunelle F, et al. US of the normal and abnormal stomach (excluding hypertrophic pyloric stenosis) in children. J Ultrasound Med 1986;5:186–8.

Teele RL, Katz AJ, Goldman H, et al. Radiographic features of eosinophilic gastroenteritis (allergic gastroenteropathy) of childhood. AJR 1979;132: 578–80.

Theoni RF, Goldberg HI, Ominsky S, et al. Detection of gastritis by single and double contrast radiography. Radiology 1983;148:621–6.

Tootla F, Lucas RJ, Bernacki EG, et al. Gastroduodenal Crohn's disease. Arch Surg 1976;3:857–8.

Turner CJ, Lipitz LR, Pastore RA. Antral gastritis. Radiology 1974;113:308–12.

Udassin R, Aviad I, Vinograd I, et al. Isolated emphysematous gastritis in an infant. Gastrointest Radiol 1984;9: 9–12.

Vuthibhagdee A, Harris NF. Antral stricture as a delayed complication of iron intoxication. Radiology 1972;103: 163–4.

Watanabe H, Magota S, Shiiba S, et al. Coarse areae gastricae in the proximal body and fundus: a sign of gastric hypersecretion. Radiology 1983;146:303–6.

Wilton GP, Wahl RL, Juni JE, et al. Detection of gastritis by (99m)Tc-labelled red-blood-cell scintigraphy. AJR 1984;143:759–60.

Gastric Ulcer

Amaral NM. Radiographic diagnosis of shallow gastric ulcers: a comparative study of technique. Radiology 1978;129:597–600.

Ament ME, Christie DL. Upper gastrointestinal fiberoptic endoscopy in pediatric patients. Gastroenterol 1977; 72:1244–8.

Block WM. Chronic gastric ulcer in childhood. A critical analysis of the literature with report of a case in an eleven year old boy. Am J Dis Child 1963;85:566–74.

Cello JP. *Helicobacter pylori* and peptic ulcer disease. AJR 1995;164:283–6.

Daryabeigi J, Kane PE, Johnson LM. Pseudotumor acute gastric ulcer in a child. JAMA 1977;238:512–3.

Dooley CP, Larson AW, Stace NH, et al. Double contrast barium meal and upper gastrointestinal endoscopy. Ann Intern Med 1984;101:538–45.

Drumm B, Perez-Perez GI, Blaser MJ, et al. Intrafamilial clustering of *Helicobacter pylori* infection. N Engl J Med 1990;322:359–63.

Drumm B, Rhoads M, Stringer DA, et al. Etiology, presentation and clinical course of endoscopically diagnosed peptic ulcer disease in children. Pediatrics 1988;82:410–4.

Gohel VK, Kressel HY, Laufer I. Double-contrast artifacts. Gastrointest Radiol 1978;3:139–46.

Hayden CK, Swischuk LE, Rytting JE. Gastric ulcer disease in infants: US findings. Radiology 1987;164:131–4.

Laufer I, Mullins JE, Hamilton J. The diagnostic accuracy of barium studies of the stomach and duodenum—correlation with endoscopy. Radiology 1975;115:569–73.

Marshall BJ, Warren JR. Unidentified curved bacilli in the stomach of patients with gastritis and peptic ulceration. Lancet 1984;8390:1311–5.

McNulty CAM, Wise R. Gastric microflora. BMJ 1985; 291:367–8.

Mougenot JF, Montagne JPH, Faure C. Gastrointestinal fibro-endoscopy in infants and children. Ann Radiol 1976;19:23–34.

Ott DJ, Gelfand DW, Wu WC. Detection of gastric ulcer: comparison of single and double contrast examinations. AJR 1982;139:93–7.

Peterson WL. *Helicobacter pylori* and peptic ulcer disease. N Engl J Med 1986;324:1043–8.

Seagram CGF, Stephens CA, Cumming WA. Peptic ulceration at the Hospital for Sick Children, Toronto, during the 20 year period 1949–1969. J Pediatr Surg 1973;8:407–13.

Singleton EB, Faykus MH. Incidence of peptic ulcer as determined by radiological examinations in the pediatric age group. J Pediatr 1964;65:858–62.

Stringer DA, Daneman A, Brunelle F, et al. US of the normal and abnormal stomach (excluding hypertrophic stenosis) in children. J Ultrasound Med 1986;5:186–8.

Neoplasms

Batik YW, Ahn JS, Choi HJ. Lymphoid hyperplasia of the stomach presenting as umbilicated polypoid lesions. Radiology 1971;100:277–80.

Bisset RAL, Gupta SC, Zammit-Maempel I. Radiographic and ultrasound appearances of an intra-mural haematoma of the pylorus. Clin Radiol 1988;39:316–8.

Bowen B, Ros PR, McCarthy MJ, et al. Gastrointestinal teratomas: CT and US appearance with pathologic correlation. Radiology 1987;162:431–3.

Denzler TB, Harned RK, Pergam CJ. Gastric polyps in familial polyposis coli. Radiology 1979;130:63–6.

Dixon WL, Fazzari PJ. Carcinoma of the stomach in a child. JAMA 1976;235:2414–5.

Feczko JP, Halpert RD, Ackerman LV. Gastric polyps: radiological evaluation and clinical significance. Radiology 1985;155:581–4.

Haley T, Dimier M, Hollier P. Gastric teratoma with gastrointestinal bleeding. J Pediatr Surg 1986;21:949–50.

Herlinger H. The recognition of exogastric tumors: report of six cases. Br J Radiol 1966;39:28–36.

Levine MS, Flmas N, Furth EF, et al. *Helicobacter pylori* and gastric MALT lymphoma. AJR 1996;166:86–8.

Lichtman S, Hayes G, Stringer DA, et al. Chronic intussusception due to antral myoepithelioma. J Pediatr Surg 1986;21:956–8.

Megibow AJ, Balthazar EJ, Hulnick DH, et al. CT evaluation of gastrointestinal leiomyomas and leiomyosarcomas. AJR 1985;144:727–31.

Odes HS, Krawiec J, Yanai-Inbar I, et al. Benign lymphoid hyperplasia of the stomach. Pediatr Radiol 1981;10:244–6.

Ou Tim L, Bank S, Marks IN, et al. Benign lymphoid

hyperplasia of the gastric antrum—another cause of "état mammelonné." Br J Radiol 1977;50:29–31.

Schroeder BA, Wells RG, Sty JR. Inflammatory fibroid polyp of the stomach in a child. Pediatr Radiol 1987;17: 71–2.

Siegel MJ, Shackelford GD. Gastric teratomas in infants: report of 2 cases. Pediatr Radiol 1978;7:197–200.

Stringer DA, Daneman A, Brunelle F, et al. US of the normal and abnormal stomach (excluding hypertrophic stenosis) in children. J Ultrasound Med 1986;5:186–8.

Wurlitzer FP, Mares JA, Isaacs H, et al. Smooth muscle tumors of the stomach in childhood and adolescence. J Pediatr Surg 1973;8:421–7.

Bezoar; Foreign Body Ingestion

Cremin BJ, Fisher RM, Stokes NJ, et al. Four cases of lactobezoar in neonates. Pediatr Radiol 1974;2:107–10.

DeBakey M, Ochsner A. Bezoars and concretions: a comprehensive review of the literature with an analysis of 303 collected cases and a presentation of 8 additional cases. Surgery 1938;4:934–63.

Desrentes M. Wizardry and radiography: a clinical case. Radiology 1990;177:116–8.

Kuiper DH. Gastric bezoar in a patient with myotonic dystrophy: a review of gastrointestinal complications of myotonic dystrophy. Am J Dig Dis 1971;16:529–34.

Malpani A, Ramani SK, Wolverson M. Role of US in trichobezoars. J Ultrasound Med 1988;7:661–3.

McCracken S, Jongeward R, Silver TM, et al. Gastric trichobezoar: US findings. Radiology 1986;161:123–4.

Naik DR, Bolia A, Boon AW. Demonstration of a lactobezoar by ultrasound. Br J Radiol 1987;60:506–8.

Ratcliffe JF. The ultraUS appearance of a trichobezoar. Br J Radiol 1982;55:166–7.

Schreiner RL, Brady MS, Franken EA Jr, et al. Increased incidence of lactobezoars in low birth infants. Am J Dis Child 1979;133:936–40.

Tennenhouse JE, Wilson SR. US detection of a small bowel bezoar. J Ultrasound Med 1990;9:603–5.

Valberg LS, McCorriston JR, Partington MW. Bezoar: an unusual cause of protein-losing enteropathy. Can Med Assoc J 1966;94:388–9.

Wolf RS, Davis LA. Lactobezoar: a foreign body formed by the use of undiluted powdered milk substance. JAMA 1963;184:782.

Spontaneous Rupture of the Stomach in Neonates

Lloyd JR. The etiology of gastrointestinal perforations in the newborn. J Pediatr Surg 1969;4:77–84.

Pochaczevsky R, Bryk D. New roentgenographic signs of neonatal gastric perforation. Radiology 1972;102: 147–8.

Shaw A, Blanc WA, Santulli TV, et al. Spontaneous rupture of the stomach in the newborn: a clinical and experimental study. Surgery 1965;58:561–70.

Takebayaski H, Azada K, Tokura K, et al. Congenital atresia of the duodenum with gastric perforation: case report and review of the literature. Am J Dis Child 1975;129: 1227–9.

Gastric Rupture following Blunt Abdominal Trauma

Tu RK, Starshak RJ, Brown B. CT diagnosis of gastric rupture following blunt abdominal trauma in a child. Pediatr Radiol 1992;22:146–7.

Pneumatosis

Bell RS, Graham CB, Stevenson JK. Roentgenologic and clinical manifestations of neonatal necrotizing enterocolitis. AJR 1971;112:123–4.

Holgerson LO, Borns PF, Srouji MN. Isolated gastric pneumatosis. J Pediatr Surg 1974;9:813–6.

Leonidas JC. Gastric pneumatosis in infancy. Arch Dis Child 1976;51:398.

Radin DR, Rosen RS, Halls JM. Acute gastric dilatation: a rare cause of portal venous gas. Case report. AJR 1987;148:279–80.

Robinson AE, Grossman H, Brumley GW. Pneumatosis intestinalis in the neonate. AJR 1974; 120:333–41.

Santulli TV, Schullinger JN, Heird WC, et al. Acute necrotizing enterocolitis in infancy: a review of 64 cases. Pediatrics 1975;55:376–87.

Stone HH, Allen WB, Smith RB, et al. Infantile pneumatosis intestinalis. J Surg Res 1968;8:301–7.

Diffuse Neonatal Gastric Infarction

Johnson JF, Woisard KK, Cooper GL. Diffuse neonatal gastric infarction. Pediatr Radiol 1988;18:161–3.

Volvulus

Campbell JB. Neonatal gastric volvulus. AJR 1979;132:723–5.

Campbell JB, Rappaport LN, Skerker LB. Acute mesentero-axial volvulus of the stomach. Radiology 1972;103:153–6.

Cole BC, Dickinson SJ. Acute volvulus of the stomach in infants and children. Surgery 1971;70:707–17.

Cybulsky I, Himal HS. Gastric volvulus within the foramen of Morgagni. Can Med Assoc J 1985;133:209–10.

Dalgaard JR. Volvulus of the stomach. Acta Chir Scand 1952;103:131–53.

Kilcoyne RF, Babbitt DP, Sakaguchi S. Volvulus of the stomach: a case report. Radiology 1972;103:157–8.

Yousef S, Laberge JM, Ducharme JC. Gastric volvulus in infants and children. Ann Coll Phys Surg Can 1983;16:372.

Ziprkowski MN, Teele RL. Gastric volvulus in childhood. AJR 1979;132:921–5.

Displacement

Grossman H, Redo SF. Unusual causes of gastric displacement in children. Radiology 1966;87:728–9.

Oh KS, Strife JL, Fischer KC, et al. Pyloroduodenal deformity due to liver malformation associated with omphalocoele. AJR 1977;128:957–60.

Siegel MJ, McAlister WH, Askin FN. Lymphangiomas in children: report of 121 cases. Can Assoc Radiol J 1978;30:99–102.

Miscellaneous Procedures

Cory DA, Fitzgerald JF, Cohen MD. Percutaneous nonendoscopic gastrostomy in children. Am J Roentgenol 1988;151:995–7.

Ho CS. Percutaneous gastrostomy for jejunal feeding. Radiology 1983;149:596–8.

Ho CS, Gray RR, Goldinger M, et al. Percutaneous gastrostomy for enteral feeding. Radiology 1985;156:349–51.

Ho CS, Yeung EY. Percutaneous gastrostomy and transgastric jejunostomy [review]. AJR 1992;158:251–7.

Keller MS, Lai S, Wagner DK. Percutaneous gastrostomy in a child. Radiology 1986;160:261–2.

McLean G, Rombeau JL, Caldwell MD, et al. Transgastrostomy jejunal intubation for enteric alimentation. AJR 1982;139:1129–33.

McLoughlin RF, So CB, Gray RR. Flouroscopically guided percutaneous gastrostomy: current status. J Can Assoc Radiol 1996;47:10–5.

Tao HH, Gilies RR. Percutaneous feeding gastrostomy. AJR 1983;141:793–4.

Towbin RB, Ball WS, Bissett GS III. Percutaneous gastrostomy and percutaneous gastrojejunostomy in children: antegrade approach. Radiology 1988;168:473–6.

Vade A, Jafri SZH, Agha FP, et al. Radiologic evaluation of gastrostomy complications. AJR 1983;141:328–30.

Van Sonnenberg E, Wittich GR, Cabrera OA, et al. Percutaneous gastrostomy and gastroenterostomy. 1. Techniques derived from laboratory evaluation. 2. Clinical experience. AJR 1986;146:577–86.

Weber A, Nadel S. CT appearance of retrograde jejunoduodenogastric intussusception: a rare complication of gastrostomy tubes. AJR 1991;156:957–9.

Wills JS, Oglesby JT. Percutaneous gastrostomy: further experience. Radiology 1985;154:71–4.

Wills JS, Oglesby JT. Percutaneous gastrostomy. Radiology 1988;167:41–3.

Wojtowycz MM, Arata JA Jr. Subcutaneous emphysema after percutaneous gastrostomy. AJR 1988;151:311–2.

Wollman B, D'Agostino HB, Walus-Wigle JR, et al. Radiologic, endoscopic, and surgical gastrostomy: an institutional evaluation and meta-analysis of the literature. Radiology 1995;197:699–704.

9

SMALL BOWEL

Doug Jamieson, MB, ChB, FRCPC, and
David A. Stringer, BSc, MBBS, FRCR, FRCPC

EMBRYOGENESIS OF THE MIDGUT

The midgut extends from the bile duct orifice to the start of the distal third of the transverse colon. Prior to 6 weeks of gestation, the midgut is connected via the vitelline duct to the yolk sac. The vitelline duct divides the midgut into its cranial and caudal limbs.

Initially the midgut is a straight hollow tube. During development the gut undergoes a 270° counterclockwise rotation (in frontal view) to assume the adult configuration. This occurs in three 90° stages (Figure 9–1).

Stage 1: Prior to 6 weeks' gestation, the duodenum initially rotates 90° counterclockwise to lie to the right of the superior mesenteric artery. The cecum also rotates 90° counterclockwise to lie to the left of the superior mesenteric artery (Figure 9–1A).

Stage 2: At this point, the rapidly growing bowel herniates into the umbilical cord, remaining there from 6 to 10 weeks' gestation. This process can be seen on antenatal ultrasonography (US) as an umbilical bulge which must not be mistaken for an omphalocele (Cyr et al., 1986). During this period, the duodenum rotates another 90° to lie posterior to the superior mesenteric artery while the rest of the midgut is in the umbilical cord (Bill, 1979; Snyder and Chaffin, 1954) (Figure 9–1B).

Stage 3: At about 10 weeks of gestation, the herniated bowel re-enters the abdomen and the final 90° of duodenal and 180° of cecal rotation follow (Figures 9–1C,D).

In later fetal life, the colon and small bowel can be seen on US. The colon can be distinguished in some fetuses at 22 weeks' gestation and in all fetuses by 28 weeks (Nyberg et al., 1987). Ultrasonographically, the colon appears as a tubular continuous structure around the perimeter of the abdomen that does not peristalse. The small bowel is seen on US in only 30% of fetuses over 34 weeks' gestation and routinely shows peristalsis (Nyberg et al., 1987).

CONGENITAL AND DEVELOPMENTAL ANOMALIES OF THE SMALL BOWEL

Congenital and developmental anomalies of the small bowel may be associated with polyhydramnios if there is functional or structural obstruction, and they frequently present postnatally in the first 24 hours with clinical evidence of obstruction (bilious vomiting and abdominal distension). A list of causes for neonatal small-bowel obstruction is given in Table 9–1.

Clinically, the most important congenital and developmental condition to distinguish expeditiously is malrotation and malfixation. This entity can result in ischemia of the entire small bowel secondary to a volvulus twisting off the superior mesenteric artery. The resulting short-gut syndrome or death can be averted by timely diagnosis and surgical intervention.

Malrotation and Malfixation of the Midgut

General Considerations
Malrotation can be defined as any abnormal rotation of the gut. Malrotation often results in malfixa-

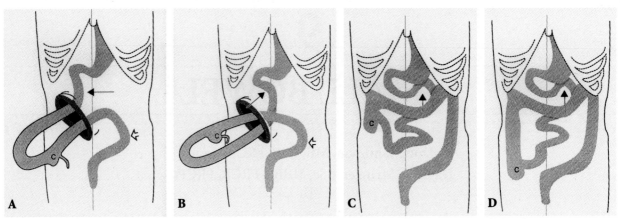

FIGURE 9–1. Stages of normal intestinal rotation. *A*, End of stage I (6 weeks of gestation). The duodenum has rotated 90° counterclockwise with the duodenojejunal junction (*arrow*) coming to lie to the right of the midline and superior mesenteric artery (SMA); the cecum (c) also rotates 90° counterclockwise to lie to the left of the midline and SMA. At this point, the rapidly growing bowel including the cecum, herniates into the umbilical cord. *B*, End of stage II (10 weeks of gestation). The duodenum has rotated another 90° counterclockwise with the duodenojejunal junction (*arrow*) coming to lie in the midline posterior to the SMA while the rest of the midgut is in the umbilical cord. No large bowel rotation has taken place. *C*, Early stage III (after 10 weeks of gestation). The duodenum has rotated its last 90° counterclockwise with the duodenojejunal junction (*arrow*) coming to lie to the left of the midline at or almost at the level of the duodenal cap, and the cecum (c) is continuing to rotate. If rotation ceases at this point, a high cecum (type 3C malrotation) results. *D*, End of stage III. Frontal view of the normally rotated bowel. The duodenojejunal junction (*arrow*) remains to the left of the midline at or almost at the level of the duodenal cap, and the cecum (c) has now reached its normal location in the right iliac fossa. The root of the mesentery extends from the duodenojejunal junction to the ileocecal valve adjacent to the cecum.

tion, which can be defined as an abnormal fixation of the gut by the mesentery. Although rotations of the duodenum and cecum have some similarities,

important differences in their timing result in abnormalities of rotation that affect solely the duodenum or solely the large bowel.

Most of the numerous anatomic variations of abnormal rotation can be related to the three normal embryologic stages of rotation described above. Malrotation can be classified according to the stage of normal rotation at which arrest or error occurred. Hence, an arrest occurring in stage I results in type 1 malrotation, also known as nonrotation. Stage II arrest results in a type 2 malrotation, and stage III arrest results in a type 3 malrotation (Figure 9–2).

Many malrotations are associated with Ladd's bands, which are abnormal condensations of peritoneal attachment. They often constrict or obstruct bowel and require surgical lysis (Ladd, 1932).

Type 1 malrotation is due to an arrest or error in stage I of rotation, i.e., before 6 weeks of gestational age and before the midgut protrudes into the yolk sac (Figure 9–2A).

The gut is always straight (nonrotated) at 4 weeks' gestation but by 5 weeks the gut has length-

---

TABLE 9–1. Congenital Anomalies and Other Causes of Neonatal Small Bowel Obstruction

Duodenal obstruction
    Malrotation, nonrotation, malfixation, Ladd's bands, volvulus
    Duodenal atresia, stenosis, or web
    Preduodenal portal vein
Jejunal/ileal obstruction
    Jejunal/ileal atresia or stenosis (multiple atresias)
    Meconium ileus or peritonitis
    Aganglionosis
    Hypoperistalsis syndromes (pseudo-obstruction)
Other causes of obstruction
    Mass lesions
        Duplications
        Tumors
        Hematomas
        Intussusception (rare)
        Meckel's band

ened to become convoluted with the duodenum lying to the right of the midline and the developing distal colon lying to the left of the midline with up to 90° of rotation having occurred. This rotation is further aided by the developing liver and left umbilical vein (Snyder and Chaffin, 1954).

Failure of rotation beyond this stage is also known as nonrotation although up to 90° of rotation of both the duodenum and large bowel has taken place. This nonrotated position is also the usual placement of bowel following malrotation surgery.

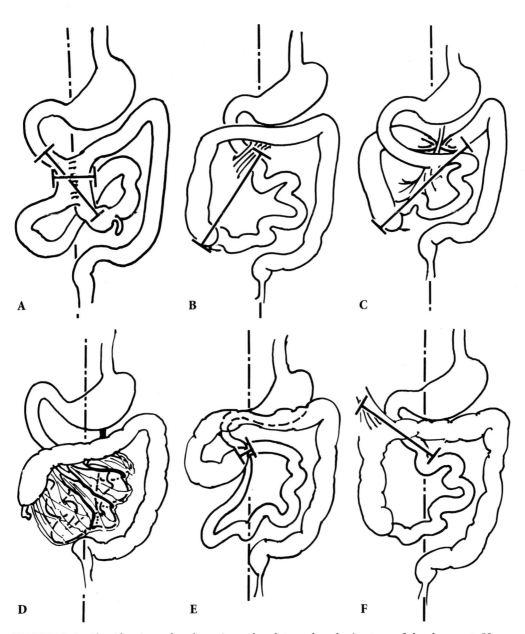

FIGURE 9–2. Classification of malrotation related to embryologic stage of development. Heavy H-shaped lines indicate the mesenteric root. *A,* Type 1A: nonrotation of colon and duodenum. *B,* Type 2A: nonrotation of duodenum only. *C,* Type 2B: reversed rotation of duodenum and colon. *D,* Type 2C: reversed rotation of duodenum only. *E,* Type 3A: colon not rotated and at greatest risk from volvulus. *F,* Type 3B: incomplete fixation of hepatic flexure. Type 3C (incomplete attachment of cecum and its mesocecum) is similar to Figure 9–1C. Type 3D (internal hernia near the ligament of Treitz) is not illustrated .

Type 2 malrotation (Figures 9–2B,C,D) is due to an arrest or error in stage II of rotation, i.e., between 6 and 10 weeks of gestational age, when the small abdominal space is overwhelmed by the rapidly lengthening gut and rapidly growing liver. The developing gut therefore herniates into the umbilical cord. During this stage, the duodenal loop normally continues to rotate counterclockwise and posteriorly so that it lies behind the superior mesenteric artery. The large bowel is relatively fixed in the umbilical cord at this time and hence cannot undergo any significant rotation during the second stage. Type 2 malrotations are rare.

Type 2A malrotation has an arrested duodenal rotation and normal colonic rotation. It is often associated with Ladd's bands constricting the right sided duodenum (Figure 9–2B).

Type 2B malrotation has the duodenum and the colon entering the abdomen in a reversed rotation (clockwise from frontal view), resulting in the duodenum anterior and the transverse colon posterior to the superior mesenteric artery. However, the cecum may be positioned in the right iliac fossa (Figure 9–2C).

Type 2C malrotation is the rarest of this group and has a reversed rotation of the duodenum with a normal counterclockwise return of large bowel to the abdomen. Entrapment of the entire small bowel with the mesentery creating an internal hernia may occur (Figure 9–2D). The entrapped small bowel may displace the colon to the left side of the abdomen (Cunningham et al., 1994).

Type 3 malrotation (Figures 9–2E,F) is due to an arrest or error in stage III of rotation, i.e., after 10 weeks of gestational age, when the midgut returns to the abdominal cavity.

In normal development the final 90° of duodenal rotation occurs very rapidly, placing the duodenum to the left of the spine completing its 270° of rotation. This is followed by a slower 180° rotation of the large bowel, bringing it to lie on the right with the cecum in the right iliac fossa. This completes the large bowel's 270° of rotation.

Type 3A malrotation (Figure 9–2E) is the commonest form of malrotation and the most likely to cause catastrophic volvulus. The term "malrotation" is often used incorrectly, especially by surgeons, to specifically designate the type 3A form of malrotation. The duodenum lying to the right of the midline and high cecum results in a very narrow mesenteric pedical which is greatly predisposed to volvulus.

Type 3B malrotation (Figure 9–2F) has the duodenum to the right of midline. The cecum may be in the right iliac fossa but the hepatic flexure is incompletely attached and there are often Ladd's bands running down from the right upper quadrant obstructing bowel (see Figure 9–1C).

Type 3C malrotation has an incompletely attached cecal mesocolon with an isolated mobile cecum, suggesting an interruption of the final stages of colon return to the abdomen. These malrotations are seldom symptomatic as they usually have a normal duodenal fixation that gives a wide mesenteric root and therefore rarely predispose to small-bowel volvulus.

Type 3D malrotation is a late occurring anomaly in which abnormal final fixation of duodenum and jejunum may result in paraduodenal hernia. These are three times more common on the left than right and are related to variations in peritoneal fixation. The left paraduodenal hernia passes into the descending mesocolon through Landzert's fossa to the left of the fourth part of the duodenum, and the right paraduodenal hernia passes into the ascending and transverse mesocolon usually through Waldeyer's fossa which is in the first part of the jejunal mesentery immediately behind the superior mesenteric artery (Myers, 1970). The placement of paraduodenal hernias in a classification of malrotation is somewhat arbitrary as they are anomalies of mesocolon fixation and development rather than true bowel malrotations.

Complications

Malrotation results in an abnormal position of the gut, which per se does not cause symptoms or clinical problems. However, the often associated abnormal mesenteric position or fixation can result in twisting or volvulus of the midgut about the superior mesenteric vessels, causing vascular occlusion and consequent bowel ischemia. Obstruction can occur due to ischemic bowel and ileus or can occasionally be mechanical, secondary to the volvulus. Obstruction can also be secondary to peritoneal (Ladd's) bands or an internal hernia. The complicating features of malrotation described below usually become manifest early in life but can present late, when the index of suspicion for midgut volvulus can be low and result in an unfortunate delay in diagnosis.

Volvulus of the Small Bowel. Malfixation of the small bowel, particularly type 3A, commonly produces volvulus in children (Berdon et al., 1970). Volvulus is the most serious complication of malrotation, and it can be fatal. The word volvulus is derived from the Latin "volvere," meaning to twist round, an apt description as the gut is twisted around the superior mesenteric artery and vein.

The normal base of the mesentery extends from the duodenojejunal junction to the cecum. The duodenojejunal junction is fixed by the ligament of Treitz, the suspensory ligament of the duodenum. This is a band of connective tissue (that may have smooth muscle fibers) arising from the region of the right diaphragmatic crus and the connective tissue around the celiac artery and inserting into the third and fourth parts of the duodenum, holding the duodenojejunal junction to the left of the second lumbar vertebral pedical and at or nearly at the level of the duodenal cap (Haley and Peden, 1943). The cecum locates in the right iliac fossa. This wide supporting base of the mesentery does not allow the small bowel to twist around the superior mesenteric artery. When the mesenteric base is short, running from a duodenojejunal junction to the right of the midline to a high-riding cecal pole in the right upper quadrant or midline, the entire small bowel is suspended from a narrow mesenteric pedical and is allowed the mobility to twist. This involves the mesenteric vessels, which twist until eventual occlusion occurs. As an analogy, if your arms are the gut and your feet are the root of the mesentery, it is easy to spin around if your feet are close together but difficult if your feet are wide apart. Approximately three and one-half twists are allowable before the vascular supply is compromised sufficiently to cause severe ischemia. Necrosis of the entire jejunum and ileum will then occur, possibly resulting in the death of the patient. A lesser number of turns may compromise the venous drainage, causing venous engorgement, edema, and even gastrointestinal hemorrhage. Obstruction to lymphatic drainage can result in lacteal engorgement and protein loss into the gut. The resulting hypoproteinemic edema and intraperitoneal lacteal rupture can cause chylous ascites (Berdon et al., 1970).

Type 3A malrotation (see Figure 9–2E) commonly undergoes volvulus as its mesenteric root is very short (Bill, 1979). Type 1 malrotation (see Figure 9–2A) may rarely volvulate, depending on its mesenteric fixation, and a type 2 malrotation (see Figure 9–2B,C,D) may occasionally present with volvulus although obstruction is more common.

Obstruction of the Small Bowel. Obstruction with bilious vomiting is a common and characteristic presenting feature in volvulus, as discussed above. Obstruction is commonly due to peritoneal (Ladd's) bands. These are condensations of mesentery which are probably an attempt by the peritoneum to fix a malpositioned bowel (Ladd, 1932; Ladd, 1936). The bands are commonly associated with type 2A or type 3B abnormal rotation. Type 2A is rare and is the result of nonrotation of the duodenum with normal rotation of the colon. Bands cross and partially compress the duodenum (see Figure 9–2B). Type 3B is more common, with incomplete attachment of the hepatic flexure. The bands arise from the peritoneum of the posterior abdominal wall adjacent to the liver and extend to the loosely attached right colon, passing anterior to the duodenum (see Figure 9–2F).

An unusual obstruction may occur in association with both types of reversed rotation of the duodenum and colon. In type 2B, the colon lies posterior to the superior mesenteric artery and the duodenum lies anterior, the opposite of normal (DePrima et al., 1985). The transverse colon may be partially obstructed by the superior mesenteric vessels and by bands from the mesentery to the small bowel (see Figure 9–2C). Volvulus occasionally develops in the partially obstructed right colon. A type 2C malrotation obstructs due to an internal hernia (Figure 9–2D).

Internal Hernia. Internal hernia is rare. It is usually due to reversed rotation of the duodenum with normal rotation and fixation of the colon, a type 2C malrotation. The duodenum rotates anterior to the superior mesenteric artery, the opposite of normal. Hence, in order for the cecum to reach its final position, it has to rotate anterior to the duodenum, which lies between it and the superior mesenteric artery. The artery and its mesentery must thus be dragged around the small bowel, encasing it in a mesenteric hernia sac (see Figure 9–2D). This is the most common form of congenital internal hernia.

Internal hernia may be asymptomatic or can cause intestinal obstruction. The diagnosis may be suggested by a rounded mass of gas-containing bowel loops seen in the right upper quadrant on a plain-film abdominal radiologic examination of a child who vomits or has abdominal pain. It is usually not possible to make the diagnosis from plain films alone.

Paraduodenal hernia classified as type 3D malrotation may be asymptomatic or present with acute high small-bowel obstruction with or without bowel ischemia. Long-standing history of indigestion, postprandial cramps, and vomiting may be elicited.

Clinical Features

The majority of neonatal patients with malrotation will present with bilious vomiting. Sixty-five to 75% will present within the first month of life, and 80 to 90% will present within the first year of life (Millar et al., 1987; Berdon et al., 1970). Bilious vomiting is the hallmark presenting symptom in malrotation with volvulus. It will be a symptom of importance in over 95% of patients although it may not be initially bile stained in up to 20% of cases (Millar et al., 1987). The vomiting may be intermittent and related to meals, and projectile vomiting and visible peristalsis may occur but abdominal distension is uncommon. The vomiting can lead to fluid and electrolyte imbalance. Most neonates presenting with malrotation symptoms are found to have volvulus at the time of operation. There is a high mortality rate among cases presenting in the first week of life if the diagnosis is at all delayed (Berdon et al., 1970). Abdominal pain is difficult to assess in infants under 1 year of age. In older children, however, abdominal pain is a major presenting symptom in nearly all patients. The abdominal physical examination may be unremarkable in 85% of patients at first presentation (Millar et al., 1987). Less than 10% of patients will present with clinical shock and ischemic bowel but this scenario can develop with catastrophic rapidity. Mural necrosis and ensuing sepsis can rapidly lead to death. A malrotation may, however, be asymptomatic through life. Symptoms from midgut volvulus or obstruction may be variable, unimpressive, and delayed in presentation.

In a malnourished child, malrotation may present with recurrent vomiting with or without distension (Silverman and Caffey, 1949). Clinically, the malnutrition may suggest celiac disease but it is secondary to chronic midgut volvulus with partial obstruction of mesenteric veins and lymphatics (Friedland et al., 1970). Dilated lacteals from lymphatic obstruction may rupture, forming either a chylous cyst in the mesentery or chylous peritoneal effusion. The presence of hypoproteinemia is further evidence of lymphatic and venous compromise.

Diarrhea may occasionally be present. Melena, due to bleeding from mesenteric and intramural varices secondary to the chronic venous obstruction rarely occurs (Silverman and Caffey, 1949).

Associated Anomalies

Congenital anomalies are commonly associated with malrotation and have been described as ubiquitous and present in 30 to 62% of cases (Stewart and Colodny, 1976; Filston and Kirks, 1981). Malrotation, especially nonrotation (type 1 malrotation), is invariably present to some degree with left-sided Bochdalek's diaphragmatic hernia, gastroschisis, and omphalocele as the abnormal position of the bowel prevents normal fixation and rotation (Bill, 1979; Snyder and Chaffin, 1954; Grob, 1963). Malrotation is commonly associated with duodenal and small-bowel stenosis or atresia, being present in 8 (Long et al., 1996) to 26% of such cases (Filston and Kirks, 1981), and 10% of duodenal webs are associated with malrotation (Richardson and Martin, 1969).

The heterotaxia syndromes, including polysplenia and asplenia, are associated with malrotation (Markowitz et al., 1977; Moller et al., 1971). A review of 25 children with heterotaxia found only 3 to have normal bowel rotation (Ditchfield and Hutson, 1998). Other anomalies associated with malrotation include intestinal pseudobstruction, Meckel's diverticulum, Hirschsprung's disease, biliary atresia, imperforate anus, intussusception (Filston and Kirks, 1981), pyloric stenosis, and absence of a kidney and ureter (Snyder and Chaffin, 1954).

Imaging

Seldom is the consequence of a delayed or missed diagnosis so potentially catastrophic as in malrotation and midgut volvulus. Appropriate radiographic consultation on a patient with suspected malrotation and midgut volvulus requires knowledge of the patient's age and exact clinical status. Imaging should identify the exact lie of bowel within the abdomen and particularly identify the location of the duodenojejunal junction and the cecum to allow inference as to the extent of the mesenteric attachment of the small bowel. A good working knowledge of the types of malrotation is required to identify abnormalities but not all patients will fit into a rigid classification, and diagnostic difficulties with subtle signs can return to haunt the diagnostician. Radiographic findings must correlate to the clinical situation and should not negate a good clinical suspicion for malrotation. Abdominal plain-film and contrast studies of the gastrointestinal tract are the mainstay of diagnosis; we do not use ultrasonography or computed tomography as primary diagnostic tools.

Plain-Film Radiography. Plain abdominal films are an initial requirement. They may be the only images obtained on an acutely ill child prior to surgery. The first plain film should be a supine view. Erect films are often helpful but not always essential and to keep radiation to a minimum, further views such as lateral, decubitus, or cross-table lateral are not routinely used although they may occasionally be helpful.

Plain abdominal film will suggest malrotation and volvulus in the majority of symptomatic cases (Berdon et al., 1970; Houston and Wittenborg, 1965). Partial duodenal obstruction is the most important plain-film finding in malrotation (Figure 9–3). If there is complete duodenal obstruction in malrotation, then the double bubble appearance may be identical to that seen in duodenal atresia. However, the degree of duodenal distention will usually be less than in duodenal atresia, and the size of the duodenal gas shadow in the right upper quadrant should be specifically evaluated to make this distinction (Figure 9–4) (Potts et al., 1985). In addition, the presence of bowel gas distal to the duodenum is rare in atresia and common in malrotation. The placement of a nasogastric tube may decompress the proximal bowel and remove evidence for obstruction as may vomiting or the infant being too sick to swallow air.

Ominous plain-film findings suggesting midgut volvulus with bowel ischemia include bowel wall thickening (Figure 9–5). A changing pattern with decreasing small-bowel gas can indicate increasing volvulus, not improvement. The absence of small-bowel gas in the presence of abdominal distension and tenderness is often associated with strangulated

midgut volvulus and bowel necrosis whereas the absence of small-bowel gas without these signs is usually associated with viable small bowel (Kassner and Kottmeier, 1975). An ileus pattern with multiple distended bowel loops and air-fluid levels, in the setting of suspected malrotation, is often a closed-loop obstruction with gangrenous bowel (Figure 9–6) (Frye et al., 1972). Intramural gas is rarely seen but if present would indicate mural necrosis.

Chronic midgut volvulus can partly occlude the mesenteric veins and lymphatics, resulting in chylous ascites of low density compared to the liver. Thus, on plain abdominal films the liver is outlined and displaced by the ascites (Berdon et al., 1970).

Neither the lack of gas nor the presence of a normal gas pattern should exclude the diagnosis of malrotation. If the diagnosis is not obvious from plain films, any infant with bilious vomiting should be investigated promptly with contrast radiography.

Contrast Radiography. In most patients, the position of the duodenum and cecum can be readily demonstrated with contrast opacification of the bowel via oral intake, nasogastric tube, or enema. Both upper gastrointestinal (GI) examination and enema may be required for adequate evaluation.

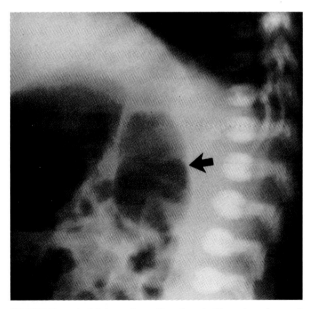

FIGURE 9–3. Malrotation. Duodenal dilatation (*arrow*) in association with a normal jejunal gas pattern indicates partial duodenal obstruction. This is most likely due to malrotation with Ladd's bands or volvulus. There are many other causes of duodenal obstruction (see Table 9–1).

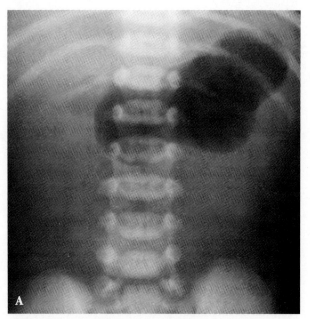 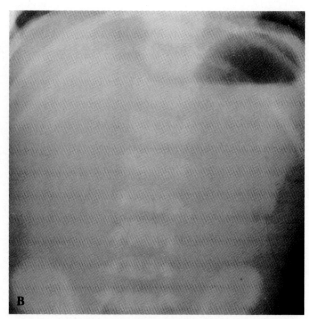

FIGURE 9–4. Malrotation with volvulus. On plain supine (*A*) or erect (*B*) films, the duodenum is often either small or absent in malrotation, unlike the appearance of duodenal dilatation seen with duodenal atresia or stenosis.

The cecum is mobile and may be normally displaced out of the right iliac fossa in up to 15% of all age groups (Snyder and Chaffin, 1954), and the cecum may be in the right iliac fossa in 16% of patients with surgically confirmed malrotation (Long et al., 1996). Duodenojejunal flexure displacement is highly indicative of malrotation. Only

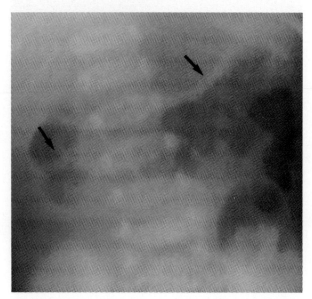

FIGURE 9–5. Malrotation with volvulus. Plain film shows the jejunum to have a thickened wall (*arrows*), suggesting ischemia.

2% of surgically confirmed malrotations may have an appropriately located duodenojejunal flexure (Long et al., 1996) and these invariably will have an abnormal cecal position to aid diagnosis. The statistical diagnostic yield from an upper GI examination is greater and more reliable than that of an enema (Steiner, 1978), and we use the former as our primary diagnostic study. A normal or equivocal duodenum in the context of a strong clinical suspicion for malrotation requires further evaluation, and we proceed to a contrast enema to identify colonic and cecal position. An enema study immediately following a duodenal study (in which the volume of administered contrast is limited) is usually diagnostic whereas the duodenal position is seldom adequately seen after contrast opacification of the colon.

There is a place for small-bowel follow-through to identify the cecum and large bowel but this is more time consuming and is regarded by some as unsatisfactory for reliably assessing cecal position (Beasley and DeCampo, 1996) especially as small and large bowel are of similar caliber in infants and hence the cecum may thus be difficult to visualize.

Historically, and particularly among surgeons, the enema was the examination of choice for malrotation (Bill, 1979; Silverman and Caffey, 1949). However, we usually reserve the enema study as our secondary investigation following a normal or equivocal upper GI examination. We use contrast enemas to investigate infants in whom distal bowel obstruction is suspected.

Upper Gastrointestinal Examination. In any pediatric upper GI examination, the delineation of the duodenum should be of primary importance; it is crucial in a context of bilious vomiting.

In 70 to 80% of the time, an upper GI examination will quickly and easily show the extent of any duodenal obstruction as well as the position of the duodenojejunal junction, thus allowing malrotation to be diagnosed—especially type 3A, the type most likely to undergo volvulus, where the duodenojejunal junction will lie in the midline (Figure 9–7). Also diagnosed will be those missed on enema examination (such as type 2A malrotation) (Figure 9–8).

The upper GI examination will demonstrate any intrinsic duodenal obstruction. Contrast should be followed beyond any duodenal obstruction if possible because in cases of malrotation and volvulus it is rare for the obstruction to be complete and

the proximal jejunum may be found lying on the right (Simpson et al., 1972). However, this is not a reliable sign by itself. When volvulus is present, a twisted ribbon or corkscrew appearance of the duodenum may be seen (Figure 9–9) as well as thickened jejunal folds indicating mucosal edema. If obstruction from volvulus is complete, a beaked appearance may be found at the site of duodenal obstruction (Figure 9–10). Occasionally the site of obstruction is not beaked but smooth and round, indistinguishable from a duodenal atresia.

Peritoneal bands usually present as obstruction in neonates; however, occasionally they may present later in childhood with intermittent pain and vomiting. A Z-shaped configuration to the distal duodenum and proximal jejunum has been described and is due to bands fixing the bowel abnormally (Ablow et al., 1983). This would be likely to occur in a type 3B malrotation with malfixation but not necessarily volvulus of bowel. Surgery is indicated to lyse the bands and ensure absence of volvulus.

The duodenum should be visualized and assessed during the first passage of a bolus of con-

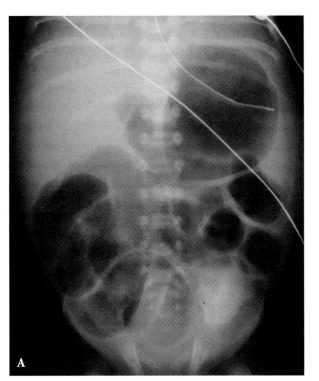 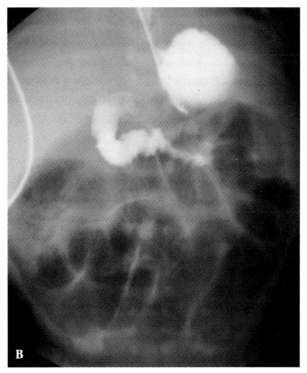

FIGURE 9–6. Malrotation and midgut volvulus with ischemic bowel. *A,* Plain radiograph in an ill neonate with an acute abdomen shows dilated bowel, suggesting ischemia. *B,* Contrast injected via a nasogastric tube demonstrated an abnormal duodenal position. At laparotomy, malrotation and midgut volvulus with ischemic bowel and areas of frank gangrene were encountered.

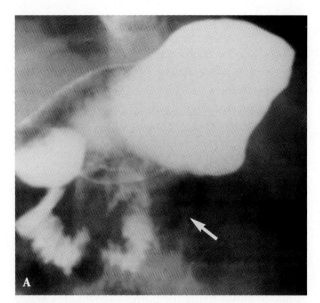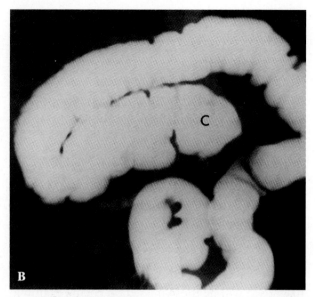

FIGURE 9–7. Type 3A malrotation with volvulus (see Figure 9–2E). *A,* On upper GI examination the supine film shows the duodenojejunal junction lying in the midline to the right of the left lumbar spine pedicles (*arrow*). This view is the most important one for making the diagnosis of malrotation. Normally the duodenojejunal junction lies to the right of the left lumbar spine pedicles as well as almost as high as the duodenal cap. *B,* The barium enema showed the cecum (c) to lie in the midline.

trast before opacification of overlying jejunal loops confound the field of view (Figure 9–11). The child may require restraint by assistants, swaddling, or appropriate restraint boards. Ingestion or nasogastric tube injection of contrast with the child in the right lateral position allows contrast to fall down the lesser curvature straight to the antrum and pylorus. The first ingested bolus should be followed through the esophagus and stomach; full concentration on the duodenum is then required. In the neonate or sick child we would use an iso-osmolar water-soluble contrast medium usually injected into the antrum or proximal duodenum via a nasogastric tube. In the older or clinically well child, oral ingestion and the use of barium is appropriate. Some radiologists initially feed the child in the left lateral position to pool contrast in the fundus; rolling the child through the supine to right lateral position then delivers the contrast to the pylorus. Once the first and second parts of the duodenum are filled, rolling the child supine then rapidly on to their left side and back on to their back (as quickly as this can be read) allows gastric contrast to flow up to the fundus, thus clearing the antrum and so enabling visualization of duodenal contrast as it passes over the vertebral bodies and up to the duodenojejunal junction. An optimal study has images of the filled duodenum in both frontal and lateral views. A well-aligned frontal view is essential and requires a field of view that allows assessment of vertebral pedicles, cardiac position, and rib symmetry (Figure 9–12). (See Chapter 3 for more information on performing an upper gastrointestinal examination.)

Much conspires against acquiring the optimal study. The fundamental problem is that radiologists visualize only bowel but it is the mesenteric fixation which is important. In particular, the ligament of Treitz *cannot* be visualized radiologically. Its position and status can therefore only be surmised from the position of the bowel. Fortunately, this is relatively reliable. However, because the consequences of missing malfixation can be catastrophic, caution should be exercised when extrapolating bowel fixation from position.

Other problems include an uncooperative child, pylorospasm, an air-filled stomach from crying displacing the duodenum in a young child, and overfilling the stomach, thus obscuring the duodenum and losing control of the child's position during the crucial first pass of contrast in the duodenum (Figure 9–13). Video capture of fluoroscopy, especially during the first pass of barium, is often invaluable for review. Fluoroscopy while rolling the patient from right decubitus to supine (and letting them rest only momentarily on their left side) will prevent missing the occasional quick transit of barium.

Where a nasogastric tube is present, aspiration of contrast at the end of the procedure reduces aspiration risks, especially important if the patient is proceeding to surgery. It is also of value when directly proceeding to an enema study (Figure 9–14).

In normal radiographic anatomy, the pylorus and first part of the duodenum (duodenal cap) are situated to the right of the midline and directed posteriorly with the duodenal cap slightly superiorly directed. An acute flexure starts the inferior descent of the second part of the duodenum. The third part crosses the vertebral column at the level of the third lumbar vertebra, passing over the inferior vena cava and aorta but under the superior mesenteric artery and vein with some upward inclination. It then ascends (in its fourth part) to the duodenojejunal junction at or almost at the level of the duodenal cap and sited just lateral to the second lumbar pedical on a true frontal view. This point is fixed

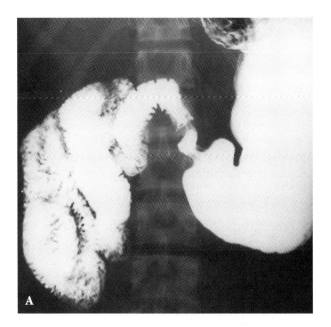

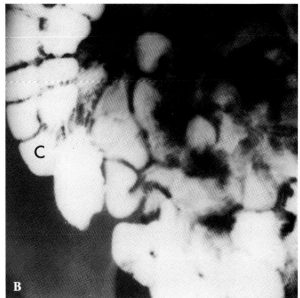

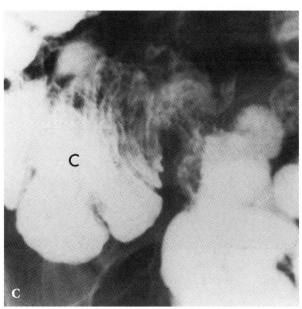

FIGURE 9–8. Type 2A malrotation (see Figure 9–2B). *A,* On upper GI examination, the position of the duodeno-jejunal junction is to the right of the spine but the cecum (c) lies in the right iliac fossa as seen on a small bowel follow-through examination (*B*) and spot films (*C*). At operation the position of the bowel was confirmed, and a volvulus was found in this 13-year-old girl who had only minor symptoms.

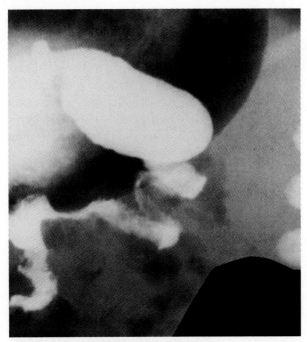

FIGURE 9–9. Malrotation with volvulus. The duodenum has the appearance of a twisted ribbon or corkscrew.

posteriorly by the ligament of Treitz, and the bowel passes anteriorly from here as jejunum. The second to fourth parts of the duodenum are retroperitoneal. This normal duodenal position must be seen

and/or recorded with confidence to report a normal study (Figure 9–15). The duodenal position should never be guessed or inferred, and if uncertain, a repeat study should be arranged, possibly as a specific duodenal intubation (see Figure 9–13).

Variations of normal duodenal position can be problematic especially in the asymptomatic child because some of them overlap subtle signs of malrotation (Katz et al., 1987; Long et al., 1996). These variations include a pylorus to the left of midline; a duodenojejunal flexure below the L1-L2 disc space or well below the level of the duodenal cap; the duodenojejunal flexure overlying the left L2 pedicle; an abnormal configuration of the triangle of the duodenal cap, inferior duodenal flexure, and duodenojejunal flexure (in the normal configuration, the inferior duodenal-to-duodenojejunal flexure is the longest side); a corkscrew or zigzag appearance to the jejunum beyond a normal duodenojejunal flexure, the entire jejunum in the right upper quadrant but a normal duodenojejunal junction (see Figure 9–11); a duodenum inversum where duodenum ascends from the cap but still crosses the midline under the mesenteric vessels and has a normal duodenojejunal flexure; and a redundant duodenum in which excessive loops of duodenum that lie distal to the duodenal cap

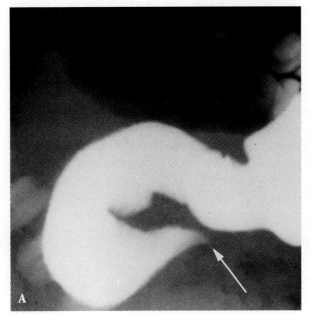

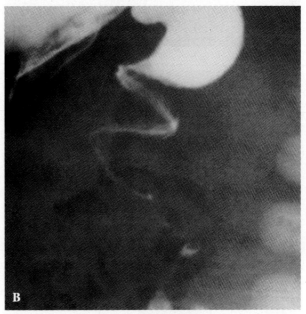

FIGURE 9–10. Malrotation with volvulus and complete obstruction. *A,* The barium has a beaked appearance at the site of obstruction (*arrow*), indicating probable volvulus. *B,* This was confirmed when a delayed film showed the typical corkscrew appearance.

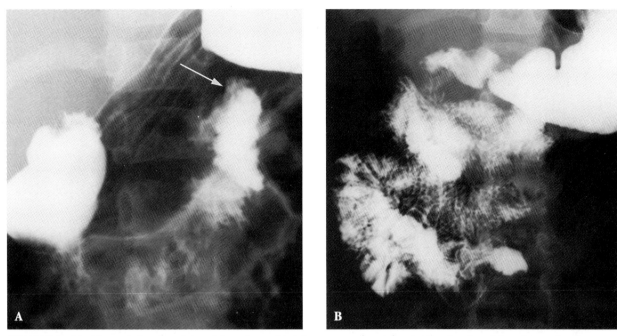

FIGURE 9–11. Normal duodenojejunal junction with jejunum on the right. *A*, The duodenojejunal junction in a true supine position is normal (*arrow*). *B*, More distal loops of jejunum lie on the right. If the duodenojejunal junction had not been accurately located, malrotation could not be excluded.

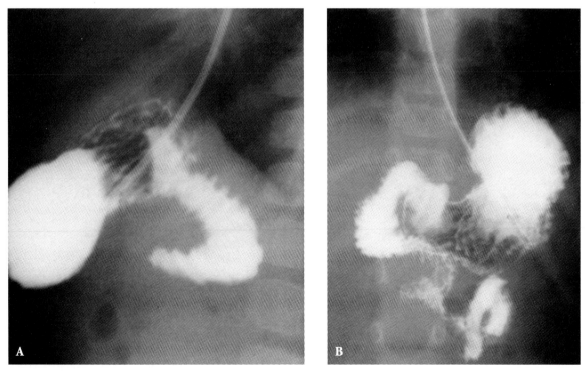

FIGURE 9–12. Malrotation with midgut volvulus. *A*, Contrast injected via a nasogastric tube with the patient in a right lateral position readily fills the proximal duodenum, which is mildly dilated with duodenal fold thickening. *B*, Rolling the patient supine shows an abnormal duodenum proceeding horizontally across the midline and spiraling into a midgut volvulus. A wide field of view, including the lower cardiac contour, allows accurate assessment of appropriate patient alignment.

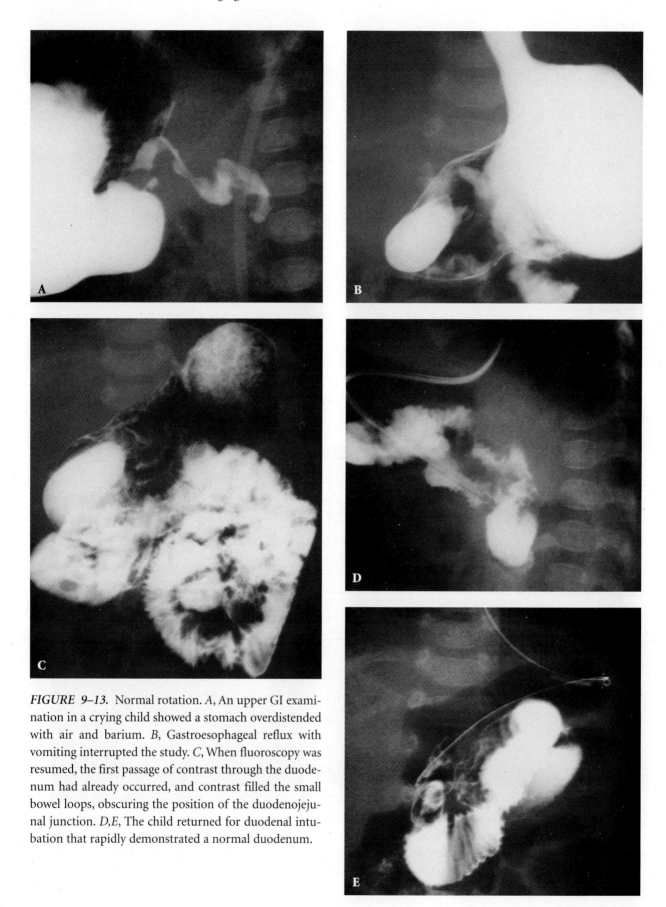

FIGURE 9–13. Normal rotation. *A,* An upper GI examination in a crying child showed a stomach overdistended with air and barium. *B,* Gastroesophageal reflux with vomiting interrupted the study. *C,* When fluoroscopy was resumed, the first passage of contrast through the duodenum had already occurred, and contrast filled the small bowel loops, obscuring the position of the duodenojejunal junction. *D,E,* The child returned for duodenal intubation that rapidly demonstrated a normal duodenum.

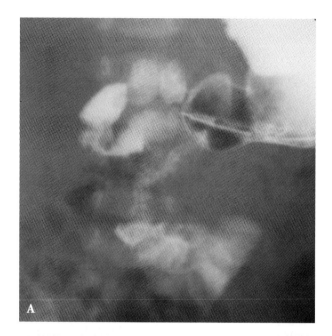

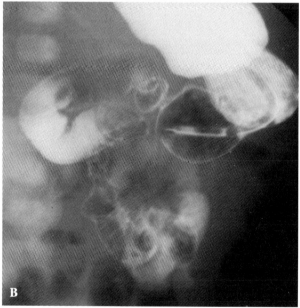

FIGURE 9–14. Malrotation. *A,B,* An upper GI examination demonstrates the fourth part of the duodenum rising to a near appropriate position just below the level of the duodenal bulb and to the left of the L2 pedicle. The abrupt descent of bowel from this high point is suspicious. *C,* Aspiration of residual gastric contrast allowed an unobscured enema which demonstrated an abnormal cecum riding high in the right upper quadrant, tucked under the transverse colon. The diagnosis of malrotation with a narrow mesenteric root was confirmed at surgery.

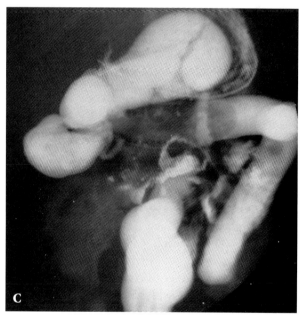

(Figure 9–16) can make identification of the true duodenojejunal junction difficult (Katz et al., 1987; Long et al., 1996). The presence of one of these variants is normal but more than two or three should increase the suspicion of malrotation. These patients require special attention to their history and clinical condition and usually require additional assessment of the colon and cecum.

Surprising mobility of the duodenum has been demonstrated especially in neonates. Virtually all infants under 4 months of age can have their duodenojejunal flexure manually displaced across the midline; this mobility decreases until about 4 years of age when the duodenum becomes fixed (Katz et al., 1987). Normally, a manually displaced duodenum will readily return to its expected position. Caution should be exercised diagnosing malrotation where a distended stomach is present (Figure 9–17) or where chronically dilated bowel from a more distal obstruction can displace the duodenum (Figure 9–18) (Taylor and Teele, 1985). Stiff nasojejunal tubes and adjacent mass lesions such as duplication cysts can occasionally cause displacement and diagnostic problems.

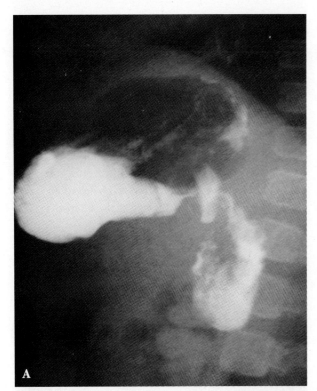 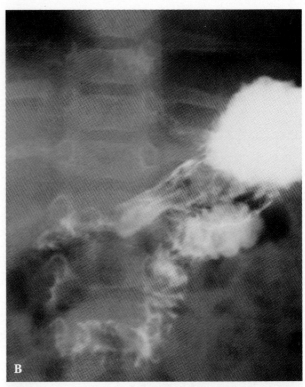

FIGURE 9–15. Normal duodenum. *A,* The right lateral position on an upper GI examination allows ready passage of contrast into the proximal duodenum. *B,* Rolling the child supine clears the gastric antrum and demonstrates contrast rising to a normal duodenojejunal junction behind the stomach, to the left of the L2 pedicle, at or near the level of the duodenal bulb. A wide field of view ensures assessment of appropriate patient alignment.

Most upper GI examinations of patients with malrotation will demonstrate an obvious abnormality and readily yield a diagnosis. Problems arise from technical inadequacy and poor recording of a study, poor appreciation of normal and normal variations in duodenal anatomy, and inadequate knowledge of the patient's clinical history. Cases of diagnostic difficulty will always arise and there should be no reluctance to repeat an inadequate study, evaluate the large bowel, and obtain all relevant history from the patient or referring doctor.

A "malfixed" bowel may occasionally end up in an apparently normal position. There is no reliable radiologic method of making the correct diagnosis in this unusual instance. Hence, the clinical status of the child should always be considered, preferably in cooperation with the referring physician.

Contrast Enema Examination. The most significant finding of malrotation on enema examination is a transverse colon that crosses the midline but doubles back so that the cecum lies near the midline in the upper abdomen (Figure 9–19) (Berdon et al., 1970) as compared to the normal cecal location overlying the right iliac crest. This is a dangerous form of malrotation, type 3A, as the root of the mesentery is short and volvulus easily occurs. Occasionally the cecum may point laterally instead of medially, and although this is most often seen with a mobile cecum, a type 3A malrotation may be present (Figure 9–20). A characteristic appearance of volvulus seen on enema examination is a beak sign at the head of the barium column either in the region of the ileocecal valve or in the distal ileum, which has filled by retrograde flow (Siegel et al., 1980).

In older children and adults, a large bowel confined to the left side of the abdomen may be discovered by chance; the cecum will be in the left iliac fossa and the duodenojejunal junction will be on the right, a type 1 malrotation (Figure 9–21). This situation is commonly called nonrotation although up to 90° of rotation has occurred; the duodenum and large bowel lie lateral to the superior mesenteric artery but on the opposite side of normal. This form of malrotation rarely undergoes volvulus and is the common placement of bowel following Ladd's procedure surgery for malrotation.

A narrowed segment of transverse colon overlying the spine has been reported on enema examination in the rare reversed rotation of a type 2B malrotation (see Figure 9–2C), and this represents a superior mesenteric artery impression (DePrima et al., 1985). The type 2C reversed malrotation of the duodenum causes entrapment of the entire small bowel, and the mesentery may displace the colon to the left side of the abdomen. Volvulus can also occur (Figure 9–22) but obstruction is more common (Cunningham et al., 1994).

A mobile cecum occurs in 15% of infants and children and is due to incomplete attachment of the cecum and its mesocolon; it has been included in the embryologic classification of malrotation as type 3C (Figure 9–23). However, in the absence of other anomalies, this finding is seldom clinically significant (Kiesewetter and Smith, 1958; Soderlund, 1962), and hence, a superiorly located cecum is not necessarily significant. Conversely, a normally positioned cecum does not always exclude malrotation and volvulus. A normally sited cecum may be found in 16% of patients with malrotation (Humphrey, 1970; Lewis, 1966; Firor and Harris, 1974; Long et al., 1996). In some cases the duodenum may be the only abnormally rotated bowel as in type 2A malrotation (see Figure 9–8). The tip of the cecum seen on an enema examination may be a considerable distance lateral to the root of the

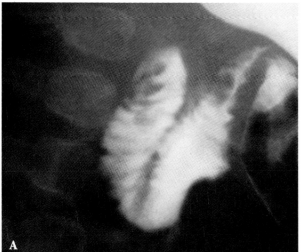

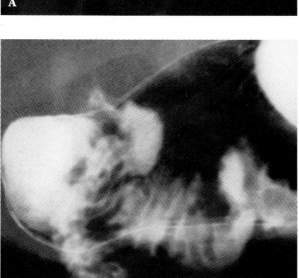

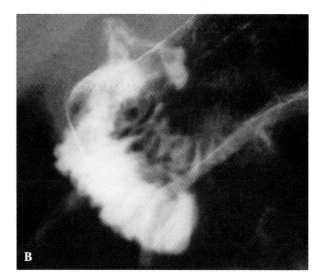

FIGURE 9–16. Redundant duodenum. *A*, Lateral view position on an upper GI examination shows contrast descending and rising back up to the level of the duodenal bulb. *B*, Supine view demonstrated that all of this portion of duodenum lay to the right of the midline. *C*, A normal position for the duodenojejunal junction was subsequently shown.

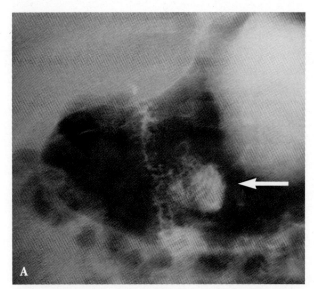

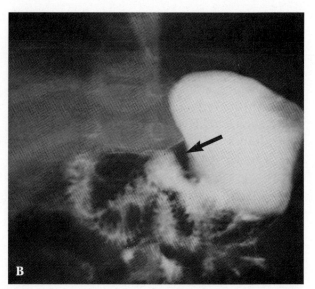

FIGURE 9–17. Duodenal mobility. *A,* A distressed crying child produced considerable gaseous overdistension of the stomach on an upper GI examination, which caused the duodenojejunal junction (*arrow*) to lie to the right of the midline. *B,* Partial gastric decompression allowed the duodenum to return to the left side (*arrow*), confirming its normal location.

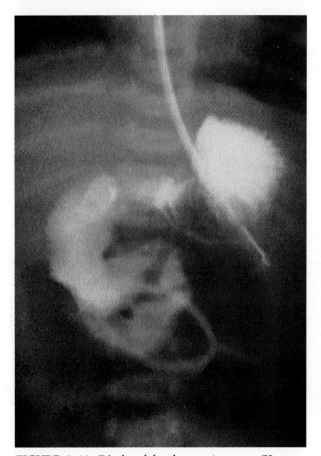

FIGURE 9–18. Displaced duodenum. An upper GI examination shows inferior displacement of the duodenojejunal junction due to distended loops of small bowel from a jejunal atresia. Normal rotation was present at surgery.

mesocolon and is a less precise marker for the root of mesocolon than the position of the duodenojejunal junction (Steiner, 1978).

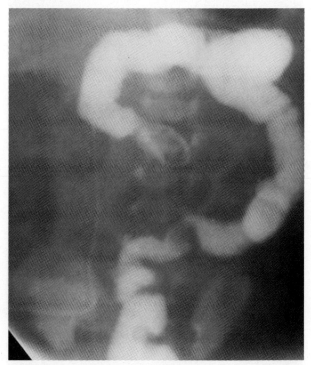

FIGURE 9–19. Type 3A malrotation with volvulus (see Figure 9–2E). Barium enema shows the transverse colon crossing the midline but then doubling back so that the cecum lies in the midline.

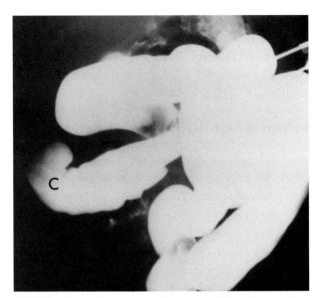

FIGURE 9–20. Type 3A malrotation with volvulus (see Figure 9–2E). Barium enema shows a high laterally pointing cecum (C). Type 3A malrotation with volvulus was found at operation.

In the larger child, an enema with barium presents few technical problems. In the neonate, iso-osmolar agents are recommended and care must be taken not to inflate balloon cuffs or use pressure likely to rupture the rectum or bowel. One must be sure contrast has indeed reached the cecum and not misjudge contrast in the hepatic flexure as an abnormally placed cecum. Occasionally redundant contrast-filled loops of sigmoid can obscure the ileocecal region.

Ultrasonography. Ultrasonographic screening of children with abdominal pain and babies with non-bilious vomiting in whom hypertrophic pyloric stenosis is suspected may sometimes show malrotation. Although operator dependent, US can be performed at the bedside expeditiously. Ultrasonography has been suggested as the initial evaluation of malrotation (Hayden et al., 1984), and in the symptomatic newborn, delineation by US of a distended duodenum indicating complete or partial obstruction will allow diagnosis and surgery. In this situation, however, clinical assessment and abdominal radiography will usually suffice. Vomiting and a nasogastric tube can remove the dilating fluids but following instillation of fluid into the stomach, the course of the duodenum can be followed by US to obtain an indication of normal rotation (Cohen et al., 1987). This is unreliable for excluding malrotation as even in an upper GI examination, where the vertebral level can be assessed, difficulty can be experienced locating the duodenojejunal flexure. Bowel dilatation associated with bowel wall thickening and peritoneal free fluid, especially if to the right

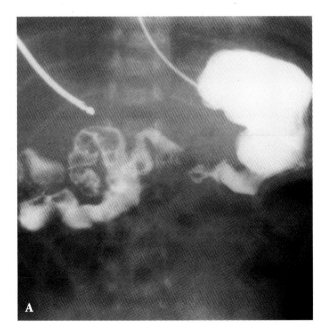

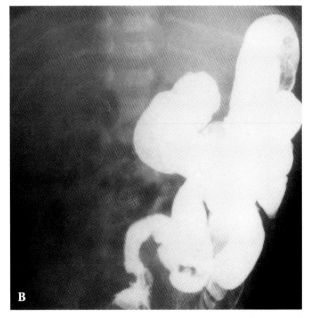

FIGURE 9–21. Type I nonrotation (see Figure 9–2A). *A,* Upper GI shows the duodenojejunal junction and proximal jejunum to lie on the right side of the abdomen. *B,* Barium enema shows all the large bowel to lie on the left.

of the midline (suggesting right-sided jejunum), would be ultrasonographic indicators of volvulus (Leonidas et al., 1991).

The relationship of the superior mesenteric artery and vein is important in malrotation. The mesenteric vein should normally lie to the right or anterior to the mesenteric artery (Zerin and DiPietro, 1991). Inversion of the mesenteric vein and artery with the vein located to the left of the artery is a sign of midgut volvulus (Figure 9–24) (Gaines et al., 1987; Loyer and Eggli, 1989; Weinberger et al., 1992). It is not pathognomonic as it has been demonstrated with normal bowel position, associat-

ed with mass lesions in the upper abdomen, and seen in patients previously operated on for malrotation (Zerin and DiPietro, 1991). The vessel inversion is of particular relevance when the vein rotates clockwise around the artery, as viewed from the feet, and has been described as the "whirlpool" sign (see Figure 9–24) (Pracos et al., 1992). The increased specificity of clockwise motion as opposed to counterclockwise motion has been emphasized (Shimanuki et al., 1996). Identifying inversion of the mesenteric artery and vein contributes to diagnosis of midgut volvulus, yet caution should be exercised if US is the only imaging or screening modality used. Bowel gas can

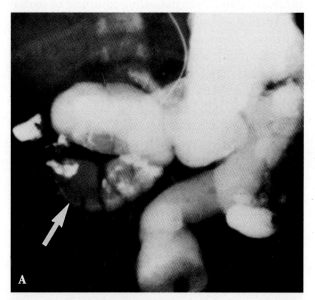

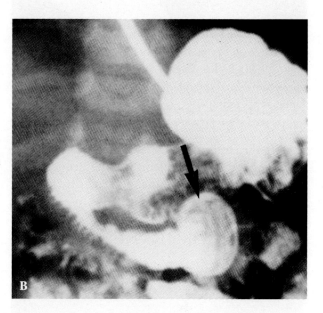

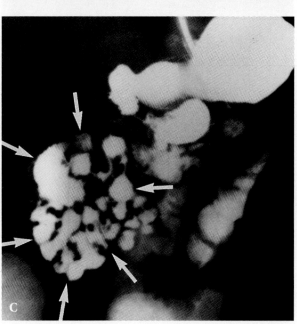

FIGURE 9–22. Reversed rotation (type 2C malrotation). *A,* Barium enema from an outside hospital shows a high cecum (*arrow*) that points laterally, a nonspecific finding. *B,* Our small bowel study the next day demonstrates a duodenojejunal junction (*arrow*) in a relatively normal location on the frontal view, on the left of the vertebral pedicles. *C,* A delayed film shows a more characteristic appearance with proximal small bowel trapped in the right upper quadrant (*arrows*), indicating an internal hernia. Some barium remains in the large bowel from the prior enema. A type 2C reversed malrotation was confirmed at operation.

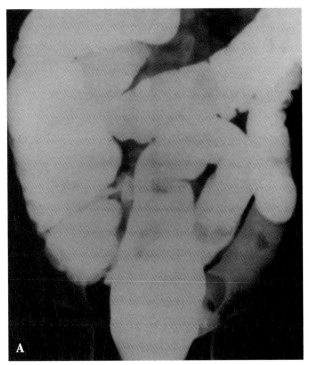 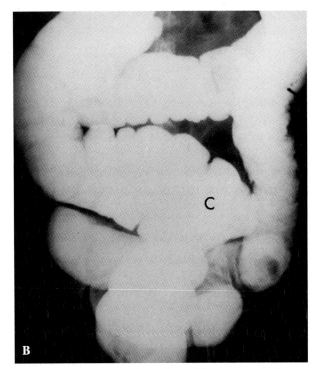

FIGURE 9–23. Mobile cecum (type 1 malrotation) (see Figure 9–1C). *A*, The normal position of the cecum. *B*, Cecum (c) moved from a normal position to a high position, mimicking a type 3A malrotation.

obscure ultrasonographic evaluation of the mesenteric vessels (Dufour et al., 1992). The vessel relationship should be assessed as caudally as possible from the splenic vein-mesenteric vein confluence; this can increase the likelihood of gas obscuring the field of view and increase the temptation to view from an oblique projection, thus misrepresenting vessel relationship (Weinberger et al., 1992). Malrotation can have a normal mesenteric vessel relationship in up to one-third of cases (Zerin and DiPietro, 1992; Dufour et al., 1992), making US a poor modality for excluding malrotation. A mesenteric vein situated directly

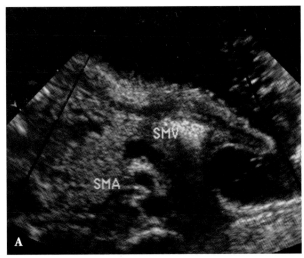 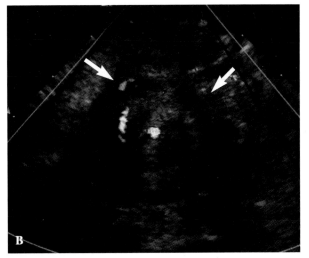

FIGURE 9–24. Malrotation and volvulus. *A*, A view on US through a fluid-filled stomach shows the superior mesenteric vein to the left of the artery. *B*, Inferior to this, a "whirl" of bowel, mesentery, and mesenteric vessels (*arrows*) represents the twisting midgut volvulus.

anterior to the mesenteric artery is associated with a higher incidence of malrotation, up to a total incidence of 28% (Dufour et al., 1992).

In the symptomatic patient, a partially obstructed duodenum or a positive "whirlpool" sign may suffice for diagnosis. We advise upper GI examination to confirm ultrasonographic findings. Assessment of the superior mesenteric vessel relationship should be included in all pediatric abdominal ultrasonographic studies but we stress that a "normal" ultrasonogram does not exclude a diagnosis of malrotation.

Other Imaging Modalities. Axial imaging is rarely indicated for evaluating rotational anomalies. Findings of malrotation may be incidental, especially if an asymptomatic type 1 nonrotation, or may be unsuspected in an older patient being investigated for abdominal pain, often mistaken as recurrent pancreatitis. Axial imaging can delineate the position of the duodenum and cecum, specific computed tomography (CT) findings of malrotation include inversion of the mesenteric artery and vein relationship and delineation of a whirl of mesentery and bowel around the superior mesenteric artery, indicative of midgut volvulus (Fisher, 1981; Nichols and Li, 1983; Paul and Dean, 1990). Computed tomography and magnetic resonance imaging (MR) can accurately and reliably demonstrate the relationship of the mesenteric artery and vein (Shatzke et al., 1990). The data for normal mesenteric vessel relationship was acquired from CT studies in which 88% of 187 patients had a mesenteric vein anterior and to the right of the artery (Zerin and DiPietro, 1991).

Computed tomography can diagnose both symptomatic and asymptomatic paraduodenal hernia, demonstrating a rounded cluster of small bowel in a retroperitoneal location to the left or (less commonly) right of the normal duodenal location (Harbin, 1982; Olazabal et al., 1992). It may also have a role in imaging the more unusual malrotation types with reversed rotational abnormalities such as types 2B and 2C. Cross-sectional imaging may help locate more accurately the duodenum and colon with respect to the mesenteric vessels (Cunningham et al., 1994).

Arteriography has no place in the evaluation of children with possible malrotation. The characteristic angiographic sign is the "barber pole sign" due to the twisted superior mesenteric artery and its branches (Buranasiri et al., 1973). Chronic volvulus can result in collateral vessel development; these have been clearly shown on angiography (Mori et al., 1987).

Surgical Treatment

Due to the frequency of volvulus with accompanying bowel ischemia, management in a symptomatic patient, especially a neonate, is urgent surgery. The surgery is based on Ladd's procedure whereby the volvulus is unraveled, peritoneal bands lysed, and the duodenum and large bowel are positioned on the right and the left, respectively. Appendectomy is routinely performed to prevent future difficulties in diagnosis. Follow-up contrast examinations are usually not indicated but if performed, will show an appearance similar to type 1 malrotation (nonrotation). Surgical treatment of the asymptomatic older child or adult, is more controversial especially if the malrotation was an incidental finding. These patients are at increased risk for potential volvulus, and careful assessment of their clinical history and (at least) a surgical consultation is required.

The risk of delayed obstruction from adhesion is the same as for any laparotomy. Specific complications from Ladd's procedure are rare but we have had one child who presented with hypoproteinemia of long duration due to partial chronic volvulus of the cecum and small bowel following a Ladd's procedure (Figure 9–25).

Atresia, Stenosis, and Duodenal Web

Clinical Features

Duodenal atresia occurs in 1 in 6000 births (Irving and Rickham, 1978), making it a common cause of neonatal small-bowel obstruction; duodenal stenosis is less common. Duodenal webs may be complete or incomplete and thus mimic atresia or stenosis. Approximately 50% of affected patients have atresia, 40% have a web, and 10% have stenosis (Fonkalsrud et al., 1969).

The mechanism that produces these anomalies is not well understood. The duodenum undergoes epithelial proliferation between 30 and 60 days of gestation, resulting in a solid tube. It then recanalizes, and interruption of this process is thought to result in atresia or stenosis (Kassner et al., 1972). The entry of biliary and pancreatic ducts, especially accessory pancreatic ducts, into the duodenum is

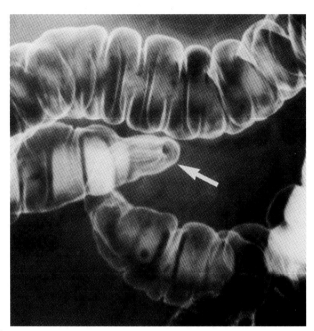

FIGURE 9–25. Chronic volvulus of the cecum, post Ladd's procedure. There is a twist or volvulus (*arrow*) in the cecum in a child with hypoproteinemia, cured by repeat Ladd's procedure.

postulated as possibly affecting recanalization (Boyden et al., 1967). This would account for atresia or stenosis invariably being at the level of the papilla of Vater, a high-risk area for developmental anomalies as complex development of pancreatic and biliary ducts and bowel rotation all occur simultaneously and in close proximity.

Associated anomalies are found in 48% of these patients (Table 9–2). Down syndrome is common and found in up to 33% of cases (Fonkalsrud et al., 1969; Farrant et al., 1981). Polyhydramnios is present antenatally in 40% of patients. In complete

TABLE 9–2. Anomalies Associated with Duodenal Atresia

Down syndrome
Esophageal atresia
Anorectal malformations
Malrotation/Ladd's bands
Renal anomalies
Biliary atresia
Congenital heart disease
Annular pancreas
Preduodenal portal vein

atresia, vomiting usually occurs soon after birth and is usually bilious, as 75% of atresias occur just distal to the papilla of Vater. Abdominal distension is often not marked. Untreated, the condition is rapidly fatal due to electrolyte loss and fluid imbalance.

Occasionally, presentation of web or stenosis may be delayed, even into adult life (Anderson and Mills, 1984).

Imaging

Ultrasonography. The diagnosis of atresia or web can be made antenatally by US (Farrant et al., 1981). Polyhydramnios is present in 40% of patients, and the stomach and duodenum of the fetus will be seen as intra-abdominal fluid-filled structures separate from normal kidneys and bladder (Figure 9–26) (Loveday et al., 1975). Confirmation of the diagnosis is possible on oblique scans, where these two fluid-filled structures may be seen to communicate (Farrant et al., 1981).

Postnatally and even in cases of stenosis or web presenting in later life, US may be diagnostic, the dilated duodenum being delineated by fluid distention (Brambs et al.,1986; Cohen et al., 1987). In esophageal atresia without fistula, an associated duodenal atresia will not be air-filled but is easily seen on US (Figure 9–27). The web itself can be seen as an echogenic band associated with proximal duodenal dilatation (Cremin and Solomon, 1987).

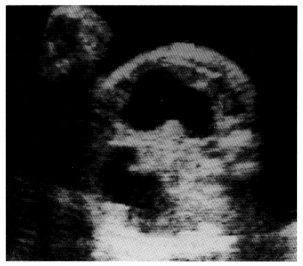

FIGURE 9–26. Antenatal US of duodenal atresia. The fluid-filled stomach and duodenum give a double bubble appearance.

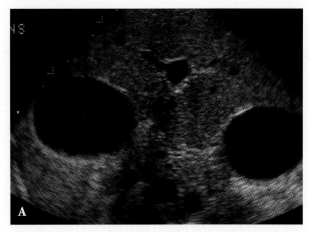
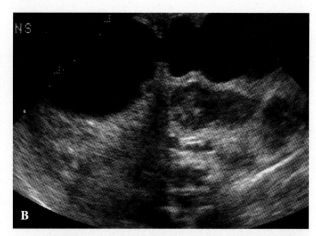

FIGURE 9–27. Duodenal atresia and esophageal atresia without a tracheoesophageal fistula in Down syndrome. *A*, Transverse US image shows the fluid-filled double bubble sign. *B*, The pylorus opening into a dilated duodenal bulb.

Plain Films. Plain abdominal films soon after birth show the characteristic double bubble appearance of duodenal atresia with air in the stomach and a dilated first part of the duodenum (Figure 9–28). A supine film is usually sufficient for diagnosis but sometimes an erect or decubitus film is necessary to delineate the duodenum (Figure 9–29). When there is little or no gas in the stomach, air may be injected through a nasogastric tube to demonstrate the obstruction. Gas is the preferred contrast medium. Other investigations are rarely needed.

Even with a complete atresia, small amounts of gas can occasionally be seen in the jejunum or ileum. This can occur via a bypass of the atresia through an accessory pancreatic duct above the atresia (duct of Santorini) to the main biliary-pancreatic duct below the atresia (Figure 9–30) (Astley, 1968; Kassner et al., 1972). Gas within the biliary tree may be present in these patients. A duodenal web may have a defect that enables gas to reach the small bowel. This is commonly called a fenestrated web. A duodenal stenosis will have distal bowel gas present.

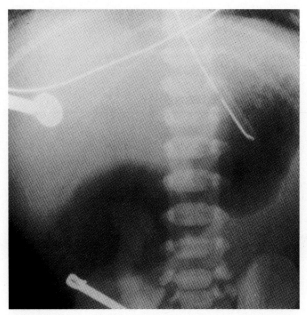

FIGURE 9–28. Duodenal atresia. Supine film shows gas only in the stomach and dilated duodenum; this double bubble appearance indicates duodenal obstruction.

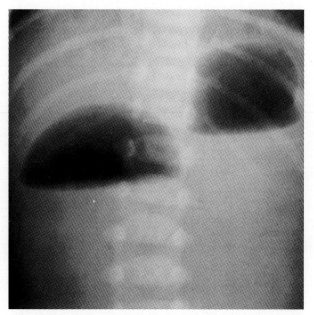

FIGURE 9–29. Duodenal atresia. On an erect film, prominent gas-fluid levels are present in the stomach and duodenum, with the double bubble appearance.

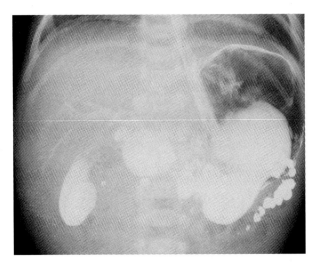

FIGURE 9–30. Duodenal atresia with accessory pancreatic duct. Contrast fills the gastric antrum and dilated duodenum proximal to an atresia. The atresia is bypassed via an accessory pancreatic duct above the atresia (duct of Santorini) to the main pancreatic duct (duct of Wirsung) below the atresia. Contrast is shown in the biliary tree and distal small bowel.

Duodenal stenosis or incomplete web usually become manifest similar to duodenal atresia although if the obstruction is minor, presentation may be delayed. Abdominal radiographs may occasionally demonstrate a dilated duodenum proximal to the stenosis (Figure 9–31). The retention of small swallowed foreign bodies in the stomach may imply a duodenal partial obstruction such as a web, stenosis, or annular pancreas (Kassner et al., 1975).

Contrast Studies. A duodenal atresia seldom needs a contrast study (Figure 9–32). A duodenal web, a stenosis, and (rarely) a complete atresia may have a defect that enables gas to reach the small bowel; such cases may require a contrast examination to show the obstruction (see Figures 9–30, 9–33). To prevent reflux and aspiration, a nasogastric tube should be used to instill only a small amount of barium, to be promptly aspirated through the tube at the end of the procedure. The examination will be safe if this precaution is followed and attention is paid to the risk of gastroesophageal reflux.

Some advise that when surgery is to be delayed, volvulus should be excluded by a colon examination. Unfortunately, the normal position of a cecum does not exclude volvulus. Conversely, an abnormal cecal position does not confirm a volvulus (see abnormal rotation and fixation of the midgut), so early operation is advisable for all such patients with duodenal obstruction (Lee et al., 1978).

With a duodenal stenosis or incomplete web, upper GI examination findings depend on the degree of obstruction. A web may appear as a linear lucency

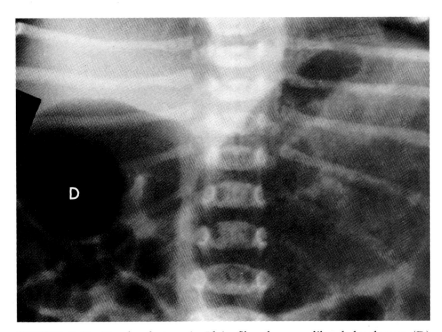

FIGURE 9–31. Duodenal stenosis. Plain film shows a dilated duodenum (D) with normal bowel gas in the rest of the small bowel.

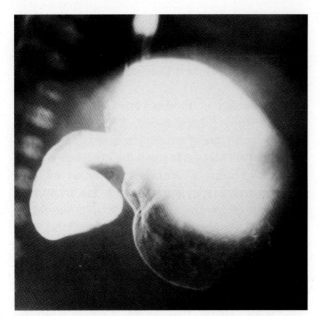

FIGURE 9–32. Duodenal atresia. Barium instilled via a nasogastric tube delineated the duodenal obstruction. However, a barium study is rarely indicated.

in the barium column and may balloon distally in the lumen of the duodenum to give the appearance of a wind sock (Figure 9–33). Occasionally the defect in the web can be seen as a jet of contrast media (Figure 9–34). The intraluminal duodenal diverticulum usually seen in adults (Heilbrun and Boyden, 1964) is now thought to be a form of duodenal web produc-

ing a windsock (Pratt, 1971). In the rare instance where the atresia has been circumvented via an accessory pancreatic duct, contrast in the biliary tree can be shown (see Figure 9–30).

Treatment

Early surgery is the treatment of choice, and the prognosis is good unless there is a serious associated anomaly. If the duodenum is very dilated, a plication of the dilated portion may be performed. This can give an unusual appearance to follow-up films (Figure 9–35).

Esophageal and Duodenal Atresia without Tracheo-esophageal Fistula. Rarely, duodenal atresia occurs with esophageal atresia in the absence of any tracheoesophageal fistula. These cases have a distinct antenatal US appearance; the stomach and duodenum are grossly distended with fluid, much more marked than in duodenal atresia alone (Hayden et al., 1983). The distal esophageal segment may also become grossly distended by secretions and appear on chest radiography examination as a posterior mediastinal mass (Crowe and Sumner, 1978).

Annular Pancreas

Annular pancreas is a rare anomaly in which the ventral anlage of the developing pancreas fails to migrate dorsally to fuse with the dorsal anlage and

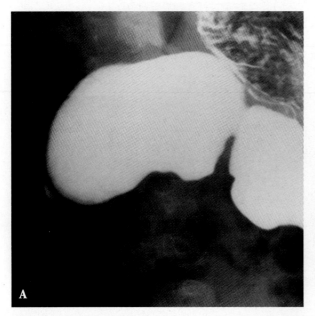

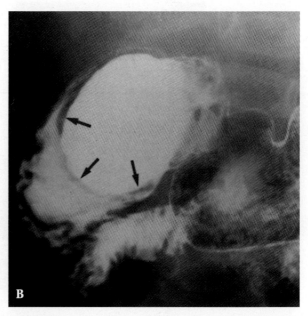

FIGURE 9–33. Duodenal web. *A,* A very dilated duodenum, shaped like a windsock, seen on early upper GI films. *B,* On delayed films, the dilated duodenum lies proximal to a linear lucency (*arrows*) that represents a duodenal web.

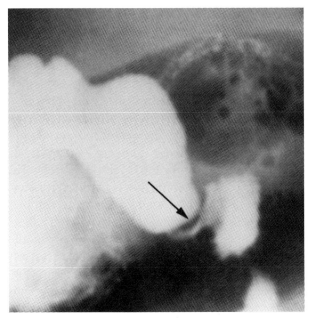

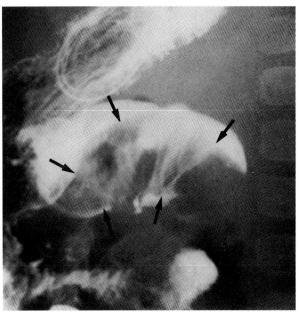

FIGURE 9–34. Duodenal web. A dilated duodenum, shaped like a windsock, lies proximal to a linear lucency (*black arrow*) that represents the duodenal web. A jet of barium passed through the defect in the web.

FIGURE 9–35. Postoperative plication of duodenal atresia. There is a large constant filling defect (*arrows*) in the proximal duodenum due to plication. There was no obstruction, however, and the child progressed well.

form the normal pancreas. The failure usually occurs at 6 weeks of gestation and causes pancreatic tissue to surround the duodenum. The underlying anomaly may be a failure of proper development of the duodenum, which therefore fails to displace the ventral anlage (Elliot et al., 1968). The anomalous pancreatic tissue is often intimately related to the muscularis of the duodenum, which makes surgical removal difficult (Salonen, 1978). A bowel bypass enterostomy is the surgical management of choice.

In the neonate, annular pancreas can be considered part of the spectrum of congenital duodenal obstruction, which includes duodenal atresia, stenosis, and web. If the ring of pancreatic tissue is complete, it produces an identical radiologic appearance to duodenal atresia (Figure 9–36), and the identification of

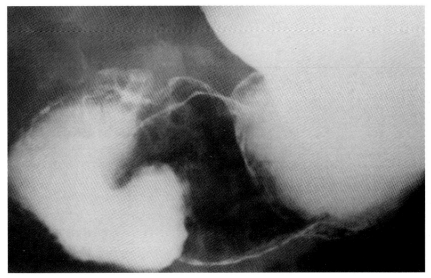

FIGURE 9–36. Annular pancreas. The obstruction mimics duodenal stenosis.

annular pancreas is only made at surgery. If the ring of pancreas is incomplete, the patient may be asymptomatic or may present either in later childhood (Figure 9–37) or as an adult with partial obstruction. It may be detected on US or on CT as a peninsula protrusion of the parenchyma from the pancreatic head (Brambs et al., 1986; Inamoto et al., 1983) but it is more often found on an upper GI examination. Annular pancreas is probably the only congenital gastrointestinal tract anomaly that is more likely to produce symptoms in adults than in children (Ravitch and Woods, 1950). The prognosis depends on the associated anomalies, which are similar to those found with duodenal atresia and include Down syndrome, malrotation, congenital heart disease, esophageal atresia, and anorectal malformations (Merrill and Raffensperger, 1976).

Preduodenal Portal Vein

Preduodenal portal vein is a rare congenital anomaly in which the portal vein lies anterior to the duodenum. The anomaly arises during growth of the embryo from 5 to 10 weeks of gestation (Bower and Ternberg, 1972). Initially, a pair of parallel vitelline veins drain the gut and are connected by three anastomotic branches. After two of these anastomotic channels disappear, the remaining channel (normally the middle channel) passes posterior to the duodenum and forms the portal vein. A preduodenal

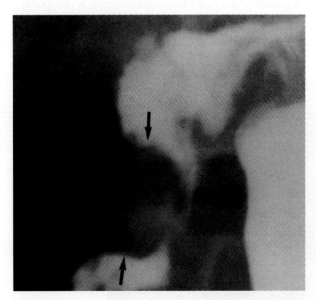

FIGURE 9–37. Annular pancreas. Extrinsic pressure by the annular pancreas of a 9-year-old boy produces a constant filling defect (*between the arrows*) on the right side of the duodenum.

portal vein results when the inferior anastomotic channel, lying anterior to the duodenum, remains patent (Figure 9–38).

Other anomalies, often multiple, occur in 83% of cases. Malrotation is the most commonly associated anomaly, and situs inversus is the next most common. Duodenal stenosis, duodenal atresia, annular pancreas, and biliary anomalies such as biliary atresia are relatively common (Braun et al., 1974; Boles and Smith, 1961; Johnson, 1971). The association of these anomalies is hardly surprising, as this region is the center of so many complex developmental interactions during embryonic life.

Radiology is rarely diagnostic of a preduodenal portal vein although US may occasionally demonstrate the anterior position of the vein (Figure 9–39), which can be confirmed with angiography (McCarten and Teele, 1978). Computed tomography and MR have similar potential to show abnormal portal venous anatomy.

Preduodenal portal vein is usually discovered in infancy during surgery for an associated anomaly. It is rarely an isolated abnormality that can cause duodenal obstruction. It is important to recognize the preduodenal portal vein during surgery because this vessel may lie hidden within a band of peritoneum, and serious hemorrhage will ensue if it is accidentally transected.

Atresia or Stenosis of the Jejunum or Ileum

Atresia or stenosis occurs more often in the jejunum and ileum than in the duodenum or colon. Atresia is more common than stenosis and denotes complete occlusion of the lumen. Atresia can be classified into four major types (Figure 9–40) (Delorimer et al., 1969).

Type I, a web, has a thin-walled diaphragm occluding the lumen and is the least common type of atresia.

Type II shows two blind ends of bowel connected by a fibrous cord of atretic bowel.

Type III, the most common form, is similar to type II but without the connecting cord and with a V-shaped deficit of variable size in the mesentery. Type III includes the type IIIB "apple peel" or "Christmas tree" atresia, where the V-shaped deficit is so large that the blind-ended distal small bowel is wrapped around a rudimentary mesentery and gives an appearance similar to an apple peel (Santulli and Blanc, 1961). The appearance has been likened also

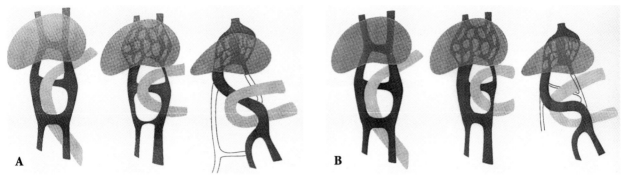

FIGURE 9–38. Preduodenal portal vein. *A*, Normal development. Of the three paired channels at 5 weeks' gestation, the middle anastomotic channel passing posterior to the duodenum remains patent and becomes the portal vein by 10 weeks' gestation. *B*, Preduodenal portal vein development. The portal vein passes anterior to the duodenum if the inferior channel remains patent.

to a Christmas tree (Weitzman and Vanderhof, 1966) and a maypole (Nixon and Tawes, 1971) but the term "apple peel" is the most accepted (Dickson, 1970; Schiavetti et al., 1984).

Type IV occurs when there are multiple atresias (El-Shafie and Rickham, 1970).

Etiology
Excluding duodenal atresia when the etiology is less clear, all types of small-bowel atresia and stenosis have an ischemic etiology; this has been shown experimentally in puppies following intrauterine surgery. Postnatal interruption of the vascular supply leads to gangrene, perforation, and peritonitis but if this occurs in the sterile fetal bowel, the avascular portion disappears with, at worst, a meconium peritonitis

(Louw and Barnard, 1955; Louw, 1966). Intrauterine ischemia may result from malrotation, volvulus, herniation, intussusception, or kinking of the fetal bowel (Louw, 1966). The cause is apparent in 25% of cases of atresia at operation (Delorimer et al., 1969).

Type IIIB occasionally has a familial incidence suggesting an autosomal recessive inheritance (Blyth and Dickson, 1969). A rare syndrome of multiple atresias, most commonly type I, affects the gastrointestinal tract from the stomach to the rectum and is associated with intraluminal calcification, which can be seen on plain films. The bile ducts may also be dilated. The condition usually but not always affects French-Canadians and has a high mortality rate (Martin et al., 1976; Daneman and Martin, 1979; Steinfield and Harrison, 1973; Guttman et al., 1973).

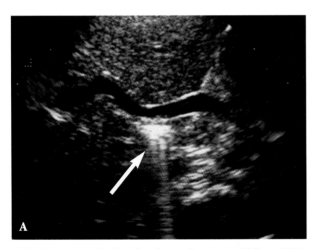
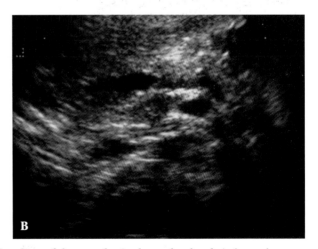

FIGURE 9–39. Preduodenal portal vein. *A*, Oblique US in the plane of the portal vein shows duodenal air (*arrow*) posterior to the portal vein. *B*, Transverse view shows an abnormal course of the portal vein over the pancreas head.

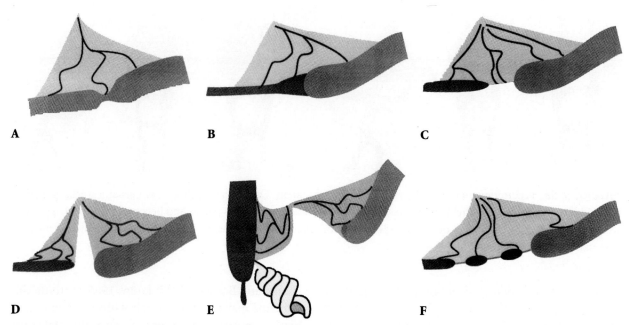

FIGURE 9–40. Types of small bowel stenosis and atresia. *A,* Stenosis of the small bowel is an incomplete occlusion of the lumen and is less common than atresia. Atresia denotes complete occlusion of the lumen and can be classified into four major types. *B,* Type I atresia, a web, has a thin-walled diaphragm occluding the lumen. *C,* Type II atresia shows two blind ends of bowel connected by a fibrous cord of atretic bowel. *D,* Type IIIA atresia, the most common form of atresia, is similar to type II atresia but without the connecting cord and with a V-shaped deficit of variable size in the mesentery. *E,* Type IIIB "apple peel" or "Christmas tree" atresia, where the V-shaped deficit is so large that the blind-ended distal small bowel is wrapped around a rudimentary mesentery. *F,* Type IV atresia occurs when there are multiple atresias.

Clinical Features

The majority of atresias present during the first day of life; stenosis may present later but usually within the first month of life. Rarely, presentation of stenosis or an incomplete diaphragm may be delayed (Agha and Jenkins, 1983). Polyhydramnios is present in approximately 25% of cases of atresia, with a higher incidence in proximal jejunal atresia and a lower incidence in distal ileal atresia (Delorimer et al., 1969).

The neonate usually presents with bilious vomiting, abdominal distension, and failure to pass meconium. Jaundice may also be present. These symptoms and signs are common whether the atresia is in the jejunum or ileum. Surprisingly, abdominal distension is present in almost as many cases of jejunal (78%) as of ileal atresia (81%), and neither the presence or absence of vomiting nor the passage of meconium will distinguish jejunal from ileal obstruction (Delorimer et al., 1969).

Associated Malformations

Jejunal or ileal atresia is associated in 25% of cases with an intra-abdominal anomaly such as malrota-tion, volvulus, gastroschisis, or intussusception, any of which could have produced an ischemic episode resulting in atresia. Malrotation occurs in 10% of cases and is the most common associated anomaly. Meconium ileus is seen in 9% and meconium peritonitis in 5%. In contrast to esophageal atresia, duodenal atresia and stenosis, and anorectal malformations, there is a low incidence of extragastrointestinal complications such as Down syndrome (Delorimer et al., 1969).

Imaging

Ultrasonography. Dilated bowel can be antenatally detected as enlarged tubular structures although distinguishing dilated aperistaltic small bowel from normal large bowel may be difficult and careful distinction from hydroureter or other intra-abdominal cystic masses is required. Antenatal diagnosis is usually made after 24 weeks of gestational age, and polyhydramnios is usually present (Nyberg, 1990). The differential diagnosis of antenatal bowel dilation includes meconium ileus, volvulus, intestinal duplication, meconium plug, and Hirschsprung's disease. Obstruction due to "apple peel" atresia has been diagnosed prenatally by US (Fletman et al., 1980). However, the diagnosis usually is not suspected until after birth. Postnatal US will show dilated small bowel with clear fluid and air-filled loops. Identifying dilated bowel with very echogenic content is suggestive of meconium and meconium ileus (Neal et al., 1997).

Plain-Film Radiography. Abdominal plain film and clinical history are the mainstays of diagnosis. The child should be at least a few hours old to allow air ingestion and delineation of the dilated loops of gas-filled small bowel down to the region of the obstruction. The site of an obstruction can be estimated by the number and distribution of the loops. When a few loops are seen in the left upper quadrant, the diagnosis is likely to be jejunal atresia (Figure 9–41), and these loops may be grossly distended (Figure 9–42). The filling of most of the abdomen with many loops favors the diagnosis of an ileal or more distal obstruction (Figure 9–43). Large bowel and dilated small bowel have a similar appearance in the neonate as the haustral pattern is not well developed. Occasionally, localized gross intestinal dilatation just proximal to the atresia may mimic gastric dilatation, a further illustration of the difficulty in accurately identifying bowel in neonates (Lee, 1982). Calcification may indicate meconium peritonitis secondary to an intrauterine perforation, and occasionally the calcification may be intraluminal or lie in the wall of the bowel. Extensive intramural calcification has been described in intestinal atresia (Steinfield and Harrison, 1973). A bubbly pattern in the right iliac fossa suggests meconium ileus; however, this pattern may occasionally be seen with an atresia where the dilated bowel proximal to the atresia is filled with meconium (Figure 9–44). Confidently separating an ileal atresia from a meconium ileus on plain-film radiography may sometimes be difficult.

Contrast Examinations. A contrast enema is the best examination to exclude large-bowel causes of obstruction, to demonstrate meconium ileus, or to show colonic position prior to surgery. An upper gastrointestinal examination is not indicated in a setting of low bowel obstruction.

Water-soluble contrast media are preferable to barium for the enema examination because an atre-

sia may rarely communicate freely with the peritoneum (Wolfson and Williams, 1970), and bowel adjacent to an atresia may be necrotic and at risk for perforation. We choose to use hypo- or iso-osmolar water-soluble contrast media for all neonatal enemas (see Chapter 3).

A microcolon is usually seen in low ileal atresia with or without a few meconium plugs (Figure 9–45). The colon is usually of more normal size in jejunal or proximal ileal atresia (see Figure 9–42). The size of the large bowel is dependent on the amount of succus entericus that is present distal to the atresia as this distends the large bowel from its small embryologic size to the size found in a normal neonate. The succus entericus, which forms meconium, is derived from stomach and small-bowel secretions, desquamated cells, and swallowed fluid and bile. The site and timing of an atresia determines whether succus entericus reaches the large bowel. Many atresias occur late in development as shown by the bile pigments, lanugo hair, and squamous cells found in the colonic contents distal to the atresia. Bile pigments, for example, are not produced until the fourth intrauterine month (Berdon et al., 1968). An "apple peel" type IIIB atresia is diagnosed if the distal ileum is shown to have a "corkscrew" or "apple peel" appearance on retrograde

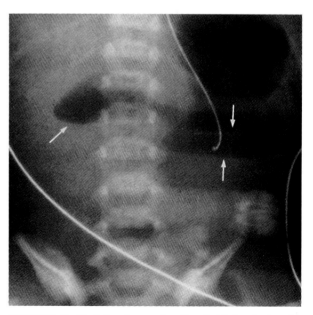

FIGURE 9–41. Jejunal atresia. Gas-fluid levels in the stomach (*arrow aimed inferiorly*), duodenum (*oblique arrow*), and proximal jejunum (*arrow aimed superiorly*) indicate high jejunal atresia and produces the triple bubble appearance.

filling, and the diagnosis is strongly suggested if the plain films suggest a high intestinal obstruction in the presence of microcolon (Schiavetti et al., 1984).

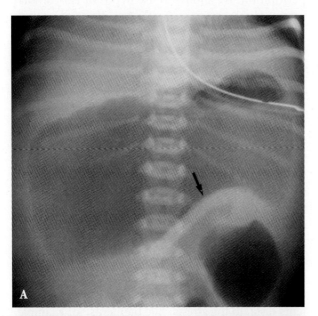

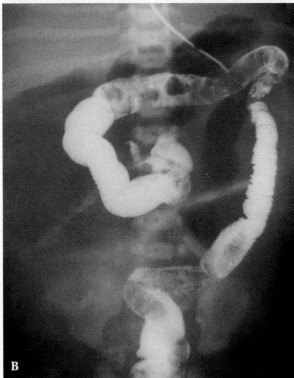

FIGURE 9–42. Jejunal atresia. *A*, Plain film shows a few grossly dilated loops of proximal small bowel with bowel wall thickening (*arrow*). *B*, Barium enema demonstrates a normal-caliber colon containing meconium pellets. Despite the location of the cecum, no volvulus was found at operation.

Treatment

Surgical resection is the treatment for atresia or stenosis of the jejunum or ileum. A distal ileal resection has a lower mortality rate than a proximal jejunal resection (Delorimer et al., 1969; Nixon and Tawes, 1971); "apple peel" (type IIIB) atresia has a high mortality rate (Leonidas et al., 1976). If a large portion of bowel has to be removed, the child can be left with a short gut. Some cases, in which the remaining gut increases its rate of growth with hypertrophy of the mucosa and dilates to increase its absorptive area, may result in surprisingly little disability. However, other patients with a markedly shortened gut do not thrive, suffer from severe chronic malabsorption, and require parenteral feeding to stay alive. After surgical resection, the atretic or stenotic segment of bowel should be examined for aganglionosis. Multiple atresias must be excluded at the time of surgery as obstruction from a missed distal atresia can result in fatal dehiscence of a bowel anastomosis (Nixon and Tawes, 1971).

Meconium Ileus/Cystic Fibrosis

Meconium ileus is a form of intestinal obstruction occurring in 10 to 20% of patients with cystic fibrosis (Leonidas et al., 1970). It is almost always a manifestation of cystic fibrosis, a condition that should be confirmed by observing the elevated level of chloride in the sweat. The exceedingly rare meconium ileus patients who do not have cystic fibrosis may have another etiology such as partial aplasia of the pancreas (Auburn et al., 1969); or it may occur secondary to stenosis of the pancreatic ducts (Hurwitt and Arnheim, 1942). Meconium ileus is rarely familial (Dolan and Touloukian, 1974).

Cystic fibrosis is an autosomal recessive disease common in the Caucasian population. A defect in the permeability of epithelium for the transport of chloride ions has been shown to be the underlying physiologic problem in cystic fibrosis (Quinton, 1983; Knowles et al., 1983), and a cystic fibrosis gene which produces the protein that regulates transmembrane ion transport has been delineated (Riordan et al., 1989). This explains how meconium ileus results in part from the abnormal production of pancreatic enzymes (Holsclaw et al., 1965) and from the presence of abnormal mucous gland secretion throughout the gastrointestinal tract. These glands produce a mucus that is high in protein and mucoprotein. Meconium in cystic fibrosis contains 85% protein with a high albu-

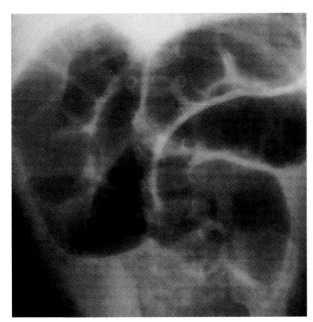

FIGURE 9–43. Ileal atresia. There are many dilated loops of bowel filling most of the abdomen.

min content whereas normal meconium contains only 7% protein (Schutt and Isles, 1968).

Clinical Features
The neonate is usually of normal birth weight but soon develops bilious vomiting, abdominal disten-

sion, and failure to pass meconium within 48 hours although a small, whitish plug of inspissated mucus may be passed. Loops of distended bowel with a thickened wall may be palpated through the abdominal wall. Sometimes there is a family history of cystic fibrosis. Simple meconium ileus may occur but up to 50% of cases are complicated by volvulus, atresia, perforation, meconium peritonitis, or pseudocyst formation (Abramson et al., 1987).

Imaging

Ultrasonography. Prenatal US can detect bowel dilatation, one-third of which cases may have meconium ileus. Other causes of antenatal bowel dilatation include atresia, stenosis, volvulus, intestinal duplication, meconium plug, and Hirschsprung's disease (Estroff et al., 1992). All will require early surgical management, so delivery in or near to a pediatric institution is indicated. Ultrasonography can also detect echogenic bowel, which may be normal prior to 20 weeks of gestation but has a reported 13% outcome of meconium ileus (Dick and Crane, 1992). The detection of fetal bowel dilatation and/or hyperechoic bowel raises the suspicion of meconium ileus, meconium peritonitis, congenital infection, neoplasm, and chromosomal trisomy. Thus, although not specific or

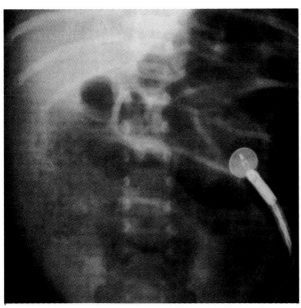

FIGURE 9–44. Ileal atresia. A bubbly pattern in the right iliac fossa suggests meconium ileus but this patient had an atresia, and the dilated distal small bowel proximal to the atresia was filled with meconium (see Figure 9–47).

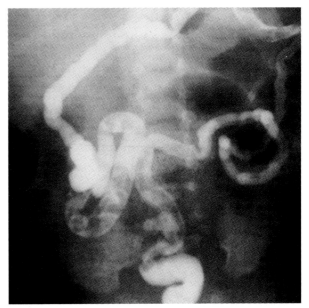

FIGURE 9–45. Ileal atresia. Water-soluble contrast enema demonstrates a microcolon with a few small meconium plugs. The presence of meconium and the size of the colon depend on the site and time of onset of the atresia.

sensitive for diagnosing cystic fibrosis, the US finding may prompt parental and amniotic DNA analysis and diligent postnatal screening for cystic fibrosis (Irish et al., 1997). The postnatal ultrasonographic appearance of meconium ileus includes distended bowel due to obstruction and hyperechogenic inspissated meconium (Figure 9–46).

Ultrasonography is capable of detecting complications of meconium ileus. If there is an associated perforation and meconium is spilt into the peritoneum, it often becomes localized as the meconium in these patients is viscous. The meconium cyst so produced can be detected by US. It appears as a well-defined fluid-filled mass with echogenic contents (Bowen et al., 1984; Carrol and Moskowitz, 1981). The rim, if calcified, will be hyperechogenic (Blumenthal et al., 1982). More diffuse spread of meconium may show as scattered dense echoes along peritoneal margins (Garb and Riseborough, 1980) or as a snowstorm effect (Lawrence and Chrispin, 1984). (See Infection and Inflammation of the Small Bowel in this chapter.)

Plain-Film Radiography. Plain abdominal films will show distal small bowel obstruction with distended loops of bowel and a granular or bubbly pattern of bowel gas usually in the right lower quadrant. This represents mixed gas and inspissated meconium (Figure 9–47) (Neuhauser, 1946). Although this is the appearance in 50 to 66% of patients, it is unfortunately nonspecific since it is also found in patients with Hirschsprung's disease, imperforate anus, meconium plug syndrome, and small bowel and ileocecal atresia without meconium ileus (see Figure

9–44) (Leonidas et al., 1970; Astley, 1977; Herson, 1957; Ein et al., 1985). It may be difficult to differentiate dilated loops of small or large bowel at this age (Astley, 1977), and if insufficient time is allowed after birth for gas to pass through the bowel, a false impression of the level of obstruction may be obtained (Holsclaw et al., 1965).

Erect or decubitus views are usually unnecessary but may show a surprising paucity of gas-fluid levels with an obvious obstructed bowel gas pattern (Figure 9–48), (Holsclaw et al., 1965; Astley, 1977). This appearance is due to the viscosity of the meconium but is seen in only 25% of cases of uncomplicated meconium ileus (Leonidas et al., 1970; Herson, 1957). A similar appearance may be found with other causes of intestinal obstruction when intestinal fluid has been vigorously suctioned from the patient prior to radiography. Conversely, the presence of gas-fluid levels does not exclude uncomplicated meconium ileus; but prominent gas-fluid levels are unusual and may suggest complications (Leonidas et al., 1970) although in our experience, not necessarily (Figure 9–49).

Plain films sometimes help detect specific complications. Intraperitoneal calcification indicates meconium peritonitis from a perforation. Meconium and consequent calcification may enter the scrotum via the patent processus vaginalis testis. If a perforation occurs, a localized pseudocyst collection of leaked meconium may develop and occasionally be outlined by a rim of calcification. (See Infection and Inflammation of the Small Bowel and Figures 9–77 to 9–79 in this chapter.)

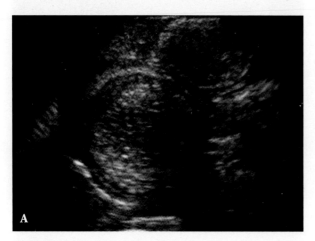 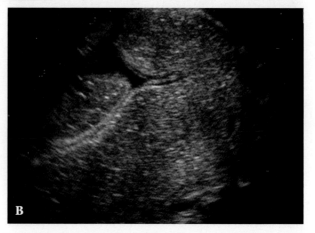

FIGURE 9–46. Meconium ileus. *A,B,* Two US views show a distended bowel with minimal free fluid and a striking echogenic intraluminal content consistent with inspissated meconium.

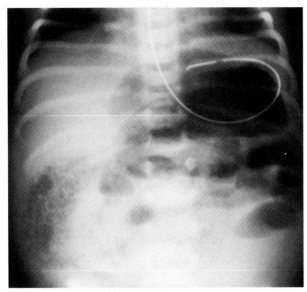

FIGURE 9–47. Meconium ileus. A typical granular pattern is in the right iliac fossa, the small bowel is dilated, and gas-fluid levels are present (see Figure 9–44).

Pseudocysts also can develop where ischemic loops of twisted bowel become adherent with loss of continuity of the intestinal lumen. A pseudocyst may be found at operation where it can mimic a mesenteric or duplication cyst (Leonidas et al.,

1970). Pseudocysts occasionally can be suspected if a large localized dilated loop is seen on plain films (Figure 9–50).

Acute perforation of the intestine is indicated by finding free intra-abdominal air, provided that sufficient time has elapsed from birth for air to reach the perforation site (Figure 9–51) (Gugliantini et al., 1979).

Contrast Examinations. A contrast enema will show a microcolon and inspissated meconium in the ileum (Figure 9–52) (Berdon et al., 1968). The choice of contrast media is controversial, and comparative data is sparse. Gastrografin and other hyperosmolar media are contraindicated, because iso-osmolar (or near-iso-osmolar) media are probably equally successful and much safer. We choose either near-iso-osmolar or non-ionic water-soluble contrast media for all neonatal enemas (see Chapter 3). If meconium is encountered, attempts to encourage its mobilization and passage are made by repeating the enema with a 15 to 20% dilution of N-acetylcysteine in a water-soluble contrast medium. Care must be taken to advance the contrast well into the meconium obstruction but not to overdistend and rupture the microcolon. The mortality rate for

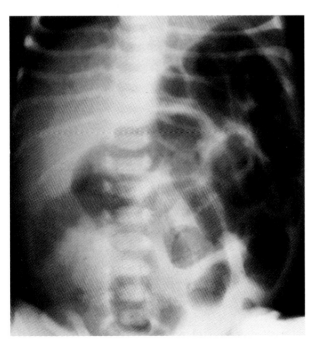

FIGURE 9–48. Meconium ileus. A faint granular pattern in the right iliac fossa accompanies dilated small bowel. Gas-fluid levels are absent on this erect film.

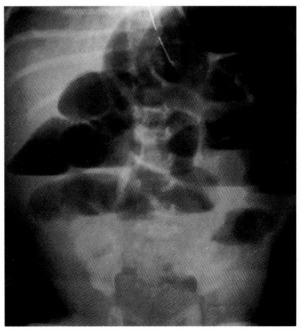

FIGURE 9–49. Meconium ileus. There are prominent air-fluid levels throughout the abdomen of a patient with uncomplicated meconium ileus.

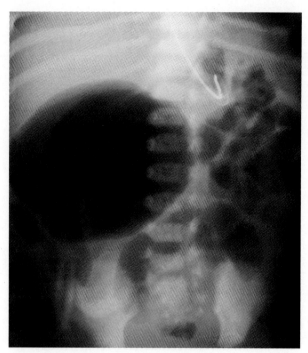

FIGURE 9–50. Pseudocyst in meconium ileus. The large gas shadow on the right represents a pseudocyst formed from ischemic loops of twisted bowel.

meconium ileus when treated by enema is lower than when treated by surgery but this is partly due to the more severe problems found in those who require surgery (Lillie and Chrispin, 1972). Approx-

imately one-third of neonates with meconium ileus can be treated successfully by a contrast enema technique. The rest are unsuccessful but half of these are found to require operation for other intra-abdominal pathology. Included in the two-thirds of unsuccessful enemas are the approximately 20% who have a perforation during the procedure. Despite this risk, the technique is worth performing as the one-third successfully treated require no further intervention and those who perforate suffer no postoperative sequelae if water-soluble contrast media is used (Ein et al., 1987).

Historically, barium was used to outline the mass of meconium in meconium ileus (Bryk, 1965; Keats and Smith, 1967). The risk of perforation and the inability of barium to mobilize meconium makes it a poor contrast medium. Diatrizoate meglumine and diatrizoate sodium solution with polysorbate 80 (Gastrografin) were introduced in 1969 (Rowe et al., 1971) and its great advantage of encouraging passage of obstructing meconium obviated the need for surgery in many patients (Noblett, 1969). However, Gastrografin is hypertonic and at full strength can cause electrolyte shifts and

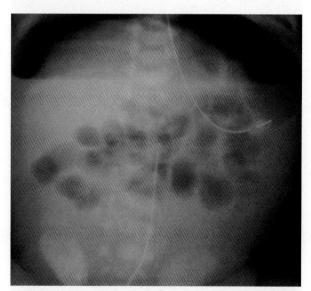

FIGURE 9–51. Meconium ileus with acute perforation. An erect film shows an air level indicating free intra-abdominal gas as sufficient time has elapsed from birth for air to traverse the gut and reach the site of the perforation.

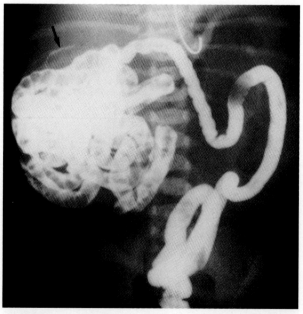

FIGURE 9–52. Meconium ileus with meconium peritonitis. Water-soluble contrast enema shows a microcolon and inspissated meconium in the ileum. Meconium peritonitis is present, and a streak of calcification (*arrow*) can be seen above loops of ileum. The rest of the calcification is obscured by overlying loops of bowel filled with contrast.

marked dehydration by drawing fluid into the bowel lumen. Intravenous fluid replacement requires attention during and after a Gastrografin enema (Wagget et al., 1970). Both Gastrografin and some of the older, more hyperosmolar ionic water-soluble contrast media were implicated in serious, sometimes fatal, side effects of dehydration, colonic irritation, perforation, and necrotizing enterocolitis (Harris et al., 1964; Leonidas et al., 1976; Rowe et al., 1971; Lutzger and Factor, 1976; Seltzer and Jones, 1978; Grantmyre et al., 1981). Therefore, the use of Gastrografin is not recommended.

Other Gastrointestinal Manifestations of Cystic Fibrosis

Duodenal Ulcer. Duodenal ulcers have been found in older children, possibly due to the failure of gastric acid neutralization as pancreatic secretions are scant (Berk and Lee, 1973). Duodenal ulcers occasionally occur in young children and can even present with pneumoperitoneum secondary to perforation (Tucker et al., 1963). In our experience, duodenal ulcers are rare in cystic fibrosis, and some of those reported may be related to stress.

Distal Intestinal Obstruction Syndrome. The distal intestinal obstruction syndrome or meconium ileus equivalent occurs in up to 15% of all patients with cystic fibrosis, primarily affecting adolescents and adults (Hanly and Fitzgerald, 1983; Matseske et al., 1972; Park and Grand, 1981; Rosentein and Langbaum, 1983). It appears to affect only the 80 to 85% of cystic fibrosis patients who have pancreatic insufficiency, manifested clinically by malabsorption, and who require pancreatic enzyme replacement therapy. The term distal intestinal obstruction syndrome is used to describe a broad range of clinical manifestations arising from partial or complete bowel obstruction and resulting from abnormally viscid mucofeculant material in the terminal ileum and right colon, where the fecal stream is usually liquid (Figure 9–53). Distal intestinal obstruction syndrome seems to be a separate entity from true constipation or distal colonic impaction, which in our experience is also common in patients with cystic fibrosis.

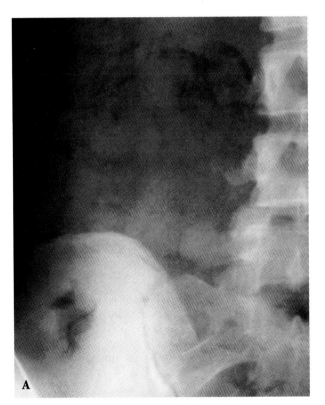 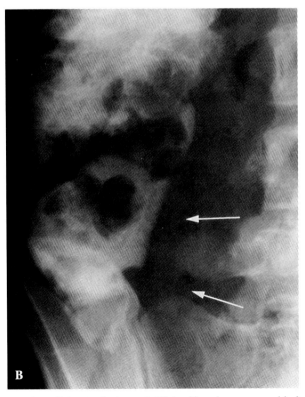

FIGURE 9–53. Distal intestinal obstruction syndrome or meconium ileus equivalent. *A*, Plain film shows a speckled fecal gas pattern in the right side of the abdomen. *B*, Contrast enema fills the large bowel and considerable speckled fecal gas shadowing is still present (*arrows*), presumably in the distal small bowel.

Distal intestinal obstruction syndrome is most commonly a chronic condition produced by partial bowel obstruction (Cleghorn et al., 1986; Hanley and Fitzgerald, 1983; Hodson et al., 1976; Park and Grand, 1981; Rosentein and Langbaum, 1983). A few patients present with complete bowel obstruction, which invariably results in acute symptoms of abdominal distension and vomiting. Typical clinical manifestations of chronic distal intestinal obstruction syndrome include recurrent episodes of colicky abdominal pain, usually in the right lower quadrant, associated with a palpable fecal mass in the right iliac fossa. Symptoms are exacerbated by food intake, and the patients are often anorexic, resulting in weight loss. Between episodes, patients may be symptom free but some complain of constant insidious abdominal pain. Clinical and radiologic examinations must be used to eliminate other causes of abdominal pain such as simple colonic constipation and intussusception. A palpable fecal mass in the right lower quadrant must be distinguished from other masses in this area, such as an appendiceal abscess and Crohn's disease. Attacks may be precipitated by a number of factors, such as sudden withdrawal of pancreatic supplements, and some seem to follow immobilization and respiratory tract infection. Plain abdominal films are useful in the patient with abdominal pain to show the extent of fecal residue or the presence of obstruction in the small bowel.

There is no single, efficacious, established treatment for chronic distal intestinal obstruction syndrome, and the cost of treatment is considerable, in terms of both medication and lost school or employment time. Management consists of increasing the dosage of pancreatic enzyme supplements and the use of mucolytic agents (N-acetylcysteine) by mouth (Hanly and Fitzgerald, 1983; Hodson et al., 1976; Rosentein and Langbaum, 1983). Some have recommended laxatives and dietary roughage for prophylaxis (Hanly and Fitzgerald, 1983; Rosentein and Langbaum, 1983). Unfortunately, these treatments do not work for all patients, and N-acetylcysteine, in particular, is expensive and unpalatable, resulting in poor patient compliance. The recurrence rate can be high. As a result, more vigorous therapy is sometimes instituted. Retention enemas containing normal saline and N-acetylcysteine have been used. We have found the above methods unreliable. Thus, a balanced electrolyte intestinal lavage solution (Golytely), given orally, is

our treatment of choice; we find it both efficacious and well tolerated (Cleghorn et al., 1986; Koletzko et al., 1989). Abdominal radiography can monitor the effectiveness of therapy, with clinical symptoms receding as the colon empties (Figure 9–54).

Miscellaneous Manifestations. Malabsorption, pancreatic insufficiency, and duodenal fold thickening are discussed later in this chapter (see Malabsorption and Chapter 13). Gastroesophageal reflux is common, occurring in over 20% of patients (Hassall et al., 1993). Large bowel complications include intussusception, appendiceal abscess, fecaloma, pneumatosis coli, fibrosing colonopathy, rectal prolapse, and constipation. Symptomatic hepatobiliary disease is more prevalent with the increasing longevity of patients. Focal biliary cirrhosis, cholestasis, and the development of portal hypertension are increasing causes of morbidity as the expected life span of cystic fibrosis patients increases (see Chapters 11 and 12).

Mesenteric and Omental Cysts

Cysts are occasionally found in the mesentery (usually the small bowel) and rarely in the omentum. Overall, they occur mostly in the fourth decade of life but approximately 25% occur in the first decade (Capropreso, 1974), and their male-to-female ratio is 1.7:1 (Arnheim et al., 1959). Many different types of cysts have been described since the initial report by a Florentine anatomist, Bienviene, in 1507 (Rifkin et al., 1983). The terms mesenteric and omental describe anatomic location. The following histologic classification has good imaging correlation and can be usefully adopted (Ros et al., 1987; Stoupis et al., 1994):

1. Enteric duplication cysts with enteric lining and muscle layer
2. Lymphangioma with endothelial lining
3. Enteric cyst with enteric lining but no muscle layer
4. Mesothelial cyst with mesothelial lining
5. Nonpancreatic pseudocyst with no lining and a fibrous wall (Ros et al., 1987)

A differential diagnosis of these cysts would require excluding cysts of renal, pancreatic, biliary, or hepatic origin and would include ovarian cysts in females, cystic neoplasm such as teratoma, and infections such as echinococcus in the appropriate geographic location.

Enteric Duplication Cyst

Clinical Features. Enteric duplication cysts are congenital and take the form of tubular or spherical lesions consisting of a muscular wall and a gastrointestinal mucosal lining (Bower et al., 1978). Ectopic gastric mucosa can be found in duplications throughout the gastrointestinal tract in a prevalence ranging from 43% in the esophagus to 2% in the colon (Macpherson, 1993). They may contain neural elements (Ros et al., 1987), and (rarely) tubular and spherical duplication cysts can coexist (Buras et al., 1986). They are typically found on the mesenteric border of the gastrointestinal tract, most often in the ileum (35%), distal esophagus (20%), stomach (8%), and duodenum (5%), with fewer occurrences elsewhere in the gastrointestinal tract. The rarest occurrence is in the mouth and pharynx (Macpherson, 1993). Spherical cysts are more common than tubular duplications, and multiple duplication cysts occur (Bisset and Towbin, 1986; Egelhoff et al., 1986). Rarely, duplication cysts communicate with the bowel lumen (Lamont et al., 1984).

The etiology of duplication cysts is uncertain. Initially it was thought to be a persistent embryonic diverticulum. Ischemia has been implicated more recently (Favara et al., 1971). A faulty recanalization of small bowel lumen, a process completed by the eighth intrauterine week, has been suggested (Bremer, 1944). Other theories include a failed attempt at twinning or an attempt at phylogenetic reversion to the double cecum of birds (Teele et al., 1980). When a duplication is present, internal secretions cause them to increase in size, thus producing a mass effect (Lamont et al., 1984).

An abdominal enteric duplication cyst usually presents during the first year of life with vomiting and abdominal pain due to obstruction. A painless abdominal mass may be palpated, and incidental detection during US can occur. If gastric mucosa is present, peptic ulceration can occur, causing gastrointestinal hemorrhage or massive melena (Inouye et al., 1965). Rectal bleeding is an uncommon but

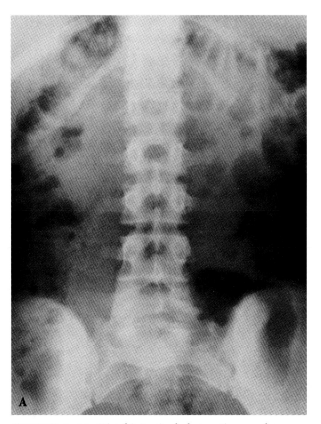 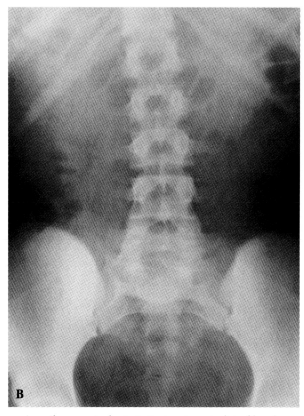

FIGURE 9–54. Distal intestinal obstruction syndrome or meconium ileus equivalent. *A*, Pretreatment plain film shows a considerable speckled fecal gas pattern in the right side of the abdomen. *B*, Post-treatment film shows the abdomen clear of feces.

well-recognized presenting sign. The differential diagnosis of rectal bleeding includes Meckel's diverticulum, juvenile polyps, colitis, intussusception, and hemorrhoids (Rose et al., 1978).

Imaging. The initial examination of any abdominal mass in a child is US. In the case of a duplication, US shows a well-defined cystic anechoic mass (Figure 9–55) (Teele et al., 1980; Ros et al., 1987), usually unilocular but occasionally multilocular with septations (Figure 9–56) (Ros et al., 1987). An echogenic inner rim (Kangarloo et al., 1979), that represents gastrointestinal mucosa is surrounded by a relatively hypoechoic layer, the muscular layer. This appearance is characteristic for a duplication cyst as it is similar to that of bowel wall (Figure 9–57). Extensive ulceration of the mucosal layer by gastric enzymes

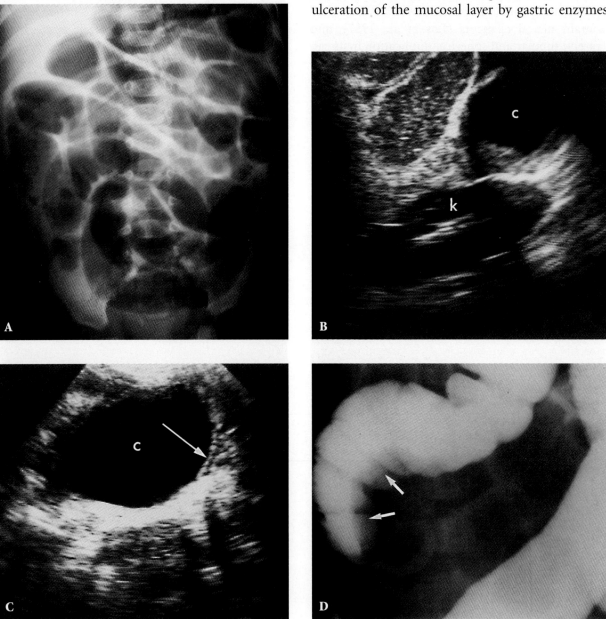

FIGURE 9–55. Duplication of the terminal ileum. *A,* Plain film shows dilated loops of small bowel, indicating distal small bowel obstruction. *B,* Longitudinal US shows a cystic mass (c) anterior to the right kidney (k) with adjacent dilated loops of hyperperistalsing small bowel. *C,* Further US views show the cyst (c) and its echogenic inner rim of gastrointestinal mucosa and hypoechoic muscular layer (arrow). *D,* Barium enema preformed prior to the US demonstrates an extrinsic impression on the cecum (*arrows*).

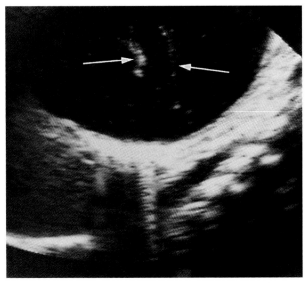

FIGURE 9–56. Duplication of the small bowel. There is partial septation with trabeculae (*arrows*) seen on US.

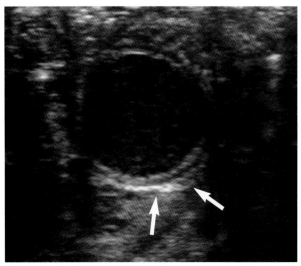

FIGURE 9–57. Enteric duplication cyst. An intraperitoneal cyst demonstrates a "gut signature" layering (*arrows*) on US.

can destroy this valuable sign, and the collection may then resemble other cystic lesions, especially ovarian cyst in a female patient. Echoic debris may be present occasionally (Figure 9–58) (Ros et al., 1987). If the cyst is subhepatic, careful US can show that it is separate from the liver and the biliary tree. Since a duplication may have interfered with fixation of the bowel, US cannot accurately reveal its site (Teele et al., 1980). The finding of a cystic abdominal mass on US with a "gut signature" lining is usually the only radiologic finding needed preoperatively. If the duplication is tubular or if the clinical context is atypical, other investigations can be used. A duplication communicating with the bowel lumen (often tubular) will not be a cystic structure readily identifiable by US.

The differential diagnosis of an enteric duplication cyst includes ovarian cyst, lymphangioma or mesenteric cyst, pancreatic pseudocyst, choledochal cyst, exophytic hepatic cyst, or a cystic tumor (Teele et al., 1980) (see Chapters 11, 12 and 13).

Plain films are seldom helpful. They may show the soft-tissue noncalcified mass of the duplication cyst displacing bowel (Figure 9–59) or evidence of intestinal obstruction (see Figure 9–55) (Ros et al., 1987). Rarely, calcification may be seen (Bastable, 1964).

A technetium Tc 99m sodium pertechnetate scan will show uptake in ectopic gastric mucosa and hence in cystic duplications which contain gastric

mucosa (Figures 9–60, 9–61) (See also Chapter 3). This test is more useful in the upper gastrointestinal tract and small bowel than the colon where the prevalence of ectopic gastric mucosa is lower (Macpherson, 1993). This scan will also demonstrate a Meckel's diverticulum, making it a good investigation for rectal bleeding (Rose et al., 1978; Ohba et al., 1981).

Gastrointestinal contrast studies may show displaced (see Figure 9–55) or obstructed loops of bowel (Figure 9–62) but only rarely does a duplication fill with barium (Bastable, 1964; Lamont et al., 1984; Ros et al., 1987). On barium upper GI series, a beaklike

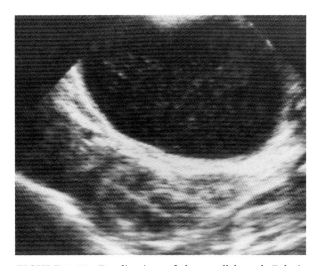

FIGURE 9–58. Duplication of the small bowel. Echoic debris is present.

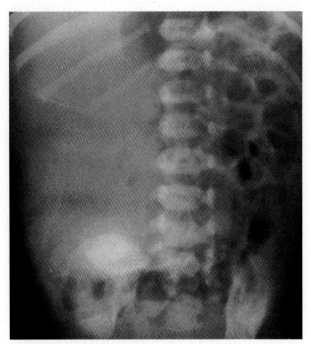

FIGURE 9–59. Duplication of the small bowel. A large soft-tissue noncalcified mass displaces bowel on the right side of the abdomen.

projection of the duodenum is described as a relatively reliable indicator of a duodenal duplication cyst (Blake, 1984) but US is still preferable for delineating

the mass. Most duplications do not communicate with the lumen of the intestine, and even those tubular ones that do communicate rarely fill. As a result, contrast examinations are not indicated unless intussusception or other pathology is suspected.

Computed tomography and MR have the ability to demonstrate and anatomically place the usually uniloculated, thick walled and fluid-filled cysts. This imaging is not routinely indicated.

Treatment. Treatment is surgical. A small bowel duplication lies in the mesentery and is intimately related to the vascular supply of the normal bowel. The wall of the duplication and that of the normal bowel may be inextricably fused. Therefore, the duplication is usually removed together with the related normal bowel. To avoid radical surgery when a large tubular duplication is present, an enteroenterostomy can be performed at the blind end of the duplication.

Duplications of the small bowel may rarely extend into the thorax through the diaphragm (Snodgrass, 1953), and the intrathoracic portion occasionally communicates with the spinal canal (see Neurenteric Cysts, Chapter 6).

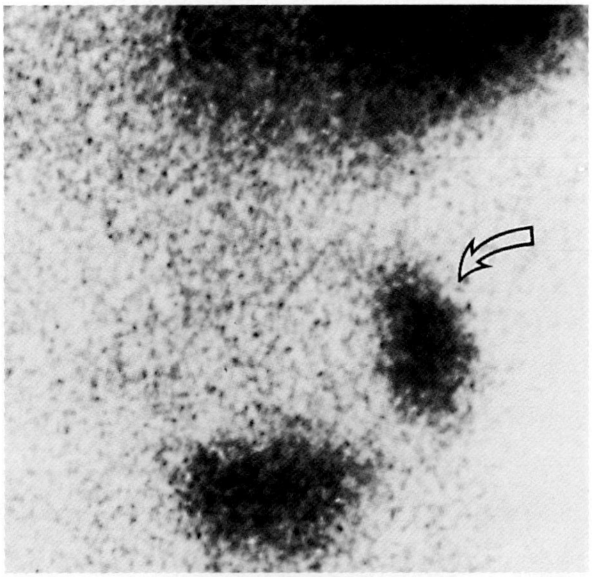

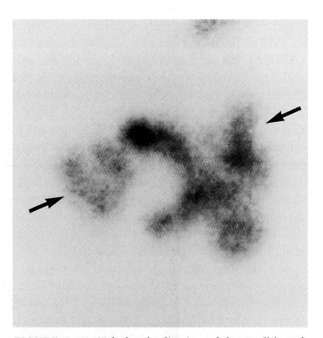

FIGURE 9–60. Cystic duplication of the small bowel. Technetium Tc 99m pertechnetate collects in a left upper abdominal duplication cyst (*arrow*). Radionuclide also accumulates in the stomach superiorly and the bladder inferiorly.

FIGURE 9–61. Tubular duplication of the small bowel. Technetium Tc 99m pertechnetate collects in a long tubular midabdominal duplication cyst (*between the arrows*). Radionuclide also accumulates in the stomach superiorly and the bladder inferiorly.

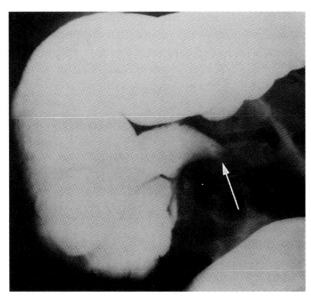

FIGURE 9–62. Duplication of the terminal ileum. There is complete obstruction to retrograde flow of barium into the terminal ileum with a beak deformity (*arrow*).

Lymphangioma

Clinical Features. Lymphangiomas are congenital malformations of the lymphatic system that result in a mass of dilated lymphatic channels with aberrant or obstructed outflow. Although usually found in the head and neck where the term cystic hygroma is often used to describe them, they can occur elsewhere, including the thorax, axilla, retroperitoneum, rarely the mesentery, and even more rarely in the omentum.

Lymphangiomas have an endothelial lining and are predominantly found in children. They most commonly present with abdominal distention although more acute presentation with pain and obstruction secondary to torsion, infection, hemorrhage, or rupture can occur (Haney and Whitley, 1984; Ros et al., 1987). Lymphangiomas are often soft and suprisingly difficult to palpate given their size, and they may displace but seldom obstruct structures (Blumhagen et al., 1987). They may occasionally cause an acute abdominal crisis that mimics appendicitis (Shackelford and McAlister, 1975).

Imaging. Ultrasonography is the best initial diagnostic modality as it reveals the cystic nature of the lesions, often with multiple thin-walled septations (Figure 9–63). The appearance will depend on the cyst's contents and on whether the cyst is uni- or multiloculated. Most commonly the cyst will have multiple thin 1- to 2-mm septations; occasionally a single thick septation is present (Blumhagen et al., 1987; Chirathivat and Shermeta, 1979; Geer et al., 1984; Ros et al., 1987). Least commonly the cyst will be unilocular (Blumhagen et al., 1987; Mittelstaedt, 1978; Ros et al., 1987; Rifkin et al., 1983). The fluid will appear either anechoic or echoic with debris (Blumhagen et al., 1987; Lucaya et al., 1978; Ros et al., 1987). The presence of debris depends on the cyst contents, i.e., chylous, serous, or hemorrhagic fluid. Chylous fluid shows as fine diffuse echoes, and hemorrhagic fluid has a coarser echogenic pattern (Blumhagen et al., 1987). The debris may appear as a layer of sediment that alters position when the patient is turned, and it may be seen in the dependent portion of the cyst (Figure

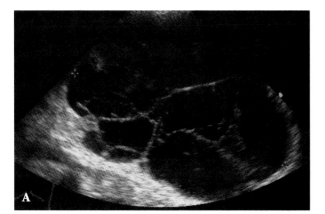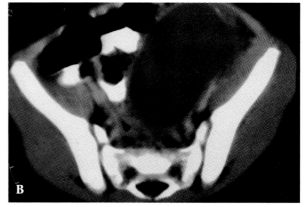

FIGURE 9–63. Lymphangioma. *A,* Ultrasonography delineates a large mass in the left lower quadrant with multiple thin septae. *B,* Computed tomography shows a thin nonenhancing rim but does not resolve the multiple septae.

9–64) (Haller et al., 1978). Hydronephrosis, deviation of the ureter, or compression of the bladder may occasionally be present and can be seen on US (Lucaya et al., 1978).

Plain films may show loops of bowel displaced by a soft-tissue mass of variable size. Barium small bowel or large bowel studies will also show displacement of the gut. Dilatation of proximal bowel will sometimes occur if the lymphangioma traps the small bowel.

Computed tomography will demonstrate the cystic abnormality with or without loculations although the septae are invariably shown better by US (see Figure 9–63). Contents are usually fluid of varying density depending on the presence of hemorrhage or infection. Occasionally, fat content as indicated by negative CT numbers is seen and can be attributed to the fatty components of chyle (Figure 9–65) (Ros et al., 1987; Stoupis et al., 1994), and a fat-fluid level may be present (Rifkin et al., 1983). Wall enhancement may be seen and will be more likely if inflamed (Ros et al., 1987). The CT features are characteristic but not specific. When the cysts are large the site of origin may be difficult to access, and the lymphangioma may mimic ascites (Haney and Whitley, 1984).

Magnetic resonance imaging with coronal and sagittal imaging planes can assist in locating the cyst. Serous contents will appear T1 hypointense and T2 hyperintense but the presence of blood or fat can cause T1 and T2 hyperintensity (Stoupis et al., 1994).

Treatment. Asymptomatic and incidentally discovered lymphangiomas should be observed. Nonradical surgical resection with marsupialization of nonresectable portions has been advised (Walker and Putnam, 1973), but the best chance for cure is complete resection at initial operation (Steyaert et al., 1996). A recurrence rate of 10% is found with incomplete resection and multiple areas of involvement (Steyaert et al., 1996). Endoscopic removal of lymphangiomas has been achieved (Hizawa et al., 1996). Identifying lymphangiomas is relevant as they are more aggressive and recur more than other mesenteric cysts (Singh et al., 1971).

Enteric Nonduplication Cyst

Enteric (nonduplication) cysts are rare and histologically different in that they have an enteric mucosal and submucosal lining but no muscular layers (Ros et al., 1987). There are no specific imaging features for a preoperative diagnosis.

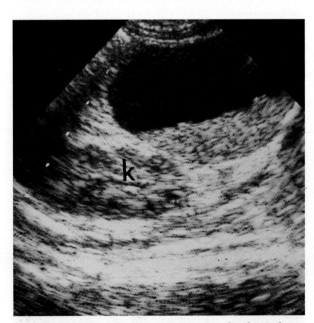

FIGURE 9–64. Mesenteric cyst. Longitudinal US shows a cystic mass lying anterior to the left kidney (k) and containing an echodense sediment that moves in response to changes in posture.

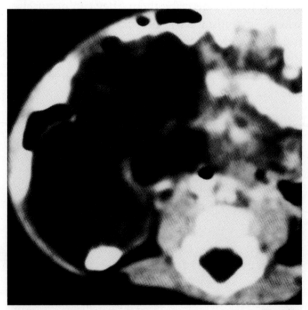

FIGURE 9–65. Mesenteric cyst. Computed tomography shows an irregular trabeculated mass of low attenuation (fat) filling a large portion of the right side of the abdomen.

Mesothelial Cysts

Mesothelial cysts are rare but may be seen in childhood (Ros et al., 1987). They contain a mesothelial lining and present with a mass that may be associated with pain.

Both US and CT will demonstrate a unilocular fluid-containing mass and thin wall. The fluid is usually anechoic.

Nonpancreatic Pseudocyst

Nonpancreatic pseudocysts have a fibrous wall with no recognizable histologic lining and are of uncertain etiology. In children, they are less common than lymphangiomas. They usually present with abdominal pain and distension. Nausea, vomiting, a palpable mass, or a history of previous trauma may occasionally be present. Some patients are asymptomatic.

Imaging is similar to that of lymphangiomas except that nonpancreatic pseudocysts are more often unilocular, and any echogenic debris is a result of hemorrhage, pus, or serous content. Computed tomography demonstrates a discernible wall not usually present with lymphangiomas. A fat-fluid level has been reported (Ros et al., 1987).

Anomalies of the Omphalomesenteric Duct

General Considerations

The omphalomesenteric (or vitelline) duct connects the primitive midgut with the embryonic yolk sac. The duct is usually obliterated in the fifth or sixth week of intrauterine life. Failure of its obliteration can result in a number of anomalies, including umbilical polyp, patent omphalomesenteric duct (omphalomesenteric fistula), omphalomesenteric sinus, omphalomesenteric duct cyst, and, most often, Meckel's diverticulum (Figure 9–66).

Cyst, Sinus, Fistula, and Band

Clinical Features. An umbilical polyp, consisting of ectopic intestinal mucosa, is the most benign manifestation unless it signals the presence of other omphalomesenteric duct anomalies. A fully patent omphalomesenteric duct is a rare finding and usually presents in the neonatal period with gastrointestinal drainage through the umbilicus. A partially patent duct will develop into a sinus when only the umbilical portion of the duct is involved. Cyst formation

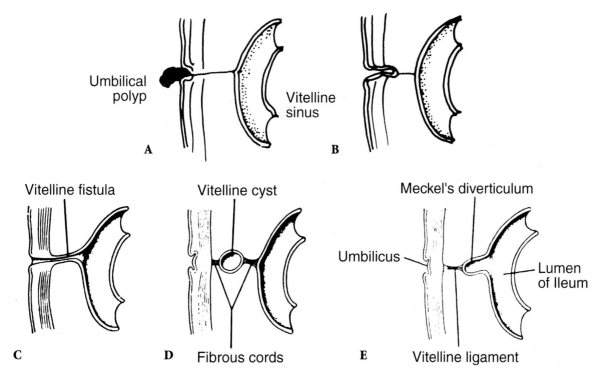

FIGURE 9–66. Diagrammatic lateral view of vitelline (omphalomesenteric duct) anomalies. *A,* Umbilical polyp, *B,* Vitelline (omphalomesenteric) sinus, *C,* Patent vitelline (omphalomesenteric) duct, *D,* Vitelline (omphalomesenteric) duct cyst, *E,* Meckel's diverticulum.

occurs when the middle portion remains patent and trapped secretions accumulate. They may be palpable. A Meckel's diverticulum develops when the intestinal portion does not involute.

A fibrous, atretic omphalomesenteric duct remnant tethers the ileum to the umbilicus and may act as an obstructing band or provide a fixation for focal volvulus. It may occur alone or with other omphalomesenteric duct anomalies.

Imaging. Prenatal US may detect umbilical omphalomesenteric duct cysts but as these are generally of little significance, only expectant obstetric management is indicated (Rosenberg et al., 1986). Postnatally, omphalomesenteric duct cysts may be palpable and US will demonstrate the cystic nature of the lesion (Figure 9–67). However, if the mass contains debris secondary to infection or hemorrhage, a definitive diagnosis may be difficult to make.

Plain radiographs seldom help but may show a soap bubble appearance or a gas-fluid level (Grosfield and Franken, 1974).

Sinuses and patent ducts are best investigated by injection of water-soluble contrast material to define the anomaly preoperatively (Figure 9–68).

A fibrous atretic omphalomesenteric duct remnant that causes volvulus or obstruction will present as a low small bowel obstruction indistinguishable from other causes of obstruction (Figure 9–69). Intermittent obstruction may occur and may have intermittent dilatation of a periumbilical bowel loop (Figure 9–70).

Meckel's Diverticulum

Clinical Features. Meckel's diverticulum results from a failure of obliteration of the intestinal end of the embryonic omphalomesenteric duct. It accounts for 90% of all omphalomesenteric duct abnormalities (Dalinka and Wunder, 1973) and has a prevalence of 1 to 3% in the general population (Rossi et al., 1996).

Meckel's diverticula lie on the antimesenteric border of the ileum 40 to 100 cm from the ileocecal valve. They are true diverticula having mucosa, submucosa, muscularis, and serosal layers identical to those of the small intestine. They are usually 5 cm in length and 2 cm in diameter although giant Meckel's diverticula are described (Rose and Pretorius, 1992). Ectopic gastric or pancreatic tissue is found in the wall of 20 to 30% of Meckel's diverticula (Enge and Frimann-Dahl, 1964).

Most Meckel's diverticula are asymptomatic with over 80% incidentally detected by imaging, laparotomy, or autopsy (Mackey and Dineen, 1978). They present when complications such as obstruction, ulceration, hemorrhage, and inflammation arise. Tumors may be found within Meckel's diverticula. They are rare and usually present in adulthood, and include benign leiomyoma, angioma, neurinoma, and lipoma as well as malignant sarcoma, carcinoid, and adenocarcinoma (Rossi et al., 1996).

Obstruction. Thirty-four to 53% of complications result in obstruction (Rossi et al., 1996). Causes include ileoileal or ileocolic intussusception with the inverted diverticulum as a lead point (see Intussus-

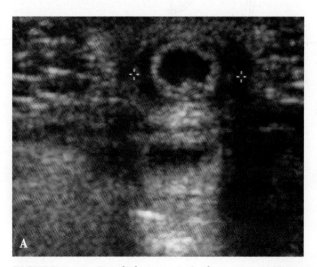 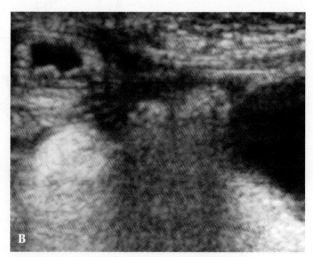

FIGURE 9–67. Omphalomesenteric duct cyst. *A,* Transverse US image just inferior to the umbilicus shows a cystic structure with surrounding inflammation. *B,* A sagittal image demonstrates no connection to the bladder apex.

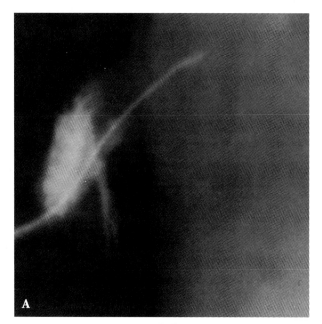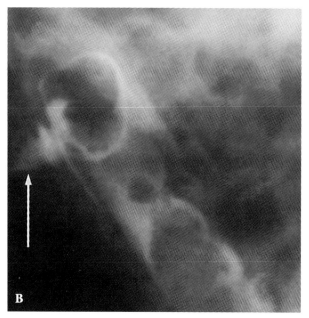

FIGURE 9–68. Patent omphalomesenteric duct. *A*, A catheter is positioned in an umbilical sinus. *B*, When contrast is injected, the bowel is opacified and the fistula is seen (*arrow*).

ception, Chapter 9). Intestinal obstruction is also caused by strangulation of an adjacent loop of small bowel by a mesodiverticular band. Focal volvulus, which occurs around the axis of a fibrous vestigial omphalomesenteric duct remnant connecting the umbilicus with the Meckel's diverticulum, results in obstruction (Gaisie et al., 1985). A less common form of obstruction is incarceration of the diverticulum in an inguinal or femoral hernia.

Obstruction may develop at any age but it often occurs at under 2 years of age and may present in the neonatal period (Rutherford and Akkers, 1966). The cause of the obstruction is generally discovered at operation. Occasionally the obstruction is only partial or intermittent, recurring over a period of years and difficult to diagnose.

Ulceration and Hemorrhage. Bleeding occurs in 12 to 25% of symptomatic Meckel's diverticula (Rossi et al., 1996). It is reported as the most common presentation in young children (Vane et al., 1987). Bleeding may be catastrophic, self limiting, or may manifest as chronic anemia. Ectopic gastric mucosa is found in 15% of Meckel's diverticula, and ectopic pancreatic tissue occurs in 5% (Dalinka and Wunder, 1973). Ectopic gastric mucosa predisposes to ulceration and hemorrhage but these complications may also occur when little or no gastric mucosa is present. Con-

versely, many Meckel's diverticula cause no symptoms despite the presence of ectopic gastric mucosa.

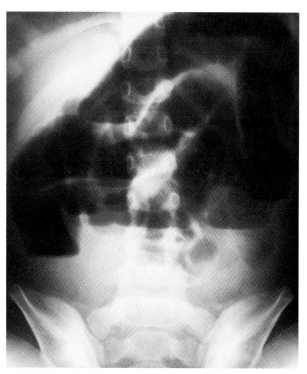

FIGURE 9–69. Fibrous atretic omphalomesenteric duct remnant causing obstruction. There are multiple air-fluid levels indicating small bowel obstruction indistinguishable from any other cause of obstruction.

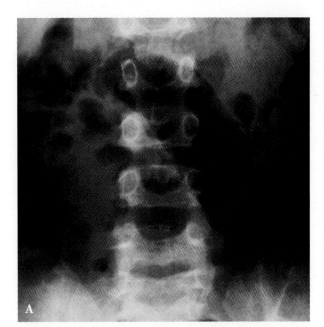 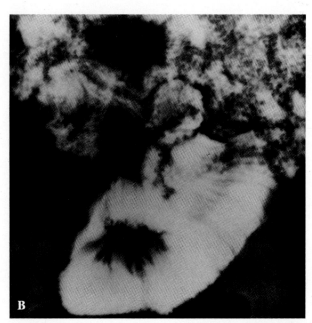

FIGURE 9–70. Fibrous atretic omphalomesenteric duct remnant causing intermittent obstruction. *A,* There is an intermittently dilated periumbilical loop of bowel on plain film. *B,* The loop was partially obstructed on barium examination, with dilatation and hyperperistalsis on fluoroscopy. The loop was found at operation to be wrapped around a fibrous atretic omphalomesenteric duct remnant.

Inflammation. Inflammation of the diverticulum can mimic appendicitis (Rutherford and Akkers, 1966). Diverticulitis can be induced by the effects of peptic acids or the diverticulum can develop an enterolith. The subsequent obstruction and inflammation is similar to appendicitis as are the sequelae of perforation, peritonitis, and inflammatory mass causing bowel obstruction (Rossi et al., 1996).

Imaging. The initial radiologic investigation of a child with a suspected Meckel's diverticulum is a technetium Tc 99m pertechnetate scan. This radionuclide is taken up by the ectopic gastric mucosa (Figure 9–71) (Rosenthal et al., 1972). Sensitivity can be improved by using a gamma camera (Sfakianakis and Haase, 1982) and premedication with cimetidine, which will decrease acid secretion but not radionuclide uptake (Diamond et al., 1991). Meckel's diverticulum may still be missed, and heterotopic gastric mucosa may occur somewhere in the gastrointestinal tract other than in the stomach or Meckel's diverticulum (most often in the duodenum) (Langkemper et al., 1980). In children, however, a complicated Meckel's diverticulum has a high probability of having ectopic gastric mucosa, giving a technetium Tc 99m pertechnetate scan an 85%

sensitivity and a 95% specificity for diagnosis (Cooney et al., 1982; Sfakianakis and Conway, 1981). In an actively bleeding patient with at least a 0.1 mL per minute rate of bleeding, a technetium Tc 99m sulfur colloid or labeled erythrocyte study can identify the site of hemorrhage.

The diagnosis may occasionally be made from plain films if the diverticulum is outlined by gas or contains an enterolith. A large diverticulum may be seen as a mass lesion (Galifer et al., 1981). If a Meckel's band, a fibrous atretic omphalomesenteric duct remnant, causes an obstructive band or provides an axis for focal volvulus, then the plain films will show air-fluid levels and dilated loops of small bowel, indicating a distal small bowel obstruction (see Figure 9–69) (Gaisie et al., 1985). In addition to the obstruction, occasionally a soft tissue mass will indicate a closed loop obstruction (Johnson and Verhagen, 1977). Extremely rarely, there may be portal vein gas from volvulus (Gaisie et al., 1985). The patient with intermittent or partial obstruction can be diagnostically difficult. The presence of a dilated central abdominal loop of bowel on plain film combined with a barium study may aid diagnosis. In the patient illustrated (see Figure 9–70), symptoms had occurred intermittently over a 5-year period with no clinical or

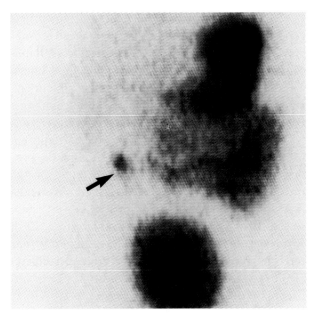

FIGURE 9–71. Meckel's diverticulum. Radionuclide accumulates in a Meckel's diverticulum (*arrow*) as well as in the stomach, jejunum, and bladder, 30 minutes after injection of technetium Tc 99m pertechnetate.

radiographic findings. The radiologic findings during an acute episode greatly aided the decision to operate, and the slightly dilated loop of small bowel was found to be caught around the omphalomesenteric duct remnant. His symptoms have not recurred postoperatively. Barium follow-through examinations are

rarely helpful although occasionally large and even small Meckel's diverticula may be seen (Figure 9–72), especially with enteroclysis techniques (Maglinte et al., 1980; Salomonowitz et al., 1983). Meckel's diverticulum on enteroclysis shows a specific appearance with a triangular fold pattern at its base and an antimesenteric location (Salomonowitz et al., 1983). An inverted diverticulum as a lead point of an intussusception can be identified during attempted air reduction as a bulbous filling defect in the air column (Kim et al., 1997) (see Intussusception, Chapter 9).

Ultrasonography can identify a complicated Meckel's diverticulum. This is most likely to occur in the setting of intussusception. The inverted diverticulum acting as the lead point appears as a blind-ended tubular structure, often bulbous, arising from the intussusceptum. The inner or serosal surface characteristically contains fluid or echogenic mesenteric fat (Daneman et al., 1997). A double target sign has been reported representing the diverticulum within the ileum within the colon (Itagaki et al., 1991) (see Intussusception, Chapter 9).

Axial imaging with CT or MR has little use in the pediatric detection of Meckel's diverticulum although an inflammatory mass in the appropriate location may suggest the diagnosis (Nigogosyan and Dolinskas, 1990). Computed tomography can demonstrate an intussusception due to an inverted diverticulum, and the presence of fat in the center

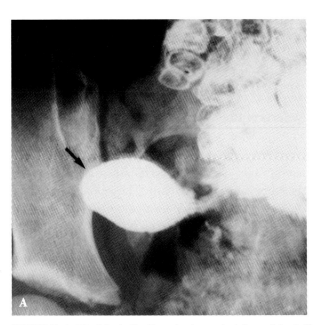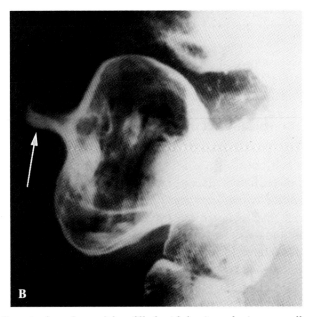

FIGURE 9–72. Meckel's diverticulum. *A*, A large Meckel's diverticulum (*arrow*) has filled with barium during a small bowel follow-through examination. *B*, Occasionally, even a small Meckel's diverticulum (*arrow*) may fill with barium.

of an ileal intraluminal mass has been described as specific for an inverted Meckel's diverticulum (Black et al., 1987).

Meckel's diverticulum may be demonstrated angiographically but this is rarely indicated (Faris and Whitely, 1973; Bree and Reuter, 1973). Findings include an anomalous feeding artery, tortuous irregular small vessels, and a dense capillary stain due to heterotopic gastric mucosa. Accumulation of contrast medium in the diverticulum may occur in the setting of acute hemorrhage. Angiographic detection requires a blood loss of at least 0.5 mL per minute in an adult and probably a greater rate in children (Meyerowitz and Fellows, 1984).

Segmental Ileal Dilatation, Ileal Dysgenesis, and Giant Meckel's Diverticulum. A rare cause of intestinal obstruction in the neonate is segmental ileal dilatation or ileal dysgenesis (Brown and Carty, 1984). The condition is a rare developmental abnormality of the ileum which may affect any portion of the gut and give a localized dilatation of a single well-defined segment of intestine with a sharp transition to normal bowel. There is no evidence of obstruction as a cause of dilatation and the ganglia cells are normal. If the affected bowel affects the ileum at the junction of the omphalomesenteric duct, there may be an associated giant Meckel's diverticulum (Orenstein et al., 1984). The segmental dilatation may be demonstrated on a barium follow-through (Morewood and Cunningham, 1985). Anemia and growth failure possibly due to bacterial growth have been described in this unusual condition (Orenstein et al., 1984). Occasionally a giant Meckel's diverticulum may be present without ileal dysgenesis and may cause volvulus (Galifer et al., 1981).

Diverticulosis of the Small Bowel

The most common form of diverticulum of the small bowel is Meckel's diverticulum. Other small bowel diverticula are rare and usually solitary; if multiple, they may constitute diverticulosis. Intestinal diverticulosis can present with malabsorption and macrocytic anemia, which results when bacterial overgrowth in the diverticula produces a form of blind-loop syndrome.

Plain erect films may show multiple gas-fluid levels if multiple diverticula are present but the diverticula usually remain occult until a barium study is performed.

Diverticula may be congenital or acquired. The congenital form can be single or multiple and is probably a variant of cystic or tubular small bowel duplication; they may communicate with the bowel lumen. These are true diverticula as they contain all four layers of bowel wall, namely, mucosa, submucosa, muscularis, and serosa (Caplan and Jacobson, 1964).

Acquired diverticula are rare in children. Mucosa can herniate through the muscularis, producing false diverticula along the course of the mesenteric vessels. Traction or pseudodiverticula may occur secondary to inflammatory bowel disease such as Crohn's disease (Caplan and Jacobson, 1964; Parulekar, 1972). Small bowel diverticulosis may rarely be found in association with cutis laxa, Ehlers-Danlos syndrome, or Noonan's syndrome (Taybi and Lachman, 1996; Cumming and Simpson, 1977).

Congenital Short Gut

The average length of a normal full-term infant gut is approximately three to seven times the crown-to-heel length of the baby irrespective of the baby's age or weight (Tiu et al., 1984). A short gut is usually a result of intestinal atresia or surgical intervention. It is rare to have a congenital short gut without atresia. The first two patients reported to have a congenital short gut without atresia were from a family of nonconsanguineous parents and other normal children (Hamilton et al., 1969). These and similar babies have presented with vomiting and intractable diarrhea (Tiu et al., 1984). Peritoneal bands may cause obstruction.

The diagnosis can be made radiologically by demonstrating an extremely short gut with very rapid transit.

Defects of the Anterior Abdominal Wall

The anterior abdominal wall is formed by the circumferential folding of the cephalic, caudal, and two lateral folds. These four folds are condensations of the embryonic mesenchyme. The cephalic fold forms the anterior wall of the thorax and epigastrium, the caudal fold forms the anterior wall of the hypogastrium, and the lateral folds fill in the anterior abdominal wall laterally. The apices of these four folds meet at the umbilicus. The rapidly elongating midgut herniates into the umbilical cord while these folds develop during the sixth to tenth intrauterine weeks. Any failure of development of the folds will result in abdominal wall defects. In addition, defects unrelated to these folds can occur, such as gastroschisis. These defects occur in between 1 in 2000 and 1 in 4000 births (Colomban and Cunningham, 1977; Lindham, 1981). Clinical studies indicate that gastroschisis is twice as common as omphalocele (Moore, 1977; Seashore, 1978; Mayer et al., 1980). Omphalocele is often associated with severe congenital heart disease, however, and when stillbirths are considered, omphalocele has a greater incidence than gastroschisis (Lindham, 1981).

Omphalocele

Omphalocele is a herniation of viscera into the base of the umbilical cord. It is contained within a translucent avascular membranous sac of peritoneum-amnion and is grossly different in appearance from the paraumbilical defect of gastroschisis. Omphaloceles arise as a result of failure of the lateral folds to develop normally prior to the tenth week. The return of the herniated bowel to the abdomen may be the stimulus necessary to promote proper development of the lateral folds, and this stimulus is deficient in those who develop an omphalocele (Mahour, 1976).

Imaging. Ultrasonography is a valuable tool in the detection of omphaloceles in utero. Physiologic herniation of bowel into the umbilicus should not persist beyond 12 weeks. It is one of the most important fetal abnormalities readily identified by US (Fink and Filly, 1983). The omphalocele sac containing herniated loops of bowel and other viscera can be seen with the umbilicus inserting directly into the sac and the sac arising from the midline (Figure 9–73). This is different from the appearance in gastroschisis, where the defect arises more laterally, the herniation is not contained by any sac, and the umbilicus is seen to insert in a normal abdominal location (Bair et al., 1986). Herniation of liver and ectopia cordis are suggestive of omphalocele and additional evidence is the presence of ascites. Ascites in a patient with gastroschisis will escape into the amniotic fluid via the abdominal defect whereas ascites in a patient with omphalocele is contained within the abdomen, enabling detection by US (Bair et al., 1986).

Pitfalls in the prenatal US diagnosis of omphalocele include rupture of the omphalocele sac, transient compression of the fetal abdomen between the placenta and uterine walls (Salzman et al., 1986), oligohydramnios (Lindfors et al., 1986; Salzman et al., 1986), and confusion of extruded bowel with umbilical cord (Lindfors et al., 1986).

The detection of an omphalocele helps to plan a rational approach to the delivery of the fetus and will alert the radiologist to look carefully for cardiac anomalies that are often present. Umbilical cord allantoic cysts may be ultrasonographically identified (Fink and Filly, 1983). Omphaloceles are otherwise discovered at birth, usually in term infants, and the diagnosis is made clinically.

Abdominal radiographs will demonstrate the herniated bowel enclosed in a sac (Figure 9–74).

Associated Anomalies. Associated anomalies are common in omphalocele. The poor survival compared to gastroschisis, only 33% in neonates (Bair et al., 1986), is due to associated anomalies and, in particular, to cardiac malformations. Cardiac malformations are more common and more serious in omphalocele than in gastroschisis; the tetralogy of Fallot accounts for one-third of associated cardiac anomalies (Moore et al., 1977).

There is incomplete small bowel rotation and fixation in almost all cases, and small bowel atresia or stenosis may occur (Mahour, 1976) although much less commonly than in gastroschisis (Moore, 1977). Meckel's diverticulum or other omphalomesenteric duct anomalies may occur. The liver may

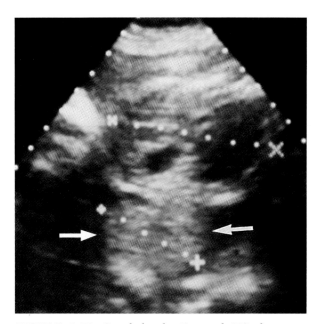

FIGURE 9–73. Omphalocele. Prenatal US shows an anterior abdominal wall sac (*between arrows*).

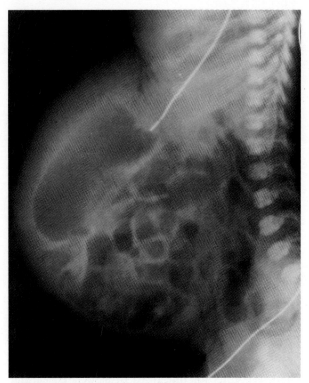

FIGURE 9–74. Omphalocele. Herniated bowel is contained within an anterior abdominal wall sac.

herniate into the sac if the defect is large. Associated chromosomal abnormalities include trisomy 13 and 18 and Beckwith-Wiedeman syndrome, facial clefts and CNS anomalies, diaphragmatic hernia, tracheoesophageal fistula, and skeletal anomalies are reported.

Management. The management of omphaloceles is determined by the size of the omphalocele and the presence of any associated abnormalities. If there are no complicated associations, small omphaloceles can be treated with primary repair. Large defects require different management as forcing the contents of the hernial sac into a small abdomen can result in respiratory distress, inferior vena cava obstruction, and even bowel ischemia (Rubin and Ein, 1976). Hence, a variety of techniques using Silon pouches, polymer membranes, or skin flaps are usually necessary (Ein et al., 1970; Ein and Shandling, 1978; Rubin and Ein, 1976). A primary repair has a better prognosis possibly because the defect is usually smaller (Ein and Rubin, 1980). The eventual prognosis is usually determined by the extent of associated abnormalities, and the prognosis is good if these abnormalities are absent or minimal.

Gastroschisis

Gastroschisis is a herniation of intraperitoneal contents through a paraumbilical defect; half of cases occur in premature infants (Moore, 1977). It is rare, with a prevalence of 1 in 10,000 live births (Tucker et al., 1992). The pathogenesis of gastroschisis is uncertain but the cause may be intrauterine interruption of the omphalomesenteric artery, with premature regression of one of the two omphalomesenteric arteries which connect the yolk sac with the dorsal aorta in the earliest embryonal phase (Hoyme et al., 1981). The resulting ischemia could account for the increased incidence of intestinal atresia. However, experimental evidence on chicken embryos has not substantiated this theory (Tibboel et al., 1986). Clinical differentiation from an omphalocele is easily made by observing the normal appearance of the umbilical cord and the lack of a covering membranous sac in gastroschisis (Touloukian and Spackman, 1971).

Imaging. In gastroschisis, fetal US can demonstrate the lack of a covering membranous sac. The loops of bowel lie in the amniotic fluid, and a normal umbilical cord can be seen entering the abdomen in the midline (Fink and Filly, 1983); this allows differentiation from omphalocele. The abdominal wall defect is usually on the right side of the umbilicus although left-sided gastroschisis has been reported (Toth and Kimura, 1993).

Abdominal radiographs will show that the herniated bowel is not enclosed by a sac (Figure 6–75).

Associated Features. The herniated loops of bowel are edematous and have a fibrogelatinous coating resulting from contact with amniotic fluid. There is gross shortening of the intestines and mesentery. Malrotation often of nonrotation type and jejunoileal atresias are common. Protracted ileus occurs in 50% of cases. This dysmotility may be due to reversible mechanical interference with normal peristalsis and possible damage to the myenteric ganglion cells caused by the thick peel that forms on the serosal surfaces in contact with amniotic fluid (Blane et al., 1985). This fibrous coating of herniated bowel is probably a late intrauterine event directly related to changes of the amniotic fluid secondary to the onset of renal function (Tibboel et al., 1986). Cardiac anomalies may be present but are less common than in omphalocele. Herniated loops of bowel may become auto-amputated if the defect is small, a serious, sometimes fatal complication (Hoffman, 1984; Moore, 1977).

Management. The combination of prematurity, contamination of the matted loops of bowel at birth, and the small size of the abdominal cavity produces serious surgical problems in gastroschisis. Advances in parenteral nutrition and the use of prosthetic materials such as Silon pouches for temporary abdominal wall closure have led to some improvement in the prognosis (Blane et al., 1985; Ein et al., 1970; Ein and Shandling, 1978; Ein and Rubin, 1980; Rubin et al., 1978). Surgical application is similar to that for omphalocele, and if possible, primary repair is preferable and has improved prognosis (Rubin et al., 1978).

In those who survive, parenteral nutrition is vital to allow the intestine to recover function; surprisingly, this often seems to occur rapidly. The length of the bowel also increases, approaching normal (Touloukian and Spackman, 1971). As prolonged survival has developed, other more long-term complications have been found (Blane et al., 1985). These complications include necrotizing enterocolitis and gastroesophageal reflux. The gastroesophageal reflux may be related to the generalized dysmotility of the gastrointestinal tract (Hillemeier et al., 1983), further compounded by distortion of the gastroesophageal junction secondary to the surgery (Blane et al., 1985). Excessive rises in intragastric pressure are not present to explain the high incidence of gastroesophageal reflux (Wesley et al., 1981).

Necrotizing enterocolitis is difficult to diagnose in babies with gastroschisis and may not be suspected clinically until perforation occurs (Blane et al., 1985). Because of this risk and the slightly later onset of necrotizing enterocolitis in these infants, a high degree of suspicion should be maintained (Blane et al., 1985).

Combined Defects of the Anterior Abdominal and Thoracic Wall

Thoracoabdominal ectopia cordis is a rare syndrome and is an extreme form of omphalocele in which not only the lateral folds but also the cephalic fold fails to develop properly. Thoracoabdominal ectopia cordis in its full extent consists of five associated anomalies: a congenitally abnormal heart and defects in the supraumbilical midline, lower ster-

num, pericardium, and anterior part of the diaphragm (Toyama, 1972). The syndrome may have all five features or be incomplete. The diagnosis is obvious at birth. Plain films may help to show the preoperative position of gas-filled bowel and the condition of the lungs.

INFECTION AND INFLAMMATION OF THE SMALL BOWEL

Meconium Peritonitis

Meconium contains lipases, proteases, bile salts, and bile acids that are very irritating to the peritoneum, resulting in an aseptic chemical peritonitis if leakage of meconium into the peritoneum occurs. Meconium peritonitis has been seen in a fetus as early as 6 months of gestation (Finkel and Slovis, 1982) and is found in approximately 1 in 35,000 live births (Payne and Neilson, 1962).

Intraperitoneal meconium leak may result in three types of peritonitis, namely, fibroadhesive, cystic, or generalized. The fibroadhesive type results from an intense fibroblastic reaction which may seal the leak but cause obstructive bands. The cystic type

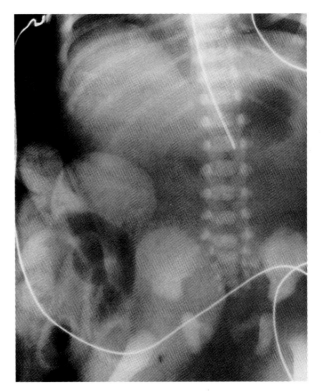

FIGURE 9–75. Gastroschisis. Herniated bowel arises from the right side of the abdomen and is not enclosed by a sac.

results from a continuing leak which is eventually sealed off by adhesions and bowel loops, forming a thickly walled cyst. The generalized form spreads throughout the peritoneal cavity and in males may reach the scrotum. Meconium peritonitis usually results in intraperitoneal calcification, which can develop within 24 hours of a meconium leak.

Intraperitoneal meconium leak can result from obstruction or malformation. A definite obstructive lesion is found in only 50% of patients, most commonly volvulus or small bowel atresia (Day and Allen, 1985). Other lesions such as intussusception, stenosis, duplication, congenital bands, Meckel's diverticulum, anorectal malformation, meconium ileus, meconium plugs, Hirschsprung's disease, or hyperplastic lymphoid tissue may be present (Day and Allen, 1985).

Cystic fibrosis is found in a significant minority of patients with meconium peritonitis and hence should be actively excluded by a sweat chloride test. The viscous meconium found in cystic fibrosis tends to become localized when it leaks with cyst formation but the finding of a cyst is not always associated with cystic fibrosis.

Clinical presentation will depend on the underlying cause and the presence of any obstruction. Rarely, the calcification is discovered serendipitously, and presumably the infant had an intrauterine perforation which has healed.

Treatment and prognosis depend on the cause of the meconium leakage. Meconium peritonitis, being sterile, has few sequelae. Rarely, adhesions can form and cause obstructive symptoms in later childhood (Moore, 1973).

Imaging

Ultrasonography. Meconium peritonitis can be diagnosed prenatally and postnatally by US (Blumenthal et al., 1982; Bowen et al., 1984; Brugman et al., 1979; Carroll and Muskowitz, 1981; Dillard et al., 1987; Fleischer et al., 1983; Garb and Reisborough, 1980; Lawrence and Chrispin, 1984; McGahan and Hansen, 1983; Nancarrow et al., 1985). Findings include a cystic mass with a hyperechogenic rim or scattered areas of hyperechogenicity with or without shadowing indicating areas of calcification (Figure 9–76). A widespread highly echogenic pattern giving a "snowstorm" effect within a few hours of birth is described and is probably due to meconium and other particulate matter in the sterile peritoneal fluid (Lawrence and Chrispin, 1984). Hydramnios is present in 50% of patients (Dillard et al., 1987) and ascites in 70%. Abdominal wall thickening has been reported, which in the absence of ascites or acoustic shadowing may lead to the erroneous diagnosis of fetal hydrops (Dillard et al., 1987).

Plain-Film Radiology. Evidence of ascites or bowel obstruction may be present but the major finding in meconium peritonitis is usually calcification (Figures 9–76, 9–77). Calcification may extend into the scrotum (Figure 9–78) or rarely, into the chest. Though most calcification seen radiologically lies within the peritoneum, it can occasionally be intramural (Van Buskirk et al, 1965) or very rarely intraluminal (Neuhauser, 1944). If a pseudocyst is present, the calcification can outline part of the pseudocyst (Figures 9–76, 9–79). The fibroadhesive type gives scattered intraperitoneal calcific plaques and the generalized type gives fainter or even absent calcification. However, if no calcification is present, there are usually ascites and bowel obstruction. Calcification is gradually reabsorbed and will disappear over a period of months or years (Tucker and Isant, 1971; Shija, 1987).

Osseous growth arrest lines have been found in association with meconium peritonitis (Wolfson and Engel, 1969).

Gastroenteritis

Gastroenteritis is a major cause of illness in infants and children; it is caused by bacterial, viral, or parasitic agents. Many millions of children die worldwide each year from gastroenteritis, with the vast majority of these deaths occurring in underdeveloped countries (Nelson, 1983).

Bacterial Gastroenteritis

Gastroenteritis in children in North America has a bacterial etiology in 10% of patients. The most common bacteria are *Salmonella*, *Shigella*, *Escherichia coli*, and *Yersinia enterocolitica*. In Asia, *Vibrio cholera* is a major cause of bacterial enteritis. *Campylobacter fetus* is increasingly implicated as a cause of enteritis. Both *Yersinia* and *Campylobacter* may be overlooked on stool cultures unless great care is taken (Hodes, 1980; Kohl et al., 1976). *Campylobacter* occurs at all ages but is found particularly in older children and young adults.

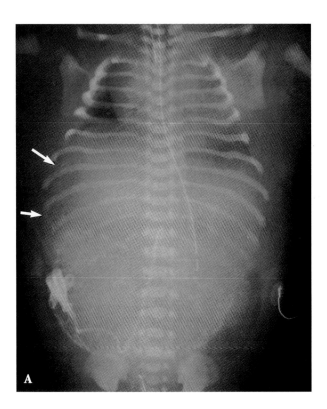

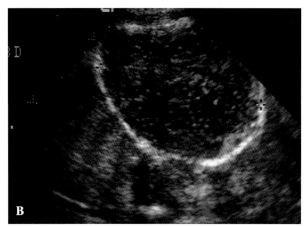

FIGURE 9–76. Meconium peritonitis and pseudocyst. *A*, Plain-film radiograph shows extensive pseudocyst wall calcification across the central abdomen as well as peritoneal spread with calcification adjacent to the lateral edge of the liver (*arrows*). *B*, Sagittal midline US shows the pseudocyst with wall calcification and echogenic content typical of meconium.

Escherichia coli is as important as *Shigella* and *Salmonella* in producing chronic malnutrition in children of underdeveloped countries due to repeated episodes of gastroenteritis. Certain strains of *Escherichia coli* are a major cause of traveler's diarrhea. Bacteria of these strains have surface pili by which they adhere to the intestinal mucosa for sufficient time to produce an exotoxin (enterotoxin) that causes diarrhea (Hodes, 1980).

Viral Gastroenteritis

In North America, the human *Rotavirus* is responsible for approximately 40% of acute diarrhea in summer and up to 80% in winter. Most infections occur between 2 to 6 years of age but infants can also be affected. The illness usually lasts 3 to 8 days and in advanced countries is usually not life threatening. However, in infants, when good care is not available, there is the risk of death from dehydration or aspiration of vomitus. Other viruses that have been implicated include astroviruses, adenoviruses, and calciviruses (Hodes, 1980).

Imaging

Plain abdominal films frequently show dilated loops of gas-filled small bowel which often contain gas-fluid levels and may mimic obstruction or ileus (Fig-

ure 9–80). These signs are nonspecific and radiology is not usually important in the diagnosis or management of gastroenteritis. In typhoid fever, irregular narrow loops of gas-filled distal small bowel may be seen (Bohrer, 1966). The ileum is said to perforate in 2 to 4% of cases, and free intraperitoneal gas may be seen. This perforation is a major cause of death.

Yersinia enterocolitica may produce irregularity or nodularity of the terminal ileum and colitis with irregular spiculation of the cecum (Shrago, 1976) (Figure 9–81). Occasionally *Yersinia enterocolitica* may present with large mesenteric lymph nodes and may initially be thought to be tuberculosis or lymphoma (Figure 9–82).

Tuberculous Enteritis/Peritonitis

One-third of the earth's population is infected with *Mycobacterium tuberculosis* (Bloom and Murray, 1992), and there has been an alarming increase in tuberculosis incidence in both the United Kingdom and the United States, especially in childhood infection (Watson, 1993; Starke et al., 1992).

Abdominal tuberculosis can involve solid organs, the gastrointestinal tract, and the peritoneum. Infection occurs via hematogenous seeding in disseminated tuberculosis or via oral ingestion of sputum from a pulmonary focus (Abrams and Holden, 1964).

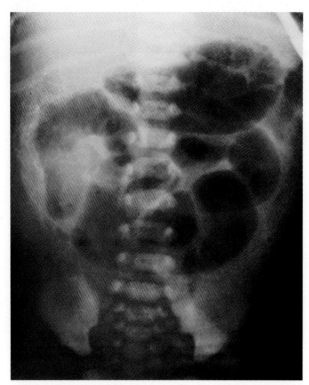

FIGURE 9–77. Meconium peritonitis. Faint intraperitoneal calcification indicates meconium peritonitis.

A chest radiograph should always be obtained if gastrointestinal tuberculosis is suspected and will show evidence of tuberculosis in the majority of cases (Nagi et al., 1987). Contact screening is important as a child with a normal chest radiograph will invariable have a diseased caregiver, and transfer of bacilli from infected sputum to the child via a moistened bottle, teat, or

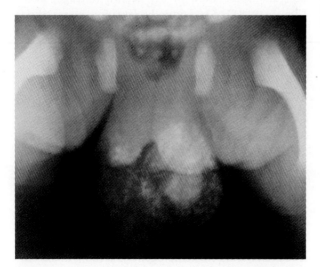

FIGURE 9–78. Meconium peritonitis. Calcification extends into the processus vaginalis within the scrotum.

soother is a ready mechanism for primary inoculation of the pharynx or gastrointestinal tract.

Children presenting with gastrointestinal tuberculosis are invariably malnourished with fever, loss of weight, abdominal pain, vomiting, and diarrhea (Millar et al., 1990). They may present as a protein-losing enteropathy. Common physical signs are abdominal distention (often described as feeling doughy on palpation), abdominal mass, and complications that include obstruction, abscess, fistula, and perforation. The most common diagnostic problem is excluding early ileocecal lymphoma. Differential diagnosis includes inflammatory bowel disease, protein-losing enteropathy, malabsorption syndromes, and infection with giardiasis, amebiasis, or yersinia.

Diagnosis requires a high clinical awareness as symptoms are usually of insidious onset and nonspecific. Marasmus, kwashiorkor, measles, whooping cough, and HIV infection/AIDS all predispose to tuberculous infection by reducing immune response in the host, and these diseases may overshadow the developing tuberculosis (Kibel, 1995). Other manifestations of acute disseminated tuberculosis such as progressive primary pulmonary disease or meningeal disease may mask gastrointestinal involvement. Bacterial confirmation of disease from gastric aspirate, sputum, and bronchial lavage have widely reported yields but are seldom higher in incidence than 25% (Kibel, 1995). Positive tuberculin skin testing, especially with the Mantoux test (intradermal injection of 5 tuberculin units of purified protein derivative), indicates infection but not necessarily the presence of active disease. Induration at the injection site is measured at 48 to 72 hours, and 5 to 9 mm of induration indicates infection with *Mycobacterium tuberculosis*, a previous BCG immunization, or atypical mycobacterium infection. If BCG has not been given, 10 to 15 mm of induration indicates tuberculous infection; 15 mm or greater indicates infection even if BCG has been given. However, a negative test does not exclude infection. False-negative results from subcutaneous (not intradermal) injection are common with inexperienced operators, and anergy resulting in poor immune response can occur from overwhelming tuberculous infection and the many conditions which predispose to infection, such as malnutrition, measles, rubella, pertussis, infectious mononucleosis, influenza, malaria, and HIV/AIDS (Kibel, 1995). The role of radiology in supporting the clinical diagnosis of tuberculosis is thus extremely important.

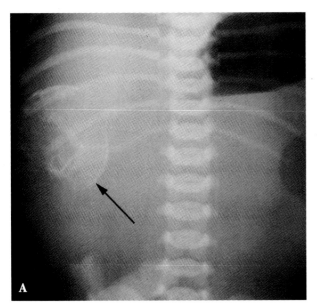

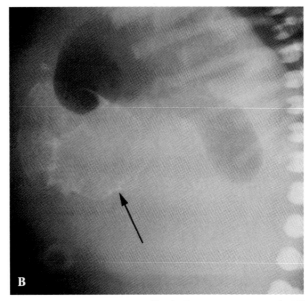

FIGURE 9–79. Calcified pseudocyst in meconium ileus. *A*, A localized cystic collection of leaked meconium is outlined by a rim of calcification (*arrow*) on supine plain film. *B*, The above as it appears on lateral plain film.

Imaging

Three components need to be evaluated: enteric involvement, adenopathy, and peritoneal disease. There is much variability and overlap in the involvement of these components. Any site in the gastrointestinal tract can be affected but there is a strong predilection for ileocecal disease. Adenopathy is a hallmark of the disease in children and may be present without identified enteric disease. It is typically related to the mesenteric root extending to the para-aortic region and the porta hepatis as one expects from GI lymphatic drainage. Peritonitis can be

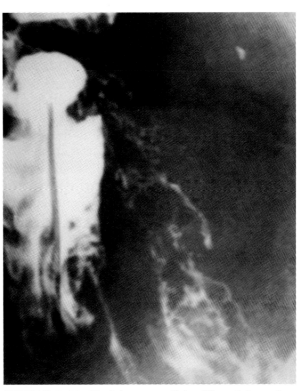

FIGURE 9–81. *Yersinia enterocolitica.* There is irregularity and nodularity of the terminal ileum. (Reprinted, with permission, from Stringer DA. Radiol Clin North Am 1987;25:107.)

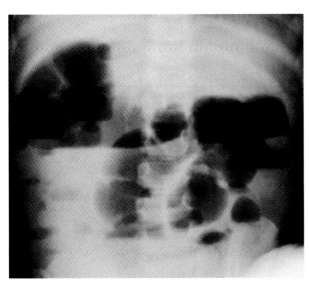

FIGURE 9–80. Gastroenteritis. Multiple gas-fluid levels mimic intestinal obstruction.

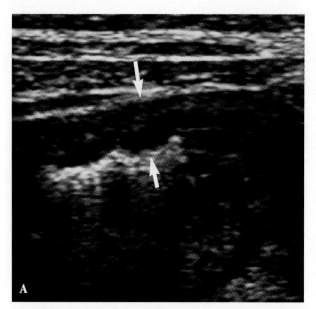 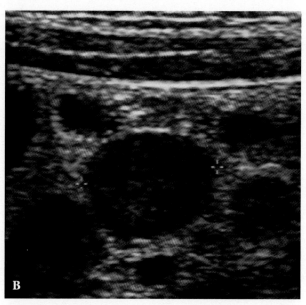

FIGURE 9–82. Yersinia enterocolitis. *A,* Image on US from the right iliac fossa shows thick-walled bowel (*arrows*), probably representing terminal ileum. *B,* Enlarged regional mesenteric lymph nodes demonstrated on US.

"wet" with free fluid or "dry" with fibrosis and adhesion, also called "plastic peritonitis."

Plain-Film Radiography. Abdominal plain films are usually nonspecific, suggesting ascites and showing fluid levels of obstruction and occasionally free air from perforation. Foci or diffuse flocculent calcification of the mesenteric adenopathy is typical when present (Figure 9–83).

Barium Studies. Small bowel follow-through studies are simple and available and show anatomic sites of involvement which may be multiple. Findings include mucosal ulceration, strictures, matted bowel loops that palpation cannot separate, and a fibrotic-appearing terminal ileum emptying through a widely open ileocecal valve into a rigid contracted cecum (Thoeni and Margulis, 1979; Werbeloff et al., 1973). The appearance may be indistinguishable from that of idiopathic inflammatory bowel disease (Figure 9–84).

Ultrasonography. Ultrasonography is useful in suspected disease as enteritis, adenopathy, and peritoneal disease can be imaged (Figure 9–85). Bowel wall thickening, often ileocecal, can be seen. Adenopathy is usually well demonstrated with typically large, matted, and hypoechoic nodes but with variable central echogenic foci reflecting caseous necrosis or calcification. Ascites is well seen; it may be clear but is usual-ly turbid with debris and stranding, and high-resolution linear probes can demonstrate a thickened irregular peritoneal lining (Denton and Hossain, 1993; Kedar et al., 1994; Lee et al., 1991; Ozkan et al., 1987).

Computed Tomography. Cross-sectional imaging demonstrates enteric disease, adenopathy, and peritoneal disease in addition to assessing the abdominal solid organs. Calcification and its location is more sensitively identified (see Figure 9–83). Oral and intravenous contrast enhancement is recommended. Bowel wall thickening may have associated inflammatory mesenteric streaking. Adenopathy can occur anywhere but typically follows the bowel lymphatic drainage to the mesenteric root and up to the para-aortic/peripancreatic region and the porta hepatis (Figure 9–86). The nodes are typically prominent, may cluster and demonstrate rim enhancement with low density, nonenhancing centers correlating to central caseous necrosis (Figure 9–87) (Pombo et al., 1992). Ascites of varying density is common and often loculated. Peritoneal thickening which may be nodular can enhance (Ablin et al., 1994; Balthazar et al., 1990; Dahlene et al., 1984; Denath, 1990; Epstein and Mann, 1982; Hanson and Hunter, 1985).

Helminth Infestations

Many parasitic infestations affect the intestine (Table 9–3). Helminth infestations affect hundreds of mil-

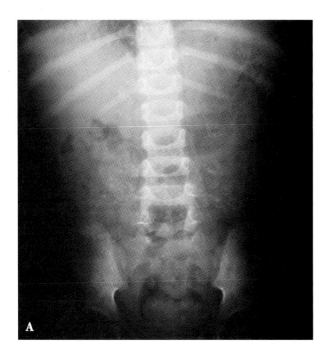

FIGURE 9–83. Abdominal tuberculosis. *A*, Typical diffuse, flocculent calcification of mesenteric adenopathy is present on plain-film radiograph. *B,C*, Computed tomography demonstrates the extensive calcified adenopathy affecting the right iliac fossa, mesenteric, and peripancreatic nodes, including the porta hepatis nodes.

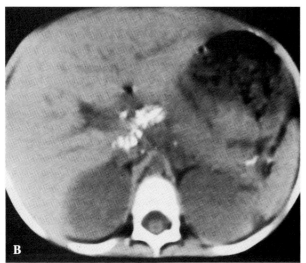

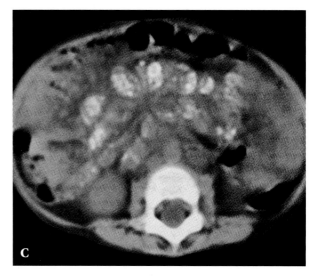

lions of people in the world. Only certain of these infestations are of importance to the radiologist.

Ascariasis

Ascariasis (roundworm infection) is the most common parasitic infection in the world; it occurs most frequently in the tropics but is common throughout North America. *Ascaris lumbricoides* is a type of nematode (roundworm) that lives in the small intestine of humans. The eggs are passed in the stool and incubate in soil for 2 to 3 weeks. Infection takes place by swallowing of the incubated eggs, which hatch and then penetrate the small intestine to pass via the liver to the lung capillaries. As the larvae enlarge, they rupture from the capillaries into the alveoli, migrate along the tracheobronchial tree to the glottis, and are swallowed. They become mature worms in the small intestine. In the 2 weeks of migration, most patients are asymptomatic but if infestation is heavy, fever, general malaise, and eosinophilia may occur. Adult worms in small numbers are asymptomatic but malnutrition or intestinal obstruction may develop if worms are present in large numbers. Worms can lodge in the appendix or migrate cephalad and be found in the esophagus; rarely, they can perforate the intestine and cause peritonitis (Katz, 1975).

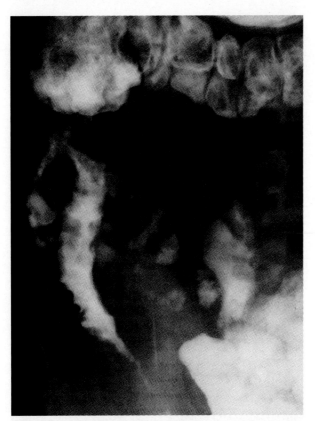

FIGURE 9–84. Tuberculous enteritis. A small bowel follow-through examination shows a rigid contracted cecum indicating terminal ileal and cecal disease. In the absence of calcific foci, this appearance may be indistinguishable from other causes of inflammatory bowel disease.

Radiologic signs of infestation may be seen during the migration phase as areas of pulmonary consolidation, often associated with eosinophilia (Bean, 1965). More direct plain-film evidence may show single worms clearly outlined by bowel gas or masses of worms outlined to give the appearance of a Medusa head. Barium examinations may clearly outline single or multiple worms (Figure 9–88) and may fill their threadlike intestine.

Strongyloidiasis

Strongyloides (roundworm infection) is a disease of tropical and subtropical areas including the southern United States but which also occurs further north (Smith et al., 1977).

Strongyloides stercoralis is a parasite whose noninfectious larvae are found in the human stool. These larvae mature in soil within 2 to 3 days and develop the ability to penetrate intact human skin. Once in the bloodstream, they pass to the lung cap-

illaries, rupture into the alveoli, and migrate along the tracheobronchial tree until they can be swallowed. They grow into mature worms and live within, but not attached to, the small bowel, in contradistinction to the closely related hookworms. However, the larvae and (less likely) the worms can invade the mucosa; the duodenum and proximal jejunum are usually the areas most affected.

The patient is asymptomatic when infestation is light but protracted mucoid diarrhea and, occasionally, malabsorption occur with heavy infection (Katz, 1975). Symptoms include abdominal pain, nausea, and vomiting (Berkmen and Rabinowitz, 1972). Perforation due to granulomatous necrotizing enterocolitis is a rare presentation (Smith et al., 1977).

In the migratory phase, transient pulmonary infiltrates occur; pleural effusions are unusual. Findings on barium examination will depend on the severity of the infection. The earliest signs are those of duodenal dilatation and mucosal edema as shown by thickening of mucosal folds. Intramural defects secondary to intramural granuloma are seen as infection increases. The lumen becomes increasingly narrowed as the bowel wall becomes rigid due to diffuse fibrosis. Gastric emptying may be delayed due to gastric involvement. Reflux of barium into the pancreatic or biliary tree may occur due to fibrosis around Oddi's sphincter. The colon is rarely affected but the picture may simulate colitis.

Trichuriasis

Trichuriasis (whipworm infection) is found particularly in the tropics but also in other areas such as the southern United States. It was estimated that over 350 million people worldwide were affected by the disease in 1947 (Reeder et al., 1968). The ova are deposited in soil from human feces and become infectious in 1 month. They have to be swallowed, hatch in the small intestine, and penetrate the villi. When mature, they re-enter the bowel lumen having produced no symptoms since little migration through host tissue takes place. The worms then pass to the large bowel and bury their heads in the colonic mucosa, where the cecum is preferentially colonized. With heavier infestation, more of the large bowel is colonized. This leads to diarrhea and tenesmus, often associated with rectal prolapse (Katz, 1975). The diarrhea tends to be watery with copious amounts of mucous.

Various radiologic signs may be present. The colonic mucosa may be granular, and the lucent outline of the worms can be seen on double-contrast examinations. Defects in the colonic wall may be seen, perhaps due to abundant mucous secretion. A pear-shaped cecum may be seen. Radiolucent rings may develop about a central pool of barium, giving an aphthoid appearance due to barium trapped within the coiled portion of the worm as it lies in the bowel (Reeder et al., 1968; Manzano et al., 1979).

Other Worm Infestations

There are a variety of other tapeworm, roundworm, hookworm, and tongue worm infestations and radiologic aspects of these are discussed below.

Anisakiasis causes severe abdominal pain. There will be a history of eating raw fish. The plain abdominal films can show air-fluid levels compatible with ileus (Matsui et al., 1985). Barium studies may show irregular thickening of the jejunum, ileum, or colon with mucosal edema and luminal narrowing with dilatation of the proximal intestine.

Occasionally both cestodes (tapeworms) or *Anisakis* worms (roundworms) may appear as filling defects on barium investigations. Ankylostomiasis (hookworm disease) may occasionally produce thickening of mucosal folds in the proximal small bowel but this sign is usually difficult to assess. Hookworms generally produce no radiologic evidence of disease, but *Oesophagostomum* (hookworms) found in monkeys and apes occasionally

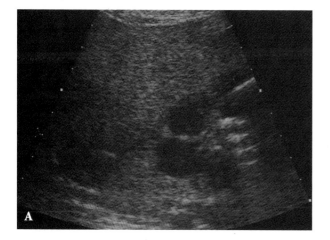

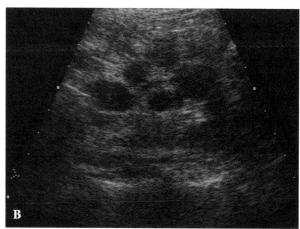

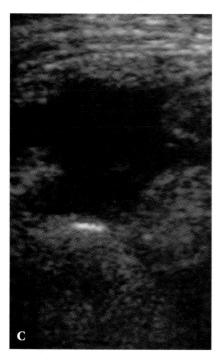

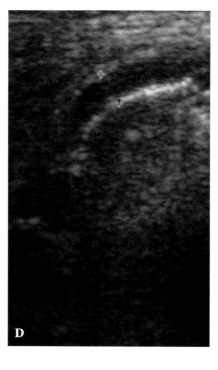

FIGURE 9–85. Abdominal tuberculosis. *A, B,* Ultrasonography demonstrates enlarged hypoechoic lymph nodes in the porta hepatis with a cluster of nodes surrounding a mesenteric vessel in the lower abdomen (*B*). *C,* Thickened irregular peritoneal lining and turbid ascites, indicating tuberculous peritonitis with bowel wall thickening in the right iliac fossa (*D*).

affect humans and may produce large bowel abscesses and nodules, which can ulcerate. When *Porocephalus armillatus* (tongue worms) die, they calcify and may be seen as C-shaped areas of calcification around the peritoneum (Figure 9–89).

Protozoal Intestinal Infections

Amebiasis
Entamoeba histolytica (pseudopodate infection) affects mainly the large bowel (see Chapter 10).

Giardiasis
Giardiasis (flagellate infection) is the other protozoal infection of the gastrointestinal tract. This disease is due to the intestinal flagellate *Giardia lamblia*, which is found especially in the tropics but is increasingly found in North America and other temperate regions. However, outbreaks of giardiasis have been reported in many parts of the world; in some communities, 10% of the population may be affected. Children and patients with dysgammaglobulinemia are commonly affected.

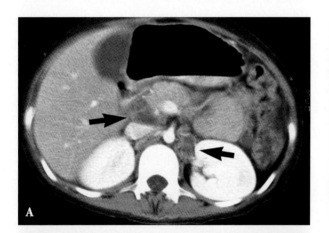

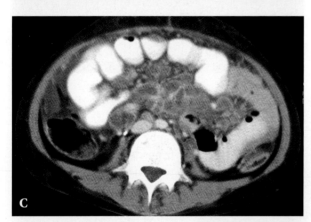

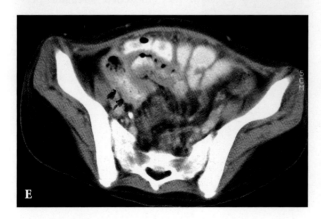

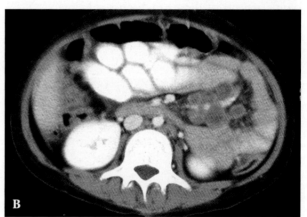

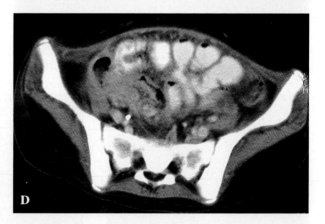

FIGURE 9–86. Abdominal tuberculosis. *A,* Nodes around the pancreas head and left renal hilum (*arrows*) on CT show the typical large, rim enhancing, clustered, low-density-center appearance of tuberculous lymph nodes. *B, C,* These nodes cluster around a mesenteric vessel (compare with Figure 9–85B) and are extensive around the mesentery (*C*). *D, E,* There is bowel wall thickening and inflammatory change in the surrounding mesentery.

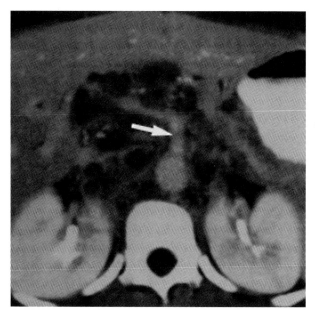

FIGURE 9–87. Tuberculosis. Computed tomography demonstrates tuberculous lymph nodes adjacent to and encasing the celiac artery (*arrow*). Central necrosis is seen in some nodes.

The infection is acquired by swallowing contaminated food or water containing cysts which develop into trophozoites in the proximal small bowel. The trophozoites attach themselves by suction discs to the intestinal mucosa, usually between the villi. Occasional invasion of the mucosa may occur. Cysts are passed in the stool to complete the cycle.

Many people remain asymptomatic despite the presence of *Giardia*; others develop severe protracted diarrhea often associated with fever. Malabsorption frequently occurs and can result in weight loss. Villous atrophy may be seen on small bowel biopsy. The diagnosis is made by finding the protozoa on small bowel biopsies, in the stool, or in duodenal aspirate (Katz, 1975).

Many patients with giardiasis show no radiologic abnormalities. Others have evidence of proximal small bowel inflammation with mucosal fold thickening and irritability. Since barium passes quickly through the irritable proximal small bowel, it may be difficult to see the changes that occur. Increased secretions may give the mucosal edge an ill-defined appearance (Figure 9–90), and a small bowel malabsorption pattern occasionally prevails (Figure 9–91).

The finding of a progression from relatively normal jejunum to abnormal later in the examination should suggest giardiasis (Brandon et al., 1985).

TABLE 9–3. Parasitic Intestinal Infections

Helminths
    Ascariasis (roundworm)
    Strongyloidiasis (roundworm)
    Trichuriasis (whipworm)
    Cestodiasis (tapeworm)
    Ankylostomiasis (hookworm)
    Enterobiasis (pinworm)
    Esophagostomiasis (hookworm)
    Toxocariasis (roundworm)
Protozoa
    Giardiasis (flagellate)
    Amebiasis (pseudopodate)
    Balantidiasis (ciliate)

The abnormalities include dilution, segmentation, and apparent fold thickening (Brandon et al., 1985).

Candidal Infection

Candida affecting the small bowel is rare but may occur in immunodeficiency states such as malignancy or AIDS. The clinical findings are of watery, sometimes explosive, diarrhea with occasional cramps and tenderness. Symptoms may last for 3 months.

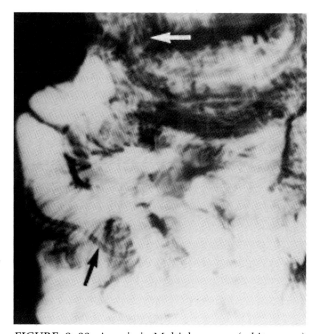

FIGURE 9–88. Ascariasis. Multiple worms (*white arrow*) are seen in the proximal bowel. A solitary worm, whose alimentary tract is outlined by barium, is seen more distally (*black arrow*).

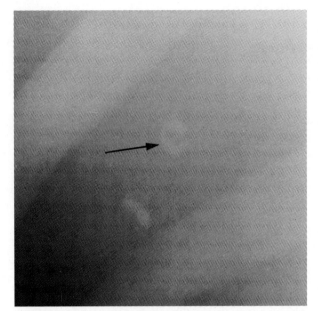

FIGURE 9–89. *Porocephalus armillatus* (tongue worms). C-shaped areas of calcification around the peritoneum (*arrow*) indicate dead *Porocephalus armillatus*.

Barium studies may show nonspecific thickened folds and dilatation of jejunum or ileum (Joshi et al., 1981; Radin, 1983). Aphthae have also been found in the terminal ileum and proximal large bowel (Gedgaudas-McClees, 1983).

Duodenal Ulcer

Duodenal ulcers are rare in children but more frequent than gastric ulcers (Drumm, Sherman et al., 1987; Seagram et al., 1973; Singleton and Faykus, 1964). They reportedly occur in approximately 1 per 2500 hospital admissions and are 2.8 times more common than gastric ulcers (Deckelbaum et al., 1974; Drumm, Sherman et al., 1987; Williams and Ahmed, 1977). It should be remembered that most series of peptic ulcer disease in children have predated the routine use of endoscopy in younger patients, and reliance upon single-contrast barium meals for diagnosis may have produced spurious results (Deckelbaum et al., 1974; Kumar and Spitz, 1984; Seagram et al., 1973; Sultz et al., 1970).

The low incidence of peptic ulcer disease in the newborn is confirmed by various reports (Adeyemi et al., 1979; Dunn et al., 1983) in which the diagnosis was established only after a serious complication such as hemorrhage or perforation. The severity of complications in this age group may account for the high mortality rate. It is reasonable to assume, however,

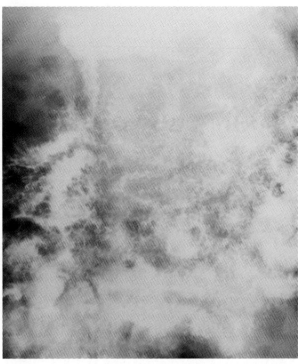

FIGURE 9–90. Giardiasis. Mucosal fold thickening is present, with rapid transit of barium through the irritable jejunum. The barium is diluted by increased secretions.

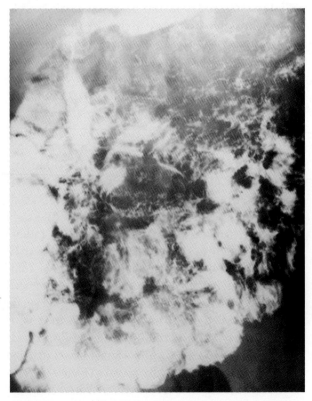

FIGURE 9–91. Giardiasis. The barium column is fragmented and the mucosal folds are thickened.

that stress ulcers uncomplicated by perforation may be more common in the neonatal period than our experience suggests (Drumm, Sherman et al., 1987).

Primary peptic ulcer disease is relatively rare in childhood; this appears to be particularly true for children under the age of 10 years. In our experience, excluding the neonatal age group, primary peptic ulcer disease has not been diagnosed in children under 10 years of age. It should be noted, however, that Deckelbaum and colleagues (1974) reported six primary gastric ulcers but no primary duodenal ulcers among 18 patients under 6 years of age.

Abdominal pain and gastrointestinal bleeding are considered to be the major presenting symptoms of primary or secondary ulcer disease in children outside the neonatal period (Kumar and Spitz, 1984; Nord et al., 1981). In children under 10 years of age, bleeding may occur without obvious manifestation of abdominal pain. In children over 10 years of age, abdominal pain is the major presenting symptom, and half of them have abdominal pain alone (Drumm, Sherman et al., 1987).

There are major age-related differences in the clinical course which appear to correlate with the apparent etiology of the ulcer disease. Among younger children, most of whom have secondary ulcers, there is a high mortality rate (15%), and many require emergency surgery for perforation or intractable bleeding (60%) (Adeyemi et al., 1979; Drumm et al., 1987). It should be emphasized that these patients are often gravely ill at diagnosis due to the severity of their underlying illness. The high mortality rate among young children with secondary peptic ulcer disease was also acknowledged by Deckelbaum and colleagues (1974), who reported a mortality rate of 33%, 12% as a direct complication of ulcer disease. This observation contrasts with children over 10 years of age, who have a negligible mortality rate and a low incidence (4%) of acute surgical emergencies (Drumm, Sherman et al., 1987). Symptoms from childhood may persist into adult life (Puri et al., 1984; White et al., 1984). Children with secondary gastric or duodenal peptic ulcer disease do not commonly suffer from recurrent disease (Deckelbaum et al., 1974; Drumm, Sherman et al., 1987). In contrast, a large proportion of patients with primary duodenal ulcers appear to suffer from recurrences even after adequate medical therapy (Puri et al., 1978). As a result, some of these children may require surgical treatment. There is often a strong family history of peptic ulcer disease in children with primary duodenal ulceration (Deckelbaum et al., 1974; Drumm, Sherman et al., 1987; Michener et al., 1960; Seagram et al., 1973).

The role of *Helicobacter pylori* (previously called *Campylobacter pylori*) in the pathophysiology of peptic ulcer disease was first recognized in 1983 (Warren and Marshall, 1983). *Helicobacter pylori* is commonly present in asymptomatic adults but is detectable in 60 to 80% of gastric ulcers and 90 to 100% of duodenal ulcers in adults (Levine and Rubesin, 1995). The presence of this organism in association with primary unexplained antral gastritis and peptic ulcer disease has been confirmed in children (Drumm et al., 1988). A triple regimen of bismuth, metronidazole, and amoxicillin or tetracycline has been shown to successfully eradicate *Helicobacter pylori* (Chiba et al., 1992). The National Institutes of Health (NIH) now recommends antacids, histamine receptor blockers (H₂ blockers), and triple therapy to treat and reduce recurrent rates of disease (NIH Conference, 1994).

Imaging

Ultrasonography. Ultrasonography may occasionally detect duodenal ulcers, especially if large (Derchi et al., 1986; Purelekar and Lubert, 1983; Stringer et al., 1986). This can be aided by giving clear fluid to the patient to fill the stomach and duodenum (Stringer et al., 1986). However, US is unreliable for diagnosis, and further investigation such as barium study or endoscopy is needed in most cases.

Plain Films. Plain films are rarely helpful as perforation with free air is uncommon.

Contrast Studies/Endoscopy. The comparative accuracy of upper GI examination and endoscopy in detecting peptic ulcer disease has been extensively evaluated among adults (Belber, 1971; Dooley et al., 1984; Gelfand et al., 1985b; Herlinger et al., 1977; Laufer, 1976; Ott et al., 1985) but has rarely been addressed for the pediatric age group (Ament and Christie, 1977; Drumm et al., 1988; Nord et al., 1981). In a pediatric series, single-contrast upper GI examinations failed to detect 33% of duodenal ulcers and was even less reliable in diagnosing gastric ulcer disease (Drumm et al., 1988). Ament and Christie (1977) came to similar conclusions regarding the efficacy of single-contrast studies, and in their series, barium studies were normal in 75% of cases with endoscopically proven gastric ulcers and in 50% of those with duodenal ulcers. There is little or no role for single-contrast barium studies in the evaluation of children with suspected peptic ulcer disease. Endoscopy may also fail to detect peptic ulcer disease in 8% of patients in whom radiology and endoscopy are performed concomitantly (Drumm et al., 1988). As a result, a small number of patients with strong clinical evidence of peptic ulcer disease may require repeat endoscopy if the initial study is normal (Drumm et al., 1988). *Helicobacter pylori* is reliably diagnosed by histologic evaluation of endoscopic brushings or biopsy. More recently, a noninvasive breath test for *Helicobacter pylori*, measuring urease activity via orally administered carbon-14-labeled urea, and a serologic test for immunoglobulin G antibodies to *Helicobacter pylori* have been shown to be highly accurate (Levine and Rubesin, 1995).

A barium double-contrast upper GI examination is more sensitive than a single-contrast study in adults (Laufer, 1976). A number of ulcers, including gastric lesions, are now detected at pediatric institutions with this technique. Double-contrast barium studies require more radiation, are more time consuming, and are difficult to perform. A degree of cooperation is required from the patient, and usually children over 8 years of age are sufficiently cooperative, but for those under 5 years of age it may be necessary to use a nasogastric tube to obtain satisfactory gaseous distension. Between 5 and 8 years of age, patient cooperation is less certain, and the procedure may not be performed satisfactorily. Even if an adequate study can be performed it is likely that the sensitivity may not be greater than that reported for adults. Disagreement exists regarding the accuracy of the barium double-contrast examination in adults. Some reports claim it is effective and capable of diagnosing up to 96% of ulcers (Herlinger et al., 1977; Laufer, 1976) but in a large prospective study, Dooley and colleagues (1984) found that double-contrast barium studies failed to demonstrate 55% and 30% of gastric and duodenal ulcers, respectively while endoscopy detected 96% of these cases. No truly comparative study between double-contrast barium meals and endoscopy has been performed in children. Where there is an appropriate pediatric endoscopy service available, radiology will very rarely be required to contribute imaging evaluation except for complications.

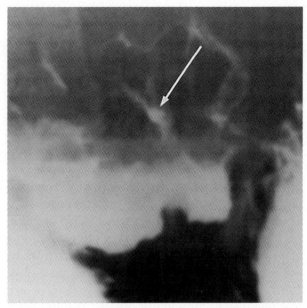

FIGURE 9–92. Acute posterior duodenal ulcer. An erect spot film shows a small constant collection of barium (*arrow*) lying in a posterior ulcer crater. This ulcer was confirmed endoscopically.

The normal duodenal cap may have a smooth coating of barium but a fine reticular or "small-dot" pattern is also normal and is probably due to barium collecting in the sulci around the villi (Bova et al., 1985).

A collection of barium lying in the ulcer crater is the most commonly seen abnormality with an acute duodenal ulcer (Figure 9–92). When the ulcer

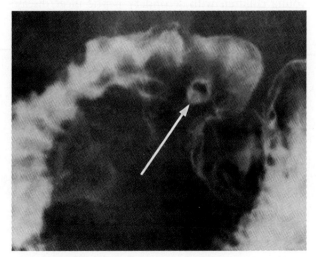

FIGURE 9–93. Acute anterior duodenal ulcer. Barium outlines an ulcer (*arrow*) on the nondependent (anterior) wall of the duodenal cap.

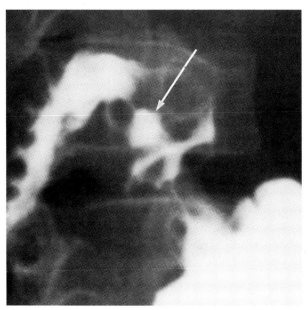

FIGURE 9–94. Chronic duodenal ulcer. There is a large ulcer crater (*arrow*) in a deformed duodenal cap.

wall of the duodenum as the duodenum is often best seen in the right anterior oblique projection.

With chronic ulceration, the duodenum may become deformed (Figure 9–94) although this is unusual in childhood. However, a degree of pyloric spasm is relatively common in children and causes contraction of the pylorus which can mimic, and should not be mistaken for, the deformity of the duodenum secondary to chronic duodenal ulceration. With chronic duodenal ulceration, perforation can result in free peritoneal air which on occasions may be massive (Figure 9–95).

Duodenitis

Duodenitis is a relatively uncommon diagnosis in childhood but is being made more often due to endoscopy. Other than peptic ulcer diseases, the differential diagnosis for duodenitis includes inflammatory bowel disease, celiac disease, viral bacterial or parasitic infection, eosinophilic enteritis, Zollinger-Ellison syndrome, and graft-versus-host disease. In a pediatric study of 75 patients with 24 biopsy-proven cases of duodenitis, the sensitivity and specificity of an upper GI examination was 46% and 98%, respectively while endoscopy

is on the nondependent wall of the duodenum, the barium does not collect in the crater and a double-contrast view is then seen (Figure 9–93). This latter appearance is seen usually in ulcers of the anterior

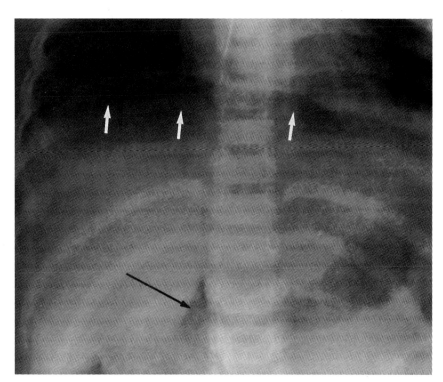

FIGURE 9–95. Perforation from an acute duodenal ulcer. There is free peritoneal air in the subhepatic space (*black arrow*) and below the diaphragm (*white arrows*).

sensitivity and specificity was 54% and 92%, respectively (Long et al., 1998). In adult studies, the sensitivity of upper GI examinations is 72% (Gelfand et al., 1985b). Mucosal fold thickening is the most common sign of duodenitis, and a measurement in excess of 4 mm (3 mm under 1 year) is used (Long et al., 1998). Care should be taken to evaluate the duodenum on nondistended and distended views as collapsed normal duodenal folds may appear thickened. Diffuse fold thickening can be found in hypoproteinemia and protein-losing enteropathy. Focal fold thickening can be found in bowel wall hemorrhage from trauma or Schönlein-Henoch purpura. Bulb deformity and ulceration are seen in duodenitis. Nodularity and erosions are best seen on double-contrast studies and are not commonly identified in children (Long et al., 1998; Gelfand et al., 1985b).

Dermatomyositis

Dermatomyositis in childhood is a different disease, clinically and pathologically, from that seen in adults. In children, dermatomyositis is a necrotizing vasculitis which involves skin, subcutaneous tissues, and musculature and often affects the gastrointestinal tract. Bowel involvement is variable with motility disorders, ulceration, perforation, hemorrhage, pneumatosis, and pneumoperitoneum (Magill et al., 1984). Bowel involvement can result in malabsorption states.

Perforation occurs infrequently but is a serious complication that can affect the esophagus, small bowel, or colon (Magill et al., 1984). Perforation is probably secondary to necrotizing vasculitis involving small vessels in the bowel wall which thrombose and result in ischemia. This may be further aggravated by infection, steroid therapy, and disordered gut motility.

Radiologic imaging may help in assessing these complications. Plain films can show the pneumatosis or pneumoperitoneum. Contrast studies can demonstrate the ulceration or perforation of the bowel and may show that it is more conical and irregular than the more usual form of peptic ulceration.

IDIOPATHIC INFLAMMATORY BOWEL DISEASE OF THE SMALL BOWEL

In children, the term inflammatory bowel disease is generally applied to the idiopathic forms of bowel disease such as ulcerative colitis, Crohn's disease, Behçet syndrome, and eosinophilic gastroenteritis. However, many other conditions can mimic these illnesses (Table 9–4).

Idiopathic inflammatory bowel disease in childhood was once considered rare but is now increasingly recognized. Although ulcerative colitis and Crohn's disease, the two most common types, have many features in common with the adult forms, the differential diagnoses, presentation, and therapy may differ in important ways from those in adults.

(Ulcerative colitis and a comparison between Crohn's disease and ulcerative colitis will be found in Chapter 10).

Regional Enteritis (Crohn's Disease)

This disease primarily affects young adults. Close questioning of many young adults with regional enteritis will reveal a long history of symptoms; in 14% of a series of 600 patients, symptoms started before 15 years of age (Van Patter et al., 1954).

The overall incidence of Crohn's disease, including in children, appears to be increasing although age of onset does not appear to be decreasing (Brahme et al., 1975; Hofley and Piccoli, 1994; Whelan, 1990). In children 16 years old and younger, an incidence of 6.1 in 100,000 and a prevalence of 41 in 100,000 is reported (Lindquist et al., 1984).

An extensive survey found that 3.8% of patients with Crohn's disease were less than 10 years old; the disease is rare under 6 years of age but has been diagnosed in a small number of infants (Miller et al., 1971; Rubin et al., 1967). There is an increased incidence in Caucasian, especially Jewish, populations and some families (Hamilton et al., 1979; Kelts and Grand, 1980), and a 56% familial incidence of inflammatory bowel disease with onset at under 5 years of age has been reported (Hofley and Piccoli, 1994).

As in adults, the ileocolic region is the most likely area to be involved although isolated proximal small bowel disease and skip lesions occur. Microscopically the mucosa may appear to be normal or to have minimal chronic inflammation. Noncaseating granulomata are present in approximately 50% although this depends on the number and type of biopsies taken. In contrast with the predominant mucosal involvement of ulcerative colitis, all layers of the bowel wall are affected with edema, lymphoid aggregates, fissures, deep undermining ulceration, and fibrosis (Kelts and Grand, 1980). All regions of the gastrointestinal tract may be involved.

The etiology of Crohn's disease is still uncertain, with multiple factors resulting in intestinal inflammation being likely. Etiologic factors that have been considered and investigated include infection (mycobacteria, *Yersinia*, *Campylobacter*, chlamydia, measles virus); abnormal intestinal immunologic and inflammatory response to bacteria, toxins, or metabolites; genetic factors (familial incidence, occurrence in twins, incidence in human leukocyte antigen (HLA) halotypes); toxins (toothpaste, tobacco, oral contraceptives); and even psychogenic factors (Ramchandani et al., 1994).

Clinical Features, Extraintestinal Effects, and Complications

Children with inflammatory bowel disease may present with symptoms similar to adults but, importantly, can present with systemic and extraintestinal symptoms that may dominate or precede gastrointestinal symptoms by years. Mistaken diagnoses include juvenile rheumatoid arthritis, systemic lupus erythematosus, iron deficiency anemia, acute rheumatic fever, idiopathic growth failure, idiopathic amenorrhea, and eating disorders (Grand and Homer, 1975; Kirschner, 1995).

Five main categories of presenting symptoms are described: recurrent gastrointestinal complaints, pseudoappendicitis, pyrexia of unknown origin or associated with arthralgia, unexplained growth failure, and anorexia nervosa-type symptoms (Silverman, 1966).

The recurrent gastrointestinal complaints are most commonly abdominal pain and diarrhea, then rectal bleeding, bowel obstruction, anorectal fistula, and stomatitis (Grand and Homer, 1975; Silverman, 1966). Perianal disease is indicative of Crohn's disease in childhood, is present in 40% of patients, and is often the earliest physical sign of disease (Guttman, 1974; Kirschner, 1995). Crohn's disease may present with bloody diarrhea and mimic ulcerative colitis so closely that differentiation may be impossible in up to 20% of cases. However, abdominal pain is a common early symptom, and the presence of perianal disease, fever, and failure to thrive are all more common with Crohn's disease than with ulcerative colitis (Hamilton et al., 1979).

TABLE 9–4. Conditions Which May Mimic Idiopathic Inflammatory Bowel Disease

Enteric infections
  Bacterial
    Campylobacter
    Clostridium difficile (pseudomembranous colitis)
    Escherichia coli
    Histoplasmosis
    Salmonella
    Shigella
    Tuberculosis
    Yersinia
  Viral
    Cytomegalovirus
  Parasites
    Entamoeba histolytica
Neutropenic colitis
Necrotizing enterocolitis
Hirschsprung's enterocolitis
Ischemic colitis
Lymphoma / lymphoproliferative disease
Schönlein-Henoch purpura
Cow's milk allergy colitis
Detergent, caustic, and herbal enema colitis

Acute regional enteritis presenting with abdominal pain, leukocytosis, fever, and tenderness in the right iliac fossa may lead to an operation for appendicitis. A normal appendix is found but part of the terminal ileum is inflamed and thickened. The affected area is often clearly demarcated from normal bowel and associated with enlarged lymph nodes. Some of these cases of acute regional enteritis do not recur but others will recur after a symptom-free period of some years. The remainder are acute exacerbations of underlying unsuspected chronic disease (Moseley et al., 1960). *Yersinia enterocolitica* infection may mimic acute Crohn's disease clinically, radiographically (see Figures 9–81, 9–82), and at laparotomy.

Fever in combination with gastrointestinal symptoms is suggestive of regional enteritis. Difficulty arises when the fever presents before gastrointestinal complaints as a pyrexia of unknown origin or when it accompanies other symptoms such as arthralgia or growth failure.

Seronegative spondyloarthropathy is the most common extraintestinal manifestation in Crohn's disease (Hofley and Piccoli, 1994). Arthritis of a few large joints may be a presenting symptom (Figure 9–96), and arthritis or spondylitis affects 10% of children and teenagers with Crohn's disease. The peripheral arthritis is benign and improves with regression of the underlying bowel disease but spondylitis is progressive, and supportive measures will be required to prevent deformity (Lindsley and Schaller, 1974). Sacroileitis may be present and be detectable on plain films (Figure 9–97).

There are many causes of growth failure in children. Poor growth and development are common findings in children with any chronic disease. However, growth failure without gastrointestinal symptoms is a common pediatric presentation of Crohn's disease. Early diagnosis and treatment is important to prevent stunted growth.

Regional enteritis may be overlooked when the combination of anorexia, weight loss, and personality change suggests anorexia nervosa.

Erythema nodosum is sometimes present and is the commonest skin manifestation of Crohn's disease. Pyoderma gangrenosum is a less common skin manifestation and is often associated with pancolitis (Hofley and Piccoli, 1994).

The major complication of regional enteritis is perforation which develops into fistula formation, phlegmon, abscess, or peritonitis. Fistulae are most often between adjacent loops of bowel but tracts to the skin (abdominal wall and perineum) and the urogenital system also occur.

Obstruction usually results from severe longstanding disease but acute obstruction from severe inflammation can occur.

Gastrointestinal bleeding from regional enteritis is rare but can be catastrophic and require surgery (Cirocco et al., 1995).

Sclerosing cholangitis is a rare complication of Crohn's disease and is more commonly associated with ulcerative colitis (Werlin et al., 1980).

Renal calculus disease is found in 5% of children with inflammatory bowel disease and is especially likely if ileostomy has been required following surgical intervention (Hofley and Piccoli, 1994).

The risk for malignancy is less than in ulcerative colitis and does not occur in childhood. Compared with the general population, patients with Crohn's disease have 20 times the incidence of adenocarcinoma of the colon (Weedon et al., 1973), a small increase in the incidence of small bowel ade-

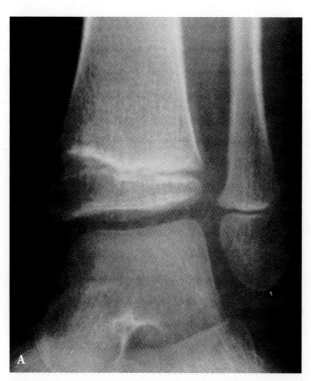 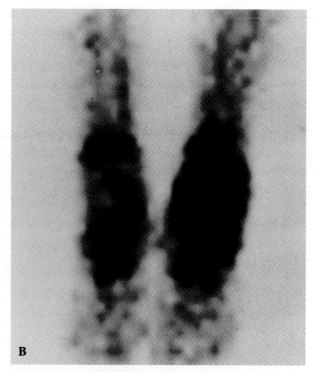

FIGURE 9–96. Crohn's disease with arthritis. *A*, Ankles show mild osteopenia on plain films. *B*, Ankles show asymmetrical increased activity on bone scan, a nonspecific appearance.

nocarcinoma (Kerber and Frank, 1984), and possibly, lymphoma (Gardiner and Stevenson, 1982). Surveillance for colorectal cancer by endoscopy, as recommended for long-standing ulcerative colitis, is not generally recommended unless severe and persistent disease has been present (Bachwich et al., 1994).

Crohn's Disease in Infancy

Crohn's disease has seldom been reported in infancy and may present acutely with development of intestinal obstruction which requires surgery as steroids do not appear helpful. The rapid improvement and lack of recurrence of any disease is in distinct contrast to adult Crohn's disease and strongly suggests a different etiology or even a different disease (Miller et al., 1971).

Imaging

Upper GI examination, small bowel follow-through examination, and contrast enema have traditionally been used for evaluating Crohn's disease. Endoscopic evaluation with flexible fiber-optic equipment is now routinely used for the upper GI and colon as superb visualization of mucosal surfaces combined with biopsy information provide a powerful diagnostic tool and increased sensitivity for disease detection (Wills et al., 1997). Cross-sectional imaging, mainly with US and CT but also MR, has been established as an excellent modality for imaging beyond the mucosa, with particular value in assessing complications.

Plain-Film Radiography. Abdominal radiography provides an overview of the abdomen and can often provide important diagnostic information or indication of complication (Taylor et al., 1986). Bowel wall thickening (thumbprinting) can indicate colitis, displaced bowel may indicate an inflammatory mass in the right iliac fossa, and evidence of small bowel obstruction may be apparent. Extraintestinal disease such as sacroileitis and/or spondylitis may be seen (see Figure 9–97), and abnormal gas collections in the abdomen or urinary system may indicate abscess or fistula tract.

Contrast Studies/Endoscopy. Since Crohn's disease can affect any part of the gastrointestinal tract from the mouth to the anus, specific investigation should be aimed at that part in which disease is clinically suspected.

Data from adult hospitals suggests a high incidence of esophageal, gastric, or duodenal involvement found endoscopically. We find inflammatory bowel disease rarely symptomatic in the upper gastrointestinal tract of children. Children with symptoms suggesting upper GI involvement will usually undergo upper GI endoscopy where direct mucosal visualization and biopsy will provide diagnosis. If an appropriate pediatric endoscopy service is not available, an upper GI examination can demonstrate pathology (Figure 9–98). A double-contrast barium study would, however, usually be recommended.

Where small bowel disease is suspected, a single-contrast small bowel follow-through examination is the best routine examination (see Chapter 3). We abbreviate the upper GI component of the study and may exclude it entirely if there has been a recent upper GI endoscopy. Encouraging an adolescent

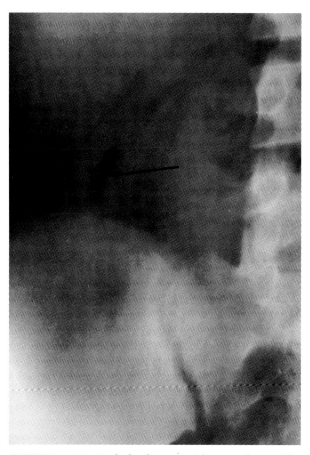

FIGURE 9–97. Crohn's disease with sacroileitis. The right sacroiliac joint was wider and less distinct than the left. The cecum and ascending colon was involved with Crohn's colitis and contains an abnormal gas pattern (*arrow*) but no feces.

who is fed up with his chronic illness and doctors in general to ingest adequate barium to fill and demonstrate the small bowel can be a challenge. The threat of passing an orogastric tube is seldom constructive. Time spent gaining the patient's confidence before the study is time well spent. We obtain serial abdominal radiographs, immediately fluoroscope sites of pathology, and always specifically interrogate the terminal ileum. The terminal ileum is often the most difficult portion of the gut to visualize. If it is seen incompletely on the small bowel study, a peroral pneumocolon (rectal insufflation of air) may be performed (Figure 9–99); it is tolerated well and requires little additional radiation (Stringer et al., 1986b) (see Chapter 3). Air and contrast can be refluxed into the terminal ileum during double-contrast colon studies (Figures 9–100, 9–101). The small bowel enema (enteroclysis) is an invasive, unpleasant procedure in children and usually requires more radiation than a small bowel meal. We reserved it for the few cases in which a conventional study or cross-sectional imaging have failed to give accurate information (Stringer et al., 1986a).

Although the terminal ileum is the most common site affected in children, small bowel disease with a normal terminal ileum may be found in up to 20% of cases, and proximal distribution of disease is more common in children than adults (Figure 9–102) (Chrispin and Tempany, 1967; Halligan et al., 1994; Kirks and Currarino, 1978). The earliest reported finding of terminal ileal disease in adults is a reticular pattern (Glick and Teplick, 1985). This has not been described in children and would be difficult to distinguish from a lymphoid follicular pattern, a normal finding. If an air contrast examination of the terminal ileum is performed, either by reflux from a double-contrast barium enema or by a peroral pneumocolon, subtle aphthae can be detected, probably the earliest form of Crohn's disease that can be seen (see Figure 9–101) (Hizawa et al., 1994).

Characteristic findings of Crohn's disease include early changes of a granular nodularity, mucosal edema, and aphthae. The translation of aphtha is ulcer and hence, the aphthoid ulceration (i.e., ulcer like ulcer) is meaningless and should be avoided. More advanced disease will have florid irregularity, widespread nodularity, or a cobblestone appearance (Figure 9–103), linear ulceration (Figure 9–104), deep "rose thorn" ulceration (Figure 9–105), a spiculated mucosal outline, and transmural thickening (Figure 9–106) (Goldberg et al., 1979). Variable narrowing and mass effect can occur due to inflammation, fibrosis, and associated spasm. Stenosis demonstrating the "string sign" may be found but occurs less frequently than in adults and usually affects the terminal ileum. When the stenosis is tight, the proximal bowel may be dilated (Figure 9–107). Skip lesions with asymmetric, discontinuous disease are typical. Fibrosis usually occurs eccentrically, causing pseudodiverticula (Figure 6–108) (Kelvin and Gedgaudas, 1981). Progressive narrowing in persistent long-standing disease will result in small bowel obstruction.

When a large mass effect suggests the possibility of a lymphoma, enteroclysis, by overcoming this spasm, may demonstrate sufficient detail to obviate laparotomy (Figure 9–109). The ability of enteroclysis to overcome spasm has been demonstrated in adults (Nolan and Piris, 1980) as well as children (Stringer et al., 1986a). Cross-sectional imaging, especially CT, can directly assess the bowel wall thickness and interloop fluid or fibrofatty proliferation and renders this application less useful. Enteroclysis may help in showing the size of a terminal ileum stricture (Figure 9–110) but this information is less important than the clinical findings.

Fistulae most often occur between adjacent loops of bowel and may be shown by barium examination (Figure 9–111). A fistulous connection to the skin can be injected directly with water-soluble contrast media (Figure 9–112).

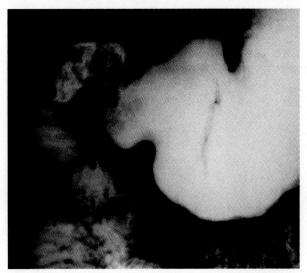

FIGURE 9–98. Crohn's disease. On upper GI examination, the duodenum has a cobblestone appearance with deep mural ulceration and rigidity.

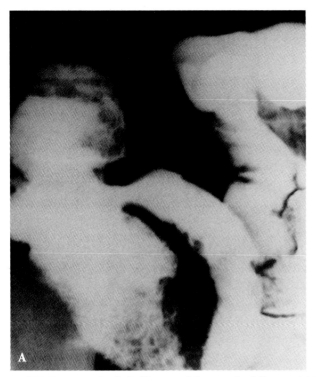
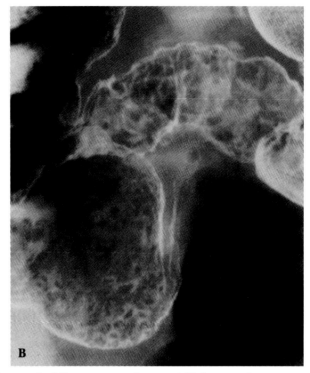

FIGURE 9–99. Crohn's disease of the terminal ileum. *A,* The terminal ileum appeared more rigid than usual on a conventional small bowel follow-through examination. *B,* A peroral pneumocolon performed immediately demonstrated extensive and unsuspected ulceration. (Reprinted with permission from Stringer DA, et al. AJR 1986;132:765.)

Ultrasonography. This modality can accurately delineate bowel wall thickening, mucosal abnormalities, strictures, fibrofatty proliferation or mesenteric "creeping fat," mesenteric nodes, and complications of inflammatory mass and abscess (Sarrazin and Wilson, 1996). The ultrasonographic features of Crohn's disease are the same for children as for adults (Dinkel et al., 1986). Bowel interrogation requires some ultrasonographic skill and experience using high-resolution linear probes and graded compression. In such hands, US has been recommended as the initial investigation of choice, with a reported sensitivity for disease detection of 87% (Sheridan et al., 1993). It is unlikely that US will displace endoscopy and biopsy for diagnosis but where up to 70% of small bowel contrast studies are normal for relatively nonspecific abdominal symptoms appropriate use of US can significantly reduce radiation exposure to the community (Sheridan et al., 1993). In patients with confirmed disease, US provides safe serial monitoring of the disease and its complications. Ultrasonography has been found effective in evaluating disease recurrence in patients who have had surgical resection (DiCandio et al., 1986).

Bowel wall thickening is typically seen in transverse section as a target lesion with central echogenicity. Normal bowel has an echogenic

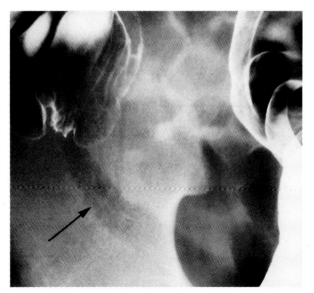

FIGURE 9–100. Crohn's disease of the terminal ileum. Reflux of air on a double-contrast barium enema shows a deformed and rigid terminal ileum (*arrow*).

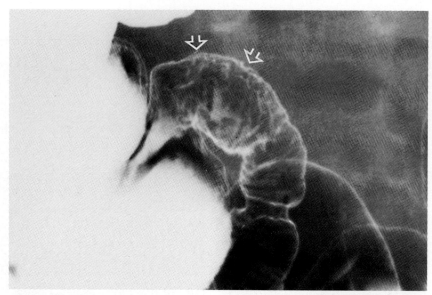

FIGURE 9–101. Crohn's disease of the terminal ileum. A double-contrast barium examination refluxed into the terminal ileum, demonstrating subtle ulceration (*arrows*), probably the earliest form of Crohn's disease that can be detected.

mucosal interface, a hypoechoic deep mucosa and muscularis mucosa, a hyperechoic submucosa, a thickened hypoechoic muscularis propria and hyperechoic serosa, and inflamed mesenteric tissue. The layering of this "gut signature" can be distorted or lost by inflammation, edema, and fibrosis

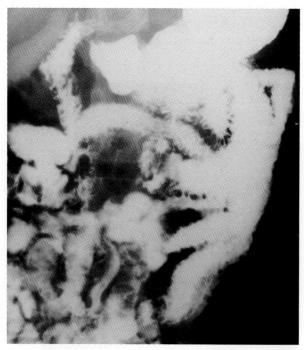

FIGURE 9–102. Crohn's disease of the jejunum. A large portion of proximal jejunum shows marked nodularity with some bowel wall thickening. The terminal ileum is normal.

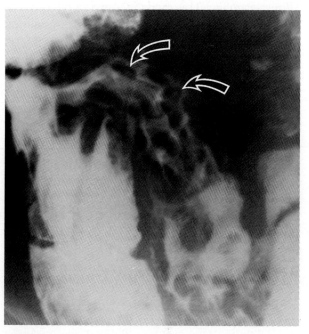

FIGURE 9–103. Crohn's disease of the terminal ileum. The terminal ileum shows florid irregularity and nodules, some of which are umbilicated or aphthous (*arrows*). (Reprinted with permission from Stringer DA. Radiol Clin North Am 1987;25:102.)

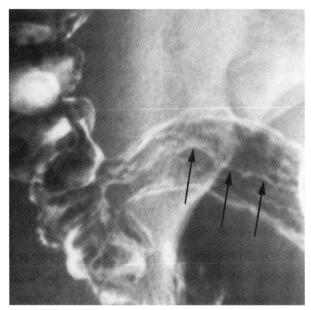

FIGURE 9–104. Crohn's disease. The terminal ileum is irregular and there are linear ulcers (*arrows*).

(Sarrazin and Wilson, 1996). In longitudinal section the affected bowel is rigid, ahaustral, noncompressible, and nonperistaltic but shows similar layering (Figure 9–113) (Dinkel et al., 1986; Kaftori et al., 1984; Khaw et al., 1991). Oblique views of diseased bowel may simulate renal tissue with central echogenic medulla and hypoechoic cortex, the "pseudokidney sign." Normal bowel wall measured from the central hyperechoic interface to outer echogenic serosal interface is 2 to 5 mm; in Crohn's disease, diseased bowel measures 5 to 15 mm and greater (Sarrazin and Wilson, 1996). Ultrasonography with graded compression can aid differentiation from appendicitis when the patient presents acutely with a tender right iliac fossa mass and fever (Puylaert, 1986).

Ultrasonography does not compete with endoscopy and contrast studies in detection of mucosal abnormalities but use of high-resolution linear probes reveals ulcers and fissures as echogenic tracts, usually due to the presence of air (see Figure 9–105B). Mucosal cobblestone appearance and postinflammatory polyps can be seen where the lumen is fluid-filled (Dinkel et al., 1986; Sarrazin and Wilson, 1996).

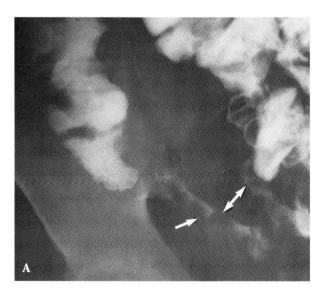

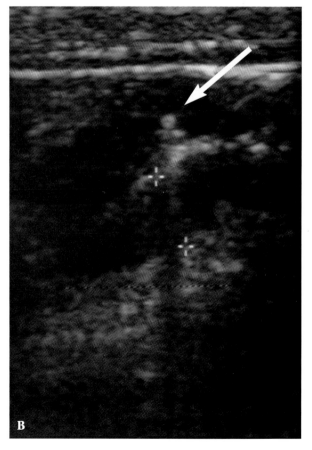

FIGURE 9 105. Crohn's disease. *A,* On small bowel follow-through examination, there is extensive terminal ileal disease with deep mural "rose thorn" ulceration (*arrow*) and wall thickening as inferred by separation between lumen contrast (*double arrow*). *B,* Ultrasonography demonstrates wall thickening and air trapped in a deep ulcer (*arrow*), which correlates well with the contrast study.

A fixed narrow lumen with proximal bowel dilatation indicates stricture and is the equivalent of the barium "string sign" (Figure 9–114).

Fibrofatty proliferation or mesenteric "creeping fat" is a response to transmural inflammation and is echogenic, surrounding the bowel and causing separation of bowel loops (see Figures 9–113, 9–114). Distinguishing a phlegmonous mass from fibrofatty proliferation may be difficult.

Mesenteric adenopathy is reactive and commonly seen in the right iliac fossa and mesenteric root. The nodes may be found in conglomerate masses and are hypoechoic and well circumscribed.

Complications of Crohn's disease, abscess in particular, can be advantageously imaged by US (Yeh and Rabinowitz, 1983). For a palpable mass, US can separate a phlegmonous mass of bowel loops

and inflamed mesentery from an abscess with its well-defined wall and echogenic content and, possibly, air (Figure 9–115). It can then be used to guide percutaneous abscess drainage (Figure 9–116), which may obviate the need for further surgery (Casola et al., 1987). A fistula to the urinary tract can result in inflammatory mass lesions of the bladder wall, intravesical gas, and debris in the bladder (Figure 9–117). Contiguity between the bladder and diseased bowel suggests pathology, and the fistula tract may be visualized rarely (Boag and Nolan, 1988; Sarrazin and Wilson, 1996).

The addition of color Doppler to the ultrasonographic evaluation of bowel can readily detect the marked hyperemia associated with inflammatory bowel disease although this finding is not specific for Crohn's disease (Quillin and Siegel, 1994).

Computed Tomography. Computed tomography accurately delineates the bowel wall thickening and the surrounding inflammatory response of inflammatory bowel disease in adults and children (Figures 9–118, 9–119, 9–120) (Goldberg et al., 1983; Gore et al., 1996; Jabra et al., 1994; Riddlesberger, 1985; Siegel et al., 1988). It is not recommended as

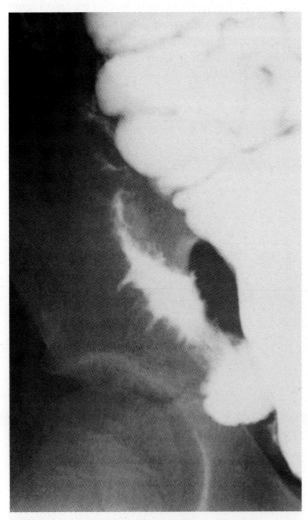

FIGURE 9–106. Crohn's disease. The terminal ileum has a spiculated appearance on barium study.

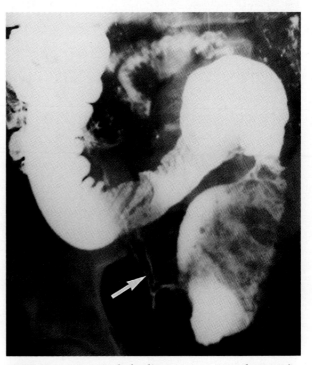

FIGURE 9–107. Crohn's disease. A narrow long stricture of the terminal ileum (*arrow*) results in dilatation of the more proximal small bowel.

enhancement. Small bowel wall thickness in adults should not exceed 2 to 3 mm, and thickening of 1 to 2 cm is commonly present with Crohn's disease (Gore et al., 1996). In healthy children the small bowel wall is usually too thin to measure, and if diseased bowel wall exceeds 1 cm, then lymphoma should be suspected (Siegel et al., 1988). Bowel wall thickening is not specific for Crohn's disease, and a

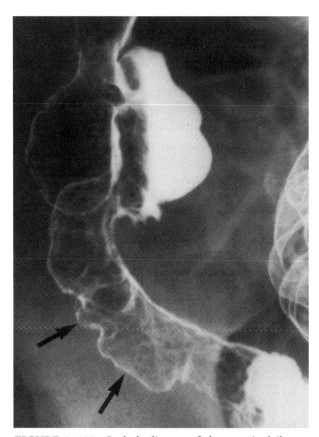

FIGURE 9–108. Crohn's disease of the terminal ileum. Eccentric pseudodiverticulae (*arrows*) form as a result of fibrosis. (Reprinted with permission from Stringer DA. Radiol Clin North Am 1987;25:103.)

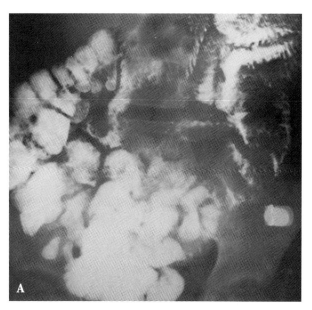

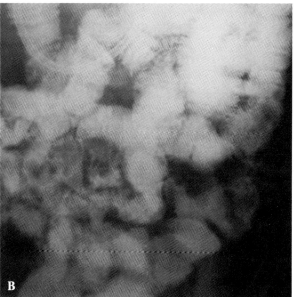

FIGURE 9–109. Crohn's disease of the jejunum. *A*, Conventional small bowel follow-through examination showed poor filling of the jejunum on outside hospital films. *B*, An enteroclysis examination overcame jejunal spasm sufficiently to allay some clinical concerns and obviated the need for rapid laparotomy.

an initial imaging modality but in patients with known disease and new or changing symptoms, it has exceptional ability to evaluate complications (Caroline and Friedman, 1994; Wills et al., 1997). Evaluation by CT of a child with inflammatory bowel disease should include assessment of bowel wall thickness; bowel obstruction; mesenteric and ischiorectal fossa abnormalities; lymphadenopathy; extraluminal fluid collections including abscess; extraluminal contrast in a fistula, sinus, or genitourinary system; and more remote complications such as gallstones, sclerosing cholangitis, hepatic steatosis, renal calculi, hydronephrosis, sacroileitis, and avascular necrosis of the femoral heads. In a study of adults with known disease, CT provided additional information which modified management in 28% of patients (Fishman et al., 1987).

Bowel CT requires attention to technical details which should include well distended, opacified bowel lumen and good intravenous contrast

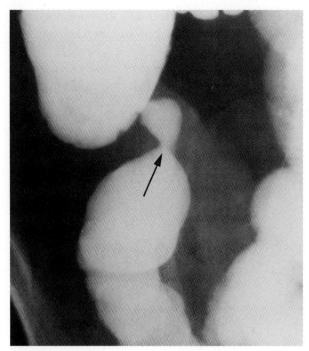

FIGURE 9–110. Crohn's disease of the terminal ileum. A tight stricture (*arrow*) of the terminal ileum is well delineated by enteroclysis.

differential diagnosis is included in Table 9–4. When viewed in transverse section, acutely diseased and inflamed bowel will show a "target" appearance with contrast enhancing inner mucosa and outer muscu-

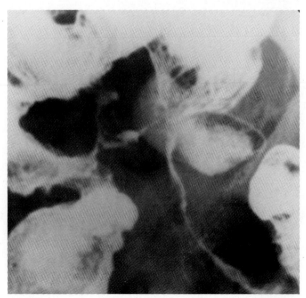

FIGURE 9–111. Crohn's disease with fistulae. Multiple fistulae between adjacent loops of bowel are well shown by barium examination.

laris propria/serosa and intervening low-attenuation edematous submucosa. More long-standing disease with onset of mural fibrosis will lose this mural stratification and appear homogeneous. The loss of bowel wall contrast enhancement suggests irreversible fibrosis (Gore et al., 1996).

Fibrofatty proliferation of the mesentery manifests as increased abundance and attenuation of the mesenteric fat with ill-defined margins and stranding down toward the mesenteric root (see Figure 9–118). The interface between the diseased bowel wall and mesentery becomes indistinct (Goldberg et al., 1983; Gore et al., 1996). This is the most common cause of bowel loop separation but it is important to distinguish it from interloop abscess or phlegmon. The increased vascularity of the mesenteric vessels with dilatation and tortuosity is more readily demonstrated with spiral scanning techniques (Meyers and McGuire, 1995).

Mesenteric lymphadenopathy is common, and nodes up to 1 cm may be found isolated or in clusters. Nodes larger than 1 cm should raise the possibility of lymphoma but certainly can be reactive.

Abscess is a common and serious complication resulting from sinus tracts, fistulae, perforations, or postoperative events (Figure 9–121, 9–122). They occur in up to 25% of patients, and their clinical presentation may be masked or altered by immunosuppressive therapy (Casola et al., 1987; Lambiase et al., 1998; Safrit et al., 1987). Abscesses are typically well circumscribed, rounded, and have strongly enhancing walls and low density content, possibly air. This air may suggest gas-forming organisms but commonly indicates communication with bowel. Computed tomography is a powerful modality for demonstrating the location, extent, and number of fluid collections. It also clearly delineates hematogenously seeded abscess as found in the liver (Safrit et al., 1987). It can accurately guide percutaneous drainage procedures, and is the imaging of choice for catheter abscess drainage in many centers (Casola et al., 1987). However, even if CT is used in diagnosis, the use of freehand ultrasonographic needle placement allows needle advancement under direct vision and does not occupy a CT scanner in a high-workload environment for extended periods of time. The traditional two-part surgical approach to an abscess from Crohn's disease was pus drainage first and then bowel and fistula resection. Percutaneous drainage can avert the first operation and can

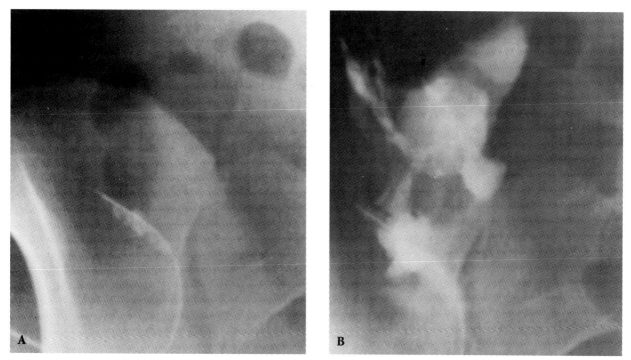

FIGURE 9–112. Crohn's disease with a fistula to the skin. *A, B,* A fistula is injected with water-soluble contrast media to demonstrate its communication with the gut (*B*).

avert surgery completely in many instances (Casola et al., 1987). Concomitant medical management with antibiotics and parenteral nutrition is essential.

Computed tomography can reliably distinguish abscess from phlegmon or inflammatory mass. A phlegmon is an ill-defined walled-off mass delineat-

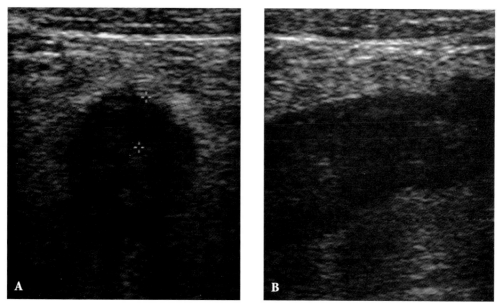

FIGURE 9–113. Crohn's disease. *A,B,* Transverse US (*A*) and longitudinal US (*B*) images of diseased bowel demonstrate marked wall thickening (between cursors), loss of mural stratification, lack of peristalsis, and rigidity. The prominent surrounding echogenicity is the mesenteric fibrofatty proliferation.

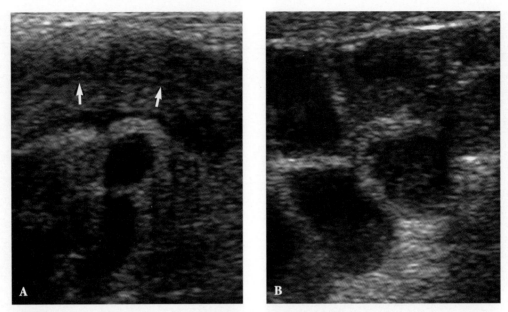

FIGURE 9–114. Crohn's disease. *A,* Longitudinal US of the terminal ileum shows a narrow lumen (*arrows*) within thickened bowel wall, the ultrasonographic equivalent of the barium "string sign." *B,* Dilated proximal small bowel is present in keeping with partial obstruction.

ed by matted loops of bowel and inflamed mesentery or omentum and no enhancement. The differentiation is important as abscess requires drainage while phlegmon does not.

Fistula and sinus tracks are hallmarks of Crohn's disease and occur in 20 to 40% of patients (Gore et al., 1996). Computed tomography can readily identify these tracks especially if contrast has

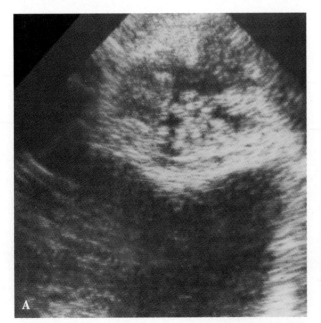

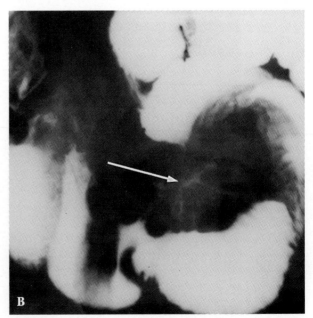

FIGURE 9–115. Crohn's disease with abscess formation. *A,* Longitudinal US shows a constant mass of mixed echogenicity in the right lower quadrant. (Reprinted with permission from Stringer DA. Radiol Clin North Am 1987;25:103.) *B,* Small bowel follow-through examination demonstrates that the right lower quadrant mass is secondary to ileal fistula formation (*arrow*).

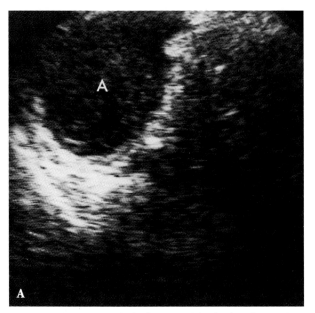
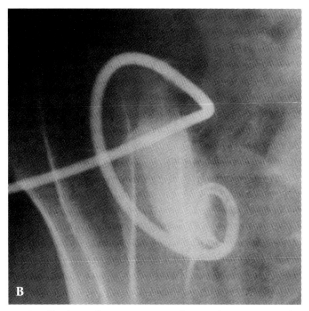

FIGURE 9–116. Crohn's disease with abscess formation. *A,* Longitudinal US shows a constant hypoechoic mass in the right iliac fossa. *B,* A 10 French pigtail catheter was inserted with ease. (Reprinted with permission from Stringer DA. Radiol Clin North Am 1987;25:93–113.)

passed down them. Fistulae unsuspected clinically may be revealed (Fishman et al., 1987), and fistulae not revealed by barium studies and sinography may be delineated (Goldberg et al., 1983). Enterovesical fistula can be delineated by CT with increased sensitivity for detection of intravesical air, bowel contrast, contiguous bowel disease, and bladder wall thickening and inflammation. If enterovesical fistula is suspected, imaging with bowel contrast before intravenous contrast is recommended so as not to confuse renal excretion of contrast with a fistula leaking contrast (Goldman et al., 1985).

Magnetic Resonance Imaging. Increasing speed and resolution have allowed MR to image bowel (Figure 9–123). The cost of MR makes it prohibitive as a routine imaging modality; yet, its lack of ionization and multiplanar imaging capacity make it appealing especially in the young girl who may require repeated imaging into her childbearing years and in patients with a history of intravenous iodinated contrast reactions. Motion artifact from arterial pulsation, respiration, and bowel peristalsis all contribute to image degradation. Saturation bands, various gating techniques, and glucagon are all required to complement fast breath-hold sequences. Adequate and uniform bowel distension remains a challenge as does communicating and gaining the coop-

eration of the preadolescent and adolescent patient. Diluted oral barium shows promise in providing a negative bowel contrast and breath hold, fat-suppressed, gadolinium-enhanced, fast multiplanar spoiled gradient-recalled images (Low and Francis, 1997). Gadolinium-enhanced fat-suppressed images

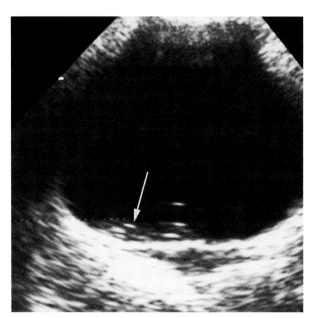

FIGURE 9–117. Crohn's disease with fistula to the bladder. Ultrasonography shows debris (*arrow*) in the bladder of a child with fecaluria.

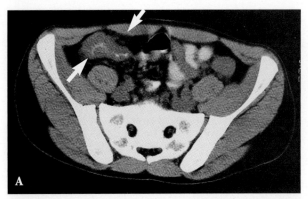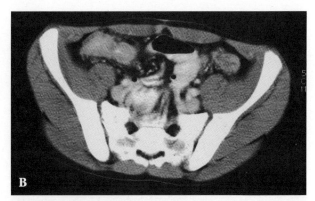

FIGURE 9–118. Crohn's disease. *A*, Computed tomography demonstrates thickened distal ileum with intraluminal contrast (*arrows*) and fibrofatty proliferation with abundance of fat and streaking of increased density. *B*, Following intravenous contrast enhancement, the serosal and mucosal layers enhance more than the muscular layer, and increased vascularity in the fibrofatty proliferation is more obvious.

are sensitive for detection of Crohn's disease, with good correlation between CT, endoscopy, and clinical evaluation (Kettritz et al., 1995; Shoenut et al., 1994). The use of half-fourier acquisition single-shot turbo spin echo sequences gives T2-weighted images in less than a second per slice and can image normal and abnormal bowel wall (Lee et al., 1998).

This technique takes advantage of the bright signal from physiologic fluid in the bowel lumen and has great potential for evaluating obstruction although its ability to evaluate soft tissue lesions is less than that of gadolinium-enhanced sequences (Regan et al., 1998). Great advances in MR of bowel pathology are expected.

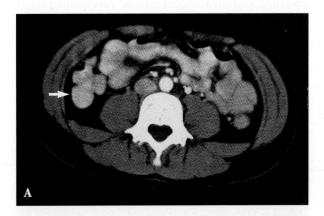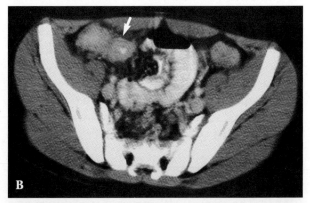

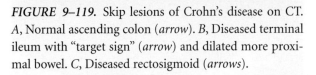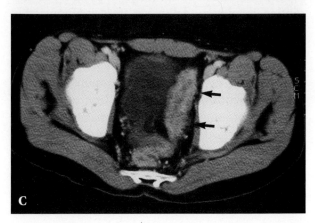

FIGURE 9–119. Skip lesions of Crohn's disease on CT. *A*, Normal ascending colon (*arrow*). *B*, Diseased terminal ileum with "target sign" (*arrow*) and dilated more proximal bowel. *C*, Diseased rectosigmoid (*arrows*).

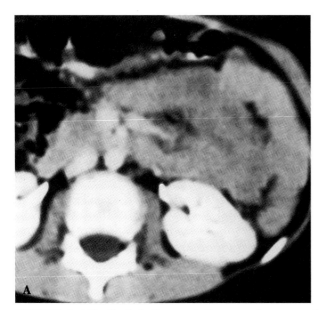 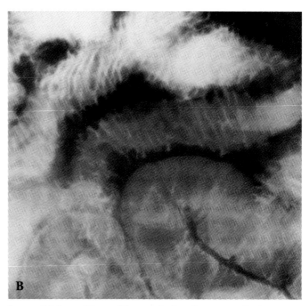

FIGURE 9–120. Crohn's disease. *A*, Computed tomography shows thickened bowel loops. *B*, On the enteroclysis examination, Crohn's disease is seen with bowel wall thickening and mucosal irregularity.

Nuclear Medicine. Leukocytes infiltrate actively diseased mucosa and are passed into the bowel lumen. Radiolabeled leukocytes accumulate in areas of active inflammation and can thus be used to assess disease activity. Indium-111-labeled white blood cells have been used in adults but technetium Tc 99m Hexamethyl: propyleneamine-oxime (HM-PAO)-labeled leukocytes is the recommended isotope in children due to its better image quality and lower radiation (Figure 9–124). Indium has a longer half-life than technetium and causes chromosomal aberrations in labeled lymphocytes (ten Berge et al., 1983) although the long-term effects of these aberrations have been debated (Thakur and McAfee, 1984).

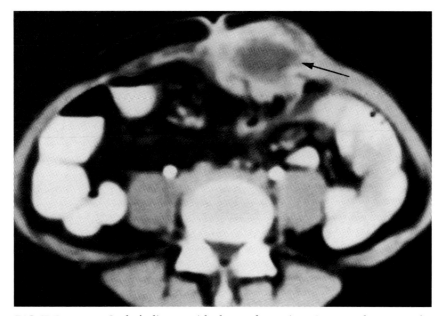

FIGURE 9–121. Crohn's disease with abscess formation. Computed tomography gives excellent delineation of a rectus sheath abscess (*arrow*) resulting from a fistula from involved gut.

Technetium Tc 99m HM-PAO-labeled leukocytes can accurately distinguish active from inactive disease and anatomically locate disease distribution (Charron, 1997; Kennan and Hayward, 1992). It has been recommended at some centers as an initial imaging modality of choice with its sensitivity and specificity (both between 80 and 90% for inflammatory bowel disease), its low radiation burden, and its easy application with no sedation or bowel preparation (Jewel et al., 1996; Jobling et al., 1996; Shah et al., 1997).

Medical Management

The goals of management should be to control acute disease, prevent relapse, attend to nutritional requirements, and ensure normal growth and development (Hofley and Piccoli, 1994). Medical therapy is aimed at inhibiting inflammatory and immune-mediated insult to bowel, controlling infection, providing appropriate nutrition (often parenteral), and attending to the emotional needs of patient and family (Wills et al., 1997). Corticosteroids and 5-aminosalicylic acid preparations are the mainstays of therapy in small bowel disease; azathioprine and 9-mercaptopurine have a place as steroid-sparing therapy in chronic disease (Hofley and Piccoli, 1994). Caloric intake calculations need to include normal growth requirement plus catch-up for any growth failure. Replacement of folate, vitamins B12, A, D, E, and K,

and trace elements is important. Elemental diets, often via percutaneous feeding tubes, can reduce dependence on steroid therapy. Parenteral nutrition may be required during acute illness, prior to surgery, or in short gut secondary to multiple resections.

Indications For Surgery

Generally, surgery is required sooner after presentation in ileocolic disease than in isolated colonic disease (Mekhjian et al., 1979). Because recurrence is so common after surgery, a conservative approach using medication and tube feeding is tried if possible (Hamilton et al., 1979). However, if there is perforation with peritonitis, unresolving bowel obstruction, uncontrolled bleeding, or draining fistulae or sinuses, surgery is usually advisable especially when the disease is localized (Grand and Homer, 1975; Hamilton et al., 1979). The value of surgery to promote growth, especially before puberty, has yet to be defined although some children have done well with surgery (Grand and Homer, 1975; Hamilton et al., 1979).

Eosinophilic Gastroenteritis

Clinical Features

Eosinophilic gastroenteritis (allergic gastroenteropathy) is a complex entity that probably encompasses a number of disorders of uncertain etiology.

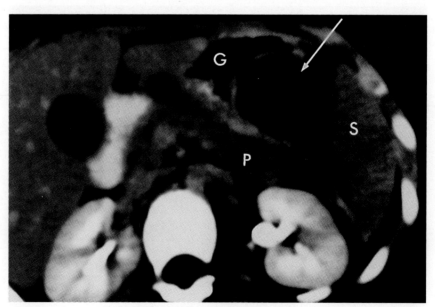

FIGURE 9–122. Crohn's disease with abscess formation. Computed tomography shows a lesser sac abscess (*arrow*) medial to the spleen (S), anterior to the pancreas (P), and posterior to the gastric antrum (G), not well delineated by US.

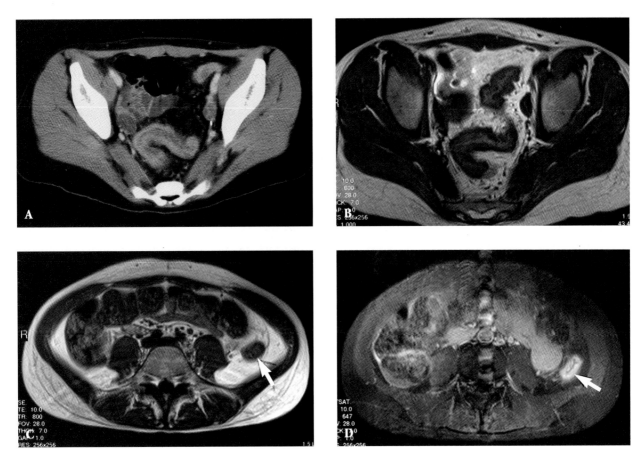

FIGURE 9–123. Crohn's disease. *A*, Computed tomography with intravenous contrast enhancement shows extensive sigmoid disease with marked fibrofatty proliferation. *B*, T1-weighted spin echo MR image shows sigmoid wall thickening and fibrofatty proliferation with signal voids of increased vasculature. *C*, T1-weighted spin echo image demonstrates descending colon disease with fibrofatty proliferation. Feces-filled colon indicates relative obstruction. Note ghosting artifact from anterior abdominal wall. *D*, Intravenous gadolinium-enhanced fat-saturated, T1 weighted image shows significant arterial pulsation artifact but good conspicuity of enhancing thickened bowel wall (*white arrow* in C and D).

Children with this condition fail to thrive, often have a history of asthma or allergies, and may develop iron deficiency anemia with peripheral eosinophilia. These patients usually respond well to steroids.

One subgroup appears distinctive, with growth retardation, abdominal pain, diarrhea, and a strong history of systemic allergy (Teele et al., 1979). Protein-losing enteropathy, iron deficiency anemia from gastrointestinal blood loss, peripheral eosinophilia, and small bowel mucosal biopsy abnormalities may also be associated (Katz et al., 1977; Waldman et al., 1967).

Imaging

Many parts of the gastrointestinal tract can be affected. The esophagus may be focally involved, resulting in stricture formation (Matzinger and Daneman, 1983). The gastric antrum may appear lacy on air-contrast barium meal examination; while this looks similar to areae gastricae, these are not usually seen in young children (Teele et al., 1979).

The small bowel pattern is radiologically normal or shows nonspecific abnormalities such as mucosal nodularity with thickening of the folds and bowel wall (Figure 9–125) (Teele et al., 1979). Occasionally, excess intraluminal bowel fluid breaks up the barium column.

Rarely, the large bowel can be affected by generalized or focal colitis, usually associated with small bowel disease (Moore et al., 1986).

Diagnosis is usually established by endoscopy, with a biopsy showing pronounced tissue eosinophil-

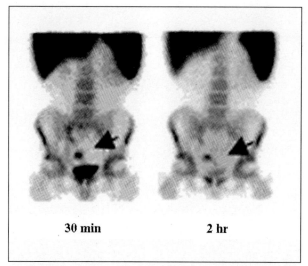

FIGURE 9–124. Crohn's disease. A technetium Tc 99m HM-PAO-labeled leukocyte study shows uptake in the terminal ileum (*arrow*) in keeping with inflammatory bowel disease.

ia in the absence of parasitic infection. The biopsy can be taken from the gastric antrum using a small bowel biopsy capsule. The degree of tissue eosinophilia is greater than that found in other forms of inflammatory bowel disease (Moore et al., 1986).

Behçet Syndrome

Clinical Features

Behçet syndrome is rare in children, especially those under 10 years of age. It is more common in Japan and Europe than North America (Stringer et al., 1986). Behçet described a triad of recurrent genital ulceration, oral ulceration (Figure 6–126), and eye inflammation (Behçet, 1937). Subsequently, others realized that the syndrome can affect many organ systems such as the gastrointestinal, cardiovascular, neurologic, and skeletal systems (Chajek and Fainaru, 1975). The diagnosis depends on a number of major or minor criteria. For the complete form of the disease, all four major criteria—buccal ulceration, genital ulceration, eye lesions, and skin lesions—have to be present but this seldom occurs in children (Stringer et al., 1986). The incomplete form requires either three major criteria or two major and two minor criteria (i.e., gastrointestinal lesions, cardiovascular lesions, thrombophlebitis, arthritis, central nervous system lesions, and family history) (Behçet, 1974; Mason and Barnes, 1969).

In children with gastrointestinal disease, three major criteria should be present before the diagnosis is made because of the difficulty in distinguishing Behçet syndrome from other forms of inflammatory bowel disease, particularly Crohn's disease. The most suggestive findings are genital ulceration or severe oral ulceration (Stringer et al., 1986). Both are uncommon in Crohn's disease and should always raise the possibility of Behçet syndrome. Skin and occular findings are less frequent than in adults (Stringer et al., 1986).

Imaging

Any part of the gastrointestinal tract from the oropharynx to the anus can be affected. Proximal gastrointestinal disease, including pharyngeal, esophageal, or duodenal ulceration and esophageal dysmotility, has been reported sporadically (Vlymen and Moskowitz, 1981). Distal small intestinal involvement, mimicking Crohn's ileitis radiologically, is not uncommon (Figure 9–127, 9–128) (James, 1979; Stanley et al., 1975). Ileal ring ulcers have been reported as a specific manifestation best seen on coned compression views of the terminal ileum (McLean et al., 1983). The US and CT findings of bowel wall thickening, a well-known feature of Crohn's disease, can be seen in Behçet syndrome. The large bowel is frequently involved in Behçet syndrome (see Chapter 10).

NEOPLASMS OF THE SMALL BOWEL OR MESENTERY

Benign Tumors

Clinical Features

Benign tumors of the small bowel are rare in childhood. When present, they may cause bleeding or intussusception or they may be part of a generalized polyposis syndrome. Mesenchymal malformations with lymphangiectasia can present with protein-losing enteropathy.

Hemangiomas can be solitary or multiple. Cutaneous and visceral hemangiomata may be present in the Klippel-Trénauney syndrome (Lewis et al., 1986). Telangiectasias are found in the bowel in Rendu-Osler-Weber syndrome (Taybi and Lachman, 1996). Neurofibromas can be associated with neurofibromatosis or occur as an isolated finding

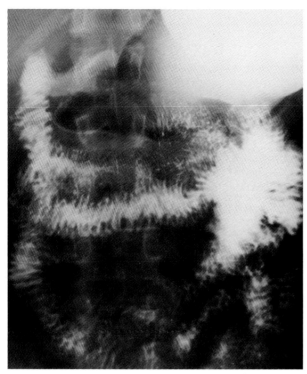

FIGURE 9–125. Eosinophilic gastroenteritis. There is marked thickening and nodularity of the jejunal mucosal folds.

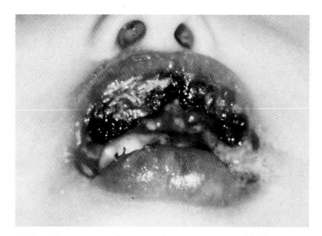

FIGURE 9–126. Behçet syndrome. Severe oral ulceration is present.

Eccentric polyposis and separation of bowel loops due to mesenteric involvement may be seen in neurofibromatosis (Figure 9–132) (Ginsburg, 1975). Megacolon secondary to neurofibromatosis may mimic Hirschsprung's disease (Hassell, 1982).

involving the mesentery, bowel wall, or both (Davis and Berk, 1973; Ginsburg, 1975; Tishler et al., 1983). Malignant transformation of neurofibromas of the gut is rare (Hochberg et al., 1974).

The polyposis syndromes usually seen in adults may be present in childhood; the Peutz-Jeghers syndrome with hamartomatous polyps is the most commonly observed in children (see Chapter 10).

Other benign mesenchymal tumors of the small bowel include fibromas, lipomas, and leiomyomas. The lipomas and related tumors have some characteristic features and so are discussed separately below.

Imaging

The benign tumor may be seen radiologically as either a lead point in an intussusception (Figure 9–129) or a polypoid lesion (Figures 9–130, 9–131). A small bowel follow-through examination is usually sufficient in children to demonstrate the lesions but if small masses are suspected or a barium follow-through examination is equivocal, enteroclysis can be performed.

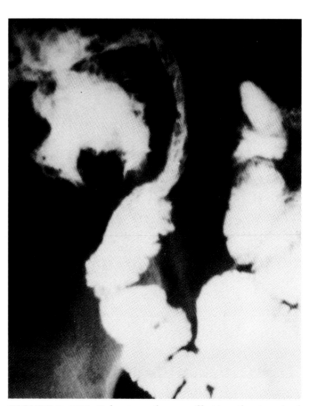

FIGURE 9–127. Behçet syndrome affecting the terminal ileum. The terminal ileum is narrow and more rigid than normal, mimicking Crohn's ileitis. (Reprinted with permission from Stringer DA. Pediatr Radiol 1986;16:132.)

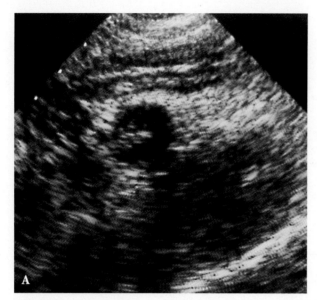

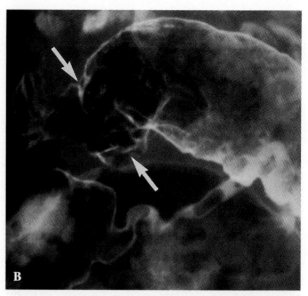

FIGURE 9–128. Behçet syndrome affecting the terminal ileum. *A,* Ultrasonography shows bowel wall thickening and a peroral pneumocolon. *B,* An irregular terminal ileum (*arrows*) on US. These are both well-known features of Crohn disease. (Reprinted with permission, Stringer DA. Pediatr Radiol 1986;16:132.)

Ultrasonography is the best initial modality if a palpable mass is present. It usually enables easy differentiation between cystic and noncystic masses. However, a solid mass occasionally contains few echoes, and a cyst may contain echoes from blood, debris, or crystals; these may cause diagnostic problems (Soderlund et al., 1986).

Although both CT and US may help delineate large neurofibromas (Figure 9–133) or other benign tumors, CT is generally reserved for those patients

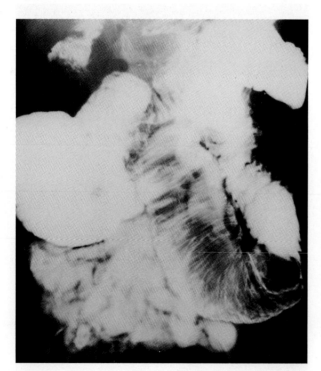

FIGURE 9–129. Small bowel intussusception in Peutz-Jeghers syndrome. Small bowel intussusception surrounded by barium gives a coiled-spring appearance in a dilated loop of jejunum on this small bowel follow-through examination. A hamartomatous polyp is the lead point.

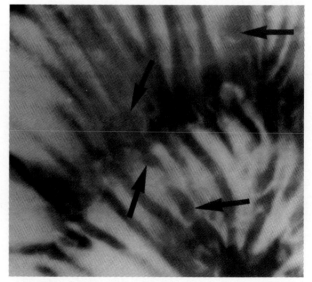

FIGURE 9–130. Small bowel hemangiomas. Multiple small filling defects are faintly seen on enteroclysis (*arrows*) and found at surgery.

in whom US is inconclusive or to better evaluate the anatomic extent of pathology. This is particularly likely when a mass is either very large or very small.

Angiography occasionally helps show vascular anomalies or bleeding sites (Fataar et al., 1981; Uflacker et al., 1985) and can lead to embolization to control hemorrhage (Chalmers et al., 1986).

Abnormal Fat Collections in the Abdomen

Lipomas, lipoblastoma, and lipoblastomatosis are rare fatty tumors in children which may occur in or adjacent to the small bowel or retroperitoneum. Lipomas in the omentum are rare and demonstrate an echoic appearance on US (Bowen et al., 1982; Haller et al., 1978). Lipomas can occur in other areas such as the retroperitoneum with displacement of adjacent organs , for example, ureters if lipomas are retroperitoneal (Bowen et al., 1982).

A form of massive fat replacement ıs a rare condition affecting the omentum and mesocolon (Hernandez et al., 1977). Gross intra-abdominal fat appears as lucencies on plain film, belying the general malnourished condition of the patient.

In addition to plain-film and ultrasonographic findings, CT and MR can be used to demonstrate the true extent and fatty nature of the lesion (Bowen et al., 1982; Ormson et al., 1985). Angiography is no longer indicated but shows an avascular mass if performed (Bowen et al., 1982).

Asymptomatic lipomas may not need specific therapy. However, there is a rare benign tumor of embryonal fat, namely, lipoblastoma or lipoblastomatosis, which has a tendency to local invasion but not to metastasize. These usually present in children under 3 years of age with a rapidly growing mass. These tumors may occur in the retroperitoneum or elsewhere but especially in limbs or intrathoracic areas (Stringel et al., 1982).

Malignant Tumors

Clinical Features

Malignant tumors are rare in children. Burkitt's and other non-Hodgkin's lymphomas are the most common of those that do occur. Lymphoma can involve the gastrointestinal tract at any site and any age (Bush and Ash, 1969; Solomons et al., 1976). In childhood, those in the first 8 years of life are most at risk (Bartram and Chrispin, 1973; Jenkin et al., 1969).

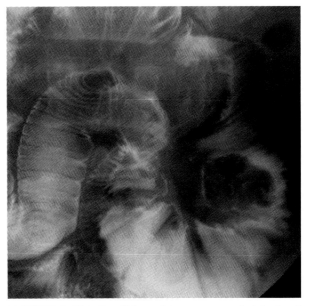

FIGURE 9–131. Small bowel hamartoma. A lobulated polyp in the distal jejunum is well delıneated by small bowel enteroclysis.

Most children with primary gastrointestinal lymphoma present with abdominal pain, vomiting, and weight loss; their symptoms are often due to a degree of distal small bowel obstruction (Cupps et al., 1969; Dunnick et al., 1979; Jenkin et al., 1969). An abdominal mass is usually palpable.

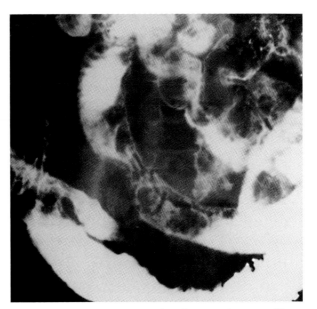

FIGURE 9–132. Mesenteric involvement in neurofibromatosis. The bowel loops are markedly separated due to neurofibromas affecting the adjacent mesentery.

Carcinoma of the small bowel and malignant peritoneal mesothelioma are extremely rare (Gutsman et al., 1976; Papadopoulos and Nolan, 1985).

Imaging

A soft-tissue mass or evidence of intussusception may be present on plain-film radiographs (Figure 9–134), and loops of adjacent bowel may show a constant appearance, suggesting involvement of contiguous bowel or mesentery (Bartram and Chrispin, 1973).

On small bowel follow-through examination, a polypoid mass or stricture may be seen (Figure 9–135). The mass may present as an intussusception and can be demonstrated by contrast examination (Figure 9–136). There may be irregular narrowed areas similar to those in Crohn's disease, and it may be difficult to differentiate these conditions (Figure 9–137) (Keller et al., 1982). Cross-sectional imaging is required to increase diagnostic confidence in separating Crohn's disease from lymphoma. Loops of bowel occasionally may be displaced by a large mesenteric mass (Figure 9–138) or may develop aneurysmal dilatation.

Ultrasonography, CT, and MR will demonstrate a tumor mass (Figure 9–139) and tumor in the bowel wall with tumor extent, particularly the extent of any adenopathy (Megibow et al., 1983). Ultrasonography may show a mass of mixed echogenicity (Figure 9–140) or a small bowel lesion with an echodense center (Figure 9–141); this appearance is due to intestinal mucosa, often eccentrically positioned, within a relatively echo-poor mass (Miller et al., 1980). Computed tomography can show thickened bowel wall and the relationship of the vascular structures (Figure 9–142). In children, bowel wall thickening in excess of 1 cm and lymph nodes in excess of 1 cm should raise suspicion for lymphoma (Siegel et al., 1988). Color Doppler interrogation of thickened bowel should be hyperemic in inflammatory bowel disease, which is helpful in differentiation from a hypovascular lymphomatous mass (Sarrazin and Wilson, 1996). Gallium-67-citrate scans will demonstrate uptake in a lymphoma mass lesion of the bowel (see Figure 9–140).

HEMORRHAGE AND TRAUMA TO BOWEL

Bowel Trauma

Clinical Features

Penetrating injury to the bowel from stabbing or gunshot requires surgical exploration, and imaging

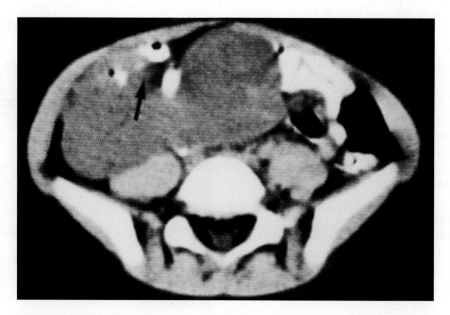

FIGURE 9–133. Neurofibromatosis. Computed tomography demonstrates a large neurofibroma flattening the right psoas muscle and separating (*arrow*) bowel loops that contain contrast.

plays little role. Blunt abdominal trauma is a major cause of bowel and mesenteric injury in which imaging plays a significant role. The incidence of bowel rupture in blunt trauma is low, under 10% in adults and even less common in children than in adults (Ford and Senac, 1993). However, early clinical signs may be occult or obscured by associated injury, making early clinical diagnosis difficult (Brown et al., 1992). Most solid organ injury now benefits from imaging delineation and expectant surgical management (Wing et al., 1985). This places great responsibility on radiologists and trauma surgeons to consider and diagnose bowel rupture early as any delay in management dramatically increases the morbidity and mortality associated with peritoneal contamination (Ford and Senac, 1993; Kovacs et al., 1986). Victims of motor vehicle accidents (especially passengers with lap belts but also pedestrians), falls from height, impalement on bicycle handlebars, crush injury, and being struck are common injuries. One should always be alert to child abuse, and a blow to the belly causing bowel injury from perforation and intramural hematoma, especially of the duodenum, are well-recognized presentations of child abuse (Kleinman, 1998). Mechanisms of injury include crushing, such as a lap belt forcing bowel against the vertebral column; shearing, as in rapid deceleration, where tearing from points of mesenteric fixation such as the ligament of Treitz or cecum occurs; and bursting, which presumes fluid-filled loops of bowel are shifted, temporarily forming closed loops and bursting in response to a rapid increase in abdominal pressures (Stevens et al., 1990).

Trauma to the bowel may result in intramural hematoma, intra- or retroperitoneal perforation, or transection. Mesenteric injuries include lacerations and rupture of mesenteric blood vessels with hematoma, possibly leading to ischemic areas of gut. The most common site of perforation in blunt abdominal trauma is the jejunum followed by the ileum, stomach, duodenum, and colon (Brown et al., 1992; Jamieson et al., 1996; Sivit et al., 1994).

Associated common intra-abdominal visceral injury includes hepatic, splenic, pancreatic, and renal injury. Blunt trauma to the abdomen is often found in the polytrauma victim with extra-abdominal injury, including head injury, spinal injury, limb fracture, pelvic fracture, and chest injury (Brown et al., 1992; Jamieson et al., 1995; Sivit et al., 1994). The lap belt injury complex merits special

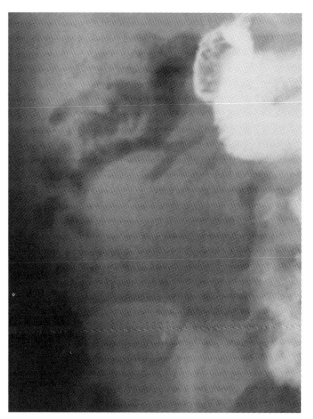

FIGURE 9–134. Non-Hodgkin's lymphoma affecting the ileum. A soft-tissue mass is displacing adjacent loops of bowel.

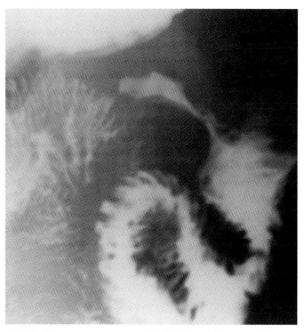

FIGURE 9–135. Non-Hodgkin's lymphoma affecting the jejunum. An irregular stricture in the jejunum is produced by encircling polypoid mass.

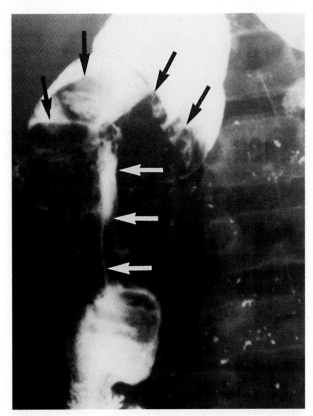

FIGURE 9–136. Non-Hodgkin's lymphoma affecting the terminal ileum. A narrow track of barium (*white arrows*) connects the distal normal small bowel to the ascending colon where the intussuscipiens is outlined by barium (*black arrows*). An intussusception of the terminal ileum was found at surgery.

attention as the presence of abdominal wall ecchymosis has a high incidence of Chance-type fractures—dislocations of the lumber spine—and bowel injuries (Hayes et al., 1991). A CT study of 61 children with lap belt ecchymosis reported that 21% had lumbar spine injury, 23% had hollow viscus injury (including two bladder ruptures), and 8% had both (Sivit et al., 1991b).

Symptoms of vomiting and obstruction can occur with intramural hematoma, especially of the duodenum. Delayed stricture of small bowel at sites of ischemia can produce bowel obstruction. This is well recognized after lap belt injury (Shalaby-Rana et al., 1992).

Imaging

Plain-Film Radiology. Radiography does have a place in assessment of the traumatized abdomen (Zahran et al., 1984) although the increasing availability and use of CT tend to reduce radiography's diagnostic value. It remains widely available and readily performed under portable circumstances in an emergency room. Pneumoperitoneum in the absence of pneumomediastinum or recent peritoneal lavage indicates bowel rupture but this is found in less than 40% of bowel perforation patients (Bulas et al., 1989; Cobb et al., 1986; Jamieson et al., 1996; Zahran et al., 1984). Retroperitoneal gas may give a mottled appearance and indicate duodenal or colonic perforation. Fractures may be more apparent on plain film, especially rib fracture and Chance-type fracture dislocation, which may shear in an axial plane and not be obvious on CT.

Contrast Examinations. These studies have little place in an acute setting. Duodenal hematoma is well demonstrated by an upper GI examination and appears as a smooth intramural mass (Figure 9–143) although thickening and crowding of the valvulae conniventes can distort the duodenal lumen and produce a picket-fence appearance. Obstruction is usually, but not always, incomplete (Figure 9–144). Rarely, contrast extravasation can be demonstrated (Figure 9–145). A coiled spring appearance is an acute phenomenon associated with

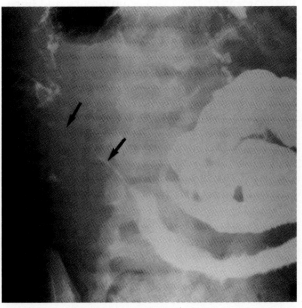

FIGURE 9–137. Non-Hodgkin's lymphoma affecting the terminal ileum. A narrow stricture in the terminal ileum (*arrows*) with mucosal irregularity and bowel loop separation of more proximal bowel mimics Crohn's disease.

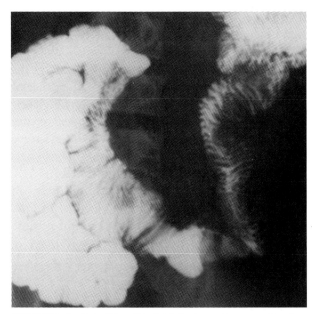

FIGURE 9–138. Non-Hodgkin's lymphoma affecting the mesentery. Loops of jejunum are fixed around a mesenteric mass.

a well-localized intramural hematoma. Ultrasonography and CT have assumed most of the diagnostic role in confirming duodenal hematoma but contrast assessment may accompany attempts to pass enteric feeding catheters past the hematoma to allow nutrition while resolution occurs.

An unusual patient who suffered localized trauma demonstrated a submucosal barium cast of the duodenum following an upper GI examination at a referring hospital (Figure 9–146). The cast was only discovered on a follow-up radiograph obtained 3 weeks later as the patient continued to vomit. A repeat examination showed complete obstruction to the duodenum, and a feeding tube was inserted with some difficulty past the obstruction. The barium cast slowly faded away over many months as the patient was fed by tube.

In the jejunum and ileum, intramural hemorrhage does not tend to cause a localized mass but more commonly gives a clearly demarcated stack-of-coins appearance due to edema or hemorrhage affecting the valvulae conniventes, similar to that seen in Schönlein-Henoch purpura. Intramural hemorrhage may occasionally act as a lead point in an intussusception.

Ultrasonography. Ultrasonography readily allows diagnosis and follow-up of duodenal hematoma

(Figures 9–144, 9–147). The mass of the hematoma is initially echogenic but evolves to a mixed echogenic lesion and later to a sonolucent lesion, indicating liquefaction (Hernanz-Schulman et al., 1989). Hematoma may be difficult to separate from the pancreas and so may be confused with a pancreatic pseudocyst (Raby and Meire, 1986). The amylase level with or without a contrast study can confirm the diagnosis. Pressure effects secondary to hematoma may affect the common bile duct and inferior vena cava (Foley and Teele, 1979).

Computed Tomography. Computed tomography is a powerful imaging modality for evaluating stable patients following blunt abdominal trauma (Berger and Kuhn, 1981; Kaufman et al., 1989; Ruess et al., 1997; Taylor et al., 1988; Wing et al., 1985). Its role in assessing bowel and mesenteric injury has also been established (Bulas et al., 1989; Jamieson et al., 1996; Sivit et al., 1994).

Demonstration of extraluminal air, intraperitoneal or retroperitoneal, indicates bowel rupture in the absence of pneumothorax/pneumomediastinum or prior diagnostic peritoneal lavage. False-positive free air has been described via a bladder rupture and urethral catheterization (Cook et al., 1989). Extraluminal air is only found in 30 to 45% of surgically proven bowel perforations (Casey et al., 1995;

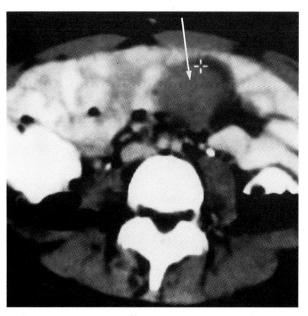

FIGURE 9–139. Neurofibrosarcoma. Computed tomography demonstrates a small relatively well-demarcated mass (*arrow*) which on histology was a neurofibrosarcoma.

Jamieson et al., 1996; Sivit et al., 1994). Similarly, extravasation of oral contrast is seldom seen as it is not routinely given in many centers. When given, ileus usually prevents it reaching the site of perforation unless it is in the upper GI tract (Clancy et al., 1993). Free air may be obvious (Figure 9–148) but small collections in mesenteric folds, held by the midrectus and pararectus recesses of the anterior abdominal wall, in the porta hepatis, along the falciform ligament and located in the retroperitoneum can be easily overlooked (Figure 9–149). Reviewing the entire CT study on wide window settings to better evaluate air collections is recommended.

The high specificity but poor sensitivity of finding extraluminal air makes it essential to look for indirect or subtle signs of bowel rupture. These

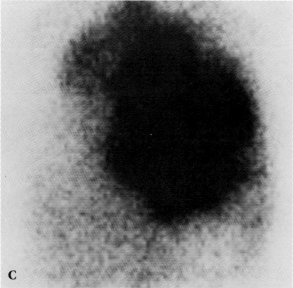

FIGURE 9–140. Burkitt's lymphoma. A large abdominal mass appears of mixed echogenicity on US (*A*), of soft-tissue density on CT (*B*), and actively takes up gallium 67 citrate (*C*).

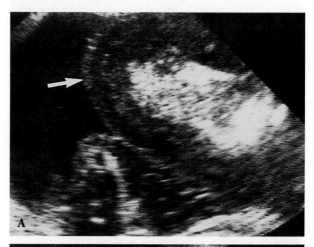

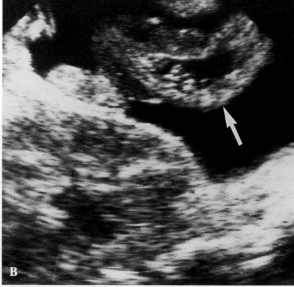

FIGURE 9–141. Non-Hodgkin's lymphoma. *A*, A loop of bowel has a thick wall (*arrow*) and an echogenic center with some adjacent ascitic fluid. *B*, Another bowel loop has a thick and irregular wall (*arrow*) outlined by surrounding ascitic fluid.

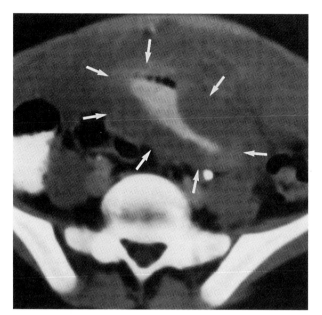 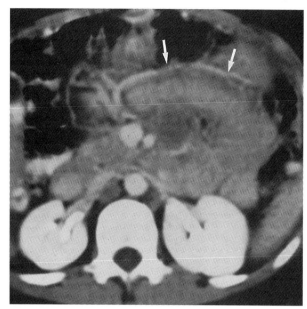

FIGURE 9–142. Burkitt's lymphoma. *A,* There is thickened bowel wall (*arrows*). *B,* The mesenteric vessels (*arrows*) are seen to pass over part of the mass.

include bowel wall thickening, bowel wall enhancement, bowel dilatation, and significant free peritoneal fluid, especially if no solid organ injury or pelvic fracture is present (Hara et al., 1992; Jamieson et al., 1996; Sivit et al., 1991a; 1994). Although common in perforation, the indirect signs of bowel rupture are not pathognomonic and can be found in nonperforating bowel and mesenteric injury (Figure 9–150) (Jamieson et al., 1996).

Mesenteric abnormality is commonly associated with bowel and abdominal trauma. It manifests as diffuse increased density in the mesenteric fat, focal density of a hematoma, and often, adjacent bowel wall thickening and free peritoneal fluid (Donohue et al., 1987; Jamieson et al., 1996; Rizzo et al., 1989).

The CT findings of severely injured children who are inadequately resuscitated and in hypovolemic shock overlap the findings of bowel rupture (Jamieson et al., 1996; Sivit et al., 1994). Known as "hypoperfusion complex" or "hypovolemic shock bowel," the findings include diffuse dilatation and enhancement of bowel wall, with free intraperitoneal fluid but also dense persistent enhancement of solid organs and diminished caliber of the aorta and inferior vena cava (Figure 9–151) (Taylor et al., 1987). This group of patients is usually clinically obvious with severe polytrauma, head injury, craniocervical disruption, and

tenuous hemodynamic stability. However, they may also have bowel perforation.

All potential bowel perforation victims require diligent and repeated clinical assessment. Fostering open and ready channels of communication between trauma surgeons and radiologists at the time of

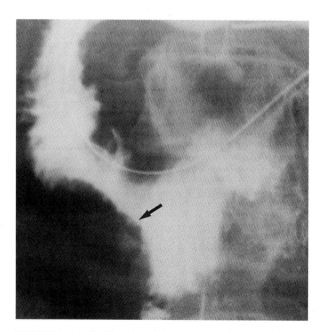

FIGURE 9–143. Duodenal hematoma. A smooth mass (*arrow*) projects into the duodenal lumen. Smaller hematomas scallop the opposite duodenal wall.

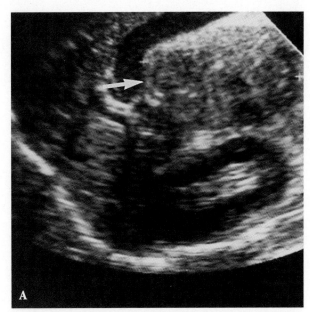
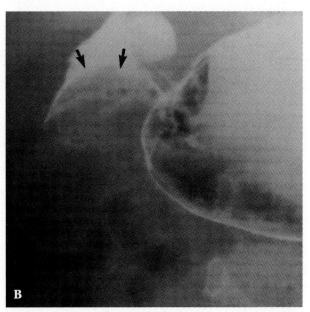

FIGURE 9–144. Duodenal hematoma. *A,* A smooth mass (*arrow*) projects into and completely obstructs the duodenal lumen. *B,* Longitudinal US shows an echogenic mass (*between arrows*) anterior to the right kidney and posteromedial to the gallbladder.

imaging is essential to integrate the clinical situation with imaged findings. This is especially important when indirect signs of bowel rupture are present and when there is overlap with mesenteric injury or

FIGURE 9–145. Duodenal hematoma and tear. A tear in the second part of the duodenum, shown as a leak on contrast study, was unsuspected at prior surgery and required prolonged drainage before it would close.

hypovolemic complex which may not benefit from laparotomy.

Signs of duodenal injury and perforation on CT merit specific attention as they are predominantly retroperitoneal where the duodenum crosses the vertebral bodies. Computed tomography depicts extraluminal air, abnormal fluid, or oral contrast adjacent to the rupture, and tracks this into retroperitoneal planes, often to the right pararenal space (Figure 9–152) (Hofer and Cohen, 1989; Kunin et al., 1993). Differentiation of a perforation from a hematoma is important as hematoma is managed conservatively whereas perforation undergoes immediate surgery.

Other Causes of Bowel Hemorrhage

Bowel wall hematoma may occur following minor trauma in a patient with a bleeding diathesis such as a hemophiliac, a thrombocytopenic leukemic patient, an oncology patient undergoing therapy, or a patient on anticoagulant therapy. Schönlein-Henoch purpura is a fairly common cause of nontraumatic bowel hematoma.

Schönlein-Henoch Purpura

Schönlein-Henoch (anaphylactoid) purpura is a nonthrombocytopenic purpura that is caused by an acute diffuse vasculitis of uncertain etiology and that affects the blood vessels of the gut, skin, joints, kidneys, and (rarely) the central nervous system. The purpura effects the body centrifugally, and the diagnosis can easily be made when gastrointestinal bleeding, nephritis, or arthritis are detected.

Schönlein-Henoch purpura is associated with hemorrhage and edema of the bowel wall. The jejunum is most commonly affected (Glasier et al., 1981). The radiologic appearance may be similar to trauma. On barium examination, the small bowel wall pathology has a localized stack-of-coins appearance (Figure 9–153) or there may be more severe involvement with gross thickening of mucosal folds, thumbprinting, and separation of bowel loops (Figure 9–154). Ultrasonography can demonstrate the bowel wall thickening caused by the hemorrhage and edema (Couture et al., 1992). Hematomas are

echogenic but become sonolucent with liquefaction (see Figure 9–147). The mucosa and bowel wall may be hyperemic on color Doppler investigation (Siegel, 1995). Reported CT findings are nonspecific but bowel wall thickening, mesenteric edema, and vascular engorgement in a young patient with acute abdominal symptoms should raise suspicion of Schönlein-Henoch purpura (Jeong, et al., 1997). In particular, CT demonstrates multifocal sites of pathology in this condition, and in a study of 7 patients, CT demonstrated lymphadenopathy in 6, a feature not previously reported (Jeong, et al., 1997).

A small hematoma may act occasionally as a lead point of an intermittent intussusception, often of small bowel (Figure 9–155), and (rarely) may even cause intestinal obstruction requiring surgery (Figure 9–156).

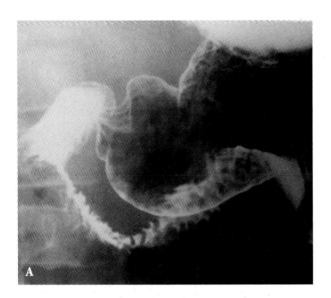

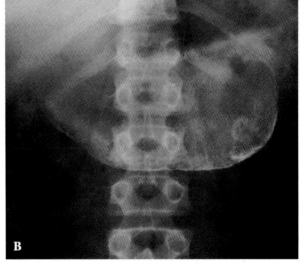

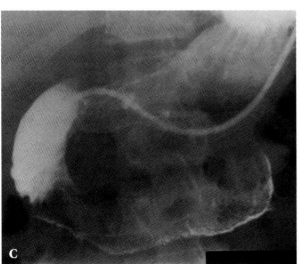

FIGURE 9–146. Duodenal hematoma and tear. *A,* An upper GI exmination at a referring hospital shows an extrinsic duodenal impression. *B,* A submucosal barium cast was present on a follow-up radiograph 3 weeks after the upper GI examination. *C,* A spot film from an upper GI examination showed complete obstruction to the duodenum, and a feeding tube was inserted with some difficulty past the obstruction. The barium cast slowly faded away over many months whilst the patient was fed by tube.

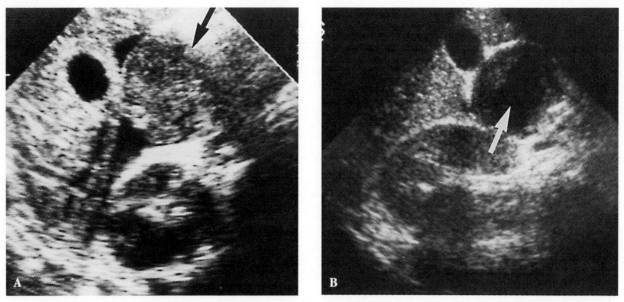

FIGURE 9–147. Duodenal hematoma. *A*, Transverse US shows an echogenic mass (*arrow*) anterior to the right kidney and medial to the gallbladder. *B*, Follow-up US shows cystic change due to early central liquefaction of the hematoma (*arrow*).

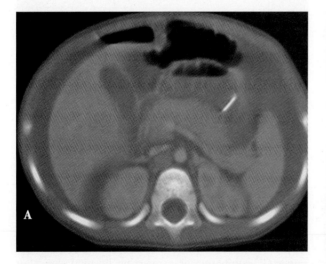

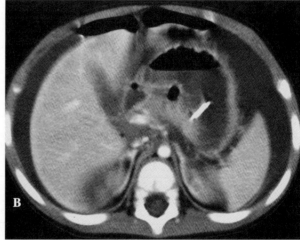

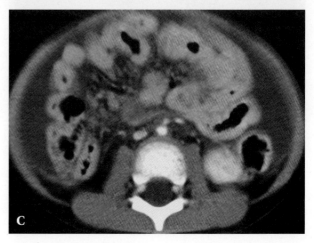

FIGURE 9–148. Jejunal perforation following nonaccidental injury. *A*, Image on CT with wide windows demonstrates free intraperitoneal air in a three-year-old child who had been punched 24 hours previously. *B*, Other images showed extensive free fluid with intact solid organs. *C*, Enhancing, thickened bowel wall with bowel dilatation is present.

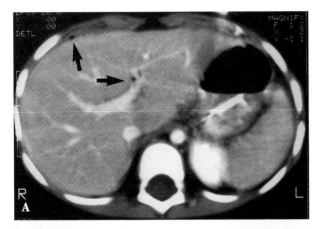

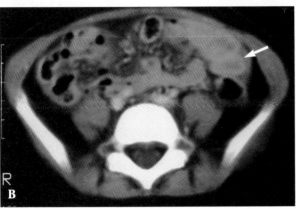

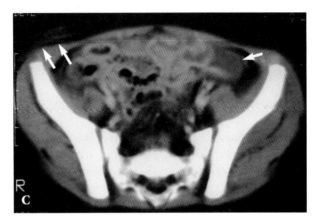

FIGURE 9–149. Jejunal perforation following a lap belt injury. *A,* Computed tomography demonstrates subtle bubbles of free air (*arrows*) and intact solid organs. *B,* Focal, thickened, enhancing bowel wall with dilatation, associated free fluid (*arrow*), and increased mesenteric fat density is present. *C,* Abdominal wall contusion from lap belt (*double arrow*) and free intraperitoneal fluid (*arrow*).

MALABSORPTION

In the past, the term *steatorrhea* was used synonymously with malabsorption since the only specific causes of malabsorption were felt to be cystic fibrosis and celiac disease. These two conditions were separated by Dorothy Anderson in 1938 (Anderson, 1938). It is now known that malabsorption is a nonspecific finding in many diseases of childhood and may be associated with fatty, watery, or normal stools. Many conditions produce malabsorption, a few of which are important to the pediatric radiologist and are considered in the following section.

A gamut of investigations are available for malabsorption. Before embarking on any of these, however, the physician must ensure that food intake has been adequate and suitable and that the child is not suffering from dietary malnutrition.

Pancreatic Enzyme Deficiency

Cystic Fibrosis

Clinical Features. A defect in the permeability of epithelium for the transport of chloride ions is the underlying physiologic problem in cystic fibrosis (Quinton, 1983; Knowles, 1985). This results in abnormal exocrine gland secretion, producing con-

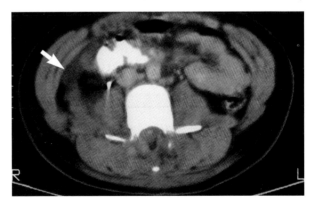

FIGURE 9–150. Chance fracture and soft tissue injury following a lap belt injury. On CT, there is tremendous posterior soft-tissue swelling associated with a "Chance-type" fracture dislocation of the lumbar spine. Thickened bowel wall in the left abdomen, increased mesenteric density and free intraperitoneal fluid (*arrow*) are also present. Laparotomy demonstrated mesenteric edema and hematoma, but no bowel perforation.

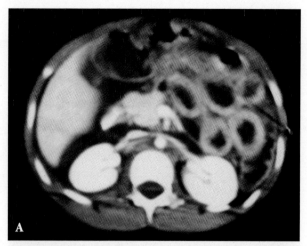
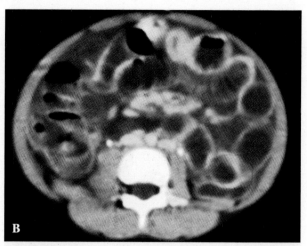

FIGURE 9–151. Hypovolemic shock bowel. *A, B,* Computed tomography shows generalized dilated, enhancing bowel wall with thickening and free intraperitoneal fluid. The solid organs show persistent dense enhancement and the caliber of major vessels is reduced. This patient had an atlanto-occipital disruption and demised. No intra-abdominal pathology showed post mortem.

centrated pancreatic secretions which inspissate and obstruct pancreatic ducts. Pancreatic inflammation, atrophy, fibrosis, duct ectasia, cyst formation, and calcification ensues (Agrons et al., 1996). When production and transport of lipase and proteolytic enzymes to the gut is less than 10% of normal, clinical manifestations of steatorrhea and malabsorption occur.

Imaging. The most striking feature of this disease is the lack of barium abnormality in a hungry child who fails to put on weight due to malabsorption. A nonspecific small bowel abnormality in which the small bowel is irregularly dilated with thick mucos-

al folds may be seen on barium examination (Harris et al., 1963). The intestinal wall may be thickened, and the transit time of barium can be prolonged. Flocculation, fragmentation, and segmentation of the barium are also nonspecific signs, more common in the past when malnutrition was usual in cystic fibrosis and when barium preparations were more likely to precipitate out of suspension. Marginal filling defects in the small bowel have been found that may be due to adherent mucus from hyperplastic goblet cells. These may be long-standing filling defects, which suggests a different but uncertain etiology (Bartram and Small, 1971; Djurhuus et al., 1973; Taussig et al., 1973).

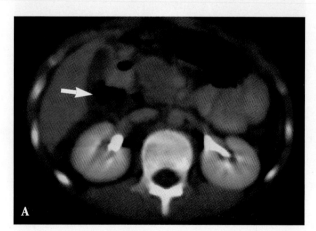
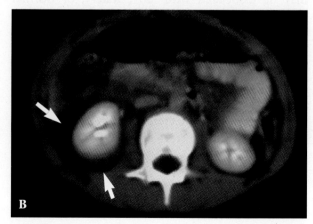

FIGURE 9–152. Duodenal rupture following blunt abdominal trauma. *A,* Computed tomography demonstrated possible extraluminal air bubbles (*arrow*). *B,* Obvious retroperitoneal fluid (*arrows*) in the right pararenal space on CT.

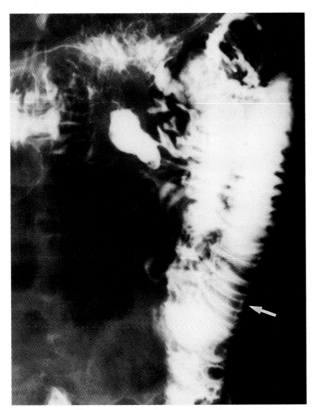

FIGURE 9–153. Schönlein-Henoch purpura. Thickened valvulae conniventes (*arrow*) give the appearance of a stack of coins.

The duodenum is especially distorted, with very thick folds (Figure 6–157) that may be distorted further by a dilated colon laden with feces. Smudging of the prominent duodenal folds may extend into the jejunum and ileum (Berk and Lee, 1973; Taussig et al., 1973). The cause of the mucosal pattern of the small bowel is uncertain. There is no correlation between it and either the abdominal symptoms, or the hypoproteinemia secondary to malabsorption, or hepatic biliary cirrhosis (Taussig et al., 1973).

The pancreas is small and echogenic on US and occasionally shows calcifications visible on plain radiographs (see Chapter 13). Cystic changes in the pancreas are rare and best shown by US and CT.

Shwachman-Diamond Syndrome

Clinical Features. Shwachman-Diamond syndrome consists of pancreatic insufficiency, neutropenia, and metaphyseal chondrodysplasia, with anemia or thrombocytopenia occasionally present (Shwachman et al., 1964). Initially, patients with this condi-

tion were thought to have cystic fibrosis but the sweat chloride test is consistently normal and the prognosis is much better. The neutropenia may be constant or intermittent; so a normal leukocyte count does not exclude the diagnosis. Occasionally there is a familial incidence of the condition, which is probably autosomal recessive (Burke et al., 1967; Shwachman et al., 1964).

Fat malabsorption due to pancreatic insufficiency is usually present but in the majority of patients, this improves with age and appears to be associated with marginal improvement in pancreatic lipase secretion (Hill et al., 1982).

Affected children often present with failure to thrive and diarrhea at a young age. Short stature becomes more obvious as the child grows older, and many children are under the third percentile for height. Respiratory function tests reveal a reduced chest wall compliance and decreased total lung volume in children under the age of 2 years (Aggett et al., 1980) which may be so severe as to mimic asphyxiating thoracic dystrophy. At the other end of

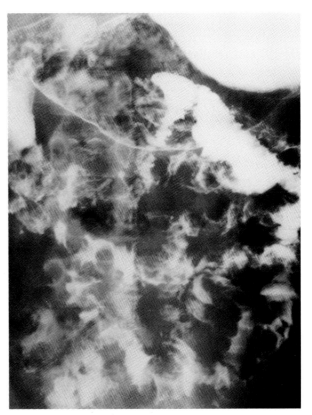

FIGURE 9–154. Schönlein-Henoch purpura. There is gross thickening of mucosal folds, thumbprinting, and separation of bowel loops.

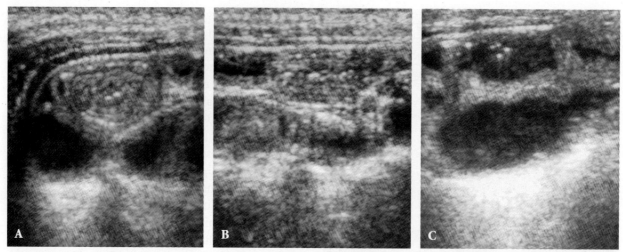

FIGURE 9–155. Schönlein-Henoch purpura, with small bowel intussusception. *A,B,* Transverse and longitudinal US images of a small bowel intussusception obtained during a period of cramping abdominal pain. *C,* Within 5 minutes, the pain resolved and only dilated loops of small bowel with minimal wall thickening remained.

the clinical spectrum, a figure skater who won an Olympic gold medal for Canada has Shwachman-Diamond syndrome.

Imaging. The first evidence of disease may be a narrow, elongated chest similar to that seen in asphyxiating thoracic dystrophy (Figure 9–158A) (Karjoo et al., 1973). Irregularity of the anterior ends of the

ribs may be seen at or before 2 years of age (Burke et al., 1967), and the rib ends may be flared (Figure 9–158B) (Aggett et al., 1980).

The slightly older child may show evidence of undertubulation of long bones and variably deficient metaphyseal ossification (chondrometaphyseal dysplasia), usually around the hips and knees (Figure 9–158C) although other areas can be involved

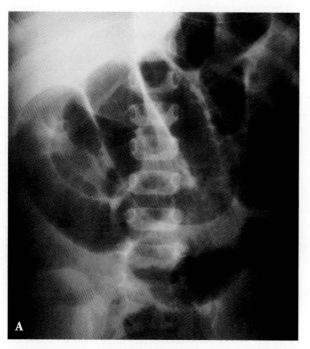

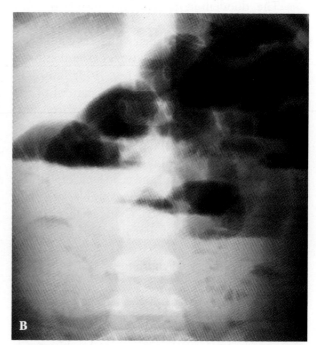

FIGURE 9–156. Intestinal obstruction due to intussusception in Schönlein-Henoch purpura. *A,* Supine film shows multiple dilated loops of proximal small bowel. *B,* Erect film demonstrates multiple air-fluid levels.

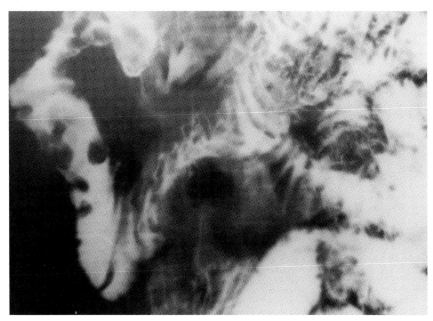

FIGURE 9–157. Cystic fibrosis. The duodenal mucosal folds are prominent.

(Fellman et al., 1972; McLennan and Steinbach, 1974; Taybi et al., 1969). The hips may develop coxa vara deformities late in childhood (Stanley and Sutcliffe, 1973). The evidence of the chondrometaphyseal dysplasia disappears in later life, leaving the bones only slightly shorter than normal. Clinodactyly due to a short hypoplastic fifth middle phalanx can be present (Aggett et al., 1980).

The small bowel pattern is often normal on barium studies or may show nonspecific changes of malabsorption such as dilatation, flocculation, and segmentation.

Mucosal Diseases

Celiac Disease

Clinical Features. Celiac disease (gluten enteropathy or nontropical sprue) results from an inherited intolerance to the gluten that is found in wheat and rye. Ten percent of patients with the disease have family members who are also affected but the exact mode of inheritance is uncertain. Celiac disease is genetically linked with dermatitis herpetiformis; there is also an increased incidence of HLA-B8.

The disease usually becomes apparent before the child reaches 2 years of age because symptoms such as chronic diarrhea, protein-losing enteropathy, irritability, vomiting, and failure to thrive occur some time after the introduction of food containing gluten. Thirty-three percent of all infants with chronic diarrhea have celiac disease (Larcher et al., 1977). Presentation is delayed sometimes for years or even decades although the child's growth is usually retarded and the child may be anemic. Other symptoms include delayed puberty, abdominal cramps, and a poor appetite.

Imaging. Radiology plays little part in the diagnosis of celiac disease, which rests on biopsy and clinical findings; barium studies are particularly of little value (Figure 9–159) (Weizman et al., 1984). The radiologic appearance is discussed below if studies are performed for other purposes.

Plain-film radiographs of patients with celiac disease show small bowel dilatation (Haworth et al., 1968). Hypoalbuminemia can cause small bowel dilatation but is probably not the cause in celiac disease (Farthing et al., 1981).

Small bowel follow-through examination shows similar dilatation with thickened transverse mucosal folds, flocculation, segmentation, and delay in transit of barium. With the newer barium preparations, flocculation and segmentation occur in less than 20% of patients, with mild small bowel dilatation in 70% and duodenal abnormalities such as erosions or thickened nodular folds in up to 80% (Marn et al., 1986). Other reported radiologic signs are reversal of the normal jejunoileal fold pattern, with a featureless jejunum and transverse folds in the ileum (Bova et al., 1985).

Enteroclysis in adults is probably more accurate in detecting abnormalities such as the fold separation in the proximal jejunum which is present in

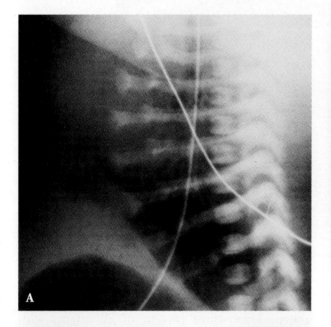

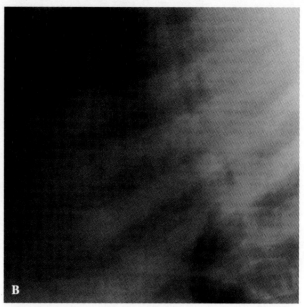

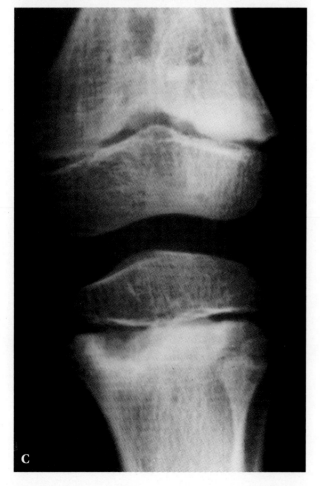

FIGURE 9–158. Shwachman-Diamond syndrome. *A*, Lateral chest radiograph shows short narrow ribs similar to those seen in asphyxiating thoracic dystrophy. This is the first radiologic evidence of disease and is present at birth but only occasionally seen. *B*, In another child, there is irregularity and flaring of the anterior ends of normal-length ribs best seen in patients between 1 and 2 years of age. At our hospital this has been the most reliable radiologic sign. *C*, A third child presented at an older age, and lucencies are present in the distal femoral and proximal tibial metaphyses, indicating deficient metaphyseal ossification. This dysplasia is best seen in patients over the age of 6 years and disappears after epiphyseal fusion.

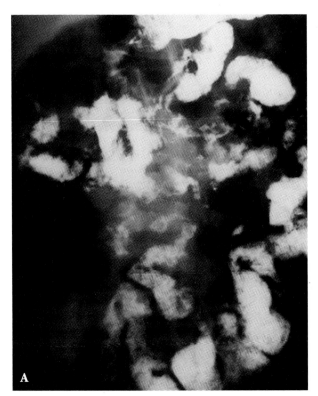 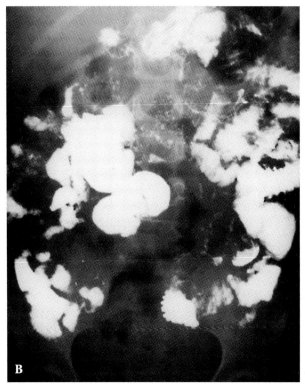

FIGURE 9–159. Malabsorption pattern. Both patients have segmentation, flocculation, and mild bowel dilatation, a nonspecific malabsorption pattern. *A*, Celiac disease. Mucosal biopsy was abnormal, and biochemically proven malabsorption was present with high fecal fat excretion. *B*, Failure to thrive due to poor intake. Small bowel biopsy was normal, and there was no biochemical evidence of malabsorption. The patient thrived when given an adequate diet.

most patients with celiac disease (Herlinger and Maglinte, 1986); however, enteroclysis is not indicated in children. Double-contrast barium meals in adult celiac patients can show a "bubbly" duodenal bulb if there is duodenitis that will aggravate the symptoms of the celiac disease (Jones et al., 1984b).

The small bowel pattern on barium follow-through examination has been used to detect celiac disease (Munyer and Moss, 1980; Tully and Feinberg, 1974) but it is normal in 5% of proven cases (Masterson and Sweeney, 1976). Unfortunately, an abnormal barium pattern is nonspecific and not diagnostic of either celiac disease or malabsorption (see Figure 9–159) (Isbell et al., 1969; Kumar and Bartram, 1979; Weizman et al., 1984). A granular barium pattern in the large bowel on follow-through examination may be seen (Duffrenne and Verdier, 1977) but is nonspecific.

Because treatment of celiac disease necessitates lifelong abstinence from gluten, the diagnosis should be made with certainty. This requires a jejunal biopsy demonstrating villous atrophy; but as

this biopsy finding may also occur in other conditions (e.g., gastroenteritis, cow's milk protein sensitivity, and giardiasis), confirmation of the diagnosis requires that the jejunal biopsy revert to normal after reintroduction of a gluten-free diet. If doubt still remains, the patient should be given a gluten challenge, and histologic relapse should be documented. Fluoroscopy can ensure accurate positioning of a biopsy capsule, and when the biopsy capsule (such as a Crosby capsule) is fired, fluoroscopy can see the knife block move, ensuring (before the capsule is withdrawn) that the biopsy has been successful (Lamont, 1983).

Small bowel intussusception is a well-recognized complication of celiac disease (Ruoff et al., 1968). It is transient and may be found in up to 20% of patients (Cohen and Lintott, 1978).

Lymphadenopathy may be seen on CT in patients with celiac disease and is a worrisome finding due to the association of celiac disease and lymphoma (Jones et al., 1984a). On a gluten free diet, however, this lymphadenopathy may regress, and only reactive hyperplasia may be found on biopsy (Jones et al., 1984a).

Celiac disease is probably associated with an increased incidence of gastrointestinal lymphoma, carcinoma, malignant histiocytosis, and ulcerative jejunitis (Brunton and Guyer, 1983) although this is debated. The small bowel and esophagus appear to be particularly affected by carcinoma (Collins et al., 1978). Megacolon is a rare association with celiac disease but evacuation of this megacolon is normal (Kappelman et al., 1977). Occasionally hyposplenism, a loss of normal hematologic and immunologic function of the spleen, may be associated with celiac disease.

Microvillus Inclusion Disease

Some infants with intractable diarrhea cannot be definitely diagnosed (Larcher et al., 1977). Among these, there are rare patients whose prognoses are very poor and who have microvillus inclusion disease (Davidson et al., 1978; Phillips et al., 1985). There are two types, congenital microvillus atrophy and acquired or autoimmune villus atrophy.

Congenital microvillus atrophy superficially resembles celiac disease but is unrelated to gluten and is associated with diarrhea from birth (unlike celiac disease) and with failure to thrive. There is a familial tendency (Davidson et al., 1978). The inclusions on electron microscopy are characteristic.

Acquired or autoimmune villus atrophy presents later in life and also superficially resembles celiac disease, with diarrhea unrelated to gluten.

Radiologic features can be similar to those of celiac disease, with dilation of bowel loops, fragmentation and segmentation of barium on follow-through examinations. Infants with the disease are at risk of gallstones and renal stones (Figure 9–160).

Tropical Sprue

Tropical sprue is widespread in some areas of the world, and many of its clinical effects and radiologic abnormalities resemble celiac disease. However, 2 weeks of treatment with tetracycline and folic acid is curative, and the presence or absence of gluten in the diet is irrelevant. Small bowel dilatation occurs when serum albumin falls below 27 g per liter even in the absence of other disease, and this has been postulated as a cause for bowel dilatation in tropical sprue. No correlation between albumin levels and bowel dilatation on barium follow-through has been found (McLean et al., 1982).

Disaccharidase Deficiency

Disaccharidase deficiency may be an inherited primary condition or secondary to an insult to the intestinal mucosa. The secondary type is more common and can follow gastroenteritis or many other gastrointestinal diseases that injure the mucosa. A number of

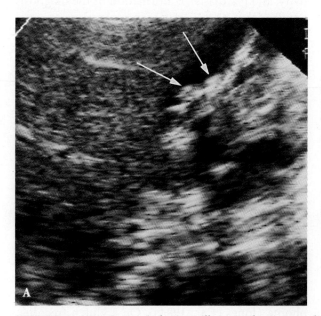 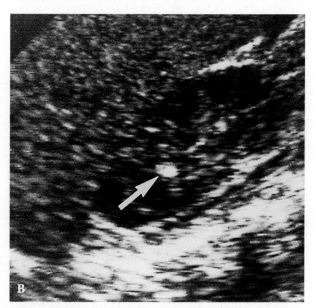

FIGURE 9–160. Congenital microvillus atrophy. Longitudinal US show echogenic opacities (*arrows*) representing gallstones (*A*) and a calculus in the right kidney (*B*) (see Chapter 8).

enzymes can be affected, and different combinations of these produce various conditions; sucrase-isomaltase deficiency and lactase deficiency are the commonest varieties. Primary lactase deficiency is especially common in Africans and Asians.

Early symptoms of lactose intolerance include watery diarrhea, abdominal distension, dehydration, and vomiting, which develop within a few hours after drinking cow's milk. In older children, crampy abdominal pain with borborygmi, nausea, and bloating may occur.

The diagnosis is made by a combination of breath hydrogen tests (Newcomer et al., 1975) or biopsy and measurements of enzyme levels; hence, the radiologic diagnosis of lactase deficiency is only of historic interest. Radiologic diagnosis was made by incorporating lactose with barium in a lactose-barium small bowel study. This mixture produces small and large bowel dilatation with dilution of barium, often with intestinal hurry causing diarrhea and abdominal cramps (Laws and Neale, 1966; Preger and Amberg, 1967). This investigation has a 10% false-negative rate when compared to assay of disaccharidase in a jejunal biopsy, which remains the definitive test. There is also a 10% false-positive rate in subjects with normal lactase levels (Morrison et al., 1974).

Cow's Milk Protein Sensitivity

Various proteins found in the milk of cows may adversely affect young children. Symptoms usually develop before the first 2 years of life and are most common under 1 year of age. The symptoms include diarrhea, vomiting, protein-losing enteropathy, and failure to thrive. Eosinophilia may be present. In some cases there may be an anaphylactic reaction to cow's milk protein resulting in shock, respiratory distress and even death.

The severity of symptoms varies. They may mimic celiac disease or become so severe that diarrhea with a fatal outcome occurs unless total parenteral alimentation is used. Radiology is seldom helpful in making the diagnosis but may be useful in excluding a structural anomaly. On US, hyperechoic tubular and round masses have been described, probably representing small bowel loops filled with malabsorbed milk (Avni et al., 1986).

Eosinophilic Gastroenteritis

Eosinophilic gastroenteritis can present with malabsorption or even with protein-losing enteropathy (Gorske et al., 1969) and is considered with other idiopathic inflammatory bowel diseases earlier in this chapter and in Chapter 10.

Hereditary Angioneurotic Edema

Hereditary angioneurotic edema is a rare autosomal dominant condition in which edema intermittently affects many organs including those of the gastrointestinal tract. The symptoms usually start in middle or late childhood. Involvement of the glottis may occur and can result in death. Abdominal pain is the most common gastrointestinal symptom. Bowel loop separation and mucosal folds thickened with edema are seen on small bowel examination with barium (Ellis and McConnel, 1969). These findings resolve after the acute attack.

Abetalipoproteinemia

Abetalipoproteinemia is an autosomal recessive condition that induces fat malabsorption but also produces retinitis pigmentosa and progressive neurologic deterioration at a late age as a result of vitamin A and E deficiencies. Fat is absorbed from the diet into cells that line the small bowel but cannot be transported out into the rest of the body due to the absence of beta lipoproteins, which gives rise to defective chylomicron formation. Acanthocytosis may be the presenting clue in an otherwise well child. Treatment consists of substituting fat with predominantly medium-chain triglycerides and oral administration of large doses of fat-soluble vitamins, particularly vitamins A and E. Barium examination shows thickening of the small bowel mucosal folds and large bowel haustra (Weinstein et al., 1973).

Intestinal Lymphangiectasia

Intestinal lymphangiectasia is a rare condition in which excessive protein is lost into the bowel lumen from abnormal small bowel lymphatics. This is often associated with steatorrhea, lymphopenia, and hypoproteinemia. A relative deficiency of the humoral and cellular immune systems is associated with lymphangiectasia although infections are rarely frequent or severe.

The disease is usually congenital and presents in infancy but occasionally occurs later, secondary to retroperitoneal fibrosis or pancreatitis (Olmsted and Madewell, 1976). Growth failure, diarrhea, vomiting, and edema are common symptoms. Abdominal distension from chylous ascites may develop early or late in the disease. Other lymphatics occasionally are also abnormal (Kingman et al., 1982) and may produce asymmetric swelling in the arms or legs. Rarely, the lymphangiectasia may be associated with pulmonary lymphangiectasia or with Noonan's syndrome (Herzog et al., 1976; Lanning et al., 1978).

Reported ultrasonographic signs include ascites, diffuse bowel wall thickening, mesenteric edema, dilated mesenteric lymphatics, and thick gallbladder and urinary bladder walls (Dorne and Jequier, 1986). These nonspecific signs may be useful as US is often used early in children.

Of affected children, 25% will have normal small bowel barium studies. The remainder have thickened valvulae conniventes, dilution of the barium column, and little if any dilatation of the bowel lumen (Figures 9–161, 9–162) (Shimkin et al., 1970). The appearance of the thickened folds has been likened to a cogwheel. The thickening of the folds is probably due to the villous lymphatic dilatation seen histologically (Olmsted and Madewell, 1976). Involvement of the large bowel is rarely detected on enema examination although polypoid lesions have been found (Marshak et al., 1979).

Lymphangiography, seldom performed, would demonstrate hypoplastic glands or ducts.

Protein loss into the small bowel may be documented with chromium-51- or iodine-131-albumin scintigraphic studies.

Immunoglobulin Deficiency Syndromes

Isolated IgA deficiency and idiopathic acquired hypogammaglobulinemia may produce a nonspecific malabsorption type of small bowel pattern on barium follow-through examination similar to that seen in celiac disease (Marshak et al., 1979). This is probably due to infections rather than a primary small bowel problem. Dysgammaglobulinemias may be associated with lymphoid hyperplasia that is most marked in the distal ileum although it may occur throughout the small bowel (Marshak et al., 1974). Lymphoma may develop and should be suspected if untoward clinical or radiologic signs are seen. Giardiasis is common in association with the immunoglobulin deficiency syndromes, especially IgA deficiency.

Graft-Versus-Host Disease

Graft-versus-host disease occurs in bone marrow transplantation patients when donor T lymphocytes damage target organs, usually skin, liver, and the gastrointestinal tract. The entire gastrointestinal tract from esophagus to rectum can be involved. It presents with watery diarrhea and a maculopapular skin rash approximately 1 to 7 weeks after bone marrow or organ transplantation (Fisk et al., 1981). The differential diagnosis includes infectious enteritis (in particular, cytomegalovirus), enteritis from radiation or chemotherapy, neutropenic colitis, pseudomembraneous colitis, and intra-abdominal abscess (Donnelly, 1996).

Plain films may show (in order of decreasing frequency) air-fluid levels, bowel wall and mucosal thickening, a gasless abdomen, bowel dilatation, pneumatosis intestinalis and/or ascites (Maile et al., 1985). In the acute phase, the small bowel mucosa on barium follow-through examination has thickened or flattened folds (Figure 9–163), a thickened bowel wall, rapid transit, and excess intraluminal fluid. The small bowel folds may disappear, especially distally (Schimmelpenninck and Zwaan, 1982). If studied with barium, the colon has mucosal irregularity and ulceration, with loss of haustral folds, thickening of the wall, and narrowing of the lumen (Fisk et al., 1981). At a later stage, these radiologic signs become strikingly segmental in distribution, and resolution finally occurs in those patients who survive (Fisk et al., 1981). With endoscopy and cross-sectional imaging, recourse to barium studies is reduced.

Cardinal CT findings are diffuse involvement and striking bowel mucosal enhancement (Donnelly and Morris, 1996). Also described are bowel dilatation, fold enlargement, and bowel wall thickening although the latter is often not present (Donnelly and Morris, 1996; Jones et al., 1986). Submucosal edema and hemorrhage can give a low attenuation area within thickened bowel wall, giving a targetlike appearance (Jones et al., 1986). There is a characteristic mucosal enhancement that corresponds to the histologic finding of mucosal replacement with a thin layer of granulation tissue. This is so characteristic that giving oral contrast is not recommended as it may obscure the finding (Donnelly and Morris, 1996). Oral contrast in this population is poorly tolerated and seldom propagates adequately through the diseased bowel and so is not routinely advocated.

Structural Abnormalities

Structural abnormalities should be actively sought in all patients with malabsorption who are referred for radiologic consultation.

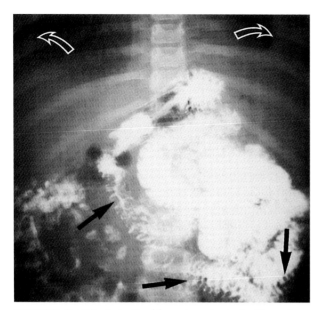

FIGURE 9–161. Intestinal lymphangiectasia. The valvulae conniventes are slightly thickened and nodular (*black arrows*). Bilateral massive pleural effusions are present (*white open arrows*).

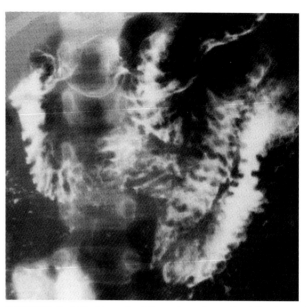

FIGURE 9–162. Intestinal lymphangiectasia. The jejunal valvulae conniventes are moderately thickened and nodular.

Malrotation is the most important condition to exclude in children because of the serious consequences if misdiagnosed. Malrotation can present in a chronic fashion.

Blind loop syndrome may be secondary to a large diverticulum or fistula but it is more often due to stasis and hence bacterial overgrowth in a segment of bowel dilated proximal to a stricture. This generates steatorrhea and interferes with vitamin B12 absorption, which produces macrocytic anemia.

Short-gut syndrome can develop in a neonate who has had large portions of the small bowel surgically removed (e.g., for multiple small bowel atresias) resulting in malabsorption. After surgery, the remaining loops of bowel tend to dilate and lengthen, and the mucosal folds tend to thicken (Bell et al., 1973). These changes increase the absorptive capacity of the bowel. The remaining bowel may demonstrate distorted motor activity. Although the presence or absence of the ileocecal valve has no appreciable effect on transit time, it is generally accepted that the prognosis is better if the valve remains untouched by surgery. In those infants with more than 20% of the small bowel remaining, an average transit time is 2 hours (Kalifa et al., 1979).

Small bowel follow-through studies will demonstrate the length of remaining bowel and indicate the transit time (Figure 9–164). Complications following ileal resection include radiopaque gallstones (Pellerin et al., 1975) and oxalate renal stones (Wise and Stein, 1975).

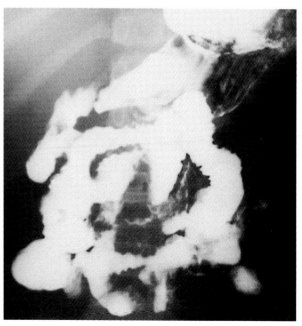

FIGURE 9–163. Graft-versus-host disease. The mucosal folds are flattened and effaced, and the bowel wall is thickened.

Rare Causes of Malabsorption

Zollinger-Ellison syndrome, mastocytosis, carcinoid (see Chapter 11), and dermatomyositis, are all extremely rare in children.

Zollinger-Ellison Syndrome

The Zollinger-Ellison syndrome is secondary to an excess of the antral hormone gastrin, produced by a pancreatic tumor such as an adenoma, adenocarcinoma, or hyperplasia of non-beta islet cells. Diarrhea is frequently present and even if absent, peristaltic activity is usually abnormal. In addition, there is hypersecretion of gastrin resulting in excess gastric acid due to the action of gastrin on the gastric parietal cells. This increase in gastric acid results in ulceration of the duodenum. Most idiopathic duodenal ulcers are found in the duodenal cap, so the finding of ulcers, especially if multiple, in other parts of the duodenum should suggest the diagnosis. In the small bowel, thickening of folds secondary to edema is one of the most characteristic features of

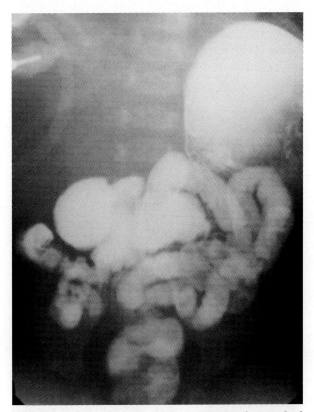

FIGURE 9–164. Short gut syndrome. Barium has reached the rectum within 15 minutes of starting an upper GI examination; it outlines the entire gut, which is shortened by previous resection because of gangrenous volvulus.

the syndrome (Zboralske and Amberg, 1968). This thickening is most pronounced in the duodenum and decreases distally, being least marked in the ileum. Flocculation due to excess intraluminal fluid may also be present (Zboralske and Amberg, 1968).

Mastocytosis

In adults the cutaneous form of mastocytosis, in which mast cells infiltrate the skin resulting in urticaria pigmentosa, is not rare. It is rare for the infiltration to be so widespread that multiple system symptoms develop, requiring radiologic evaluation. This infiltration can very occasionally occur in children.

The most common radiologic findings in children are sclerotic and/or lytic bone lesions (Huang et al., 1987; Lucaya et al., 1979). There is an equal incidence of osteoblastic and mixed osteoblastic/osteolytic lesions. However, the presence of purely osteolytic lesions is uncommon (Huang et al., 1987). Chest radiographs may show interstitial edema or rarely, pleural effusion, pulmonary edema, or cardiomegaly (Huang et al., 1987).

Gastrointestinal abnormalities are rare. The esophagus most commonly has a hiatus hernia with esophagitis and/or reflux. An abnormality of peristalsis is less common. Peptic ulcers have been described in children (Lucaya et al., 1979). Gastric and duodenal nodules may be present, and some of these may be umbilicated (Quinn et al., 1984). Localized mucosal thickening, possibly representing urticaria, and thickened folds secondary to cellular infiltration of the lamina propria are reported in all parts of the gut in adults (Huang et al., 1987), and we have seen one infant with some minor irregularity and rigidity of the terminal ileum who had systemic mastocytosis. The gallbladder may be nonfunctional with or without gallstones, and hepatosplenomegaly is not uncommon (Huang et al., 1987). Retroperitoneal lymphadenopathy is reported but unusual (Huang et al., 1987). Overall, gastrointestinal findings in children with mastocytosis are exceedingly rare.

INTESTINAL OBSTRUCTION

The causes of intestinal obstruction in children differ from those in adults (Table 9–5) (Janik et al., 1981). Hypertrophic pyloric stenosis (see Chapter 8) is the most common obstructing abnormality of the gastrointestinal tract, closely followed by intussusception.

Intussusception

Intussusception occurs when a segment of the intestine (the intussusceptum) prolapses into another segment (the intussuscipiens). Children are most commonly affected in the first 2 years of life, with a peak incidence from 3 to 9 months. Intussusception may occur in older children and even in adults (Agha, 1986) but the chance of an underlying condition acting as a lead point increases with age (Agha, 1986). Males are affected more often than females. The intussusception is ileocolic in more than 90% of cases but ileo-ileocolic, colocolic, and ileoileal intussusceptions also occur (Du, 1978; Ein and Stephens, 1971; Hutchinson et al., 1980).

Etiology

The cause of an intussusception is unknown in most cases. A temporal relationship occurs with annual outbreaks of respiratory infections and gastroenteritis but this is not a constant feature (Ein and Stephens, 1971). There is some evidence that children with intussusception, although appearing well nourished, are less so than the general population (Janik et al., 1981).

Up to 5% of cases are caused by lesions in the bowel that act as leading points (Ein,1976). Neonatal intussusceptions are rare but are invariably accompanied by lead points (Patriquin et al., 1977). The most common lead point is a Meckel's diverticulum; other lead points include polyps, duplications (Ein, 1976), and non-Hodgkin's lymphoma, where intussusception may be the presenting feature (Wayne et al., 1976). In jejunojejunal intussusceptions, the most common finding is a duplication cyst acting as a lead point (Stone et al., 1980).

Intussusceptions are also found in celiac disease (Ruoff et al., 1968), cystic fibrosis, Schönlein-Henoch purpura, hemophilia (Ein and Stephens, 1971), and rarely, Kawasaki syndrome. A rare cause of intussusception in children is polyarteritis nodosa (Fujioka et al., 1980). There is an increased incidence of ileoileal or jejunojejunal intussusception following abdominal operations, especially neuroblastoma, even in adults (Cohen et al., 1982; Cox and Martin, 1973; Dammert and Votteler, 1974; Ein and Ferguson, 1982; Franken and King, 1972; Hertz et al., 1982). The appendix may rarely intussuscept on itself (even more rarely secondary to an appendix mucocele) (Douglas et al., 1978) and can become completely invaginated within the lumen of the cecum. Alterna-

tively, it may act as a lead point resulting in a secondary ileocecal intussusception (Atkinson et al., 1976). One report suggests that appendiceal intussusception can frequently occur in asymptomatic patients as a transient phenomenon and that the majority reduce spontaneously (Levine et al., 1985). The appendiceal stump can also act in this way, giving a transient cecal intussusception; in adults, the diagnosis can be made on double-contrast barium enema when a coiled-spring appearance is seen in the cecum, with nonfilling of the appendix (Levine et al., 1985). Double-contrast barium enema studies, however, are not routinely performed in children.

Volvulus of small and large bowel have rarely been found in association with intussusception in children and possibly are related to hyperperistalsis (Leeba and Boas, 1986). Abnormalities of rotation in association with intussusception (Waugh syndrome) have been implicated in the etiology and may be more common than previously thought (Brereton et al., 1986; Waugh, 1927).

Clinical Features

The classic presentation is the sudden onset of abdominal pain that recurs intermittently in a previously well child. Initially, the child appears well between attacks but without treatment, the child progressively weakens, becomes lethargic, and may develop shock. Up to 60% of children will pass blood and mucus, causing the stool to resemble red

TABLE 9–5. Frequency of Types of Gastrointestinal Obstruction*

Type of Obstruction	Frequency (%)
Hypertrophic pyloric stenosis	25
Intussusception	18
Intestinal atresia	15
Incarcerated hernia	11
Imperforate anus	8
Hirschsprung's disease	5
Adhesion	5
Malrotation	5
Meconium plug	3
Meconium ileus	3
Annular pancreas	1
Meckel's diverticulum	0.5

*Hospital for Sick Children, Toronto, from 1968 to 1979.
Modified from Janik et al., 1981.

currant jelly. Vomiting may be present, and a palpable mass may be felt in the abdomen.

Unfortunately, many patients do not present in this manner. In particular, babies under 4 months of age often present with bleeding and vomiting without a history of abdominal pain (Newman and Schuh, 1987). Neonatal intussusception will present with obstruction often on the first day of life (Patriquin et al., 1977). Some older children also may have no pain, presenting as pale, listless children in whom a mass is often palpable (Ein et al., 1976). A few children are found to have an intussusception when long-standing atypical symptoms are investigated (Thomassen and Sutinen, 1972). In these children, the diagnosis of chronic intussusception is based on the histologic evidence of chronicity of the resected lesion (Rees and Lari, 1976).

Intussusception following laparotomy is usually atypical, commonly of small bowel, ileoileal, jejunoileal, or jejunojejunal. The clinical presentation is also atypical; usually neither rectal bleeding nor abdominal mass is present (Cox and Martin, 1973). Bowel obstruction in the immediate postoperative period is a common presenting event.

Imaging

Plain-Film Radiography. A soft-tissue mass and sparse large bowel gas are the two best predictors of an intussusception (Sargent et al., 1994). A thin curvilinear rim of air outlining the mass, the "crescent sign" (Figure 9–165), and concentric lucent rings within the mass (probably trapped mesenteric fat), the "target sign," are reliable indicators of intussusception (Figure 9–166) (Ratcliffe et al., 1991; Ratcliffe et al., 1992). A more obvious intraluminal filling defect of the intussusception may be apparent (Figure 9–167). Signs of intestinal obstruction with dilated loops of small bowel filling the abdomen are not uncommon (Figure 9–168). Small bowel may overlie the expected position of the right hemicolon. Intussusception is impossible to exclude on plain-film findings alone in 25% of normal children (Eklof and Hartelius, 1980), and only the presence of a feces- or air-filled cecum can reliably exclude it. Interobserver variability in the interpretation of plain radiograph findings of intussusception is well documented and most patients have radiographs that are abnormal but regarded as equivocal (Sargent et al., 1994; Ratcliffe et al., 1992). Additional views, including horizontal beam (cross-table lateral) and prone projections, are reported to increase diagnostic sensitivity (Johnson and Woisard, 1989; White and Blane, 1982) but in a child with an appropriate clinical history, findings on abdominal radiograph are unlikely to avert an enema study and possible reduction. Radiographic findings may, however, suggest an intussusception when it has not been clinically suspected. An equivocal clinical history with normal radiographs, which should demonstrate air or feces in the cecal pole, should not require further radiographic investigation. Abdominal radiography will only rarely provide information that contraindicates an enema. We do not think small bowel obstruction alone is a contraindication to attempted enema reduction. The detection of free air is rare and was not detected in a reported series of 1000 intussusception patients, of whom only 6 were perforated (Humphrey et al., 1981). In the appropriate clinical setting, there is a strong argument for proceeding directly to enema without preliminary abdominal radiography (Sargent et al., 1994).

Contrast/Air Enema. The enema is generally accepted as an excellent technique for both diagnosis and treatment of intussusception.

In a typical ileocolic intussusception, the enema contrast column on filling meets an intraluminal filling defect—the intussusceptum—that is the caliber of the normal colon (Figure 9–169). The intussusceptum can be found in any part of the large bowel, including the rectum (Figure 9–170). Occasionally some contrast may coat the outer surface of the intussusceptum and the inner surface of the intussuscipiens (Figure 9–171). This can cause a coiled-spring appearance. When air is used, the same findings manifest but the air provides a negative contrast that outlines the soft-tissue density of the intussusceptum (Figure 9–172). If contrast or air floods the colon with no impediment and refluxes freely into the terminal ileum, then colocolic and ileocolic intussusception is excluded. The contrast enema appearance may occasionally suggest an unreduced intussusception when the patient actually has a malrotation (Mok and Humphrey, 1982). Cecal malposition indicating gut malrotation can be detected even where reducible intussusception is present (Lobo et al., 1997). An evaluation for lead points should be done in all enemas but is especially important in the very young and in older patients (Ein, 1976). Air enema may be less sensitive for lead point detection, and contrast enema

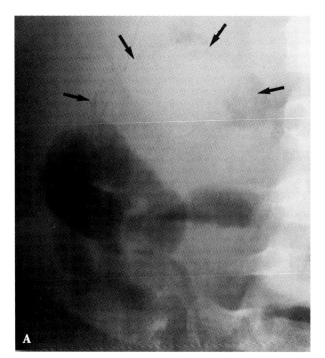 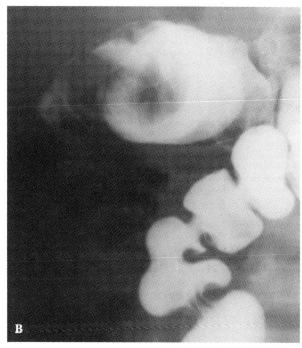

FIGURE 9–165. Ileocolic intussusception. *A*, Intussusception (*arrows*) produces a right upper quadrant mass with a faint curvilinear rim of bowel gas. *B*, Intussusception is confirmed on barium enema; the gas lucencies around the intussusceptum fill with barium.

or US may be indicated for patients of these ages and for recurrent intussusception (Miller et al., 1995; Stein et al., 1992).

Ultrasonography. Ultrasonography is a reliable investigation for diagnosing intussusception but it requires appropriate expertise. High sensitivity and negative predictive values (100%) have been reported (Pracos et al., 1987; Verschelden et al., 1992; Woo et al., 1992).

The characteristic US finding in a plane transverse to the intussusception is a hypoechoic ring surrounding an echogenic center, the "doughnut sign" (Figure 9–173) (Bowerman et al., 1982; Burke and Clark, 1977). In the longitudinal plane (Figure 9–174), the alternating hypoechogenic and echogenic layers are called the "sandwich" or "pseudokidney" sign (Swishchuk et al., 1985). The hypoechoic layer correlates to an edematous intussusceptum wall, and the echogenic central tube was felt to be intussusceptum mucosa (Swishchuk et al., 1985). Multiple concentric layering may be seen, probably representing the two layers of invaginating intussusceptum and the intussuscipiens wall or layers within the bowel wall itself (Montali et al., 1983; Swishchuk et al., 1985). These ultrasonographic fea-

tures, although characteristic, are not pathognomonic, and a differential diagnosis would include inflammatory bowel disease, enterocolitis, intramural hematoma, colonic feces, and the normal psoas muscle. A more specific sign for intussusception has been reported following experimental work in a pig model, the "crescent-in-a-doughnut" sign (del Pozo et al., 1996). The central echogenic area was identified as an eccentric crescent and found on histology to represent mesenteric fat pulled into the intussusception (Figure 9–175). This is best seen on transverse images at the base of the intussusceptum and may contain lymph nodes and blood vessels (del Pozo et al., 1996). The intussusception is invariably 3 cm or more in diameter and several centimeters in length and is most often encountered in the transverse or hepatic flexure of colon. Its peripheral location and substantial size reduce the likelihood of its being obscured by gas-filled bowel (Verschelden et al., 1992; Weinberger and Winters, 1992). The thickness of the edematous wall of the intussusception has been studied, and when in excess of 8 to 10 mm, reduction was often difficult but not contraindicated (Pracos et al., 1987). Similarly, excessive free peritoneal fluid may suggest increased difficul-

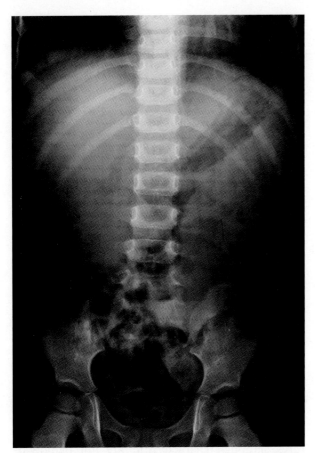

FIGURE 9–166. Ileocolic intussusception. On a plain-film radiograph, air-filled small bowel occupies the right iliac fossa. There is a soft-tissue density in the right upper quadrant which has concentric lucent rings, a reliable indicator of intussusception.

ties in reduction but does not contraindicate a reduction attempt (Pracos et al., 1987; Swischuk and Stanberry, 1990; Verschelden et al., 1992). Ultrasonography does provide a good opportunity to look for a lead point, especially important in the young or older patient (Lam and Firman, 1991). The use of color Doppler does not influence diagnosis. However, good flow in the intussusceptum suggests viable perfused bowel and correlates to successful reduction while lack of flow may indicate nonviable bowel, which, in conjunction with clinical symptoms, may suggest that reduction attempts be cautious (Lam and Firman, 1992; Lim et al., 1994).

The availability of expertise in US and the chosen method of intussusception reduction will influence the use of US. Where intussusception reduction is by fluoroscopically controlled enema, the added cost and extra examination have little validi-

ty when there is a high clinical likelihood for intussusception. In equivocal cases or patients outside the normal age range of 4 months to 2 years, when lead points may be suspected, US has a useful diagnostic role. Some institutions reduce intussusception hydrostatically with ultrasonographic control, and this has made US their imaging modality of choice.

Other Imaging Modalities. Unsuspected intussusception may be found on barium small bowel follow-through examinations. Described features include a narrow central channel surrounded by a soft tissue mass, a coiled-spring appearance around the soft tissue mass, and a mass lesion at the distal end of the narrow channel (see Figures 9–136, 9–176) (Daneman et al., 1982).

Computed tomography has little place in the routine diagnosis and management of intussusception. It may demonstrate an intussusception where the diagnosis is unsuspected, in children with a complicated presentation, or with small bowel intussusception (Merine et al., 1987). Findings include an intraluminal mass with circular layers of high and low attenuation (a "target lesion") and eccentric trapped central mesenteric fat that corresponds to the transverse ultrasonographic appearance. Also, in the longitudinal plane, the intussusceptum base is seen invaginating into the intussuscipiens (Figure

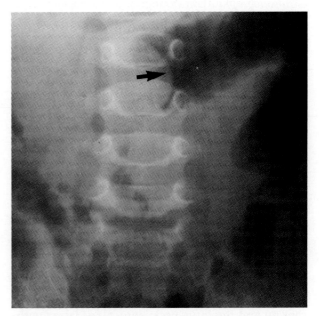

FIGURE 9–167. Ileocolic intussusception. Gas outlines a round soft-tissue density mass (*arrow*), the intussusceptum, in the transverse colon.

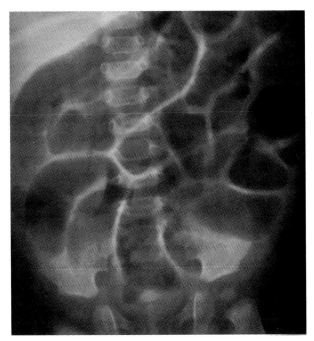

FIGURE 9–168. Ileocolic intussusception. Dilated loops of small bowel indicate obstruction.

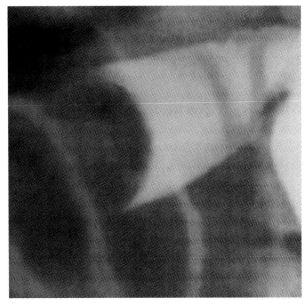

FIGURE 9–169. Ileocolic intussusception. Barium shows the intussusceptum as an intraluminal filling defect occluding the bowel lumen, and the intussusception was reduced easily.

9–177) (Cox et al., 1996; Iko et al., 1984; Mason and Quon, 1985). Free fluid and dilated obstructed bowel may be apparent, and inflammation with loss of tissue planes has been correlated to necrotic bowel at surgery (Cox et al., 1996). Pitfalls in the CT diagnosis of intussusception in children include mural hemorrhage, neutropenic colitis, and pericolic inflammation (Cox et al., 1996).

Treatment

Historic Background. The history of intussusception reduction makes fascinating reading (Frush et al., 1995; McDermott, 1994). Rectal enema and insufflations were recorded in the time of Hippocrates, 400 BC. Introsusception was described by John Hunter in 1789, and late-19th-century medical and surgical texts on both sides of the Atlantic advocated enema procedures for management of intussusception. These included "A Treatise on the Disease of Infancy and Childhood" by J. Lewis Smith from New York, who wrote in 1869, on page 435: "The medical journals contain reports of cases of intussusception successfully treated both by liquid injections and by inflation, but the latter is now commonly recommended, as it is believed to produce a more equable and effectual distention of the external or incarcerating portion of intestine and upward pressure of the

internal or that which is incarcerated. Besides, cases of cure by inflation have been reported after liquid injections had failed." How the wheel has been reinvented! The early 20th century saw a revolution in anesthesia and sepsis control, and surgical manage-

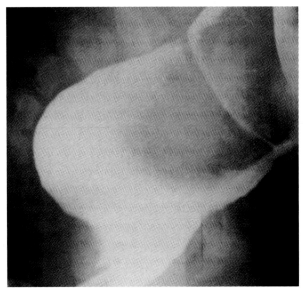

FIGURE 9–170. Ileocolic intussusception. Barium shows the intussusceptum as an intraluminal filling defect occluding the rectum. This intussusception was successfully reduced hydrostatically.

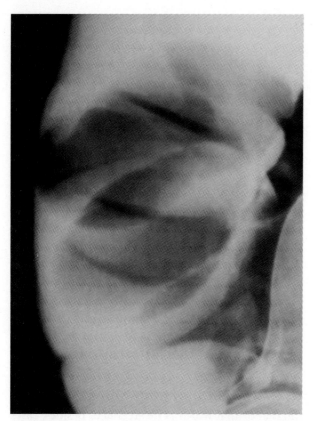

FIGURE 9–171. Ileoileocolic intussusception. Barium outlines loops of small bowel coiled within the ascending colon.

ment of intussusception dominated. The arrival of radiography provided mostly diagnostic studies in this period. Images of a successful barium enema reduction were published in 1928 although it was also claimed that manual manipulation was most fundamental to the reduction (Stevens, 1928). A surgeon, Mark Ravitch, lead a re-evaluation of intussusception reduction and established fluoroscopic control of a barium enema as the treatment of choice (Ravitch and McCune, 1948). Images of an air reduction enema were published in 1959 (Fiorito and Cuestas, 1959) but air reduction enemas were reintroduced to North America only in the 1980s, when a Chinese radiologist, L. Gu, brought her Shanghai experience to Toronto. This work won the John Caffey Gold Medal in 1987 (Gu et al., 1988). Interestingly, a series of 6396 cases of air enema reductions performed in China was published just as American enthusiasm was increasing (Guo et al., 1986). Nonetheless, the rekindling of intussusception issues resulted in much scientific investigation and critical study of colonic pressures, Valsalva's effect,

outcome analyses, and peritoneal effects of barium versus air in perforation.

General Information. The treatment of intussusception should be considered a pediatric emergency even though presentation may have been delayed or protracted. The goal of nonoperative reduction is to return the invaginated bowel by controlled application of distal intraluminal pressure. Success will spare the affected child a laparotomy.

Absolute contraindications to an attempted intussusception reduction are few, mostly clinical, and related to gangrenous bowel and bowel perforation. The radiographic demonstration of free intra-abdominal air is a rare occurrence but indicates perforation, and the clinical presence of peritonitis or a sick child who displays pallor, lethargy, dehydration, shock, and skin mottling may mandate surgery (Humphry et al., 1981). Young age, small bowel obstruction, delay in diagnosis, recurrent intussusception, rectal bleeding, free peritoneal fluid, and poor Doppler flow in the intussusceptum may indicate an increased risk of perforation and lower rates of reduction but do not contraindicate enema reduction attempts per se (Katz et al., 1993; Leonidas, 1985; Stephensen et al., 1984).

All patients require appropriate surgical consultation before an attempt at reduction. Full resuscitation of the patient should precede arrival in the radiology department, and a secure, large-bore intravenous access should be maintained. Attendance at reduction by surgical staff is recommended as it will ensure rapid management of any arising complication. Analgesia and sedation may be required for clinical or humane reasons but are not routinely given as they may reduce voluntary Valsalva's maneuvers. Glucagon is neither helpful nor indicated (Franken et al., 1983). Intravenous antibiotics are often given by the attending surgery staff although bacteremia following air enema is negligible (Somekh et al., 1996). Parents or caregivers should be appropriately informed about the procedure's risks and benefits, and their consent should be obtained.

Technical Factors. Enema reduction can be hydrostatic, using barium or an iodinated water-soluble contrast agent with fluoroscopic control; hydrostatic, using saline and ultrasonographic control; or air or carbon dioxide, using fluoroscopic control.

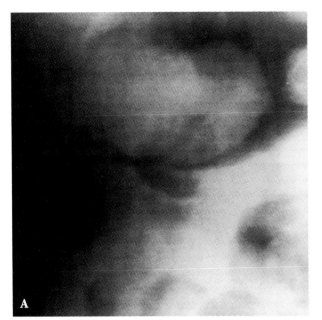
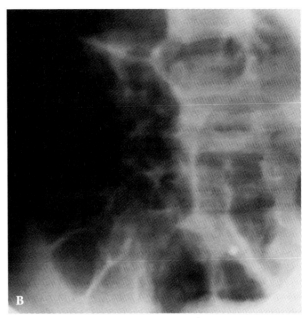

FIGURE 9–172. Ileocolic intussusception. *A,* Air enema shows the intussusceptum as an intraluminal filling defect occluding the bowel lumen. The right iliac fossa is relatively gasless. *B,* After easy reduction, the right iliac fossa is full of large and small bowel gas.

Reduction rates of 55 to 70% for hydrostatic reduction and 80 to 90% for air reduction have been reported (Kirks, 1994). A 3-foot column of barium generates 80 to 90 mm Hg pressure whereas air pressures of up to 120 mm Hg are readily used (Sargent and Wilson, 1991). This may also explain the higher rate of perforations initially seen in air reductions (Stein et al., 1992). The use of barium has been

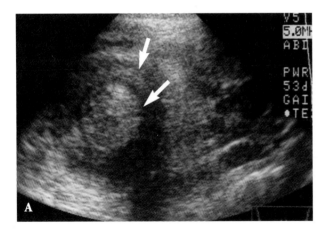
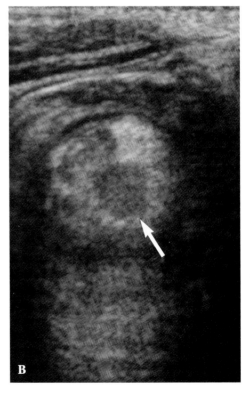

FIGURE 9–173. Ileocolic intussusception. *A,* Transverse US images shows concentric rings of intussuscepted bowel wall (*arrows*), the "target sign." *B,* More inferior at the base of the intussusceptum, transverse US shows echogenic mesenteric fat and a lymph node (*arrow*) drawn into the intussusception.

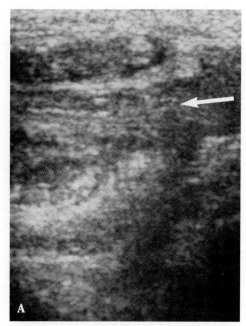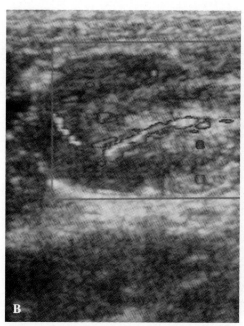

FIGURE 9–174. Ileocolic intussusception. *A*, Longitudinal US view shows the base of the intussusceptum invaginating into the intussuscipiens (*arrow*). *B*, Color Doppler interrogation of the head of the intussusception indicates wall vascularity and a prominent mesenteric vessel, centrally located.

entrenched since the work of Ravitch and McCune in 1948 (Ravitch and McCune, 1948), and in the

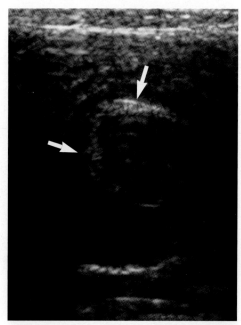

FIGURE 9–175. Ileocolic intussusception. "Crescent-in-a-doughnut" sign of an eccentric echogenic crescent of mesenteric fat (*arrows*) seen in transverse plane on US.

early 1990s remained the most widely used agent (Katz and Kolm, 1992; Meyer, 1992). Another John Caffey Gold Medal-winning presentation compared colonic perforation by liquid and air in a pig model and demonstrated air to produce smaller, more punctate perforations with localized peritoneal contamination, compared to diffuse fecal spillage with liquids (Shiels et al., 1993). Retrospective evaluation of clinical, radiologic, and pathologic records of children with perforation from both barium and air confirms that significantly less morbidity and less surgical resection of bowel occurs following air enema perforation (Daneman et al., 1995). Air enemas have also been reported as more rapidly performed and giving lower radiation dosages than hydrostatic enemas (Phelan et al., 1988; Shiels et al., 1991). Air is certainly the cheapest of the contrast media and by far the cleanest.

In patients between 6 months and 4 years of age with presumed intussusception, we have no hesitation in using air enema to diagnose and reduce intussusception. In the young or old patient in whom a lead point is likely, a positive contrast medium (Stringer and Ein, 1990) or US is considered.

The interface between enema equipment and patient is often a source of frustration and failure.

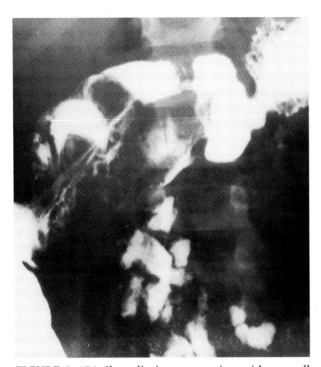

FIGURE 9–176. Ileocolic intussusception with a small lymphosarcoma as lead point. Small bowel follow-through examination shows a narrow channel of barium connecting the dilated distal ileum to the transverse colon. The surrounding soft-tissue mass is partly outlined by streaks of barium and can also be seen adjacent to the distal end of the narrow channel.

Each institution seems to have its own tricks for rectal catheter insertion and retention. Experimental work has identified Valsalva's maneuver to increase intracolonic pressure as well as intra-abdominal pressure, allowing higher reduction pressure on the intussusceptum but no increase in differential pressure across the colonic wall, and thus no increased risk of perforation (Bramson et al., 1995; Shiels et al., 1993; Shiels et al., 1991). To use Valsalva's effect, we attempt to seal the tube in the rectum. This can be done by strapping a rectal catheter and pushing the strapping cuff up against the anus and then taping the buttocks, or by pulling an underinflated large Foley bulb down on the internal anal sphincter and taping the buttocks. Both prone and supine positions are effective. The key to success is experienced staff and operators.

The appeal of ultrasonographically controlled enema reduction is the lack of ionizing radiation but the necessary expertise is not universally available. Where fluoroscopy is still used, reduction in radiation dosage should be sought. Modern digital systems with pulsed fluoroscopy and image storage ability can dramatically reduce dosage. We fluoroscope during pressure application (and automatically capture this on video for review if necessary) and use a wide field of view to ensure rapid detection of perforation. We

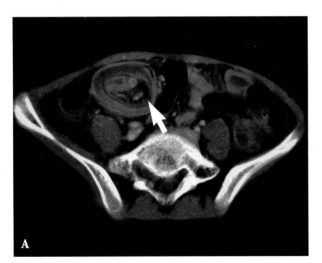
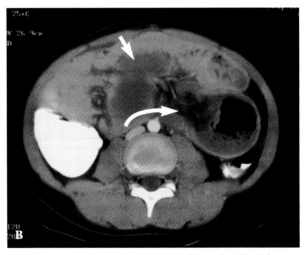

FIGURE 9–177. Ileocolic intussusception. *A*, Computed tomography shows concentric layers of bowel wall with central mesenteric fat (*large arrow*) and some air trapped between intussuscipiens and intussusceptum. This examination was done on a 14-year-old patient with neutropenic colitis and severe abdominal pain. Air reduction was successful. *B*, Longitudinal view shows mesentery drawn into the intussusception (*curved arrow*); dilated proximal bowel (*arrow*) indicates obstruction. This was a 13-year-old patient with a 1 week history of cramping abdominal pain. At laparotomy, a jejunojejunal intussusception was resected. No lead point was present although preoperative concern for a possible lymphoma as a lead point was high.

acquire one image when the intussusception is encountered and another following reduction and ileal reflux. Obtaining postreduction, postevacuation radiographs has been recommended (Eklof and Hugoosson, 1976) but we do not find this of value. Thus, we rely on clinical re-evaluation of the child.

Air Enema. Air is delivered through an airtight sump to prevent backflow contamination of the pump. The pump can be a simple handheld sphygmomanometer or an electric pump. The system must have an immediate pressure release mechanism in case of perforation. Pump pressures of only 20 to 30 mm Hg are required for diagnostic enemas (Shiels et al., 1991). On encountering an intussusception, increasing pressure to 80 mm Hg usually allows reduction (see Figure 9–172). A pressure increase of 120 mm Hg is an accepted upper limit although much higher pressures may occur during Valsalva's maneuver. Colonic perforation pressures in the pig model are around 130 mm Hg (Shiels et al., 1993). Most experienced radiologists will continue to apply a constant pressure as long as the intussusceptum is reducing and will continue reduction attempts as long as some headway is made with each attempt. This usually occurs in a stop/start fashion with hold-ups often occurring at the ileocecal valve (see Figure 9–176). When no movement occurs in 1 to 2 minutes, pressure is relieved, and after another 1 to 2 minutes, another attempt is made to gradually increase pressure to the maximum of 120 mm Hg. Successful reduction is manifest by copious air reflux into the small bowel (see Figure 9–172). Reduction attempts are abandoned if perforation occurs, the patient's clinical condition deteriorates, or no movement of the intussusceptum occurs using 120 mm Hg pressure for up to 3 minutes on more than one occasion. Reflux of air into the terminal ileum before ileocolic intussusception reduction has been reported but is rare (Fitch et al., 1985).

It is essential to have a sheathed needle of at least 18 gauge at hand during all air enema procedures as perforation can lead to rapid tension pneumoperitoneum embarrassing inferior vena cava return and causing rapid decompensation and collapse. Simple puncture of the peritoneum, leaving the sheath in place to decompress the pneumoperitoneum, allows stabilization of the patient (Stein et al., 1992).

Contrast Enema. A contrast enema has the rectal tube connected to a simple closed-loop bag elevated above the patient to generate a head of pressure. When electing a contrast enema, barium is the cheaper agent and has a good track record, yet when perforation occurs, the effects of a barium-feces mix provokes a granulomatous reaction that exacerbates and prolongs peritonitis, compared to water-soluble agents (Cochran et al., 1963; Ginai, 1985; Sisel et al., 1972). The water-soluble agents we use are one-to-one dilutions of Hypaque 150 or Cystoconray as we do not stock Gastrografin. When extravasated, these agents may cause fluid shifts and electrolyte imbalance and so are not completely benign; they are nontheless our contrast agents of choice in this setting. For the child under the age of 4 months, a one-to-one dilution of a nonionic agent such as Omnipaque is a justifiable expense.

Barium enema for diagnosis and treatment was entrenched by the work of Ravitch and McCune (Ravitch and McCune, 1948), out of which grew the dictum of three attempts for 3 minutes from 3 feet. Using these guidelines in the 1970s, reduction rates of 45% were reported in a series of 354 cases (Ein and Stephens, 1971). The same institution improved its barium reduction rate to 75% 20 years later (Palder et al., 1991). This was largely due to more aggressive reduction attempts with greater pressures, the bag limited by the ceiling, and repeated reduction attempts for times exceeding the 3-minute rule (Ein et al., 1981). Studies have shown that the delivery of pressure to the colon depends on fluid viscosity and flow as well as head of pressure. A 1-m column of barium delivers a pressure of 89 mm Hg while the same column of Urografin delivers a pressure of 78 mm Hg, and the fluid level drops during delivery, lowering the delivered pressure by at least 10 mm Hg (Sargent and Wilson, 1991). To attain pressures of 120 mm Hg would require a barium column of 1.35 m and a water-soluble agent column of 1.54 m (Sargent and Wilson, 1991). This will vary according to viscosity of media and diameter of enema tube.

Reduction is complete only when a good portion of distal ileum is filled by barium, thus excluding ileoileal intussusception (Wayne et al., 1973). Excessive barium surrounding the intussusceptum, the so called "dissection sign," indicates that it may be more difficult and occasionally impossible to reduce an ileocolic intussusception (Fishman et al., 1984) but in our experience many intussusceptions showing this sign can be reduced, and so a full attempt should be made.

Ileoileocolic intussusceptions may be more difficult to reduce as barium often percolates among the loops of ileum in the colon (see Figure 9–171), dissipating the effective pressure of the enema. The radiologic signs of ileoileocolic intussusceptions are best seen on a barium enema. The cecum and ascending colon may be filled with obvious loops of bowel. On reflux of barium through the ileocecal valve, an intussusceptum may be seen in the terminal ileum (Figure 9–178). These intussusceptions may be reducible and do not necessarily recur (Cipel et al., 1977).

Diligent observation for lead point filling defects is required at initial visualization and after reduction. A postreduction filling defect at the ileocecal valve is commonly seen, probably representing edema (Figure 9–179) (Devred et al., 1984).

Complications

Perforation. Colonic perforation is the most serious complication of attempted reduction. It most commonly occurs where the intussusception was first shown by the enema, through areas of necrosis in the bowel wall (Humphrey et al., 1981). It has been suggested that entrapped bowel with swelling induces ischemia and necrosis and that reducing the intussusception uncovers the perforation (Bramson and Blickman, 1992). Yet, in a reported series of 14 perforations that occurred during enema reduction, 8 demonstrated no mural necrosis (Daneman et al., 1995). There were shearing abnormalities with disruption of muscle layers which did suggest pressure effects, and as shown in the pig model, perforations from air were smaller than from liquids. In one case with documented free air, no perforation site was found at laparotomy (Daneman et al., 1995; Shiels et al., 1993). Perforation may rarely occur distal to the intussusception (Armstrong et al., 1980).

Perforation requires immediate surgery, and having a surgical staff in attendance at reduction usually expedites this. Immediate attention to fluid and electrolyte status may be required due to the effects of peritonitis, shock, or fluid shifts from hyperosmolar contrast agents. Immediate release of a tension pneumoperitoneum with an 18-gauge needle may be lifesaving.

Increased risk factors for perforation include age of under 6 months, small bowel obstruction,

rectal bleeding, prolonged clinical history, and mostly, increasingly aggressive attempts at enema reduction (Daneman et al., 1995; Humphry et al., 1981; Leonidas 1985; Ein et al., 1981). Many infants with these findings can still be successfully reduced, and a balance between all-out attempts to reduce and the risk of perforation requires some clinical insight and judgment.

Perforation rates of 0.16% in 9028 children and 0.14% in 6396 children have been reported (Gu et al., 1988; Guo et al., 1986), and rates of up to 2.8% were reported during early North American experience with air reduction using high pressures (Stein et al., 1992). Perforation rates in experienced hands should not exceed 1% (Daneman et al., 1995).

Lead Points. The commonest lead point is probably a hyperplastic lymphoid tissue of a Peyer's patch (Figure 9–180). True surgical lead points may be seen in 2.5 to 5% of intussusceptions although half may be restricted to the small bowel (Ein, 1976; Miller et al., 1995). The most common cause is Meckel's diverticulum (Figure 9–181), followed by benign polyps (see Figure 9–129), duplications, Schönlein-Henoch purpura (see Figure 9–155), appendix, and in the older child, lymphoma (Figures 9–176, 9–182) (Ein, 1976; Ein et al., 1986). Neonatal intussusception is

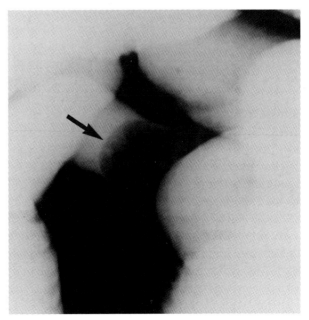

FIGURE 9–178. Ileoileocolic intussusception. Barium outlines the intussusceptum (*arrow*) within the distal ileum.

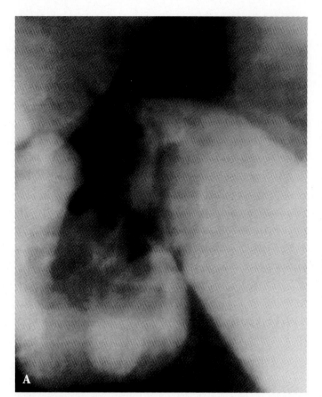 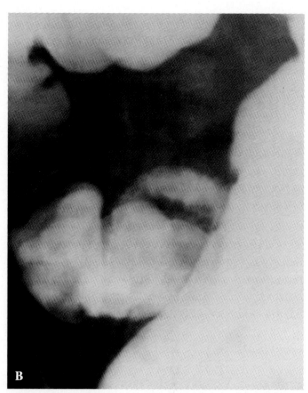

FIGURE 9–179. Ileocolic intussusception with enlarged ileocecal valve. *A,* Following intussusception reduction, the ileocecal valve is enlarged but the more significant feature is the deformity of the terminal ileum. *B,* A follow-up study 2 weeks later was normal, excluding a significant lead point. The patient has remained symptom free. The appearance was presumably due to edema.

invariably due to a lead point (Patriquin et al., 1977); otherwise, lead points tend to present in older children and with recurrent intussusception (Ein, 1976). It was believed a lead point intussusception would not be reduced by enema and thus needed surgical removal but both barium (see Figure 9–182) and air enemas have reduced lead point intussusceptions (Ein et al., 1986; Miller et al., 1995). Filling defects from lead points have been identified and missed on both air and contrast studies but many empirically feel that liquid contrast agents are better at detecting lead points and should be used where risk of lead point is high (Eklof et al., 1980; Stringer et al., 1990). An edematous ileocecal valve should not by mistaken for a lead point filling defect (see Figure 9–179). A good additional modality for identification of a lead point is US, particularly for cystic structures such as duplications and also for Meckel's diverticulum (see Figure 9–181) (Adamsbaum et al., 1989; Lam and Firman, 1991; Miller et al., 1995). If US is not routinely employed in diagnosis, then it is recommended in age groups where lead points are more likely (i.e., under 6 months and over 2 years), in recurrent intussusception, where abnormal filling defects were identified on enema study, and in atypical presentation (Miller et al., 1995). There will remain the occasional patient who will be operated on for clinical reasons; persistent small bowel obstruction in particular.

Recurrent Intussusception. Intussusception recurrence occurs in 5 to 10% of cases (Ein, 1975; Eklof and Reiter, 1978). They may occur within 12 hours or up to a year after the first event and may be multiple. Although there is an increased incidence of lead points in recurrent intussusception, the majority remain idiopathic and benefit from repeated enema reduction (Ein, 1975). Recurrent intussusception should have an ultrasonographic evaluation, and diligent assessment for a lead point is required at enema.

Failed Reduction, the Balance of Common Sense. A failed reduction is not a failure if the intussusception was necrotic at laparotomy or required resection. It is a failure if, at laparotomy, the intussusception reduced spontaneously or with minimal manipulation. Many factors affect the success-complication rates of enema reduction. A tertiary center may accrue an inherent increase in patients who are young, sick, or have delayed presentations. A peripheral center with no attending pediatric surgeon may be understandably reluctant to be aggressive with any enema reduction attempt. Close cooperation is required between surgical and radiology staff to ensure appropriate triage of patients to surgery or to enema reduction. A young or sick patient, for instance, an oncology patient with an abnormal clotting profile, may warrant a gingerly performed reduction attempt, accepting a far greater risk of

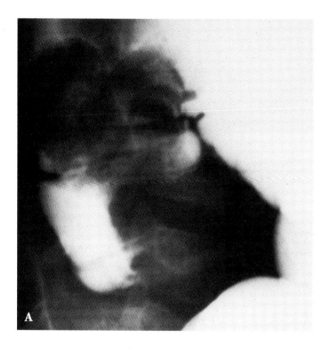

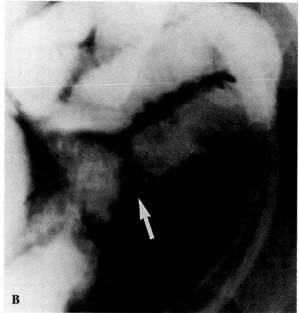

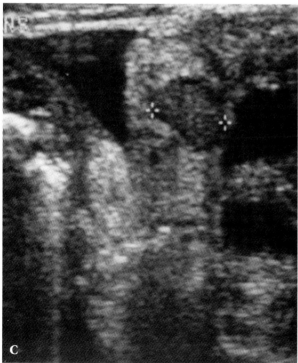

FIGURE 9–180. Ileoileocolic intussusception with lymphoid tissue (probably a Peyer's patch) as lead point. *A,* Barium outlines the coils of intussuscepting small bowel at the hepatic flexure. *B,* There was an easy reduction into the ileum, where a small mass remained (*arrow*). This small mass was still present at follow-up study; hence, surgery was performed and a small amount of lymphoid tissue was resected. This lymphoid tissue probably represented a Peyer's patch of no significance. *C,* Postreduction US in another patient shows free fluid and a mass lesion representing a Peyer's patch which was managed expectantly.

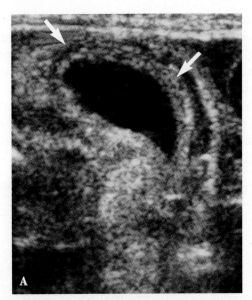
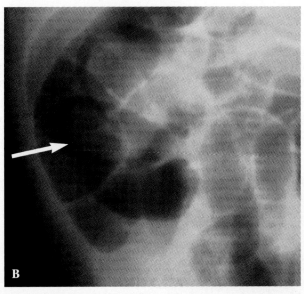

FIGURE 9–181. Intussusception with a Meckel's diverticulum as lead point. *A*, Ultrasonography detected a polypoid structure (*arrows*) as a lead point. An inverted Meckel's diverticulum containing peritoneal fluid was suggested. *B*, Air enema confirmed the lead point. This was not reduced, and a Meckel's diverticulum was surgically confirmed (*arrow*).

complication but also potentially avoiding a life-threatening surgery. A previously healthy 1-year-old child with a short history and in good condition will warrant an aggressive enema reduction using maximum pressure levels and many repeats. Such a patient, if not reduced but clinically stable or improved, may benefit from repeated delayed enema reduction, not immediate surgery (Connelly et al., 1995; Gorenstein et al., 1998). Manual manipulation of the intussusception has been frowned upon since severe warnings were made against the practice (Ravitch, 1966) but has resurfaced as a technique which has improved reduction rates in some instances (Grasso et al., 1994).

Quite how far radiologists "push the envelope" in reduction should be a balance of common sense tempered by the clinical and surgical outcomes in one's institution. Goals to strive for are reduction rates of 80 to 90% and a perforation rate of less than 1%.

Pseudo-Obstruction

The term pseudo-obstruction has been used to describe the rare clinical findings of mechanical bowel obstruction in the absence of organic occlusion of the bowel (Byrne et al., 1977). It may be primary or secondary to a wide range of conditions (Faulk et al., 1978).

Primary Idiopathic Intestinal Pseudo-Obstruction

Primary intestinal pseudo-obstruction is a heterogenous group of disorders characterized by recurrent bouts of abdominal pain and distention, resembling mechanical obstruction but due to underlying intestinal dysmotility (Byrne et al., 1977; Faulk et al., 1978; Maldonado et al., 1970; Schuffler et al., 1981; Shaw et al., 1979). Vomiting, malnutrition, diarrhea, and constipation may occur intermittently. Primary idiopathic intestinal pseudo-obstruction occurs rarely in children and often has a poor prognosis. Many patients require long-term total parenteral nutrition.

Etiology. The etiology is uncertain but a variety of histologic abnormalities have been found with variable involvement of intestinal muscle or nerve.

In many patients, there are changes in smooth muscle that are limited to fibrosis or a change in thickness of the intestinal wall. These findings are probably secondary to disuse atrophy and are of little significance; however, a primary intestinal myopathy identified on electron microscopy has been described (Bagwell et al., 1984).

Most reports in the literature have focused on neural abnormalities in the pathology of intestinal pseudo-obstruction. A familial syndrome consisting of a short small bowel, malrotation, and pyloric hypertrophy has been described in an infant with functional intestinal obstruction due to a deficiency of argyrophil neurones in the myenteric plexus, and it is thought that the hypoperistalsis was secondary to the underlying neural abnormality (Tanner et al., 1976). In other infants with intestinal pseudo-obstruction, increased nerve fibers or ganglion cells were found in the intestine (Amoury et al., 1977; Berdon et al., 1976; Tanner et al., 1976; Vezina et al., 1979; Young et al., 1981). In one case, this "hypergan-

glionosis" formed a neuromalike layer between muscle coats of the rectum (Young et al., 1981). Auerbach's plexus abnormalities have also been seen (Byrne et al., 1977; Schuffler et al., 1981; Shilkin et al., 1978). The significance of these abnormalities is unknown and the pathogenesis is poorly understood.

New histochemical stains for acetylcholinesterase and immunofluorescent markers for amine and peptide neurotransmitters may uncover a unifying pathophysiology to the present spectrum of histologic findings.

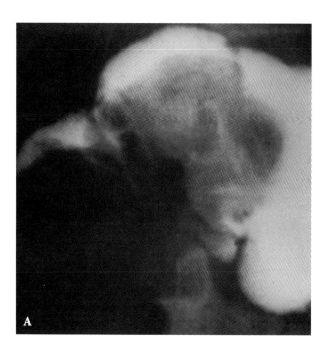

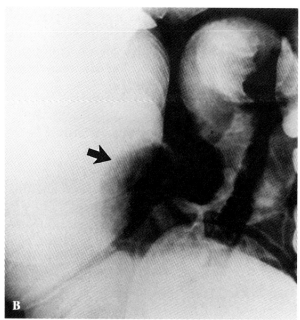

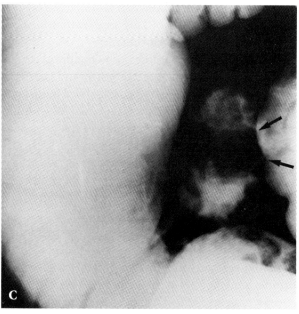

FIGURE 9–182. Ileocolic intussusception with a small lymphosarcoma as lead point. *A,* Barium outlined the intussusceptum at the hepatic flexure and easily reduced it to the ileocecal region (*B*), where a small mass (*arrow*) remains. *C,* The intussusceptum was pushed back through the ileocecal valve with difficulty and deformity, and the narrowing (*arrows*) of the terminal ileum persisted. In view of this finding and the atypical age of the patient (12 years), surgery was performed and a small lymphoma was resected.

Clinical Features. The onset of primary intestinal pseudo-obstruction generally occurs in adolescence or early adulthood; however, there have been a significant number of cases with symptoms starting in the neonatal period. These neonatal patients seem to form a distinct group.

Although intestinal peristalsis usually becomes effective within 24 hours of birth, some patients demonstrate a degree of dysmotility which produces a clinical picture of intestinal obstruction. Meconium plug syndrome and hypoplastic left hemicolon are examples of mild, short-lived forms of this dysfunction (see Chapter 10). At the other end of the spectrum, babies may have persistent ineffective peristalsis; typical examples are infants with hollow viscus myopathy, visceral neuropathy, and the megacystis-microcolon–intestinal hypomotility syndrome (Bagwell et al., 1986; Berdon et al., 1976).

Megacystis-Microcolon–Hypoperistalsis Syndrome

The megacystis-microcolon–intestinal hypomotility syndrome is a neonatal syndrome of intestinal hypomotility associated with megacystis and microcolon that was first described in female infants. It presents soon after birth and has a poor prognosis (Berdon et al., 1976; Krook, 1980; Patel and Carty, 1980; Sumner et al., 1981; Vezina et al., 1979; Wiswell et al., 1979; Young et al., 1981). Malrotation or malfixation of the bowel is common. A few affected male infants have been reported. It is occasionally familial (Berdon et al., 1976; Patel and Carty, 1980).

The cause is uncertain as ganglion cells are present. The prognosis is poor and the condition is usually fatal although hyperalimentation may delay death (Patel and Carty, 1980; Wiswell et al., 1979). The hypoperistalsis fails to respond to a gamut of medications and results in pseudo-obstruction.

Presentation occurs early with abdominal distension secondary to a thick-walled distended urinary bladder, bilious vomiting, and decreased or absent bowel sounds. These findings may mimic intestinal obstruction and lead to a laparotomy. No anatomic obstruction is found although areas of the bowel may be relatively dilated or narrow (Berdon et al., 1976). The combined small bowel and large bowel length is reduced often to one-third the normal length (Berdon et al., 1976).

Other Syndromes

Other, more undefined syndromes are thought to be caused by physiologic dysfunction of the smooth muscles or nerves of the intestinal tract. Symptoms first appear in the older child and young adult. Similarities to Hirschsprung's disease have been reported despite the presence of ganglion cells on biopsy (Kapila et al., 1975; Sieber and Girdany, 1963). A similar syndrome may involve the entire intestine (Bentley et al., 1966).

Prognosis. The literature to date has emphasized a poor prognosis for affected children, with most deaths occurring in early infancy. Of fifteen infants reported with megacystis-microcolon–hypoperistalsis syndrome, only one survived into teenage years (Young et al., 1981). In other conditions, failure of peristalsis has been stated as being incompatible with life, and so long-term parenteral support has not been advocated (Tanner et al., 1976).

We have experience of one child with primary pseudo-obstruction who is 3 years old and has progressed to full oral feeds. Others suggest a more optimistic outlook. Despite the need for lengthy periods of bowel decompression, total parenteral nutrition, and multiple operations, some patients survive with partial or complete recovery of intestinal function (Bagwell et al., 1986).

Diagnosis. Recognition of neonatal intestinal pseudo-obstruction is challenging because the initial clinical picture may resemble atresia, Hirschsprung's disease, or other nonmechanical conditions which mimic obstruction (Ueda et al., 1968). It is difficult to exclude adhesions as the cause of later obstruction in those patients who have had prior surgery.

The diagnostic studies which appear to be most helpful initially are rectal biopsy and radiologic study. Rectal manometry is not helpful in diagnosis although manometric evaluations of jejunum and esophagus have been reported as the most sensitive diagnostic tests in older age groups with suspected pseudo-obstruction (Nowak et al., 1981; Schuffler and Pope, 1976). Manometric studies of esophageal motility have been found to be abnormal in children and adults with this condition.

Total large and small bowel aganglionosis (Hirschsprung's disease) can give a similar appearance to megacystis-microcolon–hypoperistalsis syndrome; thus, biopsy is mandatory. Once the presence of ganglion cells is established by rectal biopsy, the diagnosis of neonatal intestinal pseudo-obstruction is suggested by megacystis, microcolon, and absent or ineffective peristalsis on small bowel contrast radiographs.

Additional clues to the diagnosis are the presence of a "prune belly" in a female neonate (Patel and Carty, 1980; Williams and Burkholder, 1967) and a positive family history.

Treatment. Initial management includes intestinal decompression and total parenteral nutrition, often for extended periods. Drugs are of little consistent benefit in treatment. No agent, including ceruletide, which has been shown to stimulate intestinal motility in normal adults and patients with "paralytic ileus of different origins" (Agosti et al., 1971; Bertaccini and Agosti, 1971), produces any measurable improvement in symptoms or radiographic transit time. Trials with cisapride have been disappointing in primary pseudo-obstruction but may be useful in those with a secondary disorder.

Imaging. The megacystis-microcolon–hypoperistalsis syndrome has a number of unique diagnostic features and will be considered separately from other types of pseudo-obstruction.

Imaging of Megacystis-Microcolon–Hypoperistalsis Syndrome. A large bladder and bilateral hydronephrosis may be discovered on antenatal US and, although not specific, will prompt further investigation after delivery. Polyhydramnios may be associated (Krook, 1980; Vezina et al., 1979).

The first postnatal examination of these neonates is usually a plain-film radiography, which may show the soft-tissue mass of the enlarged bladder, an abnormal and static bowel gas pattern (Figure 9–183), or a lack of bowel gas. This abnormal bowel gas pattern and failure to pass meconium often prompts a contrast study to delineate the anatomy.

Contrast enema and small bowel follow-through examination can be helpful (Figure 9–184). The enema is useful in assessing possible malrotation and demonstrating a microcolon which empties slowly. The small bowel follow-through examination is useful for assessing transit time and excluding malrotation (see Figure 9–184). Transit time may be delayed with little peristalsis and reversed peristalsis may rarely be present (Amoury et al., 1977). Transit time and peristalsis may

improve slowly in some infants, and the contrast study is a useful way to monitor progress and assess prognosis (Figure 9–185).

Ultrasonography will demonstrate the large bladder and any hydronephrosis (Figure 9–186). The megacystis and microcolon will get better with time, unlike the hypoperistalsis although there has been some improvement in a few of the infants we have seen. The renal tract can also be further investigated by renography and maybe cystography (see Figure 9–186). A cystograph may be necessary to exclude bladder outlet obstruction, though obstruction would be unusual in females. Vesicoureteric reflux is common (Berdon et al., 1976; Patel and Carty, 1980).

Imaging of Other Types of Pseudo-Obstruction. Plain films show dilated small bowel containing gas-fluid levels (Figure 9 187). This can cause a diagnostic dilemma when the child presents acutely with an exacerbation of obstructive-type symptoms because the radiologic appearance of pseudo-obstruction and mechanical obstruction are identical.

On upper GI examination, the motility of the esophagus is often abnormal, and there is delayed emptying of the stomach and erratic transit of barium. The examination can help exclude a mechanical obstruction, however. Because transit can be so

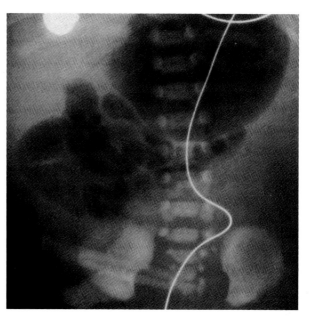

FIGURE 9–183. Megacystis-microcolon–hypoperistalsis syndrome. The plain film shows an abnormal gas pattern with dilated loops of static small bowel.

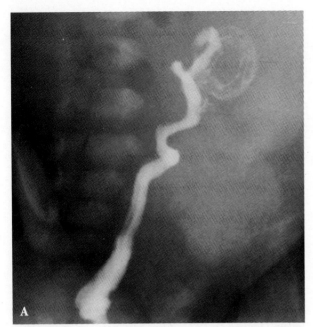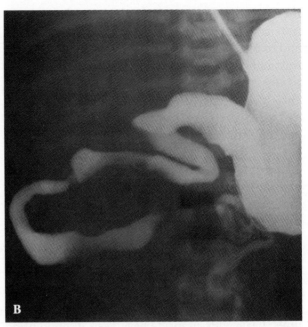

FIGURE 9–184. Megacystis-microcolon–hypoperistalsis syndrome. *A,* Barium enema demonstrates a microcolon. More proximal filling was not attempted. *B,* A small bowel follow-through examination to assess transit time showed a malrotation and almost complete stasis of barium in the duodenum.

delayed, with barium often taking many days to reach the colon, flocculation and segmentation can occur, giving such poor visualization that the study is unhelpful (see Figure 9–185). A small bowel enema is no better at showing the gut in this situation. One patient who had had multiple operations

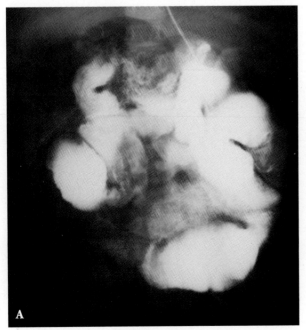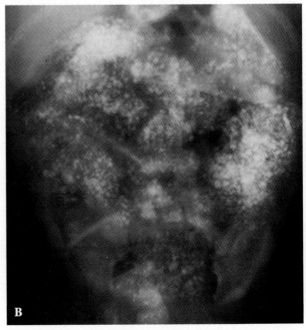

FIGURE 9–185. Neonatal intestinal pseudo-obstruction. *A,* Barium passed through the small bowel over 5 days resulting in marked flocculation of the barium on delayed films (*B*). The transit time was delayed but improved slowly over a period of 2 years.

and returned for studies because of possible mechanical obstruction was shown to have a jejunal volvulus on barium enema by refluxing barium back through the ileocecal valve (Figure 9–188). An upper GI examination and small bowel follow-through examination had both been unsuccessful in proving the need for further operation.

A contrast enema may be helpful in excluding obstruction or other abnormality. There is often poor evacuation of barium following the study.

Total large and small bowel aganglionosis (Hirschsprung's disease) can have an appearance similar to that of megacystis-microcolon–hypoperistalsis syndrome, with a marked delay in transit time and a microcolon (Figure 9–189), making biopsy mandatory.

Secondary Pseudo-Obstruction

Secondary pseudo-obstruction in children is rare and similar to that seen in adults. It has been

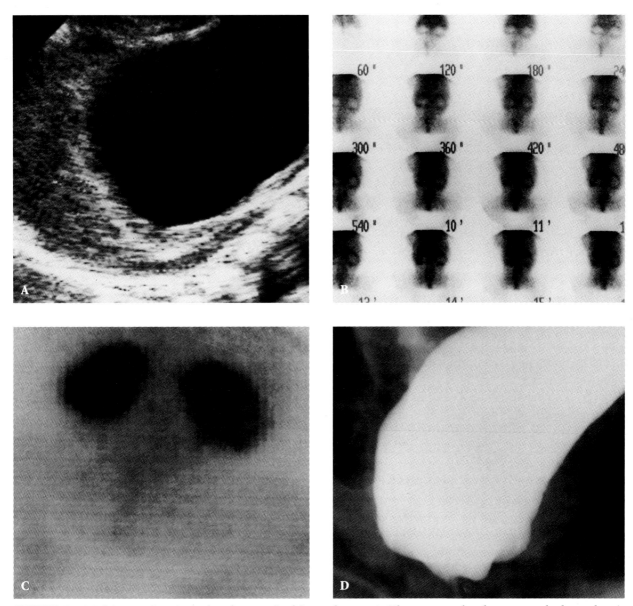

FIGURE 9–186. Megacystis-microcolon–hypoperistalsis syndrome. *A,* Ultrasonography shows gross hydronephrosis and very little renal parenchyma. *B,* There is a rim "nephrogram" effect on technetium Tc 99m DTPA renography with delayed filling of the renal pelvises (*C*) indicating poor renal function. *D,* Cystogram demonstrates the large bladder also seen on US, the preferred examination.

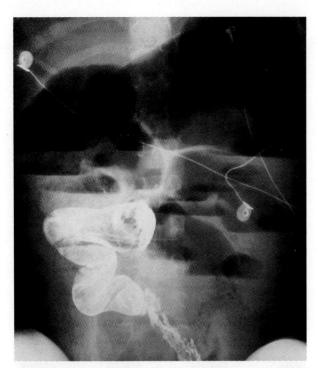

FIGURE 9–187. Pseudo-obstruction. There are marked air-fluid levels in this 8-year-old girl who has had pseudo-obstruction from birth. There was no mechanical obstruction at this time. This appearance makes diagnosis of any acute mechanical obstruction extremely difficult. Barium was present from a previous enema examination.

described in association with a variety of conditions such as potassium depletion (Lowman, 1971), autonomic nervous system incoordination or dysfunction (Melamed and Kubian, 1963), and mucocutaneous lymph node syndrome (Kawasaki disease) (Franken et al., 1979).

Bowel paralysis giving a functional obstruction can also be seen with peritonitis or other infections such as gastroenteritis, and following surgery or trauma (Clemett and Inkeles, 1971; Friman-Dahl, 1974).

Superior Mesenteric Artery and Cast Syndromes

In adults, the superior mesenteric artery has been implicated as a cause of an obstructive syndrome often producing vomiting (the superior mesenteric artery syndrome) by compression of the third, transverse, part of the duodenum. The validity of superior mesenteric artery syndrome and its possible causes has been hotly debated (Mindell and Holm, 1970).

In poorly nourished children, such as those with cerebral palsy, a similar syndrome of obstruction of the third, transverse, part of the duodenum

can occur. However, the compression is almost certainly due to the spine rather than the superior mesenteric artery (Figure 9–190) because the spine is close to the anterior abdominal wall, and the lack of mesenteric fat and the often unusual posture of these children exacerbates any compression (Vaisman et al., 1989). The radiologic placement of a nasojejunal feeding tube enables prolonged feeding so that patient bulk can increase. The obstruction may then spontaneously resolve (Vaisman et al., 1989).

Bowel obstruction sometimes occurs in children after the application of a plaster hip spica or body jacket (Berk and Coulson, 1970) or after Harrington rod placement (Figure 9–191). This is called body cast syndrome and is also probably due to compression of the duodenum as it passes anterior to the spine (Leigh, 1960). In the treatment of scoliosis, a similar syndrome can occur when Harrington rods are used to straighten the spine.

The preceding conditions have a degree of immobilization and malnutrition which are probably the most important etiologic factors.

Hernia

As in adults, certain bowel herniation results in a variable degree of intestinal obstruction in children. Some have specific manifestations in children.

Inguinal Hernia

Etiology. In children, inguinal hernias are almost always indirect. In the male fetus, the peritoneum prolapses into the inguinal canal and scrotum by the third intrauterine month. This is called the processus vaginalis. In the female fetus, a similar prolapse occurs through the inguinal canal, which ends in the labia majora and is called the canal of Nuck. If the processus vaginalis maintains an open communication with the peritoneal cavity, an inguinal hernia, herniation of bowel, can occur. Inguinal hernia is more common in male infants, outnumbering female cases by more than 9 to 1 (Gurrarino, 1974). Four out of 5 hernias occur on the right. The processus vaginalis should close within the first few months of life. The processus vaginalis may seal off in the inguinal canal, resulting in a congenital hydrocele.

Clinical Features. The majority of inguinal hernias are asymptomatic. In our experience, approximately 10% are incarcerated, suggesting that the bowel is viable but stuck. Only a very small proportion become strangulated (i.e., stuck with nonviable bowel). From the fourth day of life until the fourth month, the most common cause of intestinal obstruction is an incarcerated inguinal hernia (Gurrarino, 1974). The infant usually presents with clinical evidence of intestinal obstruction, and the diagnosis is usually obvious clinically.

Imaging. Plain films often show dilated loops of small bowel with gas-fluid levels indicating obstruction. A gas-filled loop of bowel may be seen in the inguinal canal (Figure 9–192), confirming a hernia but usually this is absent. A thickened inguinoscrotal fold may be present although this is not a specific sign (Gurrarino, 1974).

A barium enema with plentiful reflux into the ileum may show a cutoff where a loop of bowel enters the inguinal canal (Gurrarino, 1974). Herniography can be used to help detect a patent

processus vaginalis (Ekberg et al., 1984; Shackelford and McAlister, 1972). This hazardous procedure is now obsolete, with US the imaging modality of choice.

Ultrasonography with high-resolution linear probes can accurately assess the scrotum, labia, and inguinal canal structures. Fluid surrounding a testicle can be compressed back up the canal through the patent processus vaginalis under direct vision, confirming a patent processus vaginalis. Peristalsing fluid and air-filled loops of bowel or mesenteric fat passing down the canal into the scrotum are readily identified (Figure 9–193) (Siegel, 1995). In boys, bowel or omentum invariably herniates; in the female hernia, bowel, ovary, and fallopian tube often pass down the canal of Nuck, presenting as a labial mass (Figure 9–194).

Treatment. Surgery is the treatment of choice. Strangulated hernias are operated on immediately

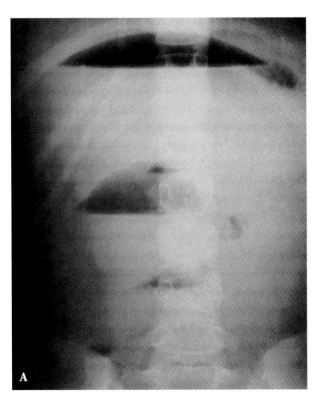
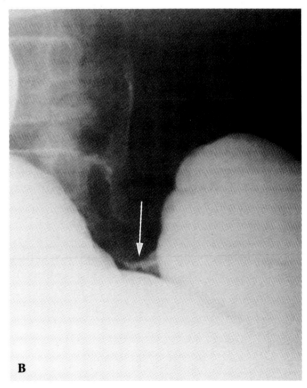

FIGURE 9–188. Pseudo-obstruction with jejunal volvulus. A 10-year-old girl with pseudo-obstruction from birth and who had had multiple operations returned for studies because of possible mechanical obstruction. *A,* Plain films showed gross dilatation of some loops of bowel but as this was not dissimilar to her previous appearance, contrast studies were performed. *B,* Barium was refluxed back through the ileocecal valve to reach the proximal small bowel and demonstrated an obstruction with a beak (arrow), suggesting a volvulus. Neither an upper GI examination nor a small bowel enema had shown the need for further operation. A jejunal volvulus was found at operation.

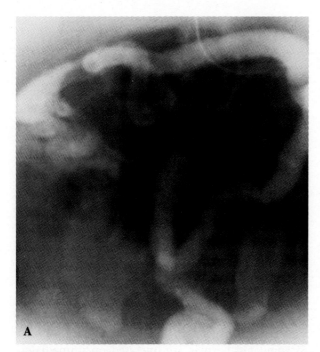
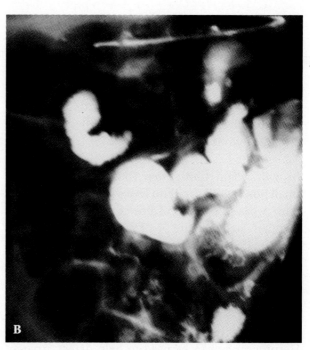

FIGURE 9–189. Hirschsprung's disease of the small and large bowel. *A,* Barium enema showed a microcolon. *B,* Small bowel follow-through examination to assess transit time showed dilated loops of small bowel and very delayed transit. No ganglia were present from duodenojejunal junction to rectum, a status incompatible with life.

but asymptomatic hernias are often left for a variable period of time if the baby is small. Incarcerated hernias may initially be reduced, followed by delayed surgery; or they may be operated on immediately depending on the status of the patient and the hernia. In male infants with an inguinal hernia, there is a strong possibility that the contralateral processus vaginalis is also open, and a hernia may develop later on that side. Consequently, many surgeons advocate exploration on both sides.

Femoral Hernia

Congenital femoral hernia is uncommon in children. Nonspecific radiologic signs of intestinal obstruction may be present. Ultrasonography and accurate anatomic location of the hernial site allows diagnosis.

Spigelian Hernia

Clinical Features. Spigelian hernias are an uncommon form of anterior abdominal wall hernia which occurs along the lateral margin of the rectus muscle, usually slightly below the umbilicus. At this point the internal oblique aponeurosis divides into two layers and proceeds to envelop the rectus muscle only anteriorly. The deep layers are weak at this level, and so hernias can develop to lie within the muscular thickness of the anterior abdominal wall, which is usually covered by the external oblique muscle. The clinical presentation depends on the hernial sac contents, namely, omentum and small or large bowel. Occasionally, unusual tissues such as stomach, ovary, or Meckel's diverticulum may be present (Arida et al., 1970). Major presenting features include intestinal obstruction with an ill-defined, slightly tender palpable mass but the features are often unusual or the condition may be asymptomatic.

Imaging. Because of their rarity and unusual presenting findings, diagnosis may be difficult. Plain films can show loops of bowel within the hernial sac. These loops may be pinched off where they enter and leave the hernial sac. These findings can also be seen on barium studies (Holder and Schneider, 1974; Hunter et al., 1977). Ultrasonography and CT may be useful, especially in the patient who has a mass but is otherwise asymptomatic. Findings include the presence of a peritoneal/muscular defect, intraparietal location of the hernial sac, and the presence of omentum and/or mesentery and loops of bowel within the sac (Balthazar et al., 1984).

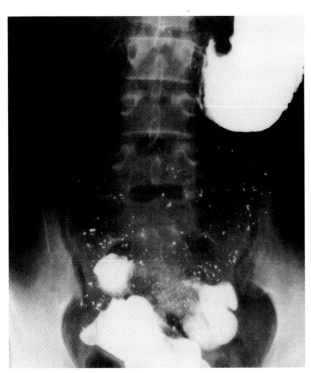

FIGURE 9–190. Superior mesenteric artery syndrome. A poorly nourished child's upper GI examination showed marked delay in gastric emptying, and most of the contrast stayed to the left of the spine, allowing filling of the ileum before more gastric emptying occurred.

Mesenteric Hernia

Paraduodenal hernia occurs with malrotation (see Embryogenesis of the Midgut and Malrotation and Malfixation of the Midgut in this chapter).

A rare internal hernia can occur in children at Treves' fold. It occurs into a defect in the mesentery of the terminal ileum between the ileocolic artery and the last ileal artery. Loops of bowel may be found in a hernial sac on barium follow-through examinations (Harbin et al., 1979). These loops of herniated bowel may undergo volvulus. Rarely, this volvulus may be chronic, to the extent of causing bleeding and anemia (Lewis and Hoskins, 1985).

Occasionally, other mesenteric defects may be a site of herniation; similarly, abdominal wall hernia is occasionally found through areas of muscular weakness that may be present at the site of a previous incision. These may be difficult to palpate if the child is fat, and if a contrast study is used for delineation (Maglinte et al., 1984), US will usually suffice. Computed tomography will also show incisional hernias as has been shown in a surprisingly large number of adults (Ghahremani et al., 1987).

Obturator Hernia

Obturator hernias are rare and may be difficult to diagnose by physical examination and clinical history. Findings are usually nonspecific although occasionally, bowel obstruction that can be easily seen on plain films may occur. Computed tomography and MR can show the hernia (Meziane et al., 1983), but the abnormality is usually demonstrated serendipitously.

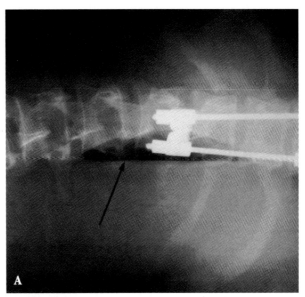

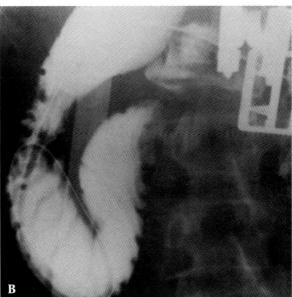

FIGURE 9–191. Superior mesenteric artery syndrome. *A,* Following Harrington rod placement for scoliosis, there is a large gastric air bubble (*arrow*) on the left-side-down decubitus film. *B,* Barium instilled via a feeding tube in the second part of the duodenum could not empty across the spine.

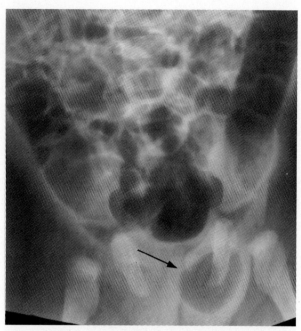

FIGURE 9–192. Left inguinal hernia. A gas-filled loop of bowel (*arrow*) is present.

Richter's Hernia

Richter's hernia is a strangulation of only part of the circumference of the intestinal wall in a hernial orifice. This can occur in children although it is uncommon (Shanbhogue and Miller, 1986). There are no specific radiologic signs.

Umbilical Protrusion

A small umbilical protrusion is commonly present at birth and is often seen on radiographic examinations of the abdomen; it should not be mistaken for a mass lesion (Figure 9–195). It is rarely a problem; the protrusion nearly always disappears spontaneously by 6 months of age although some persist until the age of 5 years. Rarely, if the protrusion is large, elective surgery is required to prevent the risk of strangulation.

Adhesions

Adhesions are a relatively common cause of intestinal obstruction in pediatrics and account for approximately 5% of all cases of intestinal obstruction (Janik et al., 1981). They usually follow abdominal surgery, and their occurrence is unpredictable and their etiology is uncertain.

Most commonly, adhesions follow appendectomy and subtotal colectomy (Janik et al., 1981). Diagnosis is usually made clinically in a child with bilious vomiting and a variably distended abdomen.

Plain-film radiography showing dilated loops of small bowel (Figure 9–196) with air-fluid levels may help the surgeon preoperatively demonstrate the approximate level of the obstruction. More detailed radiographic study is rarely indicated.

If there are subacute or intermittent symptoms, a small bowel follow-through examination can occasionally be helpful (Bartram, 1980). Enteroclysis is even more effective at detecting subtle adhesions (Caroline et al., 1984) but is rarely necessary in children because treatment depends on the severity of the symptoms (i.e., if there is small bowel obstruction then an operation is indicated; but if small bowel obstruction is absent, laparoto-

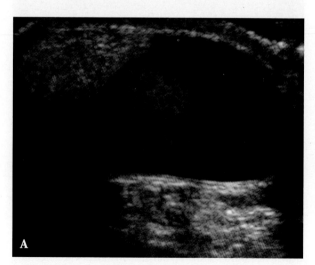

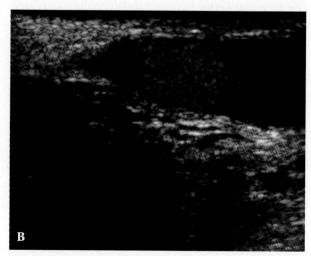

FIGURE 9–193. Inguinal hernia. *A*, Longitudinal US of the scrotum shows a normal testis, fluid, and an echogenic mass in keeping with mesenteric fat. *B*, Gentle compression reduced the mesenteric fat, confirming an inguinal hernia.

my will not be performed on the radiologic evidence alone).

In the adult population, CT has been reported as useful for assessing small bowel obstruction. Reported signs are dilated proximal bowel, caliber change at site of stricture, and causes for stricture such as malignant mass or inflammatory lesion (Megibow et al., 1991; Fukuya et al., 1992). Computed tomography is far less useful in subacute or partial obstruction than in high-grade obstruction (Megibow et al., 1983), and we do not use CT in the pediatric setting, where plain radiographs and clinical status determine surgical or expectant management.

Riley-Day Syndrome

Riley-Day syndrome (familial dysautonomia) mainly affects Ashkenazi Jews and is a recessively inherited autosomal condition. It often presents in infancy with gagging, vomiting, and aspiration of food (see Chapter 6). Autonomic dysfunction is indicated by increased sweating, decreased lacrimation, labile hypertension, and orthostatic hypotension. The small bowel may have disordered motility.

Paralytic Ileus

Paralytic ileus is uncommon in children except as a transient phenomenon after surgery. The appearance is similar to obstruction as both have dilated loops of fluid and air-filled bowel (Figure 9–197). The easiest way to differentiate these two conditions is clinical assessment.

Necrotizing Enterocolitis

Necrotizing enterocolitis is discussed in greater detail in Chapter 10 because it primarily affects the large bowel. However, it can cause perforations and produce obstructive sequelae secondary to strictures (Figure 9–198).

MISCELLANEOUS DISORDERS

Pneumoperitoneum

Pneumoperitoneum is often seen following abdominal operations and rarely can remain for up to 4 weeks (Rice et al., 1982). In blunt abdominal trauma, it signifies the rupture of a hollow abdominal viscus and usually constitutes an abdominal emergency. In older children, the causes of rupture and the radiologic signs of pneumoperitoneum

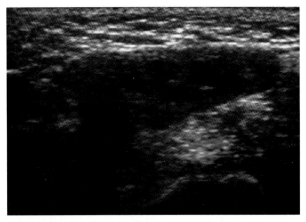

FIGURE 9–194. Inguinal hernia in a female. On US, an inguinal mass had follicular cysts, indicating an ovary herniating down the canal of Nuck.

are similar to those of adults. Causes include perforation of a gastric or duodenal ulcer, penetrating injuries, and perforation secondary to bowel obstruction or severe ulcerative colitis (Rice et al., 1982). Free perforation from Crohn's disease is rare, with most perforations walled off, developing into fistula and abscess. Perforation may be associated with steroid treatment such as is commonly prescribed for patients with rheumatoid arthritis,

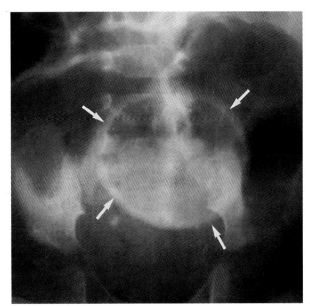

FIGURE 9–195. Umbilical protrusion. An apparent air-filled mass lesion (*arrows*) represents an umbilical protrusion. It is rarely a problem and nearly always disappears spontaneously by 6 months of age, although some persist until the age of 5 years.

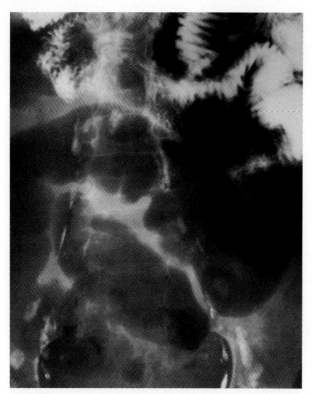
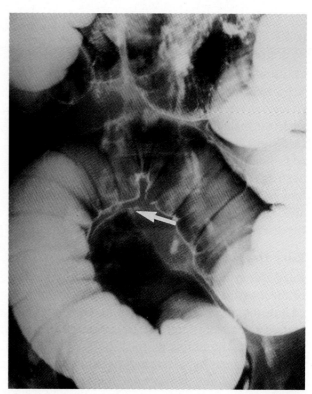

FIGURE 9–196. Adhesions causing small bowel obstruction. *A*, There are many dilated gas-filled loops of small bowel on an early film of a small bowel follow-through examination. *B*, A delayed film delineated the obstruction (*arrow*) preoperatively. There had been a previous lymphangiogram.

vasculitis, asthma, or renal transplants (ReMine and McIlrath, 1980; Rice et al., 1982; Warshaw et

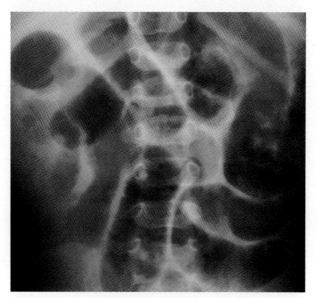

FIGURE 9–197. Paralytic ileus. There are dilated loops of fluid and air-filled bowel in a 9-month-old child who ingested medications.

al., 1976). Pneumoperitoneum may occasionally be idiopathic or related to an extra-abdominal cause such as pneumothorax/pneumomediastinum or head and neck surgery.

In infants, the clinical signs will depend on the underlying cause of the pneumoperitoneum. This may be necrotizing enterocolitis, the most common cause (see Chapter 10), or rupture of the stomach (see Chapter 8) or another viscus. In infants, as in older children, pneumoperitoneum may also be secondary to thoracic problems such as progressive tension pneumomediastinum (Campbell et al., 1975) or chronic respiratory disease (Leonidas et al., 1973). Caution must be exercised before deciding that a pneumoperitoneum is secondary to lung disease; failure to operate in the presence of a bowel perforation could have serious consequences (Leonidas et al., 1974).

Imaging

Plain-Film Radiology. Plain films may demonstrate any of the signs of pneumoperitoneum

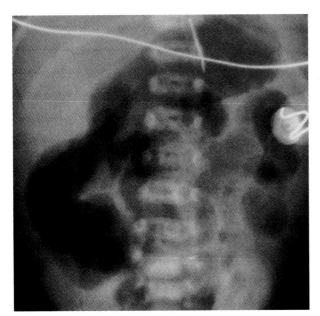

FIGURE 9–198. Jejunal obstruction secondary to necrotizing enterocolitis. Dilated loops of proximal small bowel on plain film indicate obstruction confirmed by barium study. A stricture was found at operation.

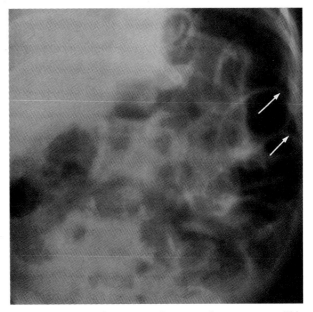

FIGURE 9–199. Pneumoperitoneum in a neonate. Triangular areas of gas (*arrows*) are seen between adjacent loops of bowel, and gas in the left upper quadrant outlines both the mucosal and serosal surfaces of the bowel wall.

described in adults. With optimum technique, and especially with the patient lying on the left lateral side for 10 minutes prior to a decubitus film, tiny amounts of free air can be seen (Rice et al., 1982). A cross-table lateral view may show a triangle of gas between loops of bowel (Seibert and Parvey, 1977) which may occasionally be seen on films taken in the supine position (Figure 9–199). As in adults, films taken in the erect position will show subdiaphragmatic air. Sometimes infants and a few older patients are too sick to be moved from the supine position; in these patients, signs are often more subtle. Findings include unusual, often linear, gas shadows in the right upper quadrant in unusual locations such as the right subhepatic space. The falciform ligament may be visualized surrounded by a relative lucency in the upper abdomen (Figure 9–200). Both outer and inner bowel wall (Rigler sign) may be seen (Bray, 1984). Less frequently, the lateral umbilical ligaments or umbilical arteries may be seen as an inverted V (Coussement et al., 1973). Considerable pneumoperitoneum is required for either of these signs. A smaller pneumoperitoneum may be seen as gas separating the liver and abdominal wall in the left-side-down decubitus position.

Contrast Studies. Studies of the bowel with water-soluble contrast media may occasionally help confirm a perforation in the upper GI tract. Low or iso-

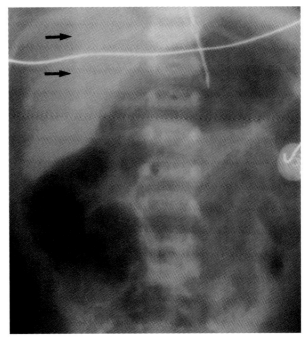

FIGURE 9–200. Pneumoperitoneum in a neonate. The falciform ligament (*arrows*) appears as a faint line of soft-tissue density within the lucency overlying the liver.

osmolar water-soluble contrast media should be used; hyperosmolar contrast media are contraindicated and may further damage an already compromised gut, such as in necrotizing enterocolitis, as well as risk aspiration leading to acute pulmonary edema or death.

Ultrasonography and CT. Abdominal radiography may be all that is required to diagnose and manage the patient. Further imaging may be indicated to evaluate the underlying condition (rather than the pneumoperitoneum) such as inflammatory bowel disease or blunt abdominal trauma.

Pneumatosis Intestinalis

Pneumatosis intestinalis (gas in the bowel wall) in the neonate is usually associated with necrotizing enterocolitis (see Chapter 10). Other implicated predisposing conditions include intestinal obstruction and lung disease, such as pneumomediastinum or cystic fibrosis (Hernanz-Shulman et al., 1986; Olmsted and Madewell, 1976; Robinson et al., 1974). In neonates, the intestinal obstruction may be due to duodenal stenosis, meconium ileus, imperforate anus, or Hirschsprung's disease (Borns and Johnson, 1973). In older children, cystic fibrosis, leukemia, or steroid or immunosuppressive treatment has been associated with pneumatosis (Gupta, 1978; Hernanz-Schulman et al., 1986; Keats and Smith, 1974). Other reported causes include carbohydrate or lactose intolerance, ischemia (secondary to intussusception, volvulus, or vessel thrombosis secondary to catheterization), and collagen diseases such as dermatomyositis or juvenile rheumatoid arthritis (Olmsted and Madewell, 1976; Robinson et al., 1974). In adults, there are additional causes of pneumatosis that could pertain to the pediatric age group; for example, pneumatosis can occur following surgery or trauma, inflammatory bowel disease, and peritoneal or bowel infections, and may be associated with transcutaneous jejunostomy feeding (Olmsted and Madewell, 1976; Strain et al., 1982).

Imaging

Plain-Film Radiography. The most important radiologic sign in pneumatosis intestinalis is gas tracking along the wall, appearing as a linear lucency of gas running parallel to a loop of bowel (Figure 9–201).

An alternative appearance is a bubbly pattern which may be difficult to distinguish from feces. Air in the portal vessels is most often seen with neonatal necrotizing enterocolitis (see Chapter 10).

Ultrasonography and CT. Pneumatosis intestinalis has a characteristic appearance with echogenic foci in bowel wall on US (Figure 9–202) and pockets of gas lying within the bowel wall on CT (Vernacchia et al., 1985). Ultrasonography is far more sensitive than plain films for detecting portal gas. Although occasionally the gas may not be visible on them, plain films remain the diagnostic modality of choice (Vernacchia et al., 1985).

Calcified Meconium in the Newborn

Calcification is rarely present within meconium lying in the bowel. It is described most commonly in association with anorectal malformations and may be related to urine passing into the bowel via rectourethral fistulae. Even more rarely, it may be found in anorectal malformations without fistulae, Hirschsprung's disease, and small bowel atresia (Cook, 1978).

Gastrointestinal Complications of Renal Transplantation in Children

Renal transplantation is now a routine pediatric surgical procedure. The operation may be technically more difficult than in adults because not only are the vessels smaller but the donated kidneys are often from adults and of disparate size to the recipient child. Associated gastrointestinal complications increasingly reported include small bowel obstruction, gastric or duodenal ulceration, pancreatitis, hepatitis, ascites, and gastroenteritis (Schnyder et al., 1979). Few deaths from these complications have been reported but there is significant morbidity. In addition, unusual infections such as cytomegalovirus typhlitis may occur (Foucar et al., 1981). We have seen one child who developed a chronic abscess with a fistula from the bowel to the renal transplant bed. Colonic perforations are also reported (Puglisi et al., 1985).

Polyarteritis Nodosa

Polyarteritis nodosa is a multisystem disease that is rare in children and is characterised by small- and medium-sized arterial inflammatory reactions which is rare in children. The kidneys are most commonly

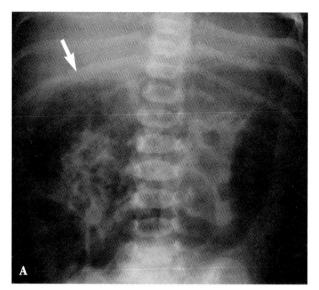
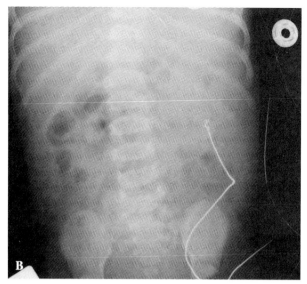

FIGURE 9–201. Pneumatosis coli. *A,* Plain-film radiographs showed extensive pneumatosis (arrow) in a term newborn who had some amniotic fluid aspiration and required initial positive pressure ventilation. The abdomen was clinically benign. *B,* By 48 hours later, the pneumatosis had resolved spontaneously.

involved, with microaneurysms, and the intestines are the second most frequently involved abdominal organ. Occasionally, the liver also shows evidence of vasculitis (Capps and Klein, 1970). Reported abdominal complications include small bowel intussusception (Fujioka et al., 1980) and retroperitoneal hemorrhage (Capps and Klein, 1970).

Anorexia Nervosa

Anorexia nervosa is progressive starvation which is self-imposed due to a psychiatric disorder. Patients are most often adolescent girls. Anorexia nervosa can result in such severe cachexia and metabolic derangement that death can result. Radiologic features are absence of subcutaneous fat and reduced muscle mass, an indication of the generalized cachexia (Haller et al., 1977). Gastrointestinal findings, like plain-film findings, are nonspecific; hence, the diagnosis of this condition depends on clinical features and not radiologic appearance.

Duodenal Diverticulum

The duodenum occasionally has a small diverticulum. It is well seen on barium study and is rarely significant (Figure 9–203).

Aerophagism

Chronic swallowing of air (aerophagia) can cause abdominal distension due to chronically dilated air-

filled loops of bowel (Figure 9–204). Children so affected usually have neurologic problems.

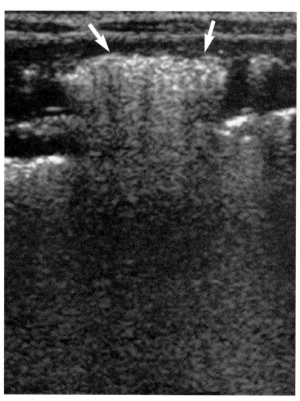

FIGURE 9–202. Pneumatosis. High-resolution linear US transducer image of bowel wall shows air (*arrows*) within the thickened wall.

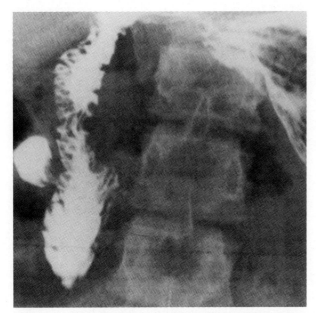

FIGURE 9–203. Duodenal diverticulum. A small diverticulum filled with barium arises from the lateral wall of the duodenum.

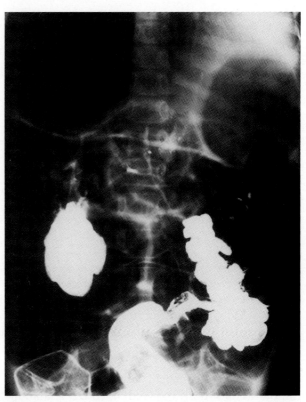

FIGURE 9–204. Aerophagism. The abdomen is distended with dilated air-filled loops of bowel from chronic air swallowing. Barium is still present from an enema performed earlier. This 11-year-old boy is autistic.

REFERENCES

EMBRYOGENESIS OF THE MIDGUT AND CONGENITAL AND DEVELOPMENTAL ANOMALIES OF THE SMALL BOWEL

Ablow RC, Hoffer FA, Seashore JH, et al. Z-shaped duodenojejunal loop: sign of mesenteric fixation anomaly and congenital bands. AJR 1983;141:461–4.

Beasley SW, DeCampo JF. Pitfalls in the radiographic diagnosis of malrotation. Australas Radiol 1996;31:376–83.

Berdon WE, Baker DH, Bull S, et al. Mid gut malrotation and volvulus: which films are most helpful? Radiology 1970;96:375–83.

Bill AH. Malrotation of the intestine. In: Ravitch MM, Welch KJ, Benson CD, et al., editors. Pediatric surgery. 3rd ed. Chicago: Year Book; 1979. p. 921–2.

Buranasiri SI, Baum S, Moreye N, Tumen H. The angiographic diagnosis of midgut malrotation with volvulus in adults. Radiology 1973;109:555–6.

Cohen HL, Haller JO, Mestel AL, et al. Neonatal duodenum: fluid-aided US examination. Radiology 1987;164:806–9.

Cunningham T, Hartman G, Bulas DI. CT findings in prearterial reversed midgut rotation. Pediatr Radiol 1994;24:537–8.

Cyr DR, Mack LA, Schonecker SA, et al. Bowel migration in the normal fetus: US detection. Radiology 1986;161:119–21.

DePrima SJ, Hardy DC, Brant WE. Reversed intestinal rotation. Radiology 1985;157:603–4.

Ditchfield MR, Hutson JM. Intestinal rotational abnormalities in polysplenia and asplenia syndromes. Pediatr Radiol 1998;28:303–6.

Dufour D, Delaet MH, Dassonville M, et al. Midgut malrotation: the reliability of sonographic diagnosis. Pediatr Radiol 1992;22:21–3.

Filston HC, Kirks DR. Malrotation, the ubiquitous anomaly. J Pediatr Surg 1981;16:614–20.

Firor HV, Harris VJ. Rotational abnormalities of the gut: reemphasis of a neglected facet; isolated incomplete rotation of the duodenum. AJR 1974;120:315–21.

Fisher JK. Computed tomographic diagnosis of volvulus in intestinal malrotation. Radiology 1981;140:145–6.

Friedland GW, Mason R, Poole GJ. Ladd's bands in older children, adolescents and adults. Radiology 1970;95:363–8.

Frye TR, Chonggi LM, Schiller M. Roentgenographic evidence of gangrenous bowel in midgut volvulus with observations in experimental volvulus. AJR 1972;114:394–401.

Gaines PA, Saunders JS, Drake D. Midgut malrotation diagnosed by ultrasound. Clin Radiol 1987;38:51–3.

Grob M. Conservative treatment of exomphalos. Arch Dis Child 1963;38:148–50.

Haley JC, Peden JK. The suspensory muscle of the duodenum. Am J Surg 1943;59:546–50.

Harbin WP. Computed tomographic diagnosis of internal hernia. Radiology 1982;143:736.

Hayden CK, Boulden TF, Swischuk LE, et al. Sonographic demonstration of duodenal obstruction with midgut volvulus. AJR 1984;143:9–10.

Houston CS, Wittenborg MH. Roentgen evaluation of anomalies of rotation and fixation of the bowel in children. Radiology 1965;84:1–8.

Humphrey A. Intestinal obstruction due to abnormal duodenal fixation in infants. J Can Assoc Radiol 1970;21:251–6.

Kassner EG, Kottmeier PK. Absence and retention of small bowel gas in infants with mid gut volvulus: mechanisms and significance. Pediatr Radiol 1975;4:28–30.

Katz ME, Siegel MJ, Shackelford GD, McAlister WH. The position and mobility of the duodenum in children. AJR 1987;148:947–51.

Kiesewetter WB, Smith JW. Malrotation of the mid gut in infancy and childhood. Arch Surg 1958;77:483–91.

Ladd WE. Congenital obstruction of the duodenum in children. N Eng J Med 1932;206:277–83.

Ladd WE. Surgical diseases of the alimentary tract in infants. N Eng J Med 1936;215:705–8.

Leonidas JC, Magid N, Soberman N, Glass TS. Midgut volvulus in infants: diagnosis with ultrasound work in progress. Radiology 1991;179:491–3.

Lewis JE. Partial duodenal obstruction with incomplete duodenal rotation. J Pediatr Surg 1966;1:47–53.

Long FR, Kramer SS, Markowitz RI, et al. Intestinal mal-

rotation in children: tutorial on radiographic diagnosis in difficult cases. Radiology 1996;198:775–80.

Loyer E, Eggli KD. Sonographic evaluation of superior mesenteric vascular relationship in malrotation. Pediatr Radiol 1989;19:173–5.

Markowitz RI, Shashikumar VL, Capitanio MA. Volvulus of the colon in a child with congenital asplenia (Ivemark's syndrome). Radiology 1977;122:442.

Millar AJW, Rode H, Brown RA, Cywes S. The deadly vomit: malrotation and midgut volvulus. A review of 137 cases. Pediatr Surg Int 1987;2:172–6.

Moller JH, Amplatz K, Wolfson J. Malrotation of the bowel in patients with congenital heart disease associated with splenic anomalies. Radiology 1971;99:393–8.

Mori H, Hayashi K, Futagawa S, et al. Vascular compromise in chronic volvulus with midgut malrotation. Pediatr Radiol 1987;17:277–81.

Myers MA. Paraduodenal hernias. Radiologic and arteriographic diagnosis. Radiology 1970;95:29–37.

Nichols DM, Li DK. Superior mesenteric vein rotation: a CT sign of midgut malrotation. AJR 1983;141:707–8.

Nyberg DA, Mack LA, Patten RM, Cyr DR. Fetal Bowel. Normal Sonographic Findings. J Ultrasound Med 1987;6:3–6.

Olazabal A, Guasch I, Casa D. Case report: CT diagnosis of non-obstructive left paraduodenal hernia. Clin Radiol 1992;46:288–9.

Paul AB, Dean DM. Computed tomography in volvulus of the midgut. Br J Radiol 1990;63:893–4.

Potts SR, Thomas PS, Garstin WIH, et al. The duodenal triangle: a plain film sign of midgut malrotation and volvulus in the neonate. Clin Radiol 1985;36:47–9.

Pracos JP, Sann L, Genin G, et al. Ultrasound diagnosis of midgut volvulus: the whirlpool sign. Pediatr Radiol 1992;22:18–20.

Richardson WR, Martin LW. Pitfalls in the surgical management of the incomplete duodenal diaphragm. J Pediatr Surg 1969;4:303–12.

Shatzke SD, Gordon DH, Haller JO, et al. Malrotation of the bowel: malalignment of the superior mesenteric artery-vein complex shown by CT and MR. J Comput Assist Tomogr 1990;14:93–5.

Shimanuki Y, Aihara T, Takano H, et al. Clockwise

whirlpool sign at colour Doppler US: an objective and definative sign of midgut volvulus. Radiology 1996;199:261–4.

Siegel MJ, Shackelford GD, McAlister WH. Small bowel volvulus in children: its appearance on the barium enema examination. Pediatr Radiol 1980;10:91–3.

Silverman FN, Caffey J. Congenital obstruction of the alimentary tract in infants and children: errors of rotation of the mid gut. Radiology 1949;53:781–7.

Simpson AJ, Leonidas JC, Krasna IH, et al. Roentgen diagnosis of mid gut malrotation: value of upper gastrointestinal radiographic study. J Pediatr Surg 1972;7:243–52.

Snyder WH, Chaffin L. Embryology of the intestinal tract: presentation of 10 cases of malrotation. Ann Surg 1954;140:368–80.

Soderlund S. Anomalies of mid gut rotation and fixation: clinical aspects based on 62 cases in childhood. Acta Paediatr 1962;51:225–38.

Steiner GM. The misplaced cecum and the root of the mesentery. Br J Radiol 1978;51:406–13.

Stewart DR, Colodny AL. Malrotation of bowel in infants and children: a 15 year review. Surgery 1976;79:716–20.

Taylor GA, Teele RL. Chronic intestinal obstruction mimicking malrotation in children. Pediatr Radiol 1985;15:392–4.

Weinberger E, Winters WD, Liddel RM, et al. Sonographic diagnosis of intestinal malrotation in infants: importance of relative positions of the superior mesenteric vein and artery. AJR 1992;159:825–8.

Zerin JM, DiPietro MA. Mesenteric anatomy at CT: normal and abnormal appearances. Radiology 1991;179:739–42.

Zerin JM, DiPietro MA. Superior mesenteric vascular anatomy at US in patients with surgically proved malrotation of the midgut. Radiology 1992;183:693–4.

Atresia, Stenosis, and Duodenal Web

Anderson JR, Mills JOM. Adult duodenal webs: a rare cause of obstruction. Clin Radiol 1984;35:223–6.

Astley R. Duodenal atresia with gas below the obstruction. Br J Radiol 1968;42:351–3.

Boyden FA, Cope JG, Bill AH. Anatomy and embryology of congenital intrinsic obstruction of duodenum. Am J Surg 1967;114:190–202.

Brambs HJ, Spamer C, Volk B, et al. Diagnostic value of ultrasound in duodenal stenosis. Gastrointest Radiol 1986;11:135–8.

Cohen HL, Haller JO, Mestel AL, et al. Neonatal duodenum: fluid-aided US examination. Radiology 1987;164:805–9.

Cremin BJ, Solomon DJ. Ultrasonic diagnosis of duodenal diaphragm. Pediatr Radiol 1987;17:489–90.

Crowe JE, Sumner TE. Combined esophageal and duodenal atresia without tracheoesophageal fistula: characteristic radiographic changes. AJR 1978;130:167–8.

Farrant P, Dewbury KC, Meire HB. Antenatal diagnosis of duodenal atresia. Br J Radiol 1981;54:633–5.

Fonkalsrud EW, deLorimier AA, Hays DM. Congenital atresia and stenosis of the duodenum: a review compiled from the members of the surgical section of the American Academy of Pediatrics. Pediatrics 1969;43:79–83.

Hayden CK, Schwartz MZ, Davis M, et al. Combined esophageal and duodenal atresia. Sonographic findings. AJR 1983;140:225–6.

Heilbrun N, Boyden EA. Intraluminal duodenal diverticula. AJR 1964;82:887–94.

Irving IM, Rickham PP. Duodenal atresia and stenosis; annular pancreas. In: Rickham PP, Lister J, Irving IM, editors. Neonatal surgery. 2nd ed. London: Butterworths; 1978. p. 335–70.

Kassner EG, Rose JS, Kottmeier PK, et al. Retention of small foreign objects in the stomach and duodenum: a sign of partial obstruction caused by duodenal anomalies. Radiology 1975;114:683–6.

Kassner EG, Sutton AL, De Groot TJ. Bile duct anomalies associated with duodenal atresia; paradoxical presence of small bowel gas. AJR 1972;116:577–83.

Lee FA, Mahour GH, Gwinn JL. Roentgenographic aspects of intrinsic duodenal obstruction. Ann Radiol 1978;21:133–42.

Loveday BJ, Barr JA, Aitken J. The intrauterine demonstration of duodenal atresia by ultrasound. Br J Radiol 1975;48:1031–2.

Pratt AD. Current concepts of the obstructing duodenal diaphragm. Radiology 1971;100:637–43.

Annular Pancreas

Brambs HJ, Spamer C, Volk B, et al. Diagnostic value of

ultrasound in duodenal stenosis. Gastrointest Radiol 1986;11:135–8.

Elliott GB, Kliman MR, Elliott KA. Pancreatic annulus: a sign or a cause of duodenal obstruction. Can J Surg 1968; 11:357–64.

Inamoto K, Ishikawa Y, Itoh N. CT demonstration of annular pancreas: case report. Gastrointest Radiol 1983;8: 143–4.

Merrill JR, Raffensperger JG. Pediatric annular pancreas: twenty year's experience. J Pediatr Surg 1976;11:921–5.

Ravitch MM, Woods AC. Annular pancreas. Ann Surg 1950;132:1116–27.

Salonen IS. Congenital duodenal obstruction: a review of the literature and a clinical study of 66 patients, including a histopathological study of annular pancreas and a follow-up study of 36 survivors. Acta Paediatr Suppl 1978;272:1–87.

Preduodenal Portal Vein

Boles ET, Smith B. Preduodenal portal vein. Pediatrics 1961;28:805–9.

Bower RJ, Ternberg JL. Preduodenal portal vein. J Pediatr Surg 1972;7:579–84.

Braun P, Collin PP, Ducharme JC. Preduodenal portal vein: a significant entity? Report of two cases and review of the literature. Can J Surg 1974;17:316–22.

Johnson GF. Congenital preduodenal portal vein. AJR 1971;112:93–9.

McCarten KM, Teele RL. Preduodenal portal vein: venography, ultrasonography, and review of the literature. Ann Radiol 1978;21:155–60.

Atresia or Stenosis of the Jejunum or Ileum

Agha FP, Jenkins JJ. Ileal mucosal diaphragm causing small bowel obstruction. Gastrointest Radiol 1983;8:57–9.

Berdon WE, Baker DH, Santulli TV, et al. Microcolon in newborn infants with intestinal obstruction. Its correlation with the level and time of onset of obstruction. Radiology 1968;90:878–85.

Blyth H, Dickson JAS. Apple peel syndrome (congenital intestinal atresia). A family history of seven index patients. J Med Genet 1969;6:275–7.

Daneman A, Martin DJ. A syndrome of multiple gastrointestinal atresias with intraluminal calcifications: a

report of a case and a review of the literature. Pediatr Radiol 1979;8:227–31.

Delorimer AA, Fonkalsrud EW, Hays DM. Congenital atresia and stenosis of the jejunum and ileum. Surgery 1969;65:819–27.

Dickson JAS. Apple peel small bowel: an uncommon variant of duodenal and jejunal atresia. J Pediatr Surg 1970; 5:595–600.

El-Shafie M, Rickham PP. Multiple intestinal atresias. J Pediatr Surg 1970;5:655–9.

Fletman D, McQuown D, Kanchanapoom V, et al. "Apple peel" atresia of the small bowel: prenatal diagnosis of the obstruction by ultrasound. Pediatr Radiol 1980;9:118–9.

Guttman FM, Braun P, Garance PH, et al. Multiple atresias and a new syndrome of hereditary multiple atresias involving the gastrointestinal tract from stomach to rectum. J Pediatr Surg 1973;8:633–9.

Lee FA. Small bowel dilatation mimicking gastric dilatation. Pediatr Radiol 1982;12:109–10.

Leonidas JC, Amoury RA, Ashcraft KW, et al. Duodenojejunal atresia with "apple-peel" small bowel: a distinct form of intestinal atresia. Radiology 1976;118:661–5.

Louw JH. Jejunoileal atresia and stenosis. J Pediatr Surg 1966;1:8–23.

Louw JH, Barnard CN. Congenital intestinal atresia: observations on its origin. Lancet 1955;2:1065–7.

Martin CE, Leonidas JC, Amoury RA. Multiple gastrointestinal atresias, with intraluminal calcifications and cystic dilatation of bile ducts: a newly recognized entity resembling "a string of pearls." Pediatrics 1976;57:268–71.

Neal MR, Siebert JJ, Vanderzalm T, Wagner CW. Neonatal ultrasonography to distinguish between meconium ileus and ileal atresia. J Ultrasound Med 1997;16:263–6.

Nixon HH, Tawes R. Etiology and treatment of small intestine atresia: analysis of a series of 127 jejunoileal atresias and comparison with 62 duodenal atresias. Surgery 1971;69:41–51.

Nyberg DA. Diagnostic ultrasound of fetal anomalies. Chicago: Year Book Medical Publishers Inc.; 1990. p. 347–8.

Santulli TV, Blanc WA. Congenital atresia of the intestine: pathogenesis and treatment. Ann Surg 1961;154:939–48.

Schiavetti E, Massotti G, Torricelli M, et al. "Apple peel"

syndrome. A radiologic study. Pediatr Radiol 1984;14: 380–3.

Steinfield JR, Harrison RB. Extensive intramural intestinal calcification in a newborn with intestinal atresia. Radiology 1973;107:405–6.

Weitzman JJ, Vanderhof RS. Jejunal atresia with agenesis of the dorsal mesentery with "Christmas tree" deformity of the small intestine. Am J Surg 1966;111:443–9.

Wolfson JJ, Williams H. A hazard of barium enema studies in infants with small bowel atresia. Radiology 1970;95:341–3.

Meconium Ileus/Cystic Fibrosis

Abramson SJ, Baker DH, Amodio JB, Berdon WE. Gastrointestinal manifestations of cystic fibrosis. Semin Roentgenol 1987;22:97–113.

Astley R. Less common disease patterns in the gastrointestinal tract with a special note on meconium ileus. In: Eklof O, editor. Current concepts in pediatric radiology. New York: Springer International; 1977. p. 48–66.

Auburn RP, Feldman SA, Gadacz TR, et al. Meconium ileus secondary to partial aplasia of the pancreas: report of a case. Surgery 1969;65:689–93.

Berdon WE, Baker DH, Santulli TV, et al. Microcolon in newborn infants with intestinal obstruction: its correlation with the level and time of onset of obstruction. Radiology 1968;90:878–85.

Berk RN, Lee FA. The late gastrointestinal manifestations of cystic fibrosis of the pancreas. Radiology 1973;106: 337–81.

Blumenthal DH, Rushovick AM, Williams RK, et al. Prenatal sonographic findings of meconium peritonitis with pathologic correlation. J Clin Ultrasound 1982;10:350–2.

Bowen A, Mazer J, Zabrabi M, Fujioka M. Cystic meconium peritonitis: ultrasonic features. Pediatr Radiol 1984; 14:18–22.

Bryk D. Meconium ileus: demonstration of the meconium mass on barium enema study. AJR 1965;95:214–6.

Carrol BA, Moskowitz PS. Sonographic diagnosis of neonatal meconium cyst. AJR 1981;137:1262–4.

Cleghorn GJ, Stringer DA, Forstner GG, et al. Treatment of distal intestinal obstruction syndrome in cystic fibrosis with a balanced intestinal lavage solution. Lancet 1986;1(8470):8–11.

Dick JM, Crane JP. Sonographically detected hyperechoic fetal bowel: significance and implications for pregnancy management. Obstet Gynecol 1992;80:778–82.

Dolan TF, Touloukian RJ. Familial meconium ileus not associated with cystic fibrosis. J Pediatr Surg 1974;9:821–4.

Ein SH, Shandling B, Reilly BJ, Stephens CA. Bowel perforation with nonoperative treatment of meconium ileus. J Pediatr Surg 1987;22(2):146–7.

Ein SH, Venugopal S, Mancer K. Ileocaecal atresia. J Pediatr Surg 1985;20:525–8.

Estroff JA, Parad RB, Benacerraf BR. Prevalence of cystic fibrosis in fetuses with dilated bowel. Radiology 1992; 183:677–80.

Garb M, Riseborough J. Meconium peritonitis presenting as fetal ascites on ultrasound. Br J Radiol 1980;53:602–4.

Grantmyre EB, Butler GJ, Gillis DA. Necrotizing enterocolitis after Renografin-76 treatment of meconium ileus. AJR 1981;136:990–1.

Gugliantini P, Caione P, Rovosecchi M, et al. Intestinal perforation in newborn following intrauterine peritonitis. Pediatr Radiol 1979;8:113–5.

Hanly JG, Fitzgerald MX. Meconium ileus equivalent in older patients with cystic fibrosis. BMJ 1983;286:1411–3.

Harris PD, Neuhauser EBD, Gerth R. The osmotic effect of water soluble contrast media on circulating plasma volume. AJR 1964;91:694–8.

Hassall E, Isreal DM, Davidson AG, Wong LT. Barrett's esophagus in children with cystic fibrosis: not a coincidental association. AJR 1993;88:1934–8.

Herson RE. Meconium ileus. Radiology 1957;68:568–71.

Hodson ME, Mearns MB, Batten JC. Meconium ileus equivalent in adults with cystic fibrosis of the pancreas: a report of six cases. BMJ 1976;2:790–1.

Holsclaw DS, Eckstein HB, Nixon HH. Meconium ileus: a 20-year review of 109 cases. Am J Dis Child 1965;109: 101–13.

Hurwitt ES, Arnheim EE. Meconium ileus associated with stenosis of the pancreatic ducts: a clinical, pathologic, and embryologic study. Am J Dis Child 1942;64:443–54.

Irish MS, Ragi H, Karamanovkian H, et al. Prenatal diagnosis of the fetus with cystic fibrosis and meconium ileus. Pediatr Surg Int 1997;12:434–6.

Keats TE, Smith TH. Meconium ileus: a demonstration of the ileal meconium mass by barium enema examination. Radiology 1967;89:1073–4.

Knowles M, Gatzy J, Boucher R. Relative ion permeability of normal and cystic fibrosis nasal epithelium. J Clin Invest 1983;71:1410–7.

Koletzko S, Stringer DA, Cleghorn GJ, Durie PR. Lavage treatment of distal intestinal obstruction syndrome in children with cystic fibrosis. Pediatrics 1989;83:727–33.

Lawrence PW, Chrispin A. Sonographic appearances in two neonates with generalized meconium peritonitis: the snowstorm sign. Br J Radiol 1984;57:340–2.

Leonidas JC, Berdon WE, Baker DH, et al. Meconium ileus and its complications: a reappraisal of plain film roentgen diagnostic criteria. AJR 1970;108:598–609.

Leonidas JC, Burry VF, Fellows RA, et al. Possible adverse effects of methylglucamine diatrizoate compounds on the bowel of newborn infants with meconium ileus. Radiology 1976;121:693–6.

Lillie JG, Chrispin AR. Investigation and management of neonatal obstruction by Gastrografin enema. Ann Radiol 1972;15:237–41.

Lutzger LG, Factor SM. Effects of some water-soluble contrast media on the colonic mucosa. Radiology 1976;118:545–8.

Matseske JW, Go VLW, DiMagno E. Meconium ileus equivalent complicating cystic fibrosis in post-neonatal children and young adults. Gastroenterology 1972;72:732–6.

Neuhauser EBD. Roentgen changes associated with pancreatic insufficiency in early life. Radiology 1946;46:319–28.

Noblett HR. Treatment of uncomplicated meconium ileus by Gastrografin enema: a preliminary report. J Pediatr Surg 1969;4:190–7.

Park RW, Grand RJ. Gastrointestinal manifestation of cystic fibrosis: a review. Gastroenterology 1981;81:1143–61.

Quinton PM. Chloride impermeability in cystic fibrosis. Nature 1993;301:421–2.

Riordan JR, Rommens JM, Kerem B, et al. Identification of the cystic fibrosis gene: cloning and characterization of complementary DNA. Science 1989;245:1066–79.

Rosentein BJ, Langbaum TS. Incidence of distal intestinal obstruction syndrome in cystic fibrosis. J Pediatr Gastroenterol Nutr 1983;2:299–301.

Rowe MI, Furst AJ, Altman DH, et al. The neonatal response to Gastrografin enema. Pediatrics 1971;48:29–35.

Schutt WH, Isles TE. Protein in meconium from meconium ileus. Arch Dis Child 1968;43:178–81.

Seltzer SE, Jones B. Cecal perforation associated with Gastrografin enema. AJR 1978;130:997–8.

Tucker AS, Mathews LW, Doershuk CF. Roentgen diagnosis of complications of cystic fibrosis. AJR 1963;89:1048–59.

Wagget J, Bishop HC, Koop CE. Experience with Gastrografin enema in the treatment of meconium ileus. J Pediatr Surg 1970;5:649–54.

Mesenteric and Omental Cysts

Arnheim EE, Schneck H, Norman A, et al. Mesentery cysts in infancy and childhood. Pediatrics 1959;24:469–76.

Bastable JRG. Intestinal duplication with calcification. Br J Radiol 1964;37:706–8.

Bisset GS, Towbin RB. Pediatric case of the day. Radiographics 1986;6:917–20.

Blake NS. Beak sign in duodenal duplication cyst. Pediatr Radiol 1984;14:232–3.

Blumhagen JD, Wood BJ, Rosenbaum DM. Sonographic evaluation of abdominal lymphangiomas in children. J Ultrasound Med 1987;6:487–95.

Bower RJ, Sieber WK, Kiesewetter WB. Alimentary tract duplications in children. Ann Surg 1978;188:669–74.

Bremer JL. Diverticula and duplications of the intestinal tract. Arch Pathol Lab Med 1944;38:132–40.

Buras RR, Guzzetta PC, Majd M. Multiple duplications of the small intestine. J Pediatr Surg 1986;21(11):957–9.

Caropreso PR. Mesenteric cysts. Arch Surg 1974;108:242–6.

Chirathivat S, Shermeta D. Recurrent retroperitoneal mesenteric cyst: a case report and review. Gastrointest Radiol 1979;4:191–3.

Egelhoff JC, Bisset GS, Strife JL. Multiple enteric duplications in an infant. Pediatr Radiol 1986;16:160–1.

Favara BE, Franciosi RA, Akers DR. Enteric duplications: thirty-seven cases: a vascular theory of pathogenesis. Am J Dis Child 1971;122:501–6.

Geer LL, Mittelstaedt CA, Staab EV, et al. Mesenteric cyst: sonographic appearance with CT correlation. Pediatr Radiol 1984;14:102–4.

Haller JO, Schneider M, Kassner EG, et al. Sonographic evaluation of mesenteric and omental masses in children. AJR 1978;130:269–74.

Haney PJ, Whitley NO. CT of benign cystic abdominal masses in children. AJR 1984;142:1279–81.

Hizawa K, Aoyagi K, Kurahara K, et al. Gastrointestinal lymphangioma: endosonographic demonstration and endoscopic removal. Gastrointest Endosc 1996;43(6):620–4.

Inouye WY, Farrell C, Fitts WT, et al. Duodenal duplication. Case report and literature review. Ann Surg 1965;162:910–6.

Kangarloo H, Sample WF, Hansen G, et al. Ultrasonic evaluation of abdominal gastrointestinal tract duplication in children. Radiology 1979;131:191–4.

Lamont AC, Starinsky R, Cremin BJ. Ultrasonic diagnosis of duplication cysts in children. Br J Radiol 1984;57:463–7.

Lucaya J, Herrera M, Espax RM, et al. Mesenteric and omental cysts in children. Ann Radiol 1978;21:161–72.

Macpherson RI. Gastrointestinal tract duplications: clinical, pathological, etiological and radiologic considerations. Radiographics 1993;13:1063–80.

Mittelstaedt C. Ultrasonic diagnosis of omental cysts. Ann Radiol 1978;21:161–72.

Ohba S, Fukuda A, Kohno S, et al. Ileal duplication and multiple intraluminal diverticula: scintigraphy and barium meal. AJR 1981;136:992–4.

Rifkin MD, Kurtz AB, Pasto ME. Mesenteric chylous (lymph-containing) cyst. Gastrointest Radiol 1983;8:267–9.

Ros PR, Olmsted WW, Moser RP, et al. Mesenteric and omental cysts: histologic classification with imaging correlation. Radiology 1987;164:327–32.

Rose JS, Gribetz D, Krasna IH. Ileal duplication cyst: the importance of sodium pertechnetate Tc 99m scanning. Pediatr Radiol 1978;6:244–6.

Shackelford GD, McAlister WH. Cysts of the omentum. Pediatr Radiol 1975;3:152–5.

Singh S, Baboo ML, Pathak IC. Cystic lymphangioma in children: report of 32 cases including lesions at rare sites. Surgery 1971;69:947–51.

Snodgrass JJ. Transdiaphragmatic duplication of the alimentary tract. AJR 1953;69:42–53.

Steyaert H, Guitard J, Moscovici J, et al. Abdominal cystic lymphangioma in children: benign lesions that can have proliferative course. J Pediatr Surg 1996;31:677–80.

Stoupis C, Ros PR, Abbitt PL, et al. Bubbles in the belly: imaging of cystic mesenteric or omental masses. Radiographics 1994;14:729–37.

Teele RL, Henschke CI, Tapper D. The radiographic and ultrasonographic evaluation of enteric duplication cysts. Pediatr Radiol 1980;10:9–14.

Walker AR, Putnam TL. Omental, mesenteric and retroperitoneal cysts: a clinical study of 33 new cases. Ann Surg 1973;178:13.

Anomalies of the Omphalomesenteric Duct

Black LM, Ros PR, Smirniotopoulos JG, et al. Intussuscepted Meckel diverticulum: radiologic-pathologic correlation. Comput Radiol 1987;11:245–8.

Bree RL, Reuter SR. Angiographic demonstration of a bleeding Meckel's diverticulum. Radiology 1973;108:287–8.

Brown A, Carty H. Segmental dilatation of the ileum. Br J Radiol 1984;57:371–4.

Cooney DR, Duszynski DO, Camboa E, et al. The abdominal technetium scan (a decade of experience). J Pediatr Surg 1982;17:611–9.

Dalinka MK, Wunder JF. Meckel's diverticulum and its complications, with emphasis on roentgenologic demonstration. Radiology 1973;106:295–8.

Daneman A, Myers M, Shuckett B, Alton DJ. Sonographic appearance of inverted Meckel diverticulum. Pediatr Radiol 1997;27:295–8.

Diamond RH, Rothstein RD, Alavi A. The role of cimetidine enhanced technetium-99m-pertechnetate imaging for visualizing Meckel's diverticulum. J Nucl Med 1991;22:647–54.

Enge I, Frimann-Dahl J. Radiology in acute abdominal disorders due to Meckel's diverticulum. Br J Radiol 1964;37:775–80.

Faris JC, Whitley JE. Angiographic demonstration of Meckel's diverticulum. Case report and review of the literature. Radiology 1973;108:285–6.

Gaisie G, Curnes JT, Scatliff HJ, et al. Neonatal intestinal obstruction from omphalomesenteric duct remnants. AJR 1985;144:109–12.

Galifer RB, Noblet D, Ferran JL. "Giant Meckel's diverticulum": report of an unusual case in a child with preoperative x-ray diagnosis. Pediatr Radiol 1981;11:217–8.

Grosfield JL, Franken EA Jr. Intestinal obstruction in the neonate due to vitelline duct cysts. Surg Gynecol Obstet 1974;138:527–34.

Itagaki A, Uchida M, Ueki K, et al. Double target sign in ultrasonic diagnosis of intussuscepted Meckel diverticulum. Pediatr Radiol 1991;21:148–9.

Johnson GF, Verhagen AD. Mesodiverticular band. Radiology 1977;123:409 12.

Kim G, Daneman A, Alton DJ, et al. The appearance of inverted Meckel diverticulum with intussusception on air enema. Pediatr Radiol 1997;27:647–50.

Langkemper R, Hoek AC, Dekker W, et al. Elevated lesions in the duodenal bulb caused by heterotopic gastric mucosa. Radiology 1980;137:621–4.

Mackey WC, Dineen P. A fifty-year experience with Meckel's diverticulum. Surg Gynecol Obstet 1978;156:56–64.

Maglinte DDT, Elmore MF, Isenberg M, et al. Meckel's diverticulum: radiological demonstration by enteroclysis. AJR 1980;134:925–32.

Meyerowitz MF, Fellows KE. Angiography in gastrointestinal bleeding in children. AJR 1984;143:837–40.

Morewood DJW, Cunningham ME. Case report: segmental dilatation of the ileum presenting with anaemia. Clin Radiol 1985;36:267–8.

Nigogosyan M, Dolinskas C. CT demonstration of inflamed Meckel's diverticulum. J Comput Assist Tomogr 1990;14:140–2.

Orenstein SR, Magill HL, Whitington PF. Ileal dysgenesis presenting with anemia and growth failure. Pediatr Radiol 1984;14:59–61.

Rose BS, Pretorius DL. A giant Meckel's diverticulum in an adult. AJR 1992;158:1408–9.

Rosenberg JC, Chervenak FA, Walker BA, et al. Antenatal sonographic appearance of omphalomesenteric duct cyst. J Ultrasound Med 1986;5:719–20.

Rosenthal L, Henry JN, Murphy DA, et al. Radiopertechnetate imaging of the Meckel's diverticulum. Radiology 1972;105:371–3.

Rossi P, Gourtsoyiannis N, Bezzi M, et al. Meckel's diverticulum: imaging dignosis. AJR 1996;166:567–73.

Rutherford RB, Akkers DR. Meckel's diverticulum: a review of 148 pediatric patients, with special reference to the pattern of bleeding and to mesodiverticular vascular bands. Surgery 1966;59:618–26.

Salomonowitz E, Wittich G, Hajek P, et al. Detection of intestinal diverticula by double contrast small bowel enema: differentiation from other intestinal diverticula. Gastrointest Radiol 1983;8:271–8.

Sfakianakis GN, Conway JJ. Detection of ectopic gastric mucosa in Meckel's diverticulum and in other aberrations by scintigraphy: pathophysiology and 10-year clinical experience. J Nucl Med 1981;22:647–54.

Sfakianakis GN, Haase GM. Abdominal scintigraphy for ectopic gastric mucosa: a retrospective analysis of 143 studies. AJR 1982;138:7–12.

Vane DW, West KW, Grosfeld JL. Vitelline duct anomalies: experience with 217 childhood cases. Arch Surg 1987;156:56–64.

Diverticulosis of the Small Bowel, Congenital Short Gut

Caplan LH, Jacobson HG. Small intestinal diverticulosis. AJR 1964;92:1048–60.

Cumming WA, Simpson JS. Intestinal diverticulosis in Noonan's syndrome. Br J Radiol 1977;50:64–5.

Hamilton JR, Reilly BJ, Morecki R. Short small intestine association with malrotation: a newly described congenital cause of intestinal malabsorption. Gastroenterology 1969;56:124–36.

Parulekar SG. Diverticulosis of the terminal ileum and its complications. Radiology 1972;103:283–7.

Taybi H, Lachman RS. Radiology of syndromes, metabolic disorders and skeletal dysplasias. 4th ed. Chicago: Mosby Year Book Publishers Inc.; 1996.

Tiu CM, Chou YH, Pan HG, et al. Congenital short gut. Pediatr Radiol 1984;14:343–5.

Defects of the Anterior Abdominal Wall

Bair JH, Russ PD, Pretorius DH, et al. Fetal omphalocele and gastroschisis: a review of 24 cases. AJR 1986;147:1047–51.

Blane CE, Wesley JR, DiPietro MA, et al. Gastrointestinal complications of gastroschisis. AJR 1985;144:589–91.

Colomban PM, Cunningham MD. Perinatal aspects of omphalocele and gastroschisis. Am J Dis Child 1977;131:1386–8.

Ein SH, Fallis JC, Simpson JS. Silon sheeting in the staged repair of massive ventral hernias in children. Can J Surg 1970;13:127–34.

Ein SH, Rubin SZ. Gastroschisis: primary closure or Silon pouch. J Pediatr Surg 1980;15:549–51.

Ein SH, Shandling B. A new non-operative treatment of large omphaloceles with a polymer membrane. J Pediatr Surg 1978;13:255–7.

Fink IJ, Filly RA. Omphalocele associated with umbilical cord allantoic cyst: sonographic evaluation in utero. Radiology 1983;149:473–6.

Hillemeier AC, Grill BB, McCallum R, et al. Esophageal and gastric motor abnormalities in gastroesophageal reflux during infancy. Gastroenterology 1983;84:741–6.

Hoffman AD. Pediatric case of the day. AJR 1984;142:1068–74.

Hoyme HE, Higginbottom MC, Jone KL. The vascular pathogenesis of gastroschisis. Intrauterine interruption of the omphalomesenteric artery. J Pediatr 1981;98:228–31.

Lindfors KK McGahan JP, Walter JP. Fetal omphalocele and gastroschisis: pitfalls in sonographic diagnosis. AJR 1986;147:797–800.

Lindham S. Omphalocele and gastroschisis in Sweden 1965–1976. Acta Paediatr 1981;70:55–60.

Mahour GH. Omphalocoele. Surg Gynecol Obstet 1976;143:821–8.

Mayer T, Black R, Matlak ME, et al. Gastroschisis and omphalocele. An eight-year review. Ann Surg 1980;192:783–7.

Moore TC. Gastroschisis and omphalocele: clinical differences. Surgery 1977;82:561–8.

Rubin SZ, Ein SH. Experience with 55 Silon pouches. J Pediatr Surg 1976;11:803–7.

Rubin SZ, Martin DJ, Ein SH. A critical look at delayed intestinal motility in gastroschisis. Can J Surg 1978;21:414–6.

Salzman L, Kuligowska E, Semine A. Pseudo-omphalocele: pitfall in fetal sonography. AJR 1986;146:1283–5.

Seashore JH. Congenital abdominal wall defects. Clin Perinatol 1978;5:61–77.

Tibboel D, Raine P, McNee M, et al. Developmental aspects of gastroschisis. J Pediatr Surg 1986;21:865–9.

Toth PP, Kimura K. Left-sided gastroschisis. J Pediatr Surg 1993;28:1543–4.

Touloukian RJ, Spackman TJ. Gastrointestinal function and radiographic appearance following gastroschisis repair. J Pediatr Surg 1971;6:427–34.

Toyama WM. Combined congenital defects of the anterior abdominal wall, sternum, diaphragm, pericardium, and heart: a case report and review of the syndrome. Pediatrics 1972;50:778–92.

Tucker JM, Brumfield CG, Davis RO, et al. Prenatal differentiation of ventral abdominal wall defects. Are amniotic fluid markers useful adjuncts? J Reprod Med 1992;37:445–8.

Wesley JR, Drongowski R, Coran AG. Intragastric pressure measurement: a guide for reduction and closure of the Silastic chimney in omphalocele and gastroschisis. J Pediatr Surg 1981;16:264–70.

Meconium Peritonitis

Blumenthall DH, Rushovick AM, Williams RK, et al. Prenatal sonographic findings of meconium peritonitis with pathologic correlation. J Clin Ultrasound 1982;10:350–2.

Bowen A, Mazer J, Zarabi M, Fujioka M. Cystic meconium peritonitis: ultrasonographic features. Pediatr Radiol 1984;14:18–22.

Brugman SM, Bjelland JJ, Thomasson JE, et al. Sonographic findings with radiologic correlation in meconium peritonitis. J Clin Ultrasound 1979;7:305–6.

Carroll BA, Muskowitz PS. Sonographic diagnosis of neonatal meconium cyst. AJR 1981;137:1262–4.

Day DL, Allan BT. Pediatric case of the day: cystic meconium peritonitis. AJR 1985;144:1296–8.

Dillard JP, Edwards DK, Leopold GR. Meconium peritonitis masquerading as fetal hydrops. J Ultrasound Med 1987;6:49–51.

Finkel LI, Slovis TL. Meconium peritonitis, intraperitoneal calcifications and cystic fibrosis. Pediatr Radiol 1982;12:92–3.

Fleischer AC, Davis RJ, Campbell L. Sonographic detection of a meconium-containing mass in a fetus: a case report. J Clin Ultrasound 1983;11:103–5.

Garb M, Riseborough J. Meconium peritonitis presenting as fetal ascites on ultrasound. Br J Radiol 1980;53:602–4.

Lawrence PW, Chrispin A. Sonographic appearances in two neonates with generalized meconium peritonitis: the snowstorm sign. Br J Radiol 1984;57:340–2.

McGahan JP, Hansen F. Meconium peritonitis with accompanying pseudocyst: prenatal sonographic diagnosis. Radiology 1983;148:125–6.

Moore TC. Internal hernia with high jejunal obstruction in infancy due to adhesions from antenatal meconium peritonitis. J Pediatr Surg 1973;8:971–2.

Nancarrow PA, Mattrey RF, Edwards DK, Skram C. Fibroadhesive meconium peritonitis: in utero sonographic diagnosis. J Ultrasound Med 1985;4:213–5.

Neuhauser EBD. The roentgen diagnosis of fetal meconium peritonitis. AJR 1944;51:421–5.

Payne RM, Neilson A. Meconium peritonitis. Am Surg 1962;28:224–31.

Shija JK. Disappearance of calcification in meconium peritonitis in a black African baby. Pediatr Radiol 1987;17:173.

Tucker AS, Isant RJ. Problems with meconium. AJR 1971;112:135–42.

Van Buskirk RW, Kurlander GJ, Samter TB. Intramural jejunal calcifiction in a newborn: a case with jejunal atresia and cystic fibrosis. Am J Dis Child 1965;110:329–32.

Wolfson JJ, Engel RR. Anticipating meconium peritonitis from metaphyseal bands. Radiology 1969;92:1055–60.

Gastroenteritis, Tuberculous, Helminth, Protozoal, Candidal

Ablin DS, Jain KA, Azouz EM. Abdominal tuberculosis in children. Pediatr Radiol 1994;24:473–7.

Abrams JS, Holden WD. Tuberculosis of the gastrointestinal tract. Arch Surg 1964;89:282–93.

Balthazar EJ, Gordon R, Hulnick D. Ileocecal tuberculosis: CT and radiologic evaluation. AJR 1990;154:499–503.

Bean WJ. Recognition of ascariasis by routine chest or abdomen roentgenograms. AJR 1965;94:379–84.

Berkmen YM, Rabinowitz J. Gastrointestinal manifestations of strongyloidiasis. AJR 1972;115:306–11.

Bloom BR, Murray CJL. Tuberculosis: commentary on a re-emergent killer. Science 1992;257:1055–64.

Bohrer SP. Typhoid perforation of the ileum. Br J Radiol 1966;39:37–41.

Brandon J, Glick SN, Teplick SK. Intestinal giardiasis: the importance of serial filming. AJR 1985;144:581–4.

Dahlene DH, Stanley RJ, Koehler RE, et al. Abdominal tuberculosis: CT findings. J Comput Assist Tomogr 1984;8:443–5.

Denath FM. Abdominal tuberculosis in children: CT findings. Gastrointest Radiol 1990;15:303–6.

Denton T, Hossain J. A radiological study of abdominal tuberculosis in a Saudi population, with special reference to ultrasound and computed tomography. Clin Radiol 1993;47:409–14.

Epstein BM, Mann JH. CT of abdominal tuberculosis. AJR 1982;139:861–6.

Gedgaudas-McClees RK. Aphthoid ulcerations in ileocolic candidiasis. AJR 1983;141:973–4.

Hanson RD, Hunter TB. Tuberculous peritonitis: CT appearance. AJR 1985;144:931–2.

Hodes HL. Gastroenteritis with special reference to rotavirus. Adv Pediatr 1980;27:195–245.

Joshi SN, Garvin PJ, Sunwoo YC. Candidiasis of the duodenum and jejunum. Gastroenterology 1981;80:829–33.

Katz M. Parasitic infections. J Pediatr 1975;87:165–78.

Kedar RP, Shah PP, Shivde RS, Malde HM. Sonographic findings in gastrointestinal and peritoneal tuberculosis. Clin Radiol 1994;49:24–9.

Kibel M. In: Cremin BJ, Jamieson DH, editors. Childhood tuberculosis—modern imaging and clinical concepts. New York: Springer Verlag; 1995. p. 105–13.

Kohl S, Jacobson JA, Nahmias A. *Yersinia enterocolitica* infections in children. J Pediatr 1976;89:77–9.

Lee DH, LIM JH, Ko YT, Yoon Y. Sonographic findings in tuberculous peritonitis of wet-ascites type. Clin Radiol 1991;44:306–10.

Manzano C, Thomas MA, Valenzuela C. Trichuriasis: roentgenographic features and differential diagnosis with lymphoid hyperplasia. Pediatr Radiol 1979;8:76–8.

Matsui T, Iida M, Murakami M, et al. Intestinal anisakiasis: clinical and radiologic features. Radiology 1985;157:299–302.

Millar AJW, Rode H, Cywes S. Abdominal tuberculosis in children: surgical management. Pediatr Surg Int 1990;5:392–6.

Nagi B, Nuggal R, Gupta R, et al. Tuberculous peritonitis in children. Pediatr Radiol 1987;17:282–4.

Nelson WE. Textbook of Pediatrics. 12th ed. Philadelphia: WB Saunders; 1983. p. 920–1.

Ozkan K, Gurses N. Ultrasound appearance of tuberculous peritonitis. J Clin Ultrasound 1987;15:350–2.

Pombo F, Rodriquez E, Mato J, et al. Patterns of contrast enhancement of tuberculous lymph nodes demonstrated by computed tomography. Clin Radiol 1992;46:13–7.

Radin DR, Fong TL, Halls JM, et al. Monilial enteritis in acquired immunodeficiency syndrome. AJR 1983;141:1289–90.

Reeder MM, Astacio JE, Theros EG. An exercise in radiologic-pathologic correlation. AJR 1968;90:382–7.

Shrago G. *Yersinia enterocolitica* ileocolitis findings observed on barium examination. Br J Radiol 1976;49:181–3.

Smith SB, Schwartzman M, Mencia LF, et al. Fatal disseminated strongyloidiasis presenting as acute abdominal distress in an unborn child. J Pediatr 1977;91:607–9.

Starke JR, Jacobs RF, Jereb J. Resurgence of tuberculosis in children. J Pediatr 1992;120:839–55.

Thoeni RF, Margulis AR. Gastrointestinal tuberculosis. Semin Roentgenol 1979;14:283–94.

Watson J. Tuberculosis in Britain today. BMJ 1993;306:221.

Werbeloff L, Novis BH, Banks S, Marks IN. Radiology of tuberculosis of the gastrointestinal tract. Br J Radiol 1973;46:329–36.

Duodenal Ulcer, Duodenitis, and Dermatomyositis

Adeyemi SD, Ein SH, Simpson JS. Perforated stress ulcer in infants. Ann Surg 1979;190:706–8.

Ament ME, Christie DL. Upper gastrointestinal fiberoptic endoscopy in pediatric patients. Gastroenterology 1977;72:1244–8.

Belber JP. Endoscopic examination of the duodenal bulb: a comparison with x-ray. Gastroenterology 1971;61:55–61.

Bova JG, Kamath V, Tio FO, et al. The normal mucosal surface pattern of the duodenal bulb: radiologic-histologic correlation. AJR 1985;145:735–8.

Chiba N, Rao BV, Rademaker JW, Hunt RH. Meta-analysis of antibiotic therapy in eradicating *Helicobacter pylori*. Am J Gastroenterol 1992;87:1716–27.

Deckelbaum RJ, Roy CC, Lussier-Lazaroff J, et al. Peptic ulcer disease: a clinical study in 73 children. Can Med Assoc J 1974;111:225–8.

Derchi LE, Ierace T, DePra L, et al. The sonographic appearance of duodenal lesions. J Ultrasound Med 1986;5:269–73.

Dooley CP, Larson AW, Stace NH, et al. Double contrast barium meal and upper gastrointestinal endoscopy. Ann Intern Med 1984;101:538–45.

Drumm B, O'Brien A, Cutz E, Sherman P. *Campylobacter pylori* associated with primary gastritis in children. Pediatrics 1987;80:192–5.

Drumm B, Rhoads JM, Stringer DA, et al. Etiology, presentation and clinical course of endoscopically diagnosed peptic ulcer disease in children. Pediatrics 1988;82:410–4.

Drumm B, Sherman P, Cutz E, Karmali M. *Campylobacter pylori* associated with primary antral gastritis and duodenal ulcers in children: a prospective study. Presented at the Annual Meeting of the American Society of Microbiology; 1987; Atlanta.

Dunn S, Weber TR, Grosfeld JL, Fitzgerald JR. Acute peptic ulcer in childhood. Arch Surg 1983;118:656–60.

Gelfand DW, Dale WJ, Ott DJ, et al. Duodenitis: endoscopic radiologic-correlation in 272 patients. Radiology 1985a;157:577–81.

Gelfand DW, Dale WJ, Ott DJ, et al. The radiologic detection of duodenal ulcers: effects of examiner variability, ulcer size and location, and technique. AJR 1985b;145:551–3.

Herlinger H, Glanville JN, Kreel L. An evaluation of the double contrast barium meal (DCBM) against endoscopy. Clin Radiol 1977;28:307–14.

Kumar D, Spitz L. Peptic ulceration in children. Surg Gynecol Obstet 1984;159:63–6.

Laufer I. Assessment of the accuracy of double contrast gastroduodenal radiology. Gastroenterology 1976;71:874–8.

Levine MS, Rubesin SE. The *Helicobacter pylori* revolution: radiographic perspective. Radiology 1995;195:593–6.

Long FR, Kramer SS, Markowitz RI, Liacouras CA. Duodenitis in children: corrolation of radiologic findings with endoscopic and pathologic findings. Radiology 1998;206:103–8.

Magill HL, Hixson SD, Whitington G, et al. Duodenal perforation in childhood dermatomyositis. Pediatr Radiol 1984;14:28–30.

Michener WM, Kennedy RLJ, DuShane JW. Duodenal ulcer in childhood: ninety-two cases with follow-up. Am J Dis Child 1960;100:814–7.

NIH Consensus Conference. *Helicobacter pylori* in peptic ulcer disease. JAMA 1994;272:65–9.

Nord KS, Rossi TM, Lebenthal E. Peptic ulcer in children. Am J Gastroenterol 1981;75:153–7.

Ott DJ, Chen YM, Gelfand DW, et al. Positive predictive value and examiner variability in diagnosing duodenal ulcer. AJR 1985;145:1207–10.

Purelekar SG, Lubert M. Ultrasound demonstration of giant duodenal ulcer. Gastrointest Radiol 1983;8:29–31.

Puri P, Boyd E, Blake N, et al. Duodenal ulcer in childhood: a continuing disease in adult life. J Pediatr Surg 1978;13:525–6.

Seagram CGF, Stephens CA, Cumming WA. Peptic ulceration at The Hospital for Sick Children, Toronto, during the 20 year period 1949–1969. J Pediatr Surg 1973;8:407–13.

Singleton EB, Faykus MH. Incidence of peptic ulcer as determined by radiologic examinations in the pediatric age group. J Pediatr 1964;65:858–62.

Stringer DA, Daneman A, Brunelle F, et al. Sonography of the normal and abnormal stomach (excluding hypertrophic pyloric stenosis) in children. J Ultrasound Med 1986;5:183–8.

Sultz HA, Schlesinger ER, Feldman JG, et al. The epidemiology of peptic ulcer in childhood. Am J Public Health 1970;60:492–8.

Warren JR, Marshall BJ. Unidentified curved bacilli on gastric epithelium in active chronic gastritis. Lancet 1983;1:1273–5.

White A, Carachi R, Young DG. Duodenal ulceration presenting in childhood. Long-term follow-up. J Pediatr Surg 1984;19:6–8.

Williams RS, Ahmed S. Peptic ulcer in childhood. Australasian Pediatric Journal 1977;13:299–301.

Regional Enteritis (Crohn's Disease)

Bachwich DR, Lichtenstein GR, Taber PG. Cancer in inflamatory bowel disease. Med Clin North Am 1994;78:1399–1412.

Boag GS, Nolan RL. Sonographic features of urinary bladder involvement in regional enteritis. J Ultrasound Med 1988;7:125–8.

Brahme F, Lindstrom C, Wenckert A. Crohn disease in defined population. An epidemiological study of incidence, prevalence, mortality and secular trends in the city of Malmo, Sweden. Gastroenterology 1975;69:342–51.

Caroline DF, Friedman AC. The radiology of inflammatory bowel disease. Med Clin North Am 1994;78:1353–85.

Casola G, van Sonnenberg E, Neff CC, et al. Abscesses in Crohn disease: percutaneous drainage. Radiology 1987;163:19–22.

Charron M. Inflammatory bowel disease in pediatric patients. Q J Nucl Med 1997;41:309–20.

Chrispin AR, Tempany E. Crohn's disease of the jejunum in children. Arch Dis Child 1967;42:631–5.

Cirrocco WC, Reilly JC, Rusin CC. Life-threatening hemorrhage and exsanguination from Crohn's disease. Dis Colon Rectum 1995;38:85–95.

DiCandio G, Mosca F, Campatelli A, et al. Sonographic detection of post surgical recurrence of Crohn disease. AJR 1986;146:523–6.

Dinkel E, Dittrich M, Peters H, Bauman W. Real-time ultrasound in Crohn's disease: characteristic features and clinical implications. Pediatr Radiol 1986;16:8–12.

Fishman EK, Wolf EJ, Jones B, et al. CT evaluation of Crohn's disease: effect on patient management. AJR 1987;148:537–40.

Gardiner R, Stevenson GW. The colitides. Radiol Clin North Am 1982;20:797–817.

Glick SN, Teplick SK. Crohn disease of the small intestine: diffuse mucosal granularity. Radiology 1985;154:313–7.

Goldberg HI, Carruthers SB Jr, Nelson JA, et al. Radiographic findings of the National Cooperation Crohn Disease Study. Gastroenterology 1979;77:925–37.

Goldberg HI, Gore RM, Margulis AR, et al. Computed tomography in the evaluation of Crohn disease. AJR 1983;140:277–82.

Goldman SM, Fishman EK, Gatewood OMB, et al. CT in the diagnosis of enterovesical fistula. AJR 1985;144:1229–33.

Gore RM, Balthazar EJ, Ghahremani GG, Miller FH. CT features of ulcerative colitis and Crohn's disease. AJR 1996;167:3–15.

Grand RJ, Homer DR. Approaches to inflammatory bowel disease in childhood and adolescence. Pediatr Clin North Am 1975;22:835–50.

Guttman FM. Granulomatous enterocolitis in childhood and adolescence. J Pediatr Surg 1974;9:115–20.

Halligan S, Nicholls S, Bartam CI, Walker-Smith JA. The distribution of small bowel Crohn's disease in children compared to adults. Clin Radiol 1994;49:314–6.

Hamilton JR, Bruce GA, Abdourhaman M, et al. Inflammatory bowel disease in children and adolescents. Adv Pediatr 1979;26:311–41.

Hizawa K, Iida M, Kohrogi N, et al. Crohn disease: early recognition and progress of apthous lesions. Radiology 1994;190:451–4.

Hofley PM, Piccoli DA. Inflammatory bowel disease in children. Med Clin North Am 1994;78:1281–1302.

Jabra AA, Fishman EK, Taylor GA. Crohn disease in the pediatric patient: CT evaluation. Radiology 1994;179:495–8.

Jewel FM, Davies A, Sandhu B, et al. Techetium-99m-HMPAO labelled leucocytes in the detection and monitoring of inflammatory bowel disease in children. Br J Radiol 1996;69:508–14.

Jobling JC, Lindley KJ, Yousef Y, et al. Investigating inflammatory bowel disease: white cell scanning, radiology, colonoscopy. Arch Dis Child 1996;74:22–6.

Kaftori JK, Pery M, Kleinhaus U. Ultrasonography in Crohn's disease. Gastrointest Radiol 1984;9:137–42.

Kelts DG, Grand RJ. Inflammatory bowel disease in children and adolescents. Curr Probl Pediatr 1980;10:1–40.

Kelvin FM, Gedgaudas RK. Radiologic diagnosis of Crohn disease (with emphasis on its early manifestations). Crit Rev Diagn Imaging 1981;16:43–91.

Kennan N, Hayward M. HMPAO-labelled white cell scintigraphy in Crohn's disease of the small bowel. Clin Radiology 1992;45:331–4.

Kerber GW, Frank PH. Carcinoma of the small intestine and colon as a complication of Crohn disease: radiologic manifestations. Radiology 1984;150:639–45.

Kettritz U, Isaacs K, Warshauer DM, Semelka RC. Crohn's disease pilot study: comparing MR of the abdomen with clinical evaluation. J Clin Gastroenterol 1995;21:249–53.

Khaw KT, Yeoman LJ, Saverymuttu SH, et al. Ultrasonic pattern in inflammatory bowel disease. Clin Radiol 1991;43:171–5.

Kirks DR, Currarino G. Regional enteritis in children: small bowel disease with normal terminal ileum. Pediatr Radiol 1978;7:10–4.

Kirschner BS. Ulcerative colitis and Crohn's disease in children. Gastroenterol Clin North Am 1995;24:99–117.

Lambiase RE, Cronan JJ, Dorfman GS, et al. Percutaneous drainage of abscesses in patients with Crohn disease. AJR 1988;150:1043–5.

Lee JKT, Marcos HB, Semelka RC. MR imaging of the small bowel using the HASTE sequence. AJR 1998;170:1457–63.

Lindquist BL, Jarnerot G, Wickbom G. Clinical and epidemiological aspects of Crohn disease in children and adolescents. Scand J Gastroenterol 1984;19:502–6.

Lindsley CB, Schaller JG. Arthritis associated with inflammatory bowel disease in children. J Pediatr 1974;84:16–20.

Low RN, Francis IR. MR imaging of the gastrointestinal tract with IV gadolinium and dilute barium oral contrast media compared with unenhanced MR imaging and CT. AJR 1997;169:1051–9.

Mekhjian HS, Switz DM, Watts HD, et al. National Cooperative Crohn Disease Study: factors determining recurrence of Crohn disease after surgery. Gastroenterology 1979;77:907–13.

Meyers MA, McGuire PV. Spiral CT demonstration of hypervascularity in Crohn disease: "vascular jejunization of the ileum" or the "comb sign." Abdom Imaging 1995;20:327–32.

Miller RC, Jackson M, Larsen E. Regional enteritis in early infancy. Am J Dis Child 1971;122:301–11.

Moseley JF, Marshak RH, Wolf BS. Regional enteritis in children. AJR 1960;84:532–9.

Nolan DJ, Piris J. Crohn disease of the small intestine: a comparative study of the radiological and pathological appearances. Clin Radiol 1980;31:591–6.

Puylaert JBCM. Mesenteric adenitis and acute terminal ileitis: US evaluation using graded compression. Radiology 1986;161:691–5.

Quillin SP, Siegel MJ. Gastrointestinal inflammation in children: colour Doppler ultrasonography. J Ultrasound Med 1994;13:751–6.

Ramchandi D, Schindler B, Katz J. Evolving concepts of psychopathology in inflammatory bowel disease: implications for treament. Med Clin North Am 1994;78:1321–30.

Regan F, Beall DP, Bohlman ME, et al. Fast MR imaging and the detection of small-bowel obstruction. AJR 1998;170:1465–9.

Riddlesberger MM. CT of complicated inflammatory bowel disease in children. Pediatr Radiol 1985;15:384–7.

Rubin S, Lambie RW, Chapman J. Regional ileitis in childhood. Am J Dis Child 1967;114:106–10.

Safrit HD, Mauro MA, Jaques PF. Percutaneous abscess drainage in Crohn's disease. AJR 1987;148:859–62.

Sarrazin J, Wilson SR. Manifestations of Crohn disease at US. Radiographics 1996;16:499–520.

Shah DB, Cosgrove M, Rees JI, Jenkin HR. The technetium white cell scan as an initial imaging investigation for evaluation of suspected childhood inflammatory bowel disease. J Pediatr Gastroenterol Nutr 1997;25:524–8.

Sheridan MB, Nicholson DA, Martin DF. Transabdominal ultrasonography as the primary investigation in patients with suspected crohn's disease or recurrence: a prospective study. Clin Radiol 1993;48:402–4.

Shoenut JP, Semelka RC, Magro CM, et al. Comparison of magnetic resonance imaging and endoscopy in distinguishing the type and severity of inflammatory bowel disease. J Clin Gastroenterol 1994;19:31–5.

Siegel M, Evans SJ, Balfe DM. Small bowel disease in children: diagnosis with CT. Radiology 1988;169:127–30.

Silverman F. Regional enteritis in children. Aust Pediatr J 1966;2:207–18.

Stringer DA, Cloutier S, Daneman A, et al. The value of the small bowel enema in children. J Can Assoc Radiol 1986a;37:13–6.

Stringer DA, Sherman P, Liu P, et al. The value of the peroral pneumocolon in pediatrics. AJR 1986b;132:763–6.

Taylor GA, Nancarrow PA, Hernanz-Schulman M, Teele RL. Plain abdominal radiographs in children with inflammatory bowel disease. Pediatr Radiol 1986;16:206–9.

ten Berge RJM, Natarajan AT, Hardeman MR, et al. Labelling with indium III has detrimental effects on human lymphocytes: concise communication. J Nucl Med 1983;24:615–20.

Thakur ML, McAfee JG. The significance of chromosomal aberrations in indium-III labelled lymphocytes. J Nucl Med 1984;25:922–7.

Van Patter WN, Bargen JA, Dockerty MB, et al. Regional enteritis. Gastroenterology 1954;26:347–50.

Weedon DD, Shorter RG, Ilstrup DM, et al. Crohn disease and cancer. N Engl J Med 1973;289:1099–1103.

Werlin SL, Glicklich M, Jona J, et al. Sclerosing cholangitis in childhood. J Pediatr 1980;96:433–6.

Whelan G. Epidemiology of inflammatory bowel disease. Med Clin North Am 1990;74:1–12.

Wills JS, Lobis IF, Dentsman FJ. Crohn disease: state of the art. Radiology 1997;202:597–610.

Yeh HC, Rabinowitz JG. Granulomatous enterocolitis: findings by ultrasonography and computed tomography. Radiology 1983;149:253–9.

Eosinophilic Gastroenteritis

Katz AJ, Goldman H, Grand RJ. Gastric mucosal biopsy in eosinophilic (allergic) gastroenteritis. Gastroenterology 1977;73:705–9.

Matzinger MA, Daneman A. Esophageal involvement in eosinophilic gastroenteritis. Pediatr Radiol 1983;13:35–8.

Moore D, Lichtman S, Lentz J, et al. Eosinophilic colitis presenting in an adolescent with isolated colonic involvement. Gut 1986;27:1219–22.

Teele RL, Katz AJ, Goldman H, et al. Radiographic features of eosinophilic gastroenteritis (allergic gastroenteropathy) of childhood. AJR 1979;132:575–80.

Waldmann TA, Wochner RD, Laster L, et al. Allergic gastroenteropathy. A cause of excessive gastrointestinal protein loss. N Engl J Med 1967;276:762–9.

Behçet Syndrome

Behçet H. Über rezidivierende, apthöse durch ein Virus verursachte Geschwüre am Mund am Auge und den Genitalien. Dermat Wchnschr 1937;105:1152–8.

Behçet's Disease Research Committee of Japan. Behçet's disease: guide to diagnosis of Behçet's disease. Jpn J Ophthalmol 1974;18:291. (In Japanese)

Chajek T, Fainaru M. Behçet's disease. Report of 41 cases and a review of the literature. Medicine 1975;54:179–96.

James DG. Behçet's syndrome. N Engl J Med 1979;301:431–2.

Mason RM, Barnes CG. Behçet's syndrome with arthritis. Ann Rheum Dis 1969;28:95–103.

McLean AM, Simms DM, Homer MJ. Ileal ring ulcers in Behçet's syndrome. AJR 1983;140:947–83.

Stanley RJ, Tedesco FJ, Melson GL, et al. The colitis of Behçet's disease: a clinical radiographic correlation. Radiology 1975;114:603–4.

Stringer DA, Cleghorn GJ, Daneman A, et al. Behçet's syndrome involving the gastrointestinal tract: a diagnostic dilemma in childhood. Pediatr Radiol 1986;16:131–4.

Vlymen WJ, Moskowitz PS. Roentgenographic manifestations of esophageal and intestinal involvement in Behçet's disease in children. Pediatr Radiol 1981;10:193–6.

NEOPLASMS OF THE SMALL BOWEL OR MESENTERY

Bartram C, Chrispin AR. Primary lymphosarcoma of the ileum and caecum. Pediatr Radiol 1973;1:28–33.

Bowen A, Gaise C, Bron K. Retroperitoneal lipoma in children: choosing among diagnostic imaging modalities. Pediatr Radiol 1982;12:221–5.

Bush RS, Ash CL. Primary lymphoma of the gastrointestinal tract. Radiology 1969;92:1349–54.

Chalmers AG, Robinson PJ, Chapman AH. Embolization in small bowel haemorrhage. Clin Radiol 1986;37:379–81.

Cupps RE, Hodgson JR, Dockerty MB, et al. Primary lymphoma in the small intestine: problems of roentgenologic diagnosis. Radiology 1969;92:1355–62.

Davis GB, Berk RN. Intestinal neurofibromas in Von Recklinghausen's disease. Am J Gastroenterol 1973;60:410–14.

Dunnick NR, Reaman GH, Head GL, et al. Radiographic manifestations of Burkitt's lymphoma in American patients. AJR 1979;132:1–6.

Fataar S, Morton P, Schulman A. Arteriovenous malformations of the gastrointestinal tract. Clin Radiol 1981;32:623–8.

Ginsburg LD. Eccentric polyposis of the small bowel: a possible radiological sign of plexiform neurofibromatosis of the small bowel and its mesentery. Radiology 1975;116:561–2.

Gutsman SI, Steinherz PG, Gray GF. Malignant peritoneal mesothelioma in a child. Am J Dis Child 1976;130:1268–9.

Haller JO, Schneider M, Kassner EG, et al. Sonographic evaluation of mesenteric and omental masses in children. AJR 1978;130:269–74.

Hassell P. Gastrointestinal manifestations of neurofibromatosis in children: a report of two cases. J Can Assoc Radiol 1982;33:202–4.

Hernandez R, Poznaski AK, Holt JF, et al. Abnormal fat collections in the omentum and mesocolon of children. Radiology 1977;122:193–6.

Hochberg FH, Da Silva AB, Galdabini J. Gastrointestinal involvement in Von Recklinghausen's neurofibromatosis. Neurology 1974;24:1144–51.

Jenkin RDT, Sonley MJ, Stephens CA, et al. Primary gastrointestinal tract lymphoma in children. Radiology 1969;92:763–7.

Keller RJ, Hertz I, Zimmerman M, et al. Carcinoma of the ileum simulating Crohn disease. AJR 1982;138:151–3.

Lewis BD, Doubilet PM, Heller VL, et al. Cutaneous and visceral hemangiomata in the Kippel-Trenaunay-Weber syndrome: antenatal sonographic detection. AJR 1986;14:598–600.

Megibow AJ, Balthazar EJ, Naidich DP, et al. Computed tomography of gastrointestinal lymphoma. AJR 1983;141:541–7.

Miller JH, Hindman BW, Lam AHK. Ultrasound in the evaluation of small bowel lymphoma in children. Radiology 1980;135:409–14.

Ormson MJ, Stephens DH, Carlson HC. CT recognition of intestinal lipomatosis. AJR 1985;144:313–4.

Papadopoulos VD, Nolan DJ. Carcinomas of the small intestine. Clin Radiol 1985;36:409–13.

Sarrazin J, Wilson SR. Manifestations of Crohn disease at US. Radiographics 1996;16:499–520.

Siegel M, Evans SJ, Balfe DM. Small bowel disease in children: diagnosis with CT. Radiology 1988;169:127–30.

Soderlund V, Mortensson W, Nybonde T. Fluid filled structures simulating solid tumours at ultrasonography: a report of five cases. Pediatr Radiol 1986;16:110–3.

Solomons NW, Wagonfeld JB, Thomsen S, et al. Leiomyosarcoma of the duodenum in a 10-year-old boy. Pediatrics 1976;58:268–73.

Stringel C, Shandling B, Mancer K, et al. Lipoblastoma in infants and children. J Pediatr Surg 1982;17:277–80.

Taybi H, Lachman RS. Radiology of syndromes, metabolic disorders and skeletal dysplasias. 4th ed. Chicago: Mosby Year Book Publishers Inc.; 1996. p. 426.

Tishler JM, Han SY, Colcher H, et al. Neurogenic tumors of the duodenum in patients with neurofibromatosis. Radiology 1983;149:51–3.

Uflacker R, Alves MA, Diehl JC. Gastrointestinal involvement in neurofibromatosis: angiographic presentation. Gastrointest Radiol 1985;10:163–5.

HEMORRHAGE AND TRAUMA TO BOWEL

Berger PE, Kuhn JP. CT of blunt abdominal trauma in childhood. AJR 1981;136:105–10.

Brown RA, Bass DH, Rode H, et al. Gastrointestinal tract perforation in children due to blunt abdominal trauma. Br J Surg 1992;79:522–4.

Bulas DI, Taylor GA, Eichelberger MR. The Value of CT in detecting bowel perforation in children after blunt abdominal trauma. AJR 1989;153:561–4.

Casey L, Vu D, Cohen AJ. Small bowel rupture after blunt trauma: computed tomographic signs and their sensitivity. Emerg Radiol 1995;2:90–5.

Clancy TV, Ragozzino MW, Ramshaw D, et al. Oral contrast is not necessary in the evaluation of blunt abdominal trauma by computed tomography. Am J Surg 1993; 166:680–4.

Cobb CM, Vinocur CD, Wagner CW, Weinstraub WH. Intestinal perforation due to blunt trauma in children in an era of increased non-operative treatment. J Trauma 1986;26:461–3.

Cook DE, Walsh JW, Vick WC, Brewer WH. Upper abdominal trauma: pitfalls in CT diagnosis. Radiology 1989;159:65–9.

Couture A, Veyrac C, Baud C, et al. Evaluation of abdominal pain in Henoch-Schönlein syndrome by high frequency ultrasound. Pediatr Radiol 1992;22:12–7.

Donohue JH, Federle MP, Griffiths BA, Trunkey DD. Computed tomography in the diagnosis of blunt intestinal and mesenteric injuries. J Trauma 1987;27:11–7.

Foley LC, Teele RL. Ultrasound of epigastric injuries after blunt trauma. AJR 1979;132:593–8.

Ford EL, Senac MO. Clinical presentation and radiographic identification of small bowel rupture following blunt abdominal trauma in children. Pediatr Emerg Care 1993;9:139–42.

Glasier CM, Siegel MJ, McAlister WH, Shackelford GD. Henoch-Schönlein syndrome in children: gastro-intestinal manifestations. AJR 1981;136:1081–5.

Hara H, Babyn PS, Bourgeois D. Significance of bowel wall enhancement on CT following blunt abdominal trauma in childhood. J Comput Assist Tomogr 1992;16:94–8.

Hayes CW, Conway WF, Walsh JW, et al. Seat belt injuries: radiologic findings and clinical correlation. Radiographics 1991;11:23–36.

Hernanz-Schulman M, Genieser NB, Ambrosino M. Sonographic diagnosis of intramural duodenal hematoma. J Ultrasound Med 1989;8:273–6.

Hofer GA, Cohen AJ. CT signs of duodenal perforation secondary to blunt abdominal trauma. J Comput Assist Tomogr 1989;13:430–2.

Jamieson DH, Babyn PS, Pearl R. Imaging gastrointestinal perforation in pediatric blunt abdominal trauma. Pediatr Radiol 1996;26:188–94.

Jeong YK, Ha HK, Yoon CH, et al. Gastro-intestinal involvement in Henoch-Schönlein syndrome: CT findings. AJR 1997;168:965–8.

Kaufman RA, Towbin R, Babcock DS, et al. Upper abdominal trauma in children after blunt abdominal trauma. AJR 1989;152:561–4.

Kleinman PK. Diagnostic imaging of child abuse. 2nd ed. Chicago: Mosby Year Book Publishers Inc.; 1998. p. 252–61.

Kovacs GZ, Davies MRQ, Saunders W, et al. Hollow viscus rupture due to blunt trauma. Surg Gynecol Obstet 1986;1163:552–4.

Kunin JR, Korobkin M, Ellis JH, et al. Duodenal injuries caused by blunt abdominal trauma: value of CT in differentiating perforation from hematoma. AJR 1993;160: 1221–3.

Raby N, Meire H. Duodenal haematoma mimicking traumatic pancreatic pseudocyst. Br J Radiol 1986;59:279–81.

Rizzo MJ, Federle MP, Griffiths BC. Bowel and mesenteric injury following blunt abdominal trauma: evaluation with CT. Radiology 1989;173:143–8.

Ruess L, Sivit CJ, Eichelberger MR, et al. Blunt abdominal trauma in children: impact of CT on operative and non-operative management. AJR 1997;169:1011–4.

Shalaby-Rana E, Eichelberger M, Kerzner B, Kapur S. Intestinal stricture due to lap-belt injury. AJR 1992;158: 63–4.

Siegel MJ. Pediatric sonography. 2nd ed. New York: Raven Press; 1995. p. 288.

Sivit CJ, Eichelberger MR, Taylor GA. CT in children with rupture of the bowel caused by blunt trauma: diagnostic efficiency and comparison with hypoperfusion complex. AJR 1994;163:1195–8.

Sivit CJ, Taylor GA, Bulas DI, et al. Blunt trauma in children: significance of peritoneal fluid. Radiology 1991a;178:185–8.

Sivit CJ, Taylor GA, Newman KD, et al. Safety-belt injuries in children with lap belt ecchymosis: CT findings in 61 patients. AJR 1991b;157:111–4.

Stevens SL, Maull KI. Small bowel injuries. Surg Clin North Am 1990;70:541–60.

Taylor GA, Fallat ME, Eichelberger MR. Hypovolemic shock in children: abdominal CT manifestations. Radiology 1987;164:479–81.

Taylor GA, Fallat ME, Potter BM, et al. The role of computed tomography in blunt abdominal trauma in children. J Trauma 1988;28:1660–4.

Wing VW, Federle MP, Morris JA, et al. The clinical impact of CT for blunt abdominal trauma. AJR 1985; 145:1191–4.

Zahran M, Eklof O, Thomasson B. Blunt abdominal trauma and hollow viscus injury in children: the diagnostic value of plain radiography. Pediatr Radiol 1984;14:304–9.

MALABSORPTION

Aggett PJ, Cavanagh NPC, Mathew DJ, et al. Shwachman's syndrome: a review of 21 cases. Arch Dis Child 1980; 55:331–47.

Agrons GA, Corse WR, Markowitz RI, et al. Gastrointestinal manifestations of cystic fibrosis: radiologic-pathologic correlation. Radiographics 1996;16:871–93.

Anderson DH. Cystic fibrosis of the pancreas and its relation to celiac disease. Am J Dis Child 1938;56:344–99.

Avni EF, Van Gansbeke DV, Rodesch P, et al. Sonographic demonstration of malabsorption in neonates. J Ultrasound Med 1986;5:85–7.

Bartram CI, Small E. The intestinal radiological changes in older people with pancreatic cystic fibrosis. Br J Radiol 1971;44:195–7.

Bell MJ, Martin LW, Schubert WK, et al. Massive small bowel resection in an infant: long term management and intestinal adaptation. J Pediatr Surg 1973;8:197–204.

Berk RN, Lee FA. The late gastrointestinal manifestations of cystic fibrosis of the pancreas. Radiology 1973;106: 337–81.

Bova JG, Friedman AC, Weser E, et al. Adaptation of the ileum in nontropical sprue: reversal of the jejunoileal fold pattern. AJR 1985;144:299–302.

Brunton FJ, Guyer PB. Malignant histiocytosis and ulcerative jejunitis of the small intestine. Clin Radiol 1983;34: 291–5.

Burke V, Colebatch JH, Anderson CM, et al. Association of pancreatic insufficiency and chronic neutropenia in childhood. Arch Dis Child 1967;42:147–57.

Cohen MD, Lintott DJ. Transient small bowel intussusception in adult coeliac disease. Clin Radiol 1978;29: 529–34.

Collins SM, Hamilton JD, Lewis TD, et al. Small bowel malabsorption and gastrointestinal malignancy. Radiology 1978;126:603–9.

Davidson GP, Cutz E, Hamilton JR, et al. Familial enteropathy: a syndrome of protracted diarrhoea from birth, failure to thrive and hypoplastic villous atrophy. Gastroenterology 1978;75:783–90.

Djurhuus MJ, Lykkegaard E, Pock-Steen OC. Gastrointestinal radiological findings in cystic fibrosis. Pediatr Radiol 1973;1:113–8.

Donnelly L. CT imaging of immunocompromised children with acute abdominal symptoms. AJR 1996;167:909–13.

Donnelly L, Morris CL. Acute graft-versus-host disease in children: abdominal CT findings. Radiology 1996;199:265–8.

Dorne HL, Jequier S. Sonography of intestinal lymphangiectasia. J Ultrasound Med 1986;5:13–6.

Duffrenne P, Verdier G. Colonic granulometry in the malabsorption syndromes. Pediatr Radiol 1977;5:14–8.

Ellis K, McConnell DJ. Hereditary angioneurotic edema involving the small intestine. Radiology 1969;92:518–9.

Farthing MJG, McLean AM, Bartram CI, et al. Radiologic features of the jejunum in hypoalbaminemia. AJR 1981;136:883–6.

Fellman K, Kozlowski K, Senger A. Unusual bone changes in exocrine pancreas insufficiency with cyclic neutropenia. Acta Radiol (Diagn) 1972;12:428–32.

Fisk JD, Shulman HM, Greening RR, et al. Gastrointestinal radiographic features of human graft-vs-host disease. AJR 1981;136:329–36.

Gorske K, Winchester P, Grossman H. Unusual protein-losing enteropathies in children. AJR 1969;92:739–44.

Harris GBC, Neuhauser EBD, Shackman H. Roentgenographic spectrum of cystic fibrosis. Postgrad Med 1963;34:251–64.

Haworth EM, Hodson CJ, Pringle EM, et al. The value of radiological investigations of the alimentary tract in children with the celiac syndrome. Clin Radiol 1968;19:65–76.

Herlinger H, Maglinte DDT. Jejunal fold separation in adult celiac disease: relevance of enteroclysis. Radiology 1986;158:605–11.

Herzog DB, Logan R, Looistra JB. The Noonan syndrome with intestinal lymphangiectasia. J Pediatr 1976;88:270–2.

Hill RE, Durie PR, Gaskin KJ, et al. Steatorrhea and pancreatic insufficiency in Shwachman syndrome. Gastroenterology 1982;83:22–7.

Huang TY, Yam LT, Li CY. Radiological features of systemic mast-cell disease. Br J Radiol 1987;60:765–70.

Isbell RG, Carlson HC, Hoffman HN. Roentgenologic-pathologic correlation in malabsorption syndromes. AJR 1969;107:158–69.

Jones B, Bayless TM, Fishman EK, Siegelman SS. Lymphadenopathy in celiac disease: computed tomographic observations. AJR 1984a;142:1127–32.

Jones B, Bayless TM, Hamilton SR, et al. "Bubbly" duodenal bulb in celiac disease: radiologic-pathologic correlation. AJR 1984b;142:119–22.

Jones B, Fishman EK, Kramer SS, et al. Computed tomography of gastrointestinal inflammation after bone marrow transplantion. AJR 1986;146:691–5.

Kalifa G, Devred P, Ricour C, et al. Radiological aspects of the small bowel after extensive resection in children. Pediatr Radiol 1979;8:70–5.

Kappelman NH, Burrill M, Toffler R. Megacolon associated with celiac sprue: report of four cases and review of the literature. AJR 1977;128:65–8.

Karjoo M, Koop CE, Cornfeld D, et al. Pancreatic exocrine enzyme deficiency associated with asphyxiating thoracic dystrophy. Arch Dis Child 1973;48:143–6.

Kingman JGC, Moriarty KJ, Furness M, et al. Lymphangiectasia of the colon and small intestine. Br J Radiol 1982;55:774–7.

Knowles M, Gatzy J, Boucher R. Relative ion permeability of normal and cystic fibrosis nasal epithelium. J Clin Invest 1983;71:1410–7.

Kumar P, Bartram CI. Relevance of the barium follow-through examination in the diagnosis of adult celiac disease. Gastrointest Radiol 1979;4:285–9.

Lamont AC. The three-stripe sign of the cocked Crosby capsule: a new radiologic sign. Br J Radiol 1983;56:307–8.

Lanning P, Simila S, Sioramo I, et al. Lymphatic abnormalities in Noonan's syndrome. Pediatr Radiol 1978;7:106–9.

Larcher VF, Shepherd R, Francis DEM, et al. Protracted diarrhoea in infancy: analysis of 82 cases with particular reference to diagnosis and management. Arch Dis Child 1977;52:597–605.

Laws JW, Neale G. Radiological diagnosis of disaccharidase deficiency. Lancet 1966;2:138–43.

Lucaya J, Perez-Candela V, Aso C, et al. Mastocytosis with

skeletal and gastrointestinal involvement in infancy. Radiology 1979;131:363–6.

Maile CW, Frick MP, Crass JR, et al. The plain abdominal radiograph in acute gastrointestinal graft-vs-host disease. AJR 1985;145:289–92.

Marn CS, Gore RM, Chahremani GG. Duodenal manifestations of nontropical sprue. Gastrointest Radiol 1986;11:30–5.

Marshak RH, Hazzi C, Lindner AE, et al. Small bowel in immunoglobulin deficiency syndromes. AJR 1974;122:227–39.

Marshak RH, Lindner AE, Maklansky D. Lymphoreticular disorders of the gastrointestinal tract: roentgenographic features. Gastrointest Radiol 1979;4:103–20.

Masterson JB, Sweeney EC. The role of small bowel follow-through examination in the diagnosis of celiac disease. Br J Radiol 1976;49:660–4.

McLean AM, Farthing MJG, Kurian G, et al. The relationship between hypoalbuminemia and the radiological appearances of the jejunum in tropical sprue. Br J Radiol 1982;55:725–8.

McLennan TW, Steinbach HL. Shwachman's syndrome: the broad spectrum of bony abnormalities. Radiology 1974;112:167–73.

Morrison WJ, Christopher NL, Bayless TM, et al. Low lactase levels: evaluation of the radiological diagnosis. Radiology 1974;111:513–8.

Munyer TP, Moss AA. Radiologic evaluation of the malabsorption syndrome. Practical Gastroenterology 1980;4:12–7.

Newcomer AD, McGill DB, Thomas PJ, et al. Prospective comparison of indirect methods for detecting lactase deficiency. N Engl J Med 1975;293:1232–6.

Olmstead WW, Madewell JE. Lymphangiectasia of the small intestine: description and pathophysiology of the roentgenographic signs. Gastrointest Radiol 1976;1:241–3.

Pellerin D, Bertin P, Nihoul-Fekete C, et al. Cholelithiasis and ileal pathology in children. J Pediatr Surg 1975;10:35–41.

Phillips AD, Jenkins P, Raafat F, et al. Congenital microvillous atrophy: specific diagnostic features. Arch Dis Child 1985;60:135–40.

Preger L, Amberg JR. Sweet diarrhea: roentgen diagnosis of disaccharidase deficiency. AJR 1967;101:287–95.

Quinn SF, Shaffer HA, Willard MR, Ross S. Bull's-eye lesions: a new gastrointestinal presentation of mastocytosis. Gastrointest Radiol 1984;9:13–5.

Quinton PM. Chloride impermeability in cystic fibrosis. Nature 1993;301:421–2.

Ruoff M, Lindner AE, Marshak RM. Intussusception in sprue. AJR 1968;104:525–8.

Schimmelpenninck M, Zwaan F. Radiographic features of small intestinal injury in graft-versus-host disease. Gastrointest Radiology 1982;7:29–33.

Shimkin PM, Waldmann TA, Krugman RL. Intestinal lymphagiectasia. AJR 1970;110:827–40.

Shwachman H, Diamond LK, Oski FA, et al. The syndrome of pancreatic insufficiency and bone marrow dysfunction. J Pediatr 1964;65:645–63.

Stanley P, Sutcliffe J. Metaphyseal chondrodysplasia with dwarfism, pancreatic insufficiency and neutropenia. Pediatr Radiol 1973;1:119–26.

Taussig LM, Saldino RM, di Sant'Agnese PA. Radiographic abnormalities of the duodenum and small bowel in cystic fibrosis of the pancreas (mucoviscidosis). Radiology 1973;106:369–76.

Taybi H, Mitchell AD, Friedman GD. Metaphyseal dystosis and the associated syndrome of pancreatic insufficiency and blood disorders. Radiology 1969;93:563–71.

Tully TE, Feinberg SB. A roentgenographic classification of diffuse diseases of the small intestine presenting with malabsorption. AJR 1974;283–90.

Weinstein MA, Pearson KD, Agus SG. Abetalipoproteinemia. Radiology 1973;108:269–73.

Weizman Z, Stringer DA, Durie PR. Radiological manifestations of malabsorption: a nonspecific finding. Pediatrics 1984;74:530–44.

Wise LW, Stein T. Biliary and urinary calculi. Pathogenesis following small bowel bypass for obesity. Arch Surg 1975;110:1043–7.

Zboralskie FF, Amberg JR. Detection of the Zollinger-Ellison syndrome: the radiologist's responsbility. AJR 1968;104:529–43.

INTESTINAL OBSTRUCTION

Janic JS, Ein SH, Filler RM, et al. An assessment of adhesive small bowel obstruction in infants and children. J Pediatr Surg 1981;16:225–9.

Intussusception

Adamsbaum C, Sellier N, Helardot P. Ileocolic intussusception with enterogenous cyst: ultrasonic diagnosis. Pediatr Radiol 1989;19:325–7.

Agha FP. Intussusception in adults. AJR 1986;146:527–31.

Armstrong AE, Dunbar JS, Graviss ER, et al. Intussusception complicated by distal perforation of the colon. Radiology 1980;136:77–81.

Atkinson GO, Gay BB, Naffis D. Intussusception of the appendix in children. AJR 1976;126:1164–8.

Bowerman RA, Silver TM, Jaffe MH. Real-time ultrasound diagnosis of intussusception in children. Radiology 1982;143:527–9.

Bramson RJ, Blickman JG. Perforation during hydrostatic reduction of intussusception: proposed mechanism and review of the literature. J Pediatr Surg 1992;27:587–91.

Bramson RT, Zambuto D, Blickman JG. Intracolonic pressure measurements during hydrostatic and air contrast barium enemas in children. Radiology 1995;195:55–8.

Brereton RJ, Taylor B, Hall CM. Intussusception and intestinal malrotation of infants: Waugh's syndrome. Br J Surg 1986;73:55–7.

Burke LF, Clark E. Ileocolic intussusception: a case report. J Clin Ultrasound 1977;5:346–7.

Cipel L, Fonkalsrud EW, Gyepes MT. Ileo-ileal intussusception in the newborn. Pediatr Radiol 1977;6:39–42.

Cochran DQ, Almond CH, Shucart WA. An experimental study of the effects of barium and intestinal contents on the peritoneal cavity. AJR 1963;89:883–7.

Cohen MD, Baker M, Grosfeld JL, et al. Post-operative intussusception in children with neuroblastoma. Br J Radiol 1982;55:197–200.

Connolly B, Alton DJ, Ein S, Daneman A. Partially reduced intussusception: when are repeated delayed reduction attempts appropriate. Pediatr Radiol 1995;25:104–7.

Cox JA, Martin LW. Postoperative intussusception. Arch Surg 1973;106:263–6.

Cox TD, Winters WD, Weinberger E. CT of intussusception in the pediatric patient: diagnosis and pitfalls. Pediatr Radiol 1996;26:26–32.

Dammert G, Votteler TP. Postoperative intussusception in the pediatric patient. J Pediatr Surg 1974;9:817–20.

Daneman A, Alton DJ, Ein S, et al. Perforation during attempted intussusception reduction in children—a comparison of perforation with barium and air. Pediatr Radiol 1995;25:81–8.

Daneman A, Reilly BJ, Silva MD, et al. Intussusception on small bowel examinations in children. AJR 1982;139:299–304.

del Pozo G, Albillos JC, Tejedor D. Intussusception: US findings with pathologic correlation—the cresent-in-a-doughnut sign. Radiology 1996;199:688–92.

Devred PH, Faure F, Padovani J. Pseudotumoural cecum after hydrostatic reduction of intussusception. Pediatr Radiol 1984;14:295–8.

Douglas NJ, Cameron DC, Nixon SJ, et al. Intussusception of a mucocele of the appendix. Gastrointest Radiol 1978;3:97–100.

Du JNH. Ten years' experience in the management of intussusception in infants and children by hydrostatic reduction. Can Med Assoc J 1978;119:1075–6.

Ein SH. Recurrent intussusception in children. J Pediatr Surg 1975;10:751–5.

Ein SH. Leading points in childhood intussusception. J Pediatr Surg 1976;11:209–11.

Ein SH, Ferguson LM. Intussusception—the forgotten postoperative obstruction. Arch Dis Child 1982;57:788–90.

Ein SH, Mercer S, Humphry A, Macdonald P. Colon perforation during attempted barium enema reduction of intussusception. J Pediatr Surg 1981;16:313–5.

Ein SH, Stephens CA. Intussusception: 354 cases in 10 years. J Pediatr Surg 1971;6:16–27.

Ein SH, Stephens CA, Minor A. The painless intussusception. J Pediatr Surg 1976;11:563–4.

Ein SH, Stephens CA, Shandling B, Filler RM. Intussusception due to lymphoma. J Pediatr Surg 1986;9:786–8.

Eklof O, Hartelius H. Reliability of the abdominal plain film diagnosis in pediatric patients with suspected intussusception. Pediatr Radiol 1980;9:199–206.

Eklof O, Hugooson C. Post evacuation findings in barium enema-treated intussusceptions. Ann Radiol 1976;19:133–9.

Eklof O, Johanson L, Lohr G. Childhood intussusception: hydrostatic reducibility and incidence of leading points in different age groups. Pediatr Radiol 1980;142:5–8.

Eklof O, Rieter S. Recurrent intussusception: analysis of a series treated with hydrostatic reduction. Acta Radiol (Diagn) 1978;19:250–8.

Fiorito ES, Cuestas LAR. Diagnosis and treatment of acute intussusception with controlled insufflation of air. Pediatrics 1959;24:241–4.

Fishman MC, Borden S, Cooper A. The dissection sign of nonreducible ileocolic intussusception. AJR 1984;143:5–8.

Fitch SJ, Magill HL, Benator RM, et al. Pseudoreduction of intussusception: is ileal reflux the end point? Gastrointest Radiol 1985;10:181–3.

Franken EA Jr, King H. Postoperative intussusception in children. AJR 1972;116:584–6.

Franken EA Jr, Smith WL, Chernish SM, et al. The use of glucagon in hydrostatic reduction of intussusception: a double blind study of 30 patients. Radiology 1983;146:687–9.

Frush PD, Zheng JY, McDermott VG, Bisset GS. Nonoperative treatment of intussusception: historical perspective. AJR 1995;165:1066–70.

Fujioka M, Bender T, Young LW, et al. Polyarteritis nodosa in children: radiological aspects and diagnostic correlation. Radiology 1980;136:359–64.

Ginai AZ. Experimental evaluation of various available contrast agents for use in the gastrointestinal tract in case of suspected leakage: effects on peritoneum. Br J Radiol 1985;58:969–78.

Gorenstein A, Raucher A, Serour F, et al. Intussusception in children: reduction with repeated delayed air enema. Radiology 1998;206:721–4.

Grasso SN, Katz ME, Presberg HJ, Croitoru DP. Transabdominal manually assisted reduction of pediatric intussusception: reappraisal of this historical technique. Radiology 1994;191:777–9.

Gu L, Alton DJ, Daneman A, et al. Intussusception reduction in children by rectal insufflation of air. AJR 1988;150:1345–8.

Guo J, Ma X, Zhou Q. Results of air pressure enema reduction of intussusception: 6,396 cases in 13 years. J Pediatr Surg 1986;21:1201–3.

Hertz I, Train J, Keller R, et al. Adult post operative enteroenteric intussusception in Crohn's disease. Gastrointest Radiol 1982;7:131–4.

Humphrey A, Ein SH, Mok PM. Perforation of the intussuscepted colon. AJR 1981;137:1135–8.

Hutchinson IF, Olayiwola B, Young DG. Intussusception in infancy and childhood. Br J Surg 1980;67:209–12.

Iko BO, Teal JS, Siram SM, et al. Computed tomography of adult colonic intussusception: clinical and experimental studies. AJR 1984;143:769–72.

Janic JS, Ein SH, Filler RM, et al. An assessment of adhesive small bowel obstruction in infants and children. J Pediatr Surg 1981;16:225–9.

Johnson JF, Woisard KK. Ileocolic intussusception: new sign on the supine cross-table radiograph. Radiology 1989;171:483–6.

Katz ME, Kolm P. Intussusception reduction 1991: an international survey of pediatric radiologists. Pediatr Radiol 1992;22:318–22.

Katz M, Phelan E, Carlin JB, Beasley SW. Gas enema for the reduction of intussusception: relationship between clinical signs and symptoms and outcome. AJR 1993;160:363–6.

Kirks DR. Diagnosis and treatment of pediatric intussusception: how far should we push our radiologic techniques? Radiology 1994;191:622–3.

Lam AH, Firman K. Ultrasound of intussusception with lead points. Australas Radiol 1991;35:343–5.

Lam AH, Firman K. Value of sonography including colour Doppler in the diagnosis and management of long-standing intussusception. Pediatr Radiol 1992;22:112–4.

Leeba JM, Boas RN. Simultaneous intussusception and sigmoid volvulus in a child. Pediatr Radiol 1986;16:248–9.

Leonidas JC. Treatment of intussusception with small bowel obstruction: application of decision analysis. AJR 1985;145:665–9.

Levine MS, Trenker SW, Herlinger H, et al. Coiled spring sign of appendiceal intussusception. Radiology 1985;155:41–4.

Lim HK, Bae SH, Lee KH, et al. Assessment of reducibility of ileocolic intussusception in children: usefulness of colour Doppler sonography. Radiology 1994;191:781–5.

Lobo E, Daneman A, Fields JM, et al. The diagnosis of malrotation during air enema procedure. Pediatr Radiol 1997;27:606–8.

Mason JT, Quon D. The inadvertent CT demonstration of intussusception. J Can Assoc Radiol 1985;36:68–70.

McDermott VGM. Childhood intussusception and approaches to treatment: a historical review. Pediatr Radiol 1994;24:153–5.

Merine D, Fishman EK, Jones B, Siegelman SS. Enteroenteric intussusception: CT findings in nine patients. AJR 1987;148:1129–32.

Meyer JS. The current radiologic management of intussusception: a survey and review. Pediatr Radiol 1992;22: 323–5.

Miller SF, Landes AB, Dautenhahn LW, et al. Intussusception: ability of fluoroscopic images obtained during air enema to depict lead points and other abnormalities. Radiology 1995;197:493–6.

Mok PM, Humphrey A. Ileo-ileocolic intussusception: radiological features and reducibility. Pediatr Radiol 1982;12:127–31.

Montali G, Croce F, De Pra L, Solbiati L. Intussusception of the bowel: a new sonographic pattern. Br J Radiol 1983;56:621–3.

Newman J, Schuh S. Intussusception in babies under 4 months of age. Can Med Assoc J 1987;136:266–72.

Palder SB, Ein SH, Stringer DA, Alton D. Intussusception: barium or air? J Pediatr Surg 1991;26:271–5.

Patriquin HB, Afshani E, Effman E, et al. Neonatal intussusception: report of 12 cases. Radiology 1977;125:463–6.

Phelan E, deCampo JF, Malecky G. Comparison of oxygen and barium reduction of ileocolic intussusception. AJR 1988;150:1349–52.

Pracos JP, Tran-Minh VA, Morin de Fine CH, et al. Acute intestinal intussusception in children. Contribution of ultrasonography (145 cases). Ann Radiol 1987;30:525–30.

Ratcliffe JF, Fong S, Cheong I, O'Connell P. Plain film diagnosis of intussusception: incidence of the target sign. AJR 1991;158:619–21.

Ratcliffe JF, Fong S, Cheong I, O'Connell P. The plain abdominal film in intussusception: the accuracy and incidence of radiographic signs. Pediatr Radiol 1992;22: 110–1.

Ravitch MM. Diagnosis and treatment of intussusception: a surgical condition. Pediatrics 1966;38:122–9.

Ravitch MM, McCune RM. Reduction of intussusception by barium enema: a clinical and experimental study. Ann Surg 1948;128:904–13.

Rees BI, Lari J. Chronic intussusception in children. Br J Surg 1976;63:33–5.

Ruoff M, Lindner AE, Marshak RM. Intussusception in sprue. AJR 1968;104:525–8.

Sargent MA, Babyn P, Alton DJ. Plain abdominal radiography in suspected intussusception: a reassessment. Pediatr Radiol 1994;24:17–20.

Sargent MA, Wilson BPM. Are hydrostatic and pneumatic methods of intussusception reduction comparable? Pediatr Radiol 1991;21:346–9.

Shiels WE, Kirks DR, Keller GL, et al. Colonic Perforation by air and liquid enemas: comparison study in young pigs. AJR 1993;160:931–5.

Shiels WE, Maves CK, Hedlund G, Kirks DR. Air enema for diagnosis and reduction of intussusception: clinical experience and pressure correlates. Radiology 1991;181: 169–72.

Sisel RJ, Donovan AJ, Yellin AE. Experimental fecal peritonitis: influence of barium sulfate or water soluble radiographic contrast material on survival. Arch Surg 1972;104:765–8.

Somekh E, Serour F, Goncalves D, Gorenstein A. Air enema for reduction of intussusception in children: risk of bacteremia. Radiology 1996;200:217–8.

Stein M, Alton DJ, Daneman A. Pneumatic reduction of intussusception: 5 year experience. Radiology 1992;183: 681–4.

Stephensen CA, Seibert JJ, Strain JD, et al. Intussusception: clinical and radiographic factors influencing reducibility. Pediatr Radiol 1984;20:57–60.

Stevens VR. Acute intussusception: manipulative reduction under fluoroscopic control. Am J Dis Child 1928;35: 61–4.

Stone DN, Kangarloo H, Graviss ER, et al. Jejunal intus-susception in children. Pediatr Radiol 1980;9:65–8.

Stringer DA, Ein SH. Pneumatic reduction: advantages, risks and indications. Pediatr Radiol 1990;20:475–7.

Swischuk LE, Hayden CK, Boulden T. Intussusception: indications for ultrasonography and an explanation of the doughnut and pseudokidney signs. Pediatr Radiol 1985;15:388–91.

Swischuk LE, Stanberry SD. Ultrasonographic detection of free peritoneal fluid in uncomplicated intussusception. Pediatr Radiol 1990;21:350–1.

Thomassen B, Sutinen S. Chronic primary intussuscep-tion in an infant. J Pediatr Surg 1972;7:299–301.

Verschelden P, Filiatrault D, Garel L, et al. Intussusception in children: reliability of US in diagnosis—a prospective study. Radiology 1992;184:741–4.

Waugh GE. Congenital malformations of the mesentery: a clinical entity. Br J Surg 1927;15:438–49.

Wayne ER, Campbell JB, Burrington JD, et al. Manage-ment of 344 children with intussusception. Radiology 1973;107:597–601.

Wayne ER, Campbell JB, Kosloske AM, et al. Intussuscep-tion in the older child—suspect lymphosarcoma. J Pedi-atr Surg 1976;11:789–94.

Weinberger E, Winters W. Intussusception in children: the role of sonography. Radiology 1992;184:601–2.

White SJ, Blane CE. Intussusception: additional observa-tions on the plain radiograph. AJR 1982;139:511–3.

Woo SK, Kim JS, Suh SJ, et al. Childhood intussusception: US-guided hydrostatic reduction. Radiology 1992;182:77–80.

Pseudo-Obstruction, Megacystis-Microcolon–Hypoperistalsis Syndrome

Agosti A, Bertaccini G, Paulucci R, et al. Caerulein treat-ment for paralytic ileus. Lancet 1971;395.

Amoury RA, Fellows RA, Goodwin CD, et al. Megacystis-microcolon–intestinal hypoperistalsis syndrome: a cause of intestinal obstruction in the newborn period. J Pediatr Surg 1977;12:1063–5.

Bagwell CE, Filler RM, Cutz E, et al. Neonatal intestinal pseudo-obstruction. J Pediatr Surg 1984;19:732–9.

Bentley JRF, Nixon HH, Ehrenpreis T, et al. Seminar on pseudo-Hirschsprung's disease and related disorders. Arch Dis Child 1966;41:143–54.

Berdon WE, Baker DH, Blanc WA, et al. Megacystis-microcolon–intestinal hypoperistalsis syndrome: a new cause of intestinal obstruction in the newborn. Report of radiologic findings in five newborn girls. AJR 1976;126:957–64.

Bertaccini G, Agosti A. Action of caerulein on intestinal motility in man. Gastroenterology 1971;60:55–63.

Byrne WJ, Cipel L, Euler AR, et al. Chronic idiopathic intestinal pseudo-obstruction syndrome in children—clinical characteristics and prognosis. J Pediatr 1977;90:585–9.

Clemett AR, Inkeles DA. Differentiation of acute and non-specific from mechanical small bowel obstruction. Radiology 1971;101:87–91.

Faulk DL, Anuras S, Christensen J. Chronic intestinal pseudo-obstruction. Gastroenterology 1978;74:922–31.

Franken EA Jr, Kleiman MB, Norins AL. Intestinal pseu-do-obstruction in mucocutaneous lymph node syn-drome. Radiology 1979;130:649–51.

Frimann-Dahl J. Roentgen examinations in acute abdom-inal diseases. 3rd ed. Springfield: Charles C Thomas; 1974.

Kapila L, Haberkorn S, Nixon HH. Chronic adynamic bowel simulating Hirschsprung's disease. J Pediatr Surg 1975;10:885–92.

Krook PM. Megacystis-microcolon–intestinal hypoperi-stalsis syndrome in a male infant. Radiology 1980;136:649–50.

Lowman RL. The potassium depletion states and postop-erative ileus: the role of the potassium ion. Radiology 1971;98:691–4.

Maldonado JE, Gregg JA, Green PA, et al. Chronic idio-pathic intestinal pseudo-obstruction in the newborn period. AJR 1970;49:203–12.

Melamed M, Kubian E. Relationship of the autonomic nervous system to "functional" obstruction of the intesti-nal tract. AJR 1963;80:22–8.

Nowak TV, Brown BP, Green JB, et al. Abnormal gas-trointestinal motility in myotonic dystrophy. Clin Res 1981;29:713A.

Patel R, Carty H. Megacystis-microcolon–intestinal

hypoperistalsis syndrome: a rare cause of intestinal obstruction in the newborn. Br J Radiol 1980;53:249–52.

Schuffler MD, Pope CE II. Esophageal motor dysfunction in idiopathic intestinal pseudo-obstruction. Gastroenterology 1976;70:677–82.

Schuffler MD, Rohrmann CA, Chaffee RG, et al. Chronic intestinal pseudo-obstruction. A report of 27 cases and review of the literature. Medicine 1981;60:173–96.

Shaw A, Shaffer H, Teja K, et al. A perspective for pediatric surgeons: chronic idiopathic intestinal pseudo-obstruction. J Pediatr Surg 1979;14:719–27.

Shilkin KB, Gracey M, Joske RA. Idiopathic intestinal pesudo-obstruction: report of a case with neuropathological studies. Aust Pediatr J 1978;14:102–6.

Sieber WK, Girdany BR. Functional intestinal obstruction in newborn infants with morphologically normal gastrointestinal tracts. Pediatr Surg 1963;53:357–61.

Sumner TE, Crowe JE, Klein A. Radiologic case of the month—megacystis-microcolon–intestinal hypoperistalsis syndrome. Am J Dis Child 1981;135:67–8.

Tanner MS, Smith B, Lloyd JK. Functional intestinal obstruction due to deficiency of argyrophil neurones in the myenteric plexus. Arch Dis Child 1976;51:837–41.

Ueda T, Okamoto E, Seki Y. Nonmechanical intestinal obstruction simulating surgical emergency in the newborn infant. J Pediatr Surg 1968;3:676–81.

Vezina WC, Morin FR, Winsberg F. Megacystic-microcolon–intestinal hypoperistalsis syndrome: antenatal ultrasound appearance. AJR 1979;133:749–50.

Williams DI, Burkholder GV. The prune belly syndrome. J Urol 1967;98:244–51.

Wiswell TE, Rawlings JS, Wilson JL, et al. Megacystis-microcolon–intestinal hypoperistalsis syndrome. Pediatrics 1979;63:805–8.

Young LW, Yunis EJ, Girdany BR, et al. Megacystis-microcolon–intestinal hypoperistalsis syndrome: additional clinical, radiologic, surgical and histopathologic aspects. AJR 1981;137:749–55.

Superior Mesenteric Artery and Cast Syndromes, Hernia, and Adhesions

Arida EJ, Joh SK, Cucolo GF. The spigelian hernia: Radiographic manifestations. Br J Radiol 1970;43:903–5.

Balthazar EJ, Subramanyam BR, Megibow A. Spigelian hernia: CT and ultrasonography diagnosis. Gastrointest Radiol 1984;9:81–4.

Bartram CI. The radiological demonstration of adhesions following surgery for inflammatory bowel disease. Br J Radiol 1980;53:650–3.

Berk RN, Coulson DB. The body cast syndrome. Radiology 1970;94:303–5.

Caroline DF, Herlinger H, Laufer I, et al. Small bowel enema in the diagnosis of adhesive obstructions. AJR 1984;142:1133–9.

Ekberg O, Fork F-Th, Fritzdorf J. Herniography in atypical inguinal hernia. Br J Radiol 1984;57:1077–82.

Fukuya T, Hawes DR, Lu CC, et al. CT diagnosis of small bowel obstruction: efficacy in 60 patients. AJR 1992;158:765–72.

Ghahremani GG, Jimenez MA, Rosenfield M, et al. CT diagnosis of occult incisional hernias. AJR 1987;148:139–42.

Gurrarino G. Incarcerated inguinal hernia in infants: plain films and barium enema. Pediatr Radiol 1974;2:247–50.

Harbin WP, Andres J, Kim SH, et al. Internal hernia into Treves field pouch. Case report and review of the literature. Radiology 1979;130:71–2.

Holder LE, Schneider HJ. Spigelian hernias: anatomy and roentgenographic manifestations. Radiology 1974;112:309–13.

Hunter TB, Freundlich IM, Zukoski CF. Preoperative radiographic diagnosis of a spigelian hernia containing large and small bowel. Gastrointest Radiol 1977;1:379–81.

Janik JS, Ein SH, Filler RM, et al. An assessment of the surgical treatment of adhesive small bowel obstruction in infants and children. J Pediatr Surg 1981;16:225–9.

Leigh TF. Acute gastric dilatation. JAMA 1960;172:1376–81.

Lewis JL, Hoskins EO. Volvulus of the small bowel into a pouch in the field of Treves presenting with anaemia. Br J Radiol 1985;58:1132–4.

Maglinte DDT, Miller RE, Lappas JC. Radiologic diagnosis of occult incisional hernias of the small intestine. AJR 1984;142:931–2.

Megibow AJ, Balthazar EJ, Medwid SW, et al. Bowel obstruction: evaluation with CT. Radiology 1991;180:313–8.

Meziane MA, Fishman EK, Siegelman SS. Computed tomographic diagnosis of obturator foramen hernia. Gastrointest Radiol 1983;8:375–7.

Mindell HJ, Holm JL. Acute superior mesenteric artery syndrome. Radiology 1970;94:299–302.

Shackelford GD, McAlister WH. Inguinal herniography. AJR 1972;115:399–407.

Shanbhogue LKR, Miller SS. Richter's hernia in the neonate. J Pediatr Surg 1986;21:881–2.

Siegel M. Pediatric sonography. 2nd ed. New York: Raven Press; 1995. p. 507.

Vaisman N, Stringer DA, Pencharz P. Functional intestinal obstruction (superior mesenteric artery or cast syndrome) in cerebral palsy. J Parenteral Enteral Nutr 1989; 13:326–8.

MISCELLANEOUS DISORDERS

Borns PF, Johnston TA. Indolent pneumatosis of the bowel wall associated with immune suppressive therapy. Ann Radiol 1973;16:163–6.

Bray FJ. The "inverted V" sign of pneumoperitoneum. Radiology 1984;151:45–6.

Campbell RE, Boggs TR, Kirkpatrick JA. Early neonatal pneumoperitoneum from progressive massive tension pneumomediastinum. Radiology 1975;114:121–6.

Capps JH, Klein RM. Polyarteritis nodosa as a cause of perirenal and retroperitoneal hemorrhage. Radiology 1970;94:143–6.

Cook PL. Calcified meconium in the newborn. Clin Radiol 1978;29:541–6.

Coussement AM, Gooding CA, Taybi H, et al. Roentgenographic visualization of the umbilical arteries in pneumoperitoneum in the newborn. AJR 1973;118:46–8.

Foucar E, Mukai K, Foucar K, et al. Colon ulceration in lethal cytomegalovirus infection. Am J Clin Pathol 1981; 136:788–801.

Fujioka M, Bender T, Young LW, et al. Polyarteritis nodosa in children: radiological aspects and diagnostic correlation. Radiology 1980;136:359–64.

Gupta A. Pneumatosis intestinalis in children. Br J Radiol 1978;51:589–95.

Haller JO, Slovis TL, Baker DH, et al. Anorexia nervosa—the paucity of radiologic findings in more than fifty patients. Pediatr Radiol 1977;5:145–7.

Hernanz-Schulman M, Kirkpatrick J, Scwachman H, et al. Pneumatosis intestinalis in cystic fibrosis. Radiology 1986;160:497–9.

Keats TE, Smith TH. Benign pneumatosis intestinalis in childhood leukemia. AJR 1974;122:150–2.

Leonidas J, Berdon WE, Baker DH, et al. Perforation of the gastrointestinal tract and pneumoperitoneum in newborns treated with continuous lung distending pressures. Pediatr Radiol 1974;2:241–6.

Leonidas J, Hall RT, Holder TM, et al. Pneumoperitoneum associated with chronic respiratory disease in the newborn. Pediatrics 1973;51:933–5.

Olmsted WW, Madewell JE. Pneumoatosis cystoides intestinalis: a pathophysiologic explanation of the roentgenographic signs. Gastrointest Radiol 1976;1:177–81.

Puglisi BS, Kauffman HM, Stewart ET, et al. Colonic perforation in renal transplant patients. AJR 1985;145:555–8.

ReMine SG, McIlrath DC. Bowel perforation in steroid-treated patients. Ann Surg 1980;192:581–6.

Rice RP, Thompson WM, Gedgaudas RK. The diagnosis and significance of extraluminal gas in the abdomen. Radiol Clin North Am 1982;20:819–37.

Robinson AE, Grossman H, Brumley GW. Pneumatosis intestinalis in the neonate. AJR 1974;120:333–41.

Schnyder PA, Brasch RC, Salvatierra O. Gastrointestinal complications of renal transplantation in children. Radiology 1979;130:361–6.

Seibert JJ, Parvey LS. The telltale triangle: use of the supine cross-table lateral radiograph in early detection of pneumoperitoneum. Pediatr Radiol 1977;5:209–10.

Strain JD, Rudikoff JC, Moore EE, et al. Pneumatosis intestinalis associated with intracatheter jejunostomy feeding. AJR 1982;139:107–9.

Vernacchia FS, Jeffrey RB, Laing FC, Wing VW. Sonographic recognition of pneumatosis intestinalis. AJR 1985;145:51–2.

Warshaw AL, Welch JP, Ottinger LW. Acute perforation of the colon associated with chronic corticosteroid therapy. Am J Surg 1976;131:442–6.

10

LARGE BOWEL

Sheila C. Berlin, MD, Carlos J. Sivit, MD, and David A. Stringer, BSc, MBBS, FRCR, FRCPC

EMBRYOGENESIS OF THE COLON

The large bowel is derived from elements of both the midgut and hindgut. The cecum, appendix, ascending colon, and proximal two-thirds of the transverse colon are midgut derivatives while the remainder of the colon arises from the hindgut. The junction between the segment of transverse colon derived from the midgut and hindgut is demarcated by a change in blood supply from the superior mesenteric artery to the inferior mesenteric artery (Gray and Skandalakis, 1972).

The cecal diverticulum, the primordium of the cecum and appendix, appears in the sixth week of gestation. This conical pouch arises on the antimesenteric border of the caudal limb of the midgut loop. Relatively slower growth of the blind sac results in formation of the appendix. The cecum and appendix move downward into the right iliac fossa as the proximal part of the colon elongates. The position of the appendix varies considerably as it may pass posterior to the cecum (retrocecal) or colon (retrocolic) or as it may descend over the brim of the pelvis (pelvic or descending). A retrocecal position of the appendix is present in about 64% of people. Only 32% of people have a pelvic position of the appendix (Moore, 1982).

Bowel derivatives of the hindgut include the left one-third to one-half of the transverse colon, the descending colon, the sigmoid colon, the rectum, and the superior part of the anal canal. The descending colon becomes retroperitoneal when its mesentery fuses with the peritoneum of the left posterior abdominal wall and then disappears. The sigmoid colon is fixed by a smaller, separate mesentery.

The cloaca (Latin: open drain or canal) is the terminal portion of the hindgut. A coronal sheet of mesenchyme, the urorectal septum, divides the cloaca.

The rectum and upper anal canal form dorsally, and the urogenital sinus forms ventrally. The urorectal septum also divides the cloacal sphincter into anterior and posterior parts. The posterior part becomes the external anal sphincter, and the anterior part becomes the urogenital diaphragm, among other structures.

The anal canal develops by the end of the eighth week, bringing the caudal part of the digestive tract into communication with the amniotic cavity. The superior two-thirds (about 25 mm) of the canal is derived from the hindgut while the inferior two-thirds (about 13 mm) develops from the proctoderm. The superior rectal artery, the continuation of the inferior mesenteric artery, supplies the superior part of the anal canal whereas the inferior rectal arteries supply the inferior part of the canal.

ANATOMY OF THE LARGE BOWEL

The anatomic position of the large bowel is relatively constant in children, with a few exceptions. If the left kidney is absent, ectopic, or excised, the splenic flexure fills the left renal fossa and may have a reversed configuration (Mascatello and Lebowitz, 1976). Rarely, the right colon may displace the right kidney (Silverman, Kelvin, and Korobkin, 1983). The right colon may lie between the liver and right hemidiaphragm, a unique configuration known as Chilaiditi syndrome (see Chapter 11). This configuration may be seen in children with gastroschisis. Interposition of the colon between the kidney and posterior abdominal wall can occur when a child is prone, an important relationship to determine prior to procedures such as renal biopsy or percutaneous nephrostomy (Hopper, Sherman, and Luethke, 1987). The large bowel elongates with age; thus, it appears more redundant and the cecum is more superiorly positioned in an infant or small child than in an older child or adult. In older children, innominate grooves may be seen on barium enema; this is a normal finding and probably represents spaces between rows of lymphoid collections (Cole, 1978). The infant colonic haustra are poorly defined, and distinction between gas in the small and large bowel may be impossible in the newborn. Gas overlying the spine on the lateral radiograph is a helpful finding as it usually lies within the colon.

A lymphoid follicular pattern on barium enema shows tiny nodular filling defects of uniform size measuring up to 2 mm in diameter (Figure 10–1). This pattern affects primarily the left colon, with progressively less involvement of more distal large bowel. Double-contrast barium enema examination shows a lymphoid follicular pattern in nearly all children under 10 years of age (Miller et al., 1987); this is particularly prominent under 5 years of age (Laufer and de Sa, 1978). Lymphoid follicles have a small, central umbilication and may appear somewhat apthoid (Capitanio and Kirkpatrick, 1970). This is a more conspicuous finding in neonates, in whom they appear relatively large. Lymphoid follicles measuring over 3 mm in diameter may be associated with inflammatory bowel disease, lymphoma (Kenney, Koehler, and Shackelford, 1982), or dysgammaglobulinemia (Figure 10–2) (Wolfson et al., 1970).

CONGENITAL AND DEVELOPMENTAL ANOMALIES OF THE LARGE BOWEL

Atresia of the Large Bowel

Congenital colonic atresia is a rare cause of neonatal intestinal obstruction. The neonate with colonic atresia typically presents with failure to pass meconium in the first days of life, abdominal distention, and vomiting. Colonic atresias can be classified according to three separate types of obstruction, similar to those in the small intestine (see Chapter 9). Type I is complete obstruction by a diaphragm and type II is obstruction by an atretic cord. Type III refers to a complete separation of the proximal and distal colon with a corresponding V-shaped defect in the mesocolon. Intrauterine vascular insufficiency is the suggested cause of colonic atresia, possibly related to thromboemboli. Sites of atresia are evenly distributed throughout the colon, supporting a random embolic event as the etiology.

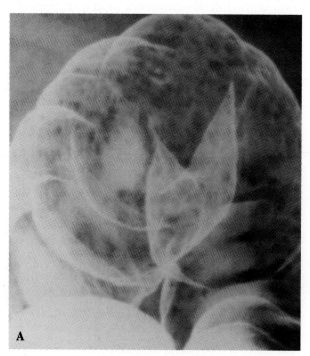 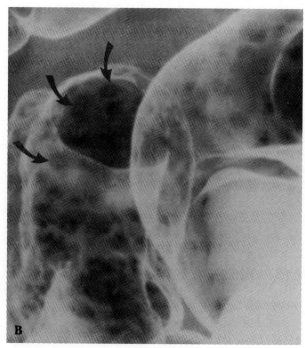

FIGURE 10–1. Normal lymphoid follicular pattern. *A,* The raised nodules at the splenic flexure are a normal feature of the colon on double-contrast examination. *B,* Some normal lymphoid follicles, with traces of barium lying in central umbilications (*arrows*), may mimic aphthae.

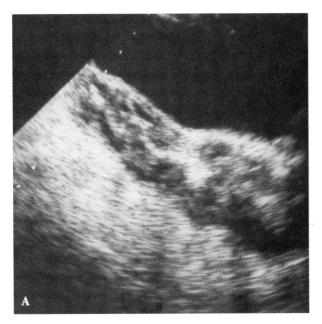

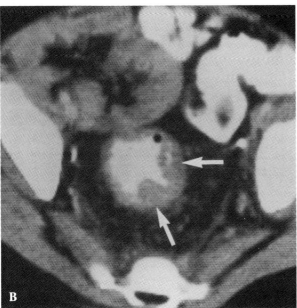

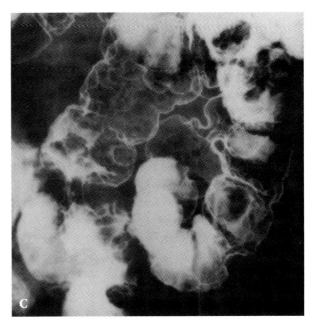

FIGURE 10–2. Lymphoid hyperplasia in a child with dysgammaglobulinemia. *A,* Longitudinal US through the bladder shows a thickened rectum that appears generally hypoechoic but with a hyperechoic central line (the mucosa) undulating over polyps. *B,* Computed tomography shows the bowel wall thickening and rectal polyps (*arrows*) outlined by rectal contrast media. The rectum is surrounded by fat. *C,* A double-contrast barium enema outlines multiple smooth polyps in a very deformed rectum. The diagnosis of lymphoid hyperplasia was made on biopsy, and there was no evidence of lymphoma or other malignant disease.

The radiographic appearance of colonic atresia is diagnostic in many cases, with a distended colon seen proximal to the atresia (Bley and Franken, 1973). While plain films show a distal intestinal obstruction (Figure 10–3), distinction between a distal small and large bowel obstruction can be difficult (Coran and Eraklis, 1960) (Figure 10–4). Occasionally, infants present with rupture of the proximal colon and pneumoperitoneum (Freeman, 1966; Lee and MacMillan, 1950).

The presumptive plain-film diagnosis is confirmed by a contrast enema. A water-soluble contrast material should be used, as iatrogenic rupture of the distal colon can occur (Staple and McAllister, 1967). Contrast enema shows a microcolon distal to the atresia, with abrupt cessation of flow at the atretic site (Figure 10–5). If the atresia is due to a web or diaphragm, the enema may show a club-shaped microcolon prolapsing into the gas-filled proximal colon, or wind-sock deformity (Winters, Weinberger, and Hatch, 1992) (Figure 10–6). Alternative causes of low bowel obstruction (ileal atresia, meconium ileus, Hirschsprung's disease, meconium plug) are identified on the contrast enema.

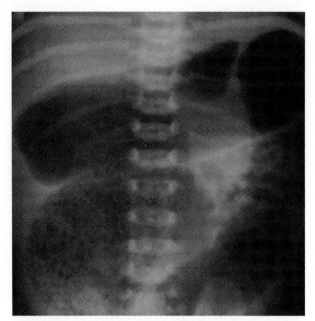

FIGURE 10–3. Colon atresia. Supine film shows specked meconium in a dilated loop of bowel in the right iliac fossa. The other very dilated loops of bowel are in the location of the transverse and descending colon, suggesting distal large bowel obstruction.

Stenosis of the Large Bowel

Congenital colonic stenosis is very rare and represents an incomplete form of atresia with a similar etiology. Acquired colonic stenosis in the pediatric population is usually secondary to necrotizing enterocolitis, but infectious, parasitic, and toxic processes must also be considered (Manzano and Barrero, 1977). The clinical and radiologic findings depend on the degree of stenosis. Contrast enema confirms the diagnosis, showing a stricture of variable length and caliber.

Anorectal Malformations

A spectrum of anorectal malformations presents in the newborn in approximately 1 in 5,000 births (Kurlander, 1967). Boys slightly outnumber girls among affected infants. An international classification system divides anorectal anomalies into four types: high, intermediate, low, and miscellaneous lesions (Table 10–1) (Figure 10–7) (Santulli, Kiesewetter, and Bill, 1970).

Failure to pass meconium and absence of an anus are the major presenting features in the newborn period. Close inspection of the perineum usually identifies the type of anorectal anomaly (Seibert

and Golladay, 1979). A perineal opening indicates a low lesion and occurs more commonly in girls in whom a fistula may be seen at the fourchette. In boys, a visible fistula appears only with an incompletely covered anus.

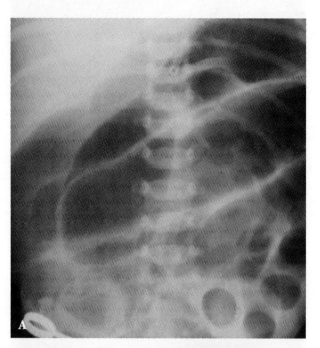

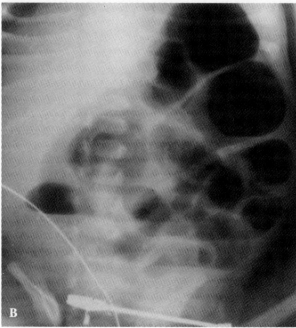

FIGURE 10–4. Colon atresia. *A,* Supine film shows multiple dilated bowel loops. *B,* Erect film shows gas-fluid levels, indicating low intestinal obstruction. However, it is not possible to determine whether the obstruction is in distal small bowel or large bowel.

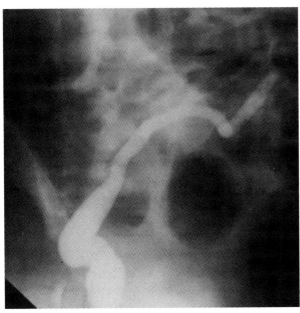

FIGURE 10–5. Type II or III colon atresia. The distal microcolon has an abrupt proximal end.

Anorectal anomalies may present as part of the association of vertebral defects, imperforate anus, tracheoesophageal fistula, and radial and renal dys-

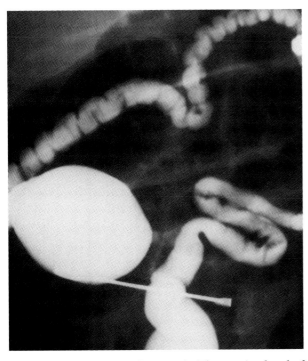

FIGURE 10–6. Type I colon atresia. The proximal end of a microcolon is dilated and has a clublike appearance due to prolapse of a diaphragm back into the proximal dilated bowel. An umbilical clamp overlies the lower abdomen.

plasia (VATER) (Quan and Smith, 1972, 1973). Vertebral anomalies are present in over 50% of patients with high malformations (Figures 10–8, 10–9) (Berdon, Baker, and Santuilli, 1968; Kurlander, 1967) and far less commonly among patients with low malformations (Thompson and Grossman, 1974).

Sacral agenesis, hemivertebrae, and fusion are common lumbosacral anomalies. Genitourinary tract anomalies are common, found in 25% of low atresias and 40% of high atresias. Anomalies include horseshoe kidney, renal agenesis and hypoplasia, hydronephrosis, and vesicoureteral reflux (Berdon, Hochberg, and Baker, 1966). Diabetes mellitus is seen in 16% of patients with sacral agenesis. When the sacrum is abnormal (Figure 10–9), the incidence of urologic anomalies is greater than 70% (Kurlander, 1967). Other rare anomalies are more striking, such as the severe caudal regression seen with sirenoform monsters. These infants also have agenesis of the urinary tract and internal genitalia as well as anomalies of the lumbosacral spine (Duhamel, 1961).

Currarino's triad consists of a complex of congenital caudal anomalies first described by Kennedy in 1926 and more clearly by Currarino in 1981 (Curranino, Coln, and Votteler, 1981; Kirks et al., 1984). The anomaly includes any one type of anorectal malformation, a presacral mass, and a

TABLE 10–1. Anorectal Malformations

Low (excluding stenosis)	Covered anus—complete
Males 42%	Anocutaneous fistula
Females 55%	(covered anus—incomplete)
	Anterior perineal anus
	Anovulvar fistula (F)
	Anovestibular fistula (F)
Intermediate (excluding stenosis)	
Males 8%	Anal agenesis without fistula
Females 25%	Anal agenesis with rectobulbar fistula (M)
	Rectovestibular fistula (F)
	Rectovaginal fistula (low) (F)
High (excluding atresia)	Anorectal agenesis without
Males 50%	fistula
Females 20%	Rectovesical fistula
	Rectourethral fistula (M)
	Rectovaginal fistula (high) (F)
	Rectocloacal fistula (F)

(F) = females only; (M) = males only.

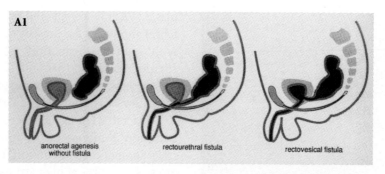

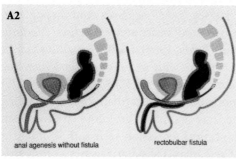

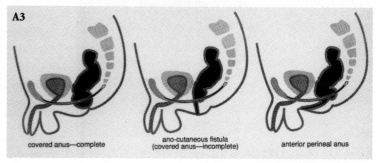

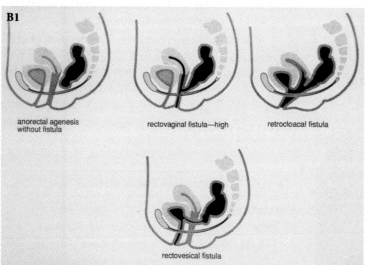

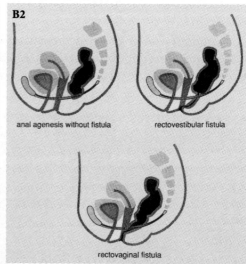

FIGURE 10–7. An international classification of anorectal malformations. Types of anorectal malformations are different for males (*A1* to *A3*) and females (*B1* to *B3*), although in each group there are 4 main types: high (*A1*, *B1*), intermediate (*A2*, *B2*), low (*A3*, *B3*), and miscellaneous. The various subcategories are listed in Table 10–1 and are indicated in this illustration except for the miscellaneous group, which includes cloacal extrophy and is beyond the scope of this book.

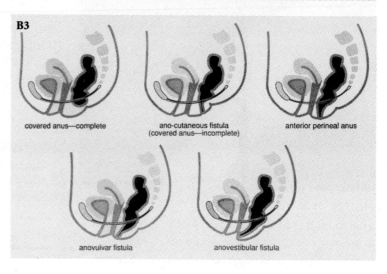

sacral bony abnormality (Kirks et al., 1984). The presacral mass may be a teratoma, anterior meningocele, enteric cyst, or a combination of any or all of these. The sacrum has a segmentation or bony cresenteric defect. The etiology is unclear but may be similar to that of neurenteric abnormalities elsewhere in the body (see Chapter 6) (Kirks et al., 1984). Radiologic assessment of the triad includes plain films of the spine and magnetic resonance imaging (MR) of the lumbosacral spine.

The type of anorectal malformation dictates therapy. Low lesions are treated by anoplasty or fistula dilatation. Intermediate and high lesions require a colostomy with definitive repair by posterior sagittal anoplasty at a later date.

Correct distinction between high and low lesions is vital, as an extended anoplasty in the patient with a high lesion is likely to result in extensive surgical deformity and possible loss of future fecal continence. In most patients, clinical and radiologic findings will establish a reliable preoperative diagnosis.

Radiography alone is unreliable for differentiating between high and low lesions (Berdon, Baker, and Santulli, 1968). Plain films obtained at least a few hours after birth typically show a distal bowel obstruction. Gas is occasionally seen in the bladder of boys, indicating a high anorectal anomaly with a rectourethral communication (see Figure 10–8).

Meconium trapped in the large bowel may calcify if there is a fistula to the urinary tract (Berdon, Baker, and Wigger, 1975), a process more common in boys than girls (Selke and Cowley, 1978). An ectopic ureter can drain directly into the colon in association with an anorectal malformation with calcified meconium (Felman et al., 1975). Meconium calcification with imperforate anus but no urinary fistula has been reported in the prune-belly syndrome and may be secondary to stasis (Morgan, Grossman, and

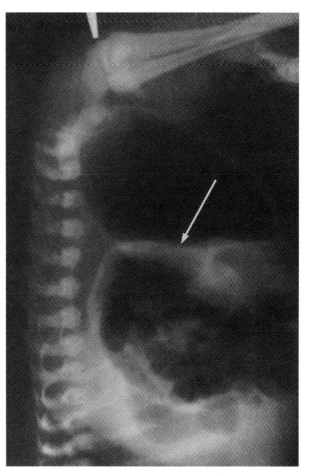

FIGURE 10–9. High anorectal anomaly. The inverted view with a marker on the anal dimple shows a large air-fluid level (*arrow*) in the distal obstructed large bowel. An assessment of the length of atresia is possible; however, the results are not reliable. The sacrum is deficient.

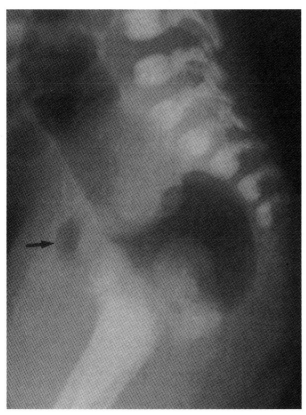

FIGURE 10–8. High anorectal anomaly with urinary tract fistula. Gas in the bladder (*arrow*) is displaced anteriorly and superiorly by a grossly dilated rectum.

Novak, 1978). Intracolonic calcification has been reported among patients with anorectal anomalies (Pouillaude et al., 1987) and may result from urine entering the bowel through a vesicoenteric fistula.

The inverted lateral view of the pelvis was historically used to demonstrate the distal extent of the colon (see Figure 10–9) (Berdon, Baker, and Santulli, 1968; Cremin, 1971). Using various bony landmarks to indicate the level of the puborectalis sling, this technique is unreliable in distinguishing between high and low lesions (Berdon, Baker, and Santulli, 1968). Inspissated meconium in the large bowel may prevent gas from reaching the distal bowel, suggesting a falsely high lesion. Conversely, a falsely low anomaly can be seen in a struggling, straining child (Figure 10–10).

Ultrasonography (US) can be used to measure the distance between the distal end of the meconium-filled large bowel and the perineum (Oppenheimer, Carroll, and Shochat, 1983) (Figure 10–11). Reports have suggested that a pouch-perineum distance of less than 1.5 cm is indicative of a low lesion, and a pouch terminating above the base of the bladder suggests a high lesion (Donaldson et al., 1989; Oppenheimer, Carroll, and Shochat, 1983). The reliability of this technique has not been established.

Other ultrasonographic signs of high lesions are intraluminal echogenic foci related to gas within the bladder or intraluminal calcifications (Morgan, Grossman, and Novak, 1978; Anderson et al., 1988). Renal US is useful in these patients to screen for associated genitourinary anomalies.

Voiding cystourethrography (VCUG) may be useful in the identification of a fistula between the large bowel and vagina, bladder, or urethra (Figure 10–12). The male urethra has a characteristic posterior kink when a rectourethral fistula is present (Figure 10–13) and is diagnostic of a high anomaly. Rare anomalies such as an unusually positioned fistula (Figure 10–14), duplicated urethra (Figure 10–15), and anal agenesis with a rectobulbar fistula are well seen by VCUG. Anal agenesis with a rectobulbar fistula occurs in less than 2% of males with anal atresia (Currarino, Votteler, and Kirks, 1978; Gupta, Bhargava, and Rohtagi, 1986). If anal atresia is present without apparent fistula and preoperative imaging of the colon is desired, percutaneous puncture of the anal dimple under fluoroscopic control may allow opacification of the distal large bowel (Murugasu, 1970). This water-soluble contrast study will demonstrate the position of the colon and may reveal a fistula (Wagner et al., 1973).

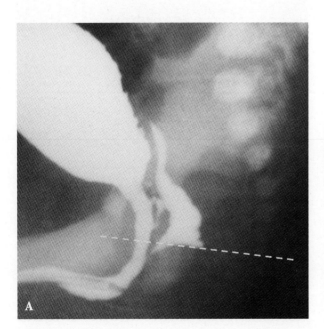 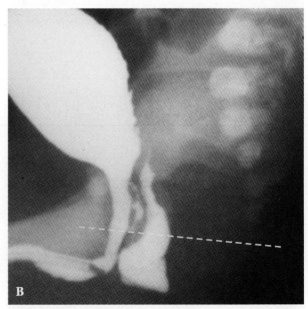

FIGURE 10–10. High anorectal anomaly. *A,* Retrograde urethrogram demonstrates a fistula to the rectum in a neonate. The distal rectum lies above the dotted line between the pubis and the sacrococcygeal joint. *B,* When the baby cries, the distal part of the large bowel descends markedly below the dotted line between the pubis and the sacrococcygeal joint. A high lesion can thus be mistaken for a low lesion on plain films.

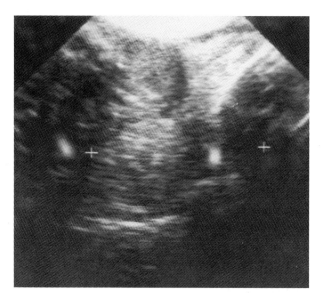

FIGURE 10–11. High anorectal anomaly. Saggital US with the transducer on the anterior abdominal wall shows the tip of the examiner's finger in the anal dimple (right-hand cursor), which is best seen in real time, and the distal meconium-filled large bowel (left-hand cursor). The accuracy of this technique is still unclear.

Magnetic resonance imaging (MR) and computed tomography (CT) may be useful in evaluating the levator sling in children with congenital anorectal anomalies (Khoda et al., 1985; Mezzacappa, Price, and Haller, 1987; Sato et al., 1988). Direct visualization of the levator mechanism and its relationship with the distal bowel not only helps the surgeon to plan the surgical approach but also predicts the degree of bowel continence the child may achieve. If the levator ani muscle is not present, it is not possible to perform a standard pull-through procedure and achieve rectal continence. T1-weighted axial, sagittal, and coronal images using 5 mm contiguous sections are the standard MR sequences for this examination. The field of view should include the lumbosacral spine, kidneys, and pelvis to detect associated genitourinary and vertebral anomalies. The puborectalis muscle and external sphincter muscle mass can be exquisitely demonstrated with MR in multiple planes. In cases of sacrococcygeal agenesis or hypoplasia, the puborectalis muscle and the external anal sphincter may be located in an eccentric position.

Prior to colostomy takedown, it may be helpful to perform a water-soluble contrast enema of the distal colonic loop to evaluate the bowel anatomy

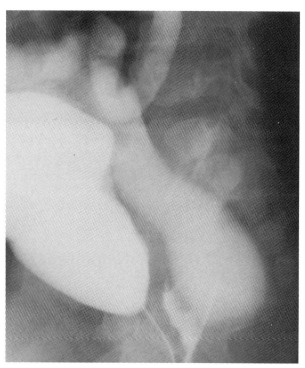

FIGURE 10–12. Anorectal malformation with rectovaginal fistula. A catheter in the vagina passes through a fistula into the rectum. Cystourethrogram shows no other fistula.

and exclude a possible fistula. Following definitive pull-through surgery, water-soluble distal colostomy loopography is often performed to evaluate for anastomotic leak and to demonstrate patency at the anal sphincter.

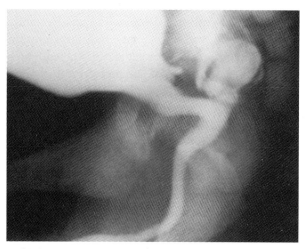

FIGURE 10–13. Anorectal malformation with a rectourethral fistula. Micturating cystourethrogram shows the characteristic posterior kink in the urethra in the region of the fistula. Contrast has entered the rectum.

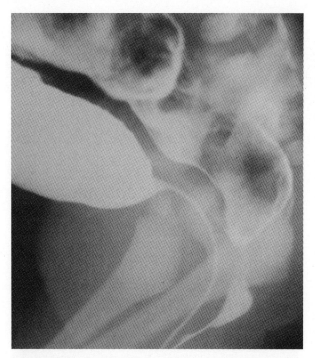

FIGURE 10–14. Anorectal malformation with a fistula from rectum to end of the penis. Micturating cystourethrogram showed no connection to the rectum. A fistulograph showed an unusual fistula from the end of the penis to the rectum.

If the large bowel has been incorrectly pulled through the levator sling, incontinence often results. Magnetic resonance imaging can accurately locate the pulled-through intestine in relation to the sphincter muscles (Sato et al., 1988) and can identify operative complications affecting rectal continence such as a misplaced neorectum, inadvertently pulled-through mesenteric fat, and implantation mucous retention cyst (Sato et al., 1988). Sequences are the same as for the preoperative examination, although coverage need not include the spine and kidneys if these have already been examined. Some authors suggest that MR should be performed in all patients considered for repeat procedures for persistent incontinence (Sato et al., 1988).

Malrotation and Malfixation of the Large Bowel

Malrotation almost always affects the small bowel as well as the colon (see Chapter 9). In this condition, the small bowel fails to enter the abdominal cavity normally, and the mesentery fails to undergo normal fixation. In patients with midgut malrotation, the cecum is usually in the midpelvis and the ascending colon is

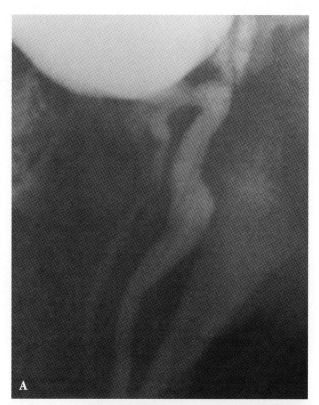

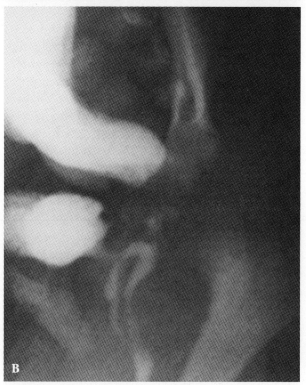

FIGURE 10–15. Anorectal malformation with a rectourethral fistula and double urethra. *A*, Micturating cystourethrogram shows a double urethra, with the major channel being posterior. *B*, Contrast has entered the rectum via a rectourethral fistula from the posterior urethra.

midline. Rarely, peritoneal bands cross anterior to the transverse colon and cause partial bowel obstruction. In nonrotation, the midgut loop fails to rotate after entering the abdomen; as a result, the caudal limb of the loop may return to the abdomen first, with the small intestine lying on the right and the entire large intestine lying on the left. This condition is generally asymptomatic, although volvulus can occur.

Failure of the proximal part of the colon to elongate during the third stage of rotation results in the cecum remaining near the inferior surface of the liver (subhepatic cecum) as the abdomen enlarges. This configuration is seen in 6% of fetuses and is more common in males. Some elongation of the colon occurs during childhood; hence, a subhepatic cecum and appendix are not as common in adults. A mobile cecum is one with an unusual degree of freedom; this anatomy occurs in 15% of people. A mobile cecum may herniate through the right inguinal canal or, rarely, result in volvulus (see Chapter 9).

Duplications of the Large Bowel

Duplications of the large bowel are rare and of uncertain etiology. Only 4 to 18% of all gastrointestinal duplications arise from the large bowel (Yucesan, Zorludemir, and Olcay, 1986). Colonic duplications are more common in girls (Kottra and Dodds, 1971).

There are two types of colonic duplication (Figure 10–16). In type I, there is duplication of a portion of the colon. The duplicated segment may be spherical (like a diverticulum) or tubular, paralleling a segment of bowel. Type II duplication is also tubular, extending the entire length of the colon from the anus to the lateral surface of the cecum; it is often associated with urogenital duplication ending in a blind pouch (Kottra and Dodds, 1971) or with a rectourinary or rectovaginal fistula (Yucesan, Zorludemir, and Olcay, 1986). Type II duplications are also associated with other anomalies such as malrotation, double or imperforate anus, fistula,

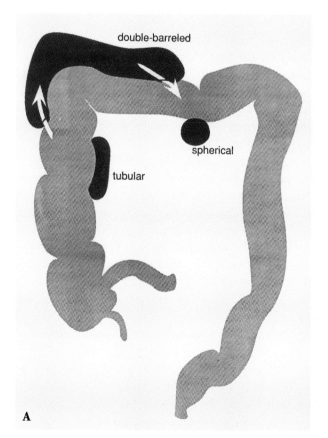
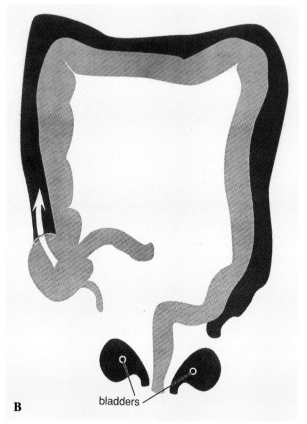

FIGURE 10–16. Large bowel duplication. There are two types of duplication. *A*, Type I may be spherical (like a diverticulum) or tubular (paralleling a segment of the bowel). The tubular variety may communicate, giving a blind-ended or double-barreled duplication. *B*, Type II extends for the entire length of the colon from the anus to the lateral surface of the cecum. In this type, the bladder may also be duplicated.

small bowel duplication, omphalocele, bladder extrophy, or spinal anomalies. When a double anus or duplication of the lower genitourinary tract is present, a type II anomaly should be suspected.

Pathologically, colonic duplications are lined with alimentary tract epithelium, most often identical to the adjoining bowel mucosa, especially if a communication exists. However, a single cyst may exhibit one or more types of mucosa from different sites in the gastrointestinal tract. The most frequently found ectopic tissues are gastric and pancreatic mucosa.

Pain, obstruction, constipation, and abdominal distention are typical presenting signs and symptoms. Rectal bleeding may result from ischemia or ectopic gastric mucosa. Duplications may intussuscept or mimic intussusception (Sonada et al., 1985). Type I duplications contain secretory mucosa that causes them to enlarge and present as an abdominal mass.

Plain films may demonstrate a soft-tissue mass displacing bowel loops (Kottra and Dodds, 1971). Calcification is a rare finding (Weber and Dixon, 1946). Occasionally, gas may be seen within the cyst. Plain films are useful in excluding associated vertebral anomalies. The diagnosis of duplication cyst is usually established by US as the appearance is virtually pathognomonic (Kangarloo et al., 1979; Barr et al., 1990). The cyst inner layer is echogenic (mucosa), the outer layer hypoechoic (muscle). The inner echogenic rim can sometimes be partly or totally destroyed as a result of pressure necrosis, peptic ulceration, or infection (Kangarloo et al., 1979). Internal echoes within the cyst result from hemorrhage, infection, or desquamated cells.

Contrast enemas may fill the duplication (Figure 10–17) or show mass effect on the large bowel (Campbell and Wolff, 1973). The mass may mimic an irreducible intussusception with a claw deformity (Sonada et al., 1985). Rectal duplications appear as retrorectal masses that cause widening of the rectosacral space and that are readily palpable (Gross, Holcomb, and Farber, 1952) unless a fistulous connection with the gut decompresses the cyst. The mass effect from other cystic masses such as mesenteric cyst are often less pronounced as they have thinner walls (Kottra and Dodds, 1971).

Computed tomography is not usually necessary in the diagnosis of duplication cyst. If performed, CT will demonstrate the cystic nature of the lesion (Ramsewak et al., 1986).

FUNCTIONAL DISORDERS OF THE LARGE BOWEL

Large bowel motility disorders result in faulty passage of stool through the colon. Generally, if the entire large bowel is involved, the small bowel dilates. If only a portion of the large bowel is involved, then the proximal large bowel dilates, leading to megacolon or megarectum.

Functional disorders can be classified according to the presence or absence of abnormalities of the myenteric plexus or smooth muscle (Table 10–2).

Hirschsprung Disease

Hirschsprung disease, or congenital aganglionic megacolon, is the most common cause of low intestinal obstruction in neonates. Harold Hirschsprung first described the classic clinical manifestations as a distinct entity in 1887. Swenson and Bill performed the first curative procedure in 1948.

The fundamental lesion in Hirschsprung disease is abnormal innervation of the bowel beginning at the anus, including the internal anal sphincter, and extending into the proximal colon for a variable distance. The rectosigmoid region is the most common transition site from normal to abnormal bowel. The transition zone is located in this region in 65% of patients. The transition zone occurs in the rectum in 8% of cases and in the more proximal large bowel in 24% of cases.

The American Academy of Pediatrics Surgical Section survey showed the overall ratio of male to female patients with Hirschsprung disease to be 3.8 to 1. The ratio was 2.8 to 1 in long segment disease and 2.2 to 1 in total colonic aganglionosis. Familial incidence was significant only in very long segment disease of the colon, where there was a 21% incidence of aganglionosis in a family member.

In most cases of Hirschsprung disease, the aganglionic segment extends from the anus to a level above which the bowel is normal. A small number of cases have been reported with skip areas, where a normal bowel segment separates aganglionic segments. Thus, a possible second site of disease should be considered in the context of postoperative colonic dysfunction (Martin et al., 1979).

Association with other serious congenital anomalies is uncommon in children with Hirschsprung disease (Berdon and Baker, 1965). Down syndrome is found in 3 to 5% of cases and cardiac disease in

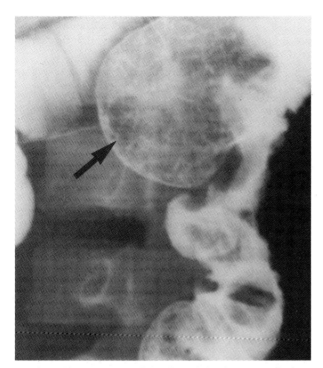

FIGURE 10–17. Type I large bowel duplication. There is a spherical duplication—like a diverticulum (*arrow*)—communicating with the proximal descending colon, which filled on barium enema.

2.5%, more common in longer segment disease. Genitourinary anomalies, particularly megaureter, are seen in 2% of cases. Colonic atresia and imperforate anus are reported associations (Johnson and Dean, 1981; Mahboubi and Templeton, 1984). Malrotation with or without facial-digital-genital (Aarskog) syndrome (Hassinger, Mulvihill, and Chandler, 1980) is reported and may result in volvulus (Tamburrini et al., 1986). Waardenburg's syndrome has been reported with total aganglionosis (Farndon and Bianchi, 1983). Other associations include cartilage hair dysplasia, congenital hearing loss, congenital rubella, hydrocephalus, cryptorchidism, hypoplastic uterus, cat's eye syndrome and Meckel diverticulum (Mahboubi and Templeton, 1984).

Unusual conditions associated with Hirschsprung disease include the congenital hypoventilation syndrome (Ondine's curse) and congenital neuroblastoma, both of which are consequences of neural crest maldevelopment (Rashkow et al., 1988). Hirschsprung disease may be considered in the spectrum of disorders that includes conditions such as pheochromocytoma, medullary carcinoma of the

TABLE 10–2. Functional Disorders of the Large Bowel*

Abnormality of myenteric plexus
    Hirschsprung disease
    Neuronal intestinal dysplasia
    Multiple endocrine neoplasia syndrome, type II
    Visceral neuropathies
        Familial
        Sporadic
    Drug-induced or anoxic damage
Normal myenteric plexus
    Neonatal functional immaturity of the large bowel
        (meconium plug/small left hemicolon syndrome)
    Microcolon of prematurity
    Megacystis-microcolon–intestinal hypoperistalsis
        syndrome
    Functional constipation
    Miscellaneous functional obstruction
        Inspissated milk or milk-curd syndrome
        Other inspissation syndromes
        Segmental dilatation of the colon
Abnormality of smooth muscle

Adapted from Krishnamurthy et al. Gastroenterology 1987;93:610–39.
*see pseudo-obstruction in the small bowel in Chapter 9.

thyroid, carcinoid tumors, and neurofibromas (Chatten and Voorhess, 1967; Gaisie, Oh, and Young, 1979; Hope, Borns, and Berg, 1965; Rashkow et al., 1988; Shocket and Teloh, 1957).

Ninety percent or more of normal neonates pass meconium in the first 24 hours of life, and 99% pass meconium by 48 hours of life. Any infant who fails to pass meconium by 48 hours of life should be considered to have Hirschsprung disease until proven otherwise. Patients with Hirschsprung disease may pass meconium in the first 2 days of life, only to have infrequent stooling later.

On examination, the child with Hirschsprung disease usually has a distended abdomen and may have palpable solid stool in the colon. Rectal examination may result in an explosive foul-smelling liquid stool, virtually pathognomonic for Hirschsprung disease with early enterocolitis. Diagnosis before the onset of enterocolitis is critical in reducing mortality (Bill and Chapman, 1962); thus, any patient in whom Hirschsprung disease is suspected should have an immediate diagnostic procedure. Enterocolitis associated with Hirschsprung disease is characterized by explosive watery diarrhea with abdominal distention, often accompanied by fever and vomiting. Distinction from infectious gastroenteritis can be difficult without a history of constipation. This frequently life-threatening complication can occur at any time, both before and after a definitive pull-through procedure (Bill and Chapman, 1962; Blane, Elhalaby, and Coran, 1994; Fraser and Berry, 1967). The postoperative enterocolitis associated with Hirschsprung disease can occur in the immediate postoperative period or later, as much as a year after corrective surgery (Blane, Elhalaby, and Coran, 1994).

In the neonatal period, conventional radiography typically shows a pattern of low intestinal obstruction, often with markedly dilated loops of bowel containing gas-fluid levels (Figure 10–18). A contrast enema is required to confirm the level of obstruction. About 5% of infants with Hirschsprung disease present with pneumoperitoneum secondary to perforation (Newman, Nussbaum, and Kirk-

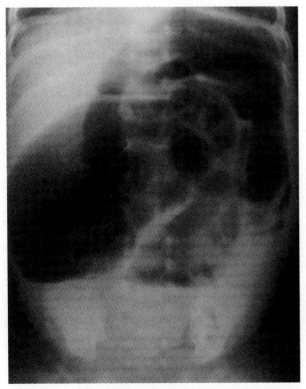

FIGURE 10–18. Hirschsprung disease in the neonate. Erect film shows multiple dilated loops of bowel, some containing gas-fluid levels.

patrick, 1987). Most of these patients have total colonic aganglionosis. Calcification in the small intestinal lumen has also been found in patients with total colonic aganglionosis (Fletcher and Yulish, 1978). This pattern of calcification resembles that which is occasionally seen in small bowel atresia and stenosis and is likely related to stasis. In the older child, conventional radiography may show stool in an obvious megacolon. Calcification in a fecaloma is rare (Campbell and Robinson, 1973). A contrast enema is necessary to establish the diagnosis.

The contrast enema performed to evaluate the patient with suspected Hirschsprung disease requires attention to some specific modifications. First, conventional teaching dictates that bowel preparation may alter the appearance of the transition zone between ganglionic and aganglionic segments. Rectal examination and cleansing enema prior to the study, however, appear not to obscure visualization of a transition zone (Rosenfield et al., 1984). Only the tip of a soft catheter should be inserted into the anus so as to insure complete visualization of the contrast-filled rectum. A balloon should not be inflated in the rectum as it may obscure the aganglionic segment or transition zone (De Bruyn, Hall, and Spitz, 1982). With the child in a lateral position, the rectum is slowly filled until contrast reaches the sigmoid colon (Cremin, 1974). A supine or prone position is satisfactory for further filling. Water-soluble contrast enema has a sensitivity and specificity equal to that of a barium enema and avoids the risk of barium spillage with perforation (O'Donovan et al., 1996). In addition, other causes of low intestinal obstruction, such as meconium plug and meconium ileus, are better studied with water-soluble contrast than with barium (see Chapter 3).

The most specific sign of Hirschsprung disease is the transition zone (Rosenfield et al., 1984), which may be abrupt or gradual (Figures 10–19 and 10–20). In long-standing cases, the aganglionic segment may become distended with stool, although the zone of transition may still be maintained (Figure 10–21). Unfortunately, not every patient has a readily identifiable transition zone (McDonald and Evans, 1954; Berman, 1956; Hope, Borns, and Berg, 1965; Schey and White, 1971; Rosenfield et al., 1984). Irregular contractions, historically termed anorectal dyskinesia, are infrequently seen in the aganglionic segment but are a

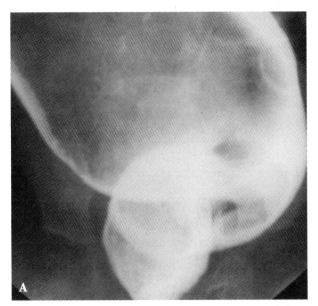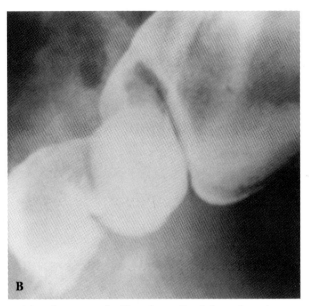

FIGURE 10–19. Hirschsprung disease. The zone of abrupt transition from grossly dilated ganglionic large bowel proximally to aganglionic large bowel distally is more easily assessed on the frontal than lateral view in this 10-month-old child. (*A*, frontal view; *B*, lateral view.)

reliable sign of Hirschspung disease (Rosenfield et al., 1984). These contractions may cause an irregular, saw-toothed appearance of the aganglionic segment (Figure 10–22). Delayed evacuation of barium on a 24-hour film is a poor predictor of Hirschsprung disease (Taxman, Yulish, and Rothstein, 1986; Rosenfield et al., 1984). A pattern of barium mixed with stool is infrequently seen on a 24-hour delayed film but has been reported as a highly reliable sign of Hirschsprung disease (Rosenfield et al., 1984). In children presenting with colitis, the enema may show mucosal edema and ulceration (Blane, Elhalaby, and Coran, 1994). The colonic mucosa has thickened folds and irregular margins due to ulceration and redundant mucosa (Figure 10–23).

Occasionally, neonatal functional immaturity of the colon (meconium plug) may mimic Hirschsprung disease with an apparent zone of transition, especially at the splenic flexure (Figure 10–24). The diagnosis is usually distinguished clinically, as these patients often have diabetic mothers, are premature, and spontaneously improve. Milk allergy colitis is also reported to mimic Hirschsprung disease with irregular narrowing of the rectum and a transition zone (Bloom, Buonome, and Fishman, 1999). Unusual imaging findings may be seen, with disease mimicking other processes such as intussus-

ception (Figure 10–25) or presentation with sigmoid volvulus (Figure 10–26).

The rectosigmoid index has been used to indicate the presence of a zone of transition (Pocharzevsky and Leonidas, 1977). This index is the maximum diameter of the rectum divided by

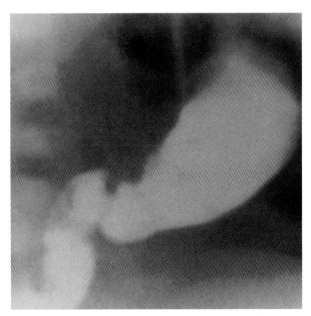

FIGURE 10–20. Hirschsprung disease. A gradual transition zone is seen from dilated ganglionic proximal bowel to aganglionic distal bowel that has a normal caliber.

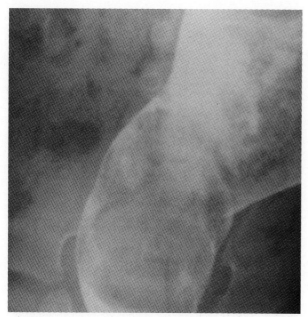

FIGURE 10–21. Hirschsprung disease. The markedly dilated rectum is full of feces, but a transition zone is seen from ganglionic sigmoid colon to aganglionic rectum.

the maximum width of the sigmoid colon. When the sigmoid colon is dilated, the index is less than 1.0 and usually less than 0.9. This index, however, is superfluous in the presence of a transition zone (Siegel, Shackelford, and McAlister, 1981).

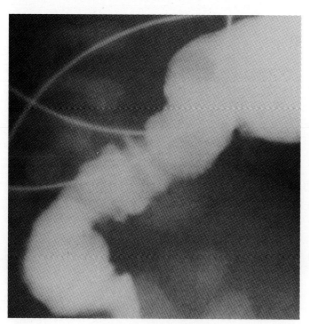

FIGURE 10–22. Hirschsprung disease. Irregular contractions are present in the aganglionic segment, best seen on fluoroscopy.

The definitive diagnosis of Hirschsprung disease is made by a full-thickness rectal biopsy to demonstrate the absence of normal ganglion cells. Because general anesthesia is required, this procedure is not benign, particularly in a neonate. The biopsy must be taken at least 1.5 cm above the dentate line since the distal 1 to 2 cm of bowel are normally hypoganglionic or aganglionic, and the specimen should be at least 2 cm long. A full-thickness biopsy also makes the major reparative procedure more difficult because of postbiopsy scarring. Thus, enema results, combined with anorectal manometry and suction biopsy, are the preferred methods for establishing or excluding the diagnosis. If there is discrepancy among the results of anorectal manometry, suction biopsy, and barium enema, the first two tests are repeated. If there is still some doubt about the exact diagnosis, a full-thickness biopsy is performed.

Total Colonic Aganglionosis

Long segment Hirschsprung disease involving at least the entire colon and often a portion of the small bowel is a difficult diagnostic problem. Since

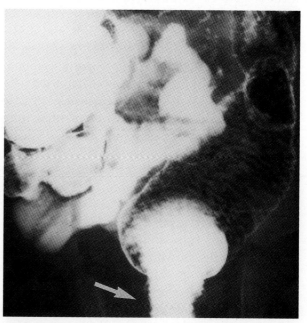

FIGURE 10–23. Enterocolitis complicating Hirschsprung disease. The mucosal pattern is abnormal, and the bowel wall margin of the left colon is irregular, found on endoscopy to be partly due to redundant mucosa and partly due to ulceration. A Soave pull-through operation has produced the narrow distal segment (*arrow*) of large bowel.

the barium enema is often normal and a small bowel transition zone is difficult to document, the diagnosis is often delayed. Approximately 30% of patients present after 1 month of age (deCampo et al., 1984). Vomiting, abdominal distention, constipation, diarrhea, and sepsis are some of the signs and symptoms at presentation. Manometry and suction biopsies confirm the presence of Hirschsprung disease, but the extent of aganglionosis is confirmed only by laparotomy with serial seromuscular biopsies.

A contrast enema may show a microcolon (23% of patients) or a normal colon (77%) (Figure 10–27). A shortened colon is seen in 23% of patients, with loss of normal hepatic and splenic flexure and sigmoid colon redundancy (deCampo et al., 1984). Meconium plug is frequently seen; unfortunately this is a nonspecific finding seen in functional immaturity of the colon, in meconium ileus, and in short segment Hirshsprung's disease as well as in normal patients.

Occasionally, a pseudotransition zone may be present, mimicking the more common form of Hirschsprung disease.

Total Intestinal Aganglionosis

Aganglionosis of the entire small and large bowel is exceedingly rare and invariably fatal. Death from intestinal obstruction is common in siblings of affected infants (Saperstein, Pollack, and Beck, 1980). The radiologic appearance is that of a small intestine pseudo-obstruction (see chapter 9).

Neuronal Intestinal Dysplasia

Neuronal intestinal dysplasia is a rare form of myenteric plexus abnormality that has been associated with neurofibromatosis and multiple endocrine neoplasia (MEN) syndrome type IIb. Clinically, colonic disease may mimic aganglionosis, but histologic examination shows hyperplastic submucosal and myenteric plexuses, giant neurons, and ganglia within the lamina propria (Krishnamurthy and Schuffler, 1987). Affected patients may have constipation, rectal bleeding, megacolon, or pseudo-obstruction. Barium enema shows a flaccid megacolon (Figure 10–28). Double-contrast barium enema may show abnormal flat or serpiginous folds or a complex lacy mucosal pattern (Demos et al., 1983). Small bowel series may show poor motility, delayed transit time and segmental intestinal dilatation (Demos et al., 1983)

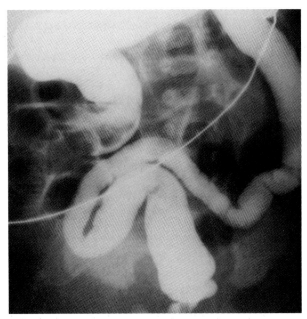

FIGURE 10–24. Hirschsprung disease. A gradual transition zone is seen from ganglionic transverse colon to aganglionic distal descending colon that has a normal caliber, mimicking meconium plug or hypoplastic left hemicolon syndrome. The transition was found to be at the splenic flexure. (see also Figure 10–29).

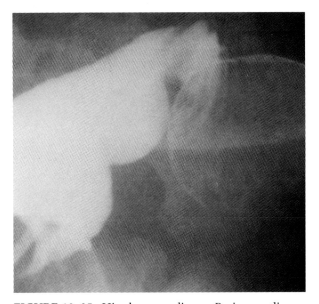

FIGURE 10–25. Hirschsprung disease. Barium outlines a normal-appearing rectum with a large filling defect in the sigmoid colon totally obstructing flow of barium and mimicking intussusception. However, irregular rectal contractions were seen on fluoroscopy, so the diagnosis was suggested preoperatively. The need for laparotomy was hence obviated, and a piece of feces was removed. Classic rectosigmoid Hirschprung disease was found on biopsy.

Visceral Neuropathies

There are groups of familial and sporadic visceral neuropathies that have an abnormal myenteric plexus (Krishnamurthy and Schuffler, 1987). The sporadic group includes the degenerative neuropathies such as those that result from Chagas' disease, a South American parasitic disease that results in a megacolon. The other groups generally present with pseudo-obstruction (see Chapter 9).

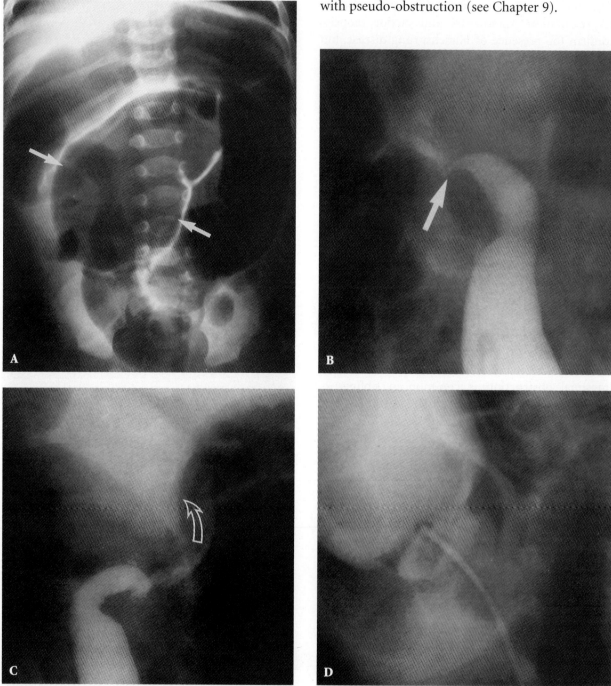

FIGURE 10–26. Hirschsprung disease and sigmoid volvulus. A 6-week-old boy presented with acute obstruction. *A*, The plain film shows dilated bowel, especially one loop in the midabdomen (between arrows). *B*, A contrast enema shows a normal-caliber rectum but a "bird of prey" or beak deformity (arrow) of the proximal rectum, indicating volvulus. *C*, Some contrast filled the dilated loop of sigmoid (in the direction of the open arrow). *D*, A catheter was gently passed through the volvulus, with prompt relief of symptoms upon evacuation of the exceedingly foul contents.

Drug-Induced or Anoxic Damage

Antineoplastic agents are the most common drugs that damage the myenteric plexus. In children, vincristine and daunorubicin are the most commonly prescribed of these drugs. Laxatives are generally not taken in high enough doses to cause colonic disease in children. The radiographic presentation is similar to that of Hirschsprung disease or pseudo-obstruction (see Chapter 9).

Neonatal Functional Immaturity of the Large Bowel (Meconium Plug/Small Left Colon Syndrome)

"Functional immaturity of the colon" is the favored term for the spectrum of disease causing transient functional neonatal intestinal obstruction (Le Quesne and Reilly, 1975). Thus, "meconium plug syndrome" and "small left colon syndrome" are labels that can be applied interchangeably for the common low intestinal obstruction speculated to be the result of abnormal motility. Affected babies are frequently premature, the infants of diabetic mothers (Davis et al., 1974; Davis and Campbell, 1975; Philippart, Reed, and Georgeson, 1975) or of mothers who have received magnesium sulfate for eclampsia (Sokal et al., 1972). Ingestion of psychotropic drugs have also

been a described association (Falterman and Richardson, 1980). Infants present with signs of bowel obstruction although they may not be critically ill. In fact, babies usually improve within hours to days of a contrast enema, and perforation is rare (Nixon, Condon, and Stewart, 1975).

Plain films show a distal obstruction (Figure 10–29) and gas-fluid levels have been reported in up to 50% of cases (Berdon et al., 1977). Water-soluble contrast use is similar to that prescribed for enema examination of meconium ileus (see Chapters 3 and 9). Contrast enema often shows a transition near the splenic flexure between dilated and narrowed colon (see Figure 10–29); occasionally, the transition is more proximal (Le Quesne and Reilly, 1975).

Microcolon of Prematurity

In very low birth-weight infants (less than 1000 g), functional immaturity of the large bowel may pre-

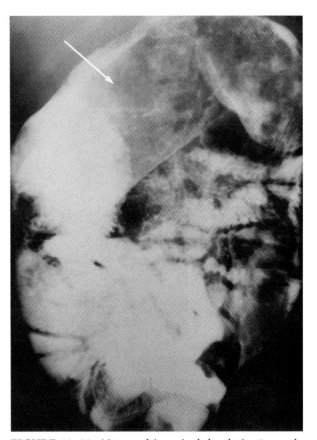

FIGURE 10–28. Neuronal intestinal dysplasia. A poorly functioning megacolon with gross fecal residue, dilatation, and abnormal haustral folds in the transverse colon (*arrow*) on single-contrast barium enema examination.

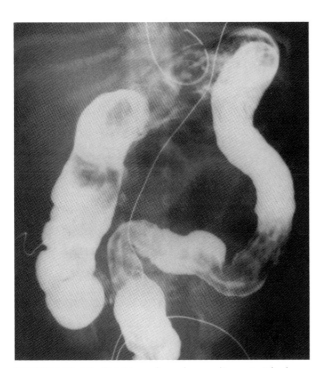

FIGURE 10–27. Total large bowel aganglionosis. The large bowel has a normal caliber.

sent as a microcolon. Toxemia and magnesium sulfate therapy appear to play a role in this functional obstruction (Amodio et al., 1986). The finding of a microcolon in a premature infant who has failed to pass meconium should raise the possibility of this diagnosis, to avoid an unnecessary procedure in these poor surgical candidates.

Megacystis-Microcolon–Intestinal Hypoperistalsis Syndrome

The megacystis-microcolon-intestinal hypoperistalsis syndrome, a rare cause of functional intestinal obstruction in the newborn, is an almost universally fatal condition described by Berdon and colleagues in 1973. Nearly all reported cases are in females (Krook, 1980; Young et al., 1981), and the syndrome is occasionally familial (Berdon et al., 1976; Patel and Carty, 1980). Newborns present with signs of obstruction and abdominal distention secondary to the large bladder and dilated bowel loops. Affected infants also usually have malrotation; thus, they may present with bilious emesis and volvulus. The generalized hypoperistalsis is unresponsive to medication and results in a pattern of pseudo-obstrution (see Chapter 9). The combined small and large bowel length is often only one-third of the normal length (Berdon et al., 1976).

Contrast enema shows a malrotated microcolon (see Chapter 9) with slow emptying. Evaluation of the urinary tract shows a markedly distended bladder and usually, dilated pelvicalyceal systems and ureters.

FUNCTIONAL CONSTIPATION

General Considerations

Constipation or obstipation occur in a spectrum of disorders, from those that require surgery (primarily congenital aganglionic megacolon, or Hirschsprung disease) to those marked by severe emotional disturbances and voluntary retention. Between these two extremes lie the bulk of patients who have no anatomic abnormalities and who are not severely emotionally disturbed (Davidson and Bauer, 1958).

Functional constipation refers to those patients who have normal ganglion cells with constipation, whether or not there is emotional disturbance. It is of prime importance to differentiate these patients, best treated medically, from those with Hirschsprung dis-

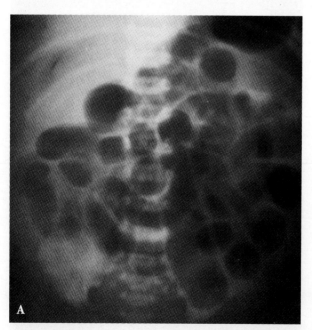
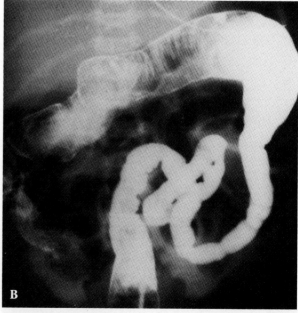

FIGURE 10–29. Functional immaturity of the large bowel (meconium plug syndrome). *A*, Plain-film radiograph in a 2-day-old boy indicates distal obstruction with many dilated loops of bowel and no rectal gas. *B*, Water-soluble contrast enema shows a distal microcolon that gently tapers proximally to the normal-sized colon. The entire colon contains many plugs of meconium. The water-soluble contrast enema aided passage of the meconium; no further treatment was necessary. The major differential diagnosis is Hirschsprung disease (see also Figure 10–24).

ease, who require surgery. In most cases, fortunately, differentiation on clinical grounds is easy. Hirschsprung disease is usually symptomatic from birth, and evidence of disease is well developed by 6 months of age, with an empty rectum on examination. In functional constipation, by contrast, the symptoms do not usually begin at birth, there is often evidence of emotional problems (such as a withdrawn temperament), the rectum is full of feces on examination, and encopresis (overflow leakage of liquid feces) is common. Encopresis rarely if ever occurs in Hirschsprung disease. This is probably related to conscious rectal sensitivity, which is increased in Hirschsprung disease but decreased in functional constipation with megarectum. (Meunier, Mollard, and Marechal, 1976). In some children, however, the diagnosis is not clear-cut. Older children rarely complain of incomplete or infrequent bowel movements, and symptoms are often few even when there is gross accumulation of feces. (Bentley, 1971). Hence, the presenting symptoms of functional constipation may include failure to thrive, poor appetite, abdominal colic, vomiting, or a variety of urinary symptoms. Chronic constipation has been known to result in chronic urinary retention. Hydronephrosis is a recognized complication and usually appears to be of uncertain etiology, but it is nonobstructive (Shopfner, 1968). Death may occur from renal failure (Bentley, 1971). If there is any concern over the diagnosis, a rectal biopsy will definitely exclude Hirschsprung disease and should be performed (Kottmeier and Clatworthy, 1965).

The cause of functional constipation is not well understood and is probably multifactorial. As the child leaves infancy, the gastrocolic reflex is less dominant, and the child becomes aware of the social taboos against indiscriminate defecation. This state of affairs occurs at a time of great emotional and intellectual development, so it is no surprise that disturbances of bowel habits sometimes occur.

Reversion to an infantile pattern of uninhibited defecation may occur; but feces are more commonly retained, resulting in chronic constipation. The retained feces accumulate and distend first the rectum and then the colon. Leakage through the anus is common, producing constant soiling, and these children may become social outcasts. Behavior problems may precede the development of constipation or occur secondary to the constipation (Bentley, 1971).

Physical impediments to defecation can also occur. Unduly hard, viscid or scanty feces will promote constipation. In patients with megarectum, the rectal sensitivity is decreased (Meunier, Mollard, and Marechal, 1976), which results in the lack of a satisfactory urge to defecate.

Imaging

Plain films and barium enema examinations will demonstrate the degree of constipation and dilatation of the large bowel. The classical barium enema finding is of megarectum dilated down to the anus with gross fecal residue, with no transition zone. Radiologic examination may help to exclude other causes of constipation such as Hirschsprung disease, although ultrashort-segment Hirschsprung disease may appear identical to functional constipation. The value of barium enemas in assessing clinical function of the large bowel is doubtful, and they are best confined to the use of helping to exclude the usual forms of Hirschsprung disease (Patriquin, Martelli, and Devroede, 1978).

MISCELLANEOUS FUNCTIONAL OBSTRUCTION

Inspissated Milk or Milk-Curd Syndrome

The "inspissated milk syndrome" is characterized by intestinal obstruction in premature infants fed on powdered milk formula (Berman and Ross, 1972; Cook and Rickham, 1969; Friedland, Rush, and Hill, 1972; Cremin, Smythe, and Cyrves, 1970; Cremin, 1973). It is probably due to excessive concentration of the powdered milk inspissating in the distal small bowel and colon. The infant presents after artificial feeding has been started, having initially passed meconium and then milk stools (Cremin, Smythe, and Cyrves, 1970).

Plain abdominal films show dense amorphous intraluminal masses often surrounded by a halo of air. The masses can be elongated or round. The appearance can mimic the ground-glass appearance of meconium and may have a paucity of air-fluid levels (Cremin, Smythe, and Cyrves, 1970).

Contrast enema examinations show a relatively narrow colon filled with multiple filling defects. The water-soluble enema enables passage of the pellets, which are found to be hardened curd.

Other Inspissation Syndromes

Rarely, other factors may cause a similar functional intestinal obstruction in infants. These include recent abdominal surgery, therapy for tetanus neonatorum (Cremin, Smythe, and Cyrves, 1970), and a variety of medications such as Resonium, an ion exchange resin (Berman, Briggs, and Thomas, 1986). The appearance is similar to the inspissated milk syndrome, except that some medications may be radiopaque and hence appear as denser opacities (Berman, Briggs, and Thomas, 1986).

Segmental Dilatation of the Colon

Segmental dilatation of the colon is a rare constipating condition that mimics Hirschsprung disease. The dilated segment may be in any part of the colon from ascending to sigmoid. The barium enema shows the dilated segment which is strikingly different from the normal caliber seen in the rest of the large bowel. Biopsy of the dilated portion shows normal ganglion cells and proximal muscular hypertrophy. Excision of the dilated segment is curative.

Abnormality of Smooth Muscle

Disorders of smooth muscle can be familial or sporadic, and the sporadic form can be primary or secondary. The familial forms are a primary visceral myopathy and are rare, presenting with pseudo-obstruction (see Chapter 6). The sporadic patients with primary visceral myopathy are similar to the familial, although primary visceral myopathy has been reported in some infants with the megacystis-microcolon–intestinal hypoperistalsis syndrome (see Chapters 9 and 10). Secondary visceral myopathy is associated with a number of disorders such as progressive systemic sclerosis, polymyositis, progressive muscular dystrophy, and amyloidosis. The clinical and radiologic appearance will depend on the underlying disease process.

INFECTION AND INFLAMMATION OF THE LARGE BOWEL

Neonatal Necrotizing Enterocolitis

Necrotizing enterocolitis (NEC) is a serious and potentially fatal acquired condition occurring primarily in premature infants. Of premature infants suffering from birth asphyxia or shock, 5 to 15% will develop NEC during their hospital stay (Kleigman, Pittard, and Fanaroff, 1979). The majority of cases occur in infants weighing less than 2000 g at birth. Symptoms are usually seen in the first week of life, often in the first few days. Extremely low birth-weight infants (less than 1000 g) may develop NEC later, some after 2 weeks. The mortality rate varies from 10 to 50% among reporting centers (Uruy et al., 1991).

Genersich first described the clinical and pathologic manifestations of NEC in 1891 (Dunn, 1963). There has been an apparent increase in the number of cases (Stevenson, Graham, and Stevenson, 1980; Berdon et al., 1964; Mizrahi et al., 1965), related to the increasing numbers of surviving premature infants. The cause of NEC is unclear, although hypoxia, acidosis, and hypotension (Cummins, 1977) as well as secondary bacterial invasion appear involved. Selective bowel ischemia has been likened to the diving reflex in aquatic mammals whereby blood is shunted away from peripheral, splanchnic, and renal tissue to the heart, brain, and adrenals in response to stress. Ischemia results in mucosal damage, endothelial damage, and small-vessel thrombosis; this may account for the thrombocytopenia frequently affecting infants with NEC. The mucosal injury is worsened by hyperosmolar feeds and infection. Necrotizing enterocolitis occurs more frequently in formula-fed infants. Fresh breast milk appears to protect the bowel in experimental animals (Cummins, 1977), but the role of these feeds in humans is unclear.

Epidemic outbreaks of NEC in newborn nurseries suggest an infectious cause. Low IgA levels in neonates predispose this population to infection (Stevenson, Graham, and Stevenson, 1980). Local infection may produce direct endothelial damage or act as a source of stress, stimulating the release of epinephrine. Endothelial damage and epinephrine release are both mechanisms for producing NEC. The role of bacterial invasion in this disease is well recognized, but such invasion is likely a secondary event after compromise of the intestinal mucosal barrier.

Pathologically, NEC can occur anywhere in the gut, with the possible exception of the duodenum (Santulli et al., 1975). The right colon and ileum are most commonly involved. Grossly, the bowel becomes dilated, gray, hemorrhagic, or friable, depending on the severity of disease. Microscopically, diseased bowel shows mucosal coagulation, ulceration, and submucosal hemorrhage in the earliest stages. Microscopic or gross strips or bubbles of gas then appear in the submucosa and subserosa (Santulli et al., 1975). Gas in the adjacent small mesenteric vessels is not uncommon at autopsy, especially in the arterioles and small submucosal arteries. The role of inflammatory mediators, such as tumor necrosis factor (TNF) alpha, platelet-activating factor, and oxygen free radicals, has also received attention (Caplan et al., 1990).

Premature, low birth-weight (less than 2000 g) infants are especially at risk. Approximately 75 to 90% of all infants with NEC weigh less than 2500 g, and approximately 80 to 90% are less than 38 weeks' gestation (Brown and Sweet, 1982). Prolonged rupture of membranes, pre-eclampsia, diabetes, maternal cocaine use, patent ductus arteriosus, umbilical vessel catheterization, and multiple births are associated with NEC. Other factors such as low Apgar score, respiratory distress syndrome, hypothermia, sepsis, heart failure, nonroutine resuscitation, and exchange transfusion have all been implicated as causes (Stevenson, Graham, and Stevenson, 1980). Twins and babies with polycythemia carry a higher risk for developing NEC (Cummins, 1977). An unusually rapid onset of NEC within 24 hours of birth may be found in neonates with severe left ventricular outflow obstruction such as hypoplastic left heart and aortic coarctation (Allen and Haney, 1984). Rapid onset of enteral feeding may be a risk factor for NEC because of changes in enteric blood flow and oxygen requirements during feeding (Anderson and Kleigman, 1991). Necrotizing enterocolitis is occasionally, but rarely, reported in infants who have never been enterally fed.

The clinical presentation of necrotizing enterocolitis varies widely. Abdominal distention is one of the earliest and most consistent signs. Other signs and symptoms include bloody stools, apnea, bradycardia, lethargy, shock, and retention of gastric contents due to poor gastric emptying. Thrombocytopenia, neutropenia, and metabolic acidosis may develop during bowel ischemia. The presence of reducing substances in the stool, caused by carbohydrate malabsorption, may be an early finding, as may increased alpha$_1$-antitrypsin levels from a protein-losing enteropathy.

Suspicion of NEC mandates that enteral feeding be discontinued. An orogastric tube is placed routinely to relieve bowel distention. Intravenous nutrition and antibiotics are begun and continued until clinical recovery. Bell and colleagues recognize three stages of NEC: stage I, early or suspected NEC; stage II, definite NEC; and stage III, advanced disease (Bell et al., 1978). Radiologists should try to interpret studies in this context.

The signs in early NEC are as nonspecific as the gastrointestinal manifestations. Diffuse gaseous distention is the most common early sign but is nonspecific (Bell, Graham, and Stevenson, 1971; Daneman, Woodward, and de Silva, 1978). Scalloping and separation of bowel loops (Figure 10–30A) due to mucosal and submucosal edema and/or hemorrhage is another early sign (Virjee et al., 1979). Loss of symmetry of the bowel gas distribution may prove somewhat more suggestive of NEC (Daneman, Woodward, and de Silva, 1978; Kogutt, 1979). When one or more of these signs is present, treatment should begin without delay. Follow-up studies include supine radiography every 12 to 24 hours, supplemented by a supine cross-table lateral or left-side-down decubitus view, both of which are sensitive for free air.

The diagnosis is confirmed by radiographic demonstration of pneumatosis intestinalis or portal venous gas. However, a wide range of interobserver variability has been shown in the radiographic diagnosis of NEC including evidence of pneumatosis (Mata and Rosengart, 1980). A foamy pattern (Figure 10–30B), similar to that seen when gas is mixed with meconium or stool, may be the earliest radiographic sign of pneumatosis. Importantly, this foamy pattern of gas mixed with stool is rare in patients under 2 weeks of age (Patriquin et al., 1984). More obvious intramural gas can be linear (Figure 10–31) or curvilinear (Figure 10–32) and confirms the presence of pneumatosis. The small bowel may be dilated with bowel wall thickening (Figure 10–33). While the terminal ileum and colon are the most frequently involved sites, the stomach may also show pneumatosis (see Figure 10–32). Extensive pneumatosis usually indicates advanced disease, but pneumatosis can be radiographically absent in severe disease (Leonidas, Hall, and Amoury, 1976). Occasionally, extensive pneumatosis occurs in patients with few clinical signs or symptoms of NEC (Bell, Graham, and Stevenson, 1971).

Portal venous gas (Figure 10–34) is usually associated with advanced disease, but it is not a fatal sign (Leonidas, Hill, and Amoury, 1976). A persistently dilated loop of bowel on sequential films over 24 to 36 hours is generally an ominous sign of impending perforation. Occasionally, perforation may follow clinical improvement of the infant (Wexler, 1978). Perforation is the only absolute indication for surgical intervention, as untreated perforation from intestinal necrosis may lead to peritonitis, sepsis, shock, and eventual death. The goal of the radiologist is to identify early perforation and thus to prevent or minimize the morbidity of peritonitis. Perforation is detected earliest with a supine cross-table lateral or left lateral decubitus view. Small collections of free air may be identified on a cross-table lateral view, where they appear as triangular lucencies, the so-called telltale triangle sign between loops of bowel immediately below the anterior abdominal wall (Seibert and Parvey, 1977). Unfortunately, plain-film radiography detects only 63% of those patients with pneumoperitoneum at the time of perforation (Frey et al., 1987). Ascites is another sign of perforation or impending perforation (Leonidas, Hill, and Amoury, 1976). The presence of intraperitoneal fluid in a context of clinical deterioration may warrant surgery.

Ultrasonography can detect bowel wall thickening (Kodroff, Hartenburg, and Goldschmidt, 1984),

ascites (Leonidas et al., 1973), and portal venous gas. The most frequent findings are thick-walled, fluid-filled loops of bowel with absent peristalsis. Intense intramural echoes with acoustic shadowing caused by pneumatosis are a more specific finding of NEC (Kodroff, Hartenburg, and Goldschmidt, 1984; Vernacchia et al., 1985). The ultrasonographic finding of portal venous gas may precede the plain-film finding. The ultrasonographic appearance of air in the portal veins can take two forms: the more common form is the highly echogenic patch in the portal veins with intermittent bursts of echoes seen with peristaltic activity; the second characteristic pattern is that of more poorly defined echogenic patches within the nondependent hepatic parenchyma (Merritt, Goldsmith, and Sharp, 1984).

Recently, the diagnosis of worsening enterocolitis has been made by CT examination of urine following enteral administration of iohexol (Patton et al., 1999). Infants with severe NEC showed increased CT attenuation coefficients in urine, corresponding to progression of NEC to an advanced stage, before evidence of perforation was visible on abdominal radiographs.

The management of NEC includes intravenous hydration and nutrition, broad spectrum

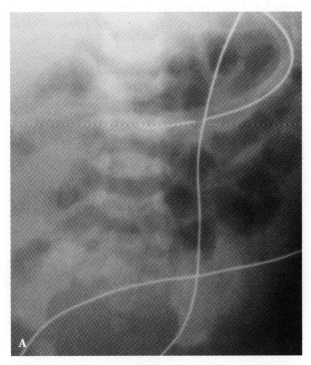 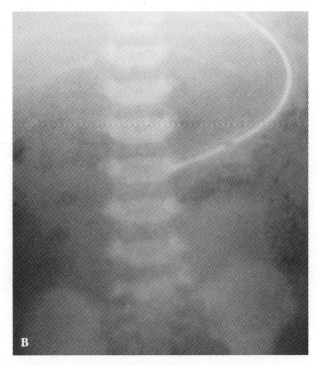

FIGURE 10–30. Necrotizing enterocolitis. *A,* Bowel loop separation is present initially. *B,* There is a foamy pattern 12 hours later due to intramural gas.

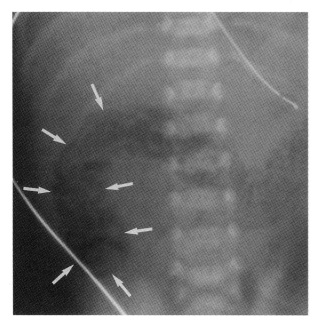

FIGURE 10–31. Extensive necrotizing enterocolitis. Intramural gas appears as linear lucencies (*arrows*) surrounding the right hemicolon and as a foamy pattern in the rest of the large bowel. The small bowel is empty, possibly due to the action of the nasogastric tube keeping the stomach gasless.

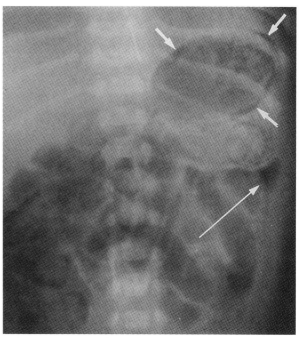

FIGURE 10–32. Extensive necrotizing enterocolitis. Intramural gas appears as curvilinear lucencies surrounding the stomach (*short arrows*) and many loops of bowel. A peripheral triangle of gas (*long arrow*) on the left suggests perforation on this supine film, but free gas was not seen on an erect film.

antibiotics, nasogastric decompression, and discontinuation of oral feeds. Indications for surgery include perforation and obstruction as well as clinical deterioration despite aggressive medical therapy. Surgery usually involves resecting the nonviable bowel while attempting to preserve as much bowel as possible, particularly the ileocecal valve. If a neonate is too small to undergo surgery, drainage of intra-abdominal abscess can be achieved with a percutaneous peritoneal drain (Ein, Marshall, and Girvan, 1977; Janik and Ein, 1980).

The most common complication of NEC is stricture formation, which may appear following medical or surgical therapy. The incidence of stricture formation may be as high as 33% (Janik, Ein, and Mancer, 1981). Strictures affect the colon in 80% of cases, most often adjacent to the splenic flexure. Strictures are multiple in 30% of cases; multiple lesions are exclusively colonic (Janik, Ein, and Mancer, 1981). Stricture should be suspected in any infant with a history of NEC and signs of obstruction or failure to thrive. A contrast enema will demonstrate colonic stricture and is indicated before a defunctioning enterostomy is closed or

when a stricture is suspected. A stricture seen soon after the acute illness (Figure 10–35A) may resolve with conservative management. Surgery is reserved for the stricture present for an extended period of time (Figure 10–35B). When a loop of bowel becomes trapped between two areas of stricture, an enterocyst may form. In this type of closed loop obstruction, US can characterize the tubular, cystic nature of the lesion as well as the internal contents of fluid and solid debris (Ball and Wylx, 1986).

Neutropenic Colitis

Neutropenic colitis, also referred to as typhlitis, is a necrotizing enterocolitis, often selectively affecting the right colon, that develops in the setting of severe neutropenia. Pathologically, it is similar to the necrotizing enterocolitis seen in NEC of infancy and in pseudomembranous enterocolitis. It most commonly occurs in leukemic children undergoing chemotherapy but may also present in the setting of disease-induced neutropenia (Kaste, Flynn, and Furman, 1997), aplastic anemia, immunosuppression related to organ transplanta-

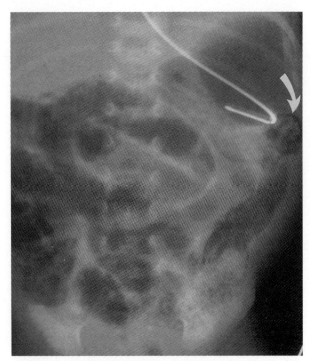

FIGURE 10–33. Extensive necrotizing enterocolitis. The splenic flexure seen end-on is outlined by a crescentic lucency (*arrow*), indicating intramural gas. There is a foamy pattern in the rest of the large bowel, and the small bowel is dilated with mild bowel wall thickening.

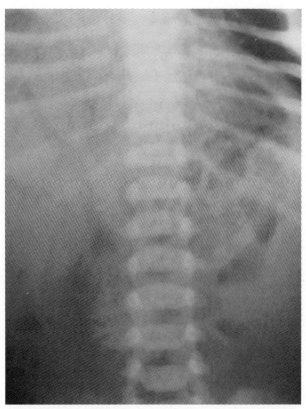

FIGURE 10–34. Severe necrotizing enterocolitis with portal venous gas. Branching lucencies within the liver parenchyma represent gas in the portal venous system. Unlike those that represent gas in the biliary tree, the lucencies extend to the periphery of the liver. Gas is rarely present in the biliary tree of infants, except after biliary tract surgery.

tion, and acquired immunodeficiency syndrome (AIDS). The frequency of neutropenic colitis has increased recently (Sloas et al., 1993), most likely as a consequence of the aggressiveness of modern chemotherapy (Ojala, Lanning, and Lanning, 1997). The mortality rate has dropped from 50 to 100% to 8 to 20% (Sloas et al., 1993; Gomez, Martino, and Rolston, 1998) over the past decade. Survival depends on prompt recognition of the condition and appropriate intervention until the normal circulating neutrophils return.

Proposed predisposing factors include severe neutropenia and cytotoxic drug-induced ileus. Bowel ileus may lead to cecal stasis, distention and ischemia with subsequent mucosal ulceration and bacterial invasion. Certain chemotherapeutic agents have been directly implicated in producing mucosal epithelial cell necrosis. The histopathologic findings of neutropenic colitis are usually limited to the terminal ileum, cecum, and ascending colon; the appendix may also be involved. The cecum may be sensitive to inflammation because of the local relative stasis of bowel contents and great

distensibility of the cecum, which can compromise blood supply. Findings include mucosal and submucosal necrosis with bacterial invasion, intramural edema, and hemorrhage. Viral and fungal infection have been noted as other causative factors. In the absence of a normal granulocytic response, intestinal necrosis may become so severe as to cause bowel wall perforation.

The clinical presentation of neutropenic colitis may be confusing, as the symptoms and signs are nonspecific. Fever, nausea, vomiting, watery or bloody diarrhea, and abdominal tenderness that frequently localizes to the right lower quadrant characterize its onset. Appendicitis, ruptured viscus, or toxic side effects of chemotherapy are frequent clinical misdiagnoses. In a review of leukemic patients with cecal and appendiceal complications, Skibber and colleagues found that appendicitis and neutropenic colitis were equal in incidence among patients with signs of right lower quadrant pain. Other mimickers of neutropenic colitis include pseudomembranous colitis, ischemic colitis, intussusception, lymphomatous or leukemic infiltration of the bowel wall, and small bowel obstruction (Frick et al., 1984).

The radiographic features of neutropenic colitis include absence of bowel gas in the right lower quadrant, dilated ascending colon, cecal intramural gas, and small bowel obstruction (Kaste, Flynn, and Furman, 1997; McNamara et al., 1986) (Figure 10–36). Plain-film abdominal radiography contributes little to distinguishing among diagnostic possibilities. Barium enema is contraindicated because of the risk of intestinal perforation and septicemia. Computed tomography is a noninvasive technique that can be useful in the evaluation of persistent right lower quadrant pain in the immunocompromised patient. The recognition of a transmural inflammatory process (Figure 10–37), in the appropriate clinical setting, is highly suggestive of the diagnosis of neutropenic colitis. However, the specificity is low because the finding can be simulated by other disorders that result in bowel wall thickening, such as leukemic infiltra-tion, intramural hemorrhage, ischemic colitis, and segmental pseudomembranous colitis. Distinguishing between neutropenic colitis and isolated proximal involvment in pseudomembranous colitis may be difficult. Helpful differentiating features include the presence of pericolonic inflammation (Figure 10–38), absence of ascites, and increased frequency of pneumatosis and subsequent perforation in neutropenic colitis. These features are unusual in pseudomembranous colitis. Ultrasonography shows wall thickening with a thickened, echogenic mucosa (Figure 10–39). Ultrasonography is advantageous because it can be a bedside technique; it is suggested by some (Sloas et al., 1993) as the imaging study for follow-up in patients with known neutropenic colitis as it is convenient, inexpensive, and does not emit radiation or require contrast material.

Idiopathic Inflammatory Bowel Disease

Idiopathic inflammatory bowel disease refers to a group of idiopathic, chronic disorders that comprises ulcerative colitis, Crohn's disease, Behçet syndrome, and eosinophilic gastroenteritis. The cause is unclear, and unpredictable exacerbations and remissions characterize the natural history. The most

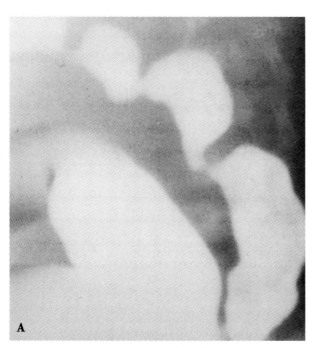
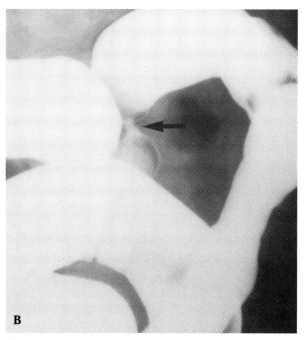

FIGURE 10–35. Strictures resulting from necrotizing enterocolitis. *A,* Multiple strictures affect the splenic flexure and descending colon 1 month after an episode of necrotizing enterocolitis. *B,* After 3 months of conservative management, only one stricture (*arrow*) remained in the splenic flexure; it required surgery.

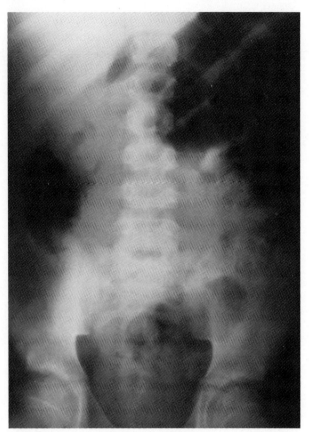

FIGURE 10–36. Neutropenic colitis in a 13-year-old girl with leukemia. Bowel gas is absent in the right lower quadrant, and there is a loss of the normal haustral pattern in the sigmoid colon.

common ages of onset are adolescence and young adulthood, but these disorders can present as early as the first year of life. There may be genetic and environmental factors that contribute to the pathogenesis of inflammatory bowel disease. The risk in family members of an affected individual is reported as in the range of 7 to 22%. Individuals migrating to developed countries appear to acquire the higher rates of disease associated with these regions.

It is usually possible to distinguish between ulcerative colitis and Crohn's disease by a combination of clinical presentation and radiologic, endoscopic, and pathologic findings. When a definitive diagnosis is impossible, as in approximately 10% of cases, it is best to refer to the chronic colitis as indeterminate colitis. The treatment of these disorders overlap greatly, but response to therapy may be incomplete if there is a misdiagnosis. Extraintestinal manifestations occur slightly more frequently with Crohn's disease than with ulcerative colitis.

Ulcerative Colitis

Ulcerative colitis is an idiopathic inflammatory disorder localized to the colon. Disease nearly always begins in the rectum and extends proximally for a variable distance without skip areas. Ulcerative colitis affects primarily adolescents and young adults, although presentation may be in infancy. The infantile form of this disease may be fulminant and fatal. The incidence of ulcerative colitis has remained stable, in contrast to the recent increase observed in Crohn's disease. Incidence rates are highest in the northern European countries and the United States and lowest in Japan. The disorder is more common in children with a family history of disease.

Symptoms of bloody diarrhea and crampy abdominal pain are typical; onset can be insidious or fulminant. Fever, anemia, hypoalbuminemia, and leukocytosis, are presenting signs and symptoms shared with acute gastroenteritis. Symptoms lasting more than 3 to 4 weeks are less likely due to infectious colitis and suggest a chronic inflammatory process such as ulcerative colitis. In establishing the diagnosis of ulcerative colitis, the stool should be sampled for enteric pathogens, ova and parasites, and in the context of antibiotic use, *Clostridium difficile*. The colitis may mimic that of hemolytic uremic syndrome, although the presence of microangiopathic hemolysis, thrombocytopenia, and renal

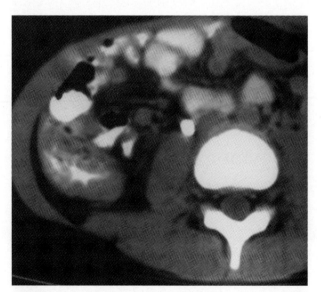

FIGURE 10–37. Neutropenic colitis in a 9-year-old boy. Shown on CT, there is transmural inflammation of the cecum and ascending colon with considerable bowel wall thickening.

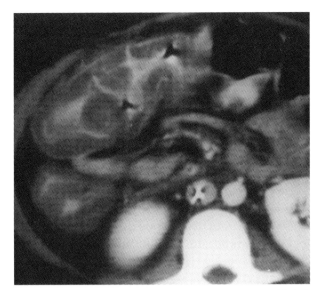

FIGURE 10–38. Neutropenic colitis in a 10-year-old girl. Transmural thickening of the ascending and proximal transverse colon is noted as well as pericolonic stranding on CT.

failure establishes the correct diagnosis. In infancy, dietary protein intolerance (e.g., cow's milk protein) is a differential consideration, although removal of the offending antigen resolves the colitis. The most difficult distinction is from Crohn's disease; correct categorization may take years until manifestations of the disease become clearer.

Generalized growth failure is present in 15% of affected children (McCaffery et al., 1970), less commonly than in children with Crohn's disease. It may precede clinical symptoms, be unaffected by steroid therapy, and be unrelated to the severity of colonic disease (Kelts and Grand, 1980). Extraintestinal manifestations are common and include pyoderma gangrenosum, sclerosing cholangitis, chronic active hepatitis, arthritis, and ankylosing spondylitis. Exacerbations and remissions characterize the clinical course. Flares may be triggered by a bout with infectious enteritis or nonsteroidal anti-inflammatory use.

The risk of colon cancer increases after the first 8 to 10 years of disease, with a subsequent increase of 0.5 to 1.0% per year (Devroede et al., 1971). Proctitis alone is associated with virtually no increased

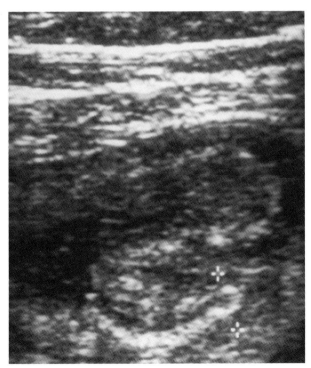

FIGURE 10–39. Typhlitis in a 16-year-old boy. Graded-compression US shows thickening cecal wall with extrusion of disease to involve the appendix (*between cursors*).

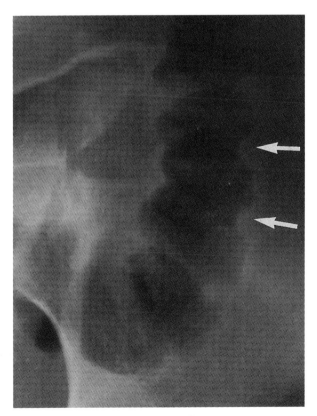

FIGURE 10–40. Ulcerative colitis. Plain-film shows haustral thickening (*arrows*) in the descending colon and proximal sigmoid colon. (Reprinted with permission from Stringer DA. Radiol Clin N Amer 1987;25:93–113.)

cancer risk. Childhood onset does not further increase this risk level.

The lesions of ulcerative colitis are confined to the mucosa, with secondary involvement of the submucosa. Fulminant colitis can be the exceptional transmural process.

No single test secures the diagnosis of ulcerative colitis. Typical endoscopic and radiologic findings, along with the appropriate history and clinical findings in a chronic disorder, suggest the proper diagnosis. Conventional radiography may show colonic thumbprinting with loss of the normal haustral pattern (Figure 10–40). With pancolitis and bowel wall thickening, the colon may be empty (Figure 10–41). In fulminant disease, a toxic megacolon may be seen.

The child with suspected ulcerative colitis undergoes colonoscopy and biopsy; thus, enemas are rarely performed. Double-contrast barium enema is comparable to colonoscopy in detecting disease, although early proctitis may be missed (Stringer, Sherman, and Jakowenko, 1986). Mild colitis shows a fine granular appearance of the mucosa. Haustral thickening secondary to edema

can be subtle in mild (Figure 10–42) or marked disease (Figure 10–43). Houston's valves may also be affected (Figure 10–44). Irregularity of the bowel wall along the mucosal line may be a more conspicuous finding than the mucosal granularity (Figure 10–45). With disease progression, granularity progresses to discrete punctate ulcerations (Figure 10–46). Submucosal tracking forms the "collar-button" ulcer (Figure 10–47). Spared or regenerating mucosa produces the so-called pseudopolyp. Characteristic of the healing phase is the filiform or inflammatory polyp (Figure 10–48). Lesions may be wormlike or rounded (Figure 10–49). Long-standing disease leads to colonic fibrosis, which may cause colonic shortening with widening of the postrectal space and loss of Houston's valves (Figure 10–50). If the ileocecal valve becomes patulous, backwash ileitis may appear (Figure 10–51).

In the fulminant variety of ulcerative colitis, usually seen in infants, NEC, Hirschsprung enterocolitis, and allergic colitis are differential considerations. The infant presents with bloody diarrhea, vomiting, and abdominal distention; the course may be fatal (Enzer and Hijmans, 1963). In many cases,

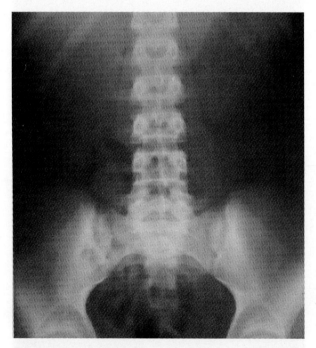

FIGURE 10–41. Ulcerative colitis. Plain film that shows no fecal residue in a patient with acute onset of bloody diarrhea indicates pancolitis. (Reprinted with permission from Stringer DA. Imaging inflammatory bowel disease in the pediatric patient. Radiol Clin N Amer 1987;25:93–113.)

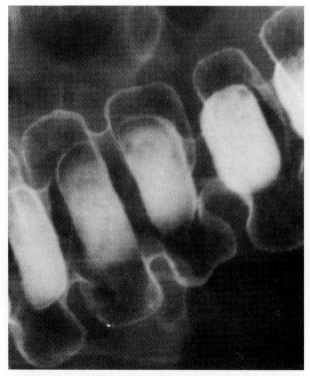

FIGURE 10–42. Ulcerative colitis. There is minor subtle haustral fold thickening of the transverse colon secondary to edema seen in the early stages of ulcerative colitis.

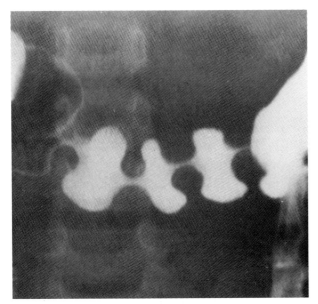

FIGURE 10–43. Ulcerative colitis. There is marked haustral fold thickening of the transverse colon as shown on a barium enema.

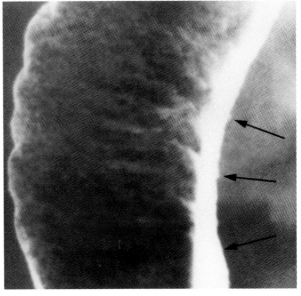

FIGURE 10–45. Mild ulcerative colitis. There is a granular mucosa and an irregular mucosal line (*arrows*), indicating early colitis.

treatment requires total colectomy. Infants show nonspecific bowel distention on plain-film radiography. The finding of a megacolon contraindicates enema examination.

Colectomy with ileostomy or resevoir construction is the surgical procedure of choice for

ulcerative colitis. An immediate postoperative water-soluble contrast enema is often performed to exclude reservoir leak or obstruction. Delayed studies for stricture formation use barium contrast.

The continent ileostomy with Kock pouch requires joining a loop of ileum at the ileostomy site.

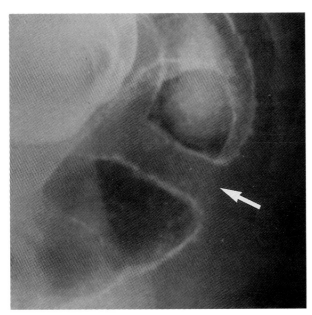

FIGURE 10–44. Ulcerative colitis. A double-contrast barium enema demonstrates irregular mucosa and thickening of Houston's valves (*arrow*) in the rectum.

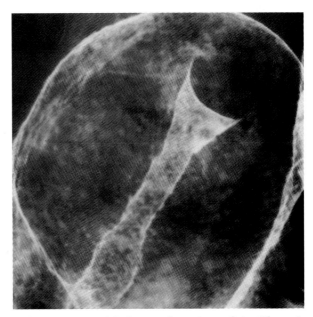

FIGURE 10–46. Moderate ulcerative colitis. There is moderate mucosal irregularity and punctate ulceration seen on double-contrast barium enema.

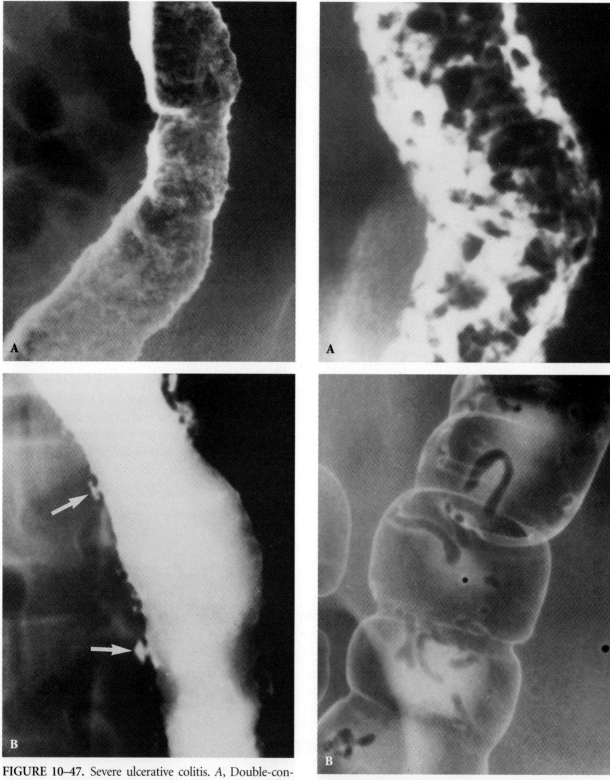

FIGURE 10–47. Severe ulcerative colitis. *A*, Double-contrast barium enema shows deep ulceration. *B*, As the disease progresses, there is submucosal tracking, with formation of "collar-button" ulcers (*arrows*). (Reprinted with permission from Stringer DA. Imaging inflammatory bowel disease in the pediatric patient. Radiol Clin N Amer 1987;25:93–113.)

FIGURE 10–48. Filiform (postinflammatory) polyps in ulcerative colitis. *A*, There is gross colitis as indicated by mucosal irregularity and nodularity seen on single-contrast barium enema. *B*, Four years later, a double-contrast study shows branching or wormlike polyps.

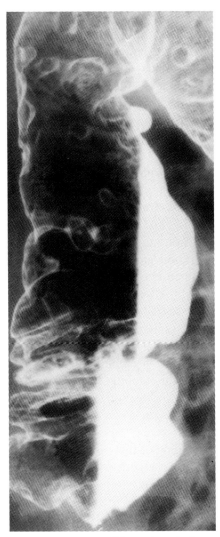

FIGURE 10–49. Filiform (postinflammatory) polyps in ulcerative colitis. There are multiple rounded polyps in the hepatic flexure seen on double-contrast barium enema.

Complications occurring in the postoperative period include stricture, fistula, pouchitis, small bowel obstruction, salt wasting, long outflow tract, and pouch prolapse (Ein, 1982). The normal appearance of the pouch on contrast examination is that of dilated ileum, sometimes irregular in shape, immediately below the ileostomy.

A simple endorectal pull-through is achieved by "pulling-through" the distal ileum into a rectal muscle cuff, anastamosed just above the anus (Figure 10–52). The pulled-through ileum loses small bowel features and appears with smoother mucosa. In addition, the postrectal space widens, although the neorectum

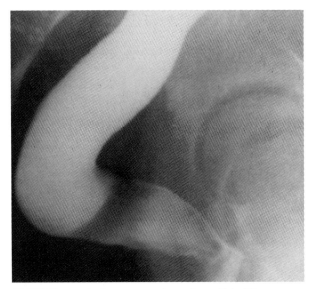

FIGURE 10–50. Late stage ulcerative colitis. The rectum is tubular, with slight widening of the postrectal space and loss of Houston's valves.

dilates over time as it adjusts to its new function as a reservoir (Bank, White, and Coran, 1986). Complications diagnosed on contrast enema include redundant ileum in the rectal sleeve, fistula, stricture, and mucosal irregularity (Bank, White, and Coran, 1986).

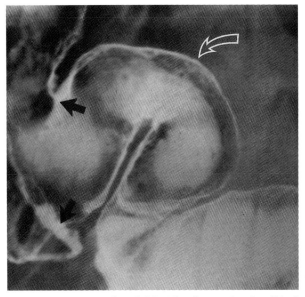

FIGURE 10–51. Reflux ileitis. The ileocecal valve (*black arrows*) becomes patulous, and reflux ileitis occurs as indicated by minor mucosal irregularity (*open white arrow*). (Reprinted with permission from Stringer DA. Imaging inflammatory bowel disease in the pediatric patient. Radiol Clin N Amer 1987;25:93–113.)

There are two major forms of ileoanal reservoir, the J-pouch and the S-pouch (Parks pouch). Both are fashioned by joining adjacent loops of ileum (see Figure 10–52). The J-pouch joins two loops of distal ileum, and the S-pouch joins three loops. Partial outlet obstruction is more common with the S-pouch (Kremer et al., 1985). Other complications include small bowel obstruction (12% of cases) and anastomotic leak (8%) (Kremer et al., 1985) and, less commonly, abscess and fistula. Contrast loopography images these pouches; water-soluble contrast is used in the immediate postoperative period, and barium is used in long-term follow-up.

Crohn Disease

Crohn disease (regional enteritis, granulomatous colitis) is an idiopathic chronic inflammatory disorder that can involve any region of the gastrointestinal tract from the mouth to the anus. Onset may be in the teenage years; infants and young children are rarely affected (Karjoo and McCarthy, 1976; Miller and Larsen, 1971; Rubin, Lambie, and Chapman, 1967). The course of disease reported in infants differs from that in older children and adults. Infants usually present with small bowel obstruction and require surgery. The rapid improvement and lack of recurrence suggests a different etiology (Miller and Larsen, 1971). The incidence of Crohn disease has increased over the past decade while that of ulcerative colitis has remained stable. A family history of inflammatory bowel disease is recognized in up to 10% of patients with Crohn disease.

The etiology of Crohn disease is uncertain, but infection and immune dysfunction have been suggested. All layers of the bowel wall may be involved, with lymphoid aggregates, deep ulceration, and fibrosis (Kelts and Grand, 1980). Disease usually involves the terminal ileum, with or without colonic involvement.

The clinical presentation varies depending on the region and degree of inflammation as well as on the presence of complications such as stricture or fistula. Children with ileocolitis usually have crampy abdominal pain and diarrhea, occasionally bloody. Right lower quadrant pain caused by ileitis may mimic appendicitis. Fever, anorexia, and fatigue are common symptoms. Failure to thrive, with delayed bone maturation and puberty, may be the initial presenting feature. Growth failure is twice as common in Crohn disease than in ulcerative colitis. Perianal disease (tag, fistula, abscess) is common in Crohn disease unlike in ulcerative colitis.

Extraintestinal manifestations include oral aphthous ulcers, peripheral arthritis, erythema nodosum, digital clubbing, renal calculi (uric acid and oxalate), and cholelithiasis. In general, the manifestation of these processes correlates with the presence of colitis.

The imaging of these patients depends on the presentation. Most patients with bloody diarrhea will have colonoscopy to evaluate the large bowel and a small bowel series to evaluate the small intestine. In the acute phase, plain films can be very helpful and may show absence of bowel gas (Figure 10–53), abnormal haustra (Figure 10–54), or toxic

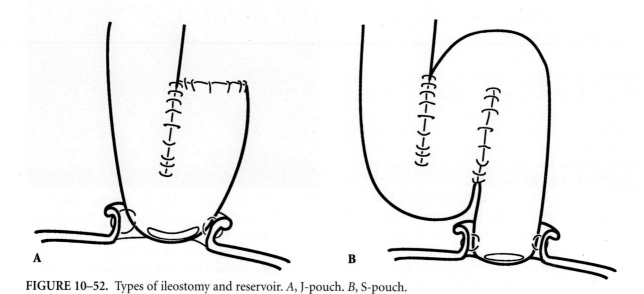

FIGURE 10–52. Types of ileostomy and reservoir. *A*, J-pouch. *B*, S-pouch.

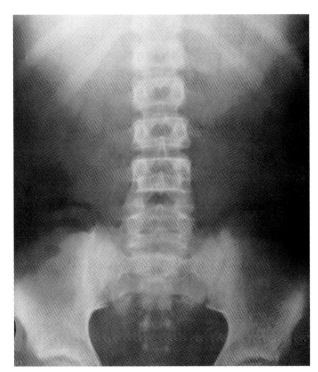

FIGURE 10–53. Crohn colitis. Plain abdominal film shows no fecal material, which in a patient with acute bloody diarrhea indicates a pancolitis.

megacolon. Enemas currently have but a small role in the diagnosis of inflammatory bowel disease. If an enema is performed, aphthae and deep mucosal ulcers will characterize this disease. These aphthae have a classic appearance as ulcers with smooth, raised edges (Figure 10–55). As disease progresses, the aphthae enlarge and coalesce (Figure 10–56) and can penetrate the deeper tissues, giving a "rose thorn" appearance (Figure 10–57). Extension of ulceration can occur along the wall of the bowel, resulting in linear ulcers (Figure 10–58) or penetration of the bowel wall, forming a sinus tract or fistula. Inflammation gives a nodular appearance, with thickening of the bowel wall (Figure 10–59).

Unlike ulcerative colitis, Crohn disease tends to involve the colon asymmetrically, with discrete ulceration separated by normal mucosa (Figure 10–60). The right colon is most commonly involved, and the rectum is usually spared. When rectal disease is present, it is often localized (Figure 10–61) but is sometimes widespread (Figure 10–62). Occasionally, pancolitis is present, and the pattern is indistinguishable from ulcerative colitis (Joffe, 1981).

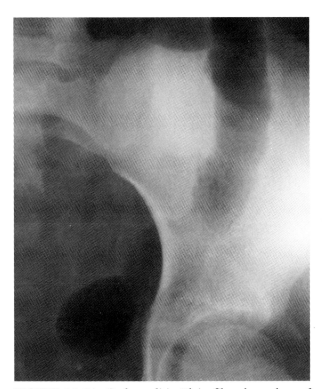

FIGURE 10–54. Crohn colitis. Plain film shows loss of the normal Haustral pattern and lack of fecal material; thickening of the bowel wall is suggested, indicating colitis affecting the sigmoid colon.

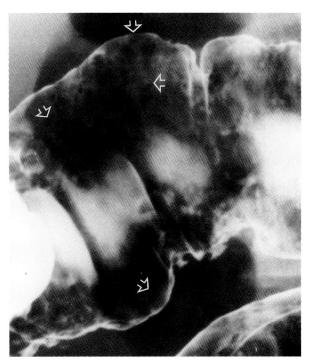

FIGURE 10–55. Early Crohn colitis. Double-contrast barium enema shows multiple aphthae that have a characteristic appearance with smooth, raised edges and a central umbilication (*arrows*). (Reprinted with permission from Stringer DA. Radiol Clin N Amer 1987;25:93–113.)

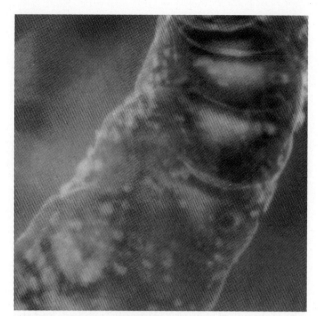

FIGURE 10–56. Moderately severe Crohn colitis. The aphthae have enlarged and coalesced, with formation of larger ulcers indicating progression of the disease.

Long-standing disease can lead to colonic stricture (Figure 10–63), which may cause bowel obstruction. Pseudodiverticula may form, although this lesion is more common in the small bowel (Figure 10–64).

Computed tomography is useful in showing abscess, phlegmon, and focal fat proliferation. While CT findings among patients with colitis are nonspecific, some features have been reported as helpful in suggesting a specific diagnosis. For example, the mean colonic wall thickness is typically greater in Crohn colitis, and isolated right colonic involvement is more common in Crohn colitis than in ulcerative colitis. In addition, abscess is associated more frequently with Crohn colitis.

The incidence of malignancy is greater in patients with Crohn disease than in the general population. Specifically, adenocarcinoma is 20 times more likely in patients with Crohn disease (Weedon et al., 1973), and there is a small increase in the incidence of small bowel adenocarcinoma (Gardiner and Stevenson, 1982).

Behçet Syndrome

Behçet syndrome is a multisystem vasculitis that is very rare in children, especially in those less than 10 years of age (Stringer et al., 1986) and in males (Kasahara et al., 1981). Aphthous stomatitis, erythema nodosum, and arthritis are among the most common

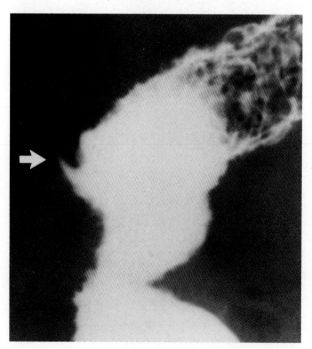

FIGURE 10–57. Severe Crohn colitis. There is extensive mucosal ulceration with great irregularity of the mucosal edge and a deep ulcer (arrow) resembling a rose thorn.

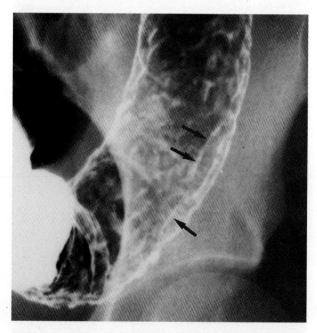

FIGURE 10–58. Crohn colitis and linear ulcers. Double-contrast barium enema shows extensive ulceration of the sigmoid colon and linear ulceration (arrows). (Reprinted with permission from Stringer DA. Imaging inflammatory bowel disease in the pediatric patient. Radiol Clin N Amer 1987;25:93–113.)

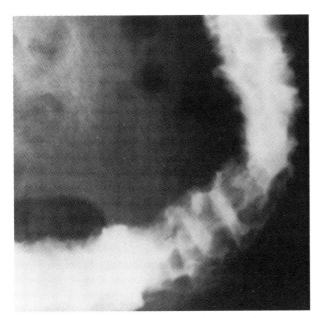

FIGURE 10–59. Severe Crohn colitis. Single-contrast enema shows gross irregularity of the mucosal wall with a nodular appearance due to the associated inflammation.

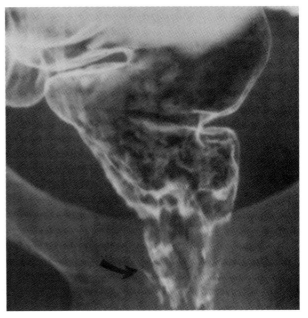

FIGURE 10–61. Rectal Crohn disease. This distal portion of rectum has an irregular mucosa, and there is a sinus tract (*arrow*) extending from just above the anus. (Reprinted with permission from Stringer DA. Radiol Clin N Amer 1987;25:93–113.)

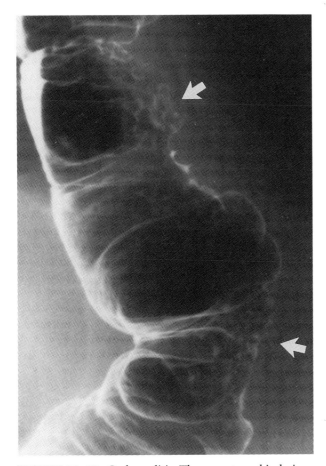

FIGURE 10–60. Crohn colitis. There are two skip lesions (*arrows*) separated by normal mucosa.

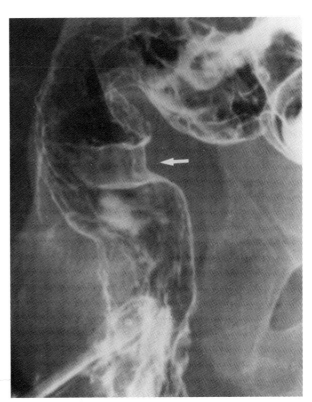

FIGURE 10–62. Rectal Crohn disease. There is gross ulceration throughout the rectum, with thickening of Houston's valves (*arrow*) and widening of the postrectal space.

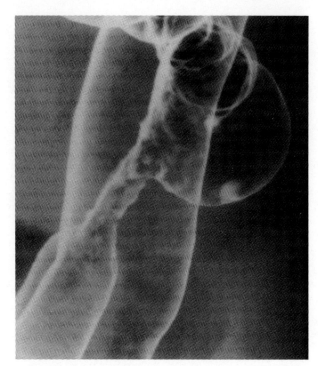

FIGURE 10–63. Crohn disease stricture. There is an irregular narrow region of large bowel in the descending colon shown on double-contrast barium enema. The mucosa is ulcerated within and adjacent to this stricture, but elsewhere the mucosa is normal.

manifestations. Gastrointestinal disease occurs in approximately 12% of cases, with ulcers forming anywhere from the mouth to the colon. Genital ulcers, myositis, and central nervous system disease define this disorder.

The diagnosis of Behçet disease should be suspected when genital ulceration or severe oral ulceration (Stringer et al., 1986) accompanies colitis. Both of these findings are uncommon in Crohn disease. Skin and ocular lesions appear less frequently than in adults with Behçet syndrome (Stringer et al., 1986). The esophagus, small bowel, and large bowel can be diseased. The bowel typically shows transmural inflammation with submucosal infiltration and edema. The ulcers are discrete and deep, often penetrating the serosal surface (Kasahara et al., 1981).

The cecum and ascending colon are the most commonly affected segments of the large bowel. The appearance on contrast enema is similar to Crohn disease (Figure 10–65), and fistulae may be present (Baba et al., 1976). Complications of colonic disease, such as hemorrhage and perforation, may be life threatening (Goldstein and Crooks, 1978). Aph-

thae similar to peptic ulcers in size and contour are the cause of these serious complications (Smith, Kime, and Pitcher, 1973; Stanley et al., 1975). Skip areas mimic the pattern of Crohn disease. Corticosteroids are the medical mainstay in the therapy of Behçet syndrome.

Eosinophilic Colitis (Allergic Gastroenteropathy)

The stomach and small bowel are the most common sites involved with eosinophilic gastroenteritis (see Chapters 6 and 9). The less common colonic disease typically occurs in the presence of small bowel disease (Teele et al., 1979; Stringer, 1987). Disease may be focal or generalized (Moore et al., 1986; Stringer,

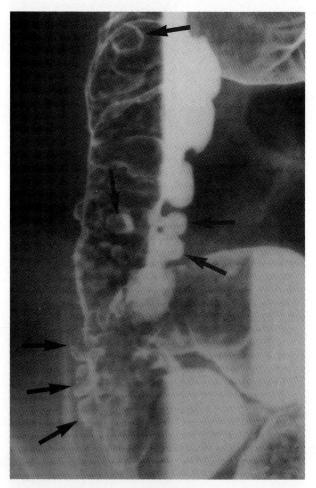

FIGURE 10–64. Crohn colitis with pseudodiverticula. There are multiple saculations or pseudodiverticula (*arrows*) in the ascending colon seen on double-contrast barium enema. (Reprinted with permission from Stringer DA. Imaging inflammatory bowel disease in the pediatric patient. Radiol Clin N Amer 1987;25:93–113.)

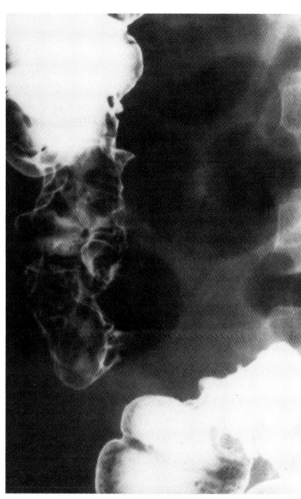

FIGURE 10–65. Behçet syndrome. There is marked deformity and irregularity of a contracted cecum on double-contrast barium enema. This appearance could also be seen in Crohn disease.

1987). The appearance on contrast enema is similar to that seen in ulcerative colitis (Figure 10–66). Biopsy, typically of the gastric antrum, establishes the diagnosis.

Infectious Colitides

Colitis-causing infectious organisms common among children in North America and Europe include *Escherichia coli, Salmonella, Shigella, Campylobacter, Yersinia,* and *Clostridium difficile.* More unusual organisms include *Entamoeba histolytica, Mycobacterium tuberculosis, Histoplasma,* and viruses.

Escherichia coli, Shigella Colitis

Hemorrhagic colitis associated with *E. coli* (015:H7) has been reported and may be more common than

has been generally accepted (Riley et al., 1983). *Salmonella* and *Shigella* are more commonly associated with enteritis, but radiologic investigation is rarely

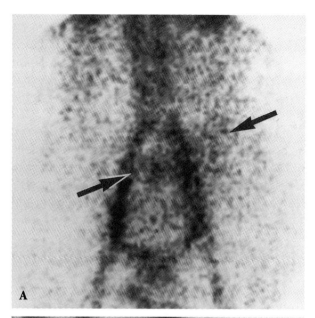

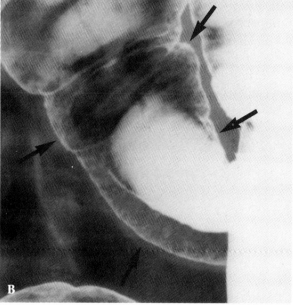

FIGURE 10–66. Eosinophilic gastroenteritis. *A,* There is a slight increase in activity in the region of the transverse colon (*between arrows*) on a technetium-99m red-blood-cell scan in a 16-year-old boy with acute rectal bleeding. *B,* Double-contrast barium enema showed an area of focal colitis in the transverse colon as indicated by mild deformity and mucosal irregularity (*arrows*). (Reprinted with permission from Moore D, et al. Eosinophilic gastroenteritis presenting in an adolescent with isolated colonic involvement. Gut 1986;27:1362–8.

necessary. Plain films show nonspecific small bowel dilatation with air-fluid levels compatible with a gastroenteritis.

Salmonella Colitis

The most common presentation of *Salmonella* infection is acute gastroenteritis. This process is usually self-limited, although bacteremic invasion and focal extraintestinal infection may develop, particularly in immunocompromised patients. *Salmonella* infections occur with exposure to undercooked poultry and poultry products (mainly eggs) as well as beef and pork. Each year, about 500 foodborne outbreaks of *Salmonella* gastroenteritis are reported, representing over 50% of all gastroenteritis outbreaks with an identifiable cause (Goldberg and Robin, 1988).

The most common clinical presentations are that of abrupt onset of nausea, vomiting, and abdominal pain and fever, followed by mild to severe watery diarrhea. The mean incubation period from the time of exposure is 24 hours. The stool, which is usually nonbloody, contains a moderate number of polymorphonuclear leukocytes and occult blood. Symptoms usually subside within 2 to 7 days in healthy children, and fatalities are rare.

The course of *Salmonella* enterocolitis is distinct among high-risk groups of children, including neonates, infants, and the immunosuppressed. In patients with acquired immunodeficiency syndrome (AIDS), the disease may become widespread and overwhelming, causing multisystem involvement, shock, and death (Sperber and Schleupner, 1987). Among patients with inflammatory bowel disease, particularly ulcerative colitis, *Salmonella* may invade the bowel wall with rapid development of a toxic megacolon, systemic toxicity, and death.

Imaging is rarely necessary in the diagnosis of infectious enterocolitis. If performed to exclude another cause of abdominal pain, plain-film radiography may show nonspecific small bowel dilatation with a pattern of ileus. Occasionally, colitis with or without toxic dilatation is seen (Figure 10–67).

Campylobacter Colitis

Campylobacter is among the most frequent causes of infectious gastroenteritis, particularly in developed countries, where the number of cases exceeds those of *Salmonella* and *Shigella* infections. The age distribution is bimodal, with a peak in small children under 4 years of age and a second peak in adolescents and young adults. The highest incidence is in the first year of life. Many infections are asymptomatic, especially in older children.

Campylobacter is cultured from the stools of 5% of children with acute diarrhea (Dekeyser et al.,

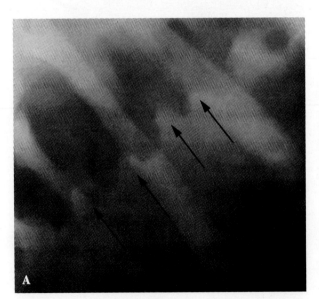
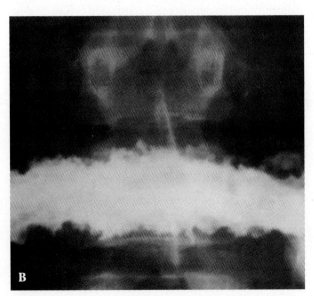

FIGURE 10–67. Salmonella colitis. *A,* Plain film shows some printing (*arrows*) of the transverse colon, indicating a severe colitis in a patient who was toxic. The barium enema was contraindicated at this time. *B,* A gentle single-contrast barium enema performed when the patient's condition had improved still demonstrated an extensive severe colitis of the transverse colon.

1972). Ninety-five percent of children with *Campy-lobacter* in their stools have diarrhea (Skirrow, 1977). Presentation may mimic acute appendicitis with severe abdominal pain (Lambert et al., 1979). Massive rectal bleeding, toxic megacolon, pseudo-membranous colitis, and acute reactive arthritis are reported complications (Lambert et al., 1979; Karmali and Tan, 1980; Gardiner, 1987). Although typically self-limiting, the infection may recur in 20% of cases (Lambert et al., 1979; Karmali and Tan, 1980; Brodey, Fertig, and Aron, 1982).

Contrast enema is rarely if ever indicated, but if performed it can show a granular mucosal pattern, aphthae, loss of haustral folds, or pancolitis (Tielbeek et al., 1985; Gardiner, 1987). Radiographic findings can mimic Crohn disease or ulcerative colitis (Gardiner, 1987).

Yersinia Colitis

Yersinia infections occur primarily in children and young adults, with most occurring in children under 7 years of age. Disease is more common in the colder months and more common in males than females. Common-source outbreaks due to contaminated food or water are reported with incubation periods ranging from 1 to 11 days. The most frequent complication in children is reactive arthritis. Joints of the extremities are usually affected, with one to four joints involved. The history may suggest enterocolitis due to *Yersinia* based on contacts with animals or ingestion of uncooked meat products, especially pork.

Children over 5 years of age tend to present with abdominal pain, fever, and watery diarrhea. This acute gastroenteritis and mesenteric adenitis can mimic acute appendicitis (Kohl, Jacobson, and Nahmias, 1976; Atkinson et al., 1983). Younger children usually present with gastroenteritis of varying severity, lasting from a few weeks to several months. Bacteremia develops in 20 to 30% of infants under 3 months of age. Occasionally, intestinal ulceration, perforation, and peritonitis result (Atkinson et al., 1983).

The primary radiologic findings are in the terminal ileum, with spasm, nodularity, edema, and superficial ulceration noted (see Chapter 9) (Gardiner and Stevenson, 1982; Vantrappen, Geboes, and Ponette, 1982). Nodularity may persist longer than other features and may relate to enlarged lymphoid follicles (Gardiner and Stevenson, 1982). Mesenteric adenopathy may be present, detectable by US (Puylaert, 1986) or CT. Cecal spasm may be associated with terminal ileal disease (Shrago, 1976).

Amebic Colitis

Human infection with *Entamoeba histolytica* is prevalent worldwide; endemic foci are particularly common in the tropics and in areas with low socioeconomic and sanitary standards. Food or drink contaminated with the organism cysts and direct fecal-oral contact are the most common means of infection. *Entamoeba histolytica* parasitizes the lumen of the gastrointestinal tract and causes few disease sequelae in most infected subjects. In a small proportion of individuals, the organism may invade the intestinal mucosa and disseminate to other organs such as the liver. *Entamoeba histolytica* is harbored by 25% of the world population. Only 1 to 17% of infected subjects acquire amebic dysentery.

Intestinal amebiasis may occur within 2 weeks of infection or may be delayed for months. Onset is usually gradual, with colicky abdominal pain and bloody diarrhea. When young children become infected, the illness tends to be rapidly progressive, with a high mortality rate. The disease primarily affects the colon and can take several different patterns. Ulcerative rectocolitis is present in 95% of patients, typhloappendicitis in 3%, ameboma in 1.5%, and fulminant colitis leading to toxic megacolon in 0.5% (Cardoso et al., 1977). Perforation may occur in the fulminant form of the disease (Clarke and Frost, 1983). Stool sampling for the organism establishes the diagnosis. If imaging studies are performed, aphthae with skip areas of involvement may be seen. When the right side of the colon is affected, distinction from Crohn colitis can be difficult. Ameboma may be plaquelike or form large, fungating necrotic masses with overhanging edges mimicking carcinoma (Gardiner and Stevenson, 1982; Martinez et al., 1982). Long-standing disease may lead to irreversible changes such as a "lead-pipe" colonic deformity or stricture (Gardiner and Stevenson, 1982; Martinez et al., 1982).

Tuberculosis and Histoplasmosis

Tuberculosis is now rare in children of developed countries (Hamilton et al., 1979) but is more common in underdeveloped areas of the world. It can mimic Crohn disease clinically and radiologically, even to the extent of having aphthae (Downey and Nakielny, 1985; Friedland and Filly, 1974). The terminal ileum and cecum are most commonly affected (see Chapter 9). The disease should be considered in patients from endemic areas. Three gross forms of intestinal involvement are seen: ulcerative, hypertrophic, and ulcerohypertrophic, with the ulcerative form being most common.

Plain-film radiography may indicate the presence of disease in extraintestinal sites such as the lungs or bones. The sacroiliac joints may be asymmetrically affected (Friedland and Filly, 1974).

On contrast studies, the earliest evidence is a change in gut motility and a stiffening of the mucosal pattern due to infiltration. Ulceration is generally linear or stellar. Mass lesions develop, and the cecum is often particularly affected (Carrera, Young, and Lewicki, 1976). Although attempts have been made to differentiate the features from those of Crohn disease, this is usually not possible.

Segmental colitis has also been reported although uncommonly. This may be associated with stenosis (Carrera, Young, and Lewicki, 1976).

Tuberculous peritonitis is a rare but serious complication and may show large exudative ascites (evident on CT) or cause lymphadenopathy (indistinguishable from lymphoma on CT) (Hanson and Hunter, 1985).

Histoplasmosis can affect the bowel in a similar way to tuberculosis but often is only a mild, self-limiting disease.

Pseudomembranous Colitis

Pseudomembranous colitis is an acute inflammatory disease of the colon that occurs following antibiotic or chemotheraputic therapy. Almost all antibiotics predispose to pseudomembranous colitis, but the disease is most common in the setting of clindamycin, ampicillin, and cephalosporin exposure (Boland et al., 1994a). Methotrexate and fluorouracil are reported chemotherapeutic agents associated with the disease (Bartlett, 1992). Pseudomembranous colitis is caused by an overgrowth of toxigenic strains of *Clostridium difficile*, a gram-positive organism that produces a spectrum of clinical illness from mild diarrhea to fulminant colitis. When severe, it can produce a life-threatening colitis named for the characteristic white pseudomembranes observed endoscopically. Though less common in children than adults, the incidence among pediatric patients is rising, probably as a result of the increasing use of antibiotics (Bartlett, 1992).

Crampy abdominal pain, fever, watery diarrhea, and leukocytosis characterize the typical presentation. The onset of symptoms may be delayed up to 8 weeks after treatment (Boland et al., 1994a). The diagnosis is established by microbiologic stool assay test to detect toxin production by *C. difficile*.

Recognized conventional radiographic findings include colonic dilatation and mucosal edema with haustral thickening and nodularity (Loughran, Tappan, and Whitehouse, 1982). Nodular haustral thickening (Figure 10–68) is the most specific finding (Stanley, Leland, and Tedesco, 1976), but it is seen in a minority (18%) of patients (Boland et al., 1994a). In as many as two-thirds of symptomatic cases, radiographs are normal (Boland et al., 1994a).

Ultrasonographic features of pseudomembranous colitis include moderate to marked thickening of the colon wall and effacement of the bowel lumen secondary to mural edema (Figure 10–69). Pathologic correlation documents the wide band of heterogeneous medium echogenicity surrounded by a narrow hypoechoic layer to represent severely edematous mucosa/submucosa and muscularis propria, respectively.

Computed tomography has a reported sensitivity for colonic abnormalities in 85% of adult cases (Boland et al., 1994b). Recognized CT abnormalities (Boland et al., 1994a; Fishman et al., 1991) include circumferential colonic wall thickening (Figure 10–70), pericolonic edema, ascites, nodular haustral thickening, and the "accordian sign," reported as a specific finding in adults with *C. difficile* colitis (Fishman et al., 1991). This term describes the appearance of contrast material trapped between thickened colonic folds in *C. difficile* colitis. A "gas accordian sign" has also been described in patients with pseudomembranous colitis (Binkovitz et al., 1999). Although classically described as a pancolitis, rectosigmoid sparing is as high as 67% (Tesdesco, Corless, and Brownstein, 1982), and isolated right colonic abnormalities are reported (Boland et al., 1994b; Fishman et al., 1991). A normal CT scan is reported in 39% of symptomatic adult cases (Boland et al., 1994b). The CT findings in children show a similar spectrum but a slightly higher frequency of abnormal findings, possibly related to errors in sampling pediatric patients with severe clinical disease. While CT findings asso-

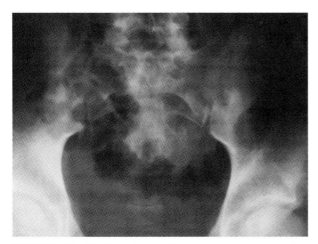

FIGURE 10–68. Pseudomembraneous colitis in a 13-year-old boy. Nodular haustral thickening gives a thumbprinting appearance to the descending and sigmoid colon on a plain-film radiograph.

ciated with pseudomembranous colitis in children may suggest the diagnosis, CT is less specific than laboratory and clinical findings (Blickman et al., 1995). The differential diagnosis includes Crohn disease, ulcerative colitis, graft-versus-host disease, neutropenic colitis, appendicitis, bowel infarct, and radiation enteritis.

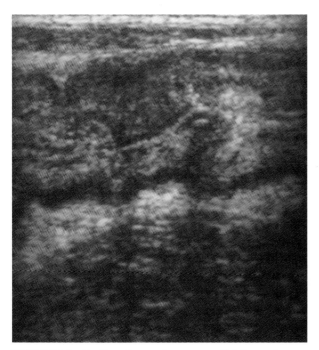

FIGURE 10–69. Pseudomembranous colitis in an 8-year-old girl. Marked thickening of the wall and obliteration of the lumen of the transverse colon are noted on US.

Miscellaneous Colitides

Hemolytic Uremic Syndrome

Hemolytic uremic syndrome (HUS) is the most common cause of acute renal failure in young children, and its incidence is increasing (Kelles, VanDyck, and Proesmans, 1994). Initially considered a renal disease, it is now known to be a systemic disorder with features common to thrombocytopenia purpura. The disease most frequently follows an episode of gastroenteritis caused by an enteric pathogen, *Escherichia coli* (0157:H7). The source of this strain is undercooked meat and unpasturized milk. Outbreaks related to ingestion of contaminated apple cider or to bathing in a contaminated swimming pool are reported. This syndrome has also been associated with other bacterial (*Shigella, Salmonella, Campylobacter, Streptococcus pneumoniae, Bartonella*), and viral (Coxsackie, influenza, varicella, human immunodeficiency virus [HIV], Epstein-Barr) infections and with endotoxemia. In addition, an association has been made with oral contraceptive use, systemic lupus erythematosus, malignant hypertension, post partum renal failure, and radiation nephritis. There are several reports of HUS among family members, but the role of genetic factors is unknown.

The syndrome is most common in children under 4 years of age. Fever, vomiting, abdominal pain, and bloody diarrhea characterize the onset of the prodromal enteritis, present in more than 80% of affected children. Sudden onset of pallor, irri-

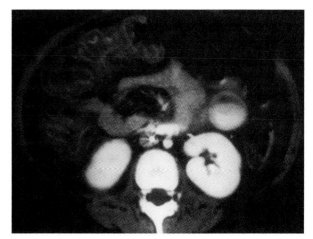

FIGURE 10–70. Pseudomembranous colitis in a 10-year-old boy. Circumferential wall thickening of the right and transverse colon as well ascites are noted on CT.

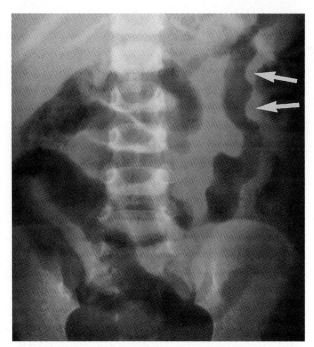

FIGURE 10–71. Hemolytic uremic syndrome. The large bowel is featureless and full of air except in the transverse colon, where there was some thumbprinting (*arrows*).

tability, weakness, lethargy, and oliguria follows in 5 to 10 days. The diagnosis is supported by the findings of microangiopathic hemolytic anemia, thrombocytopenia, and acute renal failure.

Conventional radiographic findings during the prodromal enterocolitis may show thumbprinting (Figure 10–71). Barium enema may be normal (Tocken and Campbell, 1977) or show spasm, filling defects (pseudotumors), transverse ridging, marginal serrations, or thumbprinting secondary to edema or submucosal hemorrhage (Kawanami, Bowen, and Girdany, 1984; Kirks, 1982; Peterson, Meseroll, and Shrago, 1976) (Figure 10–72). Strictures, sometimes irreversible, may be present (Peterson, Meseroll, and Shrago, 1976; Bar-Ziv, Ayoub, and Fletcher, 1974; Kirks, 1982). In the appropriate clinical context, these findings should alert the radiologist to the diagnosis (Kirks, 1982).

Ischemic Colitis

Ischemic colitis is rare in children and is usually associated with some underlying pathology such as Kawasaki disease (Fan, Lan, and Wong, 1986). The acute, subacute, or insidious presentation and radiologic appearance are similar to those seen in adults with transient crampy abdominal pain, localized

tenderness, and rectal bleeding (Anderson and Eklof, 1981).

The radiologic imaging will depend on the clinical circumstances and may include plain-film radiology, contrast studies, or nuclear medicine studies. Contrast studies may show spasm, local thickening of the intestinal wall, and coarse mucosal folds with or without ulceration (Anderson and Eklof, 1981).

Colitis of Hirschsprung Disease

Rarely, Hirschsprung disease is complicated by a life-threatening explosive bloody diarrhea from an enterocolitis. This bloody diarrhea often persists if there is not a fatal outcome (Bill and Chapman, 1962). The presence of dilated large bowel may suggest Hirschsprung disease, but toxic megacolon secondary to infantile ulcerative colitis has been reported (Karjoo and McCarthy, 1976). Hirschsprung disease usually is associated with constipation and growth failure, which aids differentiation (Hamilton et al., 1979). The colitis of Hirschsprung disease also may be characteristic on a single-contrast barium enema, with transverse barring, nodularity, and a tapering zone of transition (Berger and Wilkinson, 1974). The possibility of more subtle Hirschsprung disease can be excluded by rectal biopsy.

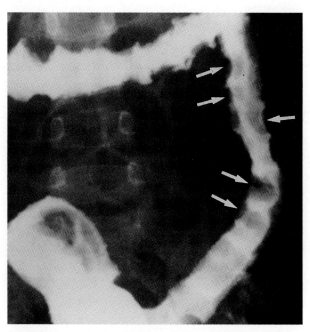

FIGURE 10–72. Hemolytic uremic syndrome. Contrast enema shows mucosal irregularity and thumbprinting (*arrow*). This type of examination is rarely required.

Allergic Colitis

Allergy to cow's milk protein is a common cause of gastrointestinal disease in infants and young children, particularly among those with a family history of allergies (Taylor, 1988). Asthma and atopic dermatitis are frequently associated extraintestinal manifestations. Whey protein is the usual offending antigen, whether in formula or breast milk. The diagnosis is usually made on clinical grounds and is confirmed by the resolution of symptoms upon the removal of milk from the diet. As patients sensitive to cow's milk may also be sensitive to soy protein, change to an elemental formula is often made (Kleinman, 1992).

Allergic colitis refers to a specific manifestation of milk protein intolerance and appears to be the most common etiology of colitis in the first year of life (Jenkins et al., 1984). Symptoms include failure to thrive, constipation, rectal bleeding or guaiac-positive stool, and abdominal distention with or without pain. Disease may affect any part of the colon, although the rectosigmoid region appears preferentially involved (Walker-Smith, 1992; Odze, Wershil, and Leichner, 1995; Odze et al., 1993). The mucosa, submucosa, and lamina propria are infiltrated with eosinophils, resulting in narrowing of the colonic lumen on barium enema (Swischuk and Hayden, 1985). Ulcerations, erosions, and crypt abscesses may be seen, sometimes in a segmental distribution (Odze et al., 1993). Allergic colitis has also been reported to mimic Hirschsprung disease, showing irregular narrowing of the rectum and a transition zone. Differentiating features show nearly constant ulceration of the rectal mucosa in allergic colitis and intact rectal mucosa in Hirschsprung disease. The location of the mucosal abnormality is typically above the transition zone in colitis of Hirschsprung disease (Elhalaby, Coran, and Blane, 1995). Last, the radiographic abnormality in the patients with allergic colitis appear out of proportion to the relatively mild clinical symptoms.

Detergent, Caustic, and Herb Enema Colitis

A variety of enema preparations have been tried in many parts of the world for a wide range of conditions. Some are prescribed by "witch doctors," others by parents (Kirchner et al., 1977; Segal, Solomon, and Mirwis, 1981). Swazi infants may receive as many as 50 enemas per year, and one South African hospital alone treats 25 patients per year for complications (Segal, Solomon, and Mirwis, 1981). Unfortunately, these numerous enemas have wide-ranging and sometimes fatal consequences.

Colitis is one common complication that can be severe (Kirchner et al., 1977; Segal, Solomon, and Mirwis, 1981). The radiologic signs are protean; the acute radiologic manifestations are of segmental toxic dilatation, necrotizing colitis, pseudopolyp formation, ulceration, and perforation (Segal, Solomon, and Mirwis, 1981). The acute phase of caustic detergent colitis has been reproduced experimentally in the dog, and the severity of the colitis is related directly to the concentration of the detergent (Kirchner et al., 1977). The chronic radiologic manifestations are loss of haustra; general loss of bowel caliber; or long, short, single or multiple strictures (Segal, Solomon, and Mirwis, 1981).

Evanescent Colitis

Evanescent colitis is an acute reversible segmental colitis unlike any other colitis and is of uncertain etiology. It is usually found in adults but can develop in childhood (Friedman and Filly, 1974).

ACUTE APPENDICITIS

Acute appendicitis is the most common condition requiring emergency abdominal surgery in children (Janik and Firor, 1979). The condition is estimated to occur in approximately 4 of every 1000 children. Acute appendicitis typically occurs in older children; it is rarely seen in children under the age of 2 years. The etiology of acute appendicitis is felt to be appendiceal luminal obstruction by hard concretions such as fecal impaction or appendiceal calculi, followed by luminal distension, ischemia, and bacterial infection. If the condition is left untreated, necrosis of the appendiceal wall can develop, resulting in appendiceal perforation, abscess formation, and peritonitis.

The optimal management of children with acute appendicitis is predicated on early diagnosis and prompt operative intervention. However, the early diagnosis of this condition in childhood remains difficult. The diagnosis of acute appendicitis has traditionally been based on clinical criteria, including right lower-quadrant pain, point tenderness in the right lower-quadrant, vomiting, and leukocytosis with a left shift. The clinical diagnosis may not be straightforward, however, and approximately one-third of children with the disease have an uncertain preoperative diagnosis (Lau et al., 1984; Sivit, 1996). This is in part due to the variable presentation of the disease and because there are no good laboratory predictors of the disorder. However, several factors account for an increased difficulty in establishing the clinical diagnosis of acute appendicitis in children when compared with adults. These include the inability of younger children to adequately communicate their complaints and localize their pain and the fact that many gynecologic disorders have a similar clinical presentation in adolescent females (Siegel, Carel, and Surratt, 1991; Sivit, 1996).

The difficulty in establishing an early diagnosis of acute appendicitis in children may lead to a delay in treatment and resulting increased morbidity. The consequences of delayed diagnosis include appendiceal perforation, abscess formation, peritonitis, and pyelephlebitis (Harrison et al., 1984; Marchildon and Dudgeon, 1977). These complications typically result in longer hospitalization and time away from school. They also result in an increased risk of infertility in females. In addition, the difficulty in establishing a clinical diagnosis of acute appendicitis has resulted in a higher prevalence of negative laparotomy in children than in adults.

There remains great variability in imaging approaches to children with suspected acute appendicitis, ranging from conventional radiography to graded-compression US and helical CT. Imaging is most helpful in the subgroup of children with suspected acute appendicitis in whom the clinical findings are equivocal. The principal imaging technique for evaluating children with suspected acute appendicitis has been graded-compression US (Ceres et al., 1990; Crady et al., 1993; Ramachandran et al., 1996; Sivit, 1996; Sivit et al., 1992; Vignault et al., 1990; Wong et al., 1994). The reported sensitivity of US for the diagnosis of appendicitis in children has ranged from 84 to 94% while the specificity has ranged from 47 to 95%. The clinical utility of US lies primarily in the subgroup of children in whom the clinical findings are equivocal, both to establish the diagnosis of acute appendicitis and to aid in the diagnosis of other abdominal and pelvic conditions that may mimic the disorder (Siegel, Carel, and Surratt, 1991; Sivit, 1996; Sivit et al., 1992).

The graded-compression ultrasonographic technique for the evaluation of acute appendicitis was first described by Puylaert (Puylaert, 1986). Graded compression is gradually applied with a linear high-frequency transducer (5 or 7 MHz) to eliminate overlying bowel gas and fluid and reduce the distance from the transducer to the appendix. Normal bowel loops and the normal appendix can be compressed with moderate pressure whereas the inflamed appendix does not compress. Visualization of the psoas muscle and iliac vessels indicates that adequate compression has been achieved. Visualization of the appendix should not be used as a criteria for a diagnostic examination, since the normal appendix is typically identified in less than one-half of children (Sivit, 1996; Sivit et al., 1992). A point of potential confusion for nonradiologists is that graded-compression US and abdominal US are different examinations. Graded-compression US looks strictly at the gastrointestinal tract, including the appendix, while abdominal US evaluates solid viscera, including the liver, spleen, pancreas, and kidneys but typically not the appendix.

The appendix is identified at graded-compression US by its tubular appearance on long axis and its blind end. The ultrasonographic criteria for the diagnosis of acute appendicitis includes visualization of an incompressible appendix that is greater than 6 mm in cross-sectional diameter (Figure 10–73), identification of an appendicolith (Figure 10–74), or demonstration of a complex mass or focal fluid collection (Figure 10–75). The latter finding represents a periappendiceal abscess following perforation. Color Doppler US is a useful adjunct in confirming the diagnosis of acute appendicitis by demonstrating blood flow in the appendiceal wall (Figure 10–76).

Potential pitfalls in the ultrasonographic diagnosis of acute appendicitis include distal appendicitis, where the inflammation may be localized to the distal appendix; retrocecal appendicitis, where the cecum may obscure visualization of the enlarged appendix; and perforated appendicitis, where the appendix may not be recognizable (Sivit, 1996; Sivit et al., 1992). It is important to image the entire length of the appendix to avoid a false-negative diagnosis in distal appendicitis. Additionally, it is important to recognize that the principal finding in perforated appendicitis is a periappendiceal or pelvic mass representing a phlegmon or abscess.

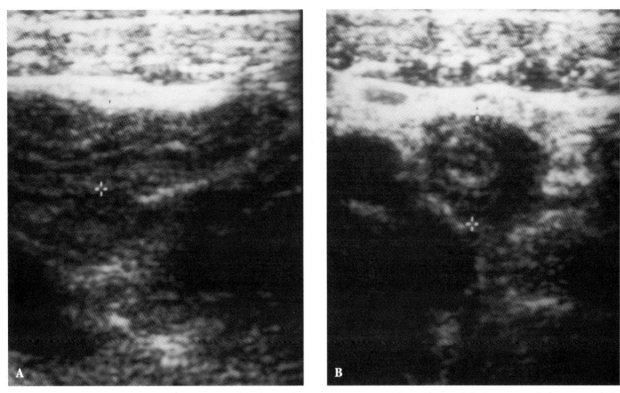

FIGURE 10–73. Acute appendicitis. Longitudinal *A* and transverse *B* views through the right lower quadrant on graded-compression US in a child with acute appendicitis demonstrate an enlarged, noncompressible appendix (*between electronic calipers*).

In recent years, there have been an increasing number of reports in adults detailing the use of helical CT for the diagnosis of acute appendicitis (Balthazar et al., 1994; Lane et al., 1997; Malone et al., 1993; Rao et al., 1997). The reported sensitivity of CT for the diagnosis of acute appendicitis in adults has ranged from 87 to 100%, and the specificity has ranged from 89 to 98%. The use of helical CT for the diagnosis in children is increasing although there are currently limited reports in the literature (Friedland and Siegel, 1997; Jabra, Shalaby-Rana, and Fishman, 1997). In spite of its higher cost and associated radiation exposure, CT may be increasingly appealing for the assessment of the older child with a larger body habitus. Due to its decreased operator dependence when compared with US, CT may also improve diagnostic accuracy in some clinical settings.

A variety of techniques have been used in the performance of appendiceal CT. These include (a) full abdominopelvic scanning after intravenous and oral contrast administration, (b) imaging limited to the lower abdomen and pelvis without any contrast material, (c) imaging of the lower abdomen and pelvis with thin collimation using oral and rectal contrast, and (d) imaging of the lower abdomen and pelvis with thin collimation using only rectal contrast. The use of rectal contrast in conjunction with thinly collimated sections has resulted in the highest reported sensitivity for the diagnosis of appendicitis in adults. Additionally, this technique eliminates the necessity of delaying scanning to opacify distal bowel loops if oral contrast is used for bowel opacification.

Signs of acute appendicitis on CT include a distended (over 6 mm) and unopacified appendix (Figure 10–77), an appendicolith (Figure 10–78), deformity of the cecal tip (also known as the arrowhead sign), stranding of pericecal fat, adjacent bowel wall thickening, periappendiceal or pelvic mass representing a phlegmon or abscess (Figure 10–79), peritoneal fluid, and mesenteric lymphadenopathy. The only CT findings that are specific for appendicitis are an enlarged appendix and an appendicolith. The remaining CT findings are nonspecific.

Computed tomography is also useful in delineating the location and extent of associated abdom-

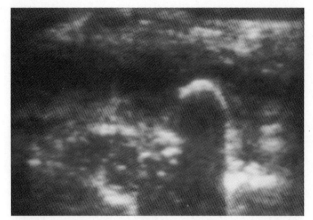

FIGURE 10–74. Acute appendicitis with an appendicolith. Longitudinal view through the right lower quadrant in a child with acute appendicitis shows an enlarged appendix with an appendicolith. Note the acoustic shadowing.

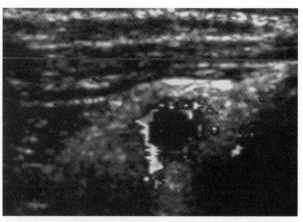

FIGURE 10–76. Acute appendicitis on color Doppler US. Transverse view through the right lower quadrant in a child with acute appendicitis demonstrates hyperemia of the appendiceal wall.

inal and pelvic fluid collections following ruptured appendicitis. Computed tomography can determine the relative size of liquefied versus nonliquefied components within the collection. These findings help guide the treatment to either percutaneous or surgical drainage following appendiceal perforation (Jeffrey, Federle, and Tolentino, 1988). Computed tomography is also useful in the postoperative evaluation of children with perforated appendcitis by demonstrating the presence and location of residual fluid collections.

Abdominal radiographs are typically normal during the early stages of acute appendicitis. They have a low sensitivity and specificity for the diagnosis and therefore should not be obtained routinely in children with suspected acute appendicitis if graded-compression US or CT is available. If abdominal radiographs are obtained, they should include supine and upright or decubitus views. Abdominal radiography is particularly useful for evaluating complications of acute appendicitis, including small bowel obstruction and pneumoperitoneum. Addi-

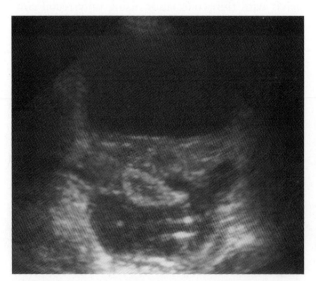

FIGURE 10–75. Perforated appendicitis. Transverse view through the pelvis in a child with perforated appendicitis demonstrates complex fluid collection in the pouch of Douglas.

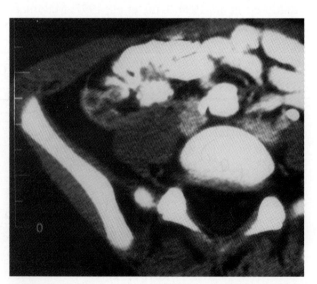

FIGURE 10–77. Acute appendicitis. Computed tomographic scan through the upper pelvis demonstrates an enlarged, fluid-filled appendix with an enhancing wall indicative of acute appendicitis.

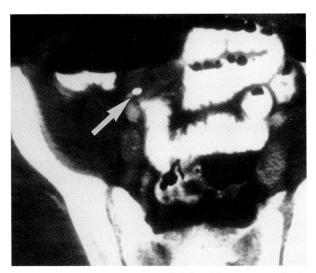

FIGURE 10–78. Acute appendicitis with an appendicolith. Computed tomographic scan through the upper pelvis demonstrates an enlarged appendix with an appendicolith (*arrow*).

tional findings associated with acute appendicitis on abdominal radiographs include a right lower-quadrant or pelvic soft-tissue mass (Figure 10–80), focally dilated small bowel loop (sentinel loop) or loops in the right lower quadrant (Figure 10–81), an indistinct right-sided psoas margin, obliteration of right-sided properitoneal or obturator internus fat, or visualization of an appendicolith. Visualization of an

appendicolith is the only specific finding for the diagnosis of acute appendicitis at abdominal radiography. However, it is seen in only 10 to 15% of patients. Very rarely, an appendicolith may be detected serendipitously in a patient without abdominal pain being examined for a reason unrelated to possible appendicitis. It has been the practice at some hospitals to watch these over time.

NEOPLASMS OF THE LARGE BOWEL

Juvenile Polyps

The juvenile colonic polyp, a retention or inflammatory polyp, is the most common tumor of the bowel in childhood, present in 3 to 4% of the population under 21 years of age. Presentation is almost always between the ages of 6 and 10 years; polyps are rarely observed before 1 year of age. Polyps are more frequent in males than females and are multiple in one-third of cases (Cremin and Louw, 1970; Pillai and Tolia, 1988). Children who have six or more juvenile polyps are considered to have juvenile polyposis, often a dominant trait in families. Between 75 to 85% of polyps arise in the rectosigmoid region, although they can affect any site in the large bowel, small bowel, or stomach (Morson and Dawson, 1972).

Juvenile polyps are likely inflammatory in etiology (Roth and Helwig, 1963). Retention cysts

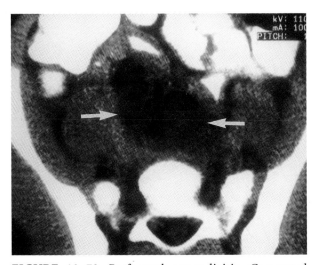

FIGURE 10–79. Perforated appendicitis. Computed tomographic scan through the pelvis demonstrates a complex collection of fluid and air (between arrows) representing an intraperitoneal abscess secondary to perforated appendicitis.

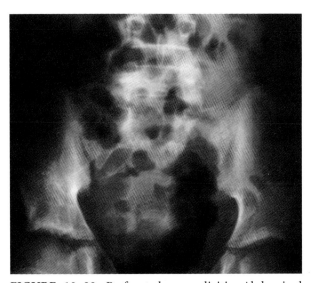

FIGURE 10–80. Perforated appendicitis. Abdominal radiograph demonstrates a soft-tissue mass in the right pelvis displacing the sigmoid colon to the left. At surgery, a perforated appendix was noted.

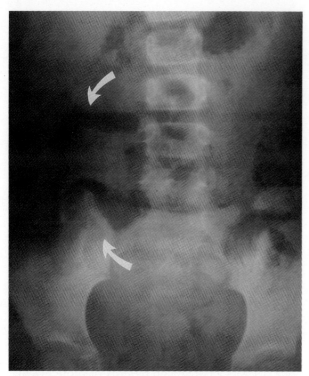

FIGURE 10–81. Acute appencicitis. Abdominal radiograph in a child with appendicitis demonstrates focally dilated bowel loops (sentinel loop) (*between arrows*) in the right lower quadrant.

form when hyperplastic mucus glands become blocked. A less favored theory is that these polyps are actually hamartomas (Morson and Dawson, 1972). Unlike adenomatous polyps, juvenile polyps are not true neoplasms, and association with carcinoma is limited to a few reports (Harned, Buck, and Sobin, 1995; Kapetanakis, Vini, and Plitsis, 1996).

Most children present with bright red painless rectal bleeding during or immediately following a bowel movement. Iron deficiency anemia may be present; colocolic intussusception is an unusual presentation. The diagnosis is often made on rectal examination, but confirmation and evaluation for additional polyps requires a complete colonoscopy.

Double-contrast barium enema, although infrequently performed, is the radiologic procedure of choice to demonstrate polyps. The juvenile polyp usually appears smooth in contour. It is of variable size but is often large, and it may be pedunculated (Figure 10–82) or sessile (Figure 10–83). Occasionally, they are very large; they then appear less regular (Figure 10–84). Treatment includes polypectomy by snare or cautery. Laparotomy is rarely indicated.

Polyposis Syndromes

Polyposis syndromes can be classified into three groups: inherited hamartomatous polyposis syndromes (juvenile polyposis, juvenile polyposis of infancy, Peutz-Jeghers syndrome, Cowden syndrome and Cronkhite-Canada syndrome); inherited adenomatous polyposis syndromes (familial polyposis, Gardner's syndrome, and Turcot syndrome); and noninherited polyposes. Some of these syndromes are discussed in more detail below. (A summary of some of these findings is shown in Table 10–3.)

INHERITED HAMARTOMATOUS POLYPOSIS SYNDROMES

Juvenile Polyposis and Juvenile Polyposis of Infancy

A child with greater than six colonic polyps (Figure 10–85) or polyps present elsewhere in the intestines

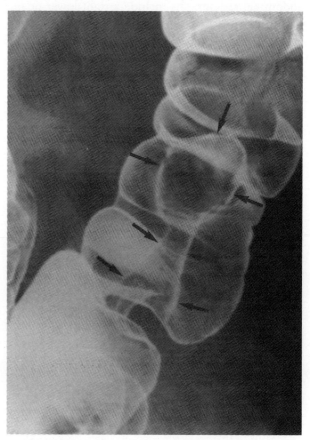

FIGURE 10–82. Pedunculated juvenile polyp. A smooth polyp on a stalk (*arrows*) arises from the wall of the sigmoid colon on a double-contrast barium enema.

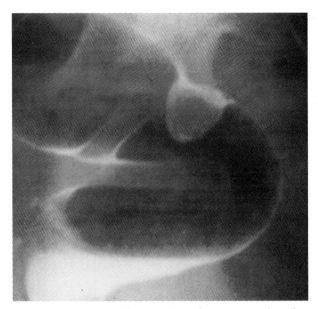

FIGURE 10–83. Sessile juvenile polyp. A smooth polyp arises from the posterosuperior wall of the rectum on a double-contrast barium enema.

or a child with a single polyp and a family history of polyposis is considered to have juvenile polyposis syndrome (Harned, Buck, and Sobin, 1995). This appears to be a heterogenous series of disorders (Sachatello, Hahn, and Carrington, 1974). A higher risk of colon carcinoma is reported in these patients. Juvenile polyposis has been associated with malrotation, hypertelorism, amyotonia congenita, hydrocephalus (Veale et al., 1966), and hypertrophic osteoarthropathy (Figure 10–86) (Baert et al., 1983; Simpson and Dalinka, 1985). Juvenile polyposis of infancy, a severe form of this disease, presents in boys in the first few months of life with diarrhea, malabsorption, and intussusception. Death is reported to occur before the age of 2 years (Ruymann, 1969; Soper and Kent, 1971; Ray and Heald, 1971).

Peutz-Jeghers Syndrome

Peutz-Jeghers syndrome is an autosomal dominant polyposis disorder defined by gastrointestinal hamartomas, mucocutaneous pigmentation, and a significant risk of development of neoplasms of the gut and other organs. The brown or black pigmentation of the lips, buccal mucosa, face, palms, and soles usually presents in early childhood. Lip pigmentation may fade (Scully, Galdsbini, and McNeely, 1978), but the buccal patches remain unchanged and are virtually pathognomonic for Peutz-Jeghers syndrome. Approximately 50% of cases are familial (Dodds, 1976).

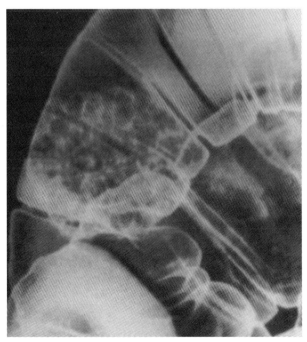

FIGURE 10–84. Juvenile polyp in an 11-year-old boy. There is a large irregular polyp in the sigmoid colon on a double-contrast barium enema.

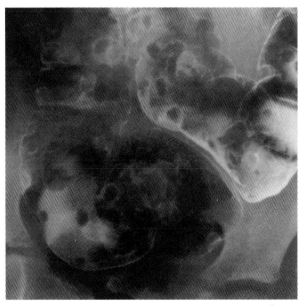

FIGURE 10–85. Juvenile polyposis coli. Multiple, moderate-sized polyps are seen in the restum and sigmoid colon. A low density barium had been used, which explains the poor coating seen. Histologically the polyps were juvenile in type.

TABLE 10–3. Intestinal Polyposis Syndromes: Polyp Distribution and Malignancy Risk

Syndrome	Inheritance	Polyp	Esophagus	Stomach	Small Bowel	Large Bowel	Site of Malignancy	Risk of Malignancy	Other Tumors and Features
Inherited Hamartomatous Polyposis Syndromes									
Juvenile polyposis	Uncertain	Juvenile hamartomas	—	—	Sometimes	100%	Usually large bowel	—	Heterogenous group of disorders with variable risk of malignancy; associated with malrotation, hypertelorism, amyotonia congenita, and hydrocephalus
Juvenile polyposis of infancy	Uncertain	Juvenile hamartomas	—	—	—	100%	—	—	Severe disease; death by age 2 years from diarrhea, malabsorption, and intussusception
Peutz-Jeghers syndrome	Autosomal dominant	Hamartomas	Rare	25%	50–95%	30%	Anywhere except esophagus	Up to 13%	Pigmentation, ovarian granulosa cell tumors
Cowden syndrome	Autosomal dominant	Juvenile hamartomas, simple hyperplastic	—	—	—	—	Thyroid, breast, ?colon cancers	?Low	Birdlike facies, circumoral papillomatosis, nodular gingival hyperplasia
Inherited Adenomatous Polyposis Syndromes									
Familial adenomatoid polyposis	Autosomal dominant	Adenoma (gastric fundus hyperplasia)	Rare	Up to 70%	Probably common	100%	Large bowel (100%)	100%	
Gardner's syndrome	Autosomal dominant	Adenoma (gastric fundus hyperplasia)	Rare	Up to 70%	Probably common	100%	Large bowel (100%)	100%	Probably a variant of familial adenomatoid polyposis, mesenchymal tumors, odontomas, desmoids, fibromas, osteomas, mesenteric fibromatosis
Turcot syndrome	Autosomal recessive	Adenoma (gastric fundus hyperplasia)	—	—	—	100%	CNS tumors	100%	Fewer polyps (< 100) of other adematous polyposis syndromes; Café au lait spots, port wine stain; sebaceous cysts, papillary thyroid carcinoma, leukemia

CNS, central nervous system
?? = probable features
AD = autosomal dominant?

The hamartomatous polyps are characterized by a smooth-muscle core arising from the muscularis mucosa and extending into the polyp, a feature specific for the syndrome. They occur primarily in the small bowel (95% of polyps), most commonly in the jejunum and ileum (Scully, Galdsbini, and McNeely, 1978). Gastric polyps occur in 25% of affected individuals and large bowel polyps in 30%. The increased incidence of adenocarcinoma of the bowel, especially of the stomach, duodenum, and colon, is not clearly related to malignant transformation of a polyp. Malignancies of the breast, lung, thyroid, skin, pancreas, uterus, and testis are reported in patients with Peutz-Jeghers.

Presentation is usually related to transient small bowel intussusception with intermittent crampy abdominal pain, bleeding, and anemia. Gastroduodenal intussusception and rectal prolapse are reported. The patient with Peutz-Jeghers is best evaluated by a small bowel follow-through examination that typically shows multiple sessile or pedunculated polyps.

Large lesions may have a multilobulated configuration. Large bowel polyps are best studied with a double-contrast barium enema (Figure 10–87); larger lesions may be evident on single-contrast examinations (Figure 10–88). Polyps are removed endoscopically when possible.

Cowden Syndrome

Cowden syndrome, or multiple hamartoma-neoplasia syndrome, is a rare autosomal dominant disease

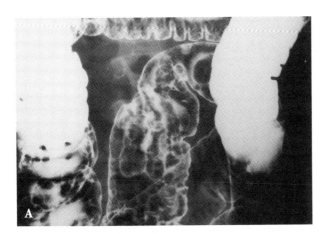

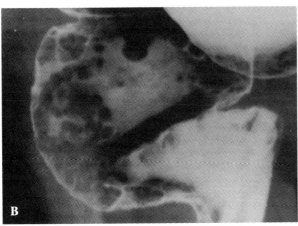

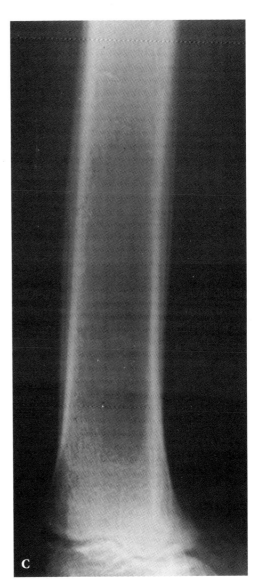

FIGURE 10–86. Generalized juvenile gastrointestinal polyposis. Double-contrast barium enema shows moderate-sized polyps scattered throughout the large bowel but particularly present in the sigmoid colon (*A*) and rectum (*B*). *C*, Periosteal reactions were present in many long bones such as the femur illustrated here.

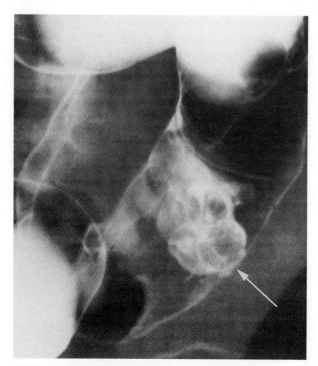

FIGURE 10–87. Peutz-Jeghers syndrome. A double-contrast barium enema demonstrates a large polyp (*arrow*) in the sigmoid colon, well coated with barium.

characterized by birdlike facies, macrocephaly, breast lesions, thyroid tumors, and gastrointestinal polyps. Alimentary tract polyps may be hamartomatous, hyperplastic, lymphomatous, inflammatory, or (rarely) adenomatous.

Cronkhite-Canada Syndrome

Cronkhite-Canada syndrome is a juvenile polyposis syndrome of poor prognosis, characterized by the presence of multiple juvenile inflammatory type of polyps. Because if affects only middle-aged adults, it will not be considered further here (Cronkhite and Canada, 1955).

INHERITED ADENOMATOUS POLYPOSIS SYNDROMES

Familial Polyposis Coli

Familial polyposis coli is an autosomal dominant syndrome characterized by carpeting of the colon by hundreds of adenomatous polyps. The risk of adenocarcinoma of the colon approaches 100%. Two-thirds of cases are familial. Symptoms related to polyps may be present in patients as young as 4 to 6

years of age (Abramson, 1967), although presentation is more typical in the third or fourth decade. With this later presentation, about two-thirds of patients have already developed colon carcinoma (Bussey, 1975); the carcinomas are often multiple and have a poor prognosis (Erbe, 1976). Extracolonic polyps are found in the stomach in 70% of patients studied by an upper gastrointestinal series (Ushio et al., 1976). These polyps are either adenomas or fundic gland hyperplasia (Watanabe et al., 1978). Adenomatous polyps are also seen in the small bowel (Ranzi et al., 1981). Patients with familial polyposis usually present with crampy abdominal pain and bloody diarrhea.

Patients suspected of having colonic polyps are generally studied by colonoscopy. On double-con-

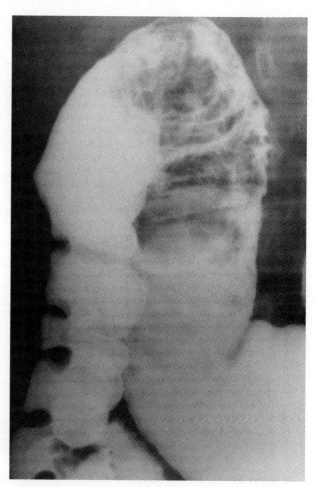

FIGURE 10–88. Peutz-Jeghers syndrome. A large polyp almost occluding the hepatic flexure is shown on a single-contrast barium enema. This polyp was asymptomatic and was not removed until the patient presented again 2 years later with intussusception.

trast barium enema examination, polyps are usually sessile and less than 1 cm in size (Bartram and Thornton, 1984); these small polyps appear to "carpet" the colon (Figure 10–89). Polyps are generally more numerous in the left colon. Lymphoid hyperplasia should not be mistaken for colonic polyposis; unlike polyps, lymphoid follicles do not have a barium rim to their margin (Kelvin et al., 1979) or project into the bowel lumen (Figure 10–90). Treatment requires total colectomy in the second decade.

Gardner Syndrome

Gardner syndrome and familial polyposis coli likely represent a spectrum of the same genetic disease, as they share the locus 5q21-q22. Classically described extraintestinal manifestations of Gardner syndrome include osteomas of the jaw, supernumery teeth, and extracolonic neoplasms such as desmoid tumors, brain tumors, papillary and follicular thyroid tumors, and carcinoid of the stomach. Jaw lesions are good predictors of polyp development in genetic kindreds with adenomatous polyposis lesions.

Clinical Features

Desmoid tumors and mesenteric fibromatosis are found in approximately 4% of patients with Gardner syndrome. The desmoid tumor is a locally invasive unencapsulated form of fibromatosis. Desmoid tumors tend to be avascular. A more diffuse fibrous tissue proliferation (mesenteric fibromatosis) may occur (Mathias et al., 1977; Naylor and Lebenthal, 1980), and the disease process may be accelerated by surgery (Bussey, Veale, and Morson, 1978). Fibrous adhesions are common in patients with Gardner syndrome postoperatively (Bussey, Veale, and Morson, 1978; Scully, Galdabini, and McNeely, 1978).

The adenomatous large bowel polyps appear at the same age and have the same malignant risks as in familial polyposis coli. In addition, patients with Gardner syndrome have a 12% risk of periampullary carcinoma, unlike those with familial polyposis coli (Bussey, 1975; Schulman, 1976). This usually develops approximately 15 years after the diagnosis of the colonic polyposis (Schuchardt and Ponsky, 1979); hence, it may represent malignant change in a previously unsuspected duodenal polyp.

Imaging

Plain-film radiography will demonstrate the osteomas in the facial bones, such as mandible, maxilla,

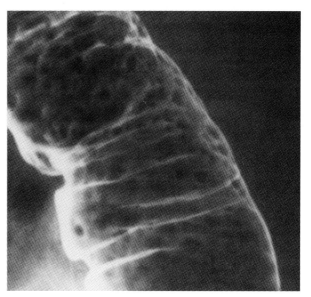

FIGURE 10–89. Familial adenomatoid polyposis coli. There are multiple small well-demarcated polypoid filling defects carpeting the large bowel seen on a double-contrast barium enema. Unlike the normal lymphoid follicular pattern, the polyps are of different sizes and their margins are somewhat better defined (see Figure 10–1).

or skull vault. In the long bones, especially the tibia and femur, localized cortical thickening is often present. Desmoid tumors involving the abdominal wall or peritoneal cavity may be present, displacing bowel loops if intra-abdominal.

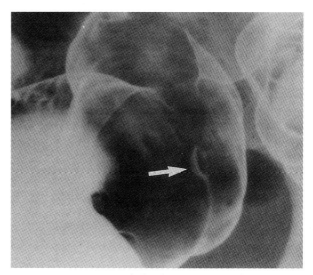

FIGURE 10–90. Familial adenomatoid polyposis coli. There are small polypoid filling defects projecting into the lumen of the large bowel (*arrow*), a feature that aids differentiation from normal lymphoid follicles.

Ultrasonography and CT can also demonstrate the desmoid masses and can be especially helpful in noninvasively investigating the postcolectomy patient who has abdominal pain. Ultrasonography shows mesenteric lesions as well-defined solid masses of relatively homogenous low echogenicity with scattered high-amplitude internal echoes that may represent mesenteric fat and vessels (Magid et al., 1984). However, US is somewhat limited by overlying bowel gas. Computed tomography will give better overall delineation in this regard. The appearance on CT is similar to lymphoma, with mesenteric desmoid lesions giving a non-enhancing mass of 50 to 69 Hounsfield units density (Magid et al., 1984). Confusion with lymphoma is unlikely in a patient with known Gardner syndrome. Computed tomography is also helpful in assessing changes in the size of the masses with therapy (such as radiotherapy), hence obviating the need for surgery, which can result in even more fibrosis.

Evaluating large bowel or small bowel polyps and gastric polyps is identical to evaluating familial adenomatoid polyposis, using double-contrast barium studies of upper and lower gastrointestinal tract and barium follow-through with endoscopy. The large bowel polyps are similar to those in familial adenomatoid polyposis, with a "carpet" of small polyps, especially in the left hemicolon (Figure 10–91). The barium follow-through may show prominent lymphoid hyperplasia in the terminal ileum, which should not be confused with polyps (Vanhoutte, 1970).

Treatment and Follow-Up
Treatment and follow-up are similar to familial polyposis coli, except that the duodenum should be regularly evaluated by double-contrast studies or endoscopy to exclude polyps or malignancy. Polyps in the duodenum may be amenable to endoscopic removal (Sweeney and Anderson, 1982).

Turcot Syndrome

Turcot syndrome, or glioma-polyposis syndrome, is characterized by colonic adenomatoid polyposis and malignancy in the central nervous system (Turcot, Despres, and St. Pierre, 1959; Radin et al., 1984). Inheritance is autosomal recessive. Presentation is usually in the second decade, with lower gastrointestinal symptoms. The central nervous system malignancy is usually diagnosed 2 to 8 years after total colonic resection (Itoh et al., 1970; Turcot, Despres, and St. Pierre, 1959; Baughman et al., 1969). Other reported abnormalities include sebaceous cysts, papillary carcinoma of the thyroid, leukemia, and spinal cord neoplasma.

Although the polyps in Turcot syndrome are adenomatous, there are rarely more than 100 polyps, in contrast to familial polyposis syndrome (Radin et al., 1984).

MISCELLANEOUS BENIGN TUMORS OF THE LARGE BOWEL

Other benign tumors of the colon include lipoma, leiomyoma, neurofibroma, and hemangioma. Hemangiomas may appear elsewhere in the body, and about 50% of patients have cutaneous hemangiomas. These rare, benign lesions can cause rapid, massive, even fatal hemorrhage. They appear as polypoid filling defects on contrast enema (Figure 10–92). Intestinal neurofibromas, also appearing as polypoid filling defects, can be multiple in von Recklinghausen's disease (Erbe, 1976).

MALIGNANT TUMORS OF THE LARGE BOWEL

Adenocarcinoma of the Colon and Rectum

Carcinoma of the colon and rectum represent fewer than 1% of malignant tumors in children. Predisposing conditions include familial multiple polyposis, ulcerative colitis, regional enteritis, and Peutz-Jeghers syndrome. Prognosis is extremely poor for adolescent patients with colorectal carcinoma because of the common spread of these tumors at the time of diagnosis (Donaldson et al., 1971). Abdominal pain, bloody stools, melena, anorexia, and weight loss are common presenting symptoms. Radiologic features of carcinoma are similar to those in adults (Ruderman, 1960). Gross bowel wall deformity, mucosal irregularity, and luminal narrowing are seen (Figure 10–93) on double-contrast barium enema. Computed tomography is performed for staging of disease.

Carcinoid

Most carcinoid tumors in children occur in the appendix and are benign. Colonic carcinoids are less

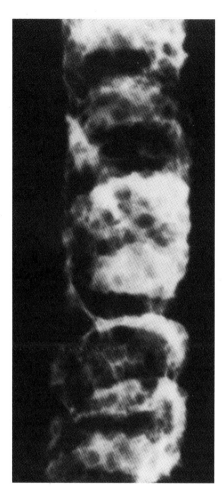

FIGURE 10–91. Gardner syndrome. There are multiple small polypoid filling defects throughout the large bowel as shown on this spot film from a barium enema.

Lymphoma

Lymphoma is the most common primary malignant tumor of the intestine in children (Rosenberg et al., 1958). Lymphoma of the large bowel is far less common than that of the small bowel. The radiographic, ultrasonographic, and CT appearances are similar to disease in the small intestine (see Chapter 9). Enema examination may show an "apple core" lesion (Figure 10–95).

Miscellaneous Malignant Large Bowel Tumors

Leimyosarcoma, an exceptionally rare malignant large bowel tumor, has been reported as early as infancy. Infants can present with intussusception or perforation (Elshafie, Spitz, and Ikeda, 1971; Ein, Beck, and Allen, 1979). As the tumor is initially of only low-grade malignancy and appears to differen-

common in children than adults (Scott, 1973; Suster, Weinberg, and Graiver, 1977; La Ferla et al., 1984) and infrequently metastasize (Chow et al., 1982). Intestinal carcinoid may present as a lead point of an intussusception or a mass lesion. Symptoms of appendiceal carcinoid may mimic those of acute appendicitis. Rarely, serotonin-producing liver metastases result in the carcinoid syndrome, characterized by diarrhea, crampy abdominal pain, skin flushing, and bronchoconstriction. These functioning neoplasms are extremely rare in children.

Ultrasonography may show a focal mass lesion originating in the bowel wall (Figure 10–94A). Computed tomography can show the regional extent of the lesion as well as evaluate for distant metastases (Figures 10–94B, C, D).

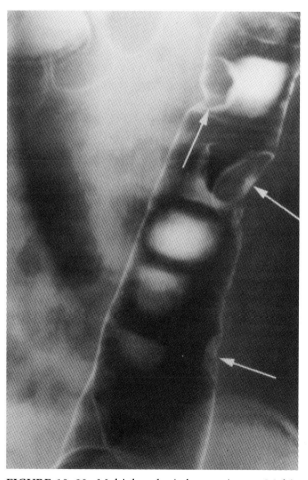

FIGURE 10–92. Multiple colonic hemangiomas. Multiple smooth sessile polyps are in the descending colon on a double-contrast barium enema in a child with hemangiomas elsewhere in the body.

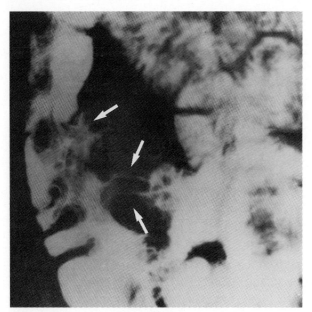

FIGURE 10–93. Carcinoma of the colon in a child with Bloom's syndrome. Single-contrast barium enema shows deformity of the cecum and terminal ileum (*arrows*). A large carcinoma was resected. Bloom's syndrome predisposes to tumors.

tiate with age, the prognosis is reported to be good (Ein, Beck, and Allen, 1979).

MUCOCELE OF THE APPENDIX

Mucocele of the appendix is relatively uncommon, occurring in approximately 0.25% of appendectomy patients (Woodruff and McDonald, 1940). This lesion affects primarily adults, but it can present in young teenagers (Dachman, Lichenstein, and Friedman, 1985). Patients may be asymptomatic, although 50% present with a palpable mass. The ratio of benign to malignant varieties is approximately 10 to 1. Inflammatory scarring or fecalith obstructs the appendiceal lumen in the benign form whereas a primary mucous cystadenoma or cystadenocarcinoma is present in the malignant form. Rupture in the malignant form can result in pseudomyxoma peritoneii, a condition seen exclusively in adult patients.

Ultrasonographically, mucoceles typically appear as large, hypoechoic, well-defined right lower-quadrant cystic masses with variable internal echogenicity, wall thickness, and calcification. Internal echoes may represent cellular material, crystals, or protein macroaggregates (Dachman, Lichenstein, and Friedman, 1985; Thurber et al., 1979).

Contrast enema may show failure of appendiceal filling or evidence of a well-defined appendiceal mass.

MALAKOPLAKIA OF THE LARGE BOWEL

Malakoplakia is a chronic inflammatory condition likely related to *Escherichia coli* infection. Although it primarily involves the urinary tract, malakoplakia may affect the large bowel in children (Akhtar et al., 1982). Symptoms include abdominal pain, diarrhea, rectal bleeding, and fever. Perianal and cutaneous fistulae, abscess, mucosal ulceration, and polyps may be seen. Double-contrast barium enema may show a nonspecific colitis with any of the above features (Radin, Chandrasoma, and Halls, 1984). The histologic finding of Michaelis-Gutmann bodies within macrophages establishes the diagnosis (Akhtar et al., 1982).

TRAUMA TO THE LARGE BOWEL

Bowel rupture is an uncommon injury following trauma in children. Blunt force injury is a more common cause of bowel rupture than perforating trauma in children. Most post-traumatic bowel ruptures occur in restrained children involved in motor vehicle crashes and demonstrate linear ecchymoses across the lower abdomen or flank (Sivit et al., 1991; Taylor and Eggli, 1988). These ecchymoses are in the pattern of the lap belt and have thus been described as "lap-belt" ecchymoses. Most injuries occur in the middle to distal small bowel. The most common site of bowel rupture is the jejunum (Sivit et al., 1991). Colonic injuries are extremely rare and are seen more commonly following penetrating injury due to gunshot or knife wounds.

Clinical findings suggestive of bowel rupture include rebound tenderness, rigidity, guarding, and absent bowel sounds. However, these findings are only present in approximately one-third of patients (Burney et al., 1983). Additionally, the appearance of these findings is often delayed for several hours following the injury.

Computed tomography is the primary modality for the evaluation of children following blunt abdominal trauma. The diagnosis of bowel rupture by CT can be challenging. The two pathognomonic findings on CT for bowel rupture are extraluminal air and extravasation of oral contrast medium. However, neither of these findings are commonly seen. The most frequent CT findings associated with bowel rupture are moderate to large amounts of unexplained peritoneal fluid and abnormally intense bowel wall enhancement (Sivit, Eichelberger, and Taylor, 1994). Additional findings include bowel dilatation, bowel wall thickening, focal hematoma surrounding a bowel loop (Figure 10–96), and infiltration of mesenteric fat (Sivit et al., 1991).

Colonic perforation has also been reported during a therapeutic contrast enema for intestinal intussusception. Perforation has been reported to occur in less than 1% of reduction attempts (Humphry, Ein, and Mok, 1981). It has been shown in an animal model that there is less fecal spillage and peritoneal contamination if colonic perforation occurs during an air enema rather than a liquid contrast enema (Shiels et al., 1993).

Rectal perforation has been reported in neonates after the use of a rectal thermometer or the placement of a rectal catheter for the performance of a contrast enema. Rectal perforation has also been reported as complicating physical examination

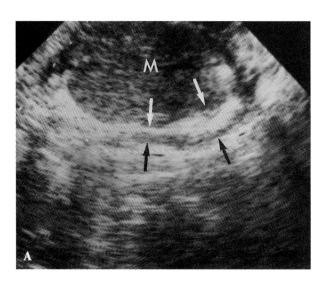

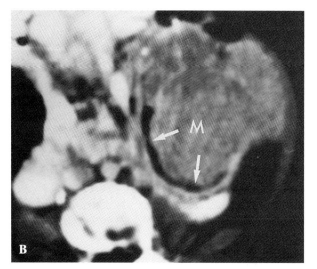

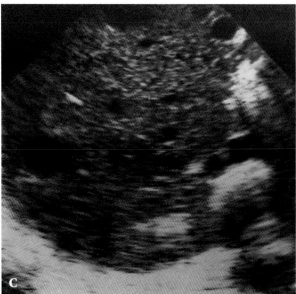

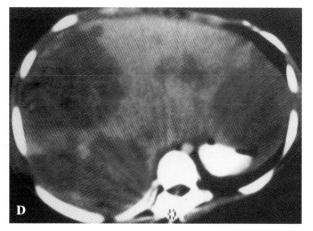

FIGURE 10–94. Malignant carcinoid of the colon. *A,* Ultrasonography shows a mass lesion (M) with a hyperechoic rim (white arrows), outside of which is a hypoechoic layer (black arrows) indicating the origin of the mass in the bowel wall. The hyperechoic line is the mucosa, which is distorted by the encroaching mass; the hypoechoic line is the muscular layer. *B,* Computed tomography demonstrates the mass (M), involving the bowel wall and projecting into the bowel lumen (arrows). *C,* Follow-up longitudinal US through the liver shows multiple hypoechoic metastases. *D,* Follow-up CT shows the metastases as well-defined areas of low attenuation.

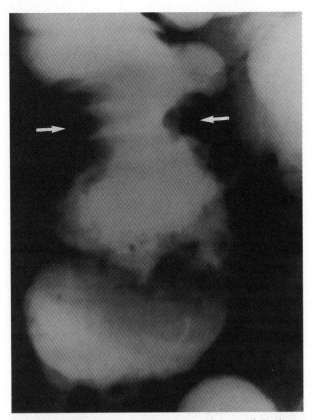

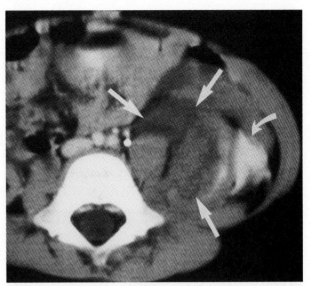

FIGURE 10–96. Colonic rupture. Computed tomographic scan through the abdomen in a child injured while sledding shows a hematoma (*between straight arrows*) in the left midabdomen in the expected location of the descending colon. Also note the high-density material (*curved arrow*) immediately lateral to the clot, representing IV contrast extravasation due to associated active hemorrhage.

FIGURE 10–95. Non-Hodgkin's lymphoma of the large bowel. Single-contrast barium enema demonstrates a mass lesion causing an "apple core" deformity on the ascending colon (*arrows*). This is associated with irregularity of the mucosa giving irregular projections indenting into the lumen.

of the rectum and anus (Fonkalsrud and Clatworthy, 1965). Rectal perforations may be intraperitoneal or extraperitoneal. The peritoneal membrane covers the anterior and lateral aspects of the rectum at the level of the third sacral segment. A rectal laceration above the peritoneal reflection can result in either peritoneal or extraperitoneal extravasation of bowel contents, while a laceration below the peritoneal reflection will be extraperitoneal.

MISCELLANEOUS DISORDERS OF THE LARGE BOWEL

Volvulus

Volvulus of the colon is rare in children. In general, malfixation, dilatation, and distention predispose to bowel volvulus. Partial midgut rotation with a high, mobile cecum may result in cecal volvulus (Snyder

and Chaffin, 1954). Volvulus has also been reported with nonrotation (Berger et al., 1982), aerophagia (Figure 10–97) (Trillis et al., 1986), pseudo-obstruction (Reinarz et al., 1985), asplenia, the so-called Ivemark syndrome (Markowitz, Shashikumar, and Capitanio, 1977), distal bowel stricture, or tumor (Martin, 1944; Lapin et al., 1973). Volvulus is reportedly more common in the institutionalized or mentally-retarded (see Figure 10–97) (Cuderman et al., 1971; Black and Cox, 1984). Males are affected more often than females (Anderson and Eklof, 1981; Allen and Nordstrom, 1964).

Conventional radiography may show intestinal obstruction, with the dilated cecum displaced to the midabdomen. The diagnosis can be confirmed by contrast enema. Enema will show tapering of the bowel lumen at the site of volvulus, an appearance likened to a bird's beak (see Figures 10–97C and 10–26).

Sigmoid volvulus is also quite rare in children and is related to a congenital abnormality of the sigmoid mesentery. Plain-film radiography may show a focal dilated loop coursing from the left lower quadrant to the right upper quadrant. Contrast enema will demonstrate the characteristic spiral torsion and may permit a therapeutic untwisting (Allen and Nordstrom, 1964) (see Figure 10–26).

Diverticulosis

Intrinsic weakness of the colonic wall, as occurs in Ehlers-Danlos or Marfan syndromes, predisposes to diverticulum formation at a young age. The adult type of diverticulosis is rare in children (Rees and Griffin, 1977). Rarely, small diverticula may be seen in teenagers, but they appear to be of little significance in this age group (Figure 10–98).

Cystic Fibrosis

Gastrointestinal manifestations of cystic fibrosis are common, occurring in 85 to 90% of patients (Park and Grand, 1981). The major intestinal complications are the result of partial or complete obstruction of the intestinal lumen. Obstruction may occur in utero or at any time during the patient's life. Recognized complications include meconium ileus, distal intestinal obstruction syndrome, intussusception, appendicitis, rectal prolapse, Crohn disease, and fibrosing colonopathy (Pickhardt, Yagan, and Siegel, 1998).

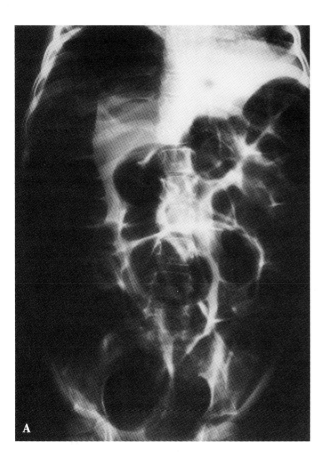

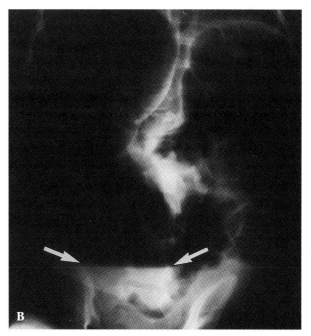

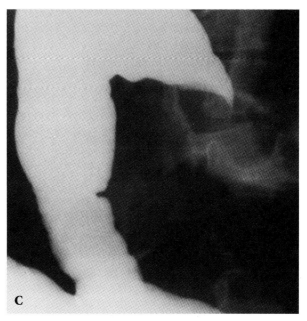

FIGURE 10–97. Volvulus of the large bowel. *A,* Plain film shows gross chronic aerophagia in a mentally retarded child. *B,* Plain film on acute admission with vomiting showed a very large dilated air-filled loop of bowel with an air-fluid level (*arrow*). *C,* Barium demonstrated a "bird of prey" deformity at the rectosigmoid junction.

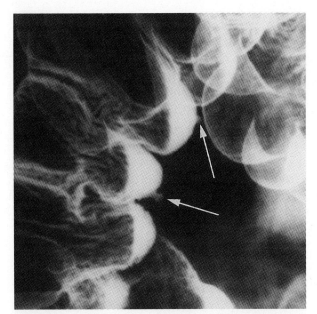

FIGURE 10–98. Small colonic diverticulum. There is a tiny diverticulum projecting from the medial aspect of the cecum. One of the authors (D. Stringer) has seen three older teenagers with this condition, and in none of the three was it felt to be clinically significant.

Meconium ileus, the earliest manifestation of cystic fibrosis, occurs in 10 to 15% of patients. In uncomplicated meconium ileus, nonsurgical relief of obstruction may be achieved with water-soluble hypertonic enema (see Chapter 3).

Children with cystic fibrosis who present with abdominal pain often have nonspecific clinical findings and are frequently referred for radiologic evaluation. Distal intestinal obstruction syndrome (DIOS) is characterized by fecal impaction in the distal ileum and proximal colon. Inspissated stool results from tenacious mucus production and steatorrhea (Hanly and Fitzgerald, 1983). Most patients have pancreatic insufficiency and require pancreatic enzyme replacement therapy. Disordered intestinal motility may also contribute to the occurrence of this condition. In most cases, the colon is involved with DIOS (Weinstein, Clemett, and Herkovic, 1968). Prevalence of DIOS is high in the second and third decades, but it is seen in only 2% of children under 5 years of age (Koletzko et al., 1989; Anderson et al., 1990). Crampy abdominal pain (often localized to the right lower quadrant), constipation, and a palpable mass are common presenting signs.

Conventional radiography assesses the degree of fecal impaction (Figure 10–99). Typically, stool is noted in the right lower quadrant, with or without evidence for bowel obstruction. A cobblestone appearance of the colonic mucosa may be seen on barium enema examination with a cornflakes pattern on double-contrast study (Figure 10–100) (Berk and Lee, 1973; Grossman, Berdon, and Baker, 1966). The finding on CT of diffuse colonic thickening has been reported in distal intestinal obstruction syndrome (Moody et al., 1990).

Treatment is usually medical and includes oral or enema administration of mucolytic agents such as acetylcysteine, water-soluble contrast such as diatrizoate sodium, and/or polyethylene glycol solutions. Surgical intervention is reserved for complications such as irreducible intussusception.

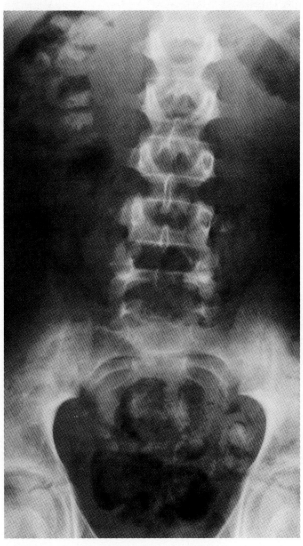

FIGURE 10–99. Cystic fibrosis. There is much fecal residue throughout the large bowel.

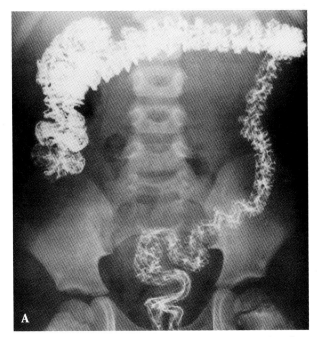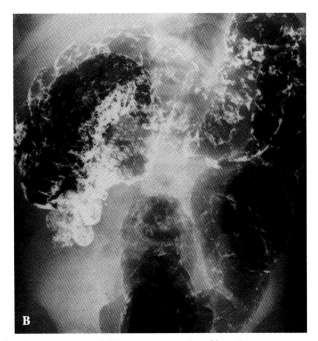

FIGURE 10–100. Cystic fibrosis. *A*, Barium coating the redundant mucosa of this postevacuation film gives a pattern similar to that of the jejunum. *B*, Insufflated air gives the so called "cornflakes" pattern of floculated barium.

The differential diagnosis of colonic disease in patients with cystic fibrosis includes fibrosing colonopathy, a condition first described in 1994 by Smyth and colleagues (Smyth, van Velzin, and Smyth, 1994). Colonic fibrosis affects the submucosa and lamina propria; inflammatory changes and intestinal obstruction characterize the disease. Patients at highest risk are those younger than 10 years of age who have been treated with high daily doses of pancreatic enzyme supplements (Campbell, Forrest, and Musgrove, 1994). Patients may present with evidence of obstruction and bloody diarrhea. Contrast enema findings include nodularity of the colonic wall, focal or long-segment narrowing and longitudinal shortening of the colon (Zerin et al., 1995). Proximal colonic wall thickening without stricture, pericolonic fat proliferation, and mesenteric infiltration are additional CT findings of colonic disease reported with cystic fibrosis patients who do not have infectious colitis or inflammatory bowel disease (Pickhardt, Yagan, and Siegel, 1998).

Rectal prolapse occurs in about 20% of patients and may be the first manifestation of cystic fibrosis (Kopelman, 1991). It is usually recurrent in the first few years of life and spontaneously resolves by 5 years of age, rarely requiring surgical intervention.

REFERENCES

EMBRYOGENESIS OF THE COLON

Gray SW, Skandalakis JE. Embryology for surgeons: the embryological basis for the treatment of congenital defects. Philadelphia: WB Saunders; 1972. p. 187–90.

Moore KL. The developing human. Philadelphia: WB Saunders; 1982. p. 239–54.

ANATOMY OF THE LARGE BOWEL

Cole FM. Innominate grooves of the colon: morphological characteristics and etiologic mechanisms. Radiology 1978;128:41–3.

Hopper KD, Sherman JL, Luethke JM, et al. The retrorenal colon in the supine and prone patient. Radiology 1987;162:443–6.

Mascatello V, Lebowitz RL. Malposition of the colon in left renal agenesis and ectopia. Radiology 1976;120:371–6.

Miller M, Stringer DA, Chui-Mei T, et al. Lymphoid follicular pattern in the colon: an indicator of barium coating. Can Assoc Radiol J 1987;38:256–8.

Silverman PM, Kelvin FM, Korobkin M. Lateral displacement of the right kidney by the colon: an anatomic variation demonstrated by CT. AJR 1983;140:313–4.

Lymphoid Follicular Pattern/Lymphoid Hyperplasia of the Large Bowel

Capitanio MA, Kirkpatrick JA. Lymphoid hyperplasia of the colon in children. Radiology 1970;94:323–7.

Kenney PJ, Koehler RE, Shackelford GD. The clinical significance of large lymphoid follicles of the colon. Radiology 1982;142:41–6.

Laufer I, de Sa D. Lymphoid follicular pattern: a normal feature of the pediatric colon. AJR 1978;130:51–5.

Miller M, Stringer DA, Chui-Mei T, et al. Lymphoid follicular pattern in the colon: an indicator of barium coating. Can Assoc Radiol J 1987;38:256–8.

Wolfson JJ, Goldstein G, Krivit W, et al. Lymphoid hyperplasia of the large intestine associated with dysgammaglobulinemia. AJR 1970;108:610–4.

Atresia and Stenosis of the Large Bowel

Bley WR, Franken EA Jr. Roentgenology of colon atresia. Pediatr Radiol 1973;1:105–8.

Coran AG, Eraklis AJ. Atresia of the colon. Surgery 1969;65:828–31.

Freeman NV. Congenital atresia and stenosis of the colon. Br J Surg 1966;53:595–9.

Lee CM, MacMillan GB. Rupture of the bowel in the newborn infant. Surgery 1950;28:48–66.

Manzano C, Barrero JL. Stenosis of the colon. Pediatr Radiol 1977;5:148–53.

Staple TW, McAllister WH. Perforation of an atretic colon during barium enema examination. AJR 1967;101:325–8.

Winters WD, Weinberger E, Hatch EI. Atresia of the colon in neonates: radiographic findings. AJR 1992;159:1273–6.

Anorectal Malformations

Anderson S, Savader B, Barnes J, Savader S. Enterolithiasis with imperforate anus. Report of two cases with sonographic demonstration and occurrence in a female. Pediatr Radiol 1988;18:130–3.

Berdon WE, Baker DH, Santulli TV, et al. The radiologic evaluation of imperforate anus: an approach correlated with current surgical concepts. Radiology 1968;90:466–71.

Berdon WE, Baker DH, Wigger HJ, et al. Calcified intraluminal meconium in newborn males with imperforate anus: enterolithiasis in the newborm. AJR 1975;125:449–55.

Berdon WE, Hochberg B, Baker DH, et al. The association of lumbosacral spine and genitourinary anomalies with imperforate anus. AJR 1966;98:181–91.

Cremin BJ. The radiological assessment of anorectal anomalies. Clin Radiol 1971;22:239–50.

Currarino G, Coln D, Votteler T. Triad of anorectal, sacral, and presacral anomalies. AJR 1981;137:395–8.

Currarino G, Votteler T, Kirks DR. Anal agenesis with rectobulbar fistula. Radiology 1978;126:457–61.

Donaldson JS, Black CT, Reynolds M, et al. Ultrasound of the distal pouch in infants with imperforate anus. J Pediatr Surg 1989;24:465–8.

Duhamel B. From the mermaid to anal imperforation: the syndrome of caudal regression. Arch Dis Child 1961; 36:152–5.

Felman AH, Walker RD, Donnelly WH, et al. Supralevator imperforate anus with unusual associated anomalies: colonic ureteral ectopy, intraluminal calcified meconium. Pediatr Radiol 1975;3:78–80.

Gupta AK, Bhargava S, Rohtagi M. Anal agenesis with recto-bulbar fistula. Pediatr Radiol 1986;16:222–4.

Kirks DR, Merten DF, Filston HC, et al. The Currarino triad: complex of anorectal malformation, sacral bony abnormality, and presacral mass. Pediatr Radiol 1984; 14:220–5.

Khoda E, Fujioka M, Ikawa H, Yokoyama J. Congenital anorectal anomaly: CT evaluation. Radiology 1985;157: 349–52.

Kurlander GJ. Roentgenology of imperforate anus. AJR 1967;100:190–201.

Mezzacappa PM, Price AP, Haller JO. MR and CT demonstration of levator sling in congenital anorectal anomalies. J Comput Assist Tomogr 1987;11(2):273–5.

Morgan CL, Grossman H, Novak R. Imperforate anus and colon calcification in association with the prune belly syndrome. Pediatr Radiol 1978;7:19–21.

Murugasu JJ. A new method of roentgenological demonstration of anorectal anomalies. Surgery 1970;68:706–12.

Oppenheimer DA, Carroll BA, Shochat SJ. Sonography of imperforate anus. Radiology 1983;148:127–8.

Pouillaude JM, Meyer P, Tran Minh V, et al. Enterolithiasis in two neonates with oesophageal and anorectal atresia. Pediatr Radiol 1987;17:419–21.

Quan L, Smith DW. The VATER association: vertebral defects, anal atresia, tracheoesophageal fistula with esophageal atresia, radial dysplasia. Birth Defects 1972; 8:75–8.

Quan L, Smith DW. The VATER association: [V]ertebral defects, [A]nal atresia, [T-E] fistula with esophageal atresia, [R]adial and [R]enal dysplasia: a spectrum of associated defects. J Pediatr 1973;82:104–7.

Santulli TV, Schullinger JN, Kiesewetter WB, et al. Imperforate anus: a survey from the members of the surgical section of the American Academy of Pediatrics. J Pediatr Surg 1971;6:484–7.

Sato Y, Pringle KC, Bergman RA, et al. Congenital anorectal anomalies: MR imaging. Radiology 1988; 168:157–62.

Seibert JJ, Golladay ES. Clinical evaluation of imperforate anus: clue to type of anorectal anomaly. AJR 1979;133: 289–92.

Selke AC, Cowley CE. Calcified intraluminal meconium in a female infant with imperforate anus. AJR 1978;130:786–8.

Thompson W, Grossman H. The association of spinal and genitourinary abnormalities with low anorectal anomalies (imperforate anus) in female infants. Radiology 1974;113:693–8.

Wagner ML, Harberg J, Kumar M, et al. The evaluation of imperforate anus utilizing percutaneous injection of water soluble iodide contrast media. Pediatr Radiol 1973;1:34–40.

Duplications of the Large Bowel

Barr LL, Hayden CK, Stansberry SD, et al. Enteric duplication cysts in children: are their ultrasonographic wall characteristics diagnostic? Pediatric Radiol 1990;20:326–8.

Campbell WL, Wolff M. Retrorectal cysts of developmental origin. AJR 1973;117:307–13.

Gross RE, Holcomb GW, Farber S. Duplications of the alimentary tract. Pediatrics 1952;9:449–67.

Kangarloo H, Sample WF, Hansen G, et al. Ultrasonic evaluation of abdominal gastrointestinal tract duplication in children. Radiology 1979;131:191–4.

Kottra JJ, Dodds WJ. Duplication of the large bowel. AJR 1971;113:310–5.

Ramsewak W, Milward S, Toi A, et al. CT guided percutaneous decompression of a rectal duplication cyst in a child. Can Assoc Radiol J 1986;37:46–7.

Sonada N, Matsuzaki S, Ono A, et al. Duplication of the caecum in a neonate simulating intussusception. Pediatr Radiol 1985;15:427–8.

Weber HM, Dixon CF. Duplication of entire large intestine (colon duplex): report of a case. AJR 1946;55:319–24.

Yucesan S, Zorludemir V, Olcay I. Complete duplication of the colon. J Pediatr Surg 1986;21:962–3.

FUNCTIONAL DISORDERS OF THE LARGE BOWEL

Berdon WE, Baker DH. The roentgenographic diagnosis of Hirschsprung disease in infancy. AJR 1965;93:432–46.

Berman CZ. Roentgenographic manifestations of congenital megacolon (Hirschsprung disease) in early infancy. Pediatrics 1956;18:227–38.

Bill AH Jr, Chapman ND. The enterocolitis of Hirschsprung disease. Am J Surg 1962;103:70–4.

Blane CE, Elhalaby E, Coran AG. Enterocolitis following endorectal pull through procedure in children with Hirschsprung disease. Pediatr Radiol 1994;24:164–6.

Bloom DA, Buonome C, Fishman SJ. Allergic colitis: a mimic of Hirschsprung disease. Pediatr Radiol 1999;29: 37–41.

Campbell JB, Robinson AE. Hirschsprung disease presenting as calcified fecaloma. Pediatr Radiol 1973;1:161–3.

Chatten J, Voorhess ML. Familial neuroblastoma. N Engl J Med 1967;277:1230–6.

Cremin BJ. The early diagnosis of Hirschprung's disease. Pediatr Radiol 1974;2:23–8.

Davis WS, Allen RP. Conditioning value of the plain film examination in the diagnosis of neonatal Hirschsprung disease. Radiology 1969;93:129–33.

de Bruyn R, Hall CM, Spitz L. Hirschsprung's disease and malrotation of the mid gut. An uncommon association. Br J Radiol 1982;55:554–7.

deCampo JF, Mayne V, Boldt DW, et al. Radiological findings in total aganglionosis coli. Pediatr Radiol 1984; 14:205–9.

Demos TC, Blonder J, Schey WL, et al. Multiple endocrine neoplasia (MEN) syndrome. Type IIB: gastrointestinal manifestations. AJR 1983;140:73–8.

Farndon PA, Bianchi A. Waardenburg's syndrome associated with total aganglionosis. Arch Dis Child 1983;58:932–3.

Fletcher DB, Yulish BS. Intraluminal calcifications in the small bowel of newborn infants with total colinic aganglionosis. Radiology 1978;126:451–5.

Fraser GC, Berry C. Mortality in neonatal Hirschsprung disease: with particular reference to enterocolitis. J Pediatr Surg 1967;2:205–11.

Gaisie G, Oh KS, Young LW. Coexistent neuroblastoma and Hirschsprung disease—Another manifestation of the neurocristopathy? Pediatr Radiol 1979;8:161–3.

Hassinger DD, Mulvihill JJ, Chandler JB. Aarskog's syndrome with Hirschsprung disease, midgut malrotation and dental anomalies. J Med Genet 1980;17:235–7.

Hope JW, Borns PF, Berg PK. Roentgenologic manifestations of Hirschsprung disease in infancy. AJR 1965;96:217–29.

Johnson JF, Cronk RL. The pseudotransition zone in long segment Hirschsprung disease. Pediatr Radiol 1980;10:87–9.

Johnson JF, Dean BF. Hirschsprung disease coexisting with colonic atresia. Pediatr Radiol 1981;11:97–8.

Krishnamurthy S, Schuffler MD. Pathology of neuromuscular disorders of the small intestine and colon. Gastroenterology 1987;93:610–39.

Leonidas JC, Krasna IH, Strauss L, et al. Roentgen appearance of the excluded colon after colostomy for infantile Hirschsprung disease. AJR 1971;112:116–22.

Mahboubi S, Templeton JM. Association of Hirschprung's disease and imperforate anus in a patient with "cat-eye" syndrome. Pediatr Radiol 1984;14:441–2.

Martin LW, Buchino JJ, LeCoutre C, et al. Hirschprung's disease with skip area (segmental aganglionosis). J Pediatr Surg 1979;14:686–7.

McDonald RG, Evans WA Jr. Hirschsprung disease—roentgen diagnosis in infants. Am J Dis Child 1954;87:575–85.

Newman B, Nussbaum A, Kirkpatrick JA Jr. Bowel perforation in Hirschsprung disease. AJR 1987;148:1195–7.

O'Donovan AN, Habra G, Somers S, et al. Bowel perforation. AJR 1996 Aug; 167(2):517–20.

Pocharzevsky R, Leonidas JC. The "rectosigmoid index"—a measurement for the early diagnosis of Hirschsprung disease. AJR 1977;123:770–7.

Rashkow JE, Haller JO, Berdon WE, Sane SM. Hirschsprungs disease, Ondine's curse and neuroblastoma—manifestations of neurocristopathy. Pediatr Radiol 1988;19:45–9.

Rosenfield NS, Ablow RC, Markowitz RI, et al. Hirschsprung disease: accuracy of the barium enema examination. Radiology 1984;150:393–400.

Saperstein L, Pollack J, Beck R. Total intestinal aganglionosis. M Sinai J Med 1980;47:72–3.

Schey WL, White H. Hirschsprung's disease. Problems in the roentgen interpretation. AJR 1971;112:105–15.

Shocket E, Teloh HA. Aganglionic megacolon, pheochromocytoma, megaloureter, and neurofibroma. Am J Dis Child 1957;94:185–91.

Siegel MJ, Shackelford GD, McAlister WH. The rectosigmoid index. Radiology 1981;139:497–9.

Tamburrini O, Iuri AB-D, Palescandolo P, et al. Hirschsprung's disease and asymptomatic malrotation: a rare association. Pediatr Radiol 1986;16:250–1.

Taxman TL, Yulish BS, Rothstein FC. How useful is the barium enema in the diagnosis of infantile Hirschsprung disease? Am J Dis Child 1986;140(9):881–4.

Neonatal Functional Immaturity of the Large Bowel

Berdon WE, Slovis TL, Campbell JB, et al. Neonatal small left colon syndrome: its relationship to aganglionosis and meconium plug syndrome. Radiology 1977;125:457–62.

Davis WS, Allen RP, Favara BE, et al. Neonatal small left colon syndrome. AJR 1974;120:322–9.

Davis WS, Campbell JB. Neonatal small left colon syndrome. Am J Dis Child 1975;129:1024–7.

Falterman CG, Richardson CJ. Small left colon syndrome associated with maternal ingestion of psychotropic drugs. J Pediatr 1980;97:308–10.

Le Quesne GW, Reilly BJ. Functional immaturity of the large bowel in the newborn infant. Radiol Clin North Am 1975;13:331–42.

Nixon GW, Condon VR, Stewart DR. Intestinal perforation as a complication of the neonatal small left colon syndrome. AJR 1975;125:75–80.

Philippart AI, Reed JO, Georgeson KE. Neonatal small left colon syndrome: intramural not intraluminal obstruction. J Pediatr Surg 1975;10:733–40.

Sokal MM, Koenigsberger MR, Rose JS, et al. Neonatal hypermagnesemia and the meconium plug syndrome. N Engl J Med 1972;286:823–5.

Microcolon of Prematurity

Amodio J, Berdon WE, Abramson S, et al. Microcolon of prematurity: a form of functional obstruction. AJR 1986; 146:239–44.

Megacystis-Microcolon–Intestinal Hypoperistalsis Syndrome

Berdon WE, Baker DH, Blanc WA, et al. Megacystis-microcolon-intestinal hypoperistalsis syndrome: a new cause of intestinal obstruction in the newborn. Report of radiologic findings in five newborn girls. AJR 1976;126:957–64.

Krook PM. Megacystis-microcolon-intestinal hypoperistalsis syndrome in a male infant. Radiology 1980;136:649–50.

Patel R, Carty H. Megacystis-microcolon-intestinal hypoperistalsis syndrome: a rare cause of intestinal obstruction in the newborn. Br J Radiol 1980;53:249–52.

Young LW, Yunis EJ, Girdany BR, et al. Megacystis-microcolon-intestinal hypoperistalsis syndrome: additional clinical, radiologic, surgical, and histopathologic aspects. AJR 1981;137:749–55.

FUNCTIONAL CONSTIPATION

Bentley JFR. Constipation in infants and children. Gut 1971;12:85–90.

Davidson M, Bauer CH. Studies of distal colonic motility in children. IV. Achalasia of the distal rectal segment despite presence of ganglia in the myenteric plexuses of this area. Pediatrics 1958;21:746–60.

Kottmeier PK, Clatworthy HW. Aganglionic and functional megacolon in children—a diagnostic dilemma. Pediatrics 1965;36:572–82.

Meunier P, Mollard P, Marechal J-M. Physiopathology of megarectum: the association of megarectum with encopresis. Gut 1976;17:224–7.

Patriquin H, Martelli H, Devroede G. Barium enema in chronic constipation: is it meaningful? Gastroenterology 1978;75:619–22.

Shopfner CE. Urinary tract pathology associated with constipation. AJR 1968;90:865–77.

MISCELLANEOUS FUNCTIONAL OBSTRUCTION

Berman EJ, Ross C. Milk curd obstruction in six week old infants. J Pediatr Surg 1972;7:342–43.

Berman L, Briggs R, Thomas RM. Case report: ion-exchange resin bezoar in a neonate. Clin Radiol 1986; 37:297–8.

Cook RCM, Rickham PP. Neonatal intestinal obstruction due to milk curds. J Pediatr Surg 1969;4:599–605.

Cremin BJ. Functional intestinal obstruction in premature infants. Pediatr Radiol 1973;1:109–12.

Cremin BJ, Smythe PM, Cyrves S. The radiological appearance of the "inspissated milk syndrome;" a cause of intestinal obstruction in infants. Br J Radiol 1970;43:856–8.

Friedland GW, Rush WA, Hill AJ. Smythe's "inspissated milk" syndrome. Radiology 1972;103:159–61.

INFECTION AND INFLAMMATION OF THE LARGE BOWEL

Allen HA, Haney PJ. Left ventricular outflow obstruction and necrotizing enterocolitis. Radiology 1984;150:401–2.

Anderson DM, Kleigman RM. The relationship of neonatal alimentation practices to the occurrence of endemic necrotizing enterocolitis. Am J Perinatol 1991;8:62.

Ball TI, Wylx JB. Enterocyst formation: a late complication of neonatal necrotizing enterocolitis. AJR 1986; 147:806–8.

Bell MJ, Ternberg JL, Feigin RD, et al. Neonatal necrotizing enterocolitis. Therapeutic decisions based upon clinical staging. Ann Surg 1978;187:1–7.

Bell RS, Graham B, Stevenson JK. Roentgenologic and clinical manifestations of neonatal necrotizing enterocolitis. Experience with 43 cases. AJR 1971;112:123–34.

Berdon WE, Grossman H, Baker DH, et al. Necrotizing enterocolitis in the premature infant. AJR 1964;83:879–87.

Brown EG, Sweet AY. Neonatal necrotizing enterocolitis. Pediatr Clin N Am 1982;29:1149–70.

Caplan MS, Sun XM, Hsueh W, et al. Role of platelet activating factor and tumor necrosis factor alpha in neonatal necrotizing enterocolitis. J Pediatr 1990;116:960.

Cummins GE. Necrotising enterocolitis. Med J Aust 1977;1:376–8.

Daneman A, Woodward S, de Silva M. The radiology of neonatal necrotizing enterocolitis. A review of 47 cases and the literature. Pediatr Radiol 1978;7:70–7.

Dunn P. Intestinal obstruction in the newborn with special reference to transient functional ileus associated with respiratory distress syndrome. Arch Dis Child 1963;389:459.

Ein SH, Marshall DG, Girvan D. Peritoneal drainage under local anesthesia for perforations from necrotizing enterocolitis. J Pediatr Surg 1977;12:963–7.

Frey EE, Smith W, Franken EA, et al. Analysis of bowel perforation in necrotizing enterocolitis. Pediatr Radiol 1987;17:380–2.

Janik JS, Ein SH. Peritoneal drainage under local anesthesia for necrotizing enterocolitis (NEC) perforation: a second look. J Pediatr Surg 1980;15:565–7.

Janik JS, Ein SH, Mancer K. Intestinal stricture after necrotizing enterocolitis. J Pediatr Surg 1981;16:438–43.

Kleigman RM, Pittard WB, Fanaroff AA. Necrotizing enterocolitis in neonates fed human milk. J Pediatr 1979; 95:450–3.

Kodroff MB, Hartenberg MA, Goldschmidt RA. Ultrasonographic diagnosis of gangrenous bowel in neonatal necrotizing enterocolitis. Pediatr Radiol 1984;14:168–70.

Kogutt MS. Necrotizing entercolitis of infancy. Early roentgen patterns as a guide to prompt diagnosis. Radiology 1979;130:367–70.

Leonidas JC, Hall RT, Amoury RA. Critical evaluation of the roentgen signs of neonatal necrotizing enterocolitis. Ann Radiol 1976;19:123–32.

Leonidas JC, Krasna IH, Fox HA, et al. Peritoneal fluid in necrotizing enterocolitis: a radiologic sign of clinical deterioration. J Pediatr 1973;82:672–5.

Mata AG, Rosengart RM. Interobserver variability in the radiographic diagnosis of necrotizing enterocolitis. Pediatrics 1980;66:68–71.

Merritt CRB, Goldsmith JP, Sharp MJ. Sonographic detection of portal venous gas in infants with necrotizing enterocolitis. AJR 1984;143:1059–62.

Mizrahi A, Barlow O, Berdon W, et al. Necrotizing enterocolitis in premature infants. J Pediatr 1965;66:697–706.

Patriquin HB, Fisch CH, Bureau M, et al. Radiologically visible fecal gas patterns in "normal" newborns and young infants. Pediatr Radiol 1984;14:87–90.

Patton WL, Willmann JK, Lutz AM, et al. Worsening enterocolitis in neonates: diagnosis by CT examination of urine after enteral administration of iohexol. Pediatr Radiol 1999;29:95–9.

Santulli TV, Schullinger JN, Heird WC, et al. Acute necrotizing enterocolitis in infancy: a review of 64 cases. Pediatrics 1975;55:376–87.

Seibert JJ, Parvey LS. The telltale triangle: use of the supine cross-table lateral radiograph of the abdomen in early detection of pneumoperitoneum. Pediatr Radiol 1977;5:209–10.

Stevenson DK, Graham CB, Stevenson JK. Neonatal necrotizing enterocolitis: 100 new cases. Adv Pediatr 1980;27:319–40.

Uruy RD, Fanaroff AA, Korones SB, et al. Necrotizing enterocolitis in very low birth weight infants: biodemographic and clinical correlates. J Pediatr 1991;119:630.

Vernacchia FS, Jeffrey RB, Laing FC, Wing VW. Sonographic recognition of pneumatosis intestinalis. AJR 1985;145:51–2.

Virjee J, Somers S, de Sa D, et al. Changing patterns of neonatal necrotizing enterocolitis. Gastrointest Radiol 1979;4:169–75.

Wexler HA. The persistent loop sign in neonatal necrotizing enterocolitis: a new indication for surgical intervention? Radiology 1978;126:201–4.

Neutropenic Colitis

Frick MP, Maile CW, Crass JR, et al. Computed tomography of neutropenic colitis. AJR 1984;143:763–5.

Gomez L, Martino R, Rolston KV. Clin Infect Dis 1998; 27(4):695–9.

Kaste SC, Flynn PM, Furman WL. Acute lymphoblastic leukemia presenting with typhlitis. Med Pediatr Oncol 1997;28:209–12.

McNamara MJ, Chalmers AG, Morgan M, Smith SEW. Typhlitis in acute childhood leukemia: radiological features. Clin Radiol 1986;37:83–6.

Ojala AE, Lanning FP, Lanning BM. Abdominal ultrasound findings during and after treatment of childhood

acute lymphoblastic leukemia. Med Pediatr Oncol 1997;
29:266–71.

Sloas MM, Flynn PM, Kaste SC, Patrick CC. Typhlitis in
children with cancer: a 30 year experience. Clin Infect Dis
1993;17:484–90.

Ulcerative Colitis
Bank ER, White SJ, Coran G. The radiographic appearance of the endorectal pull-through. Pediatr Radiol 1986;
16:216–21.

Devroede GJ, Taylor WF, Sauer WG, et al. Cancer risk and
life expectancy of children with ulcerative colitis. N Engl
J Med 1971;285:17–21.

Ein SH. Five years of the pediatric Kock pouch. J Pediatr
Surg 1982;17:644–52.

Enzer NB, Hijmans JC. Ulcerative colitis beginning in
infancy: a report of 5 cases. J Pediatr 1963;63:437–43.

Kelts DG, Grand RJ. Inflammatory bowel disease in children and adolescents. Curr Probl Pediatr 1980;10:1–40.

Kremer PW, Scholz FJ, Schoetz DJ, et al. Radiology of the
ileoanal reservoir. AJR 1985;145:559–67.

McCaffery TD, Nasr K, Lawrence AM, et al. Severe growth
retardation in children with inflammatory bowel disease.
Pediatrics 1970;45:386–93.

Stringer DA, Sherman PM, Jakowenko N. Correlation of
double-contrast high-density barium enema, colonoscopy
and histology in children with special attention to disparities. Pediatr Radiol 1986;16:298–304.

Crohn Disease
Gardiner R, Stevenson GW. The colitides. Radiol Clin
North Am 1982;20:797–817.

Joffe N. Diffuse mucosal granularity in double-contrast
studies of Crohn disease of the colon. Clin Radiol 1981;
32:85–90.

Karjoo M, McCarthy B. Toxic megacolon of ulcerative
colitis in infancy. Pediatrics 1976;57:962–5.

Kelts DG, Grand RJ. Inflammatory bowel disease in children and adolescents. Curr Probl Pediatr 1980;10:1–40.

Miller RC, Larsen E. Regional enteritis in early infancy.
Am J Dis Child 1971;122:301–11.

Rubin S, Lambie RW, Chapman J. Regional ileitis in childhood. Am J Dis Child 1967;114:106–10.

Weedon DD, Shorter RG, Ilstrup DM, et al. Crohn disease
and cancer. N Engl J Med 1973;289:1099–1103.

Behçet Syndrome
Baba S, Maruta M, Ando K, et al. Intestinal Behçet disease:
report of five cases. Dis Colon Rectum 1976;19:428–40.

Goldstein SJ, Crooks DJM. Colitis in Behçet syndrome:
two new cases. Radiology 1978;128:321–3.

Kasahara Y, Tanada S, Nishino M, et al. Intestinal involvement in Behçet disease: Review of 136 surgical cases in
the Japanese literature. Dis Colon Rectum 1981;24:103–6.

Smith GE, Kime LR, Pitcher JL. The colitis of Behçet disease: a separate entity? Colonoscopic findings and literature review. Am J Dig Dis 1973;18:987–1000.

Stanley RJ, Tedesco FJ, Melson GL, et al. The colitis of
Behçet disease: a clinical radiographic correlation. Radiology 1975;114:603–4.

Stringer DA, Cleghorn GJ, Daneman A, et al. Behçet syndrome involving the gastrointestinal tract: a diagnostic
dilemma in childhood. Pediatr Radiol 1986;16:131–4.

Eosinophilic Colitis (Allergic Gastroenteropathy)
Moore D, Lichtman S, Lentz J, et al. Eosinophilic colitis presenting with iron deficiency anemia. Gut 1986;27:1219–22.

Stringer DA. Imaging inflammatory bowel disease in the
pediatric patient. Radiol Clin N Am 1987;25:93–113.

Teele RL, Katz AJ, Goldman H, et al. Radiographic features of eosinophilic gastroenteritis (allergic gastroenteropathy) of childhood. AJR 1979;132:575–80.

Infectious Colitides
Escherichia coli, Shigella, Salmonella

Goldberg MB, Robin RH. The spectrum of Salmonella
infection. Infect Dis Clin North Am 1988;2:571–98.

Riley LW, Remis RS, Helgerson SD, et al. Hemorrhagic
colitis associated with a rare *Escherichia coli* serotype. N
Engl J Med 1983;308:681–5.

Sperber SJ, Schleupner CJ. Salmonellosis during infection
with human immunodeficiency virus. Rev Infect Dis
1987;9:93–5

Campylobacter Colitis
Brodey PA, Fertig S, Aron JM. Campylobacter entericolitis: radiographic features. AJR 1982;139:1119–1201.

Dekeyser P, Gossuin-Detrain M, Butzlerl FP, et al. Acute enteritis due to related vibrio: first positive stool culture. J Infect Dis 1972;125:390–2.

Gardiner R. Infective enterocolitides. Radiol Clin North Am 1987;25:67–77.

Karmali MA, Tan YC. Neonatal campylobacter enteritis. Can Med Assoc J 1980;122:192–3.

Lambert ME, Tischler ME, Karmali MA, et al. Campylobacter ileocolitis: an inflammatory bowel disease. Can Med Assoc J 1979;121:1377–9.

Skirrow MB. Campylobacter enteritis: a "new" disease. BMJ 1977;2:9–11.

Tielbeek AV, Rosenbusch G, Muytjens HL, et al. Roentgenologic changes in the colon in *Campylobacter* infection. Gastrointest Radiol 1985;10:358–61.

Yersinia Colitis

Atkinson GO Jr, Gray BB Jr, Ball TI Jr, et al. *Yersinia enterocolitica* colitis in infants: radiographic changes. Radiology 1983;148:113–16.

Gardiner R, Stevenson GW. The colitides. Radiol Clin North Am 1982;20:797–817.

Kohl S, Jacobson JA, Nahmias A. *Yersinia enterocolitica* infections in children. J Pediatr 1976;89:77–9.

Puylaert JBCM. Mesenteric adenitis and acute terminal ileitis: US evaluation using graded compression. Radiology 1986;161:691–5.

Shrago G. *Yersinia enterocolitica* ileocolitis findings observed on barium examination. Br J Radiol 1976;49: 181–3.

Vantrappen G, Geboes K, Ponette E. Yersinia enteritis. Med Clin North Am 1982;66:639–53.

Amebic Colitis

Cardoso JM, Kimura K, Stoopen M, et al. Radiology of invasive amoebiasis of the colon. AJR 1977;128:935–41.

Clark RM, Frost PG. Fulminating necrotizing amebic colitis with perforation: case report and review. Can Meds Assoc J 1983;128:1424–7.

Gardiner R, Stevenson GW. The colitides. Radiol Clin North Am 1982;20:797–817.

Martinez CR, Gilman RH, Rabbani GH, et al. Amebic col-

itis: correlation of proctoscopy before treatment and barium enema after treatment. AJR 1982;138:1089–93.

Tuberculosis and Histoplasmosis

Carrera GF, Young S, Lewicki AM. Intestinal tuberculosis. Gastrointest Radiol 1976;1:147–55.

Downey DB, Nakielny RA. Aphthoid ulcers in colonic tuberculosis Br J Radiol 1985;58:561–2.

Friedland GW, Filly R. Intestinal tuberculosis in a child in an affluent society. Pediatr Radiol 1974;2:199–202.

Hamilton JR, Bruce GA, Abdourhaman M, et al. Inflammatory bowel disease in children and adolescents. Adv Pediatr 1979;26:311–41.

Hanson RD, Hunter TB. Tuberculous peritonitis: CT appearance. AJR 1985;144:931–2.

Pseudomembranous Colitis

Bartlett JG. Antibiotic associated diarrhea. Clin Infect Dis 1992;15:573–81.

Binkovitz LA, Allen E, Bloom D, et al. Atypical presentation of *Clostridium difficile* colitis in patients with cystic fibrosis. AJR 1999;172:517–21.

Blickman JG, Boland GWL, Cleveland RH, et al. Pseudomembranous colitis: CT findings in children. Pediatr Radiol 1995;25:157–9.

Boland GW, Lee MJ, Cats A, et al. Antibiotic induced diarrhea: specificity of abdominal CT for the diagnosis of *Clostridium difficile* disease. Radiology 1994a;191:103–6.

Boland GW, Lee MJ, Cats A, Muellero PR. Pseudomembranous colitis: diagnostic sensitivity of the abdominal plain radiograph. Clin Radiol 1994b;49:473–5.

Fishman EK, Kavura MK, Jones BJ, et al. Pseudomembraneous colitis: CT evaluation of 26 cases. Radiology 1991; 180:57–60.

Loughran CR, Tappin JA, Whitehouse GH. The plain abdominal radiograph in pseudomembranous colitis due to *Clostridium difficile*. Clin Radiol 1982;33:277–81.

Stanley RJ, Leland MG, Tedesco FJ, et al. Plain film findings in severe pseudomembranous colitis. Radiology 1976;118:7–11.

Tedesco FJ, Corless JK, Brownstein RE. Rectal sparing in antibiotic associated pseudomembranous colitis: a prospective study. Gastroenterology 1982;83:1259–60.

Miscellaneous Colitides

Hemolytic Uremic Syndrome

Bar-Ziv J, Ayoub JIG, Fletcher BD. Hemolytic-uremic syndrome: a case presenting with acute colitis. Pediatr Radiol 1974;2:203–6.

Kawanami T, Bowen A, Girdany BR. Enterocolitis: prodrome of the hemolytic-uremic syndrome. Radiology 1984;151:91–2.

Kelles A, VanDyck M, Proesmans W. Childhood haemolytic uraemic syndrome: long-term outcome and prognostic features. Eur J Pediatr 1994;153:38.

Kirks DR. The radiology of enteritis due to hemolytic-uremic syndrome. Pediatr Radiol 1982;12:179–83.

Peterson RB, Meseroll WP, Shrago GG, et al. Radiographic features of colitis associated with hemolytic-uremic syndrome. Radiology 1976;118:667–71.

Tocken ML, Campbell JR. Colitis in children with the hemolytic-uremic syndrome. J Pediatr Surg 1977;12: 213–19.

Ischemic Colitis

Anderson JF, Eklof O. Segmental vascular occlusion of the colon. A tentative diagnosis in two pediatric cases. Pediatric Radiology 1981;11:5–7.

Fan ST, Lan WY, Wong KK. Ischemic colitis in Kawasaki disease. J Pediatr Surg 1986;21:964–5.

Colitis of Hirschsprung Disease

Berger LA, Wilkinson D. The investigation of colitis in infancy. Pediatr Radiol 1974;2:145–54.

Bill AH Jr, Chapman ND. The enterocolitis of Hirschsprung disease: its natural history and treatment. Am J Surg 1962;103:70–4.

Hamilton JR, Bruce GA, Abdourhaman M, et al. Inflammatory bowel disease in children and adolescents. Adv Pediatr 1979;26:311–41.

Karjoo M, McCarthy B. Toxic megacolon of ulcerative colitis in infancy. Pediatrics 1976;57:962–5.

Allergic Colitis

Elhalaby EA, Coran AG, Blane CE, et al. Enterocolitis associated with Hirschsprung disease: a clinical radiological characterization based on 168 patients. J Pediatr Surg 1995;30:76–83.

Jenkins HR, Pincott JR, Soothill JF, et al. Food allergy: the major cause of infantile colitis. Arch Dis Child 1984; 59:326–9.

Kleinman RE. Cowmilk allergy in infancy and hypoallergenic formulas. J Pediatr 1992;121.

Odze RD, Wershil BK, Leichner AM. Allergic colitis in infants. J Pediatr 1995;126:163–70.

Odze RD, Bines J, Leichtner AM, et al. Allergic protocolitis in infants: a prospective clinical pathologic biopsy study. Human Pathol 1993;24:668–74.

Swischuk LE, Hayden CK. Barium enema findings (segmental colitis) in four neonates with bloody diarrhea—possible cow's milk allergy. Pediatr Radiol 1985;15:34–7.

Taylor GA. Cow's milk protein/soy protein allergy: gastrointestinal imaging. Radiology 1988;167:866.

Walker-Smith JA. Cow milk sensitivity enteropathy predisposing factors and treatment. J Pediatr 1992;121:111–5.

Detergent, Caustic, and Herb Enema Colitis

Kirchner SG, Buckspan GS, O'Neill JA, et al. Detergent enema: a cause of caustic colitis. Pediatr Radiol 1977;6: 141–6.

Segal I, Solomon A, Mirwis J. Radiological manifestations of ritual-enema-induced colitis. Clin Radiol 1981;32: 657–62.

Evanescent Colitis

Friedland GW, Filly R. Evanescent colitis in a child. Pediatr Radiol 1974;2:73–4.

ACUTE APPENDICITIS

Balthazar EJ, Birnbaum RA, Yee, J, et al. Acute appendicitis: CT and US correlation in 100 patients. Radiology 1994;190:31–5.

Ceres L, Alonso I, Lopez P, et al. Ultrasound study of acute appendicitis in children with emphasis upon the diagnosis of retrocecal appendicitis. Pediatr Radiol 1990;20:258–61.

Crady SK, Jones JS, Wyn T, et al. Clinical validity of ultrasound in children with suspected appendicitis. Ann Emerg Med 1993;22:1125–9.

Friedland JA, Siegel JA. CT appearance of acute appendicitis in childhood. AJR 1997;168:439–42.

Harrison MW, Lindner DJ, Campbell JR, et al. Acute appendicitis in children: factors affecting morbidity. Am J Surg 1984;147:605–10.

Jabra AA, Shalaby-Rana EI, Fishman EK. CT of appendicitis in children. J Comput Assist Tomogr 1997;21:661–6.

Janik JS, Firor HV. Pediatric appendicitis. A twenty year study of 1640 children at Cook County Hospital. Arch Surg 1979;114:717–19.

Jeffrey RB, Federle MP, Tolentino CS. Periappendiceal inflammatory masses: CT directed management and clinical outcome in 70 patients. Radiology 1988;167:13–16.

Lane MJ, Katz DS, Ross BA, et al. Unenhanced helical CT for suspected appendicitis. AJR 1997;168:405–9.

Lau W, Fan J, Viu T, et al. Negative findings at appendectomy. Am J Surg 1984;148:375–8.

Malone AJ, Wolf CR, Malmed AS, et al. Diagnosis of acute appendicitis: value of unenhanced CT. AJR 1993;160:763–6.

Marchildon MB, Dudgeon DL. Perforated appendicitis: Current experience in a pediatric hospital. Ann Surg 1977;185:84–7.

Puylaert JCBM. Acute appendicitis: US evaluation using graded compression. Radiology 1986;158:355–60.

Ramachandran P, Sivit CJ, Newman KD, et al. Ultrasonography as an adjunct in the diagnosis of acute appendicitis: a 4-year experience. J Pediatr Surg 1996;31:164–9.

Rao PM, Rhea JT, Novelline RA, et al. Helical CT technique for the diagnosis of appendicitis: prospective evaluation of a focused appendix CT examination. Radiology 1997;202:139–44.

Siegel MJ, Carel C, Surratt S. Ultrasonography of acute abdominal pain in children. JAMA 1991;266:1987–9.

Sivit CJ. Diagnosis of acute appendicitis in children: spectrum of sonographic findings. AJR 1996;161:147–52.

Sivit CJ, Newman KD, Boenning DA, et al. Appendicitis: usefulness of US in a pediatric population. Radiology 1992;185:549–52.

Vignault F, Filiatrault D, Brandt ML, et al. Acute appendicitis in children: evaluation with US. Radiology 1990;176:501–4.

Wong ML, Casey SO, Leonidas JC, et al. Sonographic diagnosis of acute appendicitis in children. J Pediatr Surg 1994;29:1356–60.

NEOPLASMS OF THE LARGE BOWEL

Juvenile Polyps

Cremin BJ, Louw JH. Polyps in the large bowel in children. Clin Radiol 1970;21:195–200.

Harned RK, Buck JL, Sobin LH. The hamartomatous polyposis syndromes: clinical and radiologic features. AJR 1995;164:565–71.

Kapetanakis AM, Vini D, Plitsis G. Solitary juvenile polyps in children and colon cancer. Hepatogastroenterology 1996;43(12):1530–1.

Morson BC, Dawson IMP. Gastrointestinal pathology. Oxford: Blackwell Scientific; 1972. p. 436–8.

Pillai RB, Tolia V. Colonic polyps in children: frequently multiple and recurrent. Clin Pediatr 1988;37:253–7.

Roth SI, Helwig EB. Juvenile polyps of the colon and rectum. Cancer 1963;16:468–79.

INHERITED HAMARTOMATOUS POLYPOSIS SYNDROMES

Juvenile Polyposis and Juvenile Polyposis of Infancy

Baert AL, Daele Mc-V, Brock J, et al. Generalized juvenile polyposis with pulmonary arteriovenous malformations and hypertrophic osteoarthropathy. AJR 1983;141:661–2.

Harned RK, Buck JL, Sobin LH. The hamartomatous polyposis syndromes: clinical and radiologic features. AJR 1995;164:571–656.

Ray JE, Heald RJ. Growing up with juvenile gastrointestinal polyposis: report of a case. Dis Colon Rectum 1971;14:375–80.

Ruymann FB. Juvenile polyps with cachexia. Report of an infant and comparison with Cronkhite-Canada syndrome in adults. Gastroenterology 1969;57:431–38.

Sachatello CR, Hahn IS, Carrington CB. Juvenile gastrointestinal polyposis in a female infant: report of a case and review of the literature of a recently recognized syndrome. Surgery 1974;75:107–14.

Simpson EL, Dalinka MK. Association of hypertrophic osteo-arthropathy with gastrointestinal polyposis. AJR 1985;144:983–4.

Soper RT, Kent TH. Fatal juvenile polyposis in infancy. Surgery 1971;69:692–8.

Veale AMO, McColl I, Bussey HJR, et al. Juvenile polyposis coli. J Med Genet 1966;3:5–16.

Peutz-Jeghers Syndrome

Dodds WJ. Clinical and roentgen features of the intestinal polyposis syndromes. Gastrointest Radiol 1976;1:127–42.

Scully RE, Galdsbini JJ, McNeely BV. Case records of the Massachusett's General Hospital. N Engl J Med 1978; 299:1237–44.

Cronkhite-Canada Syndrome

Cronkhite LW Jr, Canada WJ. Generalized gastrointestinal polyposis: an unusual syndrome of polyposis, pigmentation, alopecia and onychotrophia. New Engl J Med 1955;252:1011–15.

INHERITED ADENOMATOUS POLYPOSIS SYNDROMES FAMILIAL POLYPOSIS COLI

Abramson DJ. Multiple polyposis in children: a review and a report of a case in a 6-year-old child who had associated nephrosis and asthma. Surgery 1967;61:288–301.

Bartram CI, Thornton A. Colonic polyp patterns in familial polyposis. AJR 1984;142:305–8.

Bussey HJR. Familial polyposis coli. Family studies, histopathology, differential diagnosis and results of treatment. Baltimore (MD): Johns Hopkins Press; 1975.

Erbe RW. Current concepts in genetics. Inherited gastrointestinal - polyposis syndromes. N Engl J Med 1976;294:1101–4.

Kelvin FM, Max RJ, Norton GA, et al. Lymphoid follicular pattern of the colon in adults. AJR 1979;133:821–5.

Ranzi T, Castagnone D, Velio P, et al. Gastric and duodenal polyps in familial polyposis coli. Gut 1981;22:363–7.

Ushio K, Sasagawa M, Doi H, et al. Lesions associated with familial polyposis coli: studies of lesions of the stomach, duodenum, bones and teeth. Gastrointest Radiol 1976; 1:67–80.

Watanabe H, Enjoji M, Yao T, et al. Gastric lesions in familial adenomatosis coli. Hum Pathol 1978;9:269–83.

Gardner Syndrome

Bussey HJR. Familial polyposis coli. Family studies, histopathology, differential diagnosis and results of treatment. Baltimore (MD): Johns Hopkins Press; 1975.

Bussey HJR, Veale AMO, Morson BC. Genetics of gastrointestinal polyposis. Gastroenter 1978;74:1325–30.

Magid D, Fishman EK, Jones B, et al. Desmoid tumors in Gardner's syndrome: use of computed tomography. AJR 1984;142:1141–5.

Mathias JR, Smith WG. Mesenteric fibromatosis associated with familial polyposis. Dig Dis 1977;22:741–4.

Naylor EW, Lebenthal E. Gardner's syndrome. Recent developments in research and management. Dig Dis Sci 1980;25:945–59.

Schuchardt WA Jr, Ponsky JL. Familial polyosis and Gardner's syndrome. Surg Gynecol Obstet 1979;148:97–103.

Schulman A. Gastric and small bowel polyps in Gardner's syndrome and familial polyposis coli. Can Assoc Radiol J 1976;27:206–9.

Scully RE, Galdabini JJ, McNeely BV. Case records of the Massachusett's General Hospital. N Engl J Med 1978;299: 1237–44.

Sweeney BF, Anderson DS. Endoscopic removal of duodenal polyp in a patient with Gardner's syndrome. Dig Dis Sci 1982;27:557–60.

Vanhoutte JJ. Polypoid lymphoid hyperplasia of the terminal ileum in patients with familial polyposis coli and with Gardner's syndrome. AJR 1970;110:340–2.

Turcot Syndrome

Baughman FA, List CF, Williams JR, et al. The glioma-polyposis syndrome. N Engl J Med 1969;281:1345–6.

Itoh H, Ohsato K, Yao T, et al. Turcot's syndrome and its mode of inheritance. Gut 1970;20:414–19.

Radin DR, Fortgang KC, Zee CS, et al. Turcot syndrome: a case with spinal cord and colonic neoplasms. AJR 1984; 142:475–76.

Turcot J, Despres JP, St. Pierre F. Malignant tumours of the central nervous system associated with familial polyposis of the colon: report of two cases. Dis Colon Rectum 1959;2:465–8.

MISCELLANEOUS BENIGN TUMORS OF THE LARGE BOWEL

Erbe RW. Current concepts in genetics. Inherited gastrointestinal-polyposis syndromes. N Engl J Med 1976; 294:1101–4.

MALIGNANT TUMORS OF THE LARGE BOWEL

Adenocarcinoma of the Colon and Rectum

Donaldson MH, Taylor P, Ravitscher R, et al. Colon carcinoma in childhood. Pediatrics 1971;48:307–11.

Ruderman RL. Carcinoma of the colon in childhood. Can Med Assoc J 1960;83:120–2.

Carcinoid

Chow CW, Sane S, Campbell PE, et al. Malignant carcinoid tumors in children. Cancer 1982;49:802–11.

La Ferla G, Baxter RA, Tavadia HB, et al. Multiple colonic carcinoid tumours in a child. Br J Surg 1984;71:843.

Scott JE. Carcinoid tumours of the colon. Br J Surg 1973;60:684–5.

Suster G, Weinberg AG, Graiver L. Carcinoid tumor of the colon in a child. J Pediatr Surg 1977;12:739–42.

Lymphoma

Rosenberg S, Diamond H, Dargeon HW, et al. Lymphosarcoma in childhood. New Engl J Med 1958;259:505–12.

Miscellaneous Malignant Large Bowel Tumors

Ein SH, Beck R, Allen JE. Colon sarcoma in the newborn. J Pediatr Surg 1979;13:455–7.

Elshafie M, Spitz L, Ikeda S. Malignant tumours of the small bowel in neonates presenting with perforation. J Pediatr Surg 1971;6:62–4.

MUCOCELE OF THE APPENDIX

Dachman AH, Lichenstein JE, Friedman AC. Mucocele of the appendix and pseudomyxoma peritonei. AJR 1985; 144:923–9.

Thurber LA, Cooperberg PL, Clement JG, et al. Echogenic fluid: a pitfall in the ultrasonic diagnosis of cystic lesions. J Clin Ultra 1979;7:273–8.

Woodruff R, McDonald J. Benign and malignant cystic tumors of the appendix. Surg Gynecol Obstet 1940;71: 750–5.

MALAKOPLAKIA OF THE LARGE BOWEL

Akhtar M, Robinson CR, Ali MA, et al. Malacoplakia of the colon and rectum: report of two cases and review of the literature. King Faisal Spec Hosp Med J 1982;2:147–53.

Radin DR, Chandrasoma P, Halls JM. Colonic malacoplakia. Gastrointest Radiol 1984;9:359–61.

TRAUMA TO THE LARGE BOWEL

Burney RE, Mueller GL, Goon GL, et al. Diagnosis of isolated small bowel injury. Ann Emerg Med 1983;12:71–4.

Fonkalsrud EW, Clatworthy HW. Accidental perforation of the colon and rectum in newborn infants. N Engl J Med 1965;272:1097–1100.

Humphry A, Ein SH, Mok PH. Perforation of the intussuscepted colon. AJR 1981;137:1135–8.

Shiels WE II, Kirks DR, Keller GL, et al. Colonic perforation by air and liquid enemas: comparison study in young pigs. AJR 1993;160:931–6.

Sivit CJ, Eichelberger MR, Taylor GA. CT in children with rupture of the bowel caused by blunt trauma: diagnostic efficacy and comparison with hypoperfusion complex. AJR 1994;163:1195–8.

Sivit CJ, Taylor GA, Newman KD, et al. Safety-belt injuries in children with lap-belt ecchymosis: CT findings in 61 patients. AJR 1991;157:111–14.

Taylor GA, Eggli KD. Lap-belt injuries of the lumbar spine in children. AJR 1988;150:1355–8.

MISCELLANEOUS DISORDERS OF THE LARGE BOWEL

Volvulus

Allen RP, Nordstrom JE. Volvulus of the sigmoid in children. AJR 1964;91:690–3.

Anderson JF, Eklof O, Thomasson B. Large bowel volvulus in children. Pediatr Radiol 1981;11:129–38.

Berger RB, Hillemeier AC, Stahl RS, et al. Volvulus of the ascending colon: an unusual complication of nonrotation of the mid gut. Pediatr Radiol 1982;12:298–300.

Black RE, Cox JA. Volvulus of the transverse colon in children—report of a case and review of the literature. Z Kinderchir 1984;39:69–71.

Cuderman BS, Roback SA, Weintraub WH, et al. Volvulus of the transverse colon. Surgery 1971;69:797–9.

Lapin R, Kane AA, Lee CS, et al. Volvulus of the transverse colon associated with submucosal hamartoma. Am J Gastroenterol 1973;59:170–3.

Markowitz RI, Shashikumar VL, Capitanio MA. Volvulus of the colon in a child with congenital asplenia (Ivemark's syndrome). Radiology 1977;122:442.

Martin JD Jr. Megacolon associated with volvulus of the transverse colon. Am J Surg 1944;64:412–16.

Reinarz S, Smith WL, Franken EA, et al. Splenic flexure volvulus: a complication of pseudoobstruction in infancy. AJR 1985;145:1303–4.

Snyder WH, Chaffin I. Embryology and pathology of the intestinal tract: presentation of 48 cases of malrotation. Ann Surg 1954;140:368–80.

Trillis F, Gauderer MWL, Ponsky JL, et al. Transverse colon volvulus in a child with pathologic aerophagia. J Pediatr Surg 1986;21:966–8.

Diverticulosis

Rees BI, Griffin PJA. Colonic diverticulosis in a child. BMJ 1977;2:1194.

Cystic Fibrosis

Anderson HO, Hjelt K, Waever E, et al. The age related incidence of meconium ileus equivalent in a cystic fibrosis population: the impact of high energy intake. J Pediatr Gastroenterol Nutr 1990;11:356–60.

Berk RN, Lee FA. The late gastrointestinal manifestations of cystic fibrosis of the pancreas. Radiology 1973;106:377–81.

Campbell CA, Forrest J, Musgrove C. High-strength pancreatic enzyme supplements and large bowel stricture in cystic fibrosis. Lancet 1994;343:109–10.

Grossman H, Berdon WE, Baker DM. Gastrointestinal findings in cystic fibrosis. AJR 1966;97:227–38.

Hanly JG, Fitzgerald MX. Meconium ileus equivalent in older patients with cystic fibrosis. BMJ 1983;286:1411–13.

Koletzko S, Stringer DA, Cleghorn GJ, Durie PR. Lavage treatment of distal intestinal obstruction syndrome in cystic fibrosis. Pediatrics 1989;83:727–33.

Kopelman H. Gastrointestinal and nutritional aspects of cystic fibrosis. Thorax 1991;46:261–7.

Moody AR, Haddock JA, Given-Wilson R, et al. CT monitoring of therapy for meconium ileas. J Comput Assist Tomogr 1990;14:1010–12.

Park RW, Grand RJ. Gastrointestinal manifestation of cystic fibrosis: a review. Gastroenterology 1981;81:1143–61.

Pickhardt PJ, Yagan N, Siegel MJ. Cystic fibrosis: CT findings of colonic disease. Radiology 1998;206:725–30.

Smyth RL, van Velzin D, Smyth AR, et al. Strictures of the ascending colon in cystic fibrosis and high-strength pancreatic enzymes. Lancet 1994;343:85–6.

Weinstein LD, Clemett AR, Herkovic T. Morphologic and radiographic findings in cystic fibrosis [abstract]. Gastroenterology 1968;54:1282.

Zerin JM, Kuhn-Fulton J, White SJ, et al. Colonic strictures in children with cystic fibrosis. Radiology 1995;194:223–6.

11

PEDIATRIC BILIARY IMAGING

Marilyn Ranson, BSc, MD, FRCPC,
Chee Hiew, MB, BS, FRACR, and Paul S. Babyn, MDCM

EMBRYOLOGY OF THE BILIARY TRACT

The liver, gallbladder, and biliary duct system arise from the hepatic diverticulum of the foregut and develop by the fourth gestational week (Gray and Skandalakis, 1972). The hepatic diverticulum divides into two parts: the larger cranial part gives rise to the liver, while the smaller caudal part develops into the gallbladder and cystic duct (Stringer, 1989).

By the beginning of the fifth gestational week the early precursors of the gallbladder, cystic duct, hepatic ducts, and common bile duct have developed within the ventral mesentery of the duodenum. The extrahepatic parts of the biliary system elongate, becoming a solid cord of cells. Re-establishment of the lumina of the extrahepatic biliary system begins within the common bile duct during the sixth week and gradually progresses proximally. During the recanalization process, two or more lumina temporarily appear within a duct and then coalesce to form a single lumen. Failure of recanalization of the bile ducts or gallbladder can result in atresia, and failure of the two lumina to coalesce may cause some cases of duplication anomalies (Schneck, 1994).

Formation of the intrahepatic bile duct system begins around the eighth gestational week. The prevailing theory postulates that the intrahepatic biliary system is derived from hepatocyte precursor cells, which transform into ductules and ducts to join the extrahepatic biliary bud at the hilum. These hepatocytes form a layer of cells surrounding the portal vein branches like a sleeve, referred to as the ductal plate. From 12 weeks of gestation, progressive remodeling of the ductal plates takes place, with segments of the double-layered ductal plate dilating to form tubular structures. The normal development of intrahepatic ducts requires epithelial-mesenchymal interactions, which proceed from the hilum of the liver to the periphery, along the branches of the developing portal vein. By birth, the most peripheral portal vein branches are not yet accompanied by a mature bile duct, indicating incompleteness or immaturity of the intrahepatic bile duct system at this time (Desmet, 1992a; Desmet, 1998).

NORMAL ANATOMY AND IMAGING OF THE BILIARY TREE

Ultrasonography

Ultrasonography (US) is the initial modality of choice for imaging the biliary tree in children of all ages. The gallbladder is normally adjacent to the undersurface of the liver, in the plane of the interlobar fissure (Meilstrup et al., 1991). With age, there is a gradual increase in gallbladder length in normal pediatric patients (Slovis et al., 1980). The gallbladder length is at least 1.5 cm in a neonate, and the upper limits for the gallbladder size in children is 7.5 cm in length and 3.5 cm in diameter (McGahan et al., 1982). Measurements of gallbladder wall thickness are similar to adults and are normally less than 3 mm (McGahan et al., 1982).

The bile ducts within the liver travel with the hepatic artery and portal vein branches; together, they form the portal triads (Siegel, 1996). Normally, the left and right hepatic ducts join together into a common hepatic duct which lies anterolaterally to the portal vein. The cystic duct is located posterolateral to the common hepatic duct and combines with it to form the common bile duct. On ultrasonographic examination, the cystic duct is difficult to identify, and as a result, the common hepatic duct cannot be reliably distinguished from the common bile duct (Schneck, 1994). The size of the common bile duct increases linearly with age and may be slightly larger in children with contracted gallbladders (Hernanz-Schulman, 1995) or patients with previous biliary surgery (Siegel, 1996). On US, the internal diameter of the common bile duct should not exceed 2 mm in infants or 4 mm in children older than 1 year (Siegel, 1996). In adolescents and adults, the upper limit of the common bile duct is 5 to 7 mm; the upper limit for the common hepatic duct is 4 mm (Schneck, 1994; McGahan et al., 1982; Siegel, 1996). The proximal intrahepatic ducts can be seen in normal patients but should not exceed 2 mm. Evaluation of the pancreatic biliary junction is limited with US, and the distal common bile duct may be obscured by bowel gas.

Computed Tomography

Computed tomography (CT) may also be used to assess the biliary tree and may be indicated in children who have biliary dilatation without a documented cause for biliary obstruction on US. Visualization of the biliary tree is improved with the use of dynamic intravenous contrast and thin (3 to 5 mm) collimation. The course of the extrahepatic duct can usually be identified adjacent to the portal vein and within the pancreatic head (Baron, 1997). The bile duct lumen is near water attenuation and the normal duct wall is seen as a thin enhancing structure (Baron, 1997). The normal common duct ranges from 2 to 6 mm in diameter (Co et al., 1986). With current technology, intrahepatic ducts may occasionally be seen but should be less than 2 mm in size (Baron, 1997). Compared with US, CT may better demonstrate the distal common bile duct because it is not limited by bowel gas.

Magnetic Resonance Imaging

Magnetic resonance cholangiopancreatography (MRCP) is a noninvasive method of evaluating the biliary tree using heavily T2-weighted sequences. Stationary fluid within the bile ducts has a long T2 relaxation time and is seen as high signal intensity. The background is eliminated by using fat suppression and because of the extreme T2 weighting

(Arshanskiy and Vyas, 1998; Chan et al., 1998). Conventional T2 or fast spin echo T2 sequences may be utilized, and the maximum intensity projection (MIP) reformation provides a three-dimensional image of the biliary tree (Arshanskiy and Vyas, 1998). Faster imaging may be done with a half-fourier acquisition single-shot turbo spin echo (HASTE) sequence that may be completed within a few seconds and does not require breathholding, which is advantageous in children (Ernst et al., 1998; Miyazaki et al., 1998). The images are comparable to conventional cholangiography, and MRCP may demonstrate obstructed biliary ducts not visualized on other forms of cholangiography (Gembala, 1994). Currently, MRCP is limited to children with dilated biliary ducts and disorders of the extrahepatic biliary tree because of insufficient spatial resolution (Guibaud et al., 1998).

Hepatobiliary Scintigraphy

Hepatobiliary scans can be used to evaluate hepatocellular function, biliary obstruction or leak, and origin of cystic masses from the biliary tree. The technetium Tc 99m iminodiacetic acid (IDA) derivatives are used for pediatric hepatobiliary scintigraphy. The most commonly used agents are diisopropyl IDA (DISIDA;disofenin) and methyltribromoiminodiacetic acid (mebrofenin). Mebrofenin is the best agent to use with higher bilirubin levels because of greater hepatic uptake (Ben-Haim et al., 1995). In patients with decreased hepatic uptake, the accuracy of IDA scans can be improved by phenobarbital induction, which enhances excretion of the radiopharmaceutical into the bile (Majd, 1983).

VARIANTS AND GENERAL DISORDERS OF THE BILIARY TRACT

Gallbladder

The gallbladder and biliary tree may be affected by a wide range of congenital anomalies, altering their number, shape, and position (Williams and Williams, 1955; Maingot, 1980). It is estimated that 10 to 20% of the population have some anomaly of the biliary tree (Stringer, 1989).

Anomalies
Number. Congenital absence of the gallbladder is rare, with a necropsy incidence of 0.03 to 0.09% with an equal sex incidence (Maingot, 1980). Agen-

esis of the gallbladder may be associated with other anomalies including congenital heart disease, tracheoesophageal fistula, imperforate anus, and genitourinary malformations (Gray and Skandalakis, 1972). The diagnosis is difficult to make with imaging and is usually made intraoperatively. A congenitally small gallbladder is of no clinical significance.

Duplication of the gallbladder is common in domesticated mammals but is rare in humans, with an incidence of 1 in 4000. Duplication of the gallbladder can be partial or complete, with complete duplication being associated with two separate gallbladders and two cystic ducts (Diaz et al., 1991). Duplication of the gallbladder is rarely symptomatic in children but it can be associated with cholelithiasis, cholecystitis, obstructive biliary disease, and biliary cirrhosis (Granot et al., 1983; Goiney et al., 1985). Differentiation between a double gallbladder, vascular band, and a folded gallbladder may be difficult on US (Goiney et al., 1985).

Shape. There is a wide variation in gallbladder configuration, including an hourglass or dumbbell shape. There may be a diverticulum, an enlarged Hartmann's pouch, or a phrygian cap. Hartmann's pouch is an outpouching of the junction of the gallbladder neck and the cystic duct. A phrygian cap is a common variation in which there is folding of the gallbladder fundus (Figure 11–1). The gallbladder may have a junctional fold or may contain septa. Gallbladder septa can be partial or complete and may lead to stasis and stone formation (Meilstrup et al., 1991). Multiseptate gallbladder is a rare anomaly with multiple bridging septa, which create a honeycombed appearance (Figure 11–2) (Meilstrup et al., 1991; Adear and Barki, 1990; Lev-Toaff et al., 1987).

Position. Anomalous position of the gallbladder may be either congenital or acquired and can be divided into five types: left-sided, intrahepatic, suprahepatic, retrohepatic, and floating (Naganuma et al., 1998). The most common anomalous position of the gallbladder is left-sided, below the left lobe of the liver or intrahepatic within the liver parenchyma (McLoughlin et al., 1987). The gallbladder may be suprahepatic with hypoplasia of the right lobe of the liver or eventration of the diaphragm (Gansbeke et al., 1984). It may be retrohepatic with atrophy of the right lobe of the liver (Naganuma et al., 1998) and identified in a retroperitoneal location in the right renal fossa post nephrectomy (Figure 11–3) (Lang et al., 1997). The gallbladder may float or be suspend-

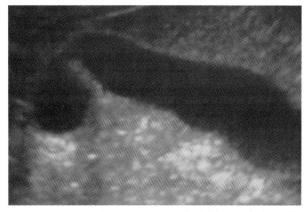

FIGURE 11–1. Phrygian cap with folding of the gallbladder fundus.

ed on a long mesentery, and rarely, it may undergo volvulus or torsion (Levard et al., 1994). In children, sudden body movements or blunt abdominal trauma may play a role in producing torsion of a mobile gallbladder (Kitagawa et al., 1997).

Cholelithiasis

The first year of life has the highest incidence of ultrasonographically detected gallstones compared to any other childhood year, with most occurring in early infancy. The incidence falls to a low level in the second year of life, gradually rising toward and into adolescence (Stringer, 1989). Gallstones in infancy are generally asymptomatic, and since they differ in a number of respects from gallstones found in older children, they will be considered separately below.

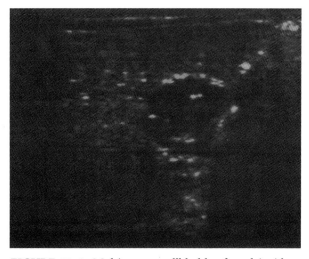

FIGURE 11–2. Multiseptate gallbladder found incidentally on ultrasonography.

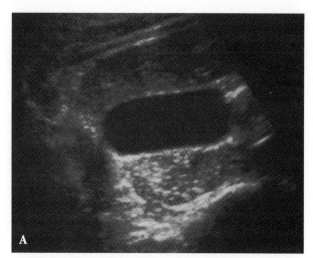
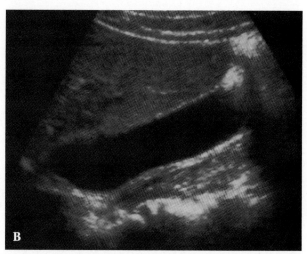

FIGURE 11–3. Gallbladder positioned ectopically between the liver and the psoas muscle after right nephrectomy for Wilms' tumor. *A,* Transverse and *B,* longitudinal ultrasonographs.

Gallstones in Infants. Neonatal gallstones are usually pigment stones (Descos et al., 1984). Immature physiologic mechanisms related to bile acid production and secretion, together with other factors, appear to lead to the formation of gallstones in this age group. Delayed oral feeding and total parenteral nutrition (TPN) may also decrease bile acid production and lead to cholestasis (Callahan et al., 1982; Brill et al., 1982). Other factors include dehydration, prematurity, and medications such as diuretics (Stringer, 1989).

Sepsis, with or without inflammation of the biliary tree, can result in cholestasis especially if there is associated dehydration and acidosis. In addition, certain bacteria such as *Escherichia coli* can cause calcium bilirubinate stones by hydrolyzation of conjugated bilirubin. The deconjugated bilirubin then combines with calcium and precipitates to form pigmented stones (Maki, 1966).

Anatomic abnormalities, congenital or secondary to surgery, may promote cholestasis. Neonates with short-gut syndrome may develop gallstones secondary to alterations of the enterohepatic bile circulation. Cardiac abnormalities have also been implicated in gallstone production (Stringer, 1989).

Hemolysis with resulting overproduction of bilirubin is a predisposing factor of gallstones but is rarely associated with cholelithiasis in infancy (Debray et al., 1993; Jonas et al., 1990).

Gallstones in infants are usually clinically silent, and spontaneous resolution may occur. The exact mechanism of their disappearance in infants is unknown. Gallstones may be broken up and dissolved as the cholestasis improves, or malleable pigment stones may be passed into the duodenum (Keller et al., 1985; Fakhry, 1982; Cooperberg and Gibney, 1987). Rarely, cholecystitis may occur or a stone may impact in the common bile duct, causing obstructive jaundice. Persistent obstruction and associated signs of cholangitis are indications for treatment (Debray et al., 1993).

Echogenic foci identified within the fetal gallbladder during the third trimester may represent gallstones. They are not usually associated with risk factors and often resolve without symptoms (Brown et al., 1992).

Gallstones in Older Children. Teenaged females continue to make up the largest group of children with gallstones (Lugo-Vicente, 1997). Gallstones in this group are associated with obesity, adolescent pregnancy, and the use of birth control pills (Rescorla, 1997). Gallstones may develop due to the lithogenic effect of estrogen on bile (Lugo-Vicente, 1997).

Hematologic disorders account for many gallstones in children. Causes include sickle cell anemia, hereditary spherocytosis, and thalassemia major (Rescorla, 1997; Senaati et al., 1993). Sickle cell disease, in particular, has a 27% incidence of gallstones in patients 2 to 18 years of age, and the incidence increases with age (Sarnaik et al., 1980).

An increasing number of children develop gallstones after prolonged TPN or following distal ileal resection (Rescorla, 1997). Ileal pathology that interferes with the normal enterohepatic cycle of bile salts is important in the formation of gallstones (Garel et al., 1981; Pellerin et al., 1975). The ileal dysfunction most commonly arises secondary to surgery or to inflammatory bowel disease, most commonly Crohn's disease.

Other predisposing conditions are sepsis, anatomic anomalies, metabolic disorders, immune deficiency, and cystic fibrosis (Lugo-Vicente, 1997). Heart transplant patients have an increased incidence of cholelithiasis that may be related to the higher rate of hemolysis and cyclosporine-induced changes in bile metabolism (Milas et al., 1996).

Gallstones that are symptomatic usually produce intermittent, mild or severe colicky pain, which in older children is localized in the right upper quadrant. Radiation to the back or shoulder is uncommon in childhood. Nausea and vomiting is present in approximately 50% of cases. There may be associated anorexia, fatigue, and listlessness. Gallstones may rarely predispose to cholecystitis (Stringer, 1989).

Imaging. Plain abdominal radiography may demonstrate radiopaque gallstones in 36 to 47% of children as opposed to 15% of adults. This difference is probably related to the increased percentage of pigmented gallstones which are radiopaque, compared with cholesterol stones more commonly found in adults (Figure 11–4) (Rescorla, 1997). Pigment stones are usually associated with a hemolytic process although some arise after ileal resection or in association with TPN (Rescorla, 1997).

Ultrasonography, with a sensitivity of 95%, is the most reliable method of diagnosing gallstones (Cooperberg and Burhenne, 1980). Gallstones typically appear as discrete echogenic foci with distal acoustic shadowing (Figures 11–5, 11–6). The acoustic shadowing is related to the size of the stone and not its calcium content; thus, small stones may not shadow (Siegel, 1996). Gallstones usually lie in the most dependent portion of the gallbladder and move with changes in the patient's position (Figure 11–7) (Cooperberg and Gibney, 1987). Occasionally, gallstones may float if they have a high cholesterol content, contain gas or fissures (Siegel, 1996), or if the specific gravity of bile is increased (Yeh et al, 1986). When the gallbladder becomes filled with stones, visualization of the gallbladder may be replaced by a highly echogenic line with distal acoustic shadowing—the so-called wall echo shadow (WES) triad (Figure 11–8) (MacDonald et al., 1981). Tumefactive sludge or sludge balls may mimic gallstones but do not typically shadow (Figures 11–9, 11–10). Biliary sludge giving low-level echoes within the gallbladder may obscure underlying gallstones (Figure 11–11) (Conrad et al., 1979).

Computed tomography may demonstrate gallstones but is not the imaging modality of choice due to its radiation exposure, lower sensitivity, and greater expense (Rebner et al., 1985). Conventional cholangiography or MRCP may be used to assess stones if there is associated biliary obstruction. (This is discussed in the section on choledocholithiasis). If surgery is indicated, intraoperative cholangiography may be performed at the time of cholecystectomy. Post-cholecystectomy recurrence of stones is unusual but may occur if there is an underlying disease (Stringer, 1989).

Cholecystitis

Acute and chronic cholecystitis in children is relatively rare but certain pediatric patients are prone to

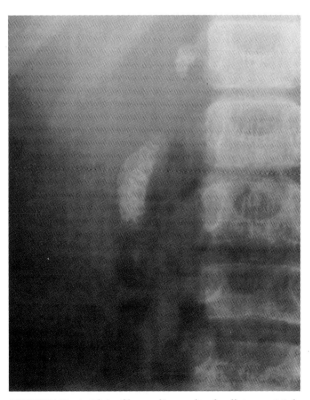

FIGURE 11–4. Plain-film radiograph of gallstones. Multiple opacities with dense rims are present in the gallbladder and cystic duct of a 1-year-old child with thalassemia.

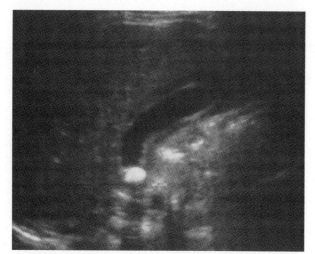

FIGURE 11-5. Infantile gallstone. Ultrasonograph shows an echogenic focus with distal acoustic shadowing.

these diseases (O'Hara, 1996; Greenberg et al., 1980; Tsakayannis et al., 1996). It can occur at any age, including infancy, and can be acalculous or calculous.

Acalculous Cholecystitis. Acalculous cholecystitis may be due to many factors, including congenital anomalies of the biliary tract, parenteral nutrition, trauma or surgery, specific infections (*Salmonella,* streptococcal group A or B, *Ascaris*), or systemic diseases such as diabetes mellitus (Tsakayannis et al., 1996; Thurston et al., 1986; Roca et al., 1988; McEvoy and Suchy, 1996; Dickinson et al., 1971; Crystal and Fink, 1971). Systemic vasculitis and Kawasaki disease may be associated with cholecystitis but are more likely to cause acute hydrops of the gallbladder (McEvoy and Suchy, 1996). Although

uncommon, acalculous cholecystitis appears to be more common in cases of acute cholecystitis in childhood than in adult life (Crystal and Fink, 1971).

The pathogenesis of acalculous cholecystitis remains unclear but probable mechanisms include gallbladder ischemia, biliary stasis, infection, and direct chemical toxicity (Tsakayannis et al., 1996;

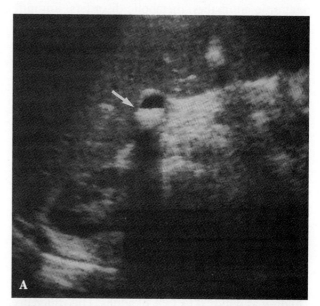

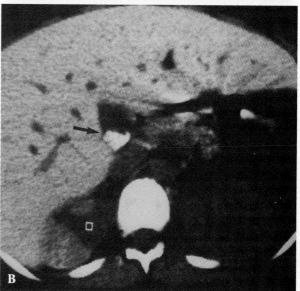

FIGURE 11-7. Multiple small gallstones in a child with thalassemia. *A,* Transverse ultrasonograph shows an echogenic fluid level with acoustic shadowing secondary to layering of multiple small gallstones (*arrow*). *B,* Computed tomography shows the multiple gallstones and increased attenuation within the liver due to iron deposition in this child with thalassemia.

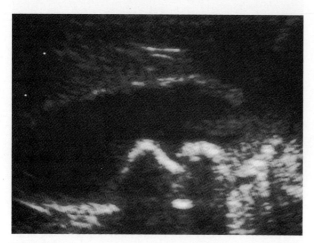

FIGURE 11-6. Adolescent with gallstones secondary to sickle cell disease.

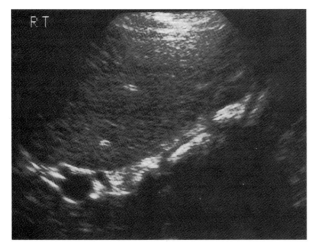

FIGURE 11–8. The gallbladder is filled with stones, producing the wall echo shadow (WES) sign.

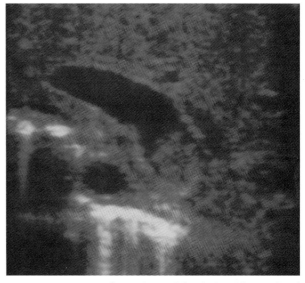

FIGURE 11–10. Echogenic mobile foci without distal acoustic shadowing consistent with a sludge ball.

Swayne, 1986). In some patients, there is congenital or inflammatory narrowing of the cystic duct or external compression from enlarged lymph nodes (McEvoy and Suchy, 1996).

Calculous Cholecystitis. Cholecystitis is a rare complication of gallstones in children (Reif et al., 1991; Nicotra et al., 1997). Unlike adult cases, at least 50% of childhood cases of cholecystitis do not have associated cholelithiasis (Greenberg et al., 1980). Inflammation of the gallbladder usually occurs when a gallstone becomes impacted in the cystic duct.

Other than the presence or absence of gallstones, acute acalculous and calculous cholecystitis have many clinical and radiologic features in common and are considered together.

Clinical Features of Acute Cholecystitis in Childhood. The triad of right upper quadrant pain, vomiting, and fever is the usual clinical presentation (Greenberg et al., 1980; Tsakayannis et al., 1996; McEvoy and Suchy, 1996). Abdominal pain can be constant or colicky and may be poorly localized by the young child. Jaundice occurs in 25 to 45% of children with cholecystitis, probably secondary to inflammation around the bile duct as choledocholithiasis is rare (Crystal and Fink, 1971). The white cell count is usually elevated in acute cholecystitis, and serum bilirubin and alkaline phosphatase levels may be increased (McEvoy and Suchy, 1996). There is right upper quadrant tender-

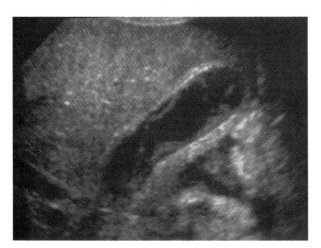

FIGURE 11–9. Echogenic material within the gallbladder consistent with sludge.

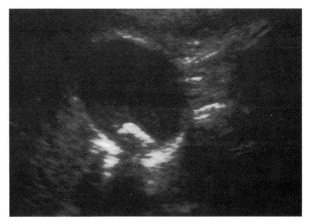

FIGURE 11–11. Mixture of sludge and stones layered in the dependent portion of the gallbladder in a patient with spherocytosis.

ness and guarding, and an enlarged, tender gallbladder is sometimes palpable.

Chronic cholecystitis is usually more indolent, with recurrent bouts of upper abdominal discomfort of varying severity being a constant feature (McEvoy and Suchy, 1996). There may be a history of fat intolerance in older children.

Differential Diagnosis. Cholecystitis and cholelithiasis should be considered in the differential diagnosis of abdominal pain in children (Greenberg et al., 1980; Bailey et al., 1989). Due to the rarity of the condition in children, it is common for an initial diagnosis of acute appendicitis, pancreatitis, bowel obstruction, or perforation to be made as the clinical features may mimic these conditions. Radiologic studies play an important role in making or excluding the diagnosis. In children with sickle cell disease, it may be difficult to differentiate acute cholecystitis from hepatic vaso-occlusive crisis and hepatitis (Taylor, 1997).

Imaging

Ultrasonography. Ultrasonography should be the primary screening test for any child with right upper quadrant pain, fever, and vomiting (Greenberg et al., 1980). The ultrasonographic findings of acute cholecystitis in children are similar to those in adults (Nicotra et al., 1997; Haller, 1991). Findings include gallbladder wall thickening and distension, and gallstones may be detected (Roca et al., 1988; Nicotra et al., 1997).

A gallbladder wall thickness of over 3 mm is abnormal (McGahan et al., 1982), and when associated with a small amount of fluid around the gallbladder, the finding is suggestive of cholecystitis (Nicotra et al., 1997; Haller, 1991; Mindell and Ring, 1979; Finberg and Birnholz, 1979; Engel et al., 1980; Mirvis et al., 1986; Ralls et al., 1985) (Figure 11–12). However, gallbladder wall thickening of over 3 mm can be present in many conditions unrelated to cholecystitis, such as hypoalbuminemia (Patriquin et al., 1983; Fiske et al., 1980), varices (Saigh et al., 1985), metachromatic leukodystrophy (Heier et al., 1983), Henoch-Schönlein purpura (Pery et al., 1990; Amemoto et al., 1994), graft-versus-host disease and hepatic venoocclusive disease in bone marrow transplant patients (Figure 11–13) (Benya et al., 1993; Day and Carpenter, 1993), portal hypertension (Saverymuttu et al., 1990), ascites, and physiologic contraction of the gallbladder (Patriquin et al., 1983). In addition, the gallbladder wall may not be thickened on US in some cases of cholecystitis (Patriquin et al., 1983). Follow-up US may help demonstrate progressive wall thickening when clinical suspicion is high, especially in acalculous cholecystitis (Jeffrey and Sommer, 1993).

A hypoechoic layer within the gallbladder wall may be found in acalculous or calculous cholecystitis (Greenberg et al., 1980; Croce et al., 1981; Cohan et al., 1987; Beckman et al., 1985; Marchal et al., 1979); this layer reflects subserosal edema, hemorrhage, inflammatory cell infiltration, or muscular hypertrophy (Figures 11–14, 11–15) (Lim et al., 1987). Striat-

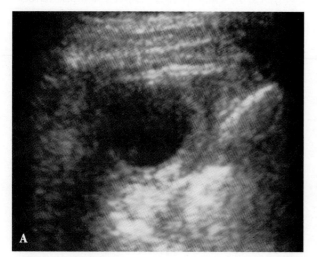 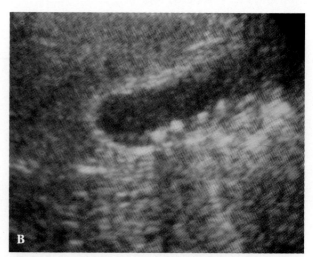

FIGURE 11–12. Acute calculous cholecystitis in a 14-year-old girl. *A*, Ultrasonograph shows thickening of the gallbladder wall with a small amount of fluid around the gallbladder. *B*, Ultrasonograph showing multiple mobile shadowing calculi in the gallbladder.

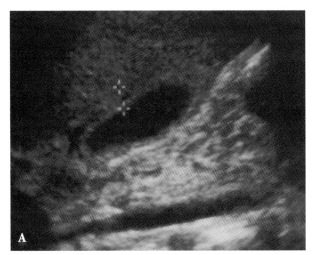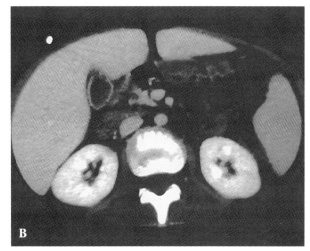

FIGURE 11–13. Graft-versus-host disease following bone marrow transplantation for acute myelogenous leukemia in a 12-year-old boy. *A,* Ultrasonograph shows thickening of the gallbladder wall. *B,* Contrast-enhanced CT shows enhancement of the gallbladder mucosa and mucosal enhancement in the colon.

ed wall thickening with alternating, irregular, and discontinuous hypo- and hyperechoic stripes has also been reported (Cohan et al., 1987). Color and power Doppler have been used recently to detect a hyper-vascularized gallbladder wall in acute cholecystitis (Uggowitzer et al., 1997; Schiller et al., 1996).

The ultrasonographic Murphy's sign, defined as maximal tenderness over the ultrasonographically localized gallbladder, is a useful secondary sign (Roca et al., 1988; Ralls et al., 1985). This sign may be difficult to elicit in the infant or young child. Absence of Murphy's sign in the presence of ultrasonographic findings of cholecystitis may indicate gangrenous cholecystitis (Simeone et al., 1989).

Complications of cholecystitis can be demonstrated on US. The presence of intraluminal membranes and echoes with or without gallbladder wall irregularity may indicate hemorrhagic or gangrenous cholecystitis (Kane, 1980; Jeffrey et al., 1983; Chinn et al., 1987). A hypoechoic area around the gallbladder wall may indicate development of a pericholecystic abscess (Bergman et al., 1979). Emphysematous cholecystitis is related to infection of the gallbladder by gas-producing organisms but may be secondary to ischemia rather than a primary infection (Blaquiere and Dewbury, 1982). Ultrasonography is characteristic, with dense echoes arising from intraluminal or intramural gas with reverberation echoes posteriorly (Blaquiere et al., 1982; Parulekar et al., 1982). These complications are rare in children (Haller, 1991).

In chronic cholecystitis resulting from cystic fibrosis or chronic irritation by gallstones, US may be normal or there may be focal or diffuse thickening of the gallbladder wall (Nicotra et al., 1997). Gallstones or sludge may also be present within the gallbladder.

Radionuclide Scintigraphy. Radionuclide scintigraphy has been effectively used in the diagnosis of acalculous and calculous cholecystitis in adults (Swayne, 1986; Weissmann et al., 1979; Weissmann et al., 1983; Samuels et al., 1983) and children (O'Hara, 1996; Nicotra et al., 1997; Coughlin and Mann, 1990). Nonvisualization of the gallbladder at 1 hour with

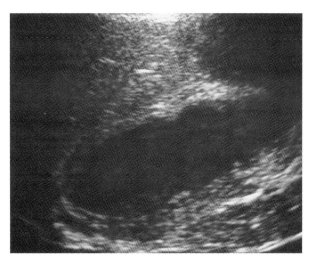

FIGURE 11–14. Acute acalculous cholecystitis in an 11-year-old girl. Ultrasonograph shows a distended gallbladder containing echogenic debris and irregular wall thickening.

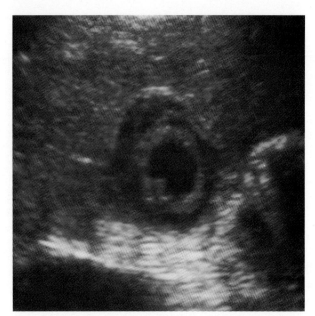

FIGURE 11–15. Acalculous cholecystitis in a 3-year-old neutropenic patient. Ultrasonograph shows thickening of the gallbladder wall which appears hypoechoic.

normal hepaticoenteric transit of tracer is highly accurate for the diagnosis of acute cholecystitis (Figure 11–16) (O'Hara, 1996; Weissmann et al., 1981). Focal increased flow to the gallbladder region, an angiographic effect, can be detected on rapid sequence imaging (Colletti et al., 1987). In addition, increased

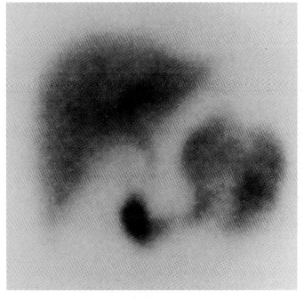

FIGURE 11–16. Acute cholecystitis. On an HIDA scan, there is excretion into the gut but nonvisualization of the gallbladder after 4 hours and even after extended imaging.

pericholecystic hepatic uptake, known as the "rim sign," is often associated with acute gangrenous cholecystitis and cholecystitis complicated by perforation (Brachman et al., 1993; Bushnell et al., 1986; Hayashi et al., 1997; Swayne and Ginsberg, 1989). This occurs due to transmural inflammation of the gallbladder wall and spread into the liver. These two signs are highly specific for acute cholecystitis when associated with nonvisualization of the gallbladder (Colletti et al., 1987; Brachman et al., 1993; Bushnell et al., 1986; Hayashi et al., 1997; Treves et al., 1995).

In children, visualization of the gallbladder on hepatobiliary scintigraphy does not rule out cholecystitis. Visualization of the gallbladder can occur with acalculous or toxic cholecystitis since the cystic duct may still be patent (Treves et al., 1995). Failure of effective gallbladder contraction following a fatty meal or injection of cholecystokinin (CCK) is usually seen in acalculous cholecystitis, chronic cholecystitis, or partial cystic duct obstruction. Delayed visualization of the gallbladder despite normal liver function may also be seen in chronic cholecystitis (O'Hara, 1996; Weissmann et al., 1981; Treves et al., 1995).

False-positive results occur in sick neonates and in patients with severe nonbiliary intercurrent illness, prolonged fasting, total parenteral nutrition, and hepatocellular dysfunction (Mirvis et al., 1986; Shuman et al., 1982; El-Shafie and Mah, 1986). The findings on hepatobiliary scintigraphy also may be difficult to interpret when the cystic duct is patent and acute cholecystitis results from calculi obstructing the common bile duct since radioisotope will appear in the gallbladder (Massie et al., 1983).

Computed Tomography and Magnetic Resonance Imaging. Computed tomography is rarely indicated since a combination of clinical, ultrasonographic, and/or radionuclide scintigraphic findings are usually sufficient to make the diagnosis (Nicotra et al., 1997). Common findings include thickening and nodularity of the gallbladder wall, poor definition of the wall, pericholecystic fluid and stranding, distension of the lumen, subserosal edema, cholelithiasis, and high-attenuation bile (Mirvis et al., 1986; Kane et al., 1983; Fidler et al., 1996). Intramural and intraluminal gas is indicative of emphysematous cholecystitis (Kane et al., 1983).

Magnetic resonance imaging appears sensitive in detecting gallbladder disease (McCarthy et al., 1986) but there is little indication for its use in diagnosing cholecystitis.

Hydrops of the Gallbladder

Acute hydrops is massive distension of the gallbladder without associated anomalies, biliary calculi, or acute inflammation. Most cases of hydrops have a prior severe illness usually infectious in etiology (Dinulos et al., 1994). Gallbladder hydrops has been reported in 5% of children with Kawasaki syndrome (mucocutaneous lymph node syndrome) (Choi and Sharma, 1989). Other associations include leukemia, burns, sepsis, upper respiratory tract infection, hepatitis, and gastroenteritis. Specific infections include leptospirosis, ascariasis, typhoid fever, scarlet fever, Epstein-Barr virus, group B streptococcal infection, and familial Mediterranean fever (Dinulos et al., 1994; Bloom and Swain, 1966; Wicks et al., 1978; Neu et al., 1980; Rumley and Rodgers, 1983; Wirth et al., 1985). Clinical features are variable; right upper quadrant pain, fever, and dehydration are the most common. However, many patients have no clinical findings.

The mechanisms involved in the development of hydrops are unknown (Rumley and Rodgers, 1983; Kumari et al., 1979). Noncalculous blockage of the cystic duct may play a role in the development of hydrops, and suspected causes include viscous bile from fasting and dehydration, and mesenteric adenitis, which may cause local pressure on the cystic duct (Siegel, 1996; Dinulos et al., 1994; Ternberg and Keating, 1975). Once distension of the gallbladder occurs, the acute angulation of the gallbladder neck may further increase obstruction.

Ultrasonography provides rapid noninvasive evaluation of hydrops and has been well demonstrated in relation to Kawasaki syndrome (Wirth et al., 1985; Ternberg and Keating, 1975) and typhoid fever (Ternberg and Keating, 1975). Diagnosis is based on clinical findings and demonstration of a massively distended gallbladder with a spherical rather than teardrop configuration (Figure 11–17). The gallbladder has a normal wall thickness, and biliary ducts are not dilated (Siegal, 1996; Madign and Teele, 1984; Cohen et al., 1986).

The clinical course of gallbladder hydrops is almost always benign, and conservative treatment is appropriate in patients who do not have acute abdominal pain (Dinulos et al., 1994). Spontaneous decompression with rehydration and resolution of the associated disease process appears to be the normal course in the absence of secondary gallbladder infection (Wirth et al., 1985; Cohen et al., 1986; Bradford et al., 1982). Most cases resolve within 5 to 15 days of diagnosis, and resolution is usually complete by 4 weeks. Rarely, complications related to perforation may develop, and cholecystostomy may be required (Choi and Sharma, 1989).

Adenomyomatosis and Cholesterolosis

Cholesterolosis and adenomyomatosis are rare noninflammatory abnormalities of the gallbladder which may occur in childhood. These disorders are of unknown etiology, and they appear to be unrelated (Berk et al., 1983). Cholesterolosis results from abnormal accumulations of triglycerides and cholesterol esters or precursors in the lamina propria of the gallbladder wall. Ultrasonography demonstrates single or multiple adherent nonshadowing echogenic masses protruding into the gallbladder's lumen. Adenomyomatosis is characterized by herniation of hyperplastic mucosa into or through a thickened muscular layer (Rokitansky-Aschoff sinuses). Findings on US include intramural diverticula that may contain cholesterol crystals, and diffuse or segmental

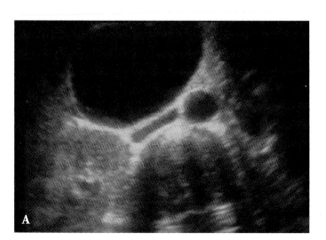

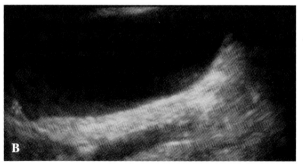

FIGURE 11–17. Hydrops of the gallbladder in a child with Kawasaki disease. *A,* Transverse and *B,* longitudinal ultrasonographs demonstrate a markedly distended gallbladder.

thickening of the gallbladder wall (Figures 11–18, 11–19) (Siegel, 1996). Although there may be some association with abdominal pain, many patients with these disorders are asymptomatic (Berk et al., 1983).

Gallbladder Polyps

Gallbladder polyps are rare in the pediatric population and may be associated with Crohn's disease, Peutz-Jeghers syndrome, and leukodystrophy (Schimpl et al., 1994). True polyps are papillomas and adenomas that result from localized overgrowth of the epithelial lining of the mucosa. Pseudopolyps include cholesterol, inflammatory polyps, and gastric heterotopia (Schimpl et al., 1994; Barzilai and Lerner, 1997). In metachromatic leukodystrophy, deposition of sulfatide in the gallbladder wall causes thickening and papilloma formation (Heier et al., 1983) (Figure 11–20). The differential diagnosis includes gallstones, sludge balls, and blood clots.

On US, polyps have the echogenicity of soft tissue and may be sessile or pedunculated. They do not usually demonstrate posterior acoustic shadowing, and they are attached to the gallbladder wall, differentiating them from gallstones. Gallbladder polyps may be incidental findings but may become symptomatic if they obstruct the gallbladder neck. Inflammatory polyps are often associated with gallstones (Barzilai and Lerner, 1997). Adenomatous and papillary gallbladder polyps are considered precancerous lesions, and cholecystectomy is recom-

mended for polyps larger than 1 cm because of the increased risk of malignancy (Schimpl et al., 1994; Mogilner et al., 1991; Sugiyama et al., 1995).

Bile Ducts

Bile Duct Anomalies

There is a wide variation in the normal anatomy of the bile ducts, with anomalies noted in 14 to 28% of necropsies (Sussman et al., 1986). Some of these anomalies can be detected with US, which may help in preoperative assessment (Sussman et al., 1986). The most common biliary anomaly is an anomalous right hepatic duct emptying into the common hepatic or cystic duct (Reid et al., 1986). It is important to recognize this anomaly on preoperative cholangiograph to prevent ligation of the duct that may result in obstructive cholangitis (Reid et al., 1986). Another biliary duct anomaly is duplication of the common bile duct (Schneck, 1994). Rarely, the cystic duct is absent, with the gallbladder attached to the common bile duct through a wide mouth.

Interposition of the gallbladder is a rare anomaly that can present with intermittent jaundice (Niemeir, 1942; Yazbeck et al., 1985). In this condition, the hepatic ducts drain, separately or together, directly into the gallbladder while the gallbladder drains directly into the common bile duct (Figure 11–21). Ultrasonography may show ducts entering a cystic mass in the region of the porta that could

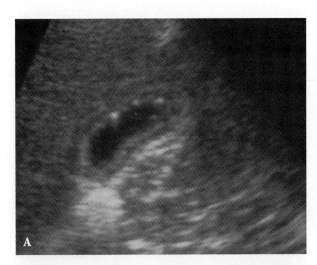

FIGURE 11–18. Adenomyomatosis. Longitudinal ultrasonograph shows tiny echogenic foci with ring down artifact within the gallbladder wall, in keeping with cholesterol deposition in Rokitansky-Aschoff sinuses.

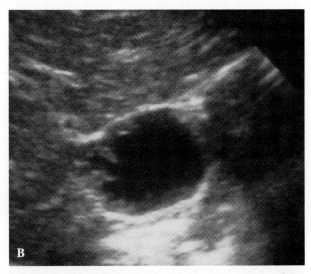

FIGURE 11–19. Adenomyomatosis. Transverse ultrasonograph shows irregular thickening of the fundus of the gallbladder.

mimic a choledochal cyst (Figure 11–22a) (Yazbeck et al., 1985). Percutaneous transhepatic cholangiography or intraoperative cholangiography can demonstrate the abnormal anatomy of the biliary tree for diagnosis and surgical planning (Figure 11–22b) (Stringer, 1987).

Congenital stenosis of the ampulla of Vater (Yousefzadeh et al., 1979) may result in obstructive jaundice; congenital stenosis or diaphragms in the biliary tree also occur (Fisher et al., 1968; Chapoy et al., 1981). Bronchobiliary fistulae are rare and may be iatrogenic (Garel et al., 1980) or congenital (Waggett et al., 1970; Sane et al., 1971). Possible causes include union of an anomalous bronchial bud with an anomalous bile duct and duplication of the upper gastrointestinal tract (Sane et al., 1971). The fistula usually arises from the right main bronchus (Chang and Guilian, 1985) but may also arise from the trachea (Stigol et al., 1966) and extends inferiorly to communicate with the biliary system. The infant usually presents with respiratory distress or aspiration pneumonia. The diagnosis can be made by cholangiography or bronchography and may be successfully treated with surgery.

Bile Plug Syndrome

Bile plug syndrome is extrahepatic obstruction of the bile ducts secondary to sludge in infants without an anatomic abnormality. Bile plug syndrome is a rare cause of obstructive jaundice in the perinatal period and is caused by inspissated or precipitated bile. The etiology is unclear but it may be related to prematurity, infection, dehydration, total parenteral nutrition, furosemide, gastrointestinal dysfunction, cystic fibrosis, and hemolysis due to Rh or ABO incompatibility (Pfeiffer et al., 1986; Davies et al., 1986a; Pariente et al., 1989; Sty et al., 1987; Taylor and Qaquandah, 1972). Bile plug syndrome often resolves spontaneously. However, persistent obstruction may require cholangiography with irrigation of the biliary system with saline or a mucolytic agent such as N-acetylcysteine (Pariente et al., 1989; Brown, 1990). If this is unsuccessful, choledochotomy and sphincterotomy or even biliary-enteric anastomosis may be necessary (Brown, 1990; Lang and Pinckney, 1991).

The best diagnostic modality is US, which shows dilatation of the biliary tree and sludge within biliary ducts and the gallbladder (Figure 11–23) (Pfeiffer et al., 1986; Davies et al., 1986a). Sludge is

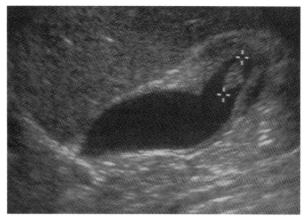

FIGURE 11–20. Gallbladder wall thickening and polypoid mass in this child with metachromatic leukodystrophy.

characteristically seen as low-level echoes without distal acoustic shadowing and may have a layered appearance or form sludge balls (Fakhry, 1982). The dilatation of the biliary ducts may be difficult to differentiate from a choledochal cyst.

Choledocholithiasis

Choledocholithiasis is uncommon in pediatric patients, occurring in 2 to 6% of children with cholelithiasis (Rescorla, 1997). Biliary stones in infants may be caused by the same factors as bile plug syndrome, including prematurity, infection, dehydration, total parenteral nutrition, furosemide, hemolytic disorders, gastrointestinal dysfunction, and cystic fibrosis (Jonas et al., 1990; Pariente et al., 1989). Biliary stones may also be seen in children with immunodeficiency and in patients with previous biliary tract surgery such as portoenterostomy

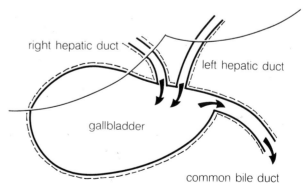

FIGURE 11–21. Interposition of the gallbladder. The diagram shows the gallbladder connected directly to the left and right intrahepatic ducts (*black arrows*) and the common bile duct (*black arrows*) without a cystic duct.

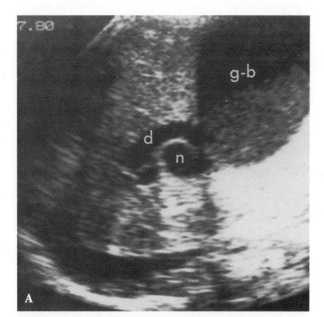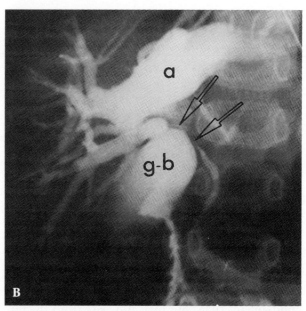

FIGURE 11–22. Interposition of the gallbladder. *A,* Longitudinal ultrasonograph shows the gallbladder (g-b) containing sludge and communicating with a normal cystic duct (n) and a dilated intrahepatic duct (d). A second dilated duct could be seen on other views. *B,* A percutaneous transhepatic cholangiograph in another patient shows the gallbladder (g-b) connecting directly to the dilated intrahepatic ducts (a) and via tight stenosis (*arrows*) to the proximal common bile duct. (Reprinted with permission from Stringer DA, Dobranowski J, Ein SH, et al. Interposition of the gallbladder—or the absent common hepatic duct and cystic duct. Pediatr Radiol 1987;17:151–3.)

for biliary atresia or liver transplantation (Enriquez et al., 1992; Sheng et al., 1996). Patients who are symptomatic and jaundiced require surgical intervention. Asymptomatic patients with normal liver function tests may be followed closely with ultrasonography (Jonas et al., 1990).

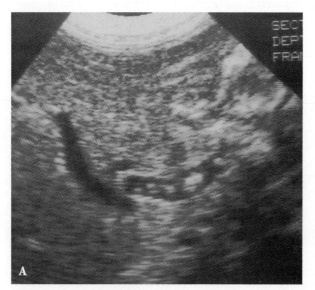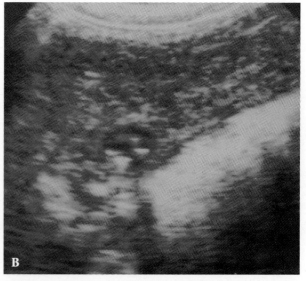

FIGURE 11–23. Bile plug syndrome in a patient with cystic fibrosis. Ultrasonograph shows multiple echogenic opacities in a dilated common bile duct (*A*) and gallbladder (*B*) in a newborn infant who rapidly developed obstructive jaundice. Tenacious, sticky bile was removed at surgery. (Reprinted with permission from Davies C, Daneman A, Stringer DA. Inspissated bile in a neonate with cystic fibrosis. J Ultrasound Med 1986;5:335–7.)

Biliary calculi are composed of bile pigments and cellular debris and may contain calcifications. On US, they are round or tubular echogenic structures, usually with posterior acoustic shadowing (Figures 11–24, 11–25). In the absence of associated typical features of biliary tract dilatation, they may be confused with other liver anomalies such as parenchymal calcification or pneumobilia. The sensitivity of US for choledocholithiasis is in the range of 60 to 90% (Siegel, 1996; Rescorla, 1997; Laing et al., 1984). Although common duct stones may be missed, US may suggest the diagnosis by demonstrating dilatation of the intrahepatic and extrahepatic bile ducts.

Computed tomography may fail to detect stones readily seen on US because some stones are only slightly higher or similar in density to bile, as is seen with cholesterol stones (Baron, 1997). Unenhanced CT scanning with thin collimation of 3 to 5 mm helps visualize biliary tract stones (Baron, 1997). The sensitivity of CT for detection of biliary stones is similar to US, ranging from 50 to 90% (Gembala, 1994).

Cholangiography may be used to assess for biliary calculi and to differentiate them from other causes of biliary obstruction if US and CT have failed to determine the etiology (Figure 11–26). Endoscopic retrograde cholangiopancreatography (ERCP) may be performed for diagnosis and stone extraction (Rescorla, 1997). The spatial resolution of magnetic resonance cholangiography is less than conventional cholangiography but stones as small as 2 to 3 mm may be detected (Chan et al., 1996; Reinhold et al., 1996). The sensitivity of MRCP for choledocholithiasis is up to 95% (Chan et al., 1996). This imaging modality will show stones as low signal intensity in contrast to the surrounding high signal intensity of bile. It is important to correlate the three-dimensional projection with the source images since false positives may be caused by pneumobilia, surgical clips, and vascular compression by the right hepatic artery (Watanabe et al., 1998).

Cholangitis

Cholangitis is rare in children and can be divided into two main forms: sclerosing cholangitis and ascending or acute cholangitis.

Primary Sclerosing Cholangitis. Primary sclerosing cholangitis is a chronic progressive disorder characterized by inflammation and fibrosis of the

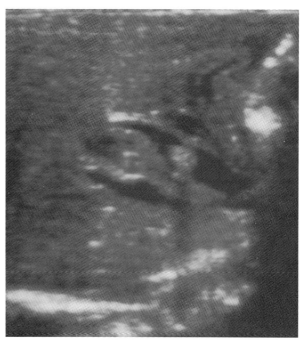

FIGURE 11–24. Increasing jaundice in a 1-month-old female. Ultrasonograph demonstrates an echogenic, acoustically shadowing stone within a dilated common hepatic duct.

intrahepatic and extrahepatic bile ducts, eventually leading to biliary cirrhosis (McEvoy and Suchy, 1996; Sisto et al., 1987; Ong et al., 1994; Classen et al., 1987). Its etiology is unknown. Primary sclerosing cholangitis in children may be associated with inflammatory bowel disease (Ong et al., 1994; Classen et al., 1987) but this association is less frequent in children than in adults (McEvoy and Suchy,

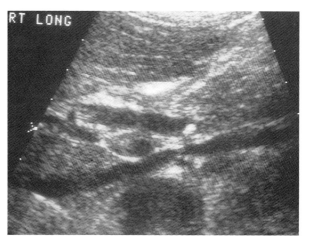

FIGURE 11–25. Biliary obstruction due to a common bile duct stone in a patient with sickle cell disease.

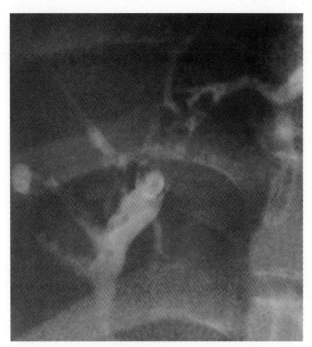

FIGURE 11–26. Multiple gallstones in the intrahepatic biliary tree after cholecystectomy. Percutaneous transhepatic cholangiography shows multiple filling defects obstructing a dilated left intrahepatic duct.

1996). Other associations include immunodeficiency and Langerhans' cell histiocytosis (McEvoy and Suchy, 1996; Sisto et al., 1987; Classen et al., 1987). It may be idiopathic (Sisto et al., 1987; Spivak et al., 1982). Primary sclerosing cholangitis affects children of all ages, including neonates and infants (McEvoy and Suchy, 1996; Sisto et al., 1987).

Clinical features may be nonspecific. Abdominal pain, jaundice, chronic diarrhea, and fever are the most frequent symptoms and signs. There may be hepatomegaly, and alkaline phosphatase and transaminase levels are usually elevated. Infants may present with neonatal cholestatic jaundice (Debray et al., 1994). Diagnosis is based on a combination of biochemical, histologic, and radiologic tests (McEvoy and Suchy, 1996).

Cholangiography is the imaging procedure of choice; ERCP or percutaneous transhepatic cholangiography can be performed to visualize the biliary tree (Nicotra et al., 1997). Typical cholangiographic findings include multifocal short annular strictures of the intrahepatic and extrahepatic ducts with intervening normal or saccular dilated segments, diverticulum-like outpouchings, and decreased arborization of the biliary tree ("pruned tree" or

"rosary" appearance) (Sisto et al., 1987; Ong et al., 1994; Classen et al., 1987; MacCarty et al., 1983; Chen and Goldberg, 1984) (Figure 11–27a). Rarely, a localized form of primary sclerosing cholangitis may present with unifocal stricture of the common bile duct (Sokal et al., 1990).

Ultrasonography shows dilatation of the intrahepatic and extrahepatic bile ducts and concentric ductal wall thickening (Figure 11–27b) (Nicotra et al., 1997). Alteration in hepatic echotexture is seen as cirrhosis develops.

Computed tomography demonstrates scattered "skip" dilatations of the intrahepatic ducts due to multiple intrahepatic duct strictures (Baron, 1997; Rahn et al., 1983). Abnormalities of the extrahepatic ducts may also show on CT, including concentric or eccentric wall thickening, mural nodularity and enhancement, and ductal dilatation and strictures (Teefey et al., 1988). Signs of portal hypertension are evident in later stages of the disease (Figure 11–28).

Diagnosis is confirmed on liver biopsy, which shows the presence of portal hepatitis, periportal fibrosis or periportal hepatitis, septal fibrosis with or without bridging necrosis, and biliary cirrhosis (Ong et al., 1994).

Clinical course is variable but usually progressive. There is no specific treatment for primary sclerosing cholangitis (Sisto et al., 1987; Classen et al., 1987). Immunosuppressive therapy with prednisone and azathioprine may be beneficial. Prognosis remains poor, and liver transplantation is an option for patients with end-stage liver disease (McEvoy and Suchy, 1996; Debray et al., 1994). Percutaneous balloon dilatation of ductal strictures has been performed as a palliative procedure in adults (Skolkin et al., 1989). Hepatocellular carcinoma may occur but bile duct carcinoma, which can develop in adults, has not been reported in children (Debray et al., 1994).

Acute or Ascending Cholangitis. Acute or ascending cholangitis, also known as obstructive suppurative cholangitis, is a potentially life-threatening condition that requires early diagnosis and treatment (Balthazar et al., 1993). It usually occurs following complete or partial biliary obstruction from gallstones, bile duct stricture, or congenital extrahepatic biliary tree anomaly, and as a complication of biliary-enteric anastomotic surgery (Kasai procedure). Treatment must aim at correcting the underlying abnormality to allow biliary drainage and prevent hepatic damage.

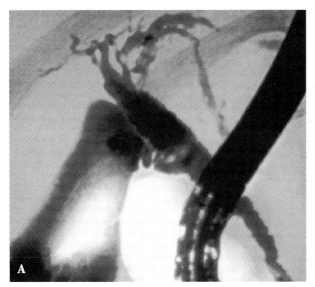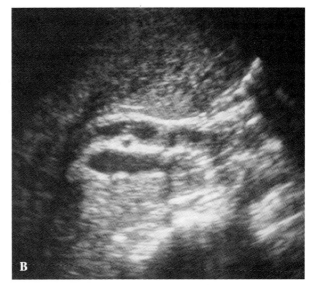

FIGURE 11–27. Primary sclerosing cholangitis and inflammatory bowel disease in an 8-year-old girl. *A,* Reduced arborization of the biliary tree shown on ERCP. There is involvement of the intra- and extrahepatic ducts with irregularity of the ducts and areas of constriction and dilatation. *B,* Ultrasonograph shows dilatation of the common duct, with mild irregularity of the ductal wall.

Most patients present with abdominal pain, tenderness, fever, chills, and jaundice. The responsible organisms are usually gram-negative organisms (Balthazar et al., 1993).

Acute cholangitis usually produces no findings on CT (Baron, 1997). Biliary dilatation may be seen but there is no correlation between the severity of ascending cholangitis and the degree of biliary dilatation (Balthazar et al., 1993). Absence of biliary dilatation on US or CT does not exclude mechanical obstruction or cholangitis. Thickening of the bile duct walls with diffuse concentric enhancement may be seen in patients with infectious cholangitis, and suppurative material in the bile ducts may be seen as increased attenuation of the bile (Bathazar et al., 1993). Biliary duct dilatation with biliary sludge as well as thickening of the wall of the common bile duct can be seen on US (Gaines et al., 1991; Mittelstaedt, 1997). Liver abscesses, biliary air, and portal venous gas are seen in patients with severe forms of cholangitis (Balthazar et al., 1993; Dennis et al., 1985).

Other Causes of Cholangitis. Recurrent pyogenic cholangitis or Oriental cholangiohepatitis is endemic to areas of southeast Asia. The cause of the disease is unknown but associations with clonorchiasis, ascariasis, and nutritional deficiency have been suggested (Lim, 1991). Pathologically, there is dilatation of the intra- and extrahepatic ducts which con-

tain soft, pigmented stones and pus, and enteric bacteria can be cultured from the bile (Lim, 1991; Lim, 1990). A spectrum of ultrasonographic and computed tomographic features are seen, including intraductal calculi, marked intrahepatic and extrahepatic biliary duct dilatation (up to 3 to 4 cm), pruning of the dilated intrahepatic ducts, segmental atrophy (particularly the left lateral segment), strictures, ductal wall enhancement, and increased periportal echogenicity

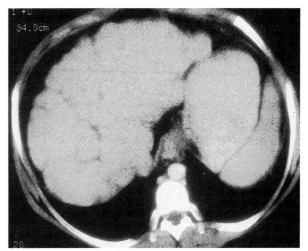

FIGURE 11–28. Primary sclerosing cholangitis in a 15-year-old girl. Contrast-enhanced CT shows hepatic cirrhosis.

(Baron, 1997; Mittelstaedt, 1997; Lim, 1991; Chan et al., 1989). Cholangiography shows similar findings.

Acquired immunodeficiency syndrome (AIDS) cholangitis is due to opportunistic infection with *Cryptosporidium*, *Cytomegalovirus*, or human immunodeficiency virus (HIV) itself (Baron, 1997; Dolmatch et al., 1987). Radiologic findings include mild biliary duct dilatation and wall thickening, ampullary stenosis, irregular strictures, and gallbladder wall thickening (Baron, 1997; Mittelstaedt, 1997; Grumbach et al., 1989; Rusin et al., 1992).

Cystic Fibrosis
General Considerations. Cystic fibrosis can have many effects upon the liver and biliary tree. Biliary tract anomalies are found in 5 to 33% of patients with cystic fibrosis (Agrons et al., 1996). There is an increased incidence of gallbladder disease with age, including cholelithiasis and cholecystitis (Anagnostopoulos et al., 1993), and biliary strictures may also occur (Schneck, 1994). Gallstones can be found in approximately 10% of patients with cystic fibrosis (L'Heureux et al., 1977). Focal biliary fibrosis is a hepatic lesion pathognomonic of cystic fibrosis found in 25% of postmortem examinations of cystic fibrosis patients. In approximately 5% of patients, this progresses to multinodular cirrhosis (di Sant'Agnese and Blanc, 1956; Oppenheimer and Esterly, 1975).

Cystic fibrosis may cause jaundice in neonates due to inspissated bile, the bile plug syndrome (Davies et al., 1986a). Impairment of biliary drainage within the intrahepatic ducts may be important in the pathogenesis of liver disease (Dogan et al., 1994). Obstruction of the bile ducts by thick tenacious bile may lead to periductal inflammation and fibrosis (Quillin et al., 1993). In severe neonatal forms, the process can be associated with hypoplasia of the biliary ducts and findings can be similar to biliary atresia (Greenholz et al., 1997).

Imaging. Ultrasonographic findings may include a microgallbladder (Figure 11–29), sludge, and gallstones (Graham et al., 1985; McHugo et al., 1987). The atrophic gallbladder may be difficult to detect on US, and hence, gallstones may not be appreciated or differentiated from bowel gas. Ultrasonography, CT, and MR can demonstrate intrahepatic ductal dilatation that may contain inspissated bile or stones (Figure 11–30) (Schneck, 1994). Biliary strictures are difficult to detect on US and CT and are best evaluated with cholangiography.

Cholangiography can depict filling defects caused by inspissated bile, mucus, or stones and may demonstrate bile duct strictures. There may be irregularity of the intrahepatic ducts secondary to recurrent cholangitis or focal biliary cirrhosis (Schneck, 1994).

On hepatobiliary scintigraphy, patients with cystic fibrosis may show nonvisualization of the gallbladder and focal areas of intrahepatic retention of tracer secondary to cholestasis (Dogan et al., 1994; O'Connor et al., 1996).

Spontaneous Perforation of the Bile Ducts in Early Infancy
This is a rare but potentially fatal occurrence during infancy that usually presents within the first 3 months of life (Siegel, 1996). The perforation most commonly occurs at the junction of cystic and common hepatic duct or just distal to this level (Fawcett et al., 1986). The etiology is uncertain but theories include a developmental weakness or focal area of infarction of the bile duct wall or a congenital luminal diverticula that perforates (Stringer, 1989). Biliary stones are sometimes associated with perforation, and it is uncertain whether they are a cause or result of perforation of the bile duct (Descos et al., 1984; Haller, 1989).

The most common findings are jaundice and abdominal distension due to bilious ascites in a full-term infant (Fawcett et al., 1986; Haller et al., 1989; Hyde, 1965; Stringel and Mercer, 1983). Failure to thrive, vomiting, and acholic stool are other common symptoms. Abdominal swelling can extend into the inguinal and scrotal regions, presenting as a hernia due to the ascites (Fawcett et al., 1986). A less common presentation is acute peritonitis without jaundice. Liver function tests are generally normal except for elevated bilirubin levels, which may help differentiation from neonatal hepatitis (Siegel, 1996; Haller et al., 1989).

Plain film radiography may show evidence of ascites. Ultrasonography may show free intraperitoneal fluid or a loculated subhepatic fluid collection and may contain echogenic debris. There is no evidence of biliary ductal dilatation (Fawcett et al., 1986; Haller et al., 1989). Hepatobiliary scintigraphy will make a definitive diagnosis by demonstrating leak of radionuclide from the duct (Fawcett et al., 1986; Stringel and Mercer, 1983). Intraoperative cholangiography is used to confirm the diagnosis at surgery. Early surgical intervention is required with drainage, and spontaneous healing usually occurs within 1 month (Haller et al., 1989).

Multiple Biliary Papillomatosis

Multiple biliary papillomatosis involves the intra- and/or extrahepatic bile ducts and is rare in children. Biliary papillomas are benign slow-growing tumors of the biliary duct epithelium that frequently present with clinical features of extrahepatic biliary obstruction. This may be caused by an increase in size, autoamputation, or excessive mucus secretions produced by the papilloma (Bines et al., 1992). Patients present with jaundice and epigastric pain, and there may be complications of biliary cirrhosis and liver failure (Khan et al. 1998). They have low-grade malignant potential, and adenocarcinoma has occurred within biliary papillomas in adults (Bines et al., 1992).

The presence of multiple sessile filling defects on percutaneous transhepatic cholangiography or ERCP is suggestive of the diagnosis. Extrahepatic biliary rhabdosarcoma should also be considered as it can present with similar clinical findings. Therapeutic approach depends on the site and extent of disease; surgical curettage and Roux-en-Y jejunal conduit may improve drainage in the young patient. There is a high rate of recurrence after surgical resection, and the condition may progress to involve other intrahepatic and extrahepatic ducts. Because of the risk of recurrence and malignant transformation, liver transplantation may be the best long-term option (Bines et al., 1992). (Other tumors arising from the biliary tract will be discussed in the section on liver tumors.)

CONGENITAL AND DEVELOPMENTAL ANOMALIES

Biliary Atresia and Idiopathic Neonatal Hepatitis

Neonatal jaundice may be caused by hemolysis, sepsis, infections (*Cytomegalovirus*, herpes simplex, rubella, *Coxsackie* B virus, echoviruses 14 and 19, congenital syphilis, and toxoplasmosis), and a variety of metabolic diseases such as alpha$_1$-antitrypsin deficiency, tyrosinemia, galactosemia, and cystic fibrosis (Table 11–1). The possibility of hepatobiliary disease must be considered in any neonate jaun-

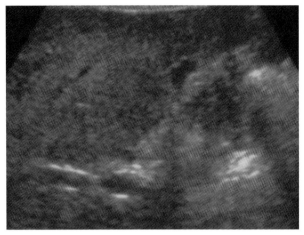

FIGURE 11–29. Longitudinal ultrasonograph. Small gallbladder in a patient with cystic fibrosis.

diced beyond 14 days (Balistreri et al., 1996). When other causes have been excluded and jaundice persists, the diagnosis is probably biliary atresia or idiopathic neonatal hepatitis.

Biliary atresia and idiopathic neonatal hepatitis are two overlapping conditions, which probably represent opposite ends of a spectrum of obstructive cholangiopathies although this is not proved (Landing, 1974). Together, they cause over 90% of the cases of neonatal obstructive jaundice (Thaler, 1968). Idiopathic neonatal hepatitis accounts for approximately 35 to 45% of infantile cholestatic liver disease. Premature and male infants are more commonly affected (Stringer, 1989). Biliary atresia accounts for approximately one-third of cases of neonatal cholestasis (Schneck, 1994). It occurs more

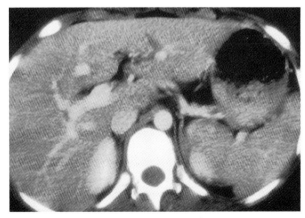

FIGURE 11–30. Computed tomography showing intrahepatic biliary ductal dilatation in a patient with cystic fibrosis.

frequently in females, and affects 1 in 8000 to 12,000 births (Balistreri et al., 1996).

Clinical Features
Biliary atresia and neonatal hepatitis are clinically similar, with persistent jaundice and hepatomegaly generally occurring in an otherwise healthy neonate. The jaundice usually starts in the first weeks of life and increases gradually along with signs of hepatomegaly.

Differentiation between these two conditions is often difficult because biliary atresia can be an evolving process in the postnatal period. In neonatal hepatitis, a fall in the elevated serum levels of conjugated bilirubin and alkaline phosphatase usually but not always occurs after 4 months of age; this does not occur in biliary atresia (Thaler, 1968). Differentiation

---

TABLE 11–1. Causes of Neonatal Jaundice

Extrahepatic disorders
  Biliary atresia
  Choledochal cyst
  Bile plug syndrome
  Choledocholithiasis
  Spontaneous perforation of CBD
Intrahepatic disorders
  Bile duct paucity
    Alagille syndrome
    Nonsyndromic paucity of bile ducts
  Parenchymal disease
    Idiopathic neonatal hepatitis
    Infection
      Cytomegalovirus
      Rubella
      Herpes simplex
      Coxsackie B virus
      Echovirus
      Congenital syphilis
      Toxoplasmosis
  Toxic/metabolic
    Total parenteral nutrition
    Alpha$_1$-antitrypsin
    Cystic fibrosis
    Galactosemia
    Tyrosinemia
  Endocrine
    Hypothyroidism
    Panhypopituitarism

CBD = common bile duct.

---

between these conditions is important because the treatment is different. Neonatal hepatitis is managed conservatively with medical therapy while patients with biliary atresia require surgical intervention.

Biliary atresia may be associated with other congenital anomalies in 10 to 30% of patients (Chandra, 1974; Karrer et al., 1991; Lefkowitch, 1998; Vazquez et al., 1995). These anomalies include polysplenia, preduodenal portal vein, hepatic arterial anomalies, azygous continuation of the inferior vena cava, situs inversus, malrotation, and intestinal atresia (Table 11–2) (Chandra, 1974; Karrer et al., 1991; Vazquez et al., 1995; Abramson et al., 1987; Yanagihara et al., 1995). Cardiac defects include anomalous pulmonary venous return, atrial septal defect (Karrer et al., 1991), and pulmonary stenosis (Silveira et al., 1991). Biliary atresia can also be seen in chromosomal abnormalities most commonly trisomy 18 but also trisomy 21, and Turner's syndrome (Silveira et al., 1991). Associated anomalies do not preclude successful biliary reconstruction with Kasai procedure or liver transplantation but preoperative evaluation is important as surgical modification may be required (Karrer et al., 1991; Vazquez et al., 1995).

Skeletal changes include osteopenia. In longstanding biliary atresia, patients may develop rickets, modeling deformities, and fractures (Figure 11–31) (Baker and Harris, 1964; Hirano et al., 1990; Katayama et al., 1975).

Etiology and Pathology
The etiology of biliary atresia remains unknown but possible causes include viral infection (*Reovirus* type 3, *Cytomegalovirus*, Epstein-Barr virus, and rubella), ischemic injury, abnormal bile acid metabolism,

---

TABLE 11–2. Anomalies Associated with Biliary Atresia

Polysplenia
Preduodenal portal vein
Hepatic arterial anomalies
Cardiac defects
Azygous continuation of IVC
Situs inversus
Malrotation
Intestinal atresia

IVC = inferior vena cava.

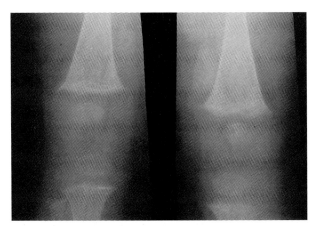

FIGURE 11–31. Biliary atresia and rickets. There is osteopenia as well as fraying and cupping of the metaphyses.

pancreaticobiliary maljunction, genetic influence, and developmental anomaly (Lefkowitch, 1998; Park et al., 1996). Classic clinical data suggest that the process of biliary atresia starts as an intrauterine phenomenon (Gautier and Eliot, 1981). In the early stages, the main interlobar bile ducts are present along their entire course (Chiba et al., 1975); with time, these ducts diminish in number and size (Landing, 1974; Kasai, 1970), a process called the "disappearing bile duct syndrome." The presence of active and progressive inflammation and fibrosis involving the intra- and extrahepatic bile ducts suggests an acquired etiology. However, association with anomalies such as the polysplenia syndrome supports a congenital origin for biliary atresia. More than one cause or pathogenesis may lead to a final common lesion (Walker et al., 1996).

Histopathologic examination of the liver is used to differentiate biliary atresia from neonatal hepatitis (Middlesworth and Altman, 1997). The main pathologic process in neonatal hepatitis is hepatocellular damage while in biliary atresia there is injury to the biliary ducts (Park et al., 1996) as well as periportal fibrosis, intrahepatic small bile duct proliferation, and hepatocellular cholestasis (Figure 11–32). Pathologic features in neonatal hepatitis include giant cell transformation, parenchymal disruption, and cirrhosis (Park et al., 1996; Kirks, 1998). Liver biopsy has been used to help distinguish between these two conditions with an accuracy of 86 to 96% (Smetana et al., 1965; Lai et al., 1994; Ohnuma et al., 1997; Park et al., 1997). However, the early pathologic changes of biliary atresia may be similar to neonatal hepatitis, and fol-

low up biopsies are recommended in equivocal cases (Park et al., 1996).

Postoperatively in long-term survivors with biliary atresia, the liver is heterogeneous, with some areas resembling normal hepatic architecture and other areas showing evidence of biliary cirrhosis (Kimura et al., 1980). In general, cirrhotic change occurs more readily in the peripheral part of the liver. The preponderance of normal or abnormal liver parenchyma seems to depend on time elapsed since operation, presence or absence of ascending cholangitis, and excellent or poor flow of bile (Kimura et al., 1980). Portal hypertension can develop secondary to the biliary cirrhosis.

Imaging of Biliary Atresia and Neonatal Hepatitis
Imaging of infants with cholestatic jaundice is geared toward demonstrating anatomy and function of the liver and biliary system to determine if operation is necessary. Preoperative imaging is usually restricted to US and radionuclide scintigraphy (Kirks et al., 1984). If biliary atresia is not excluded and if the diagnosis is still uncertain, a laparotomy and operative cholangiography are advisable before 3 months of age since operations for biliary atresia performed after this time have a poor prognosis.

Ultrasonography. Ultrasonography is the best initial radiologic investigation because it can exclude other causes of obstructive jaundice such as a choledochal cyst and other anatomic anomalies. However, US does not specifically differentiate between biliary atresia and neonatal hepatitis. It may be used to evaluate the hepatic parenchyma and

FIGURE 11–32. Histology of biliary atresia. On light micrograph, there is evidence of fibrosis with obliteration of ductal structures (×10 original magnification).

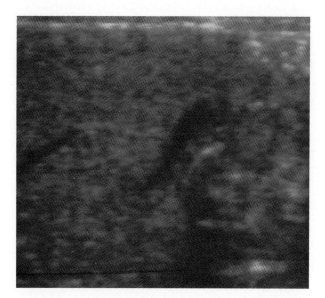

FIGURE 11–33. Ultrasonograph shows a small gallbladder in a patient with biliary atresia.

assess liver size. The parenchyma in both conditions is often inhomogeneous but in biliary atresia there may be a marked increase in periportal echoes, which may represent early periportal fibrosis. A triangular or tubular echogenic density adjacent to the portal vein bifurcation has been described on ultrasonographs of patients with biliary atresia. It has been termed the "triangular cord sign" and is felt to represent the fibrous remnant of biliary atresia (Park et al., 1997; Choi et al., 1996).

In patients with biliary atresia, the gallbladder is often small or not visualized (Figure 11–33). Failure to find a gallbladder is likely to be associated with biliary atresia but can occur occasionally in severe neonatal hepatitis where bile production is severely decreased. The finding of a "normal gallbladder" is supportive evidence for neonatal hepatitis (Figure 11–34) (Abramson et al., 1982). However, a normal (≥1.5 cm in length) or (rarely) large gallbladder may be seen in approximately 10% of infants with biliary atresia (Siegel, 1996). Contraction of the gallbladder after a meal does not eliminate the possibility of biliary atresia (Ikeda et al., 1989; Ohi and Ibrahim, 1992).

Intrahepatic bile duct dilatation occurs infrequently, but indicates atresia when it is present (Figure 11–35) (Abramson et al., 1982). Cystic changes that may be seen within the liver in the late stages of biliary atresia are related to dilatation of the biliary ducts and may be secondary to cholangitis (Betz et al., 1994).

Choledochal cysts are occasionally associated with biliary atresia and are well shown by US as cystic structures in the porta hepatis (Figure 11–36). At least five cases of antenatally diagnosed biliary atresia have been reported. All of them had type 1 cysts, and antenatal diagnosis was made between 19 and 32 weeks. The differential diagnosis includes a choledochal cyst with complete distal obstruction. If the operative cholangiograph shows hypoplastic intrahepatic ducts and no communication with the

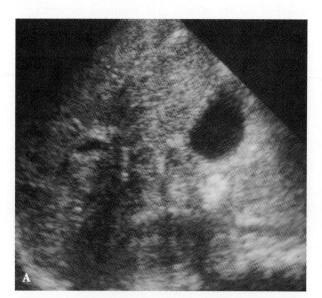

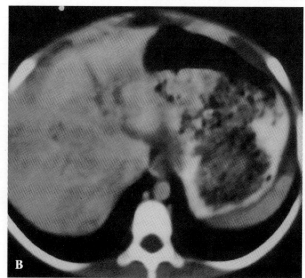

FIGURE 11–34. Neonatal hepatitis. *A,* Ultrasonograph demonstrates nonspecific heterogeneous liver parenchyma and normal-sized gallbladder. *B,* Postcontrast CT shows patchy low attenuation within the parenchyma and periportal regions.

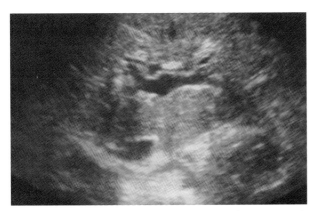

FIGURE 11–35. Biliary atresia. Transverse ultrasonograph of the liver demonstrates increased periportal echogenicity, and minimal prominence of the intrahepatic biliary ducts.

intestine, this confirms the diagnosis of biliary atresia (Tsuchida et al., 1995).

Ultrasonography is the initial imaging modality of choice for biliary atresia, and a careful search should be made for associated anomalies such as situs inversus and polysplenia. Computed tomography also can identify congenital abnormalities and acquired abnormalities related to portal hypertension (Day et al., 1989).

Radionuclide Scintigraphy. Liver uptake in biliary atresia is usually normal if the patient is under 2 months of age but can be decreased if there is severe hepatic dysfunction (Nadel, 1996). Biliary atresia prevents excretion of IDA derivatives into the bowel (Figure 11–37); however, severe neonatal hepatitis may produce poor hepatic uptake, possibly leading to diminished excretion of radionuclide into the gastrointestinal tract. Therefore, if no radiopharmaceutical is seen in the bowel on imaging up to 24 hours, the distinction between severe hepatocellular disease and biliary atresia cannot be made. If a patent biliary tree is shown with passage of activity into the bowel, biliary atresia is virtually excluded (Nadel, 1996). Rarely in biliary atresia, even technetium Tc 99m DISIDA may show apparent gut excretion because biliary atresia is an evolving process. Hence, laparotomy should not be postponed if other clinical and laboratory data strongly support atresia (Williamson et al., 1986).

Magnetic Resonance Imaging. Magnetic resonance imaging (MR) is not used routinely but preliminary studies have been done using magnetic resonance cholangiography in neonates with cholestasis. Biliary atresia can be ruled out using this technique if the complete extrahepatic biliary duct is identified on MRCP (Guibaud et al, 1998). Nonvisualization of the extrahepatic biliary tree is not specific for biliary atresia as other disorders associated with decreased biliary excretion may also have this appearance (Guibaud et al., 1998). In patients with biliary atresia, MR may also show periportal thickening that is thought to be related to periportal fibrosis (Guibaud et al., 1998).

Cholangiography. Diagnostic percutaneous transhepatic cholangiography is not usually performed for biliary atresia (Franken et al., 1978; Carty, 1977) because it is a difficult procedure in neonates and young infants and is often either unhelpful or

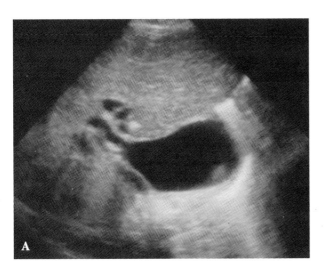
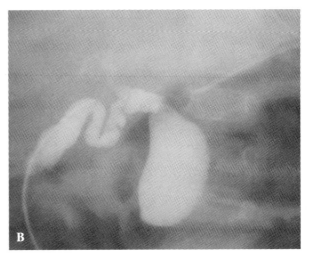

FIGURE 11–36. Biliary atresia and choledochal cyst. *A,* Oblique ultrasonograph demonstrates a large cystic structure in the porta hepatis. *B,* An intraoperative cholangiograph demonstrates filling of the cyst and some mildly dilated intrahepatic ducts but no communication with the duodenum.

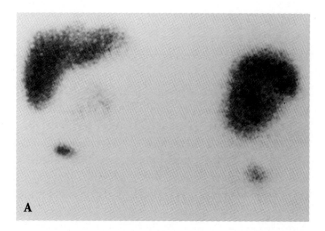

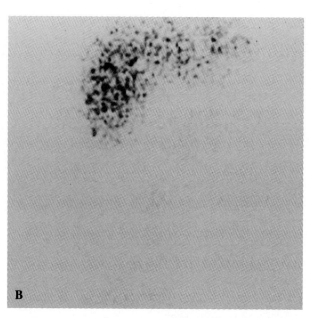

FIGURE 11–37. Diisopropyl-IDA scan in a patient with biliary atresia. Anterior and lateral views show no excretion of the radiopharmaceutical into the bowel at (A) 2 and (B) 24 hours.

unsuccessful. The bile ducts in biliary atresia are very attenuated, if present, and show variable filling (Figure 11–38). Occasionally there may be filling of a tortuous thin extrahepatic common bile duct with a relatively normal intrahepatic biliary tree, the diagnosis of biliary atresia being made only at operation (Carty, 1977). Percutaneous transhepatic cholangiography is definitive only when a normal intrahep-

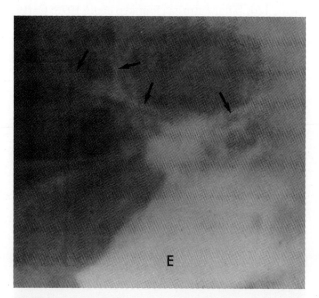

FIGURE 11–38. Biliary atresia. A preoperative percutaneous transhepatic cholangiograph shows fine attenuated ducts (*arrows*) that are disorganized and do not communicate with the extrahepatic duct. Extravasation of contrast medium (E) occurred during the procedure.

atic and extrahepatic system is shown, thereby excluding biliary atresia. In severe neonatal hepatitis, the ducts are patent but a thin common bile duct may be present (Carty, 1977), and the ducts can be distorted by the inflammation (Figure 11–39). As a result, the value of the procedure is open to question, and preoperative percutaneous transhepatic cholangiography is not generally performed.

Endoscopic retrograde cholangiopancreatography is useful for visualizing the extrahepatic biliary tree and recently has been performed in pediatric patients with smaller endoscopes. This requires a high degree of skill but with experienced operators it has been successful in 90% of patients (Ohnuma et al., 1997; Wilkinson, 1996). If only the pancreatic duct fills, the patient will require a laparotomy for presumed biliary atresia. If the intrahepatic and main bile ducts fill, biliary atresia is excluded (Ohnuma et al., 1997).

Surgery

Generally, if there is clinical doubt after ultrasonography, a nuclear medicine scan with or without biopsy is performed without delay, followed by an exploratory laparotomy with operative cholangiography. Biliary atresia is most amenable to successful surgery in the first few months of life; if untreated, the vast majority of cases progress to irreversible biliary cirrhosis and death.

In the past, biliary atresia was divided into an operable or correctable group and an inoperable

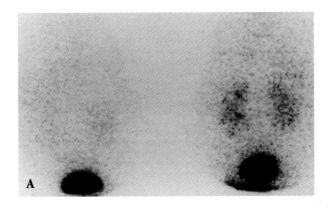

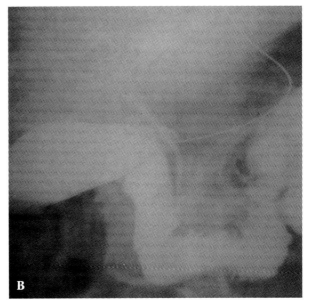

FIGURE 11–39. Severe neonatal hepatitis. *A,* Technetium Tc 99m diisopropyl-IDA (DISIDA) scan shows little hepatic activity at 4 hours. *B,* Intraoperative injection of contrast into the gallbladder demonstrates a patent biliary tree and free drainage into the duodenum.

group (Figure 11–40). The correctable group consisted of a small percentage of cases in which the distal extrahepatic biliary duct was obstructed but the proximal common hepatic duct was patent. Such a case was classified as correctable because its suffi-

ciently developed biliary system allows primary anastomosis of the bile duct to the bowel. This classification is no longer valid regarding surgical treatment but it is still sometimes useful as it gives an anatomic division of the various abnormalities.

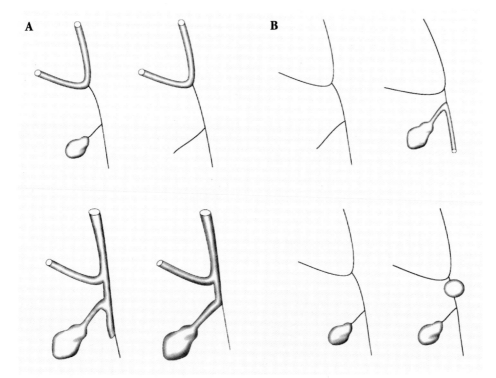

FIGURE 11–40. Types of biliary atresia. *A,* The operable, or correctable, group of patients with biliary atresia has a major portion of the common bile duct that is patent. *B,* The inoperable group does not have this patency.

Many patients with biliary atresia can now be treated surgically with the portoenterostomy developed by Kasai. After resection of the fibrous bile duct remnant, a loop of small bowel is anastomosed to the bed of the porta hepatis with a Roux-en-Y anastomosis, creating a bile drainage pathway for the small patent ductules (Schneck, 1994; Kasai et al., 1968).

The best results are obtained when the Kasai operation is performed within 2 months of birth; results are poor when surgery is delayed until after 3 months of life (Majd, 1983). The long-term success rate of the Kasai procedure is 25 to 40% (Grosfeld, 1994). Predictors of a poor outcome include the age of the patient at the time of surgery, the degree of patency of extrahepatic ducts, and the development of hepatic fibrosis (Karrer et al., 1990).

Operative cholangiography is performed through the gallbladder, which may be small and atretic. Care must be taken to ensure adequate filling of the intrahepatic biliary system (Walker et al., 1996). In neonatal hepatitis, operative cholangiography will demonstrate a patent biliary tree; in biliary atresia, no communication with the bowel will be found (Figure 11–41). It is sometimes difficult to reach a correct diagnosis (Hays et al., 1967), and if operative cholangiography does not demonstrate the extrahepatic biliary tree, exploration of the porta hepatis may be necessary.

Liver transplantation is indicated in patients with a failed Kasai operation and in those who present late with liver failure. Biliary atresia is the most common indication for pediatric liver transplantation, and more than half of the candidates for liver transplantation have biliary atresia (Ohi and Ibrahim, 1992). Any surgical procedure performed must not preclude later transplantation.

Complications and Post-Kasai Imaging

Ascending cholangitis is the most frequent complication of a Kasai procedure and usually occurs in the first 2 years after surgery (Walker et al., 1996). It may be secondary to insufficient biliary drainage, portal venous infection, or destruction of lymph drainage at the porta hepatis. Other complications include progressive cirrhosis, hepatic failure, and portal hypertension (Figures 11–42, 11–43). This may result in esophageal varices and hypersplenism (Figure 11–44) (Middlesworth and Altman, 1997; Ohi and Ibrahim, 1992; Kobayashi et al., 1976). Intrahepatic portal vein thrombosis has also been described as a complication after the Kasai procedure (Figure 11–45) (Cuffari et al., 1997). Rarely, hepatocellular carcinoma (Middlesworth and Altman, 1997) and cholangiocarcinoma can occur in association with biliary cirrhosis secondary to biliary atresia (Kulkarni and Beatty, 1977).

Percutaneous transhepatic cholangiography has been used to demonstrate the intrahepatic radicles following surgery (Chaumont et al., 1982). Both biliary ducts and hepatic lymphatics can be opacified. Bile lakes, which are intrahepatic accumulations

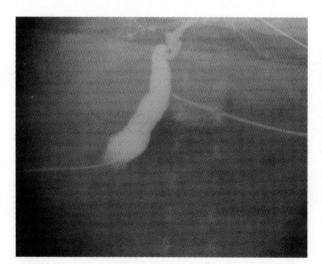

FIGURE 11–41. Biliary atresia. Intraoperative cholangiograph via injection of the gallbladder demonstrates a patent cystic duct and a few narrow intrahepatic radicles but no drainage of contrast into the duodenum.

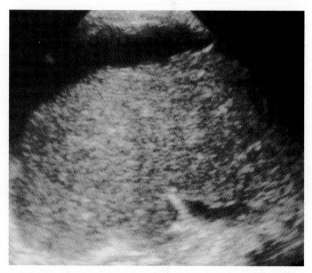

FIGURE 11–42. Biliary atresia with cirrhosis. Transverse ultrasonograph demonstrates coarse echogenic liver parenchyma with nodularity and associated ascites.

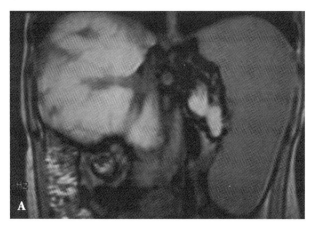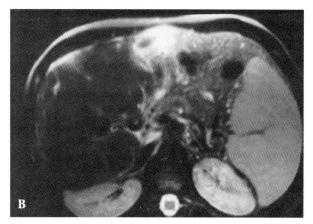

FIGURE 11–43. Cirrhosis and splenomegaly in a patient with biliary atresia demonstrated on (*A*) coronal T1-weighted and (*B*) axial T2-weighted MR.

of bile, can occur postoperatively (Fonkalsrud and Arima, 1975). Ultrasonography and percutaneous transhepatic cholangiography may help delineate the presence and site of drainage of these structures (Figure 11–46). Drainage of the bile lakes in patients with cholangitis has resulted in clinical improvement in some patients (Brunelle et al., 1985). The Roux loop may occasionally be seen as a cystic structure in the porta hepatis on US. Hepatobiliary scintigraphy can be used to demonstrate patency of the portoenterostomy as well as detect complications such as bile leak (Kirks, 1998; Nadel, 1996).

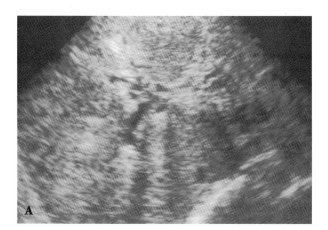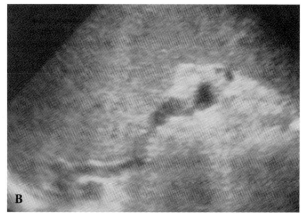

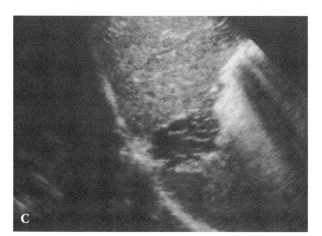

FIGURE 11–44. Biliary atresia post-Kasai procedure. *A*, Transverse ultrasonograph shows heterogeneous echogenic liver parenchyma. Longitudinal ultrasonograph demonstrates (*B*) splenomegaly and (*C*) gastroesophageal varices related to portal hypertension.

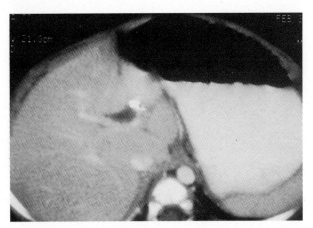

FIGURE 11–45. Biliary atresia. Axial CT demonstrates low attenuation with calcification in the porta hepatis related to portal vein thrombosis.

Alagille Syndrome (Arteriohepatic Dysplasia)

General Considerations

Alagille syndrome (also known as Watson-Alagille syndrome, syndromatic hepatic ductal hypoplasia, or arteriohepatic dysplasia) is a form of biliary hypoplasia with a paucity of bile ducts. Alagille syndrome is the most common form of familial intrahepatic cholestasis with an autosomal dominant inheritance pattern and may be related to a deletion on the short arm of chromosome 20 (Byrne et al., 1985; Elmslie et al., 1995). The syndrome complex consists of chronic intrahepatic cholestasis and peripheral pulmonary artery stenosis combined with other somatic defects that include characteristic facies, skeletal, and eye abnormalities. Other less common findings include renal abnormalities, pancreatic insufficiency, mild mental retardation, growth retardation, and hypogonadism (Alagille, 1996; Berrocal et al., 1997; Devriendt et al., 1996; Kahn, 1991; Schwarzenberg et al., 1992). The eye abnormality is an asymptomatic embryologic remnant called posterior embryotoxon. It is not specific for Alagille syndrome but is found in 90 to 95% of patients with this syndrome (Riely, 1987). The peripheral pulmonary stenosis is not clinically significant, and other cardiac anomalies encountered include patent ductus arteriosus, ventricular septal defect, tetralogy of Fallot, total anomalous venous return, and coarctation of the aorta (Riely, 1987).

Associated skeletal abnormalities include butterfly vertebrae of the thoracic spine, short distal phalanges, short ulna, radioulnar synostosis, narrowing of the interpediculate distance in the lumbar spine, and retarded bone age (Brunelle et al., 1986; Rosen-

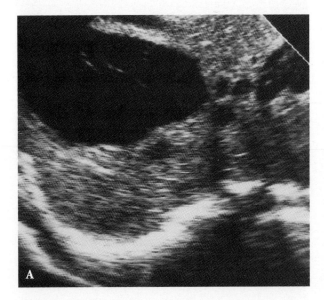

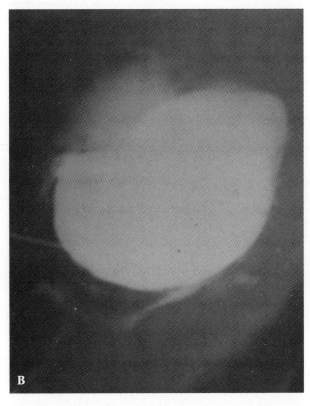

FIGURE 11–46. Bile lakes in biliary atresia following the Kasai procedure. *A*, A large intrahepatic cystic structure is seen on transverse ultrasonography. *B*, A percutaneous cholangiograph demonstrated a large bile lake.

field et al., 1980). Vertebral anomalies such as butter-fly vertebrae may be difficult to detect at birth and may no longer be present in adulthood (Figure 11–47) (Riely, 1987). In conjunction with evidence of hepatic and cardiac abnormalities, skeletal abnormalities may aid in the diagnosis of Alagille syndrome.

The hepatic abnormality is a congenital absence or hypoplasia of interlobular bile ducts in association with a patent extrahepatic biliary tree (Kahn, 1991). This results in jaundice of varying severity and duration, which usually develops during infancy (Alagille, 1996). It is considered to have a better prognosis than biliary atresia and is usually treated medically, with some patients showing improvement in cholestasis during childhood. Patients surviving into adulthood may develop late complications such as cirrhosis, liver failure, pancreatitis, and hepatocellular carcinoma (Schwartzenberg et al., 1992; Bekassy et al., 1992; Keeffe et al., 1993; Hoffenberg et al., 1995). Liver transplantation may be required in 15 to 50% of patients (Hoffenberg et al., 1995; Krantz et al., 1997). Patients may be at increased risk of postoperative complications because of the associated cardiopulmonary disease (Tzakis et al., 1993).

Imaging
Ultrasonography is of major value in excluding a surgically correctable cause of jaundice. The liver may be enlarged, predominantly affecting the left lobe (Alagille, 1996). The liver is generally of increased echogenicity and may show evidence of regenerating cirrhotic nodules (Singcharoen et al., 1986). There may be associated splenomegaly (Halvorsen et al., 1995).

Renal abnormalities include absent or hypoplastic/dysplastic kidneys and cystic disease (Berrocal et al., 1997; Martin et al., 1996; Pombo et al., 1995). There may be alteration of renal parenchymal echogenicity and nephrocalcinosis related to treatment (Berrocal et al., 1997).

Hepatobiliary scintigraphy demonstrates prolonged parenchymal transit time with patency of the extrahepatic biliary tree (Schneck, 1994; Halvorsen et al., 1995). Occasionally, there may be failure of radionuclide excretion, which reflects intrahepatic cholestasis in a similar way to biliary atresia (Figure 11–48) (Summerville et al., 1988). Intraoperative cholangiography may show nonfilling of the intrahepatic biliary tree, which may also be confused with biliary atresia (Figure 11–49).

Liver biopsy is recommended for histologic confirmation and will demonstrate paucity of interlobular bile ducts and may show evidence of fibrosis or cirrhosis. Bile duct paucity may also be seen in other nonsyndromic forms of intrahepatic cholestasis, and associated findings therefore are important in establishing the diagnosis of Alagille syndrome. Other causes of bile duct paucity include metabolic abnormalities, infection, chromosomal disorders, and Byler's syndrome (Alagille, 1996; Kahn, 1991; Alagille, 1987).

Byler's Syndrome
Byler's syndrome is the second most common form of familial intrahepatic cholestasis. It usually presents in infancy with symptoms of pruritus, hepatomegaly, and jaundice. In contrast to Alagille

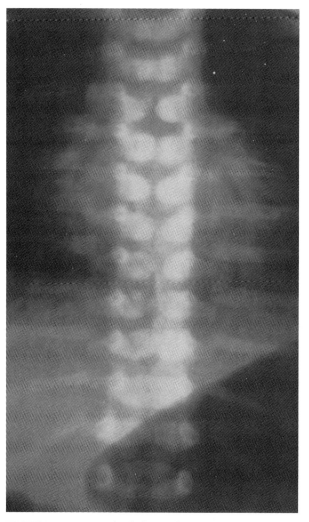

FIGURE 11–47. Multiple butterfly vertebrae are present in this patient with Alagille syndrome.

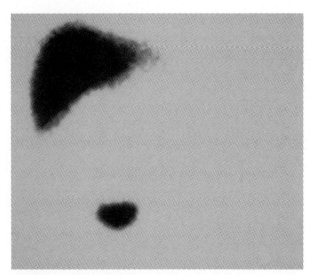

FIGURE 11–48. Alagille syndrome. The HIDA scan shows good hepatic uptake but no excretion of radiopharmaceutical into the bowel.

syndrome, this disorder is confined to the liver, without associated abnormality of other organs (Riely, 1987). Histologic findings include giant cell transformation and paucity of bile ducts; however, these findings are not specific and may occur in other cholestatic syndromes (Riely, 1987). Other pathologic findings include periportal fibrosis, cirrhosis, and cysts in the periportal region (Siegel,

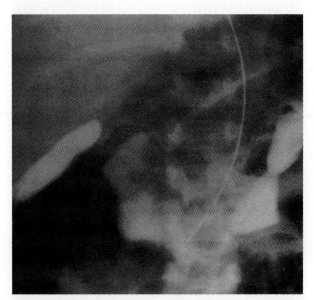

FIGURE 11–49. Alagille syndrome. Intraoperative cholangiograph fills a small galllbladder, a narrow cystic duct, and a common bile duct. No communication is seen with the liver.

1996). The prognosis is poor, and most patients die of hepatic failure during childhood. Liver transplantation is the only successful treatment. Hepatoma has been described as a complication in an adult patient (Quillin and Brink, 1992). Findings on US include multiple intrahepatic cysts that do not communicate with the dilated bile ducts (Siegel, 1996).

Choledochal Cyst

Classification
Choledochal cysts are cystic malformations of the biliary tree. They can be classified into five types according to cyst morphology and location (Figure 11–50) (Todani et al., 1977). Type I consists of fusiform dilatation of the common bile duct and is the commonest form, representing 80 to 90% of choledochal cysts (Crittenden and McKinley, 1985; Katyal and Lees, 1992; O'Neill, 1992). Type II consists of an eccentric diverticulum of the common bile duct and accounts for approximately 2% of cases. Type III is a choledochocele that is a focal dilated segment of the intraduodenal portion of the common bile duct (1.4 to 5% of cases). Type IV, the second most common form, consists of multiple cysts of the extrahepatic biliary ducts and may involve the intrahepatic biliary tract (19% of cases) (Schneck, 1994). Type V (Caroli's disease) consists of single or multiple intrahepatic biliary cysts (Todani et al., 1977). Caroli's disease is rare and probably of different etiology; it is included in the classification of choledochal cysts for convenience. Caroli's disease is considered separately in the later section, Cystic Disease of the Liver and Kidneys, as it represents a continuum with congenital hepatic fibrosis and autosomal recessive polycystic disease.

General Considerations
Choledochal cysts are rare anomalies of the biliary tract with an incidence in females four to five times greater than in males (Silberman and Glaessner, 1964; Barlow et al., 1976). It is more common in Japan than in North America (Rosenfield and Griscom, 1975).

The etiology of a choledochal cyst is uncertain. Initial theories suggested a congenital cause including a focal weakness of the bile duct wall, an obstruction of Oddi's sphincter, or a failure of recanalization of the embryonic common bile duct (Crittenden and McKinley, 1985; Barlow et al., 1976;

Yamaguchi, 1980). The most widely accepted theory is anomalous insertion of the common bile duct into the pancreatic duct with a long common channel (Babbitt et al., 1973; Miyano et al., 1979; Ono et al., 1982). The anomalous insertion is thought to result in reflux of pancreatic juice retrogradely into the common bile duct, leading to inflammation, dilatation, and scarring (Babbitt et al., 1973). High amylase levels have been found in the choledochal cyst fluid, supporting this theory (Suarez et al., 1987; Jona et al., 1979; Sherman et al., 1986). However, anomalies of the pancreaticobiliary junction are not a constant finding in all cases of choledochal cyst (Rosenfield and Griscom, 1975), being present on cholangiography only 65 to 80% of the time

(O'Neill, 1992). In addition, choledochal cysts have been identified on prenatal US as early as 15 weeks' gestational age, which is prior to excretion of pancreatic amylase (Benhidjeb et al., 1996).

Choledochal cyst in the neonate appears to be a separate entity from the choledochal cyst that presents in childhood and adolescence as they have different clinical and radiologic presentations. The pathogenesis in the neonate may be congenital whereas it may be acquired in the older child (Babbitt et al., 1973; Torrisi et al., 1990).

Clinical Features
Most cases of choledochal cyst present under the age of 10 years, with 30% under 1 year of age. Presenta-

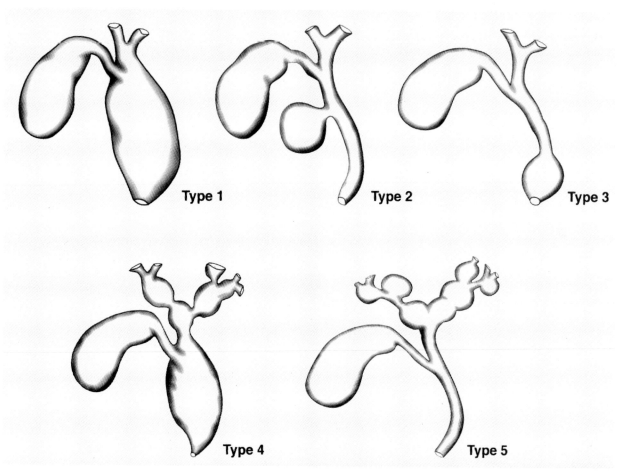

FIGURE 11–50. Types of choledochal cyst. Type I consists of fusiform dilatation of the common bile duct. Type II is an eccentric diverticulum of the common bile duct. Type III (choledochocele) consists of dilatation of the distal common bile duct as it passes through the wall of the duodenum. Type IV consists of multiple cysts of the extrahepatic ducts and possibly the intrahepatic ducts. Type V (Caroli's disease) consists of intrahepatic bile duct cysts. (Adapted from Taylor LA, Ross AJ. Abdominal masses. In: Walker AW, Devrie PR, Hamilton JR, et al., editors. Pediatric gastrointestinal disease. Philadelphia: BC Decker Inc; 1991. p. 134.)

tion is occasionally delayed into adolescence or even adulthood. The classic triad of episodic abdominal pain, jaundice, and a palpable right-sided abdominal mass occurs in only 17 to 25% of patients (Sherman et al., 1986; Bass and Cremin, 1976) or even less frequently (Barlow et al., 1976; Rosenfield and Griscom, 1975). The presence of any of the symptoms of the triad should alert the physician to the possibility of a choledochal cyst. There may also be intermittent fever and vomiting. In infants, choledochal cysts may mimic biliary atresia clinically by presenting with hepatomegaly, cholestatic jaundice, and pale stools (Sherman et al., 1986). Jaundice may be the only abnormal finding in some infants (Bass and Cremin, 1976), and 5% of cases of infantile obstructive jaundice are due to a choledochal cyst. The presenting clinical signs and symptoms of a choledochal cyst are often intermittent and may be nonspecific, resulting in a delay in diagnosis (Barlow et al., 1976; Yamaguchi, 1980; Sherman et al., 1986; Flanigan, 1975; Klotz et al., 1983; Fonkalsrud, 1973; Valayer and Alagille, 1975; Oldham et al., 1981; Nagorney et al., 1984).

Complications of choledochal cyst include stones, cholangitis (Orenstein and Whitington, 1982), malignant transformation (Rosenfield and Griscom, 1975), recurrent pancreatitis (Matsusue et al., 1982), spontaneous rupture of the cyst (Sherman et al., 1986), and biliary cirrhosis or portal hypertension. The most common complication of choledochal cyst is stone formation within the cyst, the biliary ducts, or the gallbladder (Yamaguchi,

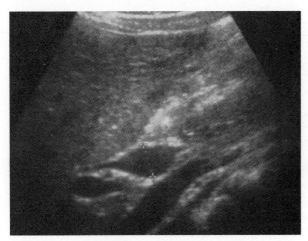

FIGURE 11–51. Small type I choledochal cyst. Longitudinal ultrasonograph demonstrates abrupt change in caliber of common bile duct with fusiform dilatation.

1980). Malignancy may arise in the wall of the choledochal cyst, gallbladder, or pancreas. The incidence of carcinomatous degeneration is related to age, with a risk of 0.7% in the first decade, 6.8% in the second, and 14.3% in adulthood (Voyles et al., 1983). It is presumed to be a result of chronic inflammation from cholangitis and/or refluxing pancreatic juice leading to epithelial metaplasia (Rha et al., 1996). Pancreatitis is uncommon but may be related to the anomalous pancreatobiliary junction with reflux of bile from the common channel into the pancreatic duct or obstruction by a stone. Rarely, there may be cholangitis, which can result in abscess formation within the liver parenchyma (Kim et al., 1995). Spontaneous rupture of a choledochal cyst with bile peritonitis is rare and usually occurs in infants less than 20 weeks of age. Perforation is often found at the junction of the cystic and common hepatic ducts (Karnak et al., 1997). Portal hypertension with varices may result from compression of the portal vein by the cyst or secondary biliary cirrhosis (Crittenden and McKinley, 1985). There has been one reported case of pseudoaneurysm of the hepatic artery complicating a choledochal cyst (Eliscu and Weiss, 1988).

Type III choledochal cyst or choledochocele is a rare anomaly in its pure form (Yamguchi, 1980). Although it can be congenital, the high incidence of presentation in later life suggests that at least some cases may be acquired (Reddy et al., 1985). Clinical manifestations are similar in most respects to other types of choledochal cyst, except that there is no female sex predominance (Venu et al., 1984) and the incidence of carcinoma is lower (Ladas et al., 1995).

Anomalies of the biliary system associated with choledochal cysts include double common bile duct or gallbladder, annular pancreas, malrotation, sclerosing cholangitis, and congenital hepatic fibrosis (Crittenden and McKinley, 1985; Akhan et al., 1994; Chaudhary et al., 1996; Evans-Jones and Cudmore, 1990). Distal atresia has been described with choledochal cysts in the neonate and may represent a separate entity (Torrisi et al., 1990).

Imaging
Ultrasonography. Ultrasonography is a simple, noninvasive diagnostic method that provides substantial information about the size, contour, position, and internal composition of choledochal cysts (Kangarloo et al., 1980).

Prenatal US may demonstrate a choledochal cyst as early as 15 to 20 weeks' gestational age (Benhidjeb et al., 1996; Rha et al., 1996; Elrad et al., 1985). Immediate postnatal US can confirm the diagnosis and expedite surgery (Dewbury et al., 1980).

Choledochal cysts appear as well-defined fluid-filled structures in the region of the porta hepatis. The cyst may measure from 2 to 35 cm, and connection with the biliary tree confirms the diagnosis (Schneck, 1994). A type I cyst is seen to be separate from the gallbladder, and the common bile duct enters the cyst (Figures 11–51, 11–52). Type II is seen as an eccentric cyst, which can appear separate from the common bile duct if the communication is narrow (Figure 11–53). With a type III choledochal cyst, there is dilatation of the lower end of the common bile duct as it passes through the duodenum. Type III cysts may be small and more diffi-cult to detect on US, and cholangiography is the diagnostic modality of choice (Figure 11–54).

In Type IV choledochal cyst there may be cystic dilatation of the intrahepatic ducts (Kangarloo et al., 1980) (Figure 11–55). Intrahepatic ductal dilatation is present in approximately 50% of patients and is limited to the central portions of the left and right main hepatic ducts (Siegel, 1996). The abrupt change in caliber of the bile duct cyst and the absence of ductal dilatation in the hepatic periphery help differentiate this from obstructive causes of dilatation of the common bile duct (Araki et al., 1981).

Ultrasonography may also show associated biliary tract stones or sludge. Stones are present within the choledochal cyst in approximately 8% of patients (Figure 11–56) (Crittenden and McKinley, 1985; Reuter et al., 1980).

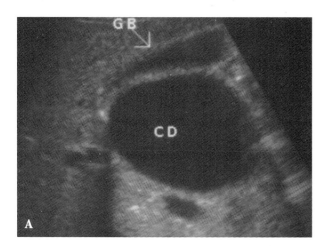

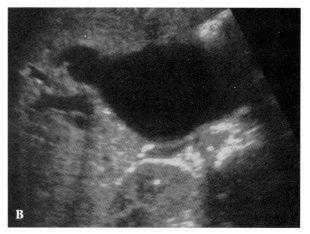

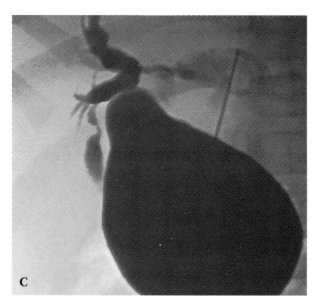

FIGURE 11–52. Large type I choledochal cyst. *A,* Transverse ultrasonograph shows choledochal cyst (CD) separate from the gallbladder (GB). *B,* Longitudinal ultrasonograph demonstrates connection to the biliary tree. *C,* Percutaneous cholangiograph demonstrates large choledochal cyst associated with intrahepatic ductal dilatation.

Ultrasonography alone gives sufficient preoperative information without the need for other modalities when a cystic right upper quadrant mass is present. Ultrasonography is usually diagnostic but when it fails to demonstrate connection to the biliary tree, other imaging modalities such as nuclear medicine, CT, or MR may help clarify the findings (Akhan et al., 1994). The differential diagnosis of choledochal cyst includes other cystic masses in the right upper quadrant such as duodenal duplication cyst, mesenteric cyst, or exophytic hepatic cyst.

Radionuclide Scintigraphy. After US, the most useful investigation is a technetium Tc 99m IDA scan, which can be used to confirm the biliary origin of the cyst. Depending on the degree of biliary obstruction, choledochal cysts have a variable appearance on scintigraphy. In the neonate presenting with obstructive jaundice, it may be seen as a photopenic defect in the porta hepatis (Figure 11–57). In older children, there may be slow accumulation of radionuclide in the choledochal cyst, followed by bowel excretion. Usually, gallbladder

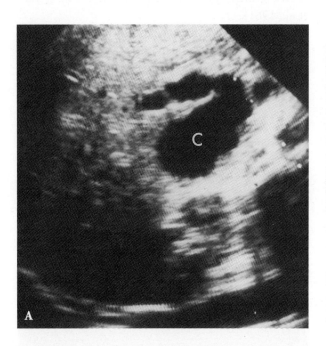

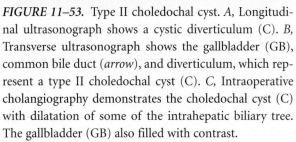

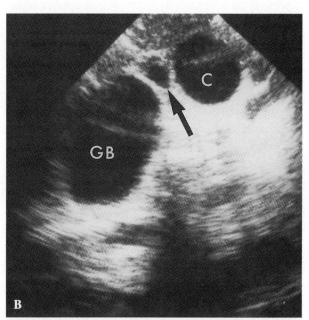

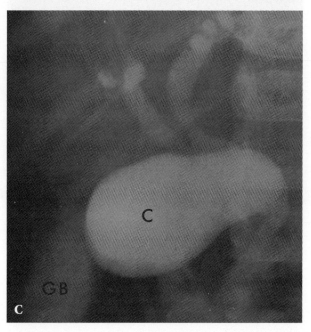

FIGURE 11–53. Type II choledochal cyst. *A,* Longitudinal ultrasonograph shows a cystic diverticulum (C). *B,* Transverse ultrasonograph shows the gallbladder (GB), common bile duct (*arrow*), and diverticulum, which represent a type II choledochal cyst (C). *C,* Intraoperative cholangiography demonstrates the choledochal cyst (C) with dilatation of some of the intrahepatic biliary tree. The gallbladder (GB) also filled with contrast.

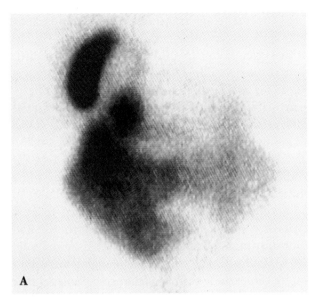
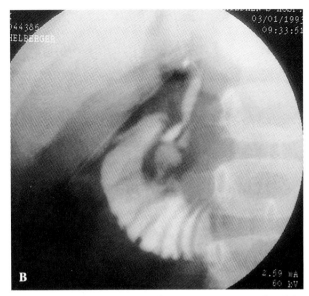

FIGURE 11–54. Type III choledochal cyst in a 5-year-old female with abdominal pain and cystic structure in the right upper quadrant of uncertain etiology demonstrated by previous ultrasonography. *A*, Hepatobiliary scan demonstrates excretion of contrast into cystic structure associated with distal common bile duct. *B*, Percutaneous cholangiograph demonstrates a choledochocele, a type III choledochal cyst. (Courtesy of Dr. Massoud Majd.)

activity is not visualized but administration of CCK may help differentiation from choledochal cyst (Grossman et al., 1991). Hepatobiliary scintigraphy may be useful in detecting complications such as cyst rupture (Figure 11–58) (Karnak et al., 1997).

Computed Tomography. Computed tomography can delineate choledochal cysts accurately but is usually unnecessary. It is more accurate in demonstrating the intrahepatic biliary tree and can be used to visualize the distal part of the common bile duct if the duct is obscured by bowel gas on US (Figure 11–59) (Katyal and Lees, 1992; Kim et al., 1995). In addition, CT may help in evaluating postoperative complications (Araki et al., 1980).

Magnetic Resonance Imaging. Magnetic resonance imaging is of value in investigating congenital anomalies of the biliary tree, and MRCP can be used to delineate the anatomy of the choledochal cyst and its relationship to structures within the porta hepatis, which may be helpful for preoperative plan-

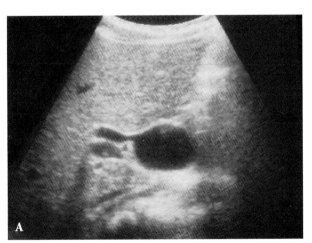
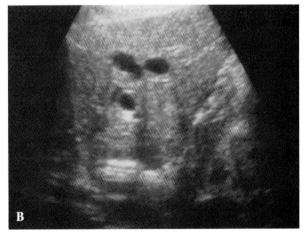

FIGURE 11–55. Type I choledochal cyst. *A*, Transverse ultrasonograph demonstrates fusiform dilatation of the extrahepatic common duct consistent with a choledochal cyst. *B*, Longitudinal ultrasonograph shows associated intrahepatic dilatation in the left lobe of the liver.

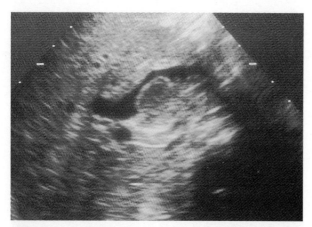

FIGURE 11–56. Type I choledochal cyst. Longitudinal ultrasonograph demonstrates sludge within a type I fusiform choledochal cyst.

ning (Figure 11–60) (Arshanskiy and Vyas, 1998; Ystgaard et al., 1992). The latter also may be useful in detecting the anomalous pancreaticobiliary duct union although it may be difficult to delineate in young children (Arshanskiy and Vyas,1998; Kubo et al., 1995; Irie et al., 1998).

Cholangiography. Although not usually indicated preoperatively in children, cholangiography will show details of cyst morphology (Figure 11–61). It can also demonstrate biliary strictures, calculi, and an anomalous pancreatobiliary duct union (Figure 11–62) that may not be seen on US (Savader et al., 1991).

Percutaneous transhepatic cholangiography may give similar information to ERCP but usually with better filling of intrahepatic ducts and little pancreatic duct filling. Choledochal cyst (Altman et al., 1978) and the presence of an anomalous biliary-pancreatic duct junction can be shown by ERCP. However, there may be insufficient bile duct filling to show the whole system (Sherman et al., 1986). The modality of choice for diagnosis of type III choledochal cysts is ERCP as these cysts are often difficult to detect using other imaging techniques. In addition, endoscopic surgery can be used to treat type III choledochal cysts with less morbidity and mortality than conventional surgery (Zimmon et al., 1978). Endoscopic retrograde cholangiopancreatography can exclude primary sclerosing cholangitis, a much rarer cause of extrahepatic biliary obstruction in childhood (Spivak et al., 1982). However, ERCP is technically more difficult to perform (especially in very young children), may require a general anesthetic, and has been associated with traumatic pancreatitis (Vanderspuy, 1978).

Surgery and Complications

Surgical management varies, depending on the type and extent of choledochal cyst that is present. Internal drainage procedures were initially used as treatment but complications including cholangitis, strictures, and malignancy occurred. Therefore, the current treatment of choice for types I and II chole-

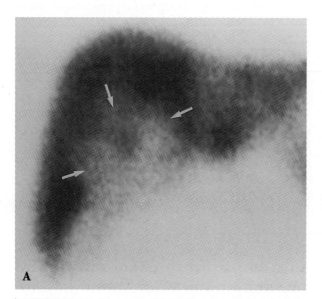
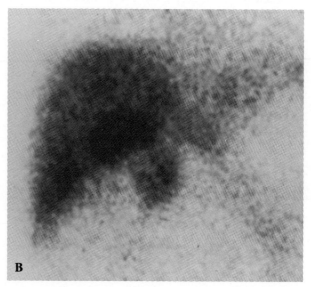

FIGURE 11–57. Type I choledochal cyst. *A,* Technetium Tc 99m sulfur colloid scan shows a defect (*arrows*) in the region of the porta hepatis. *B,* This region fills on the delayed biliary scan (technetium Tc 99m IDA) confirming a choledochal cyst.

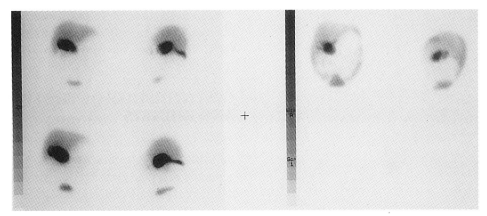

FIGURE 11–58. Spontaneous perforation of a choledochal cyst. Hepatobiliary scintigraphy demonstrates excretion of radionuclide into a choledochal cyst. There is evidence of a leak with extension of radionuclide within the peritoneal cavity on the delayed images consistent with perforation. (Courtesy of Dr. Massoud Majd.)

dochal cysts is total cyst excision, cholecystectomy, and biliary enteric anastomosis (Todani et al., 1977). Standard Roux-en-Y hepaticojejunostomy appears to be the preferred method of internal drainage (O'Neill, 1992). Type II diverticulum may be treated with simple cyst excision with preservation of the common duct (Schneck, 1994).

Type III cysts have associated stenosis of the common bile duct and pancreatic duct and have a low risk of carcinoma. As a result, they may be treated with transduodenal sphincteroplasty without cyst excision (Katyal and Lees, 1992; O'Neill, 1992).

Type IV cysts are treated with excision of the extrahepatic biliary component, and this may result in some regression in the intrahepatic dilatation. Lobectomy may be performed if the intrahepatic dilatation is confined to the left lobe (Todani et al., 1977).

The anatomy is best demonstrated by operative cholangiography. Cholangiography may be performed intraoperatively by injecting the cyst or gallbladder (Savader et al., 1991). The finding of coexistent hepatic duct abnormalities such as cystic dilatation or stenosis may modify the surgical procedure (Lilly, 1979). Cholangiography and radionuclide scintigraphy are occasionally helpful in excluding anatomic obstruction postoperatively.

The long-term prognosis is good if the diagnosis is made early, and some patients have shown

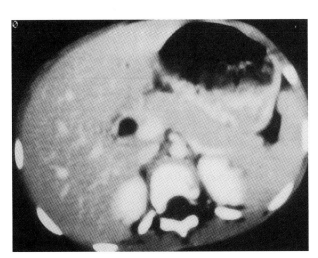

FIGURE 11–59. Transaxial CT demonstrates enlargement of the common bile duct at the level of the pancreas related to a choledochal cyst.

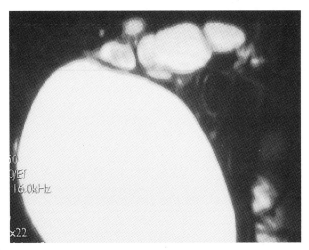

FIGURE 11–60. Magnetic resonance cholangiograph of a patient with a large type I choledochal cyst associated with dilatation of the central intrahepatic ducts.

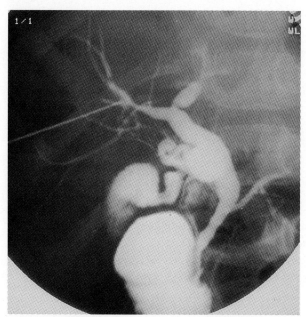

FIGURE 11–61. Percutaneous cholangiograph demonstrates fusiform dilatation of the common bile duct consistent with a Type I choledochal cyst.

regression in liver fibrosis after appropriate treatment (Rha et al., 1996). The type IV cyst is more likely to develop biliary stones and cholangitis and to remain at risk for developing intrahepatic cholangiocarcinoma (Chaudhary et al., 1996; Lipsett,

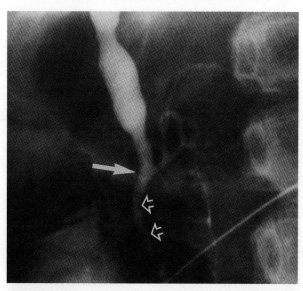

FIGURE 11–62. Type I choledochal cyst. Intraoperative cholangiography via injection of the gallbladder demonstrates an anomalous near-90-degree insertion (*large arrow*) of the common bile duct into the pancreatic duct and a long common channel (*open arrows*).

1994). Even though a permanent cure may be obtained with surgery, life-long follow-up is necessary, including ultrasonographic examination (O'Neill, 1992).

CYSTIC DISEASE OF THE LIVER AND KIDNEYS

There is a complicated spectrum of related conditions that exhibit hepatic and renal cysts. There is no generally accepted classification; three of the better-defined groups are congenital hepatic fibrosis, autosomal recessive polycystic disease, and autosomal dominant polycystic disease. In addition, since Caroli's disease (type V choledochal cyst) forms part of the spectrum, it is considered here rather than in the preceding section on choledochal cysts.

Caroli's Disease (Type V Choledochal Cyst)

Clinicopathologic Features. Caroli's disease is a rare condition primarily characterized by segmental, nonobstructive dilatation of the intrahepatic bile ducts (Caroli, 1973). The condition may be a developmental anomaly caused by a combination of overgrowth of biliary epithelium and of its supporting connective tissue. Disproportionate growth may lead to elongation and tortuosity of the bile ducts in the fetus with segmental and multiple dilatations of intrahepatic bile ducts (Nakanuma et al., 1982). Alternatively, it may be due to a ductal plate malformation where there is arrest in the fetal organogenesis of the biliary tree (Jorgensen, 1977). Insufficient resorption of ductal plates can result in large dilated segments of the primitive bile duct surrounding the portal triads (Toma et al., 1991). Another proposed mechanism is hepatic artery occlusion early in the neonatal period, leading to bile duct ischemia and cystic dilatation (Miller et al., 1995).

The initial description of the condition by Caroli and colleagues (Caroli et al., 1958) suggested that it was a rare syndrome of saccular dilatation of the intrahepatic biliary tree with normal parenchyma. However, later investigators realized that the disorder was often associated with congenital hepatic fibrosis (Fagundes-Neto et al., 1983), and a variety of subclassifications for Caroli's disease have been proposed (Bass et al., 1977; Raymond et al., 1984; Caroli, 1968; Davies et al., 1986b). Caroli's disease can be divided into two forms: a pure form which is rare and consists only of duct ectasia; and a second, more complex form associated with congenital hepatic fibrosis (Desmet, 1998; Boyle et al., 1989; Desroches et al., 1995; Zangger et al., 1995). Approximately 60 to 80% of patients with Caroli's disease and congenital hepatic fibrosis have renal disease (Sung et al., 1992). The most common renal abnormality is autosomal recessive polycystic kidney disease; others include medullary sponge, nephronophthisis, and autosomal dominant polycystic kidney disease (Miller et al., 1995; Braga et al., 1994).

Caroli's disease can also be classified as focal or diffuse. In the diffuse type, cystic dilatation of the segmental bile ducts affects the whole intrahepatic biliary tree. Focal involvement can be seen in approximately 20% of cases, and it usually involves the left lobe of the liver (Boyle et al., 1989). The diffuse type is more common than the monolobar type and is usually associated with congenital hepatic fibrosis and renal abnormalities (Bonet et al., 1996).

Patients are usually young adults who present with abdominal pain, fever, and transient jaundice (Mujahed et al., 1971; Lucaya et al., 1978). Sporadic cases of Caroli's disease presenting at birth have been described (Davies et al., 1986; Hermansen et al., 1979). There are often recurrent episodes of cholangitis with biliary calculi (Figure 11–63) and, sometimes, liver abscess formation. If congenital hepatic fibrosis is present, there may be hematemesis related to portal hypertension and esophageal varices. There is an increased incidence of hepatic adenocarcinoma and cholangiocarcinoma in patients with Caroli's disease (Merono-Cabajosa et al., 1993; Phinney et al., 1981).

Imaging

Ultrasonography. Ultrasonography is the initial imaging modality of choice. The liver may be enlarged and may contain multiple dilated tubular structures converging toward the porta hepatis (Figure 11–64). The cystic spaces represent ectatic biliary ducts and may be up to several centimeters in size (Schneck, 1994; Toma et al., 1991; Davies et al., 1986b). Gross cystic dilatation of the intrahepatic ducts is suggestive of Caroli's disease (Mittelstaedt et al., 1980). Ultrasonography may demonstrate an intraluminal central dot or protrusion in the wall of the sacculus that represents the portal radicles partially or completely surrounded by the dilated bile ducts (Figure 11–65) (Marchal et al., 1986). The portal radicles contain a portal vein and branch of the hepatic artery, and blood flow may be detected within the portal radicles with color Doppler examination (Kumakura et al., 1994; Lee et al., 1992). The differential diagnosis includes polycystic liver disease and hepatic abscesses. Demonstration of communication between the sacculi and the biliary ducts distinguishes Caroli's disease from these entities (Miller et al., 1995). Ultrasonography is useful in following patients to detect intraductal stones that have an echogenic appearance with distal acoustic shadowing (Mittelstaedt et al., 1980).

The kidneys may be normal or of variable echogenicity, depending on the extent of involvement by polycystic renal disease (Davies et al., 1986b; Marchal et al., 1986). Hyperechogenicity in the kidneys may be primarily in the renal medulla (Davies et al., 1986b) or throughout the kidney, with loss of corticomedullary differentiation (Marchal et al., 1986).

Radionuclide Scintigraphy. A HIDA nuclear medicine scan is also useful for investigation of Caroli's disease and will show that the cystic spaces are due to biliary tract dilatation (Pinos et al., 1993). There may be photon-deficient areas within the liver on the blood pool phase representing the ectatic intrahepatic ducts. As excretion of the radiopharmaceutical proceeds, these areas show marked concentration of the radionuclide (Sty et al., 1982; Sty et al., 1978). Delayed views show retention of the radiotracer within the dilated intrahepatic bile ducts that may persist after the liver parenchyma has cleared the isotope (Pinos et al., 1993). Hepatobiliary scintigraphy will distinguish Caroli's disease from polycystic liver disease but may not be able to distinguish the biliary dilatation from partial obstruction (Sung et al., 1992).

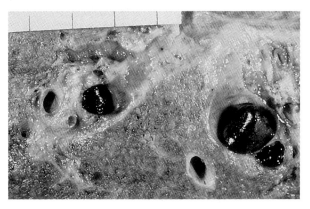

FIGURE 11–63. Pathology of patient with Caroli's disease with dilated intrahepatic ducts containing stones.

Other Modalities. Computed tomography clearly delineates the extent of intrahepatic bile duct dilatation (Araki et al., 1981), and if surgery is indi- cated, CT may be useful as a preoperative "road map" if insufficient data is obtained by US. The dilated bile ducts are visualized as low-density,

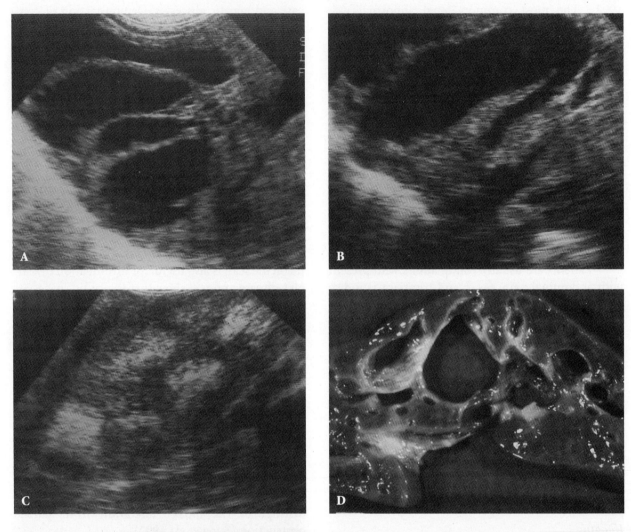

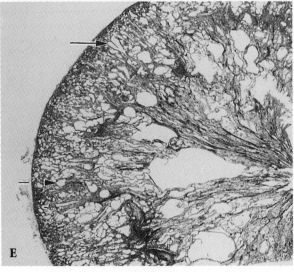

FIGURE 11–64. Caroli's disease or type V choledochal cyst. *A,* Longitudinal ultrasonography showed multiple cystic structures in the liver. *B,* Some of the cystic struc- tures appear to communicate. *C,* Longitudinal ultra- sonography through both kidneys showed marked increased echogenicity of the renal pyramids in grossly enlarged kidneys. *D,* A postmortem specimen showed gross dilatation of the biliary tree with congenital hepaic fibrosis. *E,* Sections through the kidney showed multiple tiny cysts (*arrows*). (Parts D and E reprinted with permis- sion from Davies CH, Stringer DA, Whyte H, et al. Con- genital hepatic fibrosis with saccular dilatation of intra- hepatic bile ducts and infantile polycystic kidneys. Pediatr Radiol 1986;16:302–5.)

branching tubular structures. The portal radicles may be seen on CT as a strongly enhancing dot within a dilated bile duct (central dot sign), similar to that seen on US (Kumakura et al., 1994; Choi et al., 1990). However, this sign is not specific for Caroli's disease as it may be present in patients with

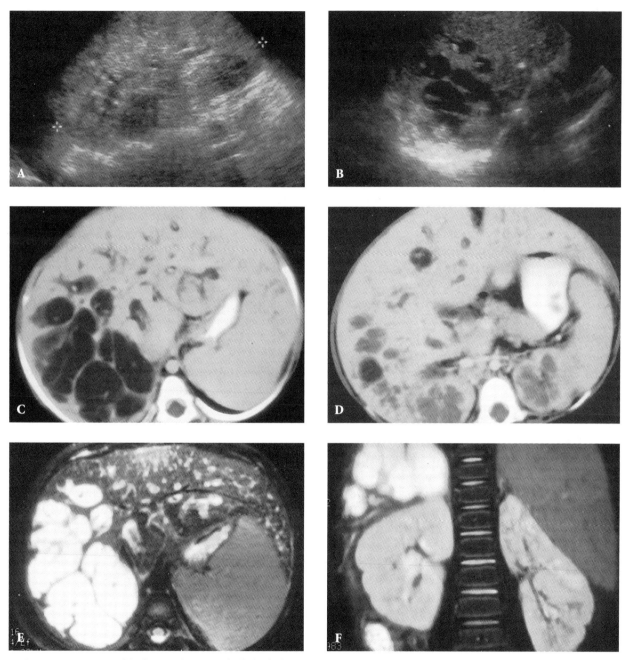

FIGURE 11–65. Caroli's disease (type V choledochal cyst) with autosomal recessive polycystic kidney disease. *A,* Longitudinal ultrasonograph of the right kidney demonstrates an enlarged echogenic kidney; the left kidney was similar in appearance. *B,* Transverse ultrasonograph through the right lobe of the liver shows marked cystic intrahepatic ductal dilatation with a central dot related to the portal radicles. *C,* Computed tomography shows corresponding abnormality in the liver with diffuse intrahepatic dilatation most marked in the right lobe of the liver with the central dot sign. *D,* At a more caudal level, the kidneys show cystic dilatation in the medullary pyramids. *E,* Axial T2-weighted MR shows the high-signal-intensity diffuse cystic dilatation of the intrahepatic ducts. *F,* Coronal T2-weighted images depict additional high-signal tubular cystic changes within the renal pyramids and splenomegaly.

periductal cysts where the vessels are surrounded by serous fluid (Herman and Siegel, 1990). Computed tomography cholangiography is a noninvasive method of confirming the biliary origin of the cysts (Musante et al., 1982).

Magnetic resonance cholangiography may be used as an alternative noninvasive method of cholangiography. Evaluation of the bile ducts in multiple planes with MIP reconstruction demonstrates high-signal intrahepatic cystic dilatations (Pavone et al., 1996). Intrahepatic calculi may be detected and are usually low signal but (rarely) may be high signal on T1- and T2-weighted images (Zangger et al., 1995).

Percutaneous transhepatic cholangiography is rarely indicated but if performed, will show the communicating nature of the dilated ducts (Mittelstaedt et al., 1980). Similar information will be given by ERCP but difficulties may be encountered in opacifying the intrahepatic biliary tree (Pavone et al., 1996). Cholangiography demonstrates sacculi of the intrahepatic biliary tree, which may vary in size, shape, and distribution in the liver. Black-pigmented calcium bilirubinate stones are commonly seen as filling defects in the biliary tree, and biliary strictures may form secondary to repeated episodes of bacterial cholangitis (Miller et al., 1995). Cholangiography may be contraindicated because of the increased risk of cholangitis (Zangger et al., 1995).

Treatment. Treatment will depend on the clinical severity of the various components. Medical treatment with litholytic therapy has been used to dissolve stones in Caroli's disease (Ros et al., 1993) but its use is limited due to the pigmentary nature of the stones and the side effects of long-term therapy (Merono-Cabajosa et al., 1993).

Surgery may be indicated if obstruction is due to biliary calculi or if associated anomalies are present, such as a choledochal cyst (Lilly, 1980). In addition, if focal disease is present, partial hepatectomy may give some relief of symptoms, especially if cholangitis is recurring (Raymond et al., 1984; Schrumpf et al., 1981). Recurrent cholangitis requires antibiotic therapy and drainage, which can be achieved by open surgery, positioning of a stent (Witlin et al., 1982), or percutaneous drainage (Rose et al., 1986). Other surgical interventions include papilloplasty and excision of the common bile duct with a Roux-en-Y hepaticojejunal anastomosis. Liver transplantation

may be considered if hepatic failure develops. Follow-up studies are indicated due to the risk of developing cholangiocarcinoma (Tsuchida et al., 1994). Except in cases cured by resection, prognosis in patients with Caroli's disease is generally poor (Schneck, 1994).

Congenital Hepatic Fibrosis

General Considerations. Congenital hepatic fibrosis (CHF), a developmental disorder usually encountered in children or young adults (Desmet, 1992b), is not a single entity but a spectrum of hepatic and renal abnormalities (Desmet, 1992b). Congenital hepatic fibrosis is present in virtually every patient with autosomal recessive polycystic kidney disease (ARPKD) and renal tubular ectasia (Patel, 1992; Kerr et al., 1961; Blyth and Ockenden, 1971; Alvarez et al., 1981). The converse is not neccessarily true since renal lesions are not always found in cases of congenital hepatic fibrosis. However, the renal lesion of autosomal recessive polycystic kidney disease is the most frequent association of congenital hepatic fibrosis and is present in over 50% of patients (Lipschitz et al., 1993; Matsuda et al., 1990). The relationship between these entities is uncertain; in spite of their similarities, congenital hepatic fibrosis, autosomal recessive polycystic disease, and renal tubular ectasia appear to be different diseases (Kerr et al., 1961; Alvarez et al., 1981; Schiff, 1982).

Congenital hepatic fibrosis and associated polycystic kidney disease are considered to be autosomal recessive in inheritance (Sty et al., 1982; Blyth and Ockenden, 1971), and the gene for ARPKD has been localized to chromosome 6 (Zerres et al., 1994). The clinical expression of congenital hepatic fibrosis varies, depending on the presence of renal abnormalities. Approximately 50% of patients with ARPKD die within the newborn period from causes usually related to pulmonary insufficiency from decreased renal function. Survival beyond this period is associated with severe hypertension, uremia, and congestive heart failure. In those children with little or no renal involvement, hepatomegaly may be present but is usually asymptomatic until at least 5 years of age. The degree of liver involvement varies, the perinatal form of ARPKD having the least involvement and the juvenile form having the most severe hepatic disease (Schneck, 1994). Patients surviving into adulthood, usually with the juvenile form, develop complications associated with liver disease, including portal hypertension with bleeding from esophageal varices and ascites (Kissane, 1990; Murray-Lyon et al., 1973). Congenital hepatic fibrosis is the second most important cause of portal venous hypertension in children (Perisic, 1995). Liver transplantation is indicated in children who develop liver failure in association with portal hypertension (Perisic, 1995).

Another major risk is ascending cholangitis with bacterial infection within dilated intrahepatic ducts (Alvarez et al., 1981). There have been reports of the development of cholangiocarcinoma, hepatocellular carcinoma (Bauman et al., 1994), and adenomatous hyperplasia (Bertheau et al., 1994) in patients with congenital hepatic fibrosis.

Other conditions may occasionally be associated with congenital hepatic fibrosis, including dysplastic kidneys, choledochal cyst, Caroli's disease, and rarely, autosomal dominant polycystic kidney disease (Davies et al., 1986b; Matsuda et al., 1990; Murray-Lyon et al., 1973; Cobben et al., 1990). Syndromes associated with congenital hepatic fibrosis include Ivemark's (Desmet, 1992b), Joubert's (Lewis et al., 1994), COACH (Barzilai et al., 1998), Laurence-Moon-Biedl, Smith-Lemli-Opitz (Lewis et al., 1994), and Meckel-Gruber syndromes (Desmet, 1992b) as well as tuberous sclerosis.

Histopathology. Liver histology shows fibrosis in the portal zones, bile duct proliferation, and agenesis of the tiny portal veins (Kerr et al., 1961; Wechsler and Thiel, 1976). Hepatocellular function is usually normal, and there is preservation of the lobular architecture of the liver. The etiology and pathogenesis of congenital hepatic fibrosis is unknown and is likely related to a spectrum of conditions rather than to a single entity. Desmet suggested that the basic lesion of congenital hepatic fibrosis corresponds to ductal plate malformation of interlobular bile ducts, resulting from faulty development. There is a progressive destructive cholangiopathy of the immature bile ducts, resulting in a fetal type of biliary fibrosis. The portal hypertension in congenital hepatic fibrosis may result from hypoplasia and paucity of intrahepatic portal vein radicles or from their compression by fibrosis (Desmet, 1992b).

The renal involvement in ARPKD is almost always bilateral, and the kidneys are large, usually smooth, and have normal fetal lobulations (Gwinn and Landing, 1968). The nephrons are normal, and the primary abnormality is at the level of the collecting ducts. Tubular ectasia is seen along the course of the ducts, with radially oriented small cysts in both the cortex and the medulla. The peripheral renal cortex is spared in patients with mild disease as it does not normally contain collecting ducts (Jain et al., 1997).

Imaging. Ultrasonography may show hepatosplenomegaly (Schneck, 1994), and the echogenicity of the liver parenchyma may be increased or heterogeneous (Figure 11–66) (Alvarez et al., 1981). Hyperechoic regions on US or hyperdense areas on CT possibly correspond to areas of fibrosis or even calcification. The gallbladder may be large, and occasionally there is intrahepatic duct dilatation (Alvarez et al., 1981). Dilatation of the intrahepatic bile ducts and biliary cysts can also be demonstrated on MRCP (Ernst et al., 1998). Intrahepatic low-signal-intensity bands corresponding to the areas of periportal fibrosis may be shown on MR (Schneck, 1994).

There may be evidence of portal hypertension with development of a portal cavernoma and large collaterals with hepatofugal flow on Doppler study (Figure 11–67). Duplication of the intrahepatic venous channels may be demonstrated on splenoportography in patients with portal hypertension and congenital hepatic fibrosis (Odievre et al., 1977). The coexistence of a cavernoma with a patent portal trunk and intrahepatic duplications may be a distinctive feature of congenital hepatic fibrosis (Besnard et al., 1994).

Radionuclide studies of the reticuloendothelial system will show hepatosplenomegaly and heterogeneous uptake in the liver, consistent with portal hypertension (Schneck, 1994).

The imaging appearance of the kidneys depends on the type and severity of involvement. Intravenous pyelography is not usually indicated but will demonstrate enlarged kidneys with delayed excretion and a streaky appearance related to the dilated tubules. Ultrasonography usually shows symmetrically enlarged kidneys with increased echogenicity resulting from the multiple acoustic interfaces of the cysts (Figure 11–68). The degree of echogenicity is variable and can be diffuse with loss of cortico-medullary differentiation (Marchal et al., 1986) or prominent, primarily in the renal medullary pyramids (Davies et al., 1986b). The severity of the echogenicity is roughly comparable to that of cystic changes, and there may be a normal peripheral cortex in patients who are less severely affected (Patel, 1992; Jain et al., 1997). Renal calcifications may be present in older or more severely affected patients and may be related to a urine acidification defect from kidney failure (Lucaya et al., 1993).

Polycystic Liver Disease

General Considerations. Polycystic disease of the liver is a congenital autosomal dominant disease. It usually presents after the age of 30 years but has been reported in children as young as 2 years of age. Polycystic liver disease is associated with polycystic kidney disease in about 50 to 60% of cases (Schneck, 1994). Approximately 33% of patients with autosomal dominant polycystic kidney disease (ADPKD) show cystic disease of the liver (Gwinn and Landing, 1968). The most common hereditary kidney disease is ADPKD, which is caused by mutations at more than one locus, the most common being chromosome 16 (Desmet, 1998; Lipschitz et al., 1993; Pirson

et al., 1996). The clinical picture is variable, and most cases present in adult life with a combination of hypertension and abdominal pain. The pain may be a feeling of fullness, pressure, or colic. Proteinuria and hematuria can be present (Chilton and Cremin, 1981), and renal failure may develop.

The liver cysts are felt to develop from Meyenburg's complexes, bile ducts that fail to undergo involution during fetal development. Subsequent cystic dilation of these bile ducts results in polycystic liver disease (Schneck, 1994; Desmet, 1998). Hepatic cysts vary in size and increase in number with age (Itai et al., 1995). These cysts are rarely of clinical significance but may occasionally be symptomatic if they hemorrhage or become infected. Patients rarely demonstrate any elevation of bilirubin or liver function tests as the intervening liver parenchyma is normal (Schneck, 1994). There are a few reports of obstructive jaundice related to compression of the biliary ducts by a cyst (Lerner et al., 1992).

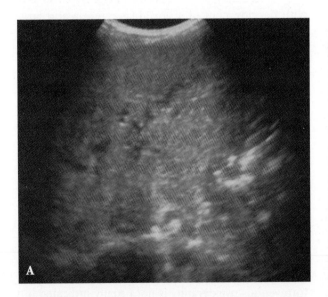

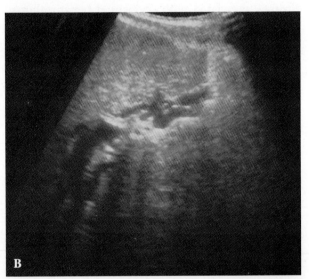

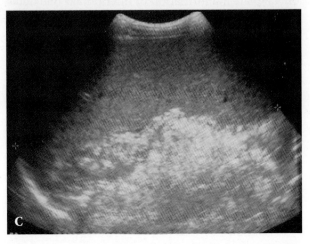

FIGURE 11–66. Congenital hepatic fibrosis with portal hypertension. *A,* Transverse ultrasonograph shows coarse echogenic liver parenchyma and mild intrahepatic duct dilatation. *B,* Longitudinal ultrasonograph shows recanalized paraumbilical veins and *C* splenomegaly.

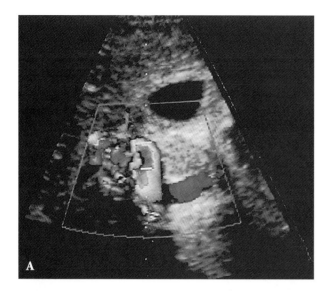

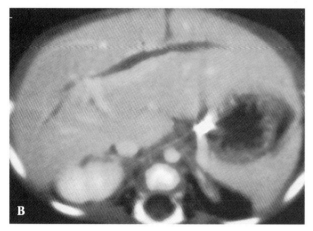

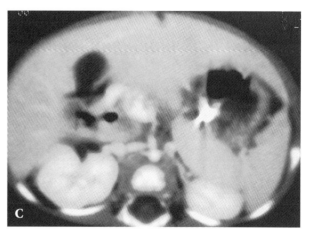

FIGURE 11–67. Congenital hepatic fibrosis with portal cavernoma. *A,* Transverse ultrasonograph shows prominent veins in the portal region. *B,* Mild intrahepatic ductal dilatation shown on CT. *C,* Enhancement of the portal cavernoma shown on CT.

In autosomal dominant kidney disease, both kidneys are affected but the disease may initially be asymmetric. The cystic changes involve both the nephron and the collecting ducts (Jain et al., 1997). The cysts are of variable size, are located in the medulla and cortex, and are separated by normal renal tissue. The cysts may contain urine, blood or exudate, and occasionally cholesterol crystals or calcium precipitates (Gwinn and Landing, 1968).

Cysts may occur in other organs, usually the pancreas, the spleen, the lung, and the parathyroid and pineal glands (Schneck, 1994; Hartman, 1992). Cerebral aneurysms (berry aneurysms) (Gwinn and Landing, 1968) occur in 10 to 30% of adult patients with ADPKD (Reuss et al., 1991). However, patients with polycystic liver disease unassociated with polycystic kidneys do not have berry aneurysms (Schneck, 1994). Other abnormalities associated with ADPKD include Caroli's disease, congenital hepatic fibrosis, and cholangiocarcinoma (Desmet, 1998).

Imaging. On US, the liver may be enlarged and may contain cysts of variable size. The hepatic cysts may contain internal echoes or have high density on CT if complicated by infection or hemorrhage, and there occasionally may be associated calcifications. On MR, uncomplicated cysts are hypointense on T1- and hyperintense on T2-weighted images. If the cysts contain protein or blood, they may be higher signal on T1-weighted images (Schneck, 1994). The biliary tree and gallbladder are normal (Schneck, 1994). Cysts may also be seen in the kidneys, pancreas, and spleen.

Ultrasonography will show variably sized cysts within the kidneys, which are often asymmetrically affected (Figure 11–69) (Blyth and Ockenden, 1971). In rare cases, the dominant type of polycystic kidney disease can occur in neonates with a clinical and radiologic picture identical to ARPKD. Therefore, family and genetic studies are important for differentiation (Patel, 1992). Normal ultrasonographic findings in childhood do not exclude ADPKD.

Isolated Congenital Hepatic Cysts

General Considerations. Simple hepatic cysts occur in 2.5% of the population, are more common in women, and are occasionally multiple (Gaines and Sampson, 1989). They can occur at any age but most present in the fourth or fifth decade (Athey et al., 1986).

The etiology of the cysts is uncertain but they probably arise from aberrant bile ducts. The cysts vary in size from a few centimeters to very large abdominal masses. The mass is usually round, well encapsulated, and lined with a simple layer of cuboidal epithelium, with three distinct connective tissue layers. A more uncommon form of congenital hepatic cyst is a duplication or foregut cyst that rarely occurs below the diaphragm (Quillin et al., 1993; Shoenut et al., 1994). Hepatic foregut cysts are solitary unilocular cysts (Kimura et al., 1980; Kadoya et al., 1990) that are lined by ciliated columnar epithelium that contains mucous-secreting glands. These cysts are secondary to abnormal budding of the primitive foregut, with the migration of the cyst into the abdomen before the fusion of the pleuroperitoneal membranes (Shoenut et al., 1994).

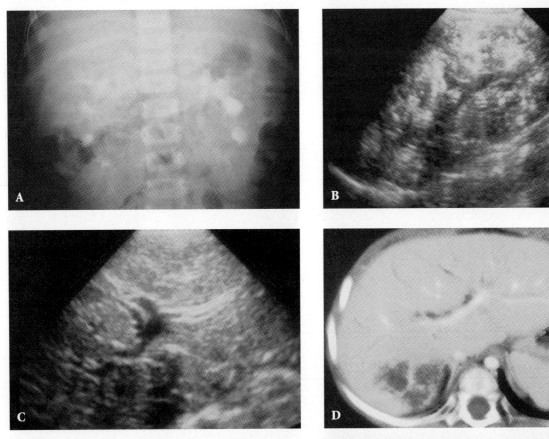

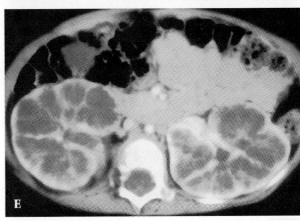

FIGURE 11–68. Autosomal recessive polycystic kidney disease and congenital hepatic fibrosis. *A,* Intravenous urography shows markedly enlarged kidneys with streaky opacification and delayed pyelograph. *B,* Longitudinal ultrasonograph of kidneys shows enlarged echogenic kidneys. *C,* Transverse ultrasonograph of liver demonstrates increased periportal echogenicity. *D* and *E,* Computed tomography shows mild intrahepatic biliary ductal dilatation and prominent cystic changes within the medullary pyramids of the kidneys, with relative sparing of the outer cortex.

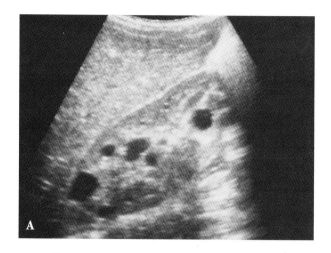

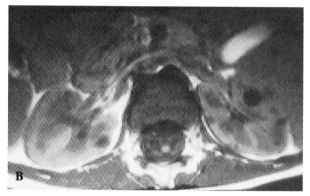

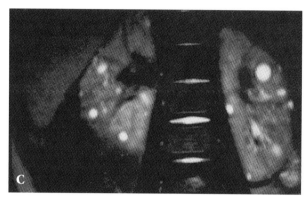

FIGURE 11–69. Autosomal dominant polycystic kidney disease. *A,* Longitudinal ultrasonograph shows multiple anechoic cysts of varied size within the renal parenchyma. Axial T1-weighted (*B*) and coronal T2-weighted (*C*) MR show the cysts to be of low signal intensity on T1 and of high signal intensity on T2, consistent with fluid.

Unlike polycystic liver disease, solitary cysts are not associated with renal or pancreatic cysts. Simple hepatic cysts may be significant if they represent a disease marker. Congenital hepatic cysts may be associated with von Hippel-Lindau disease (Gaines and Sampson, 1989), Peutz-Jeghers syndrome, and congenital diaphragmatic hernia (Pul and Pul, 1995).

The cysts are usually asymptomatic and are discovered incidentally. They may present with abdominal pain, hepatomegaly, or mass (Gaines and Sampson, 1989). Other symptoms are more variable and include nausea, vomiting, diarrhea, constipation, melena, intestinal obstruction, and even dyspnea. Rarely, the cyst may cause obstruction of the biliary tree, resulting in jaundice (Clinkscales et al., 1985).

The right lobe is affected more frequently than the left, and there is a predilection for the inferior pole of the right lobe. The cyst may be completely or partially intrahepatic or may be exophytic, hanging off the edge of the liver. Rarely, the cyst may originate in the falciform ligament (Enterline et al., 1984). The cysts may contain clear fluid or variable amounts of blood, debris, or crystals. Surgical resection is not indicated unless the cysts become infected or cause significant compression of adjacent structures (Shoenut et al., 1994). Percutaneous aspiration has been used to treat hepatic cysts with poor long-term success (Saini et al., 1983). However, injection of alcohol may be curative (Bean and Rodan, 1985).

Imaging

Ultrasonography. Ultrasonography will demonstrate the cystic nature of the hepatic cyst. Features on US include an anechoic structure with a smooth well-defined wall and posterior acoustic enhancement. The cyst may contain thin septations (Figure 11–70a) (Gaines and Sampson, 1989). If it contains protein or hemorrhage, it may be echogenic and mimic a solid lesion. Doppler US is useful in excluding flow within a solid mass or a vascular origin of the cystic mass such as a hepatic artery aneurysm.

Other causes of hepatic cysts include echinococcal cyst, amebic abscess, and cystic liver tumors such as cystadenoma (Shamsi et al., 1993). In the rare case of an exophytic cyst, other investigations may be needed to exclude other cystic anomalies such as choledochal cyst and extrinsic mass lesions.

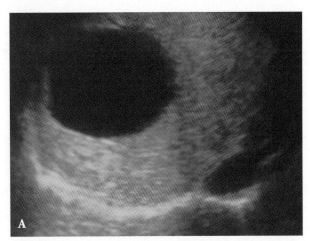
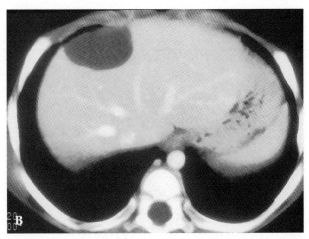

FIGURE 11–70. Hepatic cyst. *A,* Transverse ultrasonograph demonstrates a large, round anechoic lesion with increased through transmission, consistent with a simple cyst. *B,* On CT, the cyst is seen as a low-attenuation structure with no enhancement postcontrast.

Ultrasonography generally gives sufficient preoperative information to the surgeons. Other occasionally useful investigations are discussed below.

Other investigations and techniques. Magnetic resonance imaging or CT can help show the intrahepatic position and the absence of other anomalies. Generally, hepatic cysts are of low attenuation on CT, similar to water; occasionally, they may be of high density and related to hemorrhage, protein, or calcium crystals as demonstrated in ciliated hepatic foregut cysts (Kimura et al., 1980; Kadoya et al., 1990). Magnetic resonance imaging has shown variable signal intensity on T1-weighted images, low or high signal intensity if there is associated protein or hemorrhage, and high signal intensity on T2-weighted images (Shoenut et al., 1994; Shamsi et al., 1993). Administration of contrast demonstrates no enhancement on CT or MR consistent with a cyst (Figure 11–70b) (Kimura et al., 1980; Shoenut et al., 1994).

REFERENCES

Abramson SJ, Treves S, Teele RI. The infant with possible biliary atresia: evaluation by ultrasound and nuclear medicine. Pediatr Radiol 1982;1982:1–5.

Abramson SJ, et al. Biliary atresia and noncardiac polysplenic syndrome: US and surgical considerations. Radiology 1987;163:377–9.

Adear H, Barki Y. Multiseptate gallbladder in a child: incidental diagnosis on sonography. Pediatr Radiol 1990;20:192.

Agrons GA, et al. From the archives of the AFIP gastrointestinal manifestations of cystic fibrosis: radiologic-pathologic correlation. Radiographics 1996;16:871–93.

Akhan O, et al. Choledochal cysts: ultrasonographic findings and correlation with other imaging modalities. Abdom Imaging 1994;19(3):243–7.

Alagille D, et al. Syndromic paucity of interlobular bile ducts (Alagille syndrome or arteriohepatic dysplasia): review of 80 cases. J Pediatr 1987;110(2):195–200.

Alagille D. Alagille syndrome today. Clin Invest Med 1996;19(5):325–30.

Altman MS, et al. Choledochal cyst presenting as acute pancreatitis: evaluation with endoscopic retrograde cholangiopancreatography. Am J Gastroenterol 1978;70:514–9.

Alvarez F, et al. Congenital hepatic fibrosis in children. J Pediatr 1981;99:370–5.

Amemoto K, et al. Ultrasonographic gallbladder wall thickening in children with Henoch-Schönlein purpura. J Pediatr Gastroenterol Nutr 1994;19(1):126–8.

Anagnostopoulos D, et al. Gallbladder disease in patients with cystic fibrosis. Eur J Pediatr Surg 1993;3(6):348–51.

Araki T, Hai Y, Tasaka A. CT of choledochal cyst. AJR 1980;135:729–34.

Araki T, Itai Y, Tasaka A. Computed tomography of localized dilatation of the intrahepatic bile ducts. Radiology 1981;141:733–6.

Arshanskiy Y, Vyas PK. Type IV choledochal cyst presenting with obstructive jaundice: role of MR cholangiopancreatography in preoperative evaluation. AJR 1998;171:457–9.

Athey PA, Lauderman JA, King DE. Massive congenital solitary nonparasitic cyst of the liver in infancy. J Ultrasound Med 1986;5:585–7.

Babbitt DP, Starshak RJ, Clemett AR. Choledochal cyst: a concept of etiology. AJR 1973;119:57–62.

Bailey PV, et al. Changing spectrum of cholelithiasis and cholecystitis in infants and children. Am J Surg 1989;158(6):585–8.

Baker DH, Harris RC. Congenital absence of the intrahepatic bile ducts. AJR 1964;91:875–84.

Balistreri WF, et al. Biliary atresia: current concepts and research directions. Summary of a symposium. Hepatology 1996;23(6):1682–92.

Balthazar EJ, Birnbaum BA, Naidich M. Acute cholangitis: CT evaluation. J Comput Assist Tomogr 1993;17(2):283–9.

Barlow B, et al. Choledochal cyst: a review of 19 cases. J Pediatr 1976;89:934–40.

Baron R. Computed tomography of the bile ducts. Semin Roentgenol 1997;32(3):172–87.

Barzilai M, Lerner A. Gallbladder polyps in children: a rare condition. Pediatr Radiol 1997;27(1):54–6.

Barzilai M, et al. Imaging findings in COACH syndrome. AJR 1998;170(4):1081–2.

Bass EM, Cremin BJ. Choledochal cysts: a clinical and radiological evaluation of 21 cases. Pediatr Radiol 1976;5:81–5.

Bass EM, Funston MR, Shaff MI. Caroli's disease: an ultrasonic diagnosis. Br J Radiol 1977;50:366–9.

Bauman ME, Pound DC, Ulbright TM. Hepatocellular carcinoma arising in congenital hepatic fibrosis. AJG 1994;89(3):450–1.

Bean WJ, Rodan BA. Hepatic cyst: treatment with alcohol. AJR 1985;144:237–41.

Beckman I, et al. Ultrasonographic findings in acute acalculosis cholecystitis. Gastrointest Radiol 1985;10(4):387–9.

Bekassy AN, et al. Hepatocellular carcinoma associated with arteriohepatic dysplasia in a 4-year-old girl. Med Pediatr Oncol 1992;20(1):78–83.

Ben-Haim S, et al. Utility of Tc-99m mebrofenin scintigraphy in the assessment of infantile jaundice. Clin Nucl Med 1995;20(2):153–63.

Benhidjeb T, et al. Prenatal diagnosis of a choledochal cyst: a case report and review of the literature. Am J Perinatol 1996;13(4):207–10.

Benya EC, Sivit CJ, Quinones RR. Abdominal complications after bone marrow transplantation in children: sonographic and CT findings. AJR 1993;161(5):1023–7.

Bergman AB, Neiman HL, Kraut B. Ultrasonographic evaluation of pericholecystic abscesses. AJR 1979;132(2):201–3.

Berk RN, van der Vegt JH, Lichtenstein JE. The hyperplastic cholecystoses: cholesterolosis and adenomyomatosis. Radiology 1983;146:593–601.

Berrocal T, et al. Syndrome of Alagille: radiological and sonographic findings. A review of 37 cases. Eur Radiol 1997;7(1):115–8.

Bertheau P, et al. Adenomatous hyperplasia of the liver in a patient with congenital hepatic fibrosis. J Hepatol 1994;20(2):213–7.

Besnard M, et al. Portal cavernoma in congenital hepatic fibrosis. Angiographic reports of 10 pediatric cases. Pediatr Radiol 1994;24(1):61–5.

Betz BW, et al. MR imaging of biliary cysts in children with biliary atresia: clinical associations and pathologic correlation. AJR 1994;162(1):167–71.

Bines JE, et al. Multiple biliary papillomatosis in a child. J Pediatr Gastroenterol Nutr 1992;14(3):309–13.

Blaquiere RM, Dewbury KS. The ultrasound diagnosis of emphysematous cholecystitis. Br J Radiol 1982;55(650):114–6.

Bloom RA, Swain VAJ. Non-calculous distention of the gallbladder in childhood. Arch Dis Child 1966;41:503.

Blyth H, Ockenden BG. Polycystic disease of kidneys and liver presenting in childhood. J Med Genet 1971;8:257–84.

Bonet J, et al. Caroli's disease and cystic kidney disease in a woman [letter]. Nephron 1996;73(2):310–1.

Boyle MJ, Doyle GD, McNulty JG. Monolobar Caroli's disease. Am J Gastroenterol 1989;84(11):1437–44.

Brachman MB, Goodman MD, Waxman AD. The rim sign in acute cholecystitis. Comparison of radionuclide, surgical and pathologic findings. Clin Nucl Med 1993;18(10):863–6.

Bradford BF, et al. Ultrasonographic evaluation of the gallbladder in mucocutaneous lymph node syndrome. Radiology 1982;142:381–4.

Braga AC, et al. Caroli's disease with congenital hepatic fibrosis and medullary sponge kidney. J Pediatr Gastroenterol Nutr 1994;19(4):464–7.

Brill PW, Winchester P, Rosen MS. Neonatal cholelithiasis. Pediatr Radiol 1982;12:285–8.

Brown DM. Bile plug syndrome: successful management with a mucolytic agent. J Pediatr Surg 1990;25(3):351–2.

Brown DL, et al. Echogenic material in the fetal gallbladder: sonographic and clinical observations. Radiology 1992;182:73–6.

Brunelle F, et al. Sclerosing cholangitis in infancy. Proceedings of the 28th annual meeting of the Society of Pediatric Radiology; 1985; Boston.

Brunelle F, et al. Skeletal anomalies in Alagille's syndrome. Radiographic study in eighty cases. Ann Radiol 1986;29(8):687–90.

Bushnell DL, et al. The rim sign: association with acute cholecystitis. J Nucl Med 1986;27(3):353–6.

Byrne JL, et al. Del (20p) with manifestations of arteriohepatic dysplasia. Am J Med Genet 1986;24(4):673–8.

Callahan J, et al. Cholelithiasis in infants: association with total parenteral nutrition and furosemide. Radiology 1982;143(2):437–9.

Caroli J, et al. La dilatation polykystique cogenitale des voies biliares intrahepatiques. Essai de classification. Semaine Hop (Paris) 1958;34:488–95.

Caroli J. Diseases of intrahepatic bile ducts. Isr J Med Sci 1968;4:21–35.

Caroli J. Disease of the intrahepatic biliary tree. Clin Gastroenterol 1973;2:147–61.

Carty H. Percutaneous transhepatic fine needle cholangiography in jaundiced infants. Ann Radiol 1977;21:149–54.

Chan FL, et al. Evaluation of recurrent pyogenic cholangitis with CT: analysis of 50 patients. Radiology 1989;170(1 Pt 1):165–9.

Chan YL, et al. Choledocholithiasis: comparison of MR cholangiography and endoscopic retrograde cholangiography. Radiology 1996;200(1):85–9.

Chan Y, Yeung C, Lam W. Magnetic resonance cholangiography-feasibility and application in the paediatric population. Pediatr Radiol 1998;28:307–11.

Chandra R. Biliary atresia and other structural anomalies in the congenital polysplenia syndrome. J Pediatr 1974;85:649–55.

Chang CCN, Giulian BB. Congenital bronchobiliary fistula. Radiology 1985;156:82.

Chapoy PR, et al. Congenital stricture of the common hepatic duct: an unusual case without jaundice. Gastroenterology 1981;80:380–3.

Chaudhary A, et al. Choledochal cysts—differences in children and adults. Br J Surg 1996;83:186–8.

Chaumont P, et al. La cholangiographi transhepatique dans l'evaluation post-operative de l'atresie des voies bilaires extra-hepatiques de l'enfant. Ann Radiol (Paris) 1982;25:94–100.

Chen LY, Goldberg HI. Sclerosing cholangitis: broad spectrum of radiographic features. Gastrointest Radiol 1984;9(1):39–47.

Chiba T, Kasai M, Sasano N. Reconstruction of intrahepatic bile ducts in congenital biliary atresia. Tokuku J Exp Med 1975;115:99–110.

Chilton SJ, Cremin BJ. The spectrum of polycystic disease in children. Pediatr Radiol 1981;11:9–115.

Chinn DH, Miller EI, Piper N. Hemorrhagic cholecystitis. Sonographic and clinical presentation. J Ultrasound Med 1987;6(6):313–7.

Choi YS, Sharma B. Gallbladder hydrops in mucocutaneous lymph node syndrome. South Med J 1989;82(3):397–8.

Choi BS, Yeon KM, Kem SH. Caroli disease: central dot sign in CT. Radiology 1990;174:161–3.

Choi SO, et al. 'Triangular cord': a sonographic finding applicable in the diagnosis of biliary atresia. J Pediatr Surg 1996;31(3):363–6.

Classen M, et al. Primary sclerosing cholangitis in children. J Pediatr 1987;6(2):197–202.

Clinkscales NB, Trigg LP, Poklepovic J. Obstructive jaundice secondary to benign hepatic cyst. Radiology 1985;154:643–4.

Co CS, Shea WS, Goldberg HI. Evaluation of common bile duct using high resolution tomography. J Comput Assist Tomogr 1986;10:424–7.

Cobben JM, et al. Congenital hepatic fibrosis in autosomal dominant polycystic kidney disease. Kidney Int 1990;38: 880–5.

Cohan RH, et al. Striated intramural gallbladder lucencies on US studies: predictors of acute cholecystitis. Radiology 1987;164(1):31–5.

Cohen EK, et al. Hydrops of the gallbladder in typhoid fever as demonstrated by sonography. J Clin Ultrasound 1986;14:633–5.

Colletti PM, et al. Acute cholecystitis: diagnosis with radionuclide angiography. Radiology 1987;163(3):615–8.

Conrad J, et al. Significance of low level echoes within the gallbladder. AJR 1979;132:967–72.

Cooperberg PL, Burhenne HJ. Real-time ultrasonography. Diagnostic technique of choice in calculous gallbladder disease. N Engl J Med 1980;302:1277–9.

Cooperberg PL, Gibney RG. Imaging of the gallbladder. Radiology 1987;163:605–13.

Coughlin JR, Mann DA. Detection of acute cholecystitis in children. J Can Assoc Radiol 1990;41(4):213–6.

Crittenden S, McKinley MJ. Choledochal cyst-clinical features and classification. Am J Gastroenterol 1985;80:643–7.

Croce F, et al. Ultrasonography in acute cholecystitis. Br J Radiol 1981;54(647):927–31.

Crystal RJ, Fink RL. Acute acalculous cholecystitis in childhood: a report of two cases. Clin Pediatr (Phila) 1971;10:423–6.

Cuffari C, et al. Acute intrahepatic portal vein thrombosis complicating cholangitis in biliary atresia. Eur J Pediatr 1997;156(3):186–9.

Davies C, Daneman A, Stringer DA. Inspissated bile in a neonate with cystic fibrosis. J Ultrasound Med 1986a;5: 335–7.

Davies CH, et al. Congenital hepatic fibrosis with saccular dilatation of intrahepatic bile ducts and infantile polycystic kidneys. Pediatr Radiol 1986b;16:302–5.

Day DL, et al. Post-operative abdominal CT scanning in extrahepatic biliary atresia. Pediatr Radiol 1989;19(6–7): 379–82.

Day DL, Carpenter BL. Abdominal complications in pediatric bone marrow transplant recipients. Radiographics 1993;13(5):1101–12.

Debray D, et al. Cholelithiasis in infancy: a study of 40 cases. J Pediatr 1993;122(3):385–91.

Debray D, et al. Sclerosing cholangitis in children. J Pediatr 1994;124(1):49–56.

Dennis MA, et al. CT detection of portal venous gas associated with suppurative cholangitis and cholecystitis. AJR 1985;145(5):1017–8.

Descos B, et al. Pigment gallstones of the common bile duct in infancy. Hepatology 1984;4:678–83.

Desmet VJ. Congenital diseases of intrahepatic bile ducts: variations on the theme "ductal plate malformation." Hepatology 1992a;16(4):1069–83.

Desmet VJ. What is congenital hepatic fibrosis? Histopathology 1992b;20(6):465–77.

Desmet VJ. Pathogenesis of ductal plate abnormalities. Mayo Clin Proc 1998;73:80–9.

Desroches J, et al. Noninvasive diagnosis of Caroli syndrome associated with congenital hepatic fibrosis using hepatobiliary scintigraphy. Clin Nucl Med 1995;20(6): 512–4.

Devriendt K, et al. Paucity of intrahepatic bile ducts, solitary kidney and atrophic pancreas with diabetes mellitus: atypical Alagille syndrome? Eur J Pediatr 1996;155(2): 87–90.

Dewbury KC, et al. Prenatal ultrasound demonstration of a choledochal cyst. Br J Radiol 1980;53:906–7.

di Sant'Agnese PA, Blanc WA. A distinctive type of biliary cirrhosis of the liver associated with cystic fibrosis of the pancreas: recognition through signs of portal hypertension. Pediatrics 1956;15:387–408.

Diaz MJ, Fowler W, Hnatow BJ. Congenital gallbladder duplication: preoperative diagnosis by ultrasonography. Gastrointest Radiol 1991;16:198–200.

Dickinson SJ, Corley G, Santulli TV. Acute cholecystitis as a sequel of scarlet fever. Am J Dis Child 1971;121(4):331–3.

Dinulos J, et al. Hydrops of the gallbladder associated with Epstein-Barr virus infection: a report of two cases and review of the literature [comments]. Pediatr Infect Dis J 1994;13(10):924–9.

Dogan AS, Conway JJ, Lloyd-Still JD. Hepatobiliary scintigraphy in children with cystic fibrosis and liver disease. J Nucl Med 1994;35:432–5.

Dolmatch BL, et al. AIDS-related cholangitis: radiographic findings in nine patients. Radiology 1987;163(2):313–6.

El-Shafie M, Mah CL. Transient gallbladder distension in

sick premature infants: the value of ultrasonography and radionuclide scintigraphy. Pediatr Radiol 1986;16(6): 468–71.

Eliscu EH, Weiss GM. Hematobilia due to a pseudo-aneurysm complicating a choledochal cyst. AJR 1988; 151(4):783–4.

Elmslie FV, et al. Alagille syndrome: family studies. J Med Genet 1995;32(4):264–8.

Elrad H, et al. Prenatal ultrasound diagnosis of choledochal cyst. J Ultrasound Med 1985;4:553–5.

Engel JM, Deitch EA, Sikkema W. Gallbladder wall thickness: sonographic accuracy and relation to disease. AJR 1980;134(5):907–9.

Enriquez G, et al. Intrahepatic biliary stones in children. Pediatr Radiol 1992;22(4):283–6.

Enterline DS, et al. Cyst of the falciform ligament of the liver. AJR 1984;142:327–8.

Ernst O, Gottrand F, Calvo M. Congenital hepatic fibrosis: findings at MR cholangiopancreatography. AJR 1998;170(2):409–12.

Evans-Jones G, Cudmore R. Choledochal cyst and congenital hepatic fibrosis. J Pediatr Surg 1990;25(12):1259–60.

Fagundes-Neto U, et al. Caroli disease in childhood: report of two new cases. Gastroenterol Nutr 1983;2:708–11.

Fakhry J. Sonography of tumefactive biliary sludge. AJR 1982;139(4):717–9.

Fawcett HD, et al. Spontaneous extrahepatic biliary duct perforation in infancy. J Can Assoc Radiol 1986;37:206–7.

Fidler J, Paulson EK, Layfield L. CT evaluation of acute cholecystitis: findings and usefulness in diagnosis. AJR 1996;166(5):1085–8.

Finberg HJ, Birnholz JC. Ultrasound evaluation of the gallbladder wall. Radiology 1979;133(3 Pt 1):693–8.

Fisher MM, Chen S, Dekker A. Congenital diaphragm of the common hepatic duct. Gastroenterology 1968;54: 605–10.

Fiske CE, Laring FC, Brown TW. Ultrasonographic evidence of gallbladder wall thickening in association with hypoalbuminemia. Radiology 1980;135(3):713–6.

Flanigan DP. Biliary cysts. Ann Surg 1975;182:635–43.

Fonkalsrud EW. Choledochal cysts. Surg Clin North Am 1973;53:1275–80.

Fonkalsrud EW, Arima E. Bile lakes in congenital biliary atresia. Surgery 1975;77:384–90.

Franken EA, et al. Percutaneous cholangiography in infants. AJR 1978;130:1057–8.

Gaines PA, Sampson MA. The prevalence and characterization of simple hepatic cysts by ultrasound examination. Br J Radiol 1989;62:335–7.

Gaines P, et al. The thick common bile duct in pyogenic cholangitis [comments]. Clin Radiol 1991;44(3):175–7.

Gansbeke DV, et al. Suprahepatic gallbladder: a rare congenital anomaly. Gastrointest Radiol 1984;9:341–3.

Garel L, et al. An unusual iatrogenic bilio-bronchial fistula. Pediatr Radiol 1980;9:48–9.

Garel L, et al. The changing aspects of cholelithiasis in children through a sonographic study. Pediatr Radiol 1981;11:75–9.

Gautier M, Eliot N. Extrahepatic biliary atresia: morphological study of 98 biliary remnants. Arch Pathol Lab Med 1981;105:397–402.

Gembala RB. Jaundice and choledocholithiasis. In: Farrell RJ, editor. Radiology of the liver, biliary tract and pancreas. St. Louis: Mosby Year Book Inc; 1994.

Goiney RC, et al. Sonography of gallbladder duplication and differential considerations. AJR 1985;145:241–3.

Graham N, et al. Cystic fibrosis: ultrasonographic findings in the pancreas and hepatobiliary system correlated with clinical data and pathology. Clin Radiol 1985;36:199–203.

Granot E, et al. Duplication of the gallbladder associated with childhood obstructive biliary disease and biliary cirrhosis. Gastroenterology 1983;85:946–50.

Gray SW, Skandalakis JE. Extrahepatic biliary ducts and the gallbladder. In: Embryology for surgeons: the embryological basis for the treatment of congenital defects. Philadelphia: WB Saunders; 1972. p. 229.

Greenberg M, et al. The ultrasonographic diagnosis of cholecystitis and cholelithiasis in children. Radiology 1980;137(3):745–9.

Greenholz SK, et al. Biliary obstruction in infants with cystic fibrosis requiring Kasai portoenterostomy. J Pediatr Surg 1997;32(2):175–80.

Grosfeld J. Is there a place for the Kasai procedure in biliary atresia? Curr Opin Gen Surg 1994;168–72.

Grossman SA, Patel BA, Blend MJ. Use of CCK cholescintigraphy to differentiate choledochal cyst from gallbladder. Clin Nucl Med 1991;16(4):226–9.

Grumbach K, et al. Hepatic and biliary tract abnormalities in patients with AIDS. Sonographic-pathologic correlation. J Ultrasound Med 1989;8(5):247–54.

Guibaud L, Lachaud A, Touraine R. MR cholangiography in neonates and infants: feasibility and preliminary applications. AJR 1998;170:27–31.

Gwinn JL, Landing BH. Cystic diseases of the kidneys in infants and children. Radiol Clin North Am 1968;6:191–204.

Haller JO, et al. Spontaneous perforation of the common bile duct in children. Radiology 1989;172:621–4.

Haller JO. Sonography of the biliary tract in infants and children. AJR 1991;157(5):1051–8.

Halvorsen RA Jr, et al. Arteriohepatic dysplasia (Alagille's syndrome): unusual hepatic architecture and function. Abdom Imaging 1995;20(3):191–6.

Hartman DS. Renal cystic disease in multisystem conditions. Urol Radiol 1992;14:13–7.

Hayashi AK, Soudry G, Dibos PE. Rim sign. Radionuclide imaging in a patient with acute gangrenous cholecystitis and cholelithiasis after nonspecific abdominal ultrasonography. Clin Nucl Med 1997;22(6):388–9.

Hays DM, et al. Diagnosis of biliary atresia: relative accuracy of percutaneous liver biopsy, open liver biopsy, and operative biopsy. J Pediatr 1967;71:598–607.

Heier L, et al. Biliary disease in metachromatic leukodystrophy. Pediatr Radiol 1983;13(6):313–8.

Herman TE, Siegel MJ. Case report: central dot sign on CT of liver cysts. J Comput Assist Tomogr 1990;14(6):1019–21.

Hermansen MC, Starshak RJ, Werlin SL. Caroli disease: the diagnostic approach. J Pediatr 1979;94:879–82.

Hernanz-Schulman M, et al. Common bile duct in children: sonographic dimensions. Radiology 1995;195:193–5.

Hirano A, Katayama H, Shirakata A. [Bone changes in congenital biliary atresia—review of 42 cases after surgery.] Nippon Igaku Hoshasen Gakkai Zasshi 1990;50(1):29–39.

Hoffenberg EJ, et al. Outcome of syndromic paucity of interlobular bile ducts (Alagille syndrome) with onset of cholestasis in infancy. J Pediatr 1995;127(2):220–4.

Hyde GA. Spontaneous perforation of bile ducts in early infancy. Pediatrics 1965;35:453–7.

Ikeda S, Sera Y, Akagi M. Serial ultrasonic examination to differentiate biliary atresia from neonatal hepatitis—special reference to changes in size of the gallbladder. Eur J Pediatr 1989;148(5):396–400.

Irie H, et al. Value of MR cholangiopancreatography in evaluating choledochal cysts. AJR 1998;171:1381–5.

Itai Y, et al. Hepatobiliary cysts in patients with autosomal dominant polycystic kidney disease: prevalence and CT findings. AJR 1995;164(2):339–42.

Jain M, et al. High-resolution ultrasonography in the differential diagnosis of cystic diseases of the kidney in infancy and childhood: preliminary experience. J Ultrasound Med 1997;16.235–40.

Jeffrey RB, et al. Gangrenous cholecystitis: diagnosis by ultrasound. Radiology 1983;148(1):219–21.

Jeffrey RB Jr, Sommer FG. Follow-up sonography in suspected acalculous cholecystitis: preliminary clinical experience. J Ultrasound Med 1993;12(4):183–7.

Jona JZ, et al. Anatomic observations and etiologic and surgical considerations in choledochal cyst. J Pediatr Surg 1979;14:315–20.

Jonas A, et al. Choledocholithiasis in infants: diagnostic and therapeutic problems. J Pediatr Gastroenterol Nutr 1990;11(4):513–7.

Jorgensen MJ. The duct plate malformations. Acta Pathol Microbiol Immunol Scand 1977;257:1–88.

Kadoya M, et al. Ciliated hepatic foregut cyst: radiologic features. Radiology 1990;175:475–7.

Kahn E. Paucity of interlobular bile ducts. Arteriohepatic dysplasia and nonsyndromic duct paucity. Perspect Pediatr Pathol 1991;14:168–215.

Kane RA. Ultrasonographic diagnosis of gangrenous cholecystitis and empyema of the gallbladder. Radiology 1980;134(1):191–4.

Kane RA, Costello P, Duszlak E. Computed tomography in acute cholecystitis: new observations. AJR 1983;141(4):697–701.

Kangarloo H, et al. Ultrasonic spectrum of choledochal cysts in children. Pediatr Radiol 1980;9:15–8.

Karnak I, et al. Spontaneous rupture of choledochal cyst: an unusual cause of acute abdomen in children. J Pediatr Surg 1997;32(5):736–8.

Karrer FM, et al. Biliary atresia registry, 1976 to 1989. J Pediatr Surg 1990;25(10):1076–81.

Karrer FM, Hall RJ, Lilly JR. Biliary atresia and the polysplenia syndrome [comments]. J Pediatr Surg 1991;26(5): 524–7.

Kasai M, et al. Surgical treatment of biliary atresia. J Pediatr Surg 1968;3:665–75.

Kasai M. Extrahepatic bile ducts of congenital biliary atresia. J Jpn Soc Pediatr Surg (Jpn) 1970;6:251–8.

Katayama H, et al. Bone changes in congenital biliary atresia. Radiologic observation of 8 cases. AJR 1975; 124:107–12.

Katyal D, Lees GM. Choledochal cysts: a retrospective review of 28 patients and a review of the literature. Can J Surg 1992;35(6):584–8.

Keeffe EB, et al. Hepatocellular carcinoma in arteriohepatic dysplasia. Am J Gastroenterol 1993;88(9):1446–9.

Keller MS, et al. Spontaneous resolution of cholelithiasis in infants. Radiology 1985;157:345–8.

Kerr DNS, et al. Congenital hepatic fibrosis. QJM 1961; 30:91–117.

Khan AN, et al. Sonographic features of mucinous biliary papillomatosis: case report and review of imaging findings. J Clin Ultrasound 1998;26(3):151–4.

Kim OH, Chung HJ, Choi BG. Imaging of the choledochal cyst. Radiographics 1995;15(1):69–88.

Kimura S, et al. Studies on the postoperative changes in the liver tissue of long-term survivors of often sucessful surgery for biliary atresia. Z Kinderchir 1980;31:228–38.

Kirks DR, et al. An imaging approach to persistent neonatal jaundice. AJR 1984;142:461–5.

Kirks DR. Practical pediatric imaging. Diagnostic radiology of infants and children. 3rd ed. Philadelphia: Lippincott-Raven; 1998. p. 1226.

Kissane JM. Renal cysts in pediatric patients. Pediatr Nephrol 1990;4:69–77.

Kitagawa H, et al. Two cases of torsion of the gallbladder diagnosed preoperatively. J Pediatr Surg 1997;32(11): 1567–9.

Klotz D, et al. Choledochal cysts: diagnostic and therapeutic problems. J Pediatr Surg 1983;8:271–83.

Kobayashi A, et al. Congenital biliary atresia: analysis of 97 cases with reference to prognosis after hepatic portoenterostomy. Am J Dis Child 1976;130:830–3.

Krantz D, Piccoli DA, Spinner NB. Alagille syndrome. J Med Genet 1997;34:152–7.

Kubo S, et al. Choledochal cyst detected by MR cholangiopancreatography [letter]. AJR 1995;164(2):513–4.

Kulkarni PB, Beatty EC. Cholangiocarcinoma associated with biliary cirrhosis due to congenital biliary atresia. Am J Dis Child 1977;131:442–4.

Kumakura H, et al. A case of Caroli's disease: usefulness of color Doppler sonography for evaluating the malformation of the intrahepatic bile ducts. Radiat Med 1994; 12(2):75–7.

Kumari S, Lee WJ, Baron MG. Hydrops of the gallbladder in a child: diagnosis by ultrasonography. Pediatrics 1979; 63:295–7.

L'Heureux PR, et al. Gallbladder disease in cystic fibrosis. AJR 1977;128:953–6.

Ladas SD, et al. Choledochocele, an overlooked diagnosis: report of 15 cases and review of 56 published reports from 1984 to 1992. Endoscopy 1995;27(3):233–9.

Lai MW, et al. Differential diagnosis of extrahepatic biliary atresia from neonatal hepatitis: a prospective study. J Pediatr Gastroenterol Nutr 1994;18(2):121–7.

Laing FC, et al. Improved visualization of choledocholithiasis by sonography. AJR 1984;143:949–52.

Landing BH. Considerations of the pathogenesis of neonatal hepatitis, biliary atresia and choledochal cyst: the concept of infantile obstructive cholangiopathy. Prog Pediatr Surg 1974;6:113–39.

Lang EV, Pinckney LE. Spontaneous resolution of bile-plug syndrome. AJR 1991;156:1225–6.

Lang I, Connolly B, Daneman A. An unusual position of the gallbladder following nephrectomy for large neoplasms. Pediatr Radiol 1997;27:528–9.

Lee MG, et al. Hepatic arterial color Doppler signals in Caroli's disease. Clin Imaging 1992;16(4):234–8.

Lefkowitch JH. Biliary atresia. Mayo Clin Proc 1998;73(1): 90–5.

Lerner ME, et al. Polycystic liver disease with obstructive jaundice: treatment with ultrasound-guided cyst aspiration. Gastrointest Radiol 1992;17(1):46–8.

Lev-Toaff AS, et al. Multiseptate gallbladder: incidental diagnosis on sonography. AJR 1987;148:1119–23.

Levard G, et al. Torsion of the gallbladder in children. J Pediatr Surg 1994;29(4):569–70.

Lewis SME, et al. Joubert syndrome with congenital hepatic fibrosis: an entity in the spectrum of oculo-encephalo-hepato-renal disorders. Am J Med Genet 1994;52:419–26.

Lilly JR. Surgery of co-existing biliary malformations in choledochal cyst. J Pediatr Surg 1979;14:643–7.

Lilly JR. Diagnosis of Caroli disease. J Pediatr 1980;97:329–30.

Lim JII, Ko YT, Kim SY. Ultrasound changes of the gallbladder wall in the cholecystitis: a sonographic pathological correlation. Clin Radiol 1987;38(4):389–93.

Lim JH. Radiologic findings of clonorchiasis. AJR 1990;155(5):1001–8.

Lim JH. Oriental cholangiohepatitis: pathologic, clinical and radiologic features. AJR 1991;157(1):1–8.

Lipschitz B, et al. Association of congenital hepatic fibrosis with autosomal dominant polycystic kidney disease. Report of a family with review of literature. Pediatr Radiol 1993;23(2):131–3.

Lipsett PA, et al. Choledochal cyst disease. A changing pattern of presentation. Ann Surg 1994;220(5):644–52.

Lucaya J, et al. Congenital dilatation of the intrahepatic bile ducts (Caroli disease). Radiology 1978;127:746–8.

Lucaya J, et al. Renal calcifications in patients with autosomal recessive polycystic kidney disease: prevalence and cause. AJR 1993;160(2):359–62.

Lugo-Vicente HL. Trends in management of gallbladder disorders in children. Pediatr Surg Int 1997;12:348–52.

MacCarty RL, et al. Primary sclerosing cholangitis: findings on cholangiography and pancreatography. Radiology 1983;149(1):39–44.

MacDonald FR, Cooperberg PL, Cohen MM. The WES triad: a specific sonographic sign of gallstones in the contracted gallbladder. Gastrointest Radiol 1981;6:39–41.

Madign SM, Teele RL. Ultrasonography of the liver and biliary tree in children. Semin Ultrasound CT MR 1984;5:68–84.

Maingot R. Anatomical abnormalities of the biliary tract and the hepatic and cystic arteries. In: Maingot R, editor. Abdominal operations. New York: Appleton-Century-Crofts; 1980. p. 979.

Majd M. ^{99m}Tc-IDA scintigraphy in the evaluation of neonatal jaundice. Radiographics 1983;3:88–9.

Maki T. Pathogenesis of calcium bilirubinate gallstone: role of *E. coli*-glucuronidase and coagulation by inorganic ions, polyelectrolytes and agitation. Ann Surg 1966;164:90–100.

Marchal GJF, et al. Gallbladder wall sonolucency in acute cholecysittis. Radiology 1979;133(2):429–33.

Marchal GJ, et al. Caroli disease: high-frequency US and pathologic findings. Radiology 1986;158:507–11.

Martin SR, Garel L, Alvarez F. Alagille's syndrome associated with cystic renal disease. Arch Dis Child 1996;74(3):232–5.

Massie JD, Moinuddin M, Phillips JC. Acute calculus cholecystitis with patent cystic duct. AJR 1983;141(1):39–42.

Matsuda O, et al. Polycystic kidney of autosomal dominant inheritance, polycystic liver and congenital hepatic fibrosis in a single kindred. Am J Nephrol 1990;10(3):237–41.

Matsusue S, et al. Role of unusually long common pancreaticobiliary channel as a cause of relapsing pancreatitis in children. Z Kinderchir 1982;36:69–72.

McCarthy S, et al. Cholecystitis: detection with MR imaging. Radiology 1986;158(2):333–6.

McEvoy CF, Suchy FJ. Biliary tract disease in children. Pediatr Clin North Am 1996;43(1):75–98.

McGahan JP, Phillips HE, Cox KL. Sonography of the normal pediatric gallbladder and biliary tract. Radiology 1982;144(4):873–5.

McHugo JM, et al. Ultrasound findings in children with cystic fibrosis. Br J Radiol 1987;60:137–41.

McLoughlin MJ, Fnti JE, Kura ML. Ectopic gallbladder: sonographic and scintigraphic diagnosis. J Clin Ultrasound 1987;15:258–61.

Meilstrup JW, Hopper KD, Thieme GA. Imaging of gallbladder variants. AJR 1991;157:1205–8.

Merono-Cabajosa EA, et al. Caroli's disease: study of six cases, including one with epithelial dysplasia. Int Surg 1993;78(1):46–9.

Middlesworth W, Altman RP. Biliary atresia. Curr Opin Pediatr 1997;9(3):265–9.

Milas M, et al. Management of biliary tract stones in heart transplant patients. Ann Surg 1996;223(6):747–56.

Miller WJ, et al. Imaging findings in Caroli's disease. AJR 1995;165(2):333–7.

Mindell HJ, Ring BA. Gallbladder wall thickening: ultrasonic findings. Radiology 1979;133(3 Pt 1):699–701.

Mirvis SE, et al. The diagnosis of acute acalculous cholecystitis: a comparison of sonography, scintigraphy and CT. AJR 1986;147(6):1171–5.

Mittelstaedt CA, et al. Caroli disease: sonographic findings. AJR 1980;134:584–7.

Mittelstaedt CA. Ultrasound of the bile ducts. Semin Roentgenol 1997;32(3):161–71.

Miyano T, Suruga K, Suda K. Abnormal choledochopancreatic ductal junction related to the etiology of infantile obstructive jaundice diseases. J Pediatr Surg 1979;14:16–26.

Miyazaki T, Yamashita Y, Tang T. Single-shot MR cholangiopancreatography of neonates, infants, and young children. AJR 1998;170:33–7.

Mogilner JG, Dharan M, Sipiovich L. Adenoma of the gallbladder in childhood. J Pediatr Surg 1991;26(2):223–4.

Mujahed Z, Glenn F, Evans JA. Communicating cavernous ectasis of the intrahepatic ducts (Caroli disease). AJR 1971;113:21–6.

Murray-Lyon IM, Ockenden BG, Williams W. Congenital hepatic fibrosis: is it a single clinical entity? Gastroenterology 1973;64:653–6.

Musante F, Derchi LE, Bonati P. Cholangiography in suspected Caroli's disease. J Comput Assist Tomogr 1982;6:482–5.

Nadel HR. Hepatobiliary scintigraphy in children. Semin Nucl Med 1996;26(1):25–42.

Naganuma S, et al. Sonographic findings of anomalous position of the gallbladder. Abdom Imaging 1998;23:67–72.

Nagorney DM, McIlrath DC, Adson MA. Choledochal cysts in adults: clinical management. Surgery 1984;96:656–63.

Nakanuma Y, et al. Caroli disease in congenital hepatic fibrosis and infantile polycystic disease. Liver 1982;2:346–54.

Neu J, Arvin A, Ariagno RL. Hydrops of the gallbladder. Am J Dis Child 1980;134:891–2.

Nicotra JJ, et al. Congenital and acquired biliary disorders in children. Semin Roentgenol 1997;32(3):215–27.

Niemeier OW. Report of a case of unusual anomaly of the bile ducts in an adult with obstructive jaundice. Surgery 1942;12:584–90.

O'Connor PJ, et al. The role of hepatobiliary scintigraphy in cystic fibrosis. Hepatology 1996;23(2):281–7.

O'Hara SM. Pediatric gastrointestinal nuclear imaging. Radiol Clin North Am 1996;34(4):845–62.

O'Neill JA Jr. Choledochal cyst. Curr Probl Surg 1992;29(6):361–410.

Odievre M, et al. Anomalies of the intrahepatic portal venous system in congenital hepatic fibrosis. Radiology 1977;122:427–30.

Ohi R, Ibrahim M. Biliary atresia. Semin Pediatr Surg 1992;1(2):115–24.

Ohnuma N, et al. The role of ERCP in biliary atresia. Gastrointest Endosc 1997;45(5):365–70.

Oldham KT, Hart MJ, White TT. Choledochal cysts presenting in late childhood and adulthood. Am J Surg 1981;141:568–71.

Ong JC, et al. Sclerosing cholangitis in children with inflammatory bowel disease. Aust N Z J Med 1994;24(2):149–53.

Ono J, Sakoda K, Akita H. Surgical aspects of cystic dilatation of the bile duct. An anomalous junction of the pancreaticobiliary tract in adults. Ann Surg 1982;195:203–8.

Oppenheimer EH, Esterly JR. Hepatic changes in young infants with cystic fibrosis: possible relation to focal biliary cirrhosis. J Pediatr 1975;86:683–9.

Orenstein SR, Whitington PF. Choledochal cyst resulting in congenital cirrhosis. Am J Dis Child 1982;136:1025–7.

Pariente D, et al. Radiological treatment of common bile duct lithiasis in infancy. Pediatr Radiol 1989;19(2):104–7.

Park WH, et al. Electron microscopic study of the liver with biliary atresia and neonatal hepatitis. J Pediatr Surg 1996;31(3):367–74.

Park WH, et al. A new diagnostic approach to biliary atresia with emphasis on the ultrasonographic triangular cord sign: comparison of ultrasonography, hepatobiliary scintigraphy, and liver needle biopsy in the evaluation of infantile cholestasis. J Pediatr Surg 1997;32(11):1555–9.

Parulekar SG. Sonographic findings in acute emphysematous cholecystitis. Radiology 1982;145(1):117–9.

Patel PJ. Imaging of infantile polycystic kidney disease with some rare association. Urol Int 1992;48:87–94.

Patriquin H, et al. Sonography of thickened gallbladder wall: causes in children. AJR 1983;141(1):57–60.

Pavone P, et al. Caroli's disease: evaluation with MR cholangiopancreatography (MRCP). Abdom Imaging 1996;21(2):117–9.

Pellerin D, et al. Cholelithiasis and ileal pathology in childhood. J Pediatr Surg 1975;10:35–41.

Perisic VN. Long-term studies on congenital hepatic fibrosis in children. Acta Paediatr 1995;84:695–6.

Pery M, et al. The value of ultrasound in Schöenlein-Henoch purpura. Eur J Pediatr 1990;150(2):92–4.

Pfeiffer WR, Robinson LH, Balsara VJ. Sonographic features of bile plug syndrome. J Ultrasound Med 1986;5(3):161–3.

Phinney PR, Austin GE, Kadell BM. Cholangiocarcinoma arising in Caroli's disease. Arch Pathol Lab Med 1981;105:194–7.

Pinos T, et al. Caroli's disease versus polycystic hepatic disease. Differential diagnosis with Tc-99m DISIDA scintigraphy. Clin Nucl Med 1993;18(8):664–7.

Pirson Y, et al. Isolated polycystic liver disease as a distinct genetic disease, unlinked to polycystic kidney disease 1 and polycystic kidney disease 2. Hepatology 1996;23(2):249–52.

Pombo F, et al. Aortic calcification and renal cysts demonstrated by CT in a teenager with Alagille syndrome. Pediatr Radiol 1995;25(4):314–5.

Pul N, Pul M. Congenital solitary nonparasitic cyst of the liver in infancy and childhood. J Pediatr Gastroenterol Nutr 1995;21:461–2.

Quillin SP, Brink JA. Hepatoma complicating Byler disease. AJR 1992;159(2):432–3.

Quillin SP, Siegel MJ, Rothbaum R. Hepatobiliary sonography in cystic fibrosis. Pediatr Radiol 1993;23:533–5.

Rahn NHD, et al. CT appearance of sclerosing cholangitis. AJR 1983;141(3):549–52.

Ralls PW, et al. Real-time sonography in suspected acute cholecystitis. Radiology 1985;155(3):767–71.

Raymond MJ, et al. Partial hepatectomy in the treatment of Caroli disease. Dig Dis Sci 1984;29:367–70.

Rebner M, et al. CT evaluation of intracholecystic bile. AJR 1985;145:237–40.

Reddy KR, et al. Choledochocele: its clinical spectrum. Gastroenterology 1985;88:1093.

Reid SH, et al. Anomalous hepatic duct inserting into the cystic duct. AJR 1986;147:1181–2.

Reif S, Sloven DG, Lebenthal E. Gallstones in children. Characterization by age, etiology, and outcome [comments]. Am J Dis Child 1991;145(1):105–8.

Reinhold C, et al. MR cholangiopancreatography: potential clinical applications. Radiographics 1996;16(2):309–20.

Rescorla FJ. Cholelithiasis, cholecystitis, and common bile duct stones. Curr Opin Pediatr 1997;9:276–82.

Reuss A, Wladimiroff JW, Niermeyer MF. Sonographic, clinical and genetic aspects of prenatal diagnosis of cystic kidney disease. Ultrasound Med Biol 1991;17(7):687–94.

Reuter K, et al. The diagnosis of a choledochal cyst by ultrasound. Radiology 1980;136:437–8.

Rha SY, et al. Choledochal cysts: a ten year experience. Am Surg 1996;62(1):30–4.

Riely CA. Familial intrahepatic cholestatic syndromes. Semin Liver Dis 1987;7(2):119–33.

Roca M, et al. Acute acalculous cholecystitis in salmonella infection. Pediatr Radiol 1988;18(5):421–3.

Ros E, et al. Ursodeoxycholic acid treatment of primary hepatolithiasis in Caroli's syndrome. Lancet 1993;342 (8868):404–6.

Rose SC, Kumpe DA, Weil R. Percutaneous biliary drainage in diffuse Caroli disease [case report]. AJR 1986;147:159–60.

Rosenfield N, Griscom NT. Choledochal cysts: roentgenographic techniques. Radiology 1975;114:113–9.

Rosenfield NS, et al. Arteriohepatic dysplasia: radiologic features of a new syndrome. AJR 1980;135(6):1217–23.

Rumley TO, Rodgers BM. Hydrops of the gallbladder in children. J Pediatr Surg 1983;18:138–40.

Rusin JA, et al. AIDS-related cholangitis in children: sonographic findings. AJR 1992;159(3):626–7.

Saigh J, et al. Varices: a cause of focal gallbladder wall thickening. J Ultrasound Med 1985;4(7):371–3.

Saini S, et al. Percutaneous aspiration of hepatic cysts does not provide definitive therapy. AJR 1983;141:559–60.

Samuels BI, et al. A comparison of radionuclide hepatobiliary imaging and real time ultrasound for the detection of acute cholecystitis. Radiology 1983;147(1):207–10.

Sane SM, Sieber WK, Girdany BR. Congenital bronchobiliary fistula. Surgery 1971;69:599–608.

Sarnaik S, et al. The incidence of cholelithiasis in sickle cell anemia using the ultrasonic gray-scale technique. J Pediatr 1980;96(6):1005–8.

Savader SJ, et al. Choledochal cysts: role of noninvasive imaging, percutaneous transhepatic cholangiography, and percutaneous biliary drainage in diagnosis and treatment. J Vasc Interv Radiol 1991;2(3):379–85.

Saverymuttu SH, et al. Gallbladder wall thickening (congestive cholecystopathy) in chronic liver disease: a sign of portal hypertension. Br J Radiol 1990;63(756):922–5.

Schiff L. Diseases of the liver. Philadelphia: Lippincott; 1982. p. 1316.

Schiller VL, Turner RR, Sarti DA. Color Doppler imaging of the gallbladder wall in acute cholecystitis: sonographic-pathologic correlation. Abdom Imaging 1996;21(3):233–7.

Schimpl G, et al. Polypoid gastric heterotopia in the gallbladder: clinicopathological findings and review of the literature. J Pediatr Gastroenterol Nutr 1994;19(1):129–31.

Schneck CD. Part II: The gallbladder and biliary tract. Embryology, histology, gross anatomy, and normal imaging anatomy of the gallbladder and biliary tract. In: Friedman AC, Dachman AH, Farrell RJ, editors. Radiology of the liver, biliary tract, and pancreas. St. Louis: Mosby Year Book; 1994. p. 355–407.

Schrumpf E, Bergan A, Blomhoff JP. Partial hepatectomy in Caroli's disease. Scand J Gastroenterol 1981;16:581–6.

Schwarzenberg SJ, et al. Long-term complications of arteriohepatic dysplasia. Am J Med 1992;93(2):171–6.

Senaati S, et al. Gallbladder pathology in pediatric beta-thalassemic patients. Pediatr Radiol 1993;23:357–9.

Shamsi F, Deckers F, De Schepper A. Unusual cystic liver lesions: a pictorial essay. Eur J Radiol 1993;16:79–84.

Sheng R, et al. Biliary stones and sludge in liver transplant patients: a 13-year experience. Radiology 1996;198(1):243–7.

Sherman P, et al. Choledochal cysts: heterogeneity of clinical presentation. J Pediatr Gastroenterol Nutr 1986;5:867–72.

Shoenut JP, et al. Ciliated hepatic foregut cysts: US, CT, and contrast-enhanced MR imaging. Abdom Imaging 1994;19:150–2.

Shuman WP, et al. PIPIDA scintigraphy for cholecystitis: false positives in alcoholism and total parenteral nutrition. AJR 1982;138(1):1–5.

Siegel MJ. Liver and biliary tract. In: Siegel MJ, editor. Pediatric sonography. Philadelphia: Lippincott-Raven Publishers; 1996.

Silberman EL, Glaessner TS. Roentgen features of congenital cystic dilatation of the common bile duct: a report of two cases. AJR 1964;82:470–5.

Silveira TR, et al. Congenital structural abnormalities in biliary atresia: evidence for etiopathogenic heterogeneity and therapeutic implications. Acta Paediatr Scand 1991;80(12):1192–9.

Simeone JF, et al. The sonographic diagnosis of acute gangrenous cholecystitis: importance of the Murphy sign. AJR 1989;152(2):289–90.

Singcharoen T, et al. Arteriohepatic dysplasia. Br J Radiol 1986;59:509–11.

Sisto A, et al. Primary sclerosing cholangitis in children: study of five cases and review of the literature. Pediatrics 1987;80(6):918–23.

Skolkin MD, et al. Sclerosing cholangitis: palliation with percutaneous cholangioplasty. Radiology 1989;170(1 Pt 1):199–206.

Slovis TL, et al. Sonography in the diagnosis and management of hydrops of the gallbladder in children with mucocutaneous lymph node syndrome. Pediatrics 1980;65:789–94.

Smetana HF, et al. Neonatal jaundice. A critical review of persistent obstructive jaundice in infancy. Arch Pathol 1965;80:553–74.

Sokal EM, et al. Unifocal stricture of the common bile duct in two children: a localized form of primary sclerosing cholangitis. J Pediatr Gastroenterol Nutr 1990;11(2):268–74.

Spivak W, Grnd RJ, Eraklis A. A case of primary sclerosing cholangitis in childhood. Gastroenterology 1982; 82(1):129–32.

Stigol LC, Traversaro J, Trigo ER. Carinal trifurcation with congenital tracheobiliary fistula. Pediatrics 1966;37:87–91.

Stringel G, Mercer S. Idiopathic perforation of the biliary tract in infancy. J Pediatr Surg 1983;18:546–50.

Stringer DA, et al. Interposition of the gallbladder—or the absent common hepatic duct and cystic duct. Pediatr Radiol 1987;17:151–3.

Stringer DA. Pediatric gastrointestinal imaging. 1st ed. Toronto, Philadelphia: B.C. Decker Inc; 1989. p. 654.

Sty JR, et al. Hepatic scintigraphy in Caroli's disease. Radiology 1978;127:732.

Sty JR, Hubbard AM, Starshak RJ. Radionuclide hepatobiliary imaging in congenital biliary tract ectasis (Caroli disease). Pediatr Radiol 1982;12:111–4.

Sty JR, Wells RG, SB.A. Comparative imaging bile-plug syndrome. Clin Nucl Med 1987;12:489–90.

Suarez F, et al. Bilio-pancreatic common channel in children. Clinical, biological and radiological findings in 12 children. Pediatr Radiol 1987;17:207–211.

Sugiyama M, et al. Large cholesterol polyps of the gallbladder: diagnosis by means of US and endoscopic US. Radiology 1995;196(2):493–7.

Summerville DA, Marks M, Treves ST. Hepatobiliary scintigraphy in arteriohepatic dysplasia (Alagille's syndrome). A report of two cases. Pediatr Radiol 1988;18(1): 32–4.

Sung JM, et al. Caroli's disease and congenital hepatic fibrosis associated with polycystic kidney disease. A case presenting with acute focal bacterial nephritis. Clin Nephrol 1992;38(6):324–8.

Sussman SK, Hall FM, Elboim CM. Radiographic assessment of anomalous bile ducts. Gastrointest Radiol 1986;11:269–72.

Swayne LC. Acute acalculous cholecystitis: sensitivity in detection using technetium-99m iminodiacetic acid cholescintigraphy. Radiology 1986;160(1):33–8.

Swayne LC, Ginsberg HN. Diagnosis of acute cholecystitis by cholescintigraphy: significance of pericholecystic hepatic uptake. AJR 1989;152(6):1211–3.

Taylor WF, Qaquandah BY. Neonatal jaundice associated with cystic fibrosis. Am J Dis Child 1972;123:161–2.

Taylor GA. Acute hepatic disease. Radiol Clin North Am 1997;35(4):799–814.

Teefey SA, et al. Sclerosing cholangitis: CT findings. Radiology 1988;169(3):635–9.

Ternberg JL, Keating JP. Acute acalculus cholecystitis: complication of other illnesses in childhood. Arch Surg 1975;110:543–5.

Thaler MM. Studies in neonatal hepatitis and biliary atresia. Am J Dis Child 1968;116:280–4.

Thurston WA, Kelly EN, Silver MM. Acute acalculous cholecystitis in a premature infant treated with parenteral nutrition. CMAJ 1986;235(4):332–4.

Todani T, et al. Congenital bile duct cysts: classification, operative procedures, and review of thirty-seven cases including cancer arising from choledochal cyst. Am J Surg 1977;134(2):263–9.

Toma P, Lucigrai G, Pelizza A. Sonographic patterns of Caroli's disease: report of 5 new cases. J Clin Ultrasound 1991;19(3):155–61.

Torrisi JM, Haller JO, Velcek FT. Choledochal cyst and biliary atresia in the neonate: imaging findings in five cases. AJR 1990;155(6):1273–6.

Treves S, Jones A, Markisz J. Liver and spleen in pediatric nuclear medicine. New York: Springer-Verlag; 1995. p. 466–95.

Tsakayannis DE, Kozakewich HP, Lillehei CW. Acalculous cholecystitis in children. J Pediatr Surg 1996;31(1):127–31.

Tsuchida Y, Honna T, Kawarasaki H. Cystic dilatation of the intrahepatic biliary system in biliary atresia after hepatic portoenterostomy. J Pediatr Surg 1994;29(5):630–4.

Tsuchida Y, et al. Antenatal diagnosis of biliary atresia (type I cyst) at 19 weeks' gestation: differential diagnosis and etiologic implications. J Pediatr Surg 1995;30(5):697–9.

Tzakis AG, et al. Liver transplantation for Alagille's syndrome. Arch Surg 1993;128(3):337–9.

Uggowitzer M, et al. Sonography of acute cholecystitis: comparison of color and power Doppler sonography in detecting a hypervascularized gallbladder wall. AJR 1997; 168(3):707–12.

Valayer J, Alagille D. Experience with choledochal cyst. J Pediatr Surg 1975;10:65–8.

Vanderspuy S. Endoscopic retrograde cholangiopancreatography [ERCP] in children. Endoscopy 1978;10:173–5.

Vazquez J, et al. Biliary atresia and the polysplenia syndrome: its impact on final outcome. J Pediatr Surg 1995; 30(3):485–7.

Venu RP, et al. Role of endoscopic retrograde cholangiography in the diagnosis and treatment of choledochocele. Gastroenterology 1984;87:1144–9.

Voyles CR, et al. Carcinoma in choledochal cysts: age-related incidence. Arch Surg 1983;118:986–8.

Waggett J, et al. Congenital bronchobiliary fistula. J Pediatr Surg 1970;5:566–9.

Walker WA, et al. Pediatric gastrointestinal disease: pathophysiology, diagnosis, management. Vol. 2. 2nd ed. St. Louis (MO): Patterson, A.S. 1996. p. 999–2113.

Watanabe Y. et al. High-resolution MR cholangiopancreatography. Crit Rev Diagn Imaging 1998;39:115–258.

Wechsler RL, Thiel DV. Fibropolycystic disease of the hepatobiliary system and kidneys. Dig Dis 1976;21:1058–69.

Weissmann HS, et al. Rapid and accurate diagnosis of acute cholecystitis with 99m-Tc-HIDA cholescintigraphy. AJR 1979;132(4):523–8.

Weissmann HS, et al. Spectrum of 99m-Tc-IDA cholescintigraphic patterns in acute cholecystitis. Radiology 1981;138(1):167–75.

Weissmann HS, et al. The role of technetium-99m iminodiacetic acid (IDA) cholescintigraphy in acute acalculous cholecystitis. Radiology 1983;146(1):177–80.

Wicks JD, Silver TM, Bree RL. Giant cystic abdominal masses in children and adolescents: ultrasonic differential diagnosis. AJR 1978;130:853–7.

Wilkinson M. The art of diagnostic imaging: the biliary tree. J Hepatol 1996;1:5–19.

Williams C, Williams AM. Abnormalities of the bile ducts. Ann Surg 1955;141:598–605.

Williamson SL, et al. Apparent gut excretion of Tc-99m-DISIDA in a case of extrahepatic biliary atresia. Pediatr Radiol 1986;16:245–57.

Wirth S, et al. Kawasaki-Syndrome mit akutem Gallenblasenhydrops-Fallbericht und Literaturubersicht. Klin Paediatr 1985;197:68–70.

Witlin LT, et al. Transhepatic decompression of the biliary tree in Caroli disease. Surgery 1982;91:205–9.

Yamaguchi M. Congenital choledochal cyst: analysis of 1,433 patients in the Japanese literature. Am J Surg 1980; 140:653–7.

Yanagihara J, et al. An association of multiple intestinal atresia and biliary atresia: a case report. Eur J Pediatr Surg 1995;5(6):372–4.

Yazbeck S, Grignon A, Boisvert J. A pseudo-choledochal cyst. J Can Assoc Radiol 1985;36:74–5.

Yeh H, Goodman J, Rabinowitz JG. Floating gallstones in bile without added contrast material. AJR 1986;146:49–50.

Yousefzadeh DK, Soper RT, Jackson JH. Obstructive jaundice due to congenital stenosis of the ampulla of Vater. Gastrointest Radiol 1979;4:379–82.

Ystgaard B, Myrvold HE, Nilsen G. Magnetic resonance imaging in preoperative assessment of choledochal cysts. Eur J Surg 1992;158(10):567–9.

Zangger P, et al. MRI findings in Caroli's disease and intrahepatic pigmented calculi. Abdom Imaging 1995; 20(4):361–4.

Zerres K, et al. Mapping of the gene for autosomal recessive polycystic kidney disease (ARPCKD) to chromosome 6p21-cen. Nat Genet 1994;7:429–32.

Zimmon DS, et al. Choledochocele: radiologic diagnosis and endoscopic management. Gastrointest Radiol 1978;3: 349–51.

12

THE LIVER

Bruce M. Shuckett, MD, FRCPC, Chee Hiew, MB, BS, FRACR,
Tara Williams, MD, Paul S. Babyn, MDCM, Christel Wihlborg, MD,
Katherine A. Zukotynski, BASc, and David A. Stringer, BSc, MBBS, FRCR, FRCPC

EMBRYOGENESIS

Hepatic Parenchyma

Hepatic parenchyma begins development in the third to fourth week of gestation as a bud of the endodermal epithelium on the ventral surface of the distal foregut (Figure 12–1). This bud, the hepatic diverticulum, consists of rapidly proliferating cells that penetrate the septum transversum. The septum transversum is a mass of splanchnic mesoderm between the developing heart and midgut that forms the central tendon of the diaphragm and the ventral mesentary in this region. The thin, double-layered membrane of the ventral mesentary gives rise to the lesser omentum, the falciform ligament, and the visceral peritoneum of the liver (Moore and Persaud, 1998). As the hepatic diverticulum enlarges between the layers of the ventral mesentary, it divides into two parts: The larger cranial part gives rise to the liver; the smaller, caudal part develops into the gallbladder and cystic duct. The remains of the original diverticulum elongate to become the hepatic and common bile ducts. By the seventh week of gestation, both the liver and gallbladder have recognizable forms (Colon, 1990).

Interlacing cords of hepatic cells derived from the cranial bud anastomose around endothelium-lined spaces forming the primordia of hepatic sinu-

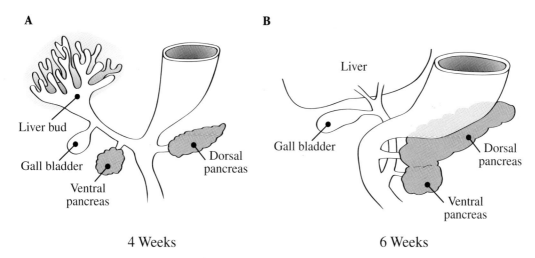

FIGURE 12–1. Liver and gallbladder embryology. *A,* The liver begins to develop in the third to fourth week of gestation as a bud of the endodermal epithelium on the ventral surface of the distal foregut that penetrates the mesodermal septum transversum. *B,* The connection between liver bud and foregut forms the bile duct, gallbladder, and cystic duct, which comes to pass posterior to the duodenum owing to the rotation and development of the bowel. (Adapted from Stringer D. Pediatric gastrointestinal imaging. B.C. Decker Inc.; 1989.)

soids. By late gestation, the ultrastructural features of hepatocytes are similar to those in the adult. However, the majority of hepatocyte plates are more than one cell thick, thereby limiting the passage of substrates. Rapidly proliferating endodermal cells form the epithelial lining of the intrahepatic portion of the biliary apparatus. Intralobular bile ducts remain sparse even in the third trimester. By the tenth week of gestation, interlobular bile ducts may be seen. Bile secretion from hepatic cells begins during the twelfth week of gestation (Mowat, 1994) Hematopoietic elements, Kupffer's cells, and fibrous tissues are derived from mesenchyme in the septum transversum (Suchy, 1994).

The liver grows so rapidly in the fetus that it comprises approximately 10% of the total body weight by the tenth week of gestation. Hematopoiesis, beginning during the sixth week of gestation, is considered responsible for the large size of the liver between the seventh and ninth weeks of development. Hematopoietic cells disappear shortly after birth by which time the liver accounts for approximately 5% of total body weight (Moore and Persaud, 1998).

Fetal Hepatic Circulation

The hepatic veins are derived from the right vitelline vein in the region of the septum transversum, whereas the portal vein develops from an anastomotic network of the vitelline veins near the duodenum (Moore and Persaud, 1998). The ductus venosus forms within the liver from anastomosis of the left umbilical vein with remnants of the vitelline veins (Strouse and Di Pietro, 1997). Most of the blood flowing from the placenta into the umbilical vein is conducted through the ductus venosus to the inferior vena cava bypassing the liver (Figure 12-2A). Existence of a physiologic sphincter regulating blood flow to the ductus venosus has been described; however, its anatomic presence is not universally accepted (Moore and Persaud, 1998). After birth, many fetal vessels become ligaments. The ductus venosus closes within 10 to 20 days after birth, forming the ligamentum venosum. The intra-abdominal part of the umbilical vein remains patent although it becomes the ligamentum teres (Figure 12-2B). The quantity of oxygenated blood flowing

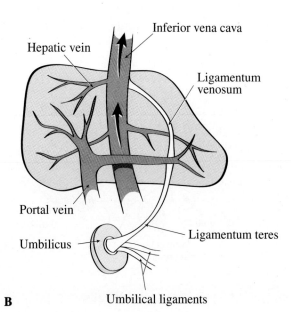

FIGURE 12–2. *A,* In fetal circulation, most of the blood in the umbilical vein flows through the ductus venosus to the inferior vena cava, bypassing the liver. A physiologic sphincter regulating blood flow to the ductus venosus has been described, however, its anatomic presence is not universally accepted. Poorly oxygenated blood returns to the placenta through umbilical arteries. B, After birth the ductus venosus closes to form the ligamentum venosum while the umbilical vein forms the ligamentum teres. (Adapted from Moore K., Persaud T. The developing human—clinically oriented embryology. 6th ed. W.B. Saunders Co.; 1998.)

into the fetal liver via the portal vein is thought to determine development and functional segmentation. Although right and left lobes are initially of comparable size, the right lobe predominates after 3 months' gestation. (Morgenstern and Mazur, 1959; Mowat, 1994). Minor variations of liver lobulation are common.

Persistence of the ductus venosus beyond the neonatal period is unusual and may involve patients with portal hypertension and cirrhosis (Strouse and Di Pietro, 1997). The ductus venosus can remain open after birth as a bypass tract of the portal vein in the case of a poorly developed intrahepatic portal system (Ikeda et al, 1999). Two-dimensional real-time gray-scale ultrasonography (US) may be used to measure the length (1 to 2 cm) and diameter (1 to 2 mm) of the ductus venosus. Duplex Doppler imaging can be used to show the waveform of flow and its velocity. Flow is typically cephalic from the left portal vein to the inferior vena cava, and initial velocity can be between 0.15 to 0.70 m per second. The closed ductus venosus may appear as a thin anechoic channel with no flow seen on color Doppler US and no signal visible on the Doppler waveform (Loberant et al., 1992). Normal cessation of umbilical vein flow leads to rapid closure of the ductus venosus (Strouse and Di Pietro, 1997). Ultrasonographic studies have shown that this occurs in approximately 90% of infants by 18 days of life. However, the exact mechanisms of closure have not been completely elucidated (Loberant et al., 1992).

Perinatal thrombosis of the ductus venosus is rare and often fatal. Incidence of umbilical cord thrombosis varies from 1 in 1300 to 1 in 1500 for normal deliveries but may rise to 1 in 250 in high-risk pregnancies. Trauma, umbilical cord abnormalities, or obstetrical complications are often responsible. Knot formation in a long cord may lead to compression, stasis, and thrombosis. Stretching of a short cord during labor may lead to vessel wall damage and thrombus formation (Hasaart et al., 1994).

NORMAL ANATOMY AND IMAGING OF THE LIVER

Anatomic Features and Imaging Appearance

The liver is the largest organ in the body, weighing approximately 1500 g in the average adult man and accounting for approximately 2.5% of total body weight (Akesson, Loeb, and Wilson-Pauwels, 1990; Rubin and Farber, 1994). Males typically have somewhat larger livers than females of the same weight (DeLand and North, 1968). The functions of the liver are numerous and include synthesis of serum proteins, detoxification of alimentary waste products, processing of dietary amino acids, carbohydrates, lipids, and vitamins; and synthesis and excretion of bile. Figure 12–3 provides an illustration of microscopic liver architecture (Cormack, 1993; Burkitt, Young, and Heath, 1997).

Situated in the right upper quadrant of the abdomen immediately below the diaphragm, the liver is roughly triangular in shape (Figure 12–4). Exact liver shape is variable, in part because of its ability to regenerate (Mould, 1972; Gazelle, Saini, and Mueller, 1998). The left hepatic border extends to the midclavicular line, and the right border

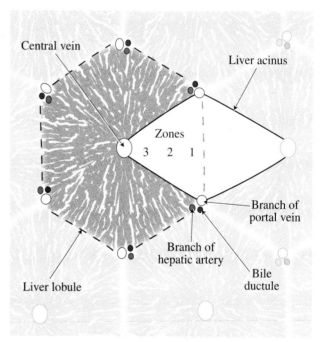

FIGURE 12–3. Hepatocytes are traditionally described as being arranged into roughly hexagonal lobules. Portal tracts located at the corners each contain a branch of the hepatic artery and portal vein, a bile ductule, and a lymphatic vessel. While each portal tract supplies many lobules, the central vein drains blood from a single lobule into the hepatic vein. More recently, the hepatic acinus has been defined in relation to hepatic vasculature. As indicated in the figure, zones 1, 2, and 3 refer to hepatocytes increasingly distant from the blood supply. (Adapted from Cotran R, Kumar V, Collins T. Robbins pathologic basis of disease. 6th ed. W.B. Saunders Co.; 1999.)

extends to the midaxillary line. The superior, anterior, and right lateral surfaces of the liver are smooth, molded against the diaphragm and abdominal wall. The inferior and posterior surfaces are grooved, resting against the inferior vena cava, right kidney, transverse colon, duodenum, pancreas, and stomach. The porta hepatis is located in the inferior hepatic surface. The portal vein, hepatic arteries, and periarterial autonomic nerves plexus enter the liver through the porta hepatis while the hepatic ducts and lymphatic channels leave it by the same route (Friedman and Dachman, 1994). The gallbladder normally extends slightly beyond the anterior inferior margin of the liver.

The liver is covered by a thin but strong connective-tissue capsule known as Glisson's capsule. Most of the capsule is covered by visceral peritoneum. The falciform ligament is a double layer of peritoneum connecting the liver with the anterior abdominal wall and the diaphragm. At the superior aspect of the liver, one layer of peritoneum passes to the right while the other passes to the left, forming the coronary ligament. That part of the liver not covered by peritoneum is referred to as the bare area. The coronary ligament surrounds the bare area of the liver like a crown, joining the right and left triangular ligaments at its edges. The posterior aspect of the left triangular ligament becomes continuous with the lesser omentum. The lesser omentum follows the course of the ligamentum venosum along the inferior surface of the liver, connecting the liver

to the lesser curvature of the stomach. The ligamentum venosum passes through the liver from the inferior vena cava to the left branch of the portal vein. The ligamentum teres passes from the porta hepatis where it is attached to the left branch of the portal vein, to the umbilicus. It may be found in the free edge of the falciform ligament (Akesson, Loeb, and Wilson-Pauwels, 1990; Moore and Persaud, 1998).

The right and left subphrenic spaces lie between the diaphragm and the right and left lobes of the liver, respectively. The right subhepatic space is the hepatorenal recess otherwise known as Morison's pouch, while the left subhepatic space is the lesser sac (Rubenstein et al., 1983; Akesson, Loeb, and Wilson-Pauwels, 1990).

The classic anatomic division of the liver is into four lobes (Figure 12–4). Anteriorly, the falciform ligament divides the liver into right and left lobes. Inferiorly, the gallbladder fossa separates the right hepatic lobe from the quadrate lobe, and the sulcus for the inferior vena cava separates the right lobe from the caudate lobe. The caudate process connects the caudate lobe to the right hepatic lobe between the gallbladder fossa and the sulcus for the inferior vena cava. The quadrate lobe is separated from the caudate lobe by the porta hepatis. The fissure for the ligamentum teres separates the left hepatic lobe from the quadrate lobe, and the fissure for the ligamentum venosum defines the border between the left hepatic lobe and the caudate lobe. When the fissure of the ligamentum teres is deep, the left hepatic lobe may

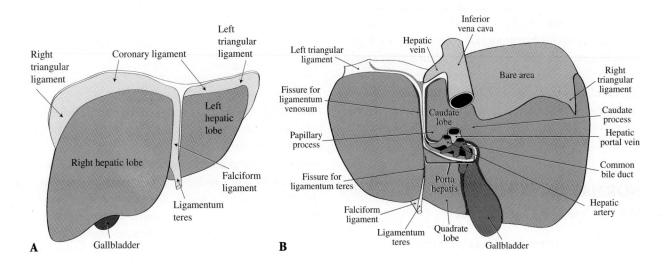

FIGURE 12–4. Outline of hepatic anatomy. *A*, Anterior view. *B*, Visceral surface. (Adapted from Netter F. Atlas of human anatomy. 2nd ed. Novartis; 1997.)

appear to be completely separated from the rest of the liver. When the fissure of the ligamentum venosum is deep, the papillary process of the caudate lobe may resemble an extrahepatic mass (Donoso et al., 1989).

This classical division into anatomic lobes is not helpful for surgical planning because resection has to follow the vascular distribution thus, a "surgical subdivision" is necessary (Michels, 1955; Daneman, 1987; Netter, 1997). This subdivision divides the liver into two lobes, four segments, and eight areas (Figure 12–5). The surgical left lobe of the liver is composed of a lateral and a medial segment. The lateral segment corresponds to the classical left hepatic lobe. The medial segment lies adjacent to the lateral segment and is demarcated to its right by the main lobar fissure, an oblique imaginary plane passing through the gallbladder and the impression for the inferior vena cava. The medial segment of the left hepatic lobe includes the quadrate lobe and the left half of the caudate lobe. The surgically defined right lobe of the liver lies to the right of the main lobar fissure and consists of anterior and posterior segments. Right and left surgical lobes define similar intrahepatic territories (Friedman and Dachman, 1994). The right hepatic artery and right portal vein supply the right surgical lobe of the liver while the right hepatic duct drains it. The left hepatic artery and left portal vein supply the left surgical lobe of the liver while the left hepatic duct drains it (Healey, 1970). Portal veins may be used to define hepatic lobes, divisions and areas because they are the most easily imaged intrahepatic portal structures (Friedman and Dachman, 1994). Another method of internally dividing the liver was developed by the French surgeon Claude Couinaud (Lafortune et al., 1991; Friedman and Dachman, 1994; Netter, 1997). There are eight Couinaud segments. The first segment denotes the caudate lobe. The second and third segments define the lateral superior and lateral inferior areas of the surgical left lobe, respectively. The fourth segment refers to the medial segment of the surgical left lobe. The sixth and seventh segments include the posterior inferior and posterior superior areas of the surgical right lobe, respectively. The fifth and eighth segments include the anterior inferior and anterior superior areas of the surgical right lobe, respectively.

Several features of normal anatomy are of note for the radiologist and are considered according to imaging modality. Anomalies of situs are discussed with the spleen (see Chapter 11).

Plain-Film Radiography

As more sophisticated imaging modalities become available, less emphasis is placed on older techniques. Nevertheless, plain-film radiography provides rapid, accessible information such as the extent

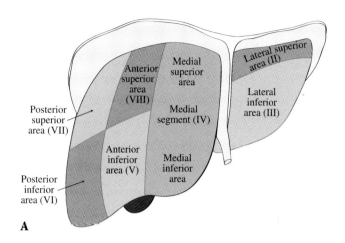

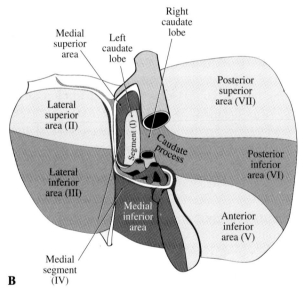

FIGURE 12–5. Surgical subdivision of the liver and Couinaud segments. *A*, Anterior view. *B*, Visceral surface. The surgical subdivision divides the liver into two lobes, four segments, and eight areas. The solid vertical line defines the border between left and right hepatic lobes. The dashed lines define the border between the medial and lateral segments of the left lobe and the anterior and posterior segments of the right lobe. The eight Couinaud segments correspond to the eight areas of the surgical subdivision, except that the first segment denotes the caudate lobe and the fourth segment includes the medial superior and inferior areas of the surgical left lobe. (Adapted from Netter F. Atlas of human anatomy. 2nd ed. Novartis; 1997.)

of air in the portal venous system or the amount of hepatobiliary calcification. Malabsorption may be suggested by a radiolucent fatty liver (Colon, 1990). Unfortunately, plain- film radiography is rarely helpful in the diagnosis of liver disease, especially since the size and shape of hepatic lobes may vary.

A Reidel lobe is a normal anatomical variant consisting of a large inferior projection from the anterior edge of the right lobe of the liver. It may be more commonly found in women, however, this is subject to debate (Gillard et al., 1998). A Reidel lobe may be mistaken for hepatomegaly on plain-film radiographs.

Ultrasonography

Normal hepatic parenchyma echogenicity is uniform, with clear delineation of hepatic vessels. Hepatic fissures appear as strongly echogenic bands on ultrasonography (US). A Reidel lobe may be present and will be relatively obvious. The liver has a characteristic appearance on US, which can be identified, even when located in an ectopic position (Newman, Bowen, and Eggli, 1994).

A variety of normal structures in the liver can give an unusual ultrasonographic appearance that should not be confused with active pathology. The falciform ligament is one of the most common pseudolesions in the liver. It appears as a focal area of increased echogenicity, especially on transverse scans (Hillman et al., 1979; Prando et al., 1979). It may be round in some projections but can be shown to be linear by altering the angle of scan. The ligamentum venosum may appear as a hyperechoic prominent round structure in transverse scans and is usually more clearly distinguished on longitudinal scans (Parulekar, 1979). The caudate lobe can mimic a hepatic tumor, and the papillary process of the caudate lobe can resemble a pancreatic mass on US (Donoso et al., 1989; Hartleb, Nowak, and Scieszka, 1995). Perihepatic fat may give the impression of an echogenic mass, particularly between the right kidney and the right lobe of the liver (Prando et al., 1979).

A dense echogenic line joins the right portal vein to the neck of the gallbladder in approximately 70% of sonograms. This line represents the fissure between the right and left lobes of the liver (Callen, Filly, and DeMartini, 1979; Fried, Kreel, and Cosgrove, 1984).

Accessory fissures, typically affecting the superior part of the right hepatic lobe, may occur and can be seen on US or computed tomography (CT).

Although they appear echodense on US, they should not be confused with pathology (Auh et al., 1984; Lim et al., 1987; Martinoli et al., 1992; Auh et al., 1994).

Measurements of liver volume are important in planning hepatic resection and transplantation as well as in the assessment of diseases and their response to treatment (Soyer et al., 1992; Itai et al., 1997). Numerous attempts have been made to measure liver size with imaging techniques (Rollo and DeLand, 1968; Carr et al., 1976; Sandrasegaran et al., 1999). Early results using radionuclide scans or US have not led to widespread clinical applications. Precise liver size is often difficult to evaluate on US. Hepatomegaly is indicated by a rounded rather than tapered inferior hepatic margin or by a right hepatic lobe that covers most of the anterior aspect of the right kidney. Methods of ultrasonographically measuring the neonatal liver have been developed, but they are generally not helpful unless serial studies are being performed with measurements taken through the same anatomic landmarks. Recent results in the literature indicate that spiral CT may allow accurate and rapid assessment of liver volume without the need for intravascular contrast media (Sandrasegaran et al., 1999). Further, magnetic resonance imaging (MR) may provide a means of estimating fetal organ volume (Garden and Roberts, 1996).

Computed Tomography

Computed tomography delineates the anatomy of the liver and adjacent structures extremely well. The porta hepatis, portocaval space, and hepatoduodenal and gastrohepatic ligaments are visible and create fewer diagnostic problems than on US. The falciform ligament and fissure for the ligamentum teres can both be seen although the ligament may be difficult to see in some patients unless there is adjacent fluid or fat (Balfe et al., 1984; Zirinsky et al., 1985; Weinstein et al., 1986). Computed tomography is effective at defining the lobes of the liver, which is particularly helpful in the preoperative assessment of liver tumors. Sectional images allow for rapid differentiation of subphrenic subhepatic and pleural fluid collections (Rubenstein et al., 1983; Daneman, 1987).

Major uses of CT include evaluation of trauma and neoplasms as well as detection of infectious lesions (Suchy, 1994). Computed tomography may be more useful than US in resolving hepatic pseudolesions seen on radionuclide scans (Morgan,

Trought, and Daffner, 1978). Portal perfusion defects may cause pseudolesions to be seen in the left hepatic lobe around the falciform ligament. Fluid collections surrounding the caudate lobe as it invaginates into the superior recess of the lesser sac may simulate intrahepatic masses (Rubenstein et al., 1983; Ohashi et al., 1995).

Magnetic Resonance Imaging

Magnetic resonance imaging (MR) is similar to CT in that it gives excellent cross-sectional images of the liver and depicts the anatomy of the liver and adjacent structures extremely well. It may permit characterization of soft-tissue masses when other imaging modalities are inconclusive. Both MR and CT can detect focal fatty hepatic changes suggested on plain-film radiographs (Friedman and Dachman, 1994). New contrast agents are being developed to enhance liver lesion conspicuity. Pulse sequences have been designed to reduce scan time and help overcome motion artifact (Mahfouz, Hamm, and Taupitz, 1997; Clement et al., 1998; Ferrucci, 1998; Laing and Gibson, 1998). Currently, MR may be used to guide needle aspiration biopsies of hepatic masses or as an imaging tool in laparoscopic interstitial laser therapy of the liver (Klotz et al., 1997; Rofsky et al., 1998). It is particularly useful in evaluating hepatic vascular supply from the portal vein, hepatic artery, and hepatic veins to the liver. This is important prior to liver transplantation and may be helpful for patients with portal hypertension (Rodgers et al., 1994; Silverman et al., 1995; Ward et al., 1997; Teo, Strouse, and Prince, 1999). Magnetic resonance imaging is a relatively new technology that provides important information about liver anatomy and pathology. It is continuing to evolve with developments in scanner hardware and software performance. Spectroscopy is possible in the liver, but further experience is required before its clinical value is known.

Normal Variants of Vascular Supply

Approximately 75% of the blood to the liver is derived from the portal vein, with the remaining 25% coming from the hepatic artery (Cormack, 1993). The hepatic artery is typically a branch of the celiac artery that ascends in the free margin of lesser omentum. Hepatic arterial variations are common and well known to angiographers but can also be visualized by US and on CT or MR. A hepatic artery is considered to be aberrant when it does not arise from the terminal end of the celiac trunk. Aberrant hepatic arteries may be either replaced or accessory. An artery is termed "replaced" if it originates from a nontypical vessel. An artery is said to be "accessory" if there is an extra hepatic artery originating from another source. This term has a more limited sense in the context of the liver, because each

---

TABLE 1. Michel's Classification of Hepatic Artery Anatomy

Type I	The right, left and middle hepatic arteries arise from the celiac axis (55%).
Type II	The right and middle hepatic arteries arise from the celiac axis. Replaced left hepatic artery arising from the left gastric artery (10%).
Type III	The left and middle hepatic arteries arise from the celiac axis. Replaced right hepatic artery arising from the superior mesenteric artery (11%).
Type IV	The middle hepatic artery arises from the celiac axis. Replaced right hepatic artery arising from the superior mesenteric artery. Replaced left hepatic artery arising from the left gastric artery (1%).
Type V	The right, left and middle hepatic arteries arise from the celiac axis. Accessory left hepatic artery arising from the left gastric artery (8%).
Type VI	The right, left and middle hepatic arteries arise from the celiac axis. Accessory right hepatic artery arising from the superior mesenteric artery (7%).
Type VII	The right, left and middle hepatic arteries arise from the celiac axis. Accessory right hepatic artery arises from the superior mesenteric artery. Accessory left hepatic artery arises from the left gastric artery (1%).
Type VIII	Combination patterns of (a) a replaced right hepatic artery and an accessory left hepatic artery or (b) an accessory right hepatic artery with a replaced left hepatic artery (2%).
Type IX	The entire hepatic trunk is derived from the superior mesenteric artery (4.5%).
Type X	The entire hepatic trunk is derived from the left gastric artery (0.5%).

hepatic artery, whether accessory or not, supplies a specific area and is essential (Michels, 1955; Healey, 1970). Table 12–1 indicates Michel's classification of hepatic artery anatomy (Michels, 1955). Right and left branches of the hepatic artery each supply approximately half of the liver parenchyma (Akesson, Loeb, and Wilson-Pauwels, 1990). Hepatic arteries and their segmental branches tend to be end arteries without anastomoses beyond the porta hepatis (Friedman and Dachman, 1994).

The portal vein is formed behind the neck of the pancreas by the convergence of the splenic and superior mesenteric veins and receives venous blood from the spleen, pancreas, and intestinal tract. It typically runs behind the first part of the duodenum and ascends in the free margin of the lesser omentum to the porta hepatis, where it divides into left and right branches supplying the liver. Variations of the hepatic portal vein are rare (Gazelle, Saini, and Mueller, 1998). They may include (1) anterior positioning of the portal vein with respect to the head of the pancreas and duodenum and (2) linkage of the portal vein to a pulmonary vein or inferior vena cava. In approximately half of the population, the inferior mesenteric vein drains into the splenic vein. In the remainder, it either joins the superior mesenteric vein or enters at the junction of the splenic and superior mesenteric veins (Friedman and Dachman, 1994; Netter, 1997). Tributaries of the portal vein provide important anastomotic connections. Among these, the left gastric vein is a direct tributary of the portal vein that communicates with the superior vena cava through the submucosal esophageal plexus. Veins surrounding the ligamentum teres form connections between the portal vein and superficial abdominal veins draining into either the superior or inferior vena cava. The superior rectal branch of the inferior mesenteric vein is linked to the inferior vena cava via the submucosal rectal venous plexus. Finally, the left and right colic veins anastomose with renal and lumbar tributaries of the inferior vena cava in the retroperitoneal fat about the kidneys. Thus, among other things, portal obstruction may lead to esophageal varices, caput medusae, and hemorrhoids.

All venous drainage of the liver occurs via hepatic veins that empty into the inferior vena cava. Two to three hepatic veins are common (Akesson, Loeb, and Wilson-Pauwels, 1990); they may be found coursing through the planes that separate the four major segments of the liver (Michels, 1955;

Healey, 1970). In higher-level axial images, hepatic veins typically appear to run longitudinally while they tend to be cut in cross section in lower-level axial images. (Friedman and Dachman, 1994). The left hepatic vein drains the lateral division and part of the medial division of the surgical left lobe. The middle hepatic artery drains the medial divisions of the surgical right and left lobes. In approximately 85% of the population, the middle hepatic vein joins the left hepatic vein just prior to entering the inferior vena cava; in the remainder, it empties into the inferior vena cava directly (Nakamura and Tsuzuki, 1981). The right hepatic vein runs between the lateral and medial divisions of the surgical right lobe passing between the bifurcation of the right portal vein into its anterior and posterior segmental branches. Thus, axial images obtained near the porta hepatis show the right hepatic vein in cross section between the limbs of the "Y" associated with the right portal vein and its branches. The intersegmental plane of the surgical right lobe of the liver is defined by the line joining the right hepatic vein with the point of bifurcation of the portal vein (Friedman and Dachman, 1994). Many small dorsal hepatic veins drain areas of the liver adjacent to the inferior vena cava. Accessory hepatic veins may also be seen, including a right inferoposterior hepatic vein entering the inferior vena cava distal to the right renal vein, a right superior hepatic vein, or minor hepatic veins running parallel to main trunks (Gazelle, Saini, and Mueller, 1998).

Ultrasonographically, portal veins inside the liver demonstrate hyperechoic margins in 99% of patients while hepatic veins have hyperechoic margins in only 29% of patients. In conjunction with anatomic location, this assists radiologic differentiation between portal and hepatic veins. (Chafetz and Filly, 1979). Further, periarterial echogenicity visualized on US may result from the fact that autonomic nerves typically follow hepatic arteries to reach the liver (Friedman and Dachman, 1994).

Color Doppler US is very helpful in assessing the presence and direction of blood flow in hepatic arteries, hepatic veins and portal veins, (Shapiro et al., 1998). Normal vascular flow patterns can be readily seen at all ages. Doppler studies are discussed in more detail in the sections on portal hypertension and liver transplantation.

Ultrasonographic and Doppler evaluation of hepatic vasculature, though often sufficient, may be technically challenging in certain cases, and magnetic resonance angiography (MRA) can be used (Teo, Strouse, and Prince, 1999). Several MRA sequences are currently available. Spin echo sequences cause rapidly flowing blood to appear black since it is not within a selected slice long enough to obtain both the 90° and 180° pulse. Time-of-flight MRA uses short repetition times and rapidly repeated pulses to saturate proton spins, causing stationary tissue to appear dark while flowing blood appears bright (Teo, Strouse, and Prince, 1999). The technique is rapid and sensitive to slow blood flow but may be subject to poor spatial resolution and slice misregistration. Three-dimensional gadolinium-enhanced MRA is based on the principle of rendering T1 of blood shorter than that of surrounding tissues via the injection of gadolinium (Prince, Grist, and Debatin, 1999). Images may be obtained using a T1-weighted sequence and then interpreted on a computer with three-dimension reconstruction capabilities. The images are confounded by respiration but remain interpretable subject to shallow breathing (Lam et al., 1998). Three-dimensional gadolinium-enhanced MRA (3D Gd MRA) is particularly useful in assessing portal vein patency. It is typically not required to visualize hepatic anatomy, the former MR techniques being adequate (Rodgers et al., 1994; Hughes et al., 1996; Teo, Strouse, and Prince, 1999).

CONGENITAL AND DEVELOPMENTAL ANOMALIES

Major anomalous structural variations associated with the liver are rare (Morgenstern and Mazur, 1959; Champetier et al., 1985). Those described in the literature include presence of accessory lobes, abnormal fissures and lobulation, agenesis or hypoplasia of hepatic lobes, vascular abnormalities, and Chilaiditi syndrome.

Agenesis or Hypoplasia of a Hepatic Lobe

Agenesis or hypoplasia of a hepatic lobe is unusual (Morgenstern and Mazur, 1959). The left lobe may be small or completely atrophic as a result of selective left portal vein obstruction, with streaming of blood to the right lobe, biliary duct obstruction, or severe malnutrition. In many cases, congenital variation is likely (Morgenstern and Mazur, 1959). The right lobe is rarely the site of atrophy or hypoplasia. Agenesis may be due to failure of the right portal

vein to develop and may be found in conjunction with right hemidiaphragm deformity, intestinal malrotation, and absence of the gallbladder (Friedman and Dachman, 1994). It is normally accompanied by hypertrophy of other hepatic segments (Radin et al., 1987; Kakitsubata et al., 1991; Kakitsubata, Kakitsubata, and Watanabe, 1995). The caudate lobe may also be absent, and this can be associated with biliary tract disease, portal hypertension, and other congenital anomalies, or it can be discovered as an incidental finding (Radin et al., 1987).

Hepatic lobe anomalies may be detected radiologically and are often associated with ectopy of the gallbladder. On plain-film radiographs, agenesis may mimic Chilaiditi syndrome, with the hepatic flexure lying under the right hemidiaphragm (Makanjuola et al., 1996). Absence of a hepatic lobe or segment may be seen on liver/spleen scintigraphy and may resemble a space-occupying mass (Makler et al., 1980; Burton, Amin, and Tisdale, 1987). Reduction in amount of arterial supply to the affected lobe is indicated by angiography (Ham, 1979). Ultrasonography, CT, MR, and cholecystography will show a gallbladder in an abnormally superior, lateral, posterior, or inferior position (Radin et al., 1987; Kakitsubata, Kakitsubata, and Watanabe, 1995). Several cases of anomalous hepatic lobes have been detected with US, CT, and MR (Radin et al., 1987; Demirci, Diren, and Selcuk, 1990; Kanematsu et al., 1991, 1993; Harada et al., 1995; Kakitsubata, Kakitsubata, and Watanabe, 1995). Absence of the right hepatic vein, right portal vein, and dilated right intrahepatic ducts is required for the diagnosis of agenesis of the right hepatic lobe with CT (Chou et al., 1998).

Accessory hepatic lobes are typically small and located on the inferior hepatic surface. They may be ectopic if separated from the liver and may cause confusion on imaging (Fitzgerald, Hale, and Williams, 1993). They occur with a frequency of less than 1% in the population (Sato et al., 1998). Detection with CT may be confirmed with liver scintigraphy (Hashimoto, Oomachi, and Watarai, 1997). Although generally of limited clinical import, torsion of an accessory lobe may require surgical intervention (Friedman and Dachman, 1994).

Vascular Abnormalities

Intrahepatic vascular fistulae are typically associated with trauma, malignant tumor, and rupture of a hepatic artery aneurysm. Developmental shunts and fistulae have been reported in the literature, but their overall frequency is unknown (Paley et al., 1997). Clinical manifestations and radiologic appearances vary, depending on the type and impact of the congenital anomaly.

Arteriohepatic venous shunts are associated with hepatic hemangioendotheliomas (DeLorimier et al., 1967). Angiography may portray pooling in vascular lakes, early filling of hepatic veins, and dilation of the hepatic artery. Enlargement of the proximal aorta, hepatic artery, and hepatic veins may be seen on Doppler studies. Hemangioendotheliomas have a characteristic appearance on several imaging modalities (Paley et al., 1997).

Arterioportal fistulae frequently present with malabsorption and are a rare cause of childhood portal hypertension (Heaton et al., 1995). They are less common than arteriovenous shunts and may be diffuse or solitary. Diffuse arterioportal shunts are normally congenital while solitary arterioportal shunts are often acquired (Van Way et al., 1971). Doppler US may portray evidence of portal hypertension with high flow in the hepatic artery and reversed flow in the portal vein. Angiography is essential in defining hepatic arterial anatomy (Hazebroek et al., 1995; Paley et al., 1997).

Portocaval shunts usually result from continued patency of the ductus venosus although they may be secondary to elevated sinusoidal vascular resistance in the context of underlying liver disease. Although potentially asymptomatic for many years, the deformity may lead to hepatic encephalopathy and liver atrophy in adulthood (Farrant, Meir, and Karani, 1996). Existence of portocaval shunts may be confirmed with US and angiography.

Diagnosis of arteriohepatic venous shunts, arterioportal fistulae, and portocaval shunts is indicated by clinical features and may be confirmed by US, CT, MR, or angiography. Potential interventional therapy includes hepatic resection, hepatic artery ligation, and embolization (DeLorimier et al., 1967; Routh et al., 1992; Hazebroek et al., 1995).

Other vascular developmental anomalies include absence, atresia, or stenosis of the portal vein. When the portal vein is absent, the mesenteric venous return may drain into the inferior vena cava while the splenic vein drains into the left renal vein (Howard, 1991; Gazelle, Saini, and Mueller, 1998). Congenital diaphragms in the hepatic veins or inferior vena cava may produce Budd-Chiari syndrome,

a syndrome in which hepatic venous drainage is obstructed by thrombosis of the hepatic veins, of the inferior vena cava, or of both (Friedman and Dachman, 1994). Congenital disease such as Ehlers-Danlos syndrome may result in hepatic artery aneurysm. The latter topics are discussed under Miscellaneous Disorders later in the chapter.

Hepatodiaphragmatic Interposition of the Colon

Hepatodiaphragmatic interposition of the colon, or Chilaiditi syndrome, is a rare congenital anomaly in which the colon interposes between the liver and the right hemidiaphragm. Its frequency in children is unknown but appears to increase with age. Its incidence in the general population is less than 2.5%, and it is more common in men than in women (Prassopoulos, Raissaki, and Gourtsoyiannis, 1996).

The mobility of the ascending colon and the hepatic flexure is usually limited superiorly by attachments of the posterior extraperitoneal surfaces to the renal fascia. Hence, the hepatic flexure rarely lies above the L1-L2 level. Occasionally, the ascending colon is not fixed and is on a mesentery (see Chapter 6, sections on malrotation and mobile cecum). When mobile, the colon can rise anteriorly to lie anterior and superior to the liver. This hardly ever causes symptoms although it has been implicated as a cause of abdominal pain and vomiting (Waldman et al., 1966). Quite uncommonly, the colon may pass posteriorly behind the liver and above a normally positioned kidney to lie between the liver and hemidiaphragm. This is of no clinical significance but may be the cause of unusual symptoms in and inflammatory disease, such as appendicitis (Cumming and Kays, 1994). It is also possible to find a combination of anterior and posterior interposition of the colon (Oubenaissa et al., 1999). The etiology is uncertain because the colon is usually not mobile.

Normal treatment of Chilaiditi syndrome is based on dietary management. However, surgical treatment may be required in cases of intestinal obstruction, internal hernias, or disease of the colon (Risaliti et al., 1993; Oubenaissa et al., 1999).

The abnormal location of the bowel can be detected on US, plain-film radiography, contrast studies, CT, and MR. Of major importance is that this syndrome must not be confused radiologically with pathology. On plain-film radiographs, the air in the colon may be mistaken for extraluminal air if haustra are not visible. On US, the echogenicity of the collapsed bowel may be mistaken for a tumor or other mass lesion. Computed tomography with contrast medium in the gut easily makes the correct diagnosis, often detected as an unsuspected finding.

INFECTION AND INFLAMMATION OF THE LIVER

Pyogenic Hepatic Abscess

General Considerations

Pyogenic hepatic abscesses are rare in children (Chusid, 1978; Arya et al., 1982; Altman and Stolar, 1985; Liu, Fitzgerald, and Blake, 1990; Kays, 1992) and occur predominantly in the first 5 years of life (Dehner and Kissane, 1969; Goldenring and Flores, 1986). However, the incidence appears to be rising, and this may be related to increasing awareness of the disease and better diagnostic techniques (Brook and Fraizer, 1993).

Bacteria can invade the liver by a number of routes (Dehner and Kissane, 1969; Puck, 1991): (1) via the portal vein, (2) by direct spread from contiguous structures, (3) by direct inoculation (surgical or trauma), (4) through hepatic arterial blood flow, and (5) by unknown or cryptogenic mechanisms. Cryptogenic liver abscesses were thought to account for up to 20% of cases (Chusid, 1978), but as diagnostic techniques improve, the percentage is getting smaller (Puck, 1991). The most common mechanism in adults is biliary obstruction (Branum et al., 1990). This is uncommon in children (Dehner and Kissane, 1969) but may occur secondary to ascending septic cholangitis in patients with congenital biliary obstruction and choledochoenterostomy (Kasai procedure for biliary atresia). In infants, hepatic abscesses are usually associated with sepsis or umbilical infection secondary to vascular catheters, and abscesses are often multiple or miliary (Dehner and Kissane, 1969; Altman and Stolar, 1985; Kays, 1992). In older children, there is usually an underlying predisposing process such as chronic granulomatous disease or immunosuppression (Dehner and Kissane, 1969; Chusid, 1978; Altman and Stolar, 1985; Kays, 1992). Hepatic abscesses as sequelae of complicated inflammatory disease of the appendix still occur (Slovis et al., 1989) (Figure 12–6), but these and other infections, such as osteomyelitis, were more important causes in the

preantibiotic era (Dehner and Kissane, 1969). Systemic sepsis with hematogenous dissemination of organisms to the liver is now the most common cause of hepatic abscesses in patients with no underlying predisposing disorders (Dehner and Kissane, 1969; Chusid, 1978; Altman and Stolar, 1985).

The clinical findings are nonspecific, with fever, abdominal pain, hepatomegaly, and leukocytosis (Dehner and Kissane, 1969; Chusid, 1978; Larsen and Raffensperger, 1979; Kays, 1992). Fever and leukocytosis are the most common findings, with abdominal pain being infrequent (Dehner and Kissane, 1969; Chusid, 1978; Larsen and Raffensperger, 1979; Kays, 1992; Huang et al., 1996). Jaundice and abnormalities of liver function tests are unusual (Dehner and Kissane, 1969; Larsen and Raffensperger, 1979; Goldenring and Flores, 1986; Kays, 1992). The diagnosis of liver abscess in the neonate is particularly difficult to establish from the clinical picture alone (Altman and Stolar, 1985; Kays, 1992). A high index of suspicion must therefore be maintained, as mortality remains relatively high (Chusid, 1978; Liu, Fitzgerald, and Blake, 1990; Kays, 1992): the mortality rate in infants less than 1 month of age approaches 75% (Chusid, 1978).

Staphylococcus aureus is the most common causative bacteria (Dehner and Kissane, 1969; Chusid, 1978; Arya et al., 1982; Liu, Fitzgerald, and Blake, 1990). Gram-negative organisms, including Enterobacter, *Escherichia coli*, Klebsiella, and Pseudomonas, are other important pathogens (Dehner and Kissane, 1969; Chusid, 1978; Kays, 1992; Brook and Fraizer, 1993). With improved anaerobic culture techniques, the increasing importance of anaerobic organisms is also being recognized (Kays, 1992; Brook and Fraizer, 1993).

Abscesses are variable in size and can be single or multiple. Multiple abscesses are common and occur in 40 to 80% of patients (Dehner and Kissane, 1969; Chusid, 1978; Arya et al., 1982; Branum et al., 1990). The majority of hepatic abscesses are found in the right lobe (Arya et al., 1982; Kuligowska and Noble, 1983; Halvorsen et al., 1984; Laurin and Kaude, 1984; Branum et al., 1990; Hochbergs et al., 1990; Marn, Bree, and Silver, 1991; Vassiliades, Bree, and Korobkin, 1992; Seeto and Rockey, 1996).

Imaging of Pyogenic Abscesses

Better radiologic diagnosis and interventional management of hepatic abscesses have contributed to an improvement in mortality rates from hepatic abscesses in recent years (Goldenring and Flores, 1986; Marn, Bree, and Silver, 1991; Puck, 1991; Kays, 1992; Huang et al., 1996; Rintoul et al., 1996). The advent of abdominal US and CT has allowed rapid, early, and accurate diagnosis of hepatic abscesses.

Plain-Film Radiography. Initial chest radiographs may show abnormalities in 50% of patients (Goldenring and Flores, 1986; Seeto and Rockey, 1996). Findings are nonspecific and include right-sided atelectasis, pneumonia and pleural effusion, and an elevated right hemidiaphragm.

Ultrasonography. Ultrasonography can provide an early diagnosis. It is highly accurate and is the least invasive diagnostic procedure (Altman and Stolar, 1985). It does not require sedation of the patient, and its portability makes it the first-line investigation in many centers (Kuligowska and Noble, 1983; Laurin and Kaude, 1984; Kays, 1992; Rintoul et al., 1996).

Findings on US are variable and nonspecific but are diagnostic in the correct clinical setting. Pyogenic abscesses are usually spherical or ovoid in shape, and the wall is irregular or thick but can be well defined (Vassiliades, Bree, and Korabkin, 1992; Nisenbaum and Rowling, 1995). The ultrasonographic pattern

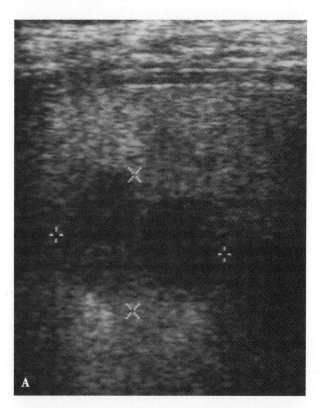

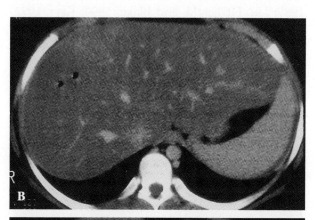

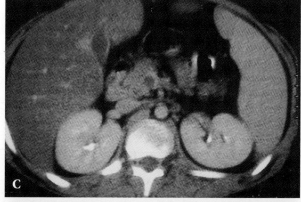

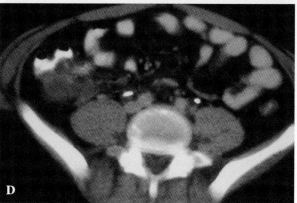

FIGURE 12–6. A 13-year-old boy with appendicitis complicated by ascending thrombophlebitis and Escherichia coli liver abscess. *A,* Ultrasonography demonstrates an ill-defined hypoechoic lesion with posterior enhancement. *B,* Contrast-enhanced CT following aspiration of the abscess shows air within the residual abscess cavity. Diffuse low attenuation of the liver due to fatty change may make detection of the abscess difficult. *C,* Filling defect in the superior mesenteric vein with *D,* inflammatory appendiceal mass in the right side of the lower abdomen.

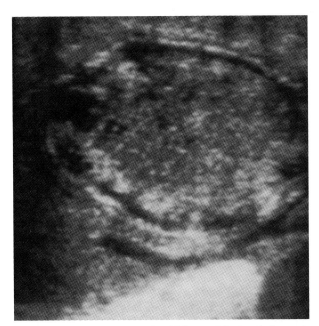

FIGURE 12–7. A 1-month-old boy with *Staphylococcus aureus* liver abscess. Ultrasonography shows a well-defined avascular mass with a hypoechoic rim. The mass is predominantly hyperechoic but contains multiple hypoechoic areas. Note mass effect on the adjacent hepatic vein. Diagnosis was confirmed with needle aspiration.

can vary from purely anechoic to highly echogenic (Kuligowska, Connors, and Shapiro, 1982; Vassiliades, Bree, and Korabkin, 1992; Nisenbaum and Rowling, 1995) (Figures 12–7, 12–8A). The typical appearance of an irregular, thick-walled, anechoic mass is often not seen (Kressel and Filly, 1978; Kuligowska, Connors, and Shapiro, 1982) (Figure 12–9B). Internal septations, fluid levels, and debris may be present (Kuligowska and Noble, 1983; Nisenbaum and Rowling, 1995). Intensely echogenic foci within the abscess due to gas bubbles may be seen (Kuligowska and Noble, 1983). Increased through transmission is common in echo-poor lesions (Kuligowska, Connors, and Shapiro, 1982) (Figure 12–10) but is not a consistently reliable finding (Laurin and Kaude, 1984). The variability in appearance will depend on the age of the abscess, which can evolve from a small solid inflammatory mass to a well-defined fluid-filled cavity over a period of time (Kuligowska and Noble, 1983; Wilson and Arenson, 1984) (Figure 12–11A; see Figure 12–8B). The major limitation of US is that parenchymal heterogeneity from pre-existent liver disease may make detection of small or early abscesses difficult (Marn, Bree, and Silver, 1991).

Computed Tomography. Computed tomography is more sensitive than US and should be used when the sonogram is negative but clinical suspicion remains high (Halvorsen et al., 1988; Branum et al., 1990; Kays, 1992; Kinnard et al., 1995; Huang et al.,

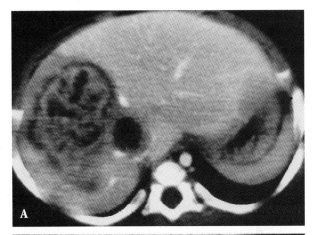

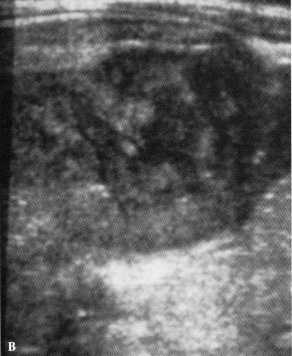

FIGURE 12–8. A 4-month-old girl with pyogenic liver abscess. *A,* Contrast-enhanced CT shows a large, irregular multiloculated mass in the right lobe of the liver. Posteriorly, adjacent to the inferior vena cava, is a well-defined rounded low-attenuation region more typical in appearance for a pyogenic abscess. *B,* Recurrent abscess in the same patient 2 months later. Ultrasonography shows an ill-defined heterogenous mass in the left lobe, corresponding to early abscess formation.

1996). Extremely sensitive, CT can detect abscesses as small as 3 to 5 mm (Miller et al., 1997). As on US, the appearance of hepatic abscesses on CT is variable and non-specific (Halvorsen et al., 1984; Kinnard et al., 1995).

The appearance on CT varies from well-defined, rounded cavities containing near water- density contents similar to hepatic cysts, to higher-density lesions mimicking neoplasms (Halvorsen et al., 1984) (see Figure 12–8A). Typically, abscesses appear of lower attenuation than the adjacent hepatic parenchyma on unenhanced images and are commonly surrounded by a thickened, enhancing wall (Jacobs and Birnbaum, 1995) (see Figure 12–9C). However, not all abscesses will demonstrate rim enhancement (Halvorsen et al., 1984). The attenuation of the abscess varies, depending on the viscosity of the pus, debris and associated hemorrhage (Foley and Jochem, 1991). Internal septations and mural nodules may also be seen (Vassiliades, Bree, and

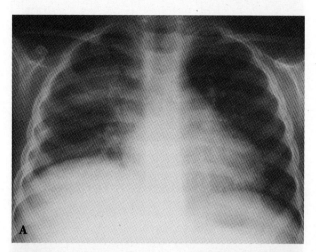

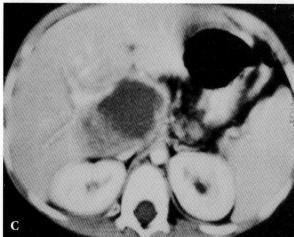

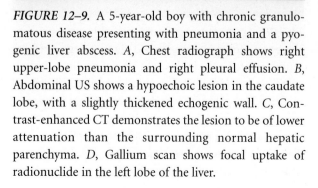

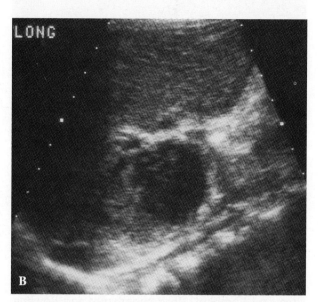

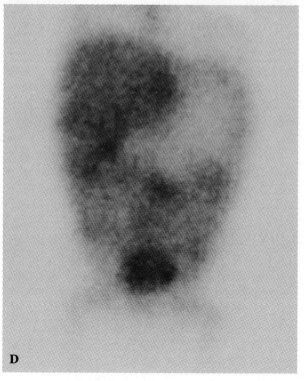

FIGURE 12–9. A 5-year-old boy with chronic granulomatous disease presenting with pneumonia and a pyogenic liver abscess. *A,* Chest radiograph shows right upper-lobe pneumonia and right pleural effusion. *B,* Abdominal US shows a hypoechoic lesion in the caudate lobe, with a slightly thickened echogenic wall. *C,* Contrast-enhanced CT demonstrates the lesion to be of lower attenuation than the surrounding normal hepatic parenchyma. *D,* Gallium scan shows focal uptake of radionuclide in the left lobe of the liver.

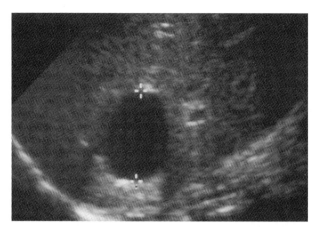

FIGURE 12–10. A 12-year-old boy with a pyogenic liver abscess in the right lobe of the liver. Ultrasonography shows a well-defined rounded hypoechoic lesion with posterior acoustic enhancement.

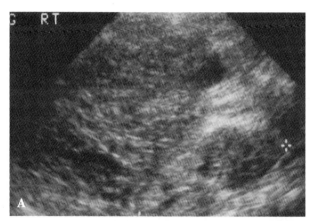

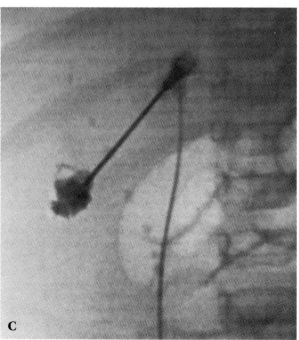

Korobkin, 1992) (see Figure 12–11B). Gas is well demonstrated on CT but is present in only 15 to 30% of cases (Halvorsen et al., 1984; Halvorsen, Foster, and Wilkinson, 1988; Vassiliades, Bree, and Korobkin, 1992; Lee, Wan, and Tsai, 1994).

A "double target sign" on dynamic CT, consisting of a hypodense central area surrounded by hyperdense rings, has been described as possibly specific

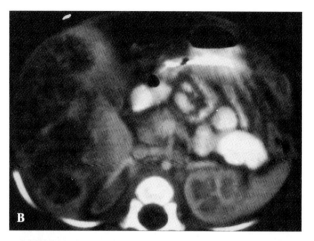

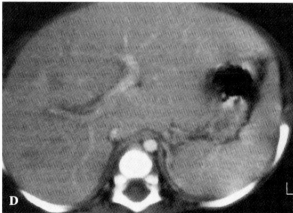

FIGURE 12–11. An 8-month-old girl with underlying congenital heart disease, *Staphylococcus aureus* septicemia, and hepatomegaly. *A*, Ultrasonography shows diffuse abnormality in the right lobe of the liver. Normal hepatic parenchyma is replaced by an ill-defined heterogenous mass containing small hypoechoic areas. *B*, Contrast-enhanced CT demonstrates the mass replacing almost the entire right lobe. The lesion appears multiseptated, with irregular peripheral enhancement. *C*, Percutaneous aspiration under ultrasonographic and fluoroscopic guidance confirmed the diagnosis of a pyogenic abscess. *D*, Computed tomography 1 month later after successful antibiotic treatment demonstrates almost complete resolution of the abscess.

for a small proportion of hepatic abscesses (Mathieu et al., 1985). Others have described the "cluster sign" (in which small abscesses appear to aggregate in a pattern that suggests the beginning of coalescence into a single larger abscess cavity) as being suggestive of a pyogenic abscess (Jeffrey et al., 1988). Dynamic CT with contrast enhancement can make hypodense abscesses more readily perceptible (Halvorsen et al.,

1984), but even multiple abscesses occasionally may become isodense with contrast (Laurin and Kaude, 1984); hence, an unenhanced study should be performed prior to intravenous contrast.

Computed tomography can also demonstrate extrahepatic pathology and thus help to identify the origin of hepatic abscesses (Kinnard et al., 1995) (Figures 12–12B; see Figures 12–6C and D).

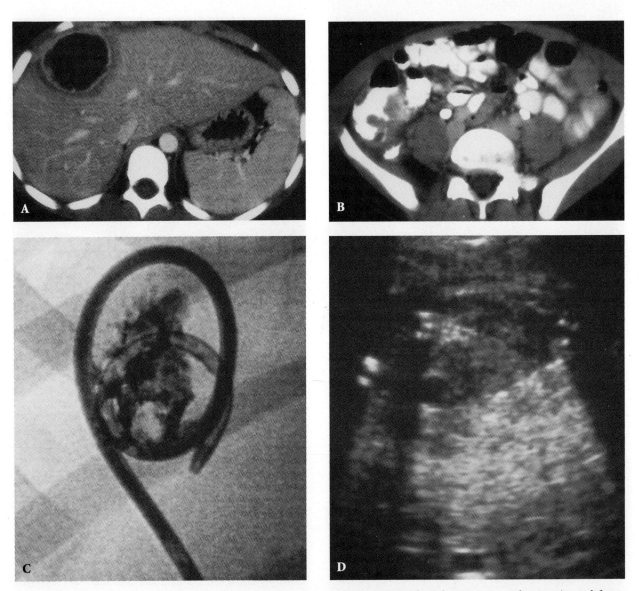

FIGURE 12–12. An 11-year-old boy with amebic liver abscess presenting with right upper- quadrant pain and fever. *A*, Contrast-enhanced CT shows a rounded low-attenuation lesion contiguous with the liver capsule and with a thin irregular enhancing wall surrounded by a rim of low attenuation. *B*, Irregular thickening of the bowel wall involving the cecum and ascending colon is also seen although there was no history of diarrhea. *C*, Percutaneous drainage was performed under US and fluoroscopic guidance with a 10 French catheter. *D*, Ultrasonography demonstrates the catheter and air (intense echogenic foci) within the residual cavity. Culture of the aspirates was negative but the diagnosis of amoebiasis was made from a positive serologic test.

Magnetic Resonance Imaging. Magnetic resonance imaging has the advantage over CT of multiplanar imaging, which allows better localization of abscesses. Magnetic resonance imaging also provides better delineation of the extent of surrounding inflammatory changes (Wall et al., 1985). However, the high cost, length of examination, and lack of easy access for interventional procedures have limited the usefulness of MR in the management of patients with hepatic abscesses (Huang et al., 1996; Mergo and Ros, 1997).

The appearances of pyogenic abscesses on MR are nonspecific (Wall et al., 1985; Mergo and Ros, 1997). Typically, abscesses appear low signal on T1-weighted and high signal on T2-weighted images (Wall et al., 1985; Schnall, 1995; Mergo and Ros, 1997). The wall is of intermediate signal (Schnall, 1995). Fluid within the abscess may occasionally show a varied signal due to the presence of blood products and high-protein contents (intermediate to high signal on T1-weighted, and intermediate to low signal on T2-weighted images). The use of gadolinium is thus important to detect and characterize liver abscesses (Schnall, 1995). A rim of enhancement is seen surrounding the abscess, but with delayed imaging, contrast in the periphery of abscess will diffuse slowly into the necrotic debris, with resultant central enhancement (Mergo and Ros, 1997).

Radionuclide Scintigraphy. Scintigraphy is now uncommonly used to diagnose hepatic abscesses, but sulfur colloid scanning is diagnostic in the appropriate clinical setting (Kinnard et al., 1995). Technetium-99m-sulfur colloid liver/spleen scanning shows an abscess as a photopenic area (Treves, Jones, and Markisz, 1995). Patchy uptake of sulfur colloid may indicate multiple tiny abscesses. A rim of increased activity surrounding a photopenic defect may be seen on hepatobiliary scan (McDonald and Davani, 1997). An abscess can also be demonstrated as an area that actively takes up gallium67citrate (O'Hara, 1996) (see Figure 12–9D), but lesions may be missed on gallium scans since normal liver uptake of radionuclide may mask small foci of infection (Laurin and Kaude, 1984; O'Hara, 1996).

Angiography. Angiography is no longer indicated, but if performed, it will show larger lesions as a hypovascular or avascular area, occasionally with a hypervascular rim. Small abscesses, even when mul-tiple, may not be appreciated (Laurin and Kaude, 1984).

Treatment of Pyogenic Abscesses

Antibiotic therapy with percutaneous drainage of macroscopic abscesses is now the treatment of choice for most pyogenic liver abscesses (Kuligowska, Connors, and Shapiro, 1982; Kuligowska and Noble, 1983; Hochbergs et al., 1990; Juul et al., 1990; Kays, 1992; Philips, 1994; Rintoul et al., 1996; Miller et al., 1997) (see Figures 12–11C and D). Microscopic and miliary abscesses are undrainable and are treated with antiobiotics alone. Both CT and US may be used to guide needles for diagnostic aspiration or for the placement of percutaneous drainage catheters (Kinnard et al., 1995). Percutaneous aspiration for definitive diagnosis and for culture material may be needed when imaging findings are equivocal or when blood cultures are negative (Taguchi et al., 1988; Hochbergs et al., 1990; Seeto and Rockey, 1996).

Surgical drainage is usually reserved for patients who have failed percutaneous drainage, for those who require surgical treatment for an underlying disease, or for those with ascites (Hashimoto, Herrman, and Grundfest-Broniatowski, 1995; Huang et al., 1996). Multiple large abscesses are not an absolute indication for surgical drainage as percutaneous drainage of these abscesses can still be performed (Hashimoto, Herrman, and Grundfest-Broniatowski, 1995).

We usually perform drainage under ultrasonographic control, with fluoroscopy to confirm catheter position (Figures 12–11, 12–12). Computed tomography is the preferred modality if sonography has been unsuccessful at demonstrating the lesion. Administration of a prophylactic antibiotic minimizes the risk of overwhelming sepsis during the procedure (Miller et al., 1997). Percutaneous techniques can be performed safely and effectively in infants and children, and the success rate for percutaneous drainage of pyogenic liver abscesses in the adult and pediatric population is high (Liu et al., 1989; Miller et al., 1997). Excellent results have also been reported with percutaneous needle aspiration of pyogenic liver abscesses (Giorgio et al., 1995).

Cat-Scratch Disease

Cat-scratch disease is a bacterial infection that usually affects children and adolescents (Larsen and

Patrick, 1992; Hopkins et al., 1996; O' Hara, 1996). Caused by a gram-negative bacillus, *Bartonella henselae*, infection follows a cat scratch. It is usually a self-limiting illness presenting with a subacute regional lymphadenitis proximal to the site of inoculation (Port and Leonidas, 1991; Hopkins et al., 1996). The disease usually resolves over 2 to 4 months (Rappaport, Cumming, and Ros, 1991). Disseminated infection occurs in 5 to 10% of cases and can involve multiple nodal sites, bones, and the liver and spleen (Larsen and Patrick, 1992; Hopkins et al., 1996). Neurologic involvement (including encephalitis) may occur, but it is uncertain whether this is related to direct bacterial invasion, bacterial toxins, or an immunologic response to infection (Hopkins et al., 1996).

Involvement of the liver is unusual but well described and includes hepatitis, hepatic granulomas, and hepatomegaly (Port and Leonidas, 1991; Rappaport, Cumming, and Ros, 1991; Larsen and Patrick, 1992; Hopkins et al., 1996). On US, hepatic granulomas range in appearance from multiple small (0.5 cm to 3.0 cm) well-defined, homogenous, hypoechoic lesions to indistinct and heterogenous lesions (Rappaport, Cumming, and Ros, 1991; Talenti et al., 1994; Hopkins et al., 1996). On CT, hepatic granulomas appear hypodense and may show peripheral or uniform enhancement with contrast (Port and Leonidas, 1991; Rappaport, Cumming, and Ros, 1991; Talenti et al., 1994) (Figure 12–13). The appearances are nonspecific, and differential diagnoses include other infectious diseases (tuberculosis, toxoplasmosis, pyogenic abscesses, and fun-

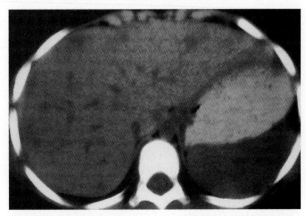

FIGURE 12–13. A 5-year-old girl with cat-scratch disease. Unenhanced CT shows multiple hypodense lesions throughout the liver and spleen.

gal infections), sarcoidosis, and malignant diseases (lymphoma, hepatoblastoma and metastatic neuroblastoma) (Port and Leonidas, 1991; Rappaport, Cumming, and Ros, 1991; Talenti et al., 1994). The lesions eventually resolve with healing but may calcify (Talenti et al., 1994).

Gallium scintigraphy may show uptake at sites of lymph node and bone involvement and may also show inhomogenous uptake in the liver without demonstrating focal hepatic lesions (Larsen and Patrick, 1992).

Chronic Granulomatous Disease of Childhood

Chronic granulomatous disease of childhood is a familial congenital defect of leukocytes in which the leukocytes are able to phagocytose catalase-positive bacteria (usually Staphylococcus aureus or Escherichia coli) but are unable to kill the bacteria effectively (Johnston and Newman, 1977; O' Shea, 1982; Forrest et al., 1988; Baehner, 1990). Several molecular defects have been identified, and each is characterized by the inability of the leukocytes to generate hydrogen peroxide and oxygen radicals in response to phagocytosis (Forrest et al., 1988). Clincally, the disease is characterized by chronic or recurrent dermatitis, lymphadenopathy, hepatosplenomegaly, and pulmonary infiltrates (O' Shea, 1982) (see Figure 12–9A). Pathologically, there are widespread suppurative and granulomatous lesions and infiltration of the viscera by pigmented histiocytes (O' Shea, 1982). Males are usually affected (80%) as the disease is X-linked, but girls may be affected through an autosomal recessive mode of transmission (Johnston and Newman, 1977; O' Shea, 1982; Baehner, 1990).

Most patients develop signs and symptoms of chronic or acute recurrent infection in the first 2 years of life although milder forms of the disease may have presentations in adolescence or adulthood (Johnston and Newman, 1977; Baehner, 1990).

Hepatic involvement is frequent (Preimesberger and Goldberg, 1974; Johnston and Newman, 1977; O' Shea, 1982; Forrest et al., 1988; Nakhleh, Glock, and Snover, 1992). Hepatic and perihepatic abscess occurs in approximately 40% of patients (Johnston and Newman, 1977), and hepatic abscess may be the first significant infection leading to the diagnosis of chronic granulomatous disease (Frayha and Biggar, 1983) (see Figures 12–9; 12–14). Ultrasonography is the investigative modality of choice (Stricof, Glazer, and Amendola, 1984). Granulomas

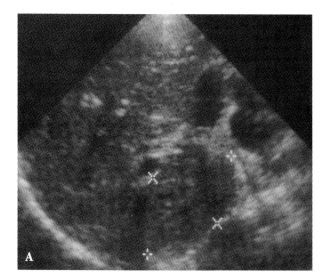 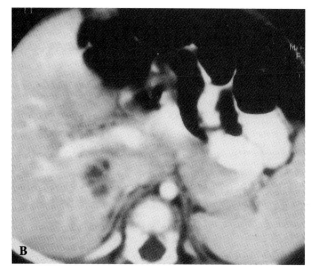

FIGURE 12–14. A 10-month-old boy with chronic granulomatous disease and pyogenic liver abscess. A, Ultrasonography shows an ill-defined hypoechoic mass in the right lobe of the liver. B, Contrast-enhanced CT shows a multiseptated low-attenuation lesion.

appear as single or multiple hypoechoic lesions, often poorly defined, that show no posterior acoustic enhancement (Garel, Pariente, and Nezelof, 1984). As the disease progresses, frank hepatic abscesses that are indistinguishable from other hepatic pyogenic abscesses can develop. Liver calcifications may be seen with US or CT following healing (Stricof, Glazer, and Amendola, 1984).

Current management includes long term antibiotic treatment with trimethoprim-sulfamethoxazole and the use of interferon gamma both prophylactically and to treat acute infective episodes (Baehner, 1990; Fischer et al., 1993). Hepatic abscesses can be treated with percutaneous drainage (Skibber et al., 1986). However, bone marrow transplantation is the only known cure at this time (Forrest et al., 1988).

Amebic Abscess

General Considerations

Amebiasis results from infection with the protozoan *Entamoeba histolytica*. It has a worldwide distribution and infects at least 10% of the world's population, an incidence rising to 30% in tropical and subtropical regions (Merten and Kirks, 1984; Aucott and Ravdin, 1993; Kimura et al., 1997; Mergo and Ros, 1997). The incidence is highest in developing countries, in areas where poor sanitary conditions and overcrowding predispose to transmission of amebic infection (Merten and Kirks, 1984; Kays,

1992; Li and Stanley, 1996; Kimura et al., 1997). In North America, the incidence is around 5%, and the organism may be endemic or may occur in scattered foci (Merten and Kirks, 1984). In developed countries, amebic infection is generally confined to high-risk groups including recent travelers to endemic areas, immigrants, inmates of mental instituitions, and sexually active male homosexuals (Aucott and Ravdin, 1993; Li and Stanley, 1996). Children, especially neonates, have an increased risk for severe disease and death (Merten and Kirks, 1984; Li and Stanley, 1996). Among parasitic diseases, only malaria and schistosomiasis result in more deaths than amebiasis (Li and Stanley, 1996).

Clinical Features. Most individuals infested with *E. histolytica* are asymptomatic (Puck, 1991; Kimura et al., 1997), and invasive amebiasis occurs in only 10% of these people (Sherlock and Dooley, 1997). Invasive amebiasis may be confined to the gastrointestinal tract; this form is more common in children (Kimura et al., 1997). Hepatic invasion is the most common extraintestinal form and usually arises as a single abscess, frequently in the right lobe (Puck, 1991; Juimo, Gervez, and Angwafo, 1992; Nisenbaum and Rowling, 1995; Li and Stanley, 1996; Kimura et al., 1997). However, the incidence of multiple abscesses involving both lobes appears to be higher in children (Merten and Kirks, 1984). Hepatic abscesses develop in one-third of amebic colitis patients and can present at any age but is 10 times more common in adults (Kimura et al., 1997).

In children, the diagnosis is often difficult to make. Presenting symptoms may be nonspecific and may mimic other febrile illnesses (Ralls et al., 1982b). Amebic liver abscesses are most common in children under 3 years of age (Haffar, Boland, and Edwards, 1982; Merten and Kirks, 1984; Nazir and Moazam, 1993), with a peak incidence in the first year of life (Merten and Kirks, 1984). Clinically, there is usually a spiking fever, a distended abdomen, and tender hepatomegaly (Merten and Kirks, 1984; Nazir and Moazam, 1993). Only 10 to 50% of patients have diarrhea (Merten and Kirks, 1984; Aucott and Ravdin, 1993; Nazir and Moazam, 1993; Li and Stanley, 1996; Sherlock and Dooley, 1997) although colitis is commonly evident pathologically in those who are examined post mortem (Merten and Kirks, 1984). Liver enzymes are usually mildly abnormal, but jaundice is very uncommon (Kays, 1992; Aucott and Ravdin, 1993; Nazir and Moazam, 1993; Sherlock and Dooley, 1997). Anemia may be present (Haffar, Boland, and Edwards, 1982; Merten and Kirks, 1984; Nazir and Moazam, 1993).

The mortality rate is less than 1% in children with intestinal amebiasis (Kimura et al., 1997), but mortality in infants and children with amebic liver abscesses is relatively high (Merten and Kirks, 1984). In infants, the course is usually fulminant and is associated with a near 50% mortality rate (Johnson et al., 1994). Most complications are related to rupture of the liver abscess into the chest (10 to 20%), the peritoneum (2 to 7%), or the pericardium (rare) (Li and Stanley, 1996). Extrahepatic complications appear to occur more frequently in children (Merten and Kirks, 1984; Porras-Ramirez, Hernandez-Herrera, and Porras-Hernandez, 1995).

Pathology. The life cycle of *E. histolytica* consists of the cyst (host-infective stage) and the trophozoite (host-tissue-invasive stage). The disease is commonly acquired by ingestion of food and water contaminated with the cyst form of the parasite. Within the intestinal tract, the cysts form trophozoites, which are the motile feeding form of the parasite and which are responsible for invasive colonic disease (Li and Stanley, 1996).

Entamoeba histolytica initially invades the intestinal wall, with resultant mucosal ulceration. Subsequent invasion into the bloodstream results in mesenteric transmission of the organism to the liver. The trophozoites produce a proteolytic enzyme in the small hepatic portal radicles leading to focal necrosis and the creation of a relatively anaerobic environment that favors growth of the amoebae and abscess formation (Merten and Kirks, 1984).

Diagnosis. Diagnosis of amebiasis can be made either by identifying the amebic trophozoites in stool, endoscopic biopsy specimens, or scrapings from the rectum, or by serologic tests that identify circulating amoeba-specific antibodies (Kimura et al., 1997). Cysts are present in the stool of only 15% of patients with hepatic amebiasis. Indirect hemagglutination assay tests are positive in 90 to 100% of patients with liver abscesses (Merten and Kirks, 1984; Li and Stanley, 1996). Currently, the enzyme-linked immunosorbent assay test is the most reliable and sensitive test, with a virtual absence of false-negative results and a low percentage (3.6%) of false-positive results (Kimura et al., 1997). Antibodies appear approximately 7 days after the onset of symptoms of invasive amebiasis, and tests may be negative early in the course of an acute infection (Li and Stanley, 1996; Kimura et al., 1997). Antibodies persist for years, and titers cannot differentiate acute infection from remote infection in highly endemic areas (Aucott and Ravdin, 1993). However, in children (especially in the very young), seropositivity may be absent or delayed, presumably because humoral antibody production is generally less efficient (Merten and Kirks, 1984); it may be negative in one-third of infants with amebic liver abscesses (Johnson et al., 1994). Hence, clinical suspicion, combined with imaging studies is important in making an early diagnosis in children.

Imaging of Amebic Abscess

Plain-Film Radiography. Plain-film findings are present in less than 50% of cases (Merten and Kirks, 1984). They are usually nonspecific and include elevation of the right hemidiaphragm, pleural effusion, and basilar atelectasis or hepatomegaly on abdominal films (Merten and Kirks, 1984; Kimura et al., 1997).

Ultrasonography. Ultrasonography is highly sensitive and is the ideal method for detection of abscesses (Ralls et al., 1982a; Ralls et al., 1987; Juimo, Gervez, and Angwafo, 1992; Kimura et al., 1997). In most instances, findings on US are not specific (Sukov, Cohen, and Sample, 1980; Ralls et al., 1982a; Merten and Kirks, 1984). Ultrasonographic features will vary, depending on the evolution of the lesion (Kimura et al., 1997). Initially, it may appear solid and hyperechoic relative to the normal hepatic parenchyma, but it eventually develops into a more echolucent area with posterior acoustic enhancement. Approximately 40% of lesions have a "suggestive sonographic pattern" (Ralls et al., 1982a; Ralls et al., 1982b). This pattern consists of (1) a lack of significant wall echoes; (2) a round or oval configuration; (3) echogenicity less than normal parenchyma with fine homogenous, low-level echoes at high gain; (4) a location contiguous with the liver capsule; and (5) distal acoustic enhancement. In contrast, pyogenic abscesses are more likely to have an irregular "honeycomb" content and ill-defined margins. However, these features are sometimes still inadequte in differentiating amebic from pyogenic abscesses; hence review, of clinical data is important (Oleszczuk-Raszke et al., 1989).

Occasionally, multiple sonolucent lesions mimicking metastatic disease are seen; this presumably represents early liver involvement-"amebic hepatitis" (Hayden et al., 1984). Multiple lesions in the same patient can have a variable appearance, and target lesions with a hypoechoic halo may be seen (Landay et al., 1980). Demonstration of perforation of the diaphragm with extension into the thorax in a nontraumatized patient is helpful in making a definitive diagnosis (Landay et al., 1980; Ralls et al., 1982; Hayden et al., 1984).

Other complications, such as obstructive jaundice or peritoneal rupture with subphrenic collection or ascites, are also well shown by US (Gupta et al., 1987). Rarer complications include cerebral, myocardial, and renal abscesses, retroperitoneal rupture, and perforation into the biliary tree (Griffin, Jennings, and Owens, 1983; Tandon et al., 1991; Juimo, Gervez, and Angwafo, 1992; Kimura et al., 1997).

Computed Tomography. Computed tomography has a sensitivity similar to that of US in the detection of abscesses (Rubinson, Isakoff, and Hill, 1980; Ralls et al., 1987b). It is especially useful in demonstrating complications and in defining the exact anatomic location and extent of lesions, especially large lesions (Merten and Kirks, 1984). Findings on CT of amebic abscesses are similar to those of pyogenic abscesses, but septations in amebic abscesses are often absent (Vassiliades, Bree, and Korobkin, 1992). Computed tomography demonstrates an avascular hypodense mass with well-defined margins and alternating hypervascular and hypovascular halos with contrast enhancement (Kimura et al., 1997) (see Figures 12–12A and B). Associated right pleural effusion and a small amount of adjacent perihepatic fluid may also be seen.

Magnetic Resonance Imaging. Magnetic resonance imaging findings of amebic abscesses are nonspecific, and lesions typically appear hypointense on T1-weighted images and hyperintense on T2-weighted images, with well-defined margins (Ralls et al., 1987b; Kimura et al., 1997; Mergo and Ros, 1997). Multiple rims of variable signal intensity are present, and surrounding edema is seen as a zone of hyperintensity on T2-weighted images. Abscesses may initially appear heterogenous on both T1- and T2-weighted images (due to necrotic debris, hemorrhage, and liquefied material in the cavity) but become more homogenously hypointense with medical therapy due to liquefaction of the abscess (Elizondo et al., 1987). With successful medical treatment, concentric rings become prominent on both T1- and T2-weighted images, reflecting maturation of the abscess wall. These correspond histologically to an inner margin of granulation tissue (isointense to liver on T1-weighted images), adjacent bands of type 1 collagen (low intensity on T1- and T2-weighted images), and an outer margin of atrophic and/or mildly inflamed liver tissue (hyperintense on T2-weighted images). Similar MR characteristics may be seen in pyogenic liver abscesses, hepatic hematomas, and necrotic tumors (Elizondo et al., 1987). Although MR is not any more specific than CT or US, it may be a useful tool for follow-up of abscesses and for documenting resolution with medical therapy (Mergo and Ros, 1997). Rarely, invasive amebiasis may result in granulomatous hepatitis in which multiple abscesses develop. Magnetic resonance imaging shows variable signal within the lesions, some of which may be of heterogenous low signal on T2W images with a double-layered wall (Giovagnoni et al., 1993).

Radionuclide Scintigraphy. The appearance on sulfurcolloid scan is usually nonspecific, with abscesses appearing as a photopenic defect. Rim enhancement around a photopenic defect on hepatobiliary scans is said to be more specific for hepatic amebic abscesses (Remedios, Colletti, and Ralls, 1986) but similar enhancement can also be seen around pyogenic abscesses (McDonald and Davani, 1997).

Treatment and Follow-up of Amebic Abscess

Antibiotic treatment alone is usually sufficient for hepatic amebiasis, but further intervention may be indicated for prevention and management of complications (van Sonnenberg et al., 1985; Ralls et al., 1987a; Aucott and Ravdin, 1993; Li and Stanley, 1996). Percutaneous aspiration or drainage is only performed if there is

- a clinical or diagnostic problem, such as imminent danger of rupture,
- a potentially fatal complication, such as large abscesses in the left lobe, with consequent risk of rupture into the pericardium,
- treatment failure, when pain and fever persists after 3 to 5 days of appropriate therapy,
- a suspicion of superimposed infection or concomitant pyogenic abscess.

(Sukov, Cohen, and Sample, 1980; Ralls et al., 1982; Ralls et al., 1987a; Saraswat et al., 1992; Porras-Ramirez, Hernandez-Herrera, and Porras-Hernandez, 1995; Li and Stanley, 1996; Kimura et al., 1997) (see Figure 12–12C). Other indications may include prenancy and noncompliance with medical therapy. (van Sonnenberg et al., 1985). The aspirated fluid is usually gray-yellow in appearance but may become pink or red-brown following subsequent aspirations. The classic "anchovy paste" appearance is unusual. Examination of the aspirate for organisms may not yield the diagnosis, but the organism is most reliably seen with a biopsy of the abscess wall (van Sonnenberg et al., 1985; Ralls et al., 1987a; Aucott and Ravdin, 1993). If an aspiration, biopsy, or drainage procedure is performed, the subcostal route is preferred to avoid lung contamination (van Sonnenberg et al., 1985). Percutaneous drainage can be of have some benefit by shortening the time of resolution of the abscess (Saraswat et al., 1992). Surgery is now indicated only for complicated abscesses or to prevent potential complications from large abscesses beneath the pericardial sac that are not accessible to percutaneous drainage (Porras-Ramirez, Hernandez-Herrera, and Porras-Hernandez, 1995; Kimura et al., 1997).

Follow-up is best performed by US (Ralls et al., 1982) (see Figure 12–12D). A variety of appearances are seen with healing. As healing progresses, the abscess may become increasingly hypoechoic, with a smooth margin; the lesion eventually disappears, leaving no residue damage (Ralls et al., 1982a; Simjee et al., 1985). Over the first few weeks, the lesions may enlarge, stay the same, or decrease in size despite adequate therapy (Ralls et al., 1983). Over months or occasionally years, the changes in the internal echogenicity are variable; most often, the lesions develop anechoic areas with focal areas of high-amplitude echoes, eventually filling in with a more normal echo pattern. Surprisingly, the length of time to resolution is not dependent on the initial size of the abscess (Ralls et al., 1983). Occasionally, residual cystic lesions, which resemble benign hepatic cysts, or slight parenchymal irregularity remain after healing is complete (Ralls et al., 1982a; Ralls et al., 1982b; Ralls et al., 1983).

Be aware that abscesses resolve slowly, with resolution occuring over 6 weeks to 18 months (Ralls et al., 1982a). Most resolve by 6 months, but 10% have an abnormal finding on US more than 1 year after therapy (Li and Stanley, 1996). The persistence of a cavity alone is not an indication for repeat aspiration or for administering another course of antibiotics (Ralls et al., 1982a; Ralls et al., 1983; Simjee et al., 1985; Ralls et al., 1987a; Aucott and Ravdin, 1993; Li and Stanley, 1996).

Hydatid Cyst

General Considerations

Hydatid disease is prevalent throughout the world and is caused by human infection with the larval forms of the tapeworms *Echinococcus granulosus* (most commonly) and *Echinococcus multilocularis* (occasionally) (Beggs, 1985; Bezzi et al., 1987; Finlay and Speert, 1992; Kammerer and Schantz, 1993; von Sinner, 1997). It occurs rarely in children in North America (Kays, 1992).

Echinococcus granulosus has the dog as its definitive host and the sheep or another ruminant as the intermediate host. Occasionally, humans may act as the intermediate host by becoming infected from contact with a definitive host or by consuming contaminated water or vegetables (Beggs, 1985; von Sinner, 1997). As a result, *E. granulosus* is endemic in sheep and cattle-raising countries (such as Australia,

New Zealand, and countries in the Mediterrranean and Baltic areas, South America, and the Middle East) and in some regions of North America (California, the Mississippi River valley, Utah, Arizona, and northern Canada) (Bret et al., 1988; Marn, Bree, and Silver, 1991; von Sinner, 1997). In addition to this pastoral form of hydatid disease, a separate biotype, the sylvatic or northern form, may be endemic in parts of Canada and Alaska, with at least one-third of cases being described in children or adolescents. The wolf is the definitive host, and in contrast to the pastoral form, the disease is usually mild and self-limited. Cysts occur in the lung and liver, but the classic radiographic signs associated with pastoral cysts are not commonly present (Finlay and Speert, 1992).

Echinococcus multilocularis has the fox as its main definitive host although dogs or cats can occasionally act as hosts. The intermediate hosts are mainly wild rodents (such as mice) that are contaminated through wild berries. Humans may occasionally become the intermediate hosts by direct contact with foxes (eg, hunters) or via contaminated plants or water (Didier et al., 1985; Ammann and Eckert, 1996). It is endemic only in the Northern Hemisphere (Ammann and Eckert, 1996).

The adult tapeworm of both species inhabits the small intestine of the definitive host, and eggs are released into the environment. Following ingestion of eggs by humans or other accidental hosts, the eggs hatch, and parasites penetrate the intestinal tract and pass via blood and lymphatics to various organs (Ammann and Eckert, 1996; von Sinner, 1997). Parasites that are filtered out by the liver can go on to produce single or multiple hydatid cysts. Because of this filtering process, 75% of human hydatid disease is found in the liver, 15% in the lungs, and 10% in the rest of the body (Beggs, 1985).

Secondary echinococcosis may develop (a) when larval tissue spreads from the primary site of infection following spontaneous or trauma-induced rupture (rupture into peritoneum, pleura, bronchial tree, or biliary ducts) or (b) with the release of viable parasitic material during invasive treatment procedures (Ammann and Eckert, 1996; von Sinner, 1997). As thee two parasites have many distinct features, they are considered separately below.

Echinococcus granulosus

Hydatid cysts due to *E. granulosus* grow very slowly, and although most are contracted in childhood, many remain undiagnosed until the third or fourth decade (Beggs, 1983; Beggs, 1985; Lewall and McCorkell, 1985; Hoff et al., 1987; Vassiliades, Bree, and Korobkin, 1992). Approximately 10 to 25% are diagnosed in childhood (Slim et al., 1971; Carcassonne et al., 1973; Bloomfield, 1980), and the peak incidence in children is between the ages of 5 and 10 years (Gharbi et al., 1981). The initial phase of the primary infection is always asymptomatic (Ammann and Eckert, 1996). Most cysts are clinically silent, but pain, discomfort, abdominal distension, or a palpable mass may be present. Infection may become symptomatic if it exerts pressure on adjacent tissue or if it induces complications (Kammerer and Schantz, 1993; Ammann and Eckert, 1996). A ruptured cyst can become an infected abscess or can rupture into biliary tree with biliary colic, jaundice, and eosinophilia. Acute immunologic reactions such as asthma or anaphylactic shock may occur when the cyst ruptures (Lewall and McCorkell, 1986; Ammann and Eckert, 1996). Complications occur in 7 to 40% of cysts (Marti-Bonmati and Menor Serrano, 1990; el-Tahir et al., 1992; Kays, 1992).

The majority of patients have single-organ involvement, with a solitary hepatic cyst most commonly in the right lobe of the liver (el-Tahir et al., 1992; Kammerer and Schantz, 1993; Ammann and Eckert, 1996). Cysts vary in size from 1 to 15 cm in diameter (Ammann and Eckert, 1996).

Pathologic Features of Echinoccus granulosis. The hydatid cyst has three layers: an outer pericyst of modified host cells only a few millimeters thick (produced by the host), a middle laminated acellular layer impervious to bacteria but not nutrients, and a thin, translucent inner germinal layer (Nisenbaum and Rowling, 1995; von Sinner, 1997). The two inner layers are formed by the parasite. The germinal layer is the living parasite; it is one cell thick and produces the laminated membrane, scolices, brood capsules, and daughter cysts. The cyst contains clear fluid, a transudate of serum. Sediment, "hydatid sand," may result from free-floating brood capsules and scolices.

In patients with hepatic hydatid disease, serologic tests using the indirect hemagglutination test or the enzyme-linked immunosorbent assay (ELISA) have false-positive or false-negative rates of 10 to 23%; thus, negative test results do not rule out disease (Beggs, 1985; Harris et al., 1986; Kammerer and Schantz, 1993; Ammann and Eckert, 1996). Diagnosis of hepatic hydatid disease thus relies on both serologic tests and documentation of lesions on imaging studies (Bret et al., 1988).

Imaging of Echinococcus granulosus. Plain films can be helpful, and various patterns of calcification of the cyst wall may be seen (von Sinner, 1997) (Figure 12–15D). Curvilinear or ringlike calcification is seen in about a quarter of cases (Beggs, 1983). Daughter cyst calcification may show as several calcific rings. Total cyst calcification with a thick, dense wall indicates that the cyst is dead or quiescent (von Sinner, 1997). Large or multiple cysts result in hepatomegaly with elevation of the hemidiaphragm. Gas or a fluid level results from infection or rupture into the bronchial tree or into the biliary tree if Oddi's sphincter is incompetent. A pleural effusion may also result from hydatid cyst rupture.

Both US and CT are sensitive in detecting hydatid cysts, which can have varied appearances depending on the evolution and maturity of the cyst (Gharbi et al., 1981; Hadidi, 1982; von Sinner, 1991; Jacobs and Birnbaum, 1995; Nisenbaum and Rowling, 1995). An uncomplicated cyst can be seen as an echolucent lesion on US or as a low-attenuation lesion on CT. This appearance can be present with other hepatic diseases, so a high index of suspicion is necessary to make the correct diagnosis. The presence of eosinophilia and the knowledge of the ethnic and geographic origins of the patient may all be helpful.

Five categories that reflect the evolutionary stages of the hydatid cyst have been described (Gharbi et al., 1981):

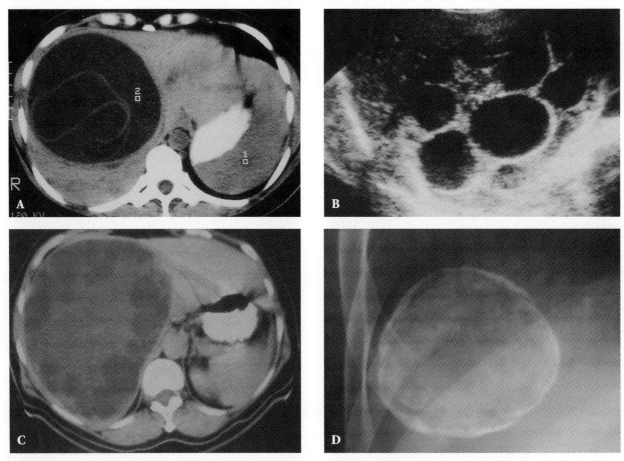

FIGURE 12–15. Hepatic hydatid disease. *A,* Unenhanced CT shows the "floating membrane" within a large hydatid cyst due to rupture of the middle membrane of the cyst. *B,* Daughter cyst formation results in a multiseptated or honeycombed appearance on ultrasonographic examination. *C,* Computed tomography shows multiple cysts within a large hepatic cyst due to daughter cyst formation. D, Radiograph shows rim calcification of a hepatic hydatid cyst. (Reproduced with the permission of Dr. Jay S. Keystone, MD, Toronto Hospital, University of Toronto.)

1. Pure fluid collection. This indicates intact membranes and is seen in the majority of cases, particularly in the first and second decades of life (Gharbi et al., 1981; Niron and Ozer, 1981; Hadidi, 1982; Hussain, 1985; Lewall and McCorkell, 1985; Gurses, Sungur, and Ozkan, 1987) (Figure 12–16). Differential diagnosis from benign hepatic cysts and abscesses may pose a problem (Harris et al., 1986; Ammann and Eckert, 1996). Echogenic debris representing hydatid sand may be seen (Lewall and McCorkell, 1985).

2. Fluid collection with a split wall. This appearance is due to internal collapse of the ruptured middle membrane of the cyst (Gharbi et al., 1981; Marti-Bonmati and Menor Serrano, 1990; von Sinner, 1991). It may be localized or become a floating membrane loose inside the cyst (Gharbi et al., 1981; Lewall and McCorkell, 1985) (see Figure 12–15A). If it collapses completely to the inferior portion of the cyst, it can give the so-called ultrasonographic water lily sign (Niron and Ozer, 1981; Lewall and McCorkell, 1986; Gurses, Sungur, and Ozkan, 1987); this has also been termed the "serpent or snake" sign (von Sinner, 1991).

3. Fluid collection with septa or multicystic appearance. Septation seen within the cyst indicates daughter cyst formation (Gharbi et al., 1981; Hussain, 1985; Lewall and McCorkell, 1985). This appears initially as wall thickening before the cyst develops (Beggs, 1985) and may give a honeycomb, polycystic, or matrix type of image (Gharbi et al., 1981; Lewall and McCorkell, 1985). Daughter cysts occur in degenerated or damaged cysts (either by trauma, toxins, or chemotherapy) (von Sinner, 1991; Mergo and Ros, 1997; von Sinner, 1997) and are characteristic of hydatid disease (von Sinner, 1991) (Figures 12–15B and C).

4. Cyst with heterogenous pattern. A heterogenous pattern can be due to many causes, including hydatid sand, infection, hemorrhage, or rupture (Niron and Ozer, 1981; Lewall and McCorkell, 1985; Gurses, Sungur, and Ozkan, 1987; Marti-Bonmati and Menor Serrano, 1990). This pseudotumoral form provides the greatest diagnostic difficulty (Gharbi et al., 1981).

5. Densely calcified lesion. These may not contain active organisms (Lewall and McCorkell, 1985), but the presence of calcification does not reliably exclude activity (Beggs, 1983). As long as only a segment of the cyst is calcified, the cyst may still contain live and infectious parasites (von Sinner, 1997).

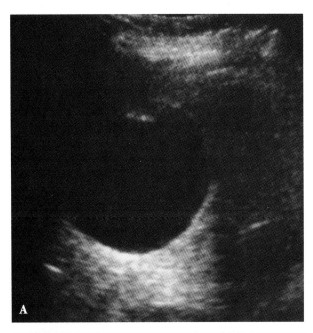

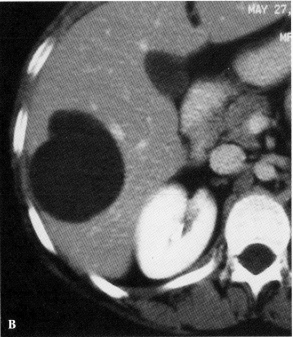

FIGURE 12–16. A 12-year-old boy with hepatic hydatid cyst. *A,* Ultrasonography shows a well-defined cystic lesion with no internal septations or debris. *B,* Contrast-enhanced CT shows a rounded lesion of uniform low attenuation.

Types 2, 3, and 5 are most characteristic of hydatid cysts (Gharbi et al., 1981; Hussain, 1985; Lewall and McCorkell, 1985; Pant and Gupta, 1987; Vassiliades, Bree, and Korobkin, 1992). However, the typical appearance of daughter cysts or features such as floating membranes or water-lily sign may be seen in only 65% of patients with hepatic hydatid cysts (Harris et al., 1986). Types 1 and 4 occur most frequently and are not specific for hydatid disease (Vassiliades, Bree, and Korobkin, 1992).

Both CT and US can show these abnormalities although CT allows better documentation of the site and size and better demonstrates calcification (de Diego Choliz et al., 1982; von Sinner et al., 1991; el-Tahir et al., 1992; Ammann and Eckert, 1996). On CT, the majority of hydatid cysts resemble simple cysts, but as they mature, daughter cysts, membrane detachment, and calcification can be detected (Scherer et al., 1978; Vassiliades, Bree, and Korobkin, 1992). Computed tomography may miss a hydatid cyst when the liver has fatty infiltration (de Diego Choliz et al., 1982). Fluid-fluid and air-fluid levels can be seen with cyst rupture and do not necessarily mean secondary infection of the cyst (Beggs, 1983; von Sinner, 1991; Vassiliades, Bree, and Korobkin, 1992). The presence of a fat-fluid level suggests a communicating rupture into the biliary tree (Mendez Montero et al., 1996). With intravenous contrast, the cyst wall and septations within the cysts may enhance (von Sinner, 1991; Jacobs and Birnbaum, 1995; Nisenbaum and Rowling, 1995).

Magnetic resonance imaging is capable of demonstrating all features of hydatid disease except small calcifications (von Sinner, 1997). Hydatid cysts appear as a hypointense lesion on T1-weighted images and as a hyperintense lesion on T2-weighted images (Vassiliades, Bree, and Korobkin, 1992; Kalovidouris et al., 1994). The layers of the cyst wall cannot be separated in intact hydatids. On T2-weighted imaging, it may appear as a low-intensity rim although this hypointense rim is not always present (Hoff et al., 1987; Lupetin and Dash, 1988; Marani et al., 1990; Marti-Bonmati and Menor Serrano, 1990; von Sinner et al., 1991; von Sinner, 1991; Taourel et al., 1993; Kalovidouris et al., 1994; von Sinner, 1997; Wojtasek and Teizidor, 1989). However, this hypointense rim is not always present. Rim enhancement may be seen with contrast (von Sinner, 1991). Calcification is seen as hypointense areas on T1-weighted images. Daughter cysts are usually isoin-

tense or slightly hypointense compared to the mother cyst on T1-weighted images (Marti-Bonmati and Menor Serrano, 1990; von Sinner et al., 1991; Taourel et al., 1993; Mergo and Ros, 1997; von Sinner, 1997).

Detached membrane is well demonstrated with MR (Taourel et al., 1993; Mergo and Ros, 1997; von Sinner, 1997). It appears as low signal on T1- and T2-weighted images - "snake or serpent" sign or "whirl" sign (von Sinner, 1991; Kalovidouris et al., 1994; von Sinner, 1997). The pericyst becomes visible as low signal on T2-weighted images and as isointense to adjacent liver tissue on T1-weighted images. With further cyst degeneration, the pericyst rupture and an area of discontinuity is seen in the cyst wall (Lupetin and Dash, 1988; von Sinner et al., 1991). Magnetic resonance imaging appears to be more sensitive than CT in detecting cyst wall irregularity, a sign of decreased parasite viability (Vassiliades, Bree, and Korobkin, 1992).

Extrinsic compression, bile stricture, or intrabiliary hydatid disease following rupture of a cyst can all cause bile duct obstruction. Both endoscopic retrograde cholangiopancreatography (ERCP) and percutaneous transhepatic cholangiography can demonstrate the exact site of obstruction or perforation, especially preoperatively (Farrelly and Lawrie, 1982; Moreira et al., 1985; Zargar et al., 1992; Ammann and Eckert, 1996; von Sinner, 1997). The presence of intraluminal material in the dilated biliary tree on US and CT is indicative of intrabiliary rupture (Marti-Bonmati, Menor, and Ballesta, 1988; Zargar et al., 1992). Biliary complications are also well demonstrated on MR (Taourel et al., 1993).

Radionuclide scintigraphy shows one or more photopenic areas but is nonspecific (Beggs, 1983; Morris et al., 1987; Treves, Jones, and Markisz, 1995). Gallium scans may show a rim of increased radionuclide uptake (Singh, Winick, and Tabarra, 1997).

Angiography is rarely helpful but if performed, may show a thin rim of enhancement in the pericyst or endocyst (Beggs, 1985), and avascular areas will be seen on the body opacification phase.

Treatment of Echinococcus granulosus. Surgical intervention is still the treatment of choice of hepatic hydatid cysts (Erdener, Ozok, and Demircan, 1992; Kammerer and Schantz, 1993; Ammann and Eckert, 1996; von Sinner, 1997). Ideally, surgery is performed to remove the intact cyst, but this is not without hazards due to the risk of intraperitoneal spill.

Medical therapy such as albendazole or mebendazole is supplementary and is given either before, during, or instead of surgery, depending on the clinical risks. However, chemotherapy may be an alternative in certain cases (inoperable cysts or high surgical risks), with reported cure rates of 30% when evaluated at 12 months (von Sinner, 1997).

Needle puncture and/or aspiration of hydatid cysts have previously been contraindicated due to the risk from potential anaphylaxis and spread of daughter cysts. However, recent reports indicate that percutaneous puncture can be performed safely in adults and children. The recently developed puncture, aspiration, injection and reaspiration (PAIR) procedure or catheter drainage offers another treatment alternative in selected cases (Mueller et al., 1985; Bret et al., 1988; Filice et al., 1990; Acunas et al., 1992; Giorgio et al., 1992; Akhan et al., 1996; Dilsiz et al., 1997; Khuroo et al., 1997). Diagnostic puncture should be used only after other diagnostic methods have failed (Kammerer and Schantz, 1993; Ammann and Eckert, 1996; von Sinner, 1997).

Ultrasonography may be used for follow-up during therapy to monitor a decrease in cyst size, detachment of cyst membrane, and disappearance of daughter cysts. It may also be used for determining the appearance of echogenic material within the cyst (Morris et al., 1984; Singcharoen et al., 1985; Bezzi et al., 1987; Caremani et al., 1996). Residual cavities after surgical treatment can also be followed with US (Marino et al., 1995). Computed tomography and MR are also effective in demonstrating response to chemotherapy or local treatment (Morris et al., 1987; von Sinner et al., 1991; von Sinner, 1997). Cysts with homogenously calcified walls usually do not need surgery or therapy, as spontaneous inactivation of larval tissue is likely to have occurred. These cysts can be followed with imaging studies (Marn, Bree, and Silver, 1991; Ammann and Eckert, 1996).

Echinococcus multilocularis

The liver is the primary site of infection in virtually 100% of cases of *Echinococcus multilocularis*. This infection is characterized by destructive tissue growth, invasion of adjacent organs, and distant metastases to other organs (heart, lungs, and brain), resembling a malignant tumor (Ammann and Eckert, 1996). Central necrosis with irregular thick and often partially calcified walls is characteristic. Lesions are poorly defined and are often prominent around the porta. Jaundice and portal hypertension can result.

Infection with *E. multilocularis* rarely affects young children but is lethal if untreated (Ammann and Eckert, 1996; Sasaki et al., 1997). Serologic tests together with US and CT are usually diagnostic.

Imaging of Echinococcus multilocularis. Several patterns are seen on US (Choji et al., 1992; Sasaki et al., 1997):

1. Granular echogenic areas with or without acoustic shadowing (areas of calcification)
2. Small hypoechoic areas with irregular margins (corresponding to small clustered parasitic vesicles)
3. Irregular echogenic region (stroma)
4. Large anechoic or hypoechoic regions (liquefied necrosis)

Lesions typically have irregular and ill-defined contours on US (Didier et al., 1985).

On CT, the appearances may be indistinguishable from those of malignant tumors (Scherer et al., 1978; Didier et al., 1985). The liver is usually enlarged, and the lesions are seen as heterogenous hypodense masses, often associated with necrotic areas, poorly defined walls, and irregular contours (Choji et al., 1992; Sasaki et al., 1997). Large lesions extend beyond the liver and invade adjacent structures (Ammann and Eckert, 1996). Clusters of microcalcification or plaquelike calcification are seen in the periphery or central parts of the lesions in nearly 70 to 90% of cases (Didier et al., 1985; Choji et al., 1992; Ammann and Eckert, 1996; Sasaki et al., 1997). Biliary duct dilatation is a common finding (Didier et al., 1985).

Angiography, if performed, may show a specific type of arterial tapering and obstruction and hence may be useful (Didier et al., 1985).

Treatment of Echinococcus multilocularis. As medical therapy has been disappointing, treatment of *Echinococcus multilocularis* infection is resection of the involved liver segments.

Ascariasis (Roundworm Infection)

Ascaris lumbricoides is heavily endemic in the Far East, Russia, Latin America, and Africa, infesting one-quarter of the world's population (Gabaldon et al., 1967). It is probably the second most common cause (after gallstones) of acute biliary symptoms. (Schulman et al., 1982). Infestation is more common under conditions of poor hygiene and in a warm, moist climate. It is therefore less common in temperate areas of Europe and North America. Children are particularly susceptible to infection (Aslam et al., 1993).

The adult roundworm lives mainly in the jejunum. Larvae penetrate the intestinal wall and migrate into the portal blood flow to reach the liver, heart, and lungs. Adult worms are also able to migrate through orifices and ducts and cause complications such as acute cholangitis, acute pancreatitis, liver abscesses, and granulomatous hepatitis (Aslam et al., 1993).

Ascariasis commonly affects the biliary tract in endemic areas (Cremin, 1982). Ascaris in the biliary tract may cause cholecystitis, or children may present with obstructive jaundice due to obstruction of the common bile duct (Cerri et al., 1983). Affected children are often restless and in severe pain (Cremin, 1982). Vomiting of worms during an episode of biliary colic can provide an important clue to the diagnosis (Aslam et al., 1993). The biliary tree becomes dilated secondary to worm infestation. Rupture of the biliary tree is a rare complication (Witcombe, 1978).

Ultrasonography may show the roundworms in the biliary tree as a bull's-eye on transverse section (Cremin, 1982); as long tubular echogenic non-shadowing structures in longitudinal section; or as coils or amorphous fragments (Schulman et al., 1982; Aslam et al., 1993). Sometimes, a thin central longitudinal echolucent line is seen, representing the digestive tract of the worm (Schulman et al., 1982; Aslam et al., 1993). Movement of the living worms on real-time US helps make the diagnosis (Cerri et al., 1983). Roundworms or their remnants are also seen well on cholangiography (Schulman et al., 1982; Aslam et al., 1993). *Ascaris lumbricoides* has also been identified as an important cause of intra-hepatic biliary calculi in endemic areas, particularly in young people (Schulman, 1987; Schulman, 1993).

Candidiasis

Candida is a common organism found on the skin and in the mouth of infants and is usually of little significance. Systemic candidiasis is a major concern in patients who are on immunosuppressive therapy or who are immunocompromised for other reasons (underlying malignancies, chronic granulamatous disease, HIV, uremia, or diabetes mellitus) (Miller, Greenfield, and Wald, 1982; Francis, Glazer, 1986; Maxwell and Mamtora, 1988; Foley and Jochem, 1991; Gorg et al., 1994). It is the most frequent cause of invasive fungal disease in neutropenic patients (Walsh, Hiemenz, and Anaissie, 1996). In addition, systemic candidiasis is being increasingly recognized in infants in neonatal intensive care units, especially those who are premature, who have long-standing vascular lines and are often receiving antibiotics. The presence of gross Candida in the mouth or Candida in the urine is suggestive, and confirmation is obtained by finding Candida on blood culture.

Disseminated candidiasis in neutropenic patients includes a spectrum of infections ranging from acute disseminated candidiasis (characterized by persistent fungemia, hypotension, multiorgan failure, and skeletal muscle and cutaneous lesions) to chronic disseminated candidiasis. Chronic disseminated candidiasis is an indolent process and commonly presents as hepatosplenic candidiasis (Walsh, Hiemenz, and Anaissie, 1996). These lesions are usually radiographically occult during neutropenia and become evident when recovery occurs (Gorg et al., 1994; Walsh, Hiemenz, and Anaissie, 1996). Occasionally, systemic candidiasis affects multiple intra-abdominal organs as well as extra-abdominal organs such as the brain, lungs, and heart.

Hepatic involvement is best evaluated by US as the examination is quick, easy, and noninvasive. It can be performed on infants, in the incubator in the neonatal intensive care unit. In the acutely sick older child, the examination can be performed at the bedside, a great advantage when the child is in reverse isolation.

Four ultrasonographic patterns of hepatic candidiasis can be recognized (Pastakia et al., 1988):

1. A "wheel-within-a-wheel" appearance is seen early in the course of the disease (Figure 12–17). This consists of a central hypoechoic nidus (a necrotic area with fungal elements) surrounded by an echogenic rim (inflammatory cells) and an outer hypoechoic zone (a ring of fibrosis).

2. The classic bull's-eye or "target" lesion (Callen, Filly, and Marcus, 1980; Miller, Greenfield, and Wald, 1982; Maxwell and Mamtora, 1988) (see Figure 12–17). These lesions are approximately 1 to 4 cm in size. The bright central focus consists of inflammatory cells.

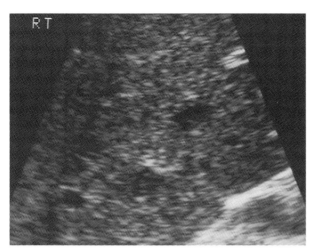

FIGURE 12–17. Hepatic candidiasis in a 13-year-old neutropenic patient with acute myelogenous leukemia. Ultrasonography shows the characteristic "wheel-within-a-wheel" appearance of an early lesion. The classic "bull's-eye" or "target" lesion is also seen.

3. A uniformly hypoechoic lesion that correlates pathologically to fibrosis and is the most common pattern (Figure 12–18).
4. Echogenic foci with variable degrees of acoustic shadowing. These lesions are small (2 to 5 mm), are seen late in the course of the disease, and represent small scars with or without calcification.

Types 1 and 2 appear only when the neutrophil count in the neutropenic patient returns to normal and suggest that the infection is active. Types 3 and 4 represent healing of the lesions.

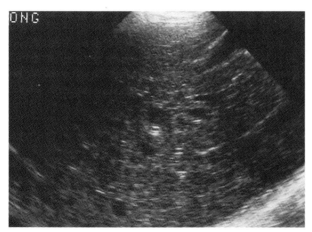

FIGURE 12–18. Fungal microabscesses in an 8-year-old boy with acute myelogenous leukemia. Ultrasonography shows multiple hypoechoic lesions in the liver.

Computed tomography shows non-enhancing focal low-density areas scattered throughout the liver and spleen (Miller, Greenfield, and Wald, 1982; Francis, Glazer, 1986; Shirkhoda, 1987; Fitzgerald and Coblentz, 1988; Maxwell and Mamtora, 1988; Pastakia et al., 1988) (Figure 12–19). Target lesions with small higher-attenuation nidi may occasionally be seen (Francis, Glazer, et al., 1986; Pastakia et al., 1988). Variable amounts of peripheral enhancement occur, depending on the size and activity of the lesions (Taylor, 1997) (Figure 12–20). Hepatic calcifications may be seen on follow-up CT (Shirkhoda, 1987).

For daily practice, it has been suggested that both US and CT (with and without contrast) should be performed to maximize detection of the disease since some lesions seen on US may not be visible on CT and vice versa (Pastakia et al., 1988). Comparison of pre- and postcontrast CT also demonstrates that some lesions are seen without enhancement while others are seen only following intravenous contrast. This aggressive approach at diagnosis is said to be justified by the high costs associated with late diagnosis and consequent delayed therapy (Pastakia et al., 1988).

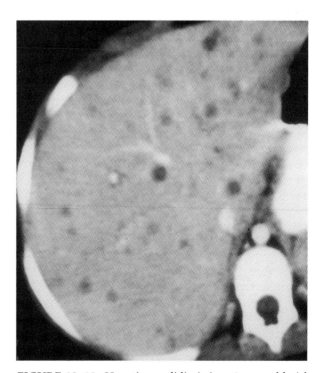

FIGURE 12–19. Hepatic candidiasis in a 9-year-old girl with dysgammaglobulinemia. Contrast-enhanced CT shows multiple non-enhancing low-attenuation lesions throughout the liver.

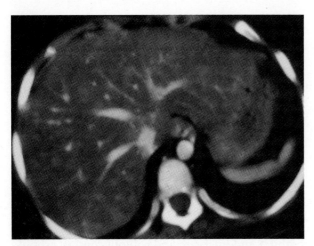

FIGURE 12–20. Hepatic fungal microabscesses in a 7-year-old neutropenic boy. Multiple ring enhancing lesions are seen throughout the liver. Diffuse low attenuation of the liver is due to fatty change.

Magnetic resonance imaging may prove to be more sensitive and may demonstrate hyperintense foci on T2-weighted images, which are hypointense relative to liver parenchyma on T1-weighted images. Diffuse enhancement may be seen early after the bolus administration of gadolinium, with peripheral rim enhancement on delayed images (Rofsky and Fleishaker, 1995) (Figure 12–21).

Although the appearances on CT and US are highly suggestive of the diagnosis, they are not specific. The differential diagnosis includes metastases, lymphoma, leukemia, and other opportunistic infections (Rofsky and Fleishaker, 1995). Tissue for histologic examination and culture may be required

for a definitive diagnosis, and US- or CT-guided biopsy can be performed (Francis, Glazer, 1986). In addition, imaging studies may demonstrate no abnormality despite a strong clinical suspicion of hepatic candidiasis. In this situation, liver biopsy is warranted to establish or exclude the diagnosis (Shirkhoda, 1987; Pastakia et al., 1988).

Hepatitis

Hepatitis commonly affects children but is not usually a radiologic diagnosis. Viral hepatitis (hepatitis A, B, C, D, or E, cytomegalovirus, Ebstein-Barr virus, herpesvirus, or HIV) is the most common cause of acute hepatic inflammation in children, but acute liver cell injury may be caused by various insults such as drugs or toxins, shock, hypoxemia, or metabolic disease (Taylor, 1997). The clinical presentation of viral hepatitis varies, with some children remaining completely asymptomatic and others presenting with nonspecific symptoms such as nausea, vomiting, or diarrhea. Viral hepatitis is often misdiagnosed as gastroenteritis (Fishman, Jonas, and Levine, 1996). Typically, patients are jaundiced at presentation.

Ultrasonography is not usually necessary for the clinical evaluation of acute hepatitis except to differentiate between obstructive and nonobstructive causes of jaundice (Blane, Jongeward, and Silver, 1983; Rofsky and Fleishaker, 1995; Zwiebel, 1995). Hepatomegaly is the most common manifestatation of acute hepatitis although imaging of the liver is often normal (Zwiebel, 1995; Taylor, 1997). In severe disease, US may demonstrate overall decreased echogenicity of the liver and increased echogencity

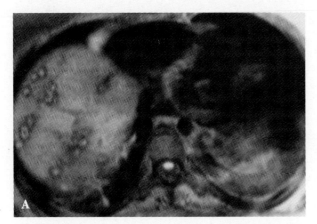
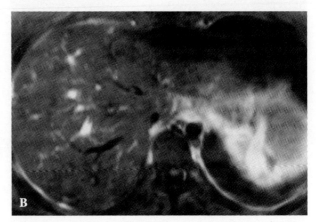

FIGURE 12–21. A 15-year-old girl with acute myelogenous leukemia and hepatic candidiasis. *A,* T1-weighted MR with fat saturation shows multiple "target" lesions throughout the liver. *B,* Contrast-enhanced T1-weighted MR with fat saturation also shows small enhancing lesions.

of the portal vein radicle walls (Kurtz et al., 1980; Needleman et al., 1986). This has been attributed to diffuse swelling of the hepatocytes and resultant increased contrast between the periportal collagenous tissue and the hypoechoic parenchyma (Kurtz et al., 1980). This appearance, which has been described as the "starry-sky" liver, is not specific and may also be seen in other conditions, including toxic shock syndrome, leukemia, and Burkitt's lymphoma (Rak, Hopper, and Parker, 1988).

Ultrasonography may also demonstrate thickening of the gallbladder wall (Zwiebel, 1995) and lymphadenopathy (particularly in the hepatoduodenal ligament) (Forsberg et al., 1987; Toppet et al., 1990; Okada et al., 1996) and ascites (Zwiebel, 1995). Parenchymal heterogeneity, which can mimic focal disease on rare occasions, may also be seen (Blane, Jongeward, and Silver, 1983; Rigauts et al., 1988).

Chronic hepatitis may be a sequela of acute hepatitis with eventual progression to cirrhosis. In chronic hepatitis, the liver appears bright on US, with increased liver echogenicity and decreased brightness and number of portal vein radicle walls (Kurtz et al., 1980; Blane, Jongeward, and Silver, 1983; Needleman et al., 1986; Rigauts et al., 1988).

Appearances of hepatitis on CT and MR are nonspecific. Findings include periportal edema (low-density tracks that parallel the portal vessels on CT and similar signal hyperintensity on T2-weighted MR images), lymphadenopathy, heterogenous parenchymal contrast enhancement on CT, and geographic zones of increased parenchymal signal intensity on T2-weighted MR images (Rofsky and Fleishaker, 1995).

Hepatobiliary scintigraphy is not routinely performed, but findings reflect underlying hepatocellular dysfunction. There is delayed radionuclide uptake by the hepatocytes, with slow clearance of blood pool radionuclide and delayed passage of radionuclide into the bowel (O' Hara, 1996). Technetium-99m-sulfurcolloid and Tc-99m-iminodiacetic acid (IDA) scans may also show hepatomegaly with heterogenous distribution of radionuclide (O' Hara, 1996).

Rare Forms of Hepatic Infection

Bacterial Infections

Tuberculosis may affect the liver, leaving sharply defined, frequently punctate calcifications in the healing phase as granulomas calcify (Rofsky and Fleishaker, 1995) (see Figure 12–18). Multiple echogenic lesions 3 to 5 mm in size, each surrounded by a hypoechoic halo, are seen on US (Mills et al., 1990). Miliary involvement of the liver in tuberculosis is not uncommon although macronodular involvement is much less common (Mills et al., 1990; Moskovic, 1990). Miliary involvement on CT appears as multiple rounded low-attenuation lesions 1 to 2 cm in size (Moskovic, 1990). Isolated tuberculous abscess of the liver is rare, and delay in diagnosis is common (Moskovic, 1990; Wilde and Kueh, 1991). The appearance resembles other pyogenic abscesses although a multiseptated (honeycomblike) appearance on US and CT has been described (Wilde and Kueh, 1991).

Actinomyces is a gram-positive anaerobic bacterium usually found in the normal colon, tonsillar crypts and teeth caries. Healthy tissue is not at risk, but damaged tissue may be at risk. The bacterium usually affects adults. Multiple hepatic abscesses can result rarely, giving an appearance on US or CT similar to that of any other pyogenic abscess (Sheth, Fishman, and Sanders, 1987).

Other Infections

Schistosamiases are granulomatous diseases that result from infection with the parasitic blood flukes called shistosomes. There are several species, but *Schistosoma japonicum* and *Schistosoma mansoni* are two species that cause significant hepatic disease (Mergo and Ros, 1997). The organisms gain entry into the bloodstream via the skin. The adult shistosome worms reside in the mesenteric veins and cause little direct damage; it is the shistosome eggs that produce the symptoms and pathology of schistosomiasis (Elliott, 1996). Eggs are released into the portal blood flow and are carried to the liver, where the eggs lodge in the portal venules and incite an intense granulomatous reaction. Hepatosplenic schistosomiasis results from development of periportal fibrosis ("pipe-stem" fibrosis) leading to presinusoidal portal hypertension.

Hepatic schistosomiasis japonica produces characteristic sonographic and pathognomonic CT changes (Cheung et al., 1996). A characteristic fish-scale network pattern with an irregular liver surface is most commonly seen on US. Echogenic branching septae separating lobules of relatively normal-appearing liver parenchyma, producing a mosaic pattern, may also be seen on US (Figures 12–22A and B). The echogenic septae represent fibrosis and dystrophic calcification where the eggs are deposited. The pathognomonic CT finding is "turtle-back" calcification (see Figure 12–22C). Septal and capsular enhancement occurring in regions of fibrosis is also characteristic (Monzawa et al., 1993) (see Figure 12–22D). Characteristic calcification may not be evident on MR, and as a result, findings may be less specific (Mergo and Ros, 1997).

The findings of hepatic schistosomiasis caused by *S. mansoni* differ, and septal calcifications are not seen (Cheung et al., 1996; Mergo and Ros, 1997). Ultrasonography demonstrates increased periportal echogenicity corresponding to areas of fibrosis (Cerri, Alwes, and Magalhaes, 1984; Fataar et al.,

1984). On CT, periportal fibrosis is seen as enhancing low-density rings (Cheung et al., 1996). On MR, the periportal zones appear isointense to normal liver on T1-weighted images and hyperintense on T2-weighted images and showed enhancement with gadolinium (Willemsen et al., 1995).

Fasciola hepatica (sheep-liver fluke) is a trematode that occasionally uses man as the definitive host. It is ingested on uncooked plants, particularly on watercress. The immature worms penetrate the intestine, migrate through the peritoneum, and penetrate the liver and hence the biliary tree. This results in granulomas in the liver that can be seen as areas of decreased attenuation on CT and that may be cystic, progressing to healed calcific areas. Branching hypodense areas caused by acute para-

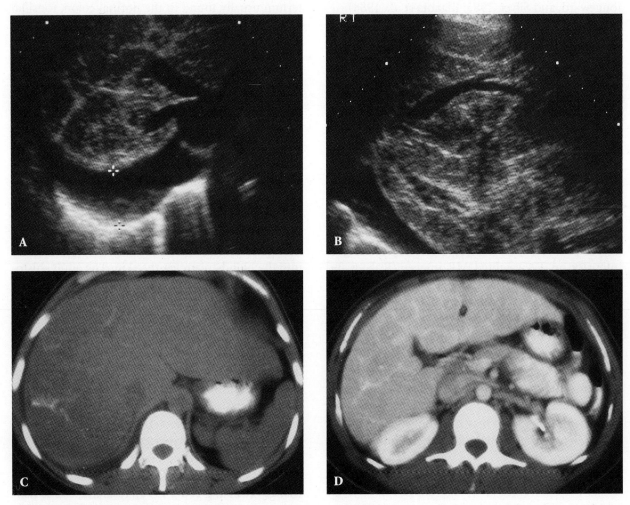

FIGURE 12–22. Hepatic schistosomiasis japonicam. *A*, Ultrasonography shows a characteristic fish-scale network pattern. An associated right pleural effusion is also seen. *B*, Ultrasonography again shows the echogenic branching septa. *C*, Unenhanced CT shows the pathognomonic "turtle-back" calcification. *D*, Enhanced CT shows an irregular liver surface with septal enhancement.

sitic migration through the liver may be seen (Liu and Harinasuta, 1996).

Toxocara in humans usually results from larval transmission through a family pet. Children are more often affected than adults and present with fever, cough, skin rashes, upper abdominal tenderness, and hepatomegaly. The CT finding of multiple areas of decreased attenuation, unchanged by contrast enhancement and simulating metastatic disease, has been described (Dupas, Barrier, and Barre, 1986). The granulomas in the liver may be seen on US as mutiple hypoechoic areas indistinguishable from multiple abscesses, malignancies, or other granulomatous diseases involving the liver (Clarke, Hinde, and Manns, 1992).

Granulomatous hepatitis may be seen in children with acquired immunodeficiency syndrome (AIDS) and can produce a diffuse hyperechoic parenchymal pattern on US (Grumbach et al., 1989). Granulomatous hepatitis in patients with AIDS may be due to mycobacterial infection, cryptococcosis, histoplasmosis, toxoplasmosis, cytomegalovirus, or drug toxicity. Multiple foci of calcification in the liver and other viscera (kidneys, spleen, lymph nodes, and adrenals) can also occur, with extrapulmonary Pneumocystis carinii infection in patients with AIDS (Lubat et al., 1990; Radin et al., 1990).

The liver is characteristically involved in congenital syphilis. Hepatosplenomegaly is the most common clinical manifestation. Rarely, fulminant hepatic failure develops, with subsequent extensive hepatic calcification. Congenital toxoplasmosis, cytomegalovirus (CMV) infection, and congenital herpes infection can also give rise to hepatic calcifications (Herman, 1995).

Abscesses around the Liver

Subphrenic, lesser sac, subhepatic, falciform ligament (Laucks, Ballantine, and Boal, 1986) and pericholecystic abscesses can all arise in children, usually as a result of adjacent infection. The radiologic appearance is similar to that in adults. Computed tomography or US are most helpful in delineating the site of the collection and facilitating percutaneous diagnostic and therapeutic aspiration or drainage (Halvorsen et al., 1982; Mueller et al., 1986). Ultrasonography most often demonstrates a fluid-filled, thick-walled mass with variable internal echoes due to the presence of debris and (possibly) gas. Abscesses on CT may appear of low density. The collection may contain air, and the wall of the abscess usually enhances with contrast (Afshani, 1981) (Figure 12–23).

NEOPLASMS OF THE LIVER

Mass Lesions

Hepatic masses account for 5 to 6% of all intra-abdominal masses in children, and primary hepatic neoplasms account for 0.5 to 2% of all pediatric malignancies. Hepatoblastoma is the third most common abdominal malignancy in childhood (after Wilms' tumor and neuroblastoma) and the most common primary malignancy of the gastrointestinal tract in children (Davey and Cohen, 1996; Donnelly and Bisset, 1998). In children less than 5 years of age, the most common tumors of the liver are hepatoblastoma, infantile hemangioendothelioma, mesenchymal hamartoma, and metastatic disease from neuroblastoma or Wilms' tumor. In children more than 5 years of age, the most common tumors are hepatocellular carcinoma, undifferentiated embryonal sarcoma (UES), hepatocellular adenoma, and metastatic disease (Davey and Cohen, 1996; Donnelly and Bisset, 1998).

Diagnostic imaging attempts to characterize lesions and distinguish benign from malignant lesions, using criteria discussed in this section. Additionally, the anatomy must be defined prior to image-guided or surgical intervention for these lesions. In the evaluation of focal hepatic masses, it is important to consider the Couinaud nomenclature (see also Normal Anatomy in this chapter), which describes hepatic segmentation based on portal venous supply and hepatic venous drainage. It is the basis for modern segmental liver surgery and subdivides the old nomenclature (lateral left, medial left, anterior right, posterior right, and caudate) by the division of the lateral segment of the left lobe into anterior and posterior subsegments by the left hepatic vein and by the division of both anterior and posterior segments of the right lobe into superior and inferior subsegments by the right portal vein (Gazelle and Haaga, 1992). This is of particular importance in the case of metastatic disease, in which metastasis resection with an adequate margin combined with maximal preservation of the liver parenchyma is the goal.

Plain films are generally not helpful as the findings are often nonspecific. Nevertheless, plain films are a common starting point and may be useful in showing calcification, bowel obstruction, and lung or osseous metastases.

Ultrasonography is generally the initial cross-sectional imaging modality of choice. Focal primary lesions are usually detectable with US, and US is particularly useful in detecting fluid spaces within lesions. In one study in adults, the sensitivity of US for liver metastases was 54%, depending on the type of primary. Sensitivity for malignant lymphoma in this group was 85% but had a large number of false-positives and therefore a low specificity (Schölmerich, Volk, and Gerok, 1987).

Doppler techniques have been evaluated with some enthusiasm as a means of increasing lesion detectability and improving specificity. Some studies have found that by using conventional pulsed (frequency-shift) Doppler, peak systolic velocity may be useful in differentiating malignant hepatic tumors from benign lesions, particularly hemangiomas (Numata et al., 1993). The authors of one large study concluded that frequency shifts of greater than 1.75 kHz gave a 68% sensitivity and a

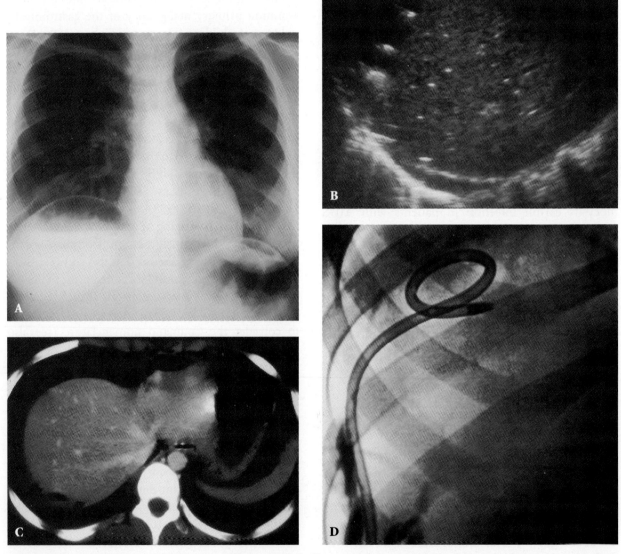

FIGURE 12–23. A 15-year-old girl on steroids for Crohn's disease with a right-sided subphrenic abscess. *A,* Erect chest radiograph shows an air-fluid level in the right upper abdomen. *B,* Ultrasonography (longitudinal image) shows the subphrenic collection containing bubbles of air (highly echogenic foci). *C,* Contrast-enhanced CT shows gas-containing collection in right subphrenic space. *D,* Percutaneous drainage of the abscess was performed with a 10 French catheter under US and fluoroscopic guidance.

94% specificity in distinguishing malignant from benign lesions in adults (Reinhold et al., 1995). The assignment of color to both frequency-shift and amplitude (power)-based Doppler has also received considerable attention (Nino-Murcia et al., 1992). Galactose-based microbubbles have been used as contrast agents to increase the sensitivity of color Doppler and correlated well in one study with angiographic findings for the evaluation of tumor vascularity (Fujimoto et al., 1994). Nevertheless, the findings of color or power Doppler remain nonspecific in distinguishing benign from malignant disease at this time.

Intraoperative US allows the use of high-frequency transducers and is a particularly sensitive means of detecting focal hepatic lesions (Baron, 1994).

In spite of advances in US, the appearance of hepatic tumors on US is still often nonspecific and generally does not allow differentiation of benign from malignant tumors (Brunelle and Chaumont, 1984). Computed tomography is usually done following US, to better delineate the hepatic mass and for staging malignant disease. The introduction of helical (spiral) CT has decreased acquisition time to a point where the entire liver may be scanned in 20 seconds or less, allowing scanning to be performed in the arterial phase during the first 20 to 30 seconds of injection and during the portal venous phase between 30 to 50 seconds. This is particularly important in hypervascular liver tumors, which have a rich arterial supply that may be seen only during hepatic arterial phase imaging (Baron, 1994). In addition to more rapid image acquisition, helical CT allows the reconstruction of images, which has been found to increase the conspicuity of focal liver lesions (Urban et al., 1993). The additional use of mechanical power injectors for rapid administration of contrast material has also contributed to the increased detection of hepatic lesions (Baron, 1994).

Certain techniques used in adults to increase in the sensitivity and specificity of CT are (1) computed tomographic arteriography, with contrast infusion directly into the hepatic artery; (2) computed tomographic arterial portography (CTAP), with injection into the superior mesenteric artery or splenic artery to opacify the portal venous system preferentially; and (3) iodized oil CT scan, whereby a small amount of iodized oil (lipiodol) is injected into the hepatic artery, followed by selective and prolonged retention of this oil within highly vascular and abnormal hepatocellular tissue, as shown by delayed CT scanning (Kemmerer, Mortele, and Ross, 1998). These highly specialized techniques are rarely if ever done in children.

Magnetic resonance imaging has advanced tremendously (Heiken, Lee, and Glazer, 1985). Prolonged scan times and resulting motion artifacts as well as limitations in spatial resolution are still significant drawbacks. Nevertheless, MR technology has improved to the point that the entire liver may be imaged with a single breathhold of as little as 12 seconds, using echo planar techniques (Goldberg et al., 1993), or 20 seconds, using gradient-echo imaging (de Lange et al., 1996; Siegelman and Outwater, 1998). Recent studies suggest that MR in its current state of development exceeds CT in the detection of focal liver lesions (Larson et al., 1994; Paulson et al., 1994). The use of intravenous gadolinium, which shortens the T1 time in the inflammatory and/or neoplastic lesions into which it diffuses, and superparamagnetic iron oxide (SPIO), which is taken up by the reticuloendothelial system of liver and spleen and which shortens the T2 time of normal liver parenchyma, have been shown to increase the detection of hepatic lesions (Larson et al., 1994; Grandin et al., 1995). Calculation of T2 times was found in one study to be 100% accurate in differentiating solid from nonsolid lesions, and 93% accurate in characterizing these lesions as benign or malignant, using a cutoff T2 time of 116 msec (Goldberg et al., 1993).

Although MR is still significantly more expensive than US and CT, it has become much more readily available over the years and can be expected to demonstrate further improved performance in lesion detection and characterization.

Although MRA is making great improvements in demonstrating the hepatic vasculature, and although US and CT are often sufficient, angiography remains the most accurate means of demonstrating the hepatic vasculature at this time (Tonkin, Wrenn, and Hollabaugh, 1988).

Radionuclide scintigraphy is still useful in the evaluation of hepatic hemangiomas with technetium-99m red-blood-cell scanning. Sulfur colloid liver/spleen scans have had a reduced role in the workup of focal hepatic lesions although they may still help in distinguishing regenerating nodules from hepatocellular carcinoma and in characterizing primary liver tumors and tumorlike conditions, particularly focal nodular hyperplasia. The use of indium-111 (In-111) octreotide, an analogue of somatostatin that binds to somatostatin receptors, has a niche role in the detection of gastrinoma and metastatic lesions of gastrinoma (Drane, 1998).

Percutaneous biopsy of hepatic masses has become a fairly commonplace technique under ultrasonographic, CT, and now, MR guidance (see Chapter , Intervention).

Benign Tumors of the Liver

Benign tumors of the liver are rare in children. They may be classified into five groups: (1) Tumorlike epithelial lesions (focal nodular hyperplasia), (2) epithelial tumors (adenoma), (3) cysts and tumorlike mesenchymal lesions (cystic mesenchymal hamartoma), (4) mesenchymal tumors (hemangiomas, hemangioendotheliomas, lipomas), and (5) benign teratomas (Edmondson, 1956). These tumors are discussed separately.

Tumorlike Epithelial Lesions (Focal Nodular Hyperplasia)

Focal nodular hyperplasia (FNH) can occur at any age, however, most are seen in women in the third to fifth decades of life (80 to 95% of cases). It is the second most common benign liver tumor, surpassed in prevalence only by hemangioma. (Mergo and Ros, 1998a). The majority of cases are diagnosed incidentally, however. Symptoms of FNH include mild epigastric pain or discomfort, and a palpable abdominal mass (Cherqui et al., 1995). The etiology is thought to be a localized hepatocyte response to an underlying congenital vascular malformation. Oral contraceptive use is associated with FNH; however, its association is different from that of hepatocellular adenoma. Unlike their behavior with hepatocellular adenoma, oral contraceptives act only to promote the growth of FNH, not to induce its formation.

Approximately 90% of FNH occurs as solitary lesions less than 5 cm in diameter. The tumor rarely grows larger than this and does not usually have internal hemorrhage or necrosis. Most FNH lesions are well defined and lack the presence of a true capsule. A distinguishing and prevalent feature is the presence of a central fibrous scar. This scar is vascular, with vessels extending outward via fibrous septae to the periphery of the tumor. The lesion contains hepatocytes and Kupffer's cells, and

although bile ducts are present, they do not communicate with the normal biliary radicles (Mergo and Ros, 1998a).

Although normal or increased uptake of technetium-99m sulfur colloid with nuclear medicine is seen in 50% of FNH and has been considered diagnostic (Welch et al., 1985), other hepatocellular neoplasms such as adenoma and hepatocellular carcinoma can also contain Kupffer's cells and demonstrate uptake. Thus, the uptake of sulfur colloid is not considered pathognomonic for FNH (Cherqui et al., 1995; Mergo and Ros, 1998a).

Ultrasonography shows a well-demarcated mass that is either hyper- or isoechoic with liver. The central scar is seen with US in approximately 20% of cases (Shamsi et al., 1993). The demonstration of arterial flow in the central scar is highly suggestive of the diagnosis (Learch, Ralls, and Johnson, 1993; Stephenson and Gibson, 1995).

With CT scanning, unenhanced imaging shows the lesion to be focally hypo- or isodense, with the central scar seen in approximately 20% of cases (Shamsi et al., 1993). When the central scar is seen on unenhanced CT, it is relatively hypodense compared to the rest of the lesion. Calcification is seen in approximately 1% of FNH, thus, its presence should suggest another diagnosis (Mergo and Ros, 1998a).

After intravenous contrast enhancement on CT, the lesion tends to be hyperdense compared to the rest of the liver in the arterial phase because of its rich hepatic arterial supply. In the portal venous phase, the lesion becomes isodense to liver. However, with diffusion of contrast material into the central scar, the scar becomes hyperdense compared to the remainder of the lesion and to normal liver. In one study, 72% of contrast-enhanced CT demonstrated the central scar (Mathieu et al., 1991).

On MR, FNH is iso- or hypointense to normal liver on T1-weighted images, with the central scar being hypointense. On T2-weighted images, the lesion demonstrates mild hyperintensity, with the central scar comparatively more hyperintense (Figure 12–24). With gadolinium enhancement, FNH is hyperintense compared to the normal liver in the early phases. With delay, the FNH becomes more isointense, and the central scar becomes more hyperintense compared to the lesion and the remainder of the liver. This enhancement pattern of the central scar may be seen in 80 to 100% of cases, using gadolinium and gradient echo techniques

(Mathieu et al., 1991; Cherqui et al., 1995). Although the MR features are considered specific for FNH, caution must be used since the enhancement pattern of the scar may be mimicked by hepatocellular adenoma, hepatocellular carcinoma, fibrolamallar carcinoma, and giant hemangioma. Other attempts to increase specificity, using reticuloendothelial agents such as superparamagnetic iron oxide, also must be regarded with caution since hepatocellular adenoma and carcinoma contain Kupffer's cells and can thus exhibit uptake of reticuloendothelial agents (Grandin et al., 1995).

Because needle biopsies of FNH can overlap with those of well-differentiated hepatocellular adenoma or carcinoma, open biopsy or surgical resection is often required (Mergo and Ros, 1998a).

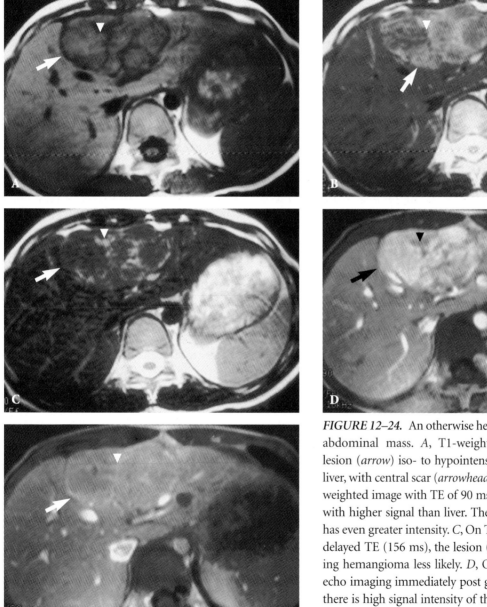

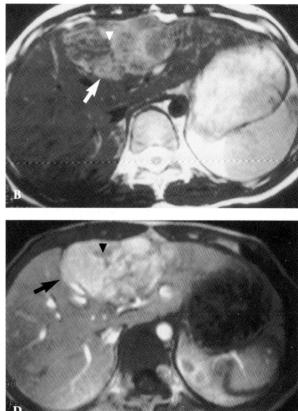

FIGURE 12–24. An otherwise healthy 11-year-old girl with abdominal mass. *A*, T1-weighted image demonstrates lesion (*arrow*) iso- to hypointense to surrounding normal liver, with central scar (*arrowhead*) hypointense. *B*, Fast T2-weighted image with TE of 90 ms shows the lesion (*arrow*) with higher signal than liver. The central scar (*arrowhead*) has even greater intensity. *C*, On T2-weighted imaging with delayed TE (156 ms), the lesion (*arrow*) loses signal, making hemangioma less likely. *D*, On T1-weighted gradient-echo imaging immediately post gadolinium enhancement, there is high signal intensity of the lesion (*arrow*), with the central scar (*arrowhead*) relatively decreased in intensity. *E*, On the 45-second delayed image, the lesion (*arrow*) has lost some of its high signal, with increasing signal in the central scar (*arrowhead*). These findings are typical of focal nodular hyperplasia, which was found at surgery.

Epithelial Tumors (Adenomas)

Hepatocellular adenoma (HCA) is a rare primary tumor of hepatocellular origin. Its incidence has increased dramatically since the introduction of oral contraceptives in 1960. Oral contraceptives and androgen steroid use have been identified as causative agents in HCA. This tumor can also occur spontaneously or be associated with type I glycogen storage disease and diabetes mellitus.

Hepatocellular adenoma presents as a solitary lesion in 80% of cases and is typically well circumscribed and encapsulated. Large subcapsular vessels are present. There are no bile ductules, portal venous tracts, or terminal hepatic veins distinguishing HCA from normal liver and FNH. The hepatocytes contain large amounts of fat. The tumor receives its vascular supply from hepatic artery branches, and as it grows to a larger size, it tends to outstrip its blood supply, resulting in hemorrhage and necrosis with occasional rupture. Contrary to FNH, which is usually an incidental finding, hepatocellular adenoma classically presents acutely with abdominal pain. Other presentations include hepatomegaly, enlarging abdominal mass, anemia, and abnormal liver function tests (Welsh et al., 1985).

The appearance on US is nonspecific. However, the high lipid content may cause a hyperechoic appearance, and internal hemorrhage or peliosis may cause an inhomogeneous appearance. When hypere-

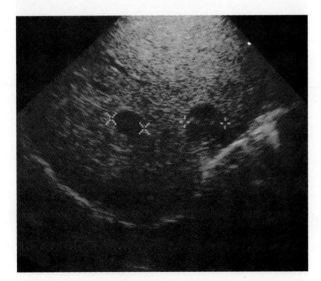

FIGURE 12–25. Axial ultrasonography of a 17-year-old male with glycogen storage disease and enlarged echogenic liver, with two hypoechoic adenomas measuring 3 cm and 2.5 cm, respectively. Both are uniformly hypoechoic.

choic, the lesions may have an echo-poor rim whereas the hypo- and isoechoic tumors have no well-defined walls (Brunelle et al., 1984) (Figure 12–25).

Color Doppler may show large subcapsular vessels. Color Doppler and pulsed wave Doppler evaluation of hepatocellular adenoma demonstrate a pattern of central venous flow and peripheral venous and arterial flow, in distinction to FNH, in which central arterial flow at the site of the central scar is more typical (Golli et al., 1994).

With nuclear medicine imaging, 20% of hepatocellular adenomas take up sulfur colloid agent due to the presence of Kupffer's cells. Hepatobiliary agents may be taken up but are not excreted due to the lack of bile ductules (Mergo and Ros, 1998a).

On non-contrast-enhanced CT, the lesions tend to be hypodense. Approximately one-half have evidence of calcification on unenhanced CT (Welch et al., 1985). With intravenous contrast, variable enhancement may be seen. In the arterial phase, the large subcapsular feeding vessels may be identified; however, this rapidly disappears in the portal venous phase (Welch et al., 1985; Mergo and Ros, 1998a).

Magnetic resonance imaging tends to show heterogeneous hyperintensity on T1-weighted images, corresponding to hemorrhagic necrosis and peliosis and/or fat; T2-weighted images are also of high signal. With intravenous gadolinium, early arterial enhancement of the subcapsular feeding vessels may be seen. (Arrivé et al., 1994; Chung et al., 1995).

A central scar as seen in FNH is rarely if ever identified, and the pattern of contrast enhancement also differs from FNH. The features of adenoma may overlap, however, with hepatocellular carcinoma, and MR cannot distinguish these entities. Moreover, percutaneous biopsy may not be sufficient to distinguish adenoma from low-grade hepatocellular carcinoma (Arrivé et al., 1994; Mergo and Ros, 1998a).

Cysts and Tumorlike Mesenchymal Lesions (Cystic Mesenchymal Hamartomas)

Mesenchymal hamartomas consist of gelatinous serous fluid in cystic spaces with bile duct and connective tissue matrix. They are considered a developmental anomaly rather than a true neoplasm (Ros et al., 1986). The patient may present with abdominal distention developing over days or weeks, or it may be a chance finding of an abdominal mass. Alphafetoprotein levels are normal. (Ros et al., 1986). There has been one case report of a ruptured cystic mesenchymal hamartoma causing neonatal ascites (George et al., 1994). These lesions are treated by excision.

Mesenchymal hamartomas may be detected as hypoechoic lesions on prenatal US (Foucor et al., 1983). Postnatal US demonstrates a predominantly cystic lesion with multiple echogenic septa (Ros et al., 1986) (Figure 12–26). Occasionally, more solid-appearing material may be identified, giving the appearance of a complex mass (Donovan et al., 1981).

On CT, the lesions are predominantly cystic-appearing. The septa may enhance with intravenous contrast.

Magnetic resonance imaging demonstrates the expected low signal intensity on T1-weighted images and cystic component high signal intensity on T2-weighted images. The septations may be seen as low signal on T2- weighted imaging.

Mesenchymal Tumors

Cavernous hemangiomas and infantile hemangioendotheliomas are mesenchymal tumors that demonstrate endothelial proliferation. These tumors demonstrate growth and involution phases that differentiate them from arterial venous malformations that grow with the child (Mulliken and Glowacki, 1982). Unlike arterial venous malformations, hemangiomas are soft-tissue tumors.

Since cavernous hemangiomas and infantile hemangioendotheliomas have different clinical and imaging features, they will be considered separately.

Cavernous Hemangioma. Cavernous hemangioma is the most common benign liver tumor in adults, with an incidence of 20% in autopsy series and a female-to-male incidence of five to one (Mergo and Ros, 1998a). The term "capillary hemangioma" is sometimes used and implies the growth stage of the hemangioma wheras cavernous hemangioma refers to the involution stage (Editorial, 1987). In this section, the term "cavernous hemangioma" will be used with reference to both growth and involution stages as appropriate. These lesions rarely present in infancy. They are usually asymptomatic (85% of cases) and are thus usually incidentally detected. However, they can cause abdominal pain, nausea, or vomiting as a result of compression of adjacent structures, rupture, hemorrhage, or thrombosis (Mergo and Ros, 1998a).

Hemangiomas are well-circumscribed blood-filled masses of variable size. Lesions that are 6 to 10 cm in diameter are referred to as giant hemangiomas. On cut section, areas of fibrosis, hemorrhage, calcification, or thrombosis are seen, particularly in larger hemangiomas. Hemangiomas may be multiple in up to 50% of cases (Mergo and Ros, 1998a).

The most common appearance on US is a well-circumscribed hyperechoic lesion with acoustic enhancement. The echogenicity may be variable due to internal fibrosis, thrombosis, necrosis, and occasionally, calcification. Compression tends to reduce the hyperechogenicity which is a finding unique to cavernous hemangioma. Color Doppler may demonstrate a large peripheral feeding vessel (Choji et al., 1988; Mergo and Ros, 1998a).

Studies following cavernous hemangiomas in adults for periods of up to 7 years have shown that growth of hemangiomas is an unexpected finding that should be treated with suspicion. In up to 20% of cases, echogenicity may decrease over time. (Gib-

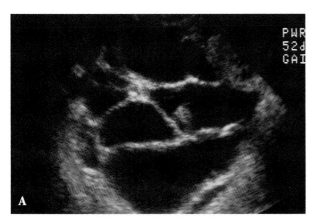 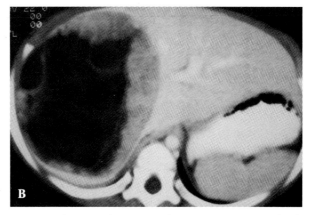

FIGURE 12–26. A 2-year-old male with a mass 10 cm in diameter, predominantly cystic with septations, seen on both *A*, ultrasonography and *B*, CT. At surgery, cystic mesenchymal hamartoma was found.

ney, Hendin, and Cooperberg, 1987; Mungovan, Cronan, and Vacarro, 1994).

Scintigraphic imaging with technetium-99m-pertechnitate-labeled red blood cells using single photon emission computed tomography (SPECT) demonstrates a photopenic defect on initial imaging that accumulates radionuclide over 30 to 50 minutes. The technique is particularly sensitive to lesions greater than 2 cm in diameter (Jacobson and Teefey, 1994; Mergo and Ros, 1998a).

With unenhanced CT, hemangioma is usually a well-defined hypodense lesion, with calcification present in approximately 10% of cases. Following intravenous contrast administration, peripheral enhancement isodense to the aorta with centripetal filling of the lesion over time is the typical enhancement pattern. The central portion of the lesion in larger hemangiomas may fail to enhance due to

fibrotic scarring (Figure 12–27). Smaller hemangiomas may enhance uniformly on early phase imaging (Mergo and Ros, 1998a).

In one large study comparing cavernous hemangioma with metastatic disease, it was found that globular or nodular peripheral enhancement isodense with the aorta (seen with cavernous hemangioma) was 67% sensitive and 100% specific in differentiating cavernous hemangiomas from hepatic metastases (Leslie et al., 1995).

Currently, MR is the most sensitive and specific imaging modality for cavernous hemangioma. On T1-weigthed images, the lesions tend to be low signal. The lesions are bright on T2-weighted images and due to their high water content have a prolonged T2 relaxation time beyond that of other soft-tissue tumors. Because of this feature, the comparison of T2 signal at an echotime (TE) of 80 ms and

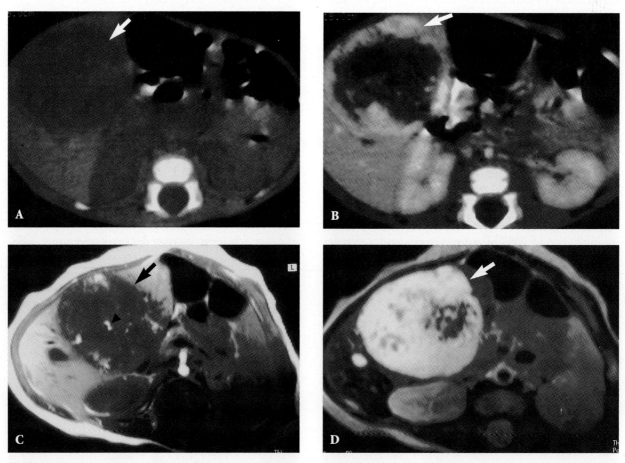

FIGURE 12–27. A 2-month-old male with abdominal mass. *A*, The lesion (*arrow*) is hypodense on non-enhanced CT. *B*, With intravenous contrast enhancement, there is peripheral enhancement typical of cavernous hemangioma (*arrow*). *C*, On T1-weighted MR, the lesion (*arrow*) is of low signal, with focal bright areas (*arrowhead*). *D*, With T2-weighting, high signal is identified (*arrow*). Needle biopsy was positive for hemangioma.

160 ms may be used with the expectation that hemangiomas will become brighter on the more heavily weighted T2 imaging whereas metastases and other tumors would lose signal on the long T2-weighted sequence. By actually calculating the T2 relaxation time and using a cutoff of 112 ms one group discriminated hemangiomas from malignant tumors with 100% sensitivity and 92% specificity (McFarland et al., 1994). Because smaller lesions may not exhibit typical findings on T2-weighted imaging and because cystic lesions may demonstrate similar T2 findings, T2 weighting alone is not considered sufficient for evaluation of hemangiomas.

Gadolinium-enhanced sequential gradient-echo imaging is highly specific for hemangioma when the pattern of nodular and peripheral enhancement is seen compared to rim enhancement seen with metastatic disease. The standard dose of gadolinium (0.1 mmol/kg) is sufficient. In a large collaborative study in four teaching hospitals, hemangiomas were subdivided by size into small (less than 1.5 cm), medium (1.5 to 5 cm), and large (greater than 5 cm) lesions. Contrast-enhanced breathhold gradient-echo imaging with T1 weighting was obtained at 1, 45, and 90 seconds and at 10 minutes after injection. Three patterns of enhancement were observed. Uniform enhancement was evident by 1 second in 35 of 81 small lesions and in no medium or large lesions. Peripheral nodular enhancement progressing centripetally to uniform enhancement was noted in 75 of 144 lesions. Peripheral nodular enhancement with persistent hypointense center (presumably due to central scarring) was seen in 44 lesions, including 16 of the 17 large lesions. All 154 lesions were hyperintense on T2-weighted imaging (Semelka et al., 1994).

Hemangioendothelioma. Hemangioendotheliomas are benign vascular tumors. Their natural history is similar to that of cutaneous hemangiomas, with a rapid proliferation phase lasting 12 to 18 months, followed by a slower involution phase lasting 5 to 8 years. Over 85% of cases present in children under 6 months of age, with a female to male ratio of 2 to 1. Before regression of the tumor, life-threatening complications such as rupture with bleeding, thrombocytopenic coagulopathy (Kasabach-Merritt syndrome), anemia, refractory congestive heart failure, and obstructive jaundice can occur. (Dachman et al., 1983). In the larger series that have been reported, solitary masses and multifocal lesions occur with approximately equal frequency. (Keslar, Buck, and Selby, 1993). Associated cutaneous hemangiomas have been reported in 9 to 87% of cases and are more frequently seen with multifocal hepatic lesions. Similar lesions may be found less commonly in the lungs, gastrointestinal tract, trachea, spleen, thymus, pancreas, and meninges. This is considered to be part of the diffuse process of hemangiomatosis rather than metastatic disease (Keslar, Buck, and Selby, 1993).

The mortality rate reported in infants symptomatic from hemangioendotheliomas ranges from 12 to 90%. A number of treatment options have been used for symptomatic hemangioendothelioma, including corticosteroid treatment, hepatic artery ligation, surgical resection, and transcatheter embolization. If the hemangioma is widespread in the liver, however, surgical resection is not possible, and in the presence of extensive portal venous and systemic arterial collaterals, transcatheter embolization may be contraindicated. Interferon alpha-2a is an antiangiogenesis factor and is currently under clinical trial as a treatment for life-threatening hemangiomas of infancy. The initial results are encouraging (Chung et al., 1996).

On plain-film radiography, hepatomegaly or abdominal mass may be noted. Finely speckled calcification is present in approximately 16% of cases, and findings of congestive heart failure may be seen on chest x-ray films (Keslar, Buck, and Selby, 1993).

On US, lesions are complex or predominantly hypoechoic, usually with well-defined margins (Figure 12–28). Although hyperechoic lesions typical of adult hemangiomas may be seen, this is unusual in hemangioendothelioma. With Doppler interrogation, the hepatic artery and proximal aorta appear enlarged, with tapering of the aorta distal to the celiac artery. Higher flow velocity than that seen in cavernous hemangiomas may be identified (Taylor et al., 1987). The hepatic veins may also be enlarged due to increased flow (Keslar, Buck, and Selby, 1993).

Unenhanced CT usually demonstrates a low-attenuation mass, with calcification seen in 40% of cases (Lucaya et al., 1985). Multifocal lesions are less likely to calcify. After injection of contrast material, peripheral enhancement is seen. Delayed scan may show filling of the central low-attenuation area, but the center often may remain hypoattenuating, particularly in the large solitary lesions. Large lesions often contain areas of infarction or hemorrhage that do not enhance at any time. Small multifocal lesions may enhance completely as they often lack hemorrhage or necrosis (Dachman et al., 1983).

On MR, small lesions tend to be homogeneous and of lower signal intensity than normal liver on T1-weighted images. Larger lesions tend to be more heterogeneous on T1-weighted images, with occasional high signal suggesting the presence of hemorrhage. On T2-weighted images, small lesions tend to be more uniformly of high signal intensity whereas large lesions typically show some degree of

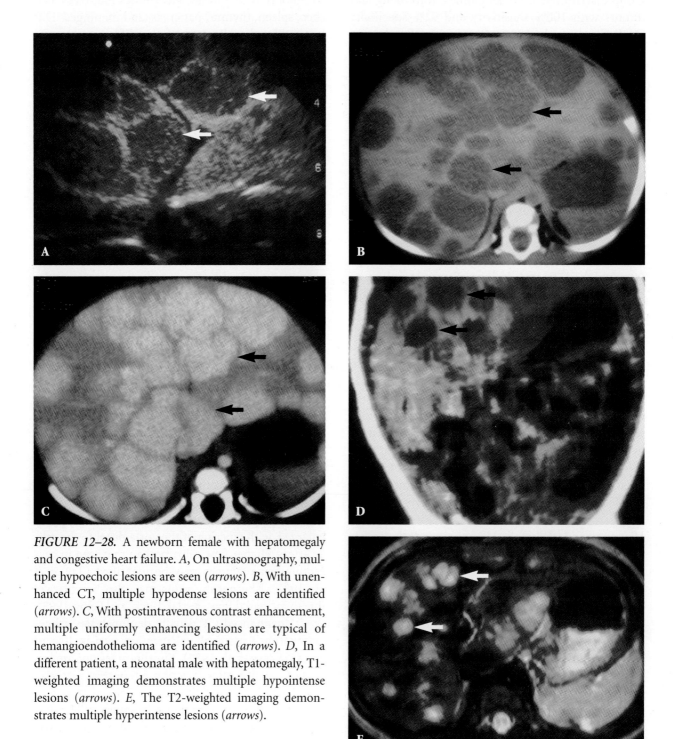

FIGURE 12–28. A newborn female with hepatomegaly and congestive heart failure. *A,* On ultrasonography, multiple hypoechoic lesions are seen (*arrows*). *B,* With unenhanced CT, multiple hypodense lesions are identified (*arrows*). *C,* With postintravenous contrast enhancement, multiple uniformly enhancing lesions are typical of hemangioendothelioma are identified (*arrows*). *D,* In a different patient, a neonatal male with hepatomegaly, T1-weighted imaging demonstrates multiple hypointense lesions (*arrows*). *E,* The T2-weighted imaging demonstrates multiple hyperintense lesions (*arrows*).

heterogeneity. On MR, the proximal abdominal aorta, celiac axis, and main hepatic artery and veins tend to be enlarged in patients with congestive failure. The presence of a high-flow lesion with or without arterial venous shunting may be noted. With successful interferon treatment, the high signal on T2-weighted images gradually decreases to the same MR signal characteristics as normal liver. The lesions also tend to become smaller, and the enlarged vessels decrease in size (Stöver et al., 1995; Chung et al., 1996).

On angiography, as expected, the abrupt decrease in the caliber of the aorta beyond the celiac axis is noted, with enlargement and tortuosity of the hepatic artery and extrahepatic feeding vessels. The portal vein may also supply the lesions. Persistent pooling of contrast material within some or all of the lesion may be seen. Arterial venous shunting with early-draining veins may also be seen, distinguishing infantile hemangioendothelioma from the adult cavernous hemangioma, in which such shunting is essentially never seen (Keslar, Buck, and Selby, 1993).

With nuclear medicine, both technetium 99m sulfur colloid and tagged red blood cells demonstrate increased flow to the viable parts of the lesion during the angiographic phase which is distinct from the appearance in the adult cavernous hemangioma which is typically photopenic in the early phase. On delayed images with sulfur colloid, after clearing of the agent, the lesions appear photopenic. On delayed red-blood-cell images, there is usually increased activity, typically seen unless large areas of hemorrhage, necrosis, or fibrosis is present (Keslar, Buck, and Selby, 1993).

Hepatoblastoma may be difficult to differentiate from hemangioendothelioma; however, hepatoblastoma is uncommonly seen in the newborn period, unlike hemangioendothelioma. As well, alphafetoprotein is usually elevated in hepatoblastoma, and hepatoblastoma tends to be more heterogeneous than hemangioendothelioma on imaging. Mesenchymal hamartoma may resemble hemangioendothelioma; however, mesenchymal hamartoma usually has multilocular cystic components. When it is solid, it appears avascular or hypovascular with imaging. Metastatic neuroblastoma usually has elevated catecholamine levels. With contrast-enhanced CT, marked enhancement is usually seen in hemangioendothelioma in the tumor itself whereas in metastatic neuroblastoma, the areas that enhance tend to represent residual liver between the metastatic lesions. (Keslar, Buck, and Selby, 1993).

Lipomatous Liver Tumors

Lipomatous liver tumors are mesenchymal tumors, classified according to their major histologic component, which may be a variable mixture of fat, muscle, and vascular and hemopoietic tissue (Cheung, Ambrose, and Po, 1993). Hepatic angiomyolipoma is rare, limited to only 5 to 10% of tuberous sclerosis cases and occasionally occurring spontaneously (Ros, 1994). The lack of detectable fat may make the diagnosis of angiomyolipoma difficult. On the other hand, the presence of fat is not pathognomonic for benign lesions in the liver (Peh et al., 1995). In tuberous sclerosis, the lesions in the liver tend to be multiple and range from almost entirely lipomatous to completely solid masses of soft-tissue density on CT (Cheung, Ambrose, and Po, 1993).

In a pure lipoma, imaging is that of a homogeneous lesion that is highly echogenic and well demarcated on US, of low radiodensity with attenuation values less than -20 Hounsfield units on CT with lack of contrast enhancement. As expected with MR, the pure lipoma is homogeneous and hyperintense on T1- and T2-weighted images, with loss of signal with fat suppression (Marti-Bonmati et al., 1989).

Patients with angiomyolipomas of the kidney may be expected to have hepatic lesions whether or not tuberous sclerosis is present. Focal fatty infiltration may simulate a focal tumor; however, in these cases, the lesion is usually not well circumscribed and is at the periphery of the liver or its segments. Blood vessels may also be seen coursing through focal fatty infiltration (Roberts et al., 1986).

Malignant Tumors of the Liver

Primary Tumors

The most important primary malignant hepatic tumors in children are hepatoblastoma, hepatocellular carcinoma (including fibrolamellar hepatocellular carcinoma), rhabdomyosarcoma, and undifferentiated embryonal sarcoma.

Hepatoblastoma. Hepatoblastoma is the most common primary malignancy of the liver in children under the age of 5 years, with a median age of 1 year. The tumor is more common in males than in females, with a two-to-one to three-to-one incidence ratio (Pobiel and Bisset, 1995). Although hepatoblastoma is usually a solitary mass, multifocal lesions may be seen. The most common presentation, in 90% of patients, is a painless mass. There is usually no history of underlying liver disease although there is an association with Beckwith-Wiedemann syndrome, hemihypertrophy, and biliary atresia. Serum alphafetoprotein levels are markedly elevated in over 90% of patients (Donnelly and Bisset, 1998). Metastatic disease occurs in 10 to 20% of cases, with pulmonary metastases being the most common (Donnelly and Bisset, 1998).

Plain films showing hepatomegaly and coarse calcification may be seen in up to 55% of patients (Dachman et al., 1987). With US, the appearance is variable, but a large well-defined primarily echogenic mass is usually seen, and a pseudocapsule may be present. Doppler imaging usually demonstrates increased hepatic arterial flow with frequency shifts over 5 kHz, much higher than in hemangioendothelioma or hemangioma (Taylor et al., 1987). Venous invasion may also be identified.

Technetium-99m-sulfur colloid scans usually demonstrate an area of absent or decreased uptake of radionuclide, but uptake may occasionally be increased, mimicking focal nodular hyperplasia (Diament et al., 1982).

On CT, calcification is well shown when present. Otherwise, the lesion is typically hypodense, with inhomogeneous enhancement. Low signal on T1-weighted images and high signal on T2-weighted images are typical with hemorrhage sometimes identified, causing inhomogeneity (Pobiel and Bisset, 1995) (Figure 12–29).

Hepatocellular Carcinoma. Hepatocellular carcinoma is the most common primary malignant tumor of the liver in children over 4 years of age and is the second most common hepatic malignancy in children, after hepatoblastoma. In adults, it is the most common primary malignant hepatic neoplasm. Unlike hepatoblastoma, pre-existing liver disease such as hepatitis B and C, glycogen storage disease, tyrosinemia, hemochromatosis, and alpha-1-antitrypsin deficiency is present in approximately 50% of cases. Other predisposing factors include hepatocarcinogens such as aflatoxin, the toxin produced by Aspergillus flavus that grows on improperly stored corn, grain, and peanuts. In North America and Europe, alcohol-related cirrhosis is the major predisposing factor whereas in Asia and Africa, hepatitis B and aflatoxin exposure are the most common etiologic factors (Donnelly and Bisset, 1998); (Fernandez and Redvanly, 1998).

Pathologically, the lesions are often multifocal, diffuse, or infiltrative. Metastatic disease is present in approximately 50% of patients at the time of diagnosis. Overall survival ranges from 0 to 29% compared to hepatoblastoma, which has an overall survival of 63 to 67% (Donnelly and Bisset, 1998). Fibrolamellar hepatocellular carcinoma will be discussed separately from hepatocellular carcinoma as it has such distinct features that it is now regarded as a distinct entity.

Hepatocellular carcinoma may be composed of multiple nodules, may be a solitary mass, or may appear as a diffusely infiltrative tumor. The latter appearance may be difficult to detect in end-stage cirrhotic liver. Hepatocellular carcinoma has a tendency for vascular invasion particularly into the portal vein (in up to 44% of cases) and less commonly into the hepatic venous system and inferior vena cava (in 4 to 6% of cases). Biliary invasion may be seen but is much less frequent than vascular invasion. The encapsulated form of hepatocellular carcinoma has a better prognosis because it does not invade the portal vein and is more readily resectable. Large hepatocellular carcinomas greater than 3 cm in diameter have a tendency to necrose and hemorrhage centrally (Fernandez and Redvanly, 1998).

The lesions of hepatocellular carcinoma are variable in appearance on US. In one study of 54 lesions of hepatocellular carcinomas less than 5 cm in diameter, a peripheral hypoechoic halo was seen in half the lesions. In lesions less than 3 cm in diameter, half the lesions were hypoechoic and commonly had posterior acoustic enhancement (Figure 12–30). The tumors between 3 and 5 cm in diameter showed a hyperechoic or mixed pattern (Choi et al., 1989).

Doppler imaging may help in evaluating hepatocellular carcinoma. In one study comparing Doppler interrogation to angiography, power Doppler detected signals related to arterial flow in 92% of angiographically hypervascular tumors compared to 73% using color Doppler. Pulsed wave Doppler was used to verify arterial flow. This was not seen in any of the angiographically hypovascular tumors (75 of 88 lesions were hypervascular; the remaining 13 were hypovascular). In addition, pulsed wave Doppler and color Doppler are highly sensitive and specific in detecting blood flow in tumor thrombus and in thereby distinguishing it from bland thrombus (Wang et al., 1991; Furuse et al., 1992). On both color Doppler and angiography, a basket pattern of a fine blood flow network around the hepatocellular carcinoma nodule has been described as a characteristic appearance (Tanaka et al., 1990).

On unenhanced CT, the lesions are poorly-defined hypo- or isodense masses. Although calcifica-

tion is more typically found in the fibrolamellar form of hepatocellular carcinoma, calcification may also be seen in untreated hepatocellular carcinoma (Teefey, Stephens, and Weiland, 1987). Encapsulated hepatocellular carcinoma is characterized by a hypodense rim on unenhanced or early enhanced CT since the capsule enhances in a delayed manner. Hepatocellular carcinoma (HCC) with fatty metamorphosis will demonstrate low attenuation within the tumor. However, the presence of a capsule and fatty metamor-

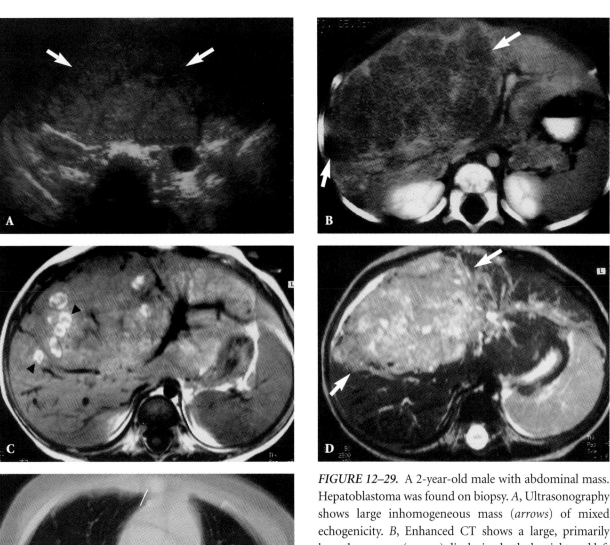

FIGURE 12–29. A 2-year-old male with abdominal mass. Hepatoblastoma was found on biopsy. *A*, Ultrasonography shows large inhomogeneous mass (*arrows*) of mixed echogenicity. *B*, Enhanced CT shows a large, primarily hypodense mass (*arrows*) displacing both the right and left portal veins. *C*, With T1-weighted MR, an isodense mass lesion with bright foci (*arrowheads*) is seen, likely representing areas of hemorrhage. *D*, With T2-weighted imaging, mainly high-signal lesion is seen (*arrows*), with areas of inhomogeneity. *E*, Multiple lung metastases (*arrows*), seen on CT examination.

phosis are rare in the non-Asian population (Fernandez and Redvanly, 1998). With dual phase CT scanning, the arterial phase may show hypervascular HCC that would be otherwise missed on portal venous phase imaging alone. Both lipidol administration and CT arterial portography are more sensitive for detecting small HCCs. Both these techniques are based on the preferential arterial supply to the tumor helping to differentiate HCC from normal hepatic parenchyma supplied primarily by the portal venous system. The presence of a central scar is not always helpful due to the presence of inflammatory and collagen scars in HCC as well as in other types of liver tumors (Fernandez and Redvanly, 1998).

Although HCC is typically hypointense on T1-weighted MR, the presence of fatty metamorphosis, necrosis, or hemorrhage may result in increased signal on T1-weighted images. Fat suppression or chemical shift sequences can distinguish fat from other causes of increased signal on T1-weighted images. The tumor is hyperintense on T2-weighted images (Itoh et al., 1987; Fernandez and Redvanly, 1998).

The fact that HCC frequently arises in chronic liver disease raises the problem of detecting such lesions in grossly abnormal hepatic parenchymal background. Gadolinium- enhanced gradient-echo MR performed in the arterial phase was found in one study to perform better than multiphase helical CT in detecting such lesions (Yamashita et al., 1996). The agent mangafodipir trisodium (Mn-DPDP) has been shown to detect hepatocellular tumors not visualized with unenhanced MR. Furthermore, the degree of tumor enhancement correlates with the degree of histologic differentiation of the tumor (Murakami et al., 1996).

Fibrolamellar Carcinoma. Fibrolamellar carcinoma (FLC) is rare neoplasm of hepatocellular origin with features so distinct from those of typical hepatocellular carcinoma that it is regarded as a separate entity. There are no known predisposing factors for FLC, and it is seen in a younger age group (ranging from 5 to 35 years of age, with a mean age of approximately 20 years). The sex incidence is equal. Alphafetoprotein levels are normal, and the 5-year survival for FLC is 60% compared to an average of 30% for typical HCC (Farhi et al., 1983; Francis, Agha, 1986; Fernandez and Redvanly, 1998).

Symptoms at presentation include abdominal mass, pain, and nausea and vomiting. The tumor usually presents as a solitary mass measuring between 4 and 17 cm in diameter, with a lobulated margin and a central fibrous scar that may be calcified. On US, the tumor is generally hyperechoic; however, the echogenicity may be variable. The central scar is hyperechoic and may demonstrate distal shadowing related to the degree of calcification.

On unenhanced CT, fibrolamellar carcinoma is usually well demarcated and hypodense compared to the remainder of the liver, with stellate areas of even greater hypodensity representing the fibrous scar. Calcification may be seen in the scar in up to 55% of cases whereas calcification may be seen in approximately 8% of typical HCC and may (rarely)

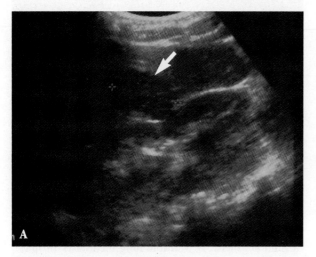
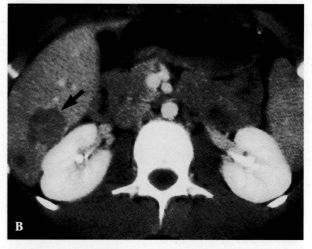

FIGURE 12–30. A 15-year-old male with antenatally acquired hepatitis B and with hepatocellular carcinoma found with surgical resection. *A*, The lesion (*arrow*) is hypoechoic on US. *B*, The lesion (*arrow*) is hypodense on contrast-enhanced CT.

be seen in focal nodular hyperplasia (FNH), either centrally or peripherally (Fernandez and Redvanly, 1998). The distinction between FLC and FNH may be difficult. Both lesions show a central scar on CT, and in approximately 40% of cases of FNH, the normally expected uptake of technetium 99m sulfur colloid does not occur. Following intravenous contrast injection in CT scanning, FLC demonstrates a moderate to marked enhancement, typically with no enhancement of the central scar. Although this helps differentiate FLC from FNH, there may be delayed accumulation of contrast by the scar in FLC (Hamrick-Turner, Shipkey, and Cranston, 1994; Fernandez and Redvanly, 1998).

Magnetic resonance imaging is helpful in distinguishing FLC from FNH. Typically on MR, FLC is hypointense relative to liver on T1 and hyperintense on T2. The central scar is characteristically of low signal on T1 and T2 without enhancement following gadolinium whereas in FNH, the central scar is of high signal on T2 and enhances with contrast. (Corrigan and Semelka, 1995). Nevertheless, exceptions may occur. In case reports, the central scar of FLC has demonstrated enhancement with gadolinium on MR, which would erroneously suggest FNH (Hamrick-Turner, Shipkey, and Cranston, 1994).

Rhabdomyosarcoma of the Biliary Tree. Between 10% and 15% of solid tumors of early childhood are rhabdomyosarcomas, but nearly all arise in the urogenital system or in the musculoskeletal system, especially of the head and neck (Friedburg et al., 1984).

Embryonal rhabdomyosarcoma of the biliary tree is a rare primary malignant tumor of childhood. It usually presents in children between 2 and 5 years of age (Arnand et al., 1987) although it may occur between infancy and as late as 17 years of age (Geoffray et al., 1987). The sex incidence is equal, and the prognosis is poor (Arnand et al., 1987). Treatment is usually surgical.

The child presents with jaundice in most cases (Arnand et al., 1987; Geoffray et al., 1987) although this may be a late complication if bile flow is not obstructed (Friedburg et al., 1984). Malaise, fever, nonspecific abdominal pain with a palpable abdominal mass, and hepatomegaly are common nonspecific symptoms and signs (Friedburg et al., 1984; Arnand et al., 1987; Geoffray et al., 1987).

Plain films are not specific. Barium studies, if performed because of a misleading presentation, may show compression of the second part of the duodenum from the extrinsic tumor.

Ultrasonography and CT are the most useful modalities. Bile duct dilatation is more common than with other tumors, and US easily demonstrates this dilatation, which is often proximal to a usually nonhomogeneous echogenic mass that may be quite hyperechoic (Miller and Greenspan, 1985). The mass is often in the porta hepatis and sometimes contains hypoechoic areas (Arnand et al., 1987; Geoffray et al., 1987). The presence of fluid (bile) around the tumor in the porta is the most specific sign (Friedburg et al., 1984), but differentiation from hepatic tumors generally is not possible (Geoffray et al., 1987).

Computed tomography will show an ill-defined or well-outlined relatively low-attenuation mass with some enhancement (Friedburg et al., 1984; Miller and Greenspan, 1985; Geoffray et al., 1987). Computed tomography is best at showing the anatomy and can show the relationship of the portal vein and bile ducts if this has not been clearly defined by US.

Technetium 99m sulfur colloid will show the tumor as a photon-deficient area whereas gallium67 will be actively taken up and will show as an area of increased uptake (Miller and Greenspan, 1985).

Cholangiography (percutaneous transhepatic, endoscopic retrograde cholangiopancreatography (ERCP), or intraoperative), will show bizarre grape-like filling defects (Geoffray et al., 1987). Intraoperative examination is useful in assessing the extent of the tumor.

Undifferentiated Embryonal Sarcoma. Undifferentiated embryonal sarcoma (also malignant mesenchymoma or hepatic mesenchymal sarcoma), although rare, is the fourth most common hepatic tumor in the pediatric age group, after hepatoblastoma, hemangioendothelioma, and hepatocellular carcinoma. Most patients present between 6 and 10 years of age (Ros et al., 1986). There may be difficulty differentiating this tumor from mesenchymal hamartoma. In both tumors, alphafetoprotein levels are not elevated. Embryonal sarcoma tends to be more solid, and also the age of presentation differs, with mesenchymal hamartomas usually presenting between 4 months and 2 years of age whereas embryonal sarcoma tends to occur after 5 years of age (Moon et al., 1994). In addition, embryonal sarcoma usually presents with pain in the right upper quadrant and with abdominal mass whereas mesenchymal hamartoma is usually asymptomatic (Newman et al., 1989). Although a relationship between mesenchymal hamartoma and undifferentiated embryonal sarcoma has been suggested, it seems unlikely since there are no reports of malignant transformation of mesenchymal hamartoma (Marti-Bonmati et al., 1993).

Embryonal sarcoma is usually quite large at presentation, with mixed cystic and solid elements. They range between 7 and 18 cm, and there is typically a solitary mass located in the right lobe of the liver (Moon et al., 1993). Long-term survival has been achieved with complete resection of the tumor and adjuvant chemotherapy (Newman et al., 1989).

On US, the tumor is predominantly echogenic, with small anechoic spaces representing cystic necrosis. Unenhanced CT demonstrates a well-circumscribed low-attenuation mass. With intravenous contrast, enhancement of septations as well as peripheral solid portions of the tumor may be seen. Punctate calcification may be seen in these tumors (Moon et al., 1994).

On MR, the mass usually presents as a low-signal lesion containing foci of high-signal areas on T1-weighted images, likely representing hemorrhage. On T2 and inversion recovery sequences, undifferentiated embryonal sarcoma (UES) is of high intensity, with hypointense septa (Marti-Bonmati et al., 1993).

Secondary Tumors

The most common hepatic secondaries in children are from neuroblastoma, Wilms' tumor, and lymphoma. Diffuse involvement of the liver by leukemia can also occur. The presence of metastases in the liver at the time of presentation is common with stage IV S neuroblastoma, and they tend to be diffusely infiltrative or multinodular (Franken et al., 1986) (Figure 12–31).

Immunosuppressed patients are at risk of posttransplantation lymphoproliferative disease (PTLD, representing a spectrum of lymphoproliferative disorders ranging from benign polyclonal B-cell hyperplasia to malignant lymphoma) that may resolve with reduction or cessation of immunosuppressive treatment. This has been described in patients who have undergone liver and heart transplantation that require relatively greater immunosuppression. Leiomyoma and leiomyosarcoma involving the gastrointestinal tract, respiratory tract, and liver have also been described in children who are immunocompromised due to HIV infection or following liver and renal transplantation (Levin et al., 1994).

Metastatic infantile choriocarcinoma is a rare entity, typically with liver involvement and a rapidly fatal course (Moon et al., 1993; Sashi et al., 1996).

Hepatic metastases from other tumors usually occur late in the disease process. This is true for Wilms' tumor, renal cell carcinoma, undifferentiated sarcoma, noninfantile neuroblastoma, and other tumors.

One large study in adults found that the sensitivity of US for liver metastases was 54% and to a large degree depended on the type of primary tumor (Schölmerich, Volk, and Gerok, 1987). In a large study of adults with pathologically proven Hodgkin's and non-Hodgkin's lymphoma, multiple well-delineated hypoechoic lesions were seen in approxi-

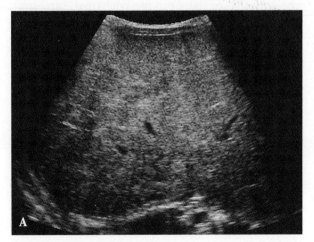
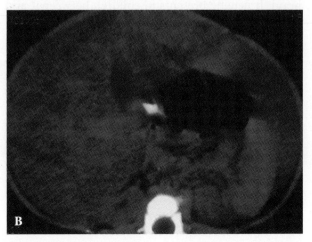

FIGURE 12–31. A 2-month-old male with stage IV S neuroblastoma with hepatomegaly. *A*, Inhomogeneity of the liver parenchyma is seen on US. *B*, The same, seen on non-contrast-enhanced CT.

mately 30% of the 68 patients with secondary hepatic lymphoma (Figure 12–32). Hepatomegaly was not a specific finding for liver involvement since only 57% of patients with hepatomegaly had histologically proven liver involvement. On the other hand, hepatomegaly is not a sensitive criterion, in that diffuse liver involvement may exist in a normal-sized liver; this study found a 44% sensitivity for hepatomegaly as a sign of involvement of the liver by secondary lymphoma (Soyer et al., 1993).

There is some controversy regarding the need for both unenhanced and enhanced CT scanning of patients with liver metastases. Up to 40% of patients with hypervascular liver metastases have lesions that become isointense with the hepatic parenchyma if imaging is not performed in the arterial phase (Bressler and Alpern, 1995).

Magnetic resonance imaging has great potential in the detection of hepatic metastases. Focal hepatic lymphoma is reliably detected with hypointensity on T1 weighting and hyperintensity on T2 weighting, relative to the remainder of the liver. Diffuse hepatic lymphoma may be undetectable either morphologically or by quantitative determination of T1 and T2 relaxation times (Weisleder et al., 1988).

The lesions of PTLD as well as spindle cell tumors (leiomyoma and leiomyosarcoma) are similar, with echo-poor lesions seen on US, hypodensity on CT, and lack of enhancement with intravenous contrast.

Metastatic infantile choriocarcinoma demonstrates a solid lesion with cystic areas due to necrosis. Red-blood-cell nuclear scanning demonstrates a large photopenic defect unlike the expected finding of a hemangioendothelioma. On T1-weighted images, the mass is hypointense with hyperintense areas in keeping with hemorrhage, and on T2-weighted images, high signal is identified. With heavy T2 weighting, the mass loses its high signal, again differentiating it from hemangioendothelioma. Beta human chorionic gonadotropin (HCG) levels are elevated and should be followed in the mother as well (maternal choriocarcinoma is observed in a majority of cases) (Moon et al., 1993; Sashi et al., 1996).

TRAUMA

Clinical Features

The liver is one of the most frequently injured abdominal organs in childhood. Motor vehicle and other accidents, falls, and child abuse cause most blunt liver injury, with hepatic injury occurring in 10 to 30% of cases of pediatric blunt abdominal trauma. Suspicion for intra-abdominal and hepatic injury is raised with abdominal wall ecchymosis, tenderness, distention, hematuria, elevated liver enzymes, and/or hypotension (Sivit et al., 1991). Hepatic parenchymal injury varies in severity, ranging from small hepatic lacerations to uncommon extensive fractures with life-threatening vascular injury that which require immediate surgery. Fortunately, most hepatic injuries are minor and hemodynamically stable and can be managed expectantly without operation. Most hepatic injuries consist of hematomas, contusions, and minor lacerations (Cooper, 1992). Blunt liver injuries predominantly

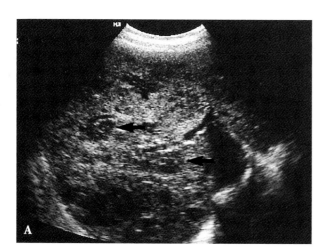
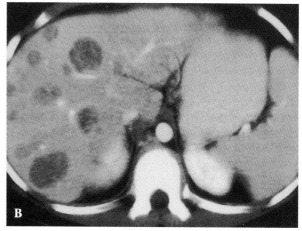

FIGURE 12–32. An 11-year-old male with non-Hodgkin's lymphoma metastatic to the liver. *A,* Multiple hypoechoic lesions (*arrows*) identified on US. *B,* Hypodense lesions seen on contrast-enhanced CT.

involve the right lobe of the liver, most often the convexity and dome of the organ, with left lobe injury being less frequent (Vock, Kehrer, and Tschaeppeler, 1986). This distribution may be related to the ligamentous fixation of the organ and pressure propagation against the diaphragm and/or the spine. The recognition of the relatively minor nature of most liver injuries, combined with the development of modern cross-sectional imaging, has led to the current trend of the routine use of expectant clinical management.

Imaging of Hepatic Trauma

Preferred Methods

The need for imaging a patient with blunt abdominal trauma is largely determined by the immediate clinical situation and the physiologic condition of the child (Brick et al., 1987). Both CT and US are commonly used in the initial assessment of children with blunt abdominal trauma, with CT being the preferred imaging modality in most centers in North America. Only hemodynamically stable patients should undergo CT imaging. Imaging does not play a major role in deciding which children with hepatic injury should go to surgery as the initial imaging appearance only rarely mandates immediate surgery (Brick et al., 1987; Ruess et al., 1995).

Computed Tomography

Initial imaging with CT is recommended for children who are hemodynamically stable and suspected of having multiple intra-abdominal injuries or severe single-organ injury or who are undergoing concomitant CT scans of the head when abdominal injury is also considered likely. Many studies have documented the superiority of CT over other imaging techniques in evaluating the severely injured child. It provides accurate information regarding the extent of hepatic injury, including its segmental distribution, its relation to major vessels and perfusion, the extent of injury to other intra-abdominal organs, and the presence of free fluid (Vock, and Tschaeppeler, 1986; Sivit et al., 1991; Taylor et al., 1994; Taylor, 1995). Additionally, CT can be used in postoperative evaluation (Vock, Kehrer, and Tschaeppeler, 1986).

Adequate CT examination for blunt abdominal trauma requires a commitment to detail. The study should be expedited as much as possible and preparations begun before the patient's arrival at the scanner. Careful patient monitoring is necessary throughout the study. All tubes and overlying wires and electrocardiography pads should be withdrawn from the scan area to avoid streak artifacts. Computed tomography can be performed with either helical or nonhelical scanning, with contiguous cuts following the intravenous administration of contrast material. Non-contrast scans are not needed. Scanning should be continued throughout the pelvis to evaluate the degree of hemoperitoneum present.

Hepatic injury appears on CT predominantly as hypodense, linear, round, or stellate areas that may occur in any portion of the liver. Hematomas or contusions are the most common liver injuries that may be intraparenchymal and/or subcapsular (Shanmuganathan and Mirvis, 1998) (Figure 12–33A). Subcapsular hematomas are often associated with parenchymal injury and are hypodense or mixed-density peripheral lenticular collections that compress or flatten the underlying parenchyma. Lacerations are linear or branching low-attenuation areas within the liver. Vascular injuries can be identified with CT and may show regions of active hemorrhage with contrast extravasation (Figure 12–34). Tearing in the capsule leads to associated hemoperitoneum that can be quantitated by CT, depending upon the amount and distribution of fluid in the peritoneal spaces. Periportal low density can be seen following trauma and may be diffuse. It may reflect hemorrhage from adjacent liver injury or (more frequently) distended periportal lymphatic vessels and accumulation of lymphedema (Shanmuganathan and Mirvis, 1998).

Several radiographic classification schemes have been proposed for children, based on the initial extent and severity of the hepatic injury (Brick et al., 1987; Becker et al., 1996). However, these schemes are limited in predicting clinical outcome or immediate need for surgery (Brick et al., 1987; Ruess et al., 1995; Taylor, 1995). Parenchymal injuries can be divided into superficial or deep lesions and simple or complex lesions (Stalker, Kaufman, and Towbin, 1986). Simple lesions are usually well defined, focal, and superficial, involving the periphery of the liver. Complex lesions are more extensive and poorly defined, often stellate in outline and deep or perihilar in location. Complex and deep lesions may be more frequently complicated in their course (Stalker, Kaufman, and Towbin, 1986). Injury to the left lobe is more likely to be complex and associated with

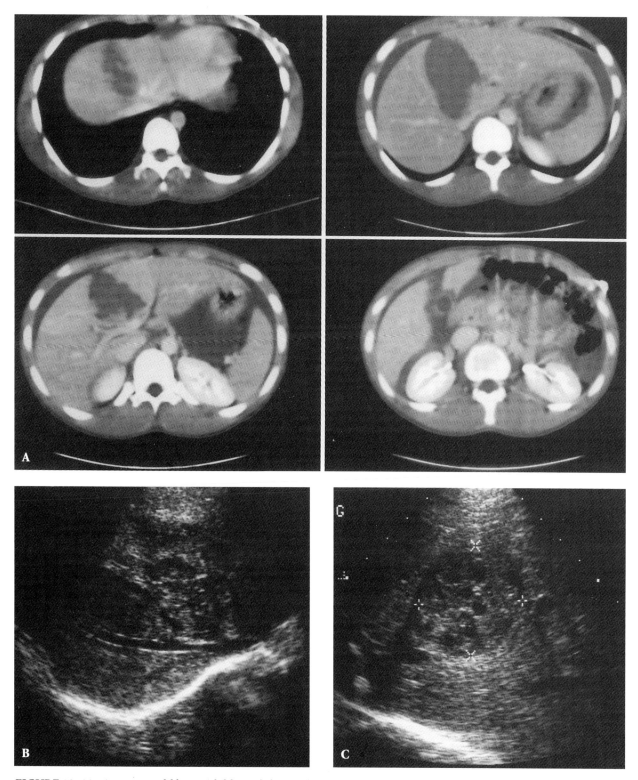

FIGURE 12–33. A 15-year-old boy with blunt abdominal trauma. *A,* Selected contrast-enhanced axial CT shows a complete transection through the anterior segment of the right lobe of the liver extending from the anterior aspect, posteriorly to the inferior vena cava. There is a significant intrahepatic hematoma and perihepatic fluid. There is fluid surrounding the gallbladder, and there is fluid within the lesser sac. *B,* Follow-up US performed a few days later indicates a complex area of echogenicity in the anterior segment of the right lobe of the liver. *C,* Ultrasonography performed 2 months later portrays interval decrease of earlier hepatic fracture and hematoma.

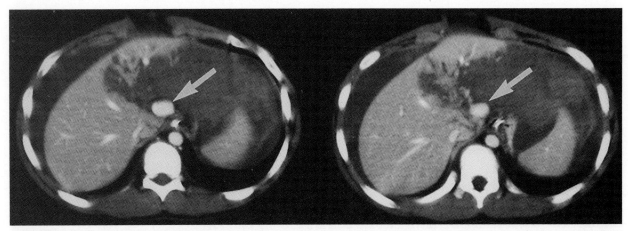

FIGURE 12–34. Selected axial CT images following contrast in a 13-year-old boy with blunt abdominal trauma. There is extensive injury to the left lobe of the liver, with marked intra-abdominal hemoperitoneum. Large intrahepatic contrast collection is evident (*arrow*) from a tear of the inferior vena cava, documented at surgery.

pancreatitis or duodenal injury. However, a left lobe injury is significantly less common than right lobe trauma.

Associated injury to the biliary system can be seen with hematobilia, biloma formation, biliary duct laceration, or even free bile leakage. Computed tomography can show increased density within the gallbladder from hemorrhage while bile leakage can be confirmed with radionuclide studies. The course of liver injury can be followed through to healing with either CT or preferably US. These studies can monitor post-traumatic cyst formation, infection and (very uncommonly) hepatic infarction. Rarely, calcification may develop.

Ultrasonography

Ultrasonography is commonly used in the initial evaluation of intra-abdominal trauma in Europe and is gaining increasing attention as a screening modality (Patrick et al., 1992). It is considered a cost-effective way to image the injured child, it is readily available and can be used immediately in the emergency unit (Patrick et al., 1992; Luks et al., 1993; Filiatrault and Garel, 1995). Ultrasonography can readily identify free intraperitoneal fluid and the majority of visceral injuries. However, not all visceral injuries are detected early on. (Patrick et al., 1992; Luks et al., 1993; Filiatrault and Garel, 1995; Richardson, Hollman, and Davis, 1997). Acutely, most intrahepatic injuries will appear echogenic. Fluid collections will appear as either echogenic or hypoechoic collections.

Other Imaging Modalities

There is currently little need for radionuclide imaging in the immediate evaluation of children with liver injury. Biliary scans can be performed in follow-up to detect suspected biliary leaks. Angiography is rarely needed and is limited to cases requiring urgent embolization.

Neonatal Trauma

In the neonate, rupture of the liver is a rare clinical diagnosis, but this complication is seen in 1 to 6% of autopsy cases (Zorzi et al, 1986). Rupture is usually caused by trauma during birth or vigorous resuscitation. Neonates usually appear normal at birth, but anemia and severe shock due to hematoma formation are seen in the second day of life. Ultrasonography can be performed at the cribside and is particularly helpful in diagnosing perinatal liver rupture. It gives excellent delineation of subcapsular hematomas (with a sonolucent band separating the liver and the diaphragm), parenchymal contusions (hyperechoic or rarely, hypoechoic areas), and dilatation of the biliary tree (Zorzi et al 1986). Other modalities are not usually required; if they are performed, the appearance of trauma in infants is similar to what is seen in older infants and children.

Role of Imaging in Follow-up of Trauma

Imaging studies are often performed in follow-up of liver injury to assess stability or healing of the liver injury and to detect possible complications. Computed tomography can show healing of hepatic injuries and resorption of hemoperitoneum within several weeks of the injury (Bulas et al., 1993; Shanmuganathan and Mirvis, 1998). Bulas showed a correlation between the grading system proposed by Brick (Brick et al., 1987) and the most appropriate timing for documenting resolution of liver injury on CT (Bulas et al., 1993). Mild injuries healed within 3 months while 3 to 6 months were required for moderate injuries, 9 months for severe injuries. However, the need to document complete healing has been questioned (Bulas et al., 1993; Allins et al., 1996). It is also uncertain whether prolonged restriction of activities until the injury has completely resolved on imaging influences the final outcome.

Complications include delayed hemorrhage, hemobilia, biloma, bile peritonitis, and infection, usually occurring within the first 2 months following injury (Karp et al., 1983; Brick et al., 1987; Cywes, Bass, and Rode, 1991; Farron, Gudinchet, and Genton, 1996). Complications are uncommon following initial nonoperative management, and not all require subsequent surgery. The routine use of follow-up imaging studies in asymptomatic patients is controversial as it often fails to impact clinical management (Allins et al., 1996; Farron, Gudinchet, and Genton, 1996). No agreement exists in the literature regarding optimum timing for follow-up studies. Generally, follow-up CT is only needed when the clinical course suggests the presence of a complication.

Although we find CT to be the most useful and cost-efficient imaging modality for initial evaluation of intra-abdominal blunt trauma, US is adequate for follow-up of any lesion previously demonstrated on CT or for documentation of post-traumatic complications (see Figures 12–33B, C). Frequently, hematomas are at first hyperechoic and ill-defined within the hepatic parenchyma, but with time and progressive liquefaction, the lesion becomes anechoic and diminishes in size. Biliary complications of hepatic trauma, including hematobilia and biloma formation, can be identified with US. Echogenic debris in the gallbladder suggests intraluminal hemorrhage. Bilomas or bile lakes can occur and may simulate a liquefied hematoma on follow-up scans.

MISCELLANEOUS DISORDERS

Cirrhosis and Portal Hypertension

Cirrhosis is the end stage of many childhood diseases of infective, metabolic, obstructive biliary, vascular, and miscellaneous etiologies (Table 12–2). Initiated by parenchymal necrosis of the liver, cirrhosis is characterized by widespread hepatic fibrosis, nodular hepatocyte regeneration, and vascular distortion (Brown, Naylor, and Yagan, 1997). The clinical manifestations of cirrhosis are primarily related to loss of liver function and to portal hypertension.

In children (as in adults), portal hypertension may be secondary to extrahepatic portal vein obstruction, hepatic venous obstruction, or hyperkinetic portal hypertension. Portal hypertension typically manifests with evidence of ascites, splenomegaly, collaterals, and altered portal venous flow (Westra et al., 1995).

Extrahepatic Portal Vein Obstruction

The majority of cases of portal hypertension in children are due to extrahepatic portal vein obstruction from portal vein thrombosis. The obstruction often develops in the neonatal period, and no cause is found in the majority of cases. Umbilical vein catheterization and infection spreading via the umbilical vein have both been implicated in the etiology. Trauma, pancreatitis, tumors, prior splenectomy (Figure 12–35), and inflammatory masses (especially from appendicitis) may all produce extrahepatic portal vein obstruction in older children on occasion (Slovis et al., 1989). An inflammatory pseudotumor of the liver has been reported as a rare cause of portal hypertension and obstructive jaundice in children. Rarely, the portal vein may be absent, as has been reported in a patient with Goldenhar's syndrome. Liver disease may be absent (Belli et al., 1989).

TABLE 12–2. Causes of Cirrhosis

Viral hepatitis
Biliary Obstruction
Venous outflow obstruction
Hemochromatosis
Wilson's disease
Autoimmune disorders
Drugs and toxins
Alpha 1 antitrypsin deficiency
Cystic fibrosis
Galactosemia
Glycogen storage disorder
Hereditary tyrosinemia
Idiopathic

Symptoms and signs usually have an insidious onset, the earliest sign being abdominal distention or splenomegaly. Ascites in the absence of cirrhosis may occasionally occur in infancy. Growth retardation is also common (Sarin et al., 1992).

Massive gastrointestinal hemorrhage from esophageal varices may be a presenting feature in children. The hemorrhage usually abates with medical management and has a better prognosis than hemorrhage from varices secondary to hepatic cirrhosis. A leash of vessels usually develops around the obstructed portal vein (a process termed "cavernous transformation") (Figure 12–37), and this is responsible for the better prognosis in this condition.

Treatment of portal hypertension is variable, with a variety of surgical shunts possible. Transjugular intrahepatic portosystemic shunt (TIPS) creation can aid the management of portal hypertension in children and appears technically feasible and safe, especially in children who need temporary relief before liver transplantation (Hackworth et al., 1998).

Imaging. Plain-Film Radiography. A chest radiograph may show an enlarged azygos vein and (rarely) a posterior mediastinal mass from varices. Plain abdominal films may show calcification in the portal vein as well as evidence of hepatosplenomegaly, especially in older children and adults.

Ultrasonography. Ultrasonographic indicators of portal hypertension include enlarged caliber of the portal vein and the presence of enlarged collaterals such as paraumbilical veins. Cavernous transformation can be detected on US as an absence of the normal portal vein in association with tortuous vessels within the porta hepatis (Figure 12–37). Occasionally, thrombus may be seen in the portal vein as a discrete echogenic structure. In some cases, cavernous transformation of the portal vein appears associated with congenital hepatic fibrosis (Bayraktar et al., 1997).

Ultrasonography may show a variety of signs of portosystemic venous collaterals. The appearance

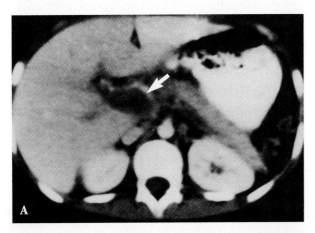
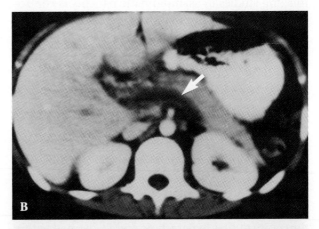
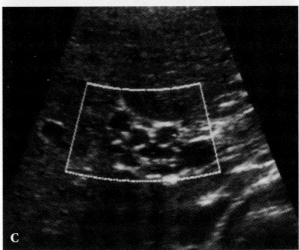

FIGURE 12–35. A 17-year-old girl following splenectomy for thalassemia with postsplenectomy thrombosis of the splenic vein and portal vein. *A* and *B*, Selected CT images following contrast demonstrating thrombus within the main portal vein and splenic vein (*arrows*). *C*, An axial ultrasonographic image obtained several months later, demonstrating interval development of cavernous transformation with numerous collaterals at the level of the porta hepatis.

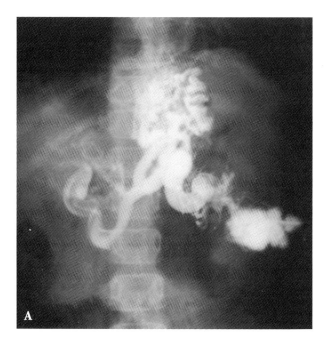

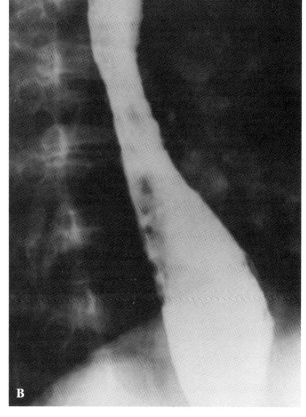

FIGURE 12–36. An 8-year-old girl with a history of umbilical vein catheterization at birth. *A,* Splenoportography (done prior to the availability of CT and MR) nicely illustrates large gastroesophageal varices with portal vein thrombosis. *B,* Barium swallow shows nodularity of the distal esophagus, in keeping with esophageal varices.

will depend on the site of the collaterals. Many collaterals pass to the base of the lesser omentum on their passage to the esophagus; hence, the base of the lesser omentum is thickened. On a longitudinal scan through the aorta at the level of the crus, the thickness of the omentum, which lies between aorta and

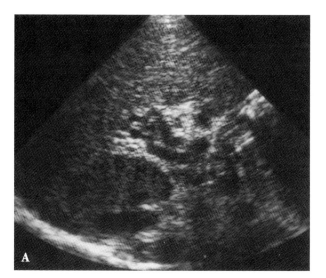

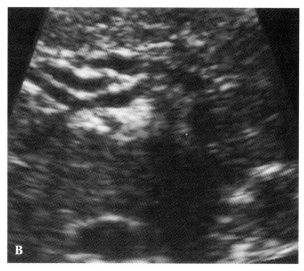

FIGURE 12–37. Selected ultrasonographic images from a 10-year-old child with cavernous transformation of the portal vein. *A,* Numerous collateral vessels are seen on the longitudinal image. *B,* Vessels are better demonstrated on detailed axial image.

liver, should be less than 1.7 times the size of the aorta at this level (Frider, Marin, and Goldberg, 1989). In addition, abnormal vessels may be seen leading to or from this area although the presence of visible vessels is less common. A coronary vein leading to this area or a vein or veins leading from the spleen are the vessels most commonly visible. The splenic vessels may appear as serpiginous anechoic structures in the splenic hilum and may be followed towards the esophagus or kidney.

Other collateral channels include splenorenal, umbilical, and pancreatoduodenal veins, gallbladder cystic duct veins, and omental veins (Kainberger et al., 1990). These shunts may occasionally be visible on US as serpiginous anechoic channels (Frider, Marin, and Goldberg, 1989). The so-called umbilical vein, if patent, is an easier vessel to visualize because it tends to be straighter. It has a characteristic position in the ligamentum teres and may have a bull's-eye appearance if fat is present in the ligament around the vessels. The vessel is likely not a recanalized umbilical vein, as autopsy studies have shown this to be a paraumbilical vessel. The patency of a portocaval anastomosis can be assessed when it is directly visualized. It is patent when there is (a) a decrease in the size of the collaterals, the portal vein, and the thickness of the omentum, and (b) an increase in size of the inferior vena cava compared with the preoperative study.

Color and power Doppler US are very useful in assessing patients for possible portal cavernoma and collateral vessels. Normal portal vein flow is toward the liver and shows respiratory variation and (infrequently) minor cardiac pulsations. Changes in portal vein flow dynamics suggestive of portal hypertension can be appreciated with color or power Doppler and include loss of normal respiratory variation, reversal of portal venous flow, and decrease of antegrade flow volume in the portal vein (Westra et al., 1995; Shapiro et al., 1998). Doppler US can also assist in assessing patency of portocaval shunts and in distinguishing blood vessels from enlarged bile ducts.

Computed Tomography and Magnetic Resonance Imaging. Computed tomography can show collaterals and the portal cavernoma, but it is usually not indicated when satisfactory US is available. Dynamic contrast-enhanced CT will show a portal cavernoma as a loss of normal vascular structures, with sinuous enhanced pathways around the outside of the porta. Rarely, a fresh thrombus may have increased attenuation prior to enhancement. Varying transient differences in hepatic attenuation may be seen in some patients. Varices are well demonstrated and may be seen extending into the thorax.

Although MR is a useful modality for assessing portal hypertension, it is usually reserved for problematic cases (Brown, Naylor, and Yagan, 1997). Magnetic resonance angiography, whether with time-of-flight sequences or contrast enhancement is a useful adjunct for demonstrating the hepatic vasculature (Hubbard, Meyer, and Mahboubi, 1992). It is sensitive in visualizing slow or absent flow in portal vessels. It may occasionally aid in the differentiation of venous occlusion from other causes of portal hypertension, and it may detect portal cavernoma. Patency of splenorenal shunts can also be assessed with MR.

Other Modalities. Varices may be seen on esophagography or endoscopically. (see Chapter 4). Although not generally required, ERCP may diagnose common bile duct varices. Angiography may rarely be needed preoperatively to demonstrate the anatomy of the portal system (Figure 12–36). It can be most safely performed with digital subtraction techniques, with a resulting reduction in the amount of contrast medium injected and a shorter examination time. The angiographic study of the portal system in children is similar to that in adults, but a general anesthetic is usually required for children under 10 years of age.

Intrahepatic Obstruction

In children, intrahepatic obstruction that produces portal hypertension is less common than extrahepatic obstruction. Intrahepatic obstruction is usually secondary to cirrhosis but can occur from uncommon liver disorders such as ciliated foregut cysts (Harty et al., 1998). The cirrhosis may be present at birth after prenatal infection, but it develops more often later in life, secondary to diseases such as biliary atresia, cystic fibrosis, Wilson's disease, or Gaucher's disease. Fatty infiltration may be present with the cirrhosis and hence is considered in this section. Most children will have evidence of hepatic disease before gastrointestinal hemorrhage occurs.

Imaging. Collaterals and varices may be present and give similar appearances to those discussed under extrahepatic obstruction, except that the portal veins are typically large if patent (Figure 12–39). The other radiologic features depend on the type and severity of the underlying hepatic disease. In cirrhosis, parenchymal nodularity is evident, whether macronodular, micronodular, or mixed due to regenerative nodules (Brown, Naylor, and Yagan, 1997) (Figures 12–40, 12–41). Other morphologic features of cirrhosis include parenchymal enlargement, altered ultrasound transmission, and heterogeneous parenchyma. Radiology is generally poor at assessing the severity of liver disease, but it may be more useful in serial studies.

Many hepatic diseases that go on to cause cirrhosis result in fat deposition. This may be detectable on plain-film radiography by increased lucency.

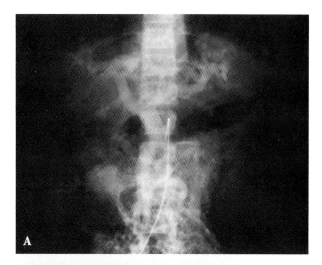

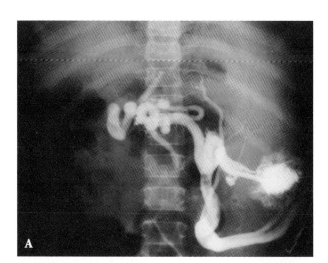

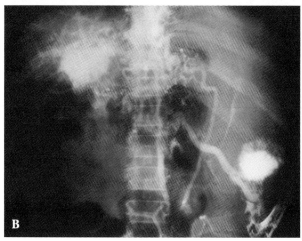

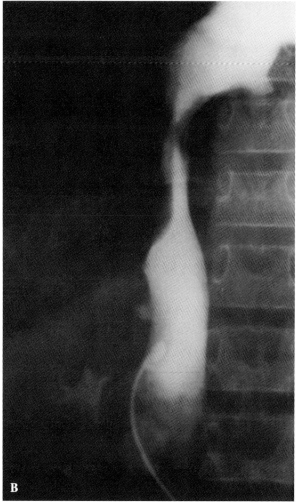

FIGURE 12–38. A 12-year-old boy with portal vein thrombosis. *A,* Early splenoportography shows extensive collateral vessels around the inferior aspect of the enlarged spleen, with portal vein thrombosis, multiple collateral vessels, and esophageal varices evident. *B,* Later film of the same patient.

FIGURE 12–39. An 11-year-old boy with cystic fibrosis and development of cirrhosis and portal hypertension. *A,* Superior mesenteric angiography with delayed imaging demonstrates patent portal vein, with collateral vessels evident. *B,* Injection of the inferior vena cava showed stenosis in the upper aspect of the intrahepatic inferior vena cava.

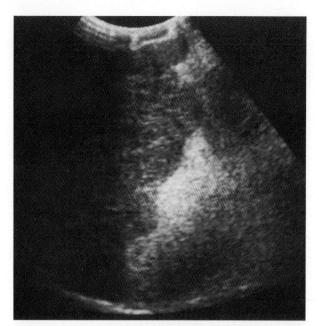

FIGURE 12–40. Longitudinal US demonstrates a nodular outline to the liver, in keeping with cirrhosis.

Ultrasonography. Sonographically, cirrhosis demonstrates altered parenchymal morphology, echogenicity, and nodularity (Brown, Naylor, and Yagan, 1997). There may be atrophy of various segments of the liver, with relative sparing of the caudate lobe, or overall enlargement of the liver. In cirrhosis, regenerative nodules can sometimes be seen as discrete islands of liver parenchyma with a thin, slightly more echogenic border corresponding to fibrous and fatty connective tissue surrounding the nodules. The outline of the liver can become very irregular owing to scarring and regeneration. This is most easily appreciated when ascites is present and with the use of a high-resolution transducer scanning over the ventral aspect of the left lobe of the liver (Simonovsky, 1999).

Fat deposition occurs commonly in cirrhosis and gives increased echogenicity on US. The increased echogenicity may be focal and mimic a mass lesion. Conversely, the increase in echogenicity

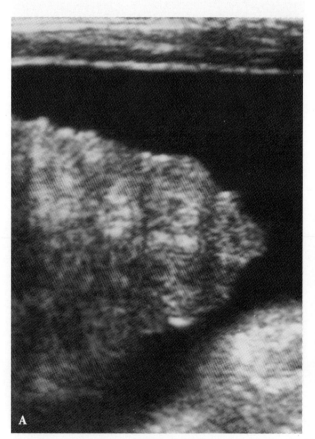

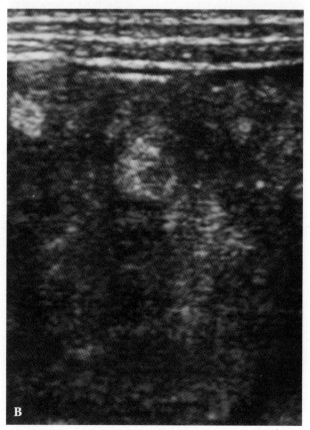

FIGURE 12–41. A $2^1/_2$-year-old girl with tyrosinemia. *A,* Diffuse irregular nodular echogenicities are evident within the liver on longitudinal US. Extensive ascites is also evident. *B,* Nodularity is also shown on the detailed high-resolution ultrasonographic image, with nodules of increased and intermediate echogenicity. Pathologic examination demonstrated hyperplastic nodules as well as several foci of hepatocellular carcinoma.

may be uniform except for a small part of the liver, such as the quadrate lobe. This can be confusing unless one realizes that the small part of the liver is the only normal portion. The increased echogenicity seen in the liver is due purely to the fatty infiltration (Figure 12–42). Fibrosis alone or in cirrhosis without fatty infiltration gives a normal echo pattern.

Alterations in portal vein dynamics are common and are generally similar to those discussed earlier for portal hypertension from extrahepatic obstruction (Shapiro et al., 1998). In patients with cirrhosis, pressure in the portal system may be so high that portal vein flow is reversed (Shapiro et al., 1998). In addition, in children with end-stage liver disease and portal hypertension, a pulsatile portal venous waveform with resistive indices greater than 0.60 is often present. Pulsatility of the portal vein may also be seen in children with tricuspid atresia and Budd-Chiari syndrome (Westra et al., 1995). Increased flow in the hepatic artery can also be noted (Shapiro et al., 1998). There is some evidence of an increase in splanchnic vein blood flow in patients with cirrhosis, as measured by splanchnic vein size or duplex Doppler blood flow measurements (Zwiebel et al., 1995). In cirrhosis, the normal phasic pulsations of the hepatic venous system can be diminished. This can also be seen in Budd-Chiari syndrome and in obstruction of the inferior vena cava.

Differential Diagnosis of Echogenic (Fatty) Liver. Diseases that can cause a fatty liver are listed in Table 12–3 and include metabolic disorders such as glycogen storage diseases (types II and III), fructose intolerance, tyrosinemia, Wilson's disease, and Reye's syndrome. In addition, malnutrition, hyperalimentation, certain drugs (such as steroids), portal tract fibrosis, severe hepatitis, and long-standing congestive heart failure can all cause a similar pattern. Careful clinical correlation with the findings is essential.

Computed Tomography and Magnetic Resonance Imaging. In cirrhosis, both CT and MR can demonstrate changes in the size and shape of the liver, whether from atrophy or parenchymal nodularity (Figure 12–43). Associated findings such as ascites, splenomegaly, and vascular alterations can also be readily visualized. On CT, heterogeneous parenchyma can be observed following contrast enhancement. Fatty infiltration is well shown on enhanced CT scans. Less commonly, enhancement can be uneven, perhaps because of vascular fibrous tissue or differential fat deposition and resorption.

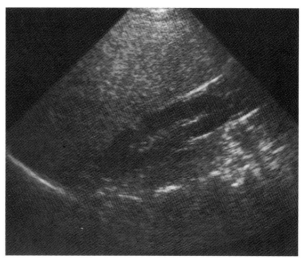

FIGURE 12–42. Fatty Infiltration. Longitudinal US shows hepatomegaly with fatty infiltration and overall increased echogenicity of the liver in this 10-year-old girl.

Nodular fatty infiltration shows no mass effect, is sharply marginated, and has a geographic pattern that enables differentiation from other mass lesions.

Both CT and MR can demonstrate fatty infiltration. Unenhanced images on CT can demonstrate focal or diffuse fatty infiltration. Chemical-shift MR with in-phase and opposed-phase gradient-echo images is used to detect fatty infiltration. Regions of fatty liver appear brighter than the spleen and uninvolved liver on in-phase T1-weighted images and show decreased signal intensity on opposed-phase images (Brown, Naylor, and Yagan, 1997).

TABLE 12–3. Differential Diagnosis of Echogenic Liver

Fat Deposition
Metabolic Disease
Glycogen Storage disease types 1 and 3
Fructose intolerance
Wilson disease
Malnutrition
Hyperalimentation
Drugs
Steroids alone or in combination
Idiopathic
Uncertain Fat Deposition
Portal tract fibrosis
Severe hepatitis
Congestive cardiac failure
Liver Transplant

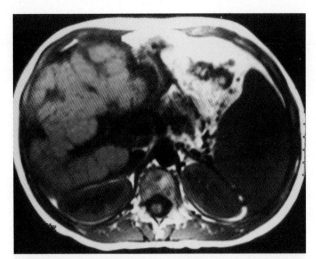

FIGURE 12–43. An 8-year-old girl with biliary atresia and history of previous Kasai repair, with ascending cholangitis. T1-weighted MR (TR 400/TE 11) demonstrates an irregular outline to the liver. There is marked distortion of the parenchyma with numerous low-signal-intensity bands, in keeping with fibrosis. Associated portal hypertension and splenomegaly is present.

Other Imaging Modalities. The nodules are characteristically active and demonstrate uptake on technetium-99m-sulfur colloid radionuclide imaging. Hepatic wedge venography with manometry has been used in the evaluation of liver disease with some predictive success but is rarely indicated.

Hepatic Venous Obstruction

Budd-Chiari syndrome is rarely seen in children. In contrast to the syndrome found in adults, hepatomegaly is usually the only clinical finding. In 70% of cases, no cause for the hepatic venous obstruction is found. The remaining 30% of cases are secondary to leukemia, sickle cell disease, or tumors such as a Wilms' tumor or HCC (Figure 12–44). Congenital diaphragms in the hepatic veins or inferior vena cava may also produce the symptom.

Imaging. Ultrasonography. Ultrasonography is a useful imaging modality in Budd-Chiari syndrome. Ultrasonographic signs reported in the hepatic veins of adults include stenosis, dilatation, thick-wall echoes, thrombosis, abnormal course, and extrahepatic anastomosis of the hepatic veins. There may be reversal of blood flow and obstruction in the inferior vena cava although this may be difficult to detect on US.

In chronic cases, hepatic veins are not seen. Caudal hepatic veins normally can be seen in children, and varying differences in size between cranial and caudal hepatic veins are normal findings. Duplex range-gated Doppler US may show slow or absent flow.

Computed Tomography and Magnetic Resonance Imaging. Although generally not indicated, CT may show ascites, hepatomegaly, and absence of visualization of hepatic veins on contrast enhancement. A fan-shaped area of increased attenuation seen initially on contrast enhancement becomes a more inhomogeneous pattern on later images.

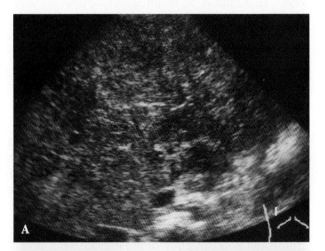

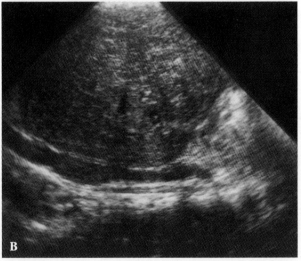

FIGURE 12–44. *A,* Longitudinal US demonstrates diffuse irregular hepatic echogenicity from diffuse involvement of the parenchyma with hepatocellular carcinoma, with thrombus of the portal vein and thrombus within the inferior vena cava. *B,* The same, on axial US. Doppler evaluation demonstrated flow in keeping with malignant thrombus (not shown).

Magnetic resonance imaging can show a striking reduction in caliber or a complete absence of hepatic veins in adults, as well as comma-shaped intrahepatic collateral vessels or marked constriction of the intrahepatic inferior vena cava. The true value of MR, especially in children, has still to be determined, but MR may eventually replace angiography.

Other Imaging Modalities. Plain-film radiography shows no specific features. Liver/spleen scintigraphy findings may be abnormal in some patients. The most specific sign is relative sparing of the caudate lobe of the liver, which may show increased activity on sulfur colloid scanning, probably because of some sparing of the separate venous drainage of the caudate lobe.

Angiography (inferior venacavography, hepatic wedge venography, or celiac or superior mesenteric artery arteriography) is the most effective radiologic investigation for precise delineation of hepatic veins or inferior vena cava. Inferior vena cavography usually shows complete occlusion, an irregular filling defect, or smooth long-segment compression. Hepatic wedge venography characteristically gives a "spider-web" pattern. In addition, an obstructing block may be seen. Celiac or superior mesenteric artery angiography may show slowing or collateral flow.

Hyperkinetic Portal Hypertension

Hyperkinetic portal hypertension is rare in children. It may occur secondary to an arteriovenous fistula such as that uncommonly seen in the spleen in association with Gaucher's disease.

Portal Vein Gas

Gas in the portal system most commonly occurs in infants with necrotizing enterocolitis (see Chapter 6). Other possible causes include inflammatory or infectious enterocolitides, diverticulitis, enterovenous fistula, closed-loop obstruction, intra-abdominal sepsis, hemorrhagic pancreatitis, hepatic artery embolization with liver infarction, peptic ulcer, gastric dilation, and gastric emphysema (Friedman and Dachman, 1994; Faberman and Mayo-Smith, 1997). Very rarely, gas in the portal veins may be related to severe bowel disease due to perforation (see Gastric Volvulus in Chapter 5), gaseous distention, or gangrene in which case it is associated with a high mortality (Benson, 1985). Portal venous gas related to umbilical venous catheters and liver transplantation

may also be present (Swaim and Gerald, 1970; King and Shuckett, 1992).

Plain-film radiography may show portal vein gas as well as indicate the presence of necrotizing enterocolitis or other gut disease. Portal vein gas can be distinguished from biliary tree gas by its more peripheral extension to the edges of the liver and by the clinical history.

Ultrasonography is more sensitive than plain-film radiography (McFadden and Dunlop, 1989). Gas may be detected as strong hyperechoic echoes in the portal vein lumen moving into the periphery of the liver. Bright linear echoes, occasionally coupled with acoustic shadowing and comet tail artifacts, may be present in the portal vein and peripheral branches or in the superior mesenteric vein and parenchyma (Friedman and Dachman, 1994).

Computed tomography is also more sensitive than radiography in detecting portal venous gas (Faberman and Mayo-Smith, 1997).

Liver Transplantation

Liver transplantation is an effective and successful treatment in children with end-stage liver disease. As a result of improved operative techniques and advances in organ preservation, immunosuppressive treatment, and imaging methods, the survival for these patients has substantially increased. Eighty to 90% 5-year survival can be expected even for infants (Baker, Dhawan, and Heaton, 1998). Surgical techniques involve whole liver grafts, segmental grafts, and split-liver transplantation. Refinements in segmented or split-liver transplantation have increased the likelihood of finding a suitable match and providing grafts to smaller children. Improvements in Doppler US and MR have led not only to improved preoperative assessment and management but also to prompt diagnosis and management of postoperative complications.

Indications for Liver Transplantation

Liver transplantation now plays a prominent role in the management of pediatric end-stage liver disease secondary to either acute or chronic disease. Biliary atresia, the most common cause of end-stage pediatric liver disease, is still the most common indication for liver transplantation, accounting for 40 to 50% of cases (Baker, Dhawan, and Heaton, 1998; Kelly, 1998). Other common causes leading to transplantation include metabolic liver disease and acute fulminant hepatic failure. Hepatic tumors, cryptogenic cirrhosis, and chronic active hepatitis are less common indications for transplantation (Westra et al., 1993; Kelly, 1998).

Preoperative Imaging

The major goal of pretransplantation imaging is to detect abnormalities that would preclude successful transplantation or alter the standard surgical approach. Since the demand for donors exceeds the supply, judicious selection of suitable recipients must be made to ensure optimal patient outcome. All recipients undergo abdominal US with color Doppler and duplex US as well as CT. Further evaluation with angiography and MR may be indicated in selected cases.

Ultrasonography. Ultrasonography is generally considered the initial imaging technique in the preoperative evaluation for potential liver transplantation. Doppler US is used to demonstrate the anatomy, size, and patency of hepatic vasculature, particularly the diameter of the extrahepatic portal vein, as well as to provide important morphologic information regarding biliary ductal dilatation, presence of any hepatic mass, and echotexture of the hepatic parenchyma (Ledesma-Medina et al., 1985; Westra et al., 1993; Bowen et al., 1996; Nghiem, 1998). Knowledge of hepatic vascular abnormalities prior to liver transplantation is crucial for the surgeon when planning the arterial and venous anastomosis. Key vascular abnormalities vital to discover preoperatively include portal vein stenosis and thrombosis, celiac axis stenosis, small-caliber hepatic arterial vessels, splenic artery aneurysms, and complete replacement of the origin of the hepatic artery by the superior mesenteric artery (Nghiem, 1998).

Patients with severe liver disease are at increased risk for portal vein stenosis and thrombosis, due to portal hypertension with venous stagnation or secondary malignant thrombosis (Abbitt, 1998). The portal vein's diameter should be carefully measured. On a long-axis ultrasonographic image, the intraluminal diameter of the portal vein is measured with calipers at its midpoint, perpendicular to the lumen. If the vein tapers, it is measured at its widest point. Patients with end-stage cirrhosis (especially due to biliary atresia) may have very small portal veins only a millimeter or two in diameter that may require operative dissection back

to the confluence of the splenic and superior mesenteric veins for anastomosis of the donor portal vein or for the interposition of a portal venous graft. If the main portal venous diameter is less than 4 mm, the vein should be traced to its origin and measured at the confluence of the splenic and superior mesenteric veins. If the portal vein is completely occluded or replaced by cavernous transformation, the superior mesenteric vein must be patent for transplantation to be feasible (Bowen et al., 1996).

Evaluation of celiac axis stenosis (usually due to impingement by the diaphragmatic crura) and detection of small recipient hepatic arteries are important to ensure adequate blood supply to the liver postoperatively. Aortohepatic interpostion graft may be necessary as an alternative inflow source to ensure viability of the graft (Nghiem, 1998). The presence of a splenic artery aneurysm in the intended pretransplant recipient warrants ligation of the artery at the time of the transplantation to prevent postoperative rupture (Ayalon et al., 1988). The anatomic variant of complete replacement of the hepatic artery of the superior mesenteric artery alters the surgical approach of the arterial reconstruction and is therefore important information.

Ultrasonography usually provides all essential anatomic information. However, if US fails to delineate the hepatic vasculature, such as with severe portovenous hypertension or cavernous transformation with prominent collateral vessels, angiography may be necessary to identify the portal vein (Westra et al., 1993; Nghiem, 1998). In addition to the portal vein, the inferior vena cava, the hepatic veins, and the hepatic artery are also evaluated with Doppler US (Skolnick and Dodd, 1993). The presence of a known liver tumor or the discovery of an unsuspected one on US mandates CT imaging to assess the extent of the disease (Bowen et al., 1996).

Computed Tomography. Contrast-enhanced helical CT scan is very useful in the pretransplantation evaluation, providing valuable information for detecting malignancy and vascular abnormalities (Nghiem, 1998). Computed tomography can detect the presence, location, and size of intrahepatic masses and is useful in estimating hepatic volume and evaluating the remainder of the abdomen for extrahepatic spread of tumors. It is also useful in patients with extrahepatic features of portal hypertension, including esophageal and periumbilical collaterals, splenomegaly, and the presence of ascites.

It has been suggested that three-dimensional CT is as accurate as angiography for assessing hepatic arterial anatomy (Nghiem, 1998). However, in most instances, conventional angiography or MRA is performed subsequent to initial abnormal or unexpected US or CT findings.

Magnetic Resonance Imaging. Like CT, MR is becoming increasingly valuable for assessing vascular abnormalities and extent of malignancy. Magnetic resonance imaging including MR angiography both arteriography (MRA) and venography (MRV) are noninvasive techniques free of radiation and therefore of benefit when imaging children. Studies done to date have shown that MR of the portal venous system is at least as accurate as angiography in evaluating the presence and extent of portosystemic collateral vessels, patency, and flow direction of the portal vein (Nghiem, Winter, and Mountford, 1995; Cheng et al., 1997; Stafford-Johnson et al., 1998; Teo, Strouse, and Prince, 1999). For these reasons, MRA/MRV is preferable to angiography if US and/or CT does not satisfactorily define the hepatic vasculature or does not show patency of the superior mesenteric veins in children with portal venous thrombosis (Bowen, Applegate, and Kanal, 1992; Teo, Strouse, and Prince, 1999).

Other Imaging Modalities. Barium meal studies are performed to assess the presence of esophageal varices and to rule out malrotation in biliary atresia (Ledesma-Medina et al., 1985). Detection of esophageal varices is important in considering prophylactic therapy such as insertion of a transjugular intrahepatic portosystemic shunt (TIPS) in waiting for transplantation (Cao et al., 1997; Steventon et al., 1997). In the adult population, the TIPS is extensively used for controlling refractory variceal bleeding before liver transplantation or as palliative care for end-stage liver disease when transplantation is excluded (Crecelius and Soulen, 1995; Kerlan et al., 1995). To date, only a few reports have documented the use of TIPS for treatment of portal hypertension in children (Cao et al., 1997; Steventon et al., 1997).

Angiography is reserved for those children in whom there has been inadequate visualization of portal vein, hepatic vessels, and inferior vena cava by other techniques or for when MR is not available.

Hepatic Transplantation

Liver transplantation may be orthotopic or auxiliary. In orthotopic transplantation, the recipient liver is removed and replaced by the donor liver. Orthotopic liver transplantation requires the grafting of four end-to-end vascular anastomoses and a biliary anastomosis. The vascular anstomoses include suprahepatic and infrahepatic inferior vena cava, the hepatic artery, and the portal vein (Nghiem, 1998). The largest portion of the liver that will fit into the recipient is usually selected. If necessary, a segment of the liver, typically the left lateral segment (segments II and III) can be resected from the donor liver, leaving the hepatic artery, portal vein, and inferior vena cava intact for transplantation into an infant. An additional modification is the split-liver technique, which uses the entire liver for two recipients; the right and left lobes are used for different patients. This technique requires reconstruction of the hepatic artery with the donor iliac artery graft and reconstruction of the portal vein with the donor iliac vein graft prior to transplantation of segments II and III into a child. The donor vessels supplying the liver remain with the right lobe and the medial segment of the left lobe, which are transplanted into an adult (Sollinger et al., 1999) (Figure 12–45). Refinements in split-liver transplantation (which initially had poor results) serve both to reduce the organ shortage and to provide grafts for smaller children (Kelly, 1998)

Auxiliary liver transplantation (ALTx) involves placement of a part of the donor liver in continuity with the native liver. This technique is technically more difficult but has the advantage of retaining the native liver in the event of graft failure or of allowing potential regeneration of the diseased liver, especially if hepatic gene therapy becomes available. It is particularly useful for patients with hepatic enzyme deficiencies in whom the liver is functionally normal but for whom transplantation is required for severe extrahepatic disease (Sollinger et al., 1999). Although its role in the management of other metabolic liver diseases is uncertain, ALTx is now the accepted therapy for Crigler-Najjar type I disease. It has also been used in patients with fulminant hepatic failure although its role in this condition is more controversial. The overall survival rate from the small studies that have been done using this treatment in children is 57%, which is less than that associated with conventional transplantation for this condition (Kelly, 1998).

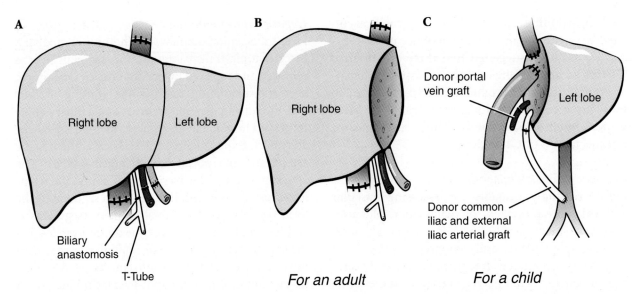

A

B

C

Right lobe

Left lobe

Right lobe

Donor portal
vein graft

Left lobe

Biliary
anastomosis

T-Tube

Donor common
iliac and external
iliac arterial graft

For an adult

For a child

FIGURE 12–45. *A,* Orthotopic transplantation. The donor hepatic artery, common bile duct, portal vein, and supra- and infrahepatic inferior vena cava are divided and anastomosed with the donor vessels. A T-tube stent has been placed in the bile duct. *B,* Right lobe reduced-size liver transplantation. The donor hepatic artery and portal vein branches to this lobe have been preserved. A choledochocholedochostomy over a T-tube was done for bile duct reconstruction. *C,* Split-liver transplantation. The left lateral segment has been reconstructed with donor arterial and venous grafts and implanted in a pediatric patient. The right branches of hepatic artery and portal vein are preserved with the right lobe for transplantation into another patient.

Postoperative Imaging

Routine postoperative imaging is done by US and supplemented by CT, angiography, and MR, as required (Westra et al., 1995). At our institution, a baseline US is performed 24 hours after transplantation, then as clinically or biochemically indicated until discharge.

Expected Postoperative Findings. The normal postoperative appearance of the graft depends on the surgical technique used. At our institution, choledochojejunostomy with placement of an internal/external stent across the anastomosis is used in young children and all patients with biliary atresia. Older children undergo choledochostomy with placement of a T-tube stent and removal of both donor and recipient gallbladders. Hepatic arterial and portal venous anastomoses are end-to-end whenever technically possible. An interposition graft is used if there is a significant size discrepancy. The hepatic segment of the recipient inferior vena cava is resected and the donor segment interposed to reconstruct the inferior vena cava. If a reduced-size or segmental liver transplant has been used, an irregular graft margin is seen (Westra et al., 1993).

Periportal edema is a normal early postoperative finding, seen in approximately 25% of all patients, most likely a result of lymphedema although it may also be seen with acute rejection (Claus and Ph, 1987; Letourneau et al., 1987; Wechsler et al., 1987; Zajko et al., 1988). Fluid collections around the falciform ligament without other fluid collections are also common and should not be confused with intrahepatic fluid collections (Westra et al., 1995) (Figure 12–46).

Complications Related to the Hepatobiliary System. Liver transplant recipients are at risk for the same postoperative complications as any other patient with a major intra-abdominal procedure as well as for complications unique to liver transplantation. Table 12–4 lists the complications of liver transplantation in descending order of frequency (Bowen et al., 1996). Table 12–5 outlines the causes of graft loss leading to retransplantation (Bowen et al., 1996).

Vascular Complications

The most common and significant vascular complication (and a major cause for retransplantation) is hepatic arterial thrombosis which typically occurs

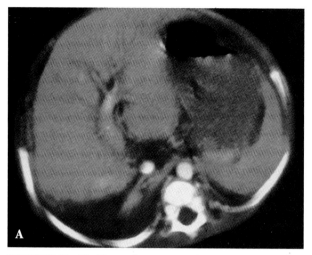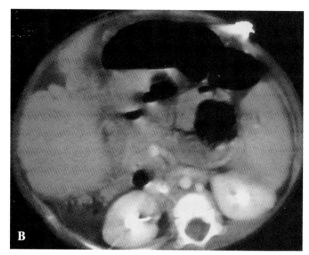

FIGURE 12–46. Normal postoperative appearance of a segmental liver transplant. *A* and *B*, Axial enhanced CT scans done immediately after left lobe segmental transplantation show periportal edema and a small amount of free fluid around the inferior edge of the liver.

within the first 2 months after surgery (Segel et al., 1986; Kaplan, Zajko, and Koneru, 1990; Nghiem, 1998). The overall rate of incidence is 16 to 26% (Westra et al., 1993; Bowen et al., 1996) although this is decreasing with the use of reduced-size grafts (Bowen et al., 1996). The diagnosis of hepatic arterial thrombosis (HAT) may be made with duplex

Doppler US. Dodd et al (Dodd et al., 1994) found that a resistive index of less than 0.5 and systolic acceleration time prolonged to greater than 0.08 seconds on spectral Doppler US were both sensitive and specific for HAT and significant stenosis of the artery. Complete absence of hepatic arterial flow may also be seen although this finding is also seen in other conditions, including severe rejection, massive hepatic necrosis, and systemic hypotension (Rollins et al., 1993; Kok et al., 1995). False-negative results may occur in patients in whom collaterals have developed. These collaterals, however, may sustain graft function indefinitely (Hall et al., 1990). Hepatic arterial thrombosis may be complicated further by fulminant hepatic necrosis, bile leak, and ischemia. Thromboses of the portal vein and inferior vena cava, in contrast, are rare (Nghiem, 1998), with reported incidences of 1 to 13% and 1 to 4% of patients, respectively (Segel

TABLE 12–4. Liver Transplant Complications

Approx. Pediatric Complication	Incidence (%)
Infection	> 60
Rejection	> 50
Vascular clot, stenosis	≤ 40
Hepatic artery thrombosis	≤ 25–40
Portal vein thrombosis/stenosis	≤ 15
Hepatic artery stenosis	≤ 10
IVC thrombosis/stenosis	≤ 5
Renal insufficiency	≤ 25
Hemorrhage	≤ 20
Biliary stenosis, leak	≤ 20
Gastrointestinal	≤ 15
Primary graft dysfunction	≤ 10
Neurologic	8
Posttransplant lymphoproliferative disorder (PTLD)	4
Recurrent liver tumor	Few data
Graft-versus host disease	Uncommon
Chronic hypoxemia	Uncommon

TABLE 5. Causes of Graft Loss in Descending Order of Frequency

Cause	Number
Vascular thromboses	40 %
Rejection	30 %
Primary graft nonfunction	20 %
Biliary tract complications	< 5 %
Hepatitis	< 5 %
Other infections	< 5 %
Other	< 5 %

et al., 1986; Kaplan, Zajko, and Koneru, 1990; Bowen et al., 1996; Nghiem, 1998).

Anastomotic narrowing of the portal vein and inferior vena cava are frequent, while anastomotic narrowing of the hepatic artery occurs less commonly (Bowen et al., 1996). Color Doppler evaluation of stenosis of the portal vein and inferior vena cava shows focal color aliasing with more than three to four times the velocity in the stenosis relative to the prestenotic segment (Nghiem, 1998). Reversal of flow in the hepatic veins or absence of periodicity in the hepatic vein on Doppler tracing are also sensitive indicators of upper inferior vena cava anastomotic stenosis. Ultrasonographic findings in the detection of arterial stenosis are a focal vessel velocity of more than 2 to 3 ms associated with turbulence immediately distal to the stenosis. If direct evaluation of the anastomosis is not possible, then a tardus-parvus waveform seen in measurement of intrahepatic arterial flow is highly suggestive of a significant hepatic artery stenosis. Balloon angioplasty of stenotic vessels has been successfully performed although high-grade hepatic artery stenosis often requires retransplantation (Nghiem, 1998).

Preliminary studies have shown MRA to be highly accurate in diagnosing the vascular complications of liver transplantation outlined above. At this time, MRA is used if US fails to satisfactorily define the hepatic vasculature (Stafford-Johnson et al., 1998).

Hepatic Parenchymal Abnormalities

Clinically, the most important complication is rejection. Current imaging is neither sensitive nor specific for rejection, and the diagnosis is made with a liver biopsy (Claus and Ph, 1987; Zajko et al., 1988; Westra et al., 1993; Holbert, Campbell, and Skolnick, 1995). Rejection is prevalent, occurring in more than half of all liver recipients although the incidence is decreasing with the use of FK506 immunosuppression (Bowen et al., 1996). Reduced portal venous flow velocity and dampening of hepatic venous pulsatility have been observed in patients experiencing acute rejection. These findings may indicate the need for biopsy or closer monitoring of response to treatment; however, the reliability of these findings requires further evaluation (Claus and Ph, 1987).

Infection is the most common postoperative complication, occurring in more than 60% of patients at some time (Bowen et al., 1996). It is most frequently superimposed on hepatic parenchymal infarction. There are three main stages of infection: early (0 to 30 postoperative days), intermediate (31 to 180 days), and late (after 180 days). Early infections are usually bacterial (usually gram-negative) in the area of the graft or are disseminated fungal infections. Intermediate infections include reactivated viruses, opportunistic organisms (including Epstein-Barr virus [EBV], and donor-transmitted organisms). Recurrent cholangitis is the most common late infection (Bowen et al., 1996).

When an abscess is suspected clinically, CT or MR is done. Patients with suspected fungal infection generally undergo both CT and US to increase sensitivity of detection. Disseminated fungal infection appears as multiple defects that may be hyper-, iso- or hypoechoic in the liver, spleen, and kidneys. On CT, these defects appear as multiple hypoattenuating areas in these organs.

Infarction occurs in approximately 10% of cases (Westra et al., 1993). It appears as areas of inhomogeneous hypoechogenicity on US and hypoattentuation on CT and may later develop calcifications. Infarcted areas may liquefy, and if they connect with the biliary tree, they develop into bile-filled cavities or bilomas within the liver parenchyma (Kaplan, Zajko, and Koneru, 1990). The diagnosis of bilomas may be confirmed with needle aspiration and radiographic or scintigraphic demonstration of communication of the cavity with the biliary tree. Complete loss of graft perfusion may be evaluated with nuclear medicine studies using iminodiacetic acid analogues, showing a decline in the functional capacity of the liver, decreased hepatocyte extraction of the radiopharmaceutical, and prolonged retention of the agent in the blood pool (Dodd et al., 1994).

Biliary Complications

Biliary complications occur in 20 to 25% of patients in most series (Westra et al., 1993; Bowen et al., 1996). Anastomotic problems such as stricture, free leakage, and perianastomotic biloma occur most often (Westra et al., 1993) (Figures 12–47, 12–48). Anastomotic narrowing can be successfully treated with balloon angioplasty (Kaplan, Zajko, and Koneru, 1990; Westra et al., 1993). Arterial ischemia (typically resulting from hepatic artery occlusion or severe stenosis) is commonly associated with biliary complications, especially when they are nonanastomotic (Westra et al., 1993). Complications related to

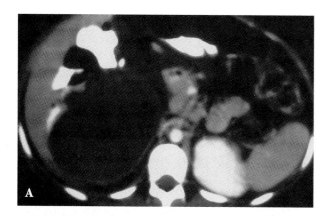

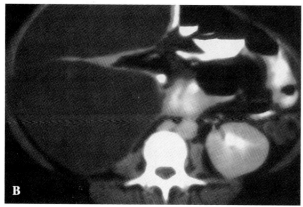

FIGURE 12–47. Biloma. *A* and *B*, Computed tomography shows a large fluid collection medial and inferior to the right lobe of the liver. *C*, Computed tomography after placement of a percutaneous drain shows nearly complete resolution of the collection.

biliary drainage tubes, such as leakage with biloma formation and dislodgment, are seen in a minority of cases. In approximately 5% of patients, progressive dilatation of the extrahepatic bile duct in the absence of clinical or biochemical obstruction may be observed (Westra et al., 1993).

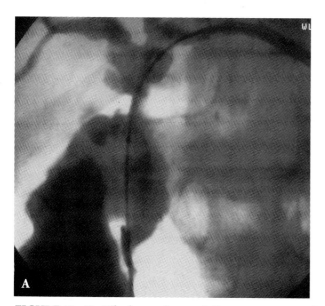

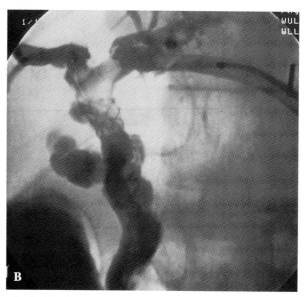

FIGURE 12–48. Bile duct stricture. *A*, Percutaneous transhepatic cholangiography (PTC) shows a stricture of the proximal common bile duct, with dilatation of the right and left intrahepatic and proximal common bile ducts. *B*, Post-balloon-angioplasty PTC demonstrates the disappearance of the bile duct stricture.

Fluid Collections

Postoperative fluid collections in the liver parenchyma and adjacent areas (including subcapsular and perihepatic areas and areas around the falciform ligament) are seen in just over one-third of patients. These collections may represent abscesses, hematomas, bilomas, seromas, or loculated ascites. If it is important clinically to differentiate among them, the diagnosis can be made with percutaneous aspiration. Every fluid collection should be investigated with color Doppler US prior to needle aspiration to ensure that it does not represent a pseudoaneurysm (Westra et al., 1993).

Extrahepatic Complications

Malignancy. Post-transplantation lymphoproliferative disorder (PTLD) is most commonly a B cell proliferation in lymph nodes and solid organs, which has been linked to immunosuppressive therapy and Epstein-Barr virus (EBV) infection (Bowen et al., 1996; Nghiem, 1998). Patients receiving immunosuppressive drugs (typically cyclosporine or tacrolimus) are prone to the formation of malignant tumors due to inhibition of suppressor T cells, allowing B cell proliferation (Nghiem, 1998).

Post-transplantation lymphoproliferative disorder typically develops within the first year of transplantation, with a reported incidence varying from 3 to 19% in pediatric recipients, depending of the age group and type of immunosuppression. Clinical presentation is that of a mononucleosis-like illness. Presentation of lymphadenopathy in the head and neck or single-organ involvement tends to regress when immunosuppression is reduced whereas disseminated or multiorgan involvement has a much worse prognosis (up to 50% mortality) (Bowen et al., 1996).

Computed tomography is most commonly used to determine disease extent. Nodules in solid organs typically appear hypoattenuating on CT scan and hypoechoic on US (Figure 12–49). Well-circumscribed pulmonary nodules with or without intrathoracic adenopathy are highly suggestive of PTLD (Dodd et al., 1992). In addition to lymphoma, unusual neoplasms such as leiomyosarcoma and spindle cell tumors occur with increased incidence, presumably as a result of immunosuppression (Bowen et al., 1996).

Other Complications. Up to 25% of patients suffer from renal insufficiency due to nephrotoxicity of immunosuppressive drugs (McDiarmid et al., 1998). Renal US may be normal or show nonspecific increased echogenicity. Computed tomography may show decreased uptake and delayed excretion of contrast (Bowen et al., 1996).

Neurologic complications occur in about 8% of recipients and include cerebral hemorrhage, ischemia, and focal infarcts (Bowen et al., 1996). They are less prevalent in children than adults but tend to be more severe and result in higher mortality.

Other rare extrahepatic complications include right adrenal hemorrhage, pancreatitis, bowel perforation, splenic infarction, and right phrenic nerve injury (Westra et al., 1993; Bowen et al., 1996). Right phrenic nerve injury occurs in less than 5% of recip-

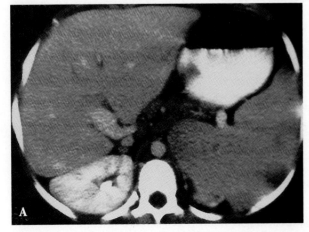 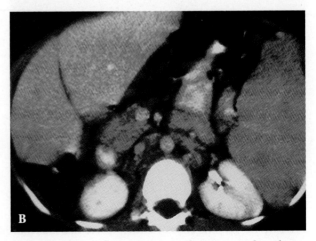

FIGURE 12–49. Post-transplantation lymphoproliferative disease. *A* and *B*, Computed tomography shows hepatosplenomegaly with a focal area of decreased attenuation in the spleen and enlarged retroperitoneal nodes.

ients and results from clamping the adrenal vein during the inferior vena cava anastomosis (Westra et al., 1993). Adrenal hemorrhages rarely require therapy. It is important to differentiate adrenal hemorrhages from more significant abnormalities such as hepatic infarction or subphrenic abscess by identifying their typical location and appearance. Pancreatitis also occurs in less than 5% of recipients but may be severe. It may be due to multiple causes, including transfusion-related hepatitis B, cytomegalovirus infection, traumatic injury during surgery, and immunosuppressive drugs (Westra et al., 1993).

Iron Disorders (Including Transfusional Hemosiderosis)

The liver is the body's main storage depot for iron. This makes the liver susceptible to iron overload. An excess of iron results in either parenchymal or reticuloendothelial deposition, depending on the underlying disease. Accumulation of iron in hepatic parenchymal cells occurs in hereditary hemochromatosis, cirrhosis, and intravascular hemolysis whereas deposition in the reticuloendothelial (RE) system is often a result of multiple transfusions. Distinguishing these two states is important due to differences in treatment and prognosis.

Hereditary Hemochromatosis

Hereditary hemochromatosis is an autosomal recessive disorder of iron metabolism characterized by increased absorption of iron from the gut, resulting in pathologic accumulation within parenchyma of the liver, pancreas, and heart. The involvement of additional organs allows its distinction from iron overload in the reticuloendothelial system (Mergo and Ros, 1998b). Early on, iron overload is confined to the liver (Siegelman et al., 1993). Unlike neonatal hemochromatosis (described below), the onset of symptoms in hereditary hemochromatosis is insidious, and the condition typically does not become clinically manifest until the second decade. Cirrhosis and portal hypertension are seen in patients with advanced hemochromatosis. Treatment is phlebotomy.

The increased density of the deposited iron results in an overall increased hepatic attenuation on CT. However, hyperdense liver on CT is not specific of iron overload since the same appearance may be seen with other disorders, including Wilson's disease, gold deposition, and glycogen storage disease

(Rofsky and Fleishaker, 1995; Mergo and Ros, 1998b). In addition, diagnosis by CT of hepatic iron overload may be limited due to confounding factors of associated steatosis (Rofsky and Fleishaker, 1995).

Findings with MR are more specific due to the paramagnetic properties of stored iron, causing marked decreased signal intensity on T2-weighted images (Figures 12–50C, D). With more severe iron overload, decreased signal on T1-weighted images may be evident. In addition, a strong correlation exists between the concentration of hepatic iron and T2 values (Gomori et al., 1991; Papakonstantinou et al., 1999). T2-weighted gradient-echo imaging is the most sensitive technique, lacking the 180° refocusing pulse, this sequence is sensitive to magnetic susceptibility effects (Siegelman, 1997). The abnormal signal should be compared to that of paraspinal muscles, where a more hypointense liver parenchyma is seen in states of iron excess.

Transfusional Hemosiderosis

Iron from lysed transfused erythrocytes is phagocytized by reticuloendothelial cells within the liver, spleen, and bone marrow. Post-transfusional hemosiderosis is the outcome of repeated transfusion required for treatment of disorders such as thalassemia, sickle cell disease, and other acute or chronic anemias.

After chronic multiple transfusions, the RE system may get saturated, resulting in the development of the more clinically important parenchymal cell iron deposit. Therefore, iron chelation therapy with deferoxamine is used in this patient population to prevent iron-induced organ damage.

The CT and MR findings of transfusional hemosisderosis are the same as in hereditary hemochromatosis, with high attenuation on CT and diffuse low hepatic signal intensity on MR T1- and T2-weighted images (Figure 12–51). Therefore, recognition of extrahepatic signals, evident on MR, can be useful in distinguishing parenchymal from RE involvement (Rofsky and Fleishaker, 1995). In transfusion-related iron overload, abnormal signal intensity is seen only in organs with significant reticuloendothelial activity, including the spleen and bone marrow as well as the liver (Rofsky and Fleishaker, 1995; Mergo and Ros, 1998b). Involvement of other parenchymal organs (such as the pancreas, adrenals, and myocardium) suggests secondary hemochromatosis.

Neonatal Hemochromatosis

Neonatal hemochromatosis, also called idiopathic neonatal iron storage disease, is an uncommon condition characterized by severe hepatic insufficiency and death usually within the first week of life (Barnard and Manci, 1991; Herman and Siegel, 1995). Fulminant hepatic failure develops, with siderosis of parenchymal cells in liver, pancreas, myocardium, thyroid gland, and oral mucosa (Hayes et al., 1992). No excess of iron is found in the RE system. This condition is not a variant of the hereditary hemochromatosis described above; instead, the infants are born with advanced cirrhosis, which becomes symptomatic within the first 24 to 48 hours of life (Barnard and Manci, 1991). Orthotopic liver transplantation seems to be the only option for these children; however, few survivors have been reported (Sigurdsson et al., 1998).

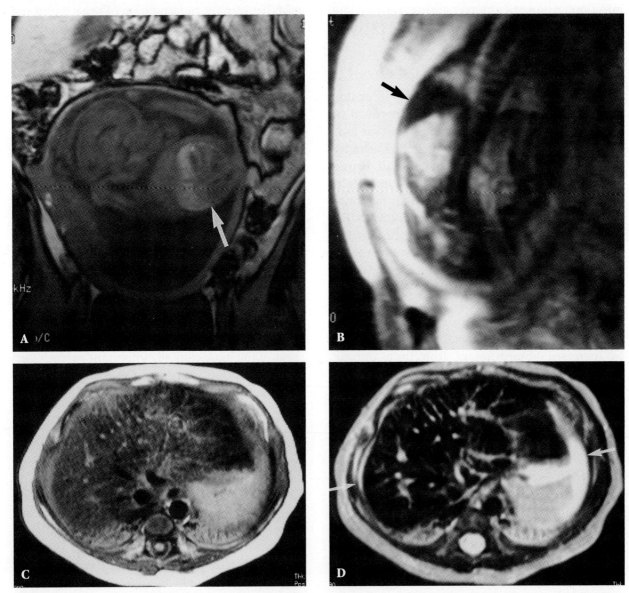

FIGURE 12–50. *A,* Coronal gradient-recalled MR scan of a 30-week fetus with a prior familial history of hemochromatosis. Signal intensity appears similar to that of the maternal liver, seen in the upper left corner. (*Arrow* points to the fetal liver.) *B,* Subsequent MR examination 4 weeks later demonstrates a significant decrease in hepatic signal intensity, in keeping with interval iron deposition. (*Arrow* points to the fetal liver.) *C* and *D,* Postnatal MR scan in the same child. Axial images through the upper abdomen (*C,* T1-weighted and *D,* T2-weighted) on the fourth day of life demonstrate marked decreased signal intensity of the liver, with evidence of ascites. High signal intensity is outlined by *arrows* in *D.*

Definitive diagnosis of neonatal hemochromatosis is usually made by biopsy of the liver or buccal mucosal glands. Magnetic resonance imaging has proved useful in the evaluation of this condition, with findings similar to those of hereditary hemochromatosis in adults (Hayes et al., 1992). Since invasive methods may be hazardous in these neonates due to their poor state of health (including coagulopathy), MR may obviate biopsy.

Prenatal diagnosis of this condition is of interest since early diagnosis and subsequent treatment is vital to prevent hepatic insufficiency. Screening for hepatic iron overload with MR is therefore indicated in a fetus with a family history of neonatal hemochromatosis (Marti-Bonmati et al., 1994) (see Figure 12–50).

Ascites

In many children, as in adults, ascites can arise as a result of many conditions, including a variety of gastrointestinal, genitourinary, cardiac, hepatic, infectious, and lymphatic abnormalities. In neonates, massive ascites as the initial presentation is most commonly thought to be urinary in nature. However, one report from a pediatric hospital shows these cases to be in minority, with bowel disease (malrotation, volvulus, atresia), cardiac arrhythmias, liver disease (cirrhosis, hepatitis), toxoplasmosis, ruptured ovarian cyst, and chylous and idiopathic ascites making up the majority (Griscom, Colodny, and Rosenberg, 1977).

Thin, clear ascitic fluid with a relatively low specific gravity is slightly more radiolucent than liver, so the lateral edge of the liver may be appreciated on plain-film radiographs (Griscom, Colodny, and Rosenberg, 1977; Love, Demos, and Reynes, 1977). Plain-film radiography is specific but not sensitive when compared with US (Bundrick, Cho, and Brewer, 1984).

Ultrasonography is the modality of choice in demonstrating ascitic fluid. Computed tomography and MR are not used to diagnose ascites unless other pathology is suspected, but these modalities will also show the ascitic fluid well.

Hepatic Artery Aneurysm

Hepatic artery aneurysms are rare in children, and their etiology is often obscure. In adults, they are usually secondary to blunt trauma, pancreatitis, or surgery (Wolinski, Gall, and Dubbins, Athey et al.,

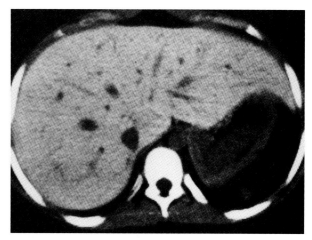

FIGURE 12–51. Iron overload in a child with thalassemia. Axial CT demonstrates prior splenectomy with marked increased parenchymal attenuation of the liver from iron overload.

1986), and preoperative diagnosis can be difficult (Athey, Sax, and Lamki, 1986).

Ultrasonography is the initial investigation of choice and will show the aneurysm as an anechoic well-cirumscribed mass with good through transmission of sound (Athey, Sax, and Lamki, 1986). Feeding vessels may be visible. Duplex Doppler US can confidently confirm the presence of blood flow and is especially useful because pulsation of the mass is unusual and feeding vessels may not be seen (Falkoff, Taylor, and Morse, 1986).

If performed, CT will show a cystic lesion that is dramatically enhanced during intravenous injection of contrast medium. Magnetic resonance imaging will show the presence of the aneurysm as a non-signal-producing mass; no signal is seen as the blood flows through the lesion. Angiography is the modality of choice for confirming the aneurysm and its anatomic location.

REFERENCES

Abbitt PL. Ultrasonography. Update on liver technique. Radiol Clin North Am 1998;36(2):299–307.

Acunas B, Rozanes I, Celik L, et al. Purely cystic hydatid disease of the liver: treatment with percutaneous aspiration and injection of hypertonic saline. Radiology 1992; 182(2):541–3.

Afshani E. Computed tomography of abdominal abscesses in children. Radiol Clin North Am 1981;19(3):515–26.

Akesson E, Loeb J, Wilson-Pauwels L. Thompson's core textbook of anatomy. 2nd ed. Philadelphia: J. B. Lippincott Co.; 1990.

Akhan O, Ozmen MN, Dincer A, et al. Liver hydatid disease: long-term results of percutaneous treatment. Radiology 1996;198(1):259–64.

Allins A, Ho T, Nguyen TH, et al. Limited value of routine followup CT scans in nonoperative management of blunt liver and splenic injuries. Am Surg 1996;62(11):883–6.

Altman RP, Stolar CJ. Pediatric hepatobiliary disease. Surg Clin North Am 1985;65(5):1245–67.

Ammann RW, Eckert J. Cestodes. Echinococcus [published erratum appears in Gastroenterol Clin North Am 1996 Dec;25(4):vii]. Gastroenterol Clin North Am 1996; 25(3):655–89.

Arnand O, Boscq M, Asquier E, et al. Embryonal rhabdomyosarcoma of the biliary tree in children: a case report. Pediatr Radiol 1987;17:250–1.

Arrivé L, Fléjou JF, Vilgrain V, et al. Hepatic adenoma: MR findings in 51 pathologically proved lesions. Radiology 1994;193:507–12.

Arya LS, Ghani R, Abdali S, et al. Pyogenic liver abscesses in children. Clin Pediatr (Phila) 1982;21(2):89–93.

Aslam M, Dore SP, Verbanck JJ, et al. Ultrasonographic diagnosis of hepatobiliary ascariasis. J Ultrasound Med 1993;12(10):573–6.

Athey PA, Sax SL, Lamki N. Sonography in the diagnosis of hepatic artery aneurysms. AJR 1986;147:725–7.

Aucott JN, Ravdin JI. Amebiasis and "nonpathogenic" intestinal protozoa. Infect Dis Clin North Am 1993; 7(3):467–85.

Auh YH, Lim JH, Kim KW, et al. Loculated fluid collections in hepatic fissures and recesses: CT appearance and potential pitfalls. Radiographics 1994;14(3):529–40.

Auh YH, Rubenstein W, Zirinsky K, et al. Accessory fissures of the liver: CT and sonographic appearance. AJR 1984;143:565–72.

Ayalon A, Wiesner RH, Perkins JD, et al. Splenic artery aneurysms in liver transplant patients. Transplantation 1988;45(2):386–9.

Baehner RL. Chronic granulomatous disease of childhood: clinical, pathological, biochemical, molecular, and genetic aspects of the disease. Pediatr Pathol 1990;10(1–2):143–53.

Baker A, Dhawan A, Heaton N. Who needs a liver transplant? (new disease specific indications). Arch Dis Child 1998;79(5):460–4.

Balfe DM, Mauro MA, Koehler RE, et al. Gastrohepatic ligament: normal and pathologic CT anatomy. Radiology 1984;150(2):485–90.

Barnard JAD, Manci E. Idiopathic neonatal iron-storage disease. Gastroenterology 1991;101(5):1420–7.

Baron RL. Detection of liver neoplasms: techniques and outcomes. Abdom Imaging 1994;19:320–4.

Bayraktar Y, Balkanci F, Kayhan B, et al. Congenital hepatic fibrosis associated with cavernous transformation of the portal vein. Hepatogastroenterology 1997;44(18):1588–94.

Becker CD, Gal I, Baer HU, et al. Blunt hepatic trauma in adults: correlation of CT injury grading with outcome. Radiology 1996;201(1):215–20.

Beggs I. The radiological appearances of hydatid disease of the liver. Clin Radiol 1983;34(5):555–63.

Beggs I. The radiology of hydatid disease. AJR 1985; 145(3):639–48.

Belli L, Romani F, Riolo F, et al. Thrombosis of portal vein in absence of hepatic disease. Surg Gynecol Obstet 1989; 169(1):46–9.

Benson MD. Case report: adult survival with intrahepatic portal venous gas secondary to acute gastric dilatation, with a review of portal venous gas. Clin Radiol 1985;36:441–3.

Bezzi M, Teggi A, De Rosa F, et al. Abdominal hydatid disease: US findings during medical treatment. Radiology 1987;162(1 Pt 1):91–5.

Blane CE, Jongeward RH Jr, Silver TM. Sonographic features of hepatocellular disease in neonates and infants. AJR 1983;141(6):1313–6.

Bloomfield JA. Hydatid disease in children and adolescents. Australas Radiol 1980;24(3):277–83.

Bowen A, Applegate GR, Kanal E. Sonography vs MR imaging in children who are candidates for liver transplantation [letter; comment]. AJR 1992;158(3):692–3.

Bowen A, Hungate RG, Kaye RD, et al. Imaging in liver transplantation. Radiol Clin North Am 1996;34(4):757–78.

Branum GD, Tyson GS, Branum MA, et al. Hepatic abscess. Changes in etiology, diagnosis, and management. Ann Surg 1990;212(6):655–62.

Bressler EL, Alpern MB. Hypervascular hepatic metastases: reevaluation of unenhanced CT scans. AJR 1995; 164:512–3.

Bret PM, Fond A, Bretagnolle M, et al. Percutaneous aspiration and drainage of hydatid cysts in the liver. Radiology 1988;168(3):617–20.

Brick SH, Taylor GA, Potter BM, et al. Hepatic and splenic injury in children: role of CT in the decision for laparotomy. Radiology 1987;165(3):643–6.

Brook I, Fraizer EH. Role of anaerobic bacteria in liver abscesses in children. Pediatr Infect Dis J 1993;12(9):743–7.

Brown JJ, Naylor MJ, Yagan N. Imaging of hepatic cirrhosis. Radiology 1997;202(1):1–16.

Brunelle F, Chaumont P. Hepatic tumors in children: ultrasonic differentiation of malignant from benign lesions. Radiology 1984;150:695–9.

Brunelle F, Tammam S, Odievre M, et al. Liver adenomas in glycogen storage disease in children. Ultrasound and angiographic study. Pediatr Radiol 1984;14:94–101.

Bulas DI, Eichelberger MR, Sivit CJ, et al. Hepatic injury from blunt trauma in children: follow-up evaluation with CT. AJR 1993; 160(2):347–51.

Bundrick TJ, Cho SR, Brewer WH. Ascites: comparison of plain film radiographs with ultrasonograms. Radiology 1984;152:503–6.

Burkitt H, Young B, Heath J. Wheater's functional histology: a text and colour atlas. 3rd ed. Churchill Livingstone; 1997.

Burton BE, Amin EA, Tisdale P. Bipartite liver: a case report. Clin Nucl Med 1987;12(8):641–3.

Callen PW, Filly RA, DeMartini WJ. The left portal vein: a possible source of confusion on ultrasonograms. Radiology 1979;130:205–6.

Callen PW, Filly RA, Marcus FS. Ultrasonography and computed tomography in the evaluation of hepatic microabscesses in the immunosuppressed patient. Radiology 1980;136(2):433–4.

Cao S, Monge H, Semba C, et al. Emergency transjugular intrahepatic portosystemic shunt (TIPS) in an infant: a case report. J Pediatr Surg 1997;32(1):125–7.

Carcassonne M, Aubrespy P, Dor V, et al. Hydatid cysts in childhood. Prog Pediatr Surg 1973;5:1–35.

Caremani M, Benci A, Maestrini R, et al. Abdominal cystic hydatid disease (CHD): classification of sonographic appearance and response to treatment. J Clin Ultrasound 1996;24(9):491–500.

Carr D, Duncan JG, Railton R, et al. Liver volume determination by ultrasound: a feasibility study. Br J Radiol 1976;49(585):776–8.

Cerri GG, Alves VA, Magalhaes A. Hepatosplenic schistosomiasis mansoni: ultrasound manifestations. Radiology 1984;153(3):777–80.

Cerri GG, Leite GJ, Simoes JB, et al. Ultrasonographic evaluation of ascaris in the biliary tract. Radiology 1983; 146(3):753–4.

Chafetz N, Filly RA. Portal and hepatic veins: accuracy of margin echoes for distinguishing intrahepatic vessels. Radiology 1979;130:725–8.

Champetier J, Yver R, Letoublon C, et al. A general review of anomalies of hepatic morphology and their clinical implications. Anat Clin 1985;7:285–99.

Cheng YF, Huang TL, Lui CC, et al. Magnetic resonance venography in potential pediatric liver transplant recipients. Clin Transplant 1997;11(2):121–6.

Cherqui D, Rahmouni A, Charlotte F, et al. Management of focal nodular hyperplasia and hepatocellular adenoma in young women. A series of 41 patients with clinical radiologic and pathologic correlation. Hepatology 1995; 22:1674–81.

Cheung H, Ambrose RE, Lee PO. Liver hamartomas in tuberous sclerosis. Clin Radiol 1993;47:421–3.

Cheung H, Lai YM, Loke TK, et al. The imaging diagnosis of hepatic schistosomiasis japonicum sequelae. Clin Radiol 1996;51(1):51–5.

Choi BI, Kim CW, Han MC, et al. Sonographic characteristics of small hepatocellular carcinoma. Gastrointest Radiol 1989;14:255–61.

Choji K, Fujita N, Chen M, et al. Alveolar hydatid disease of the liver: computed tomography and transabdominal ultrasound with histopathological correlation. Clin Radiol 1992;46(2):97–103.

Choji K, Shinohara M, Nojima T, et al. Significant reduction of the echogenicity of the compressed cavernous hemangioma. Acta Radiol 1988;29:317–20.

Chou CK, Mak CN, Lin MB, et al. CT of agenesis and

atrophy of the right hepatic lobe. Abdom Imaging 1998;23:603–7.

Chung KY, Mayo-Smith WW, Saini S, et al. Hepatocellular adenoma: MR imaging features with pathologic correlation. AJR 1995;165:303–8.

Chung T, Hoffer FA, Burrows PE, et al. MR imaging of hepatic hemangiomas of infancy and changes seen with interferon alpha-2a treatment. Pediatr Radiol 1996;26:341–8.

Chusid MJ. Pyogenic hepatic abscess in infancy and childhood. Pediatrics 1978;62(4):554–9.

Clarke HM, Hinde FR, Manns RA. Case report: hepatic ultrasound findings in a case of toxocariasis. Clin Radiol 1992;46(2):135–6.

Claus D, Ph C. Liver transplantation in children: role of the radiologist in the preoperative assessment and the postoperative follow-up. Transplantation Proc 1987;19(4):3344–57.

Clement O, Siauve N, Lewin M, et al. Contrast agents in magnetic resonance imaging of the liver: present and future. Biomed Pharmacother 1998;52:51–8.

Colon AR. Textbook of pediatric hepatology. 2nd ed. Chicago: Year Book Medical Publishers Inc.; 1990.

Cooper A. Liver injuries in children: treatments tried, lessons learned. Semin Pediatr Surg 1992;1(2):152–61.

Cormack D. Essential histology. Philadelphia: J. B. Lippincott Co.; 1993.

Corrigan K, Semelka RC. Dynamic contrast-enhanced MR imaging of fibrolamellar hepatocellular carcinoma. Abdom Imaging 1995;20:122–5.

Crecelius SA, Soulen MC. Transjugular intrahepatic portosystemic shunts for portal hypertension. Gastroenterol Clin North Am 1995;24(2):201–19.

Cremin BJ. Ultrasonic diagnosis of biliary ascariasis: "a bull's eye in the triple O." Br J Radiol 1982;55(657):683–4.

Cumming WA, Kays DW. Posterior hepatodiaphragmatic interposition of the colon complicated by appendicitis. J Pediatr Surg 1994;29(12):1626–7.

Cywes S, Bass DH, Rode H, et al. Blunt liver trauma in children. Injury 1991;22(4):310–4.

Dachman AH, Lichtenstein JE, Friedman AC, et al. Infantile hemangioendothelioma of the liver: a radiologic-pathologic-clinical correlation. AJR 1983;140:1091–6.

Dachman AH, Pakter RL, Ros PR, et al. Hepatoblastoma: radiologic-pathologic correlation in 50 cases. Radiology 1987;164:15–9.

Daneman A. Pediatric body CT. London: Springer-Verlag; 1987.

Davey MS, Cohen MD. Imaging of gastrointestinal malignancy in childhood. Radiol Clin North Am 1996;34:717–42.

de Diego Choliz J, Lecumberri Olaverri FJ, Franquet Casas T, et al. Computed tomography in hepatic echinococcosis. AJR 1982;139(4):699–702.

de Lange EE, Mugler JP III, Gay SB, et al. Focal liver disease: comparison of breath-hold T1-weighted MP-GRE MR imaging and contrast-enhanced CT-lesion detection, localization, and characterization. Radiology 1996;200:465–73.

Dehner LP, Kissane JM. Pyogenic hepatic abscesses in infancy and childhood. J Pediatr 1969;74(5):763–73.

DeLand F, North W. Relationship between liver size and body size. Radiology 1968;91:1195–8.

DeLorimier AA, Simpson EB, Baum RS, et al. Hepatic-artery ligation for hepatic hemangiomatosis. N Engl J Med 1967;277(7):333–7.

Demirci A, Diren HB, Selcuk MB. Computed tomography in agenesis of the right lobe of the liver. Acta Radiol 1990;31:105–6.

Diament MJ, Parvey LS, Tonkin ILD, et al. Hepatoblastoma: technetium sulfur colloid uptake simulating focal nodular hyperplasia. AJR 1982;139:168–71.

Didier D, Weiler S, Rohmer P, et al. Hepatic alveolar echinococcosis: correlative US and CT study. Radiology 1985;154(1):179–86.

Dilsiz A, Acikgozoglu S, Gunel E, et al. Ultrasound-guided percutaneous drainage in the treatment of children with hepatic hydatid disease. Pediatr Radiol 1997;27(3):230–3.

Dodd GD, Ledesma-Medina J, Baron RL, et al. Posttransplant lymphoproliferative disorder: intrathoracic manifestations. Radiology 1992;184:65–9.

Dodd GD, Memel DS, Zajko AB, et al. Hepatic artery stenosis and thrombosis in transplant recipients: Doppler diagnosis with resistive index and systolic acceleration time. Radiology 1994;192:657–61.

Donnelly LF, Bisset GS. Pediatric hepatic imaging. Radiol Clin North Am 1998;36(2):413–27.

Donoso L, Martinez-Noguera A, Zidan A, et al. Papillary process of the caudate lobe of the liver: sonographic appearance. Radiology 1989;173(3):631–3.

Donovan AT, Wolverson MK, de Mello D, et al. Multicystic hepatic mesenchymal hamartoma of childhood: computerized tomography and ultrasound characteristics. Pediatr Radiol 1981;11:163–5.

Drane WE. Scintigraphic techniques for hepatic imaging. Update for 2000. Radiol Clin North Am 1998;36(2):309–18.

Dupas B, Barrier J, Barre P. Detection of Toxocara by computed tomography. Br J Radiol 1986;59(701):518–9.

What is an arteriovenous malformation? [editorial]. Cardiovasc Intervent Radiol 1987;10:53–4.

Edmondson HA. Differential diagnosis of tumors and tumor-like lesions of the liver in infancy and childhood. Am J Dis Child 1956;91:168–86.

Elizondo G, Weissleder R, Stark DD, et al. Amebic liver abscess: diagnosis and treatment evaluation with MR imaging. Radiology 1987;165(3):795–800.

Elliott DE. Schistosomiasis. Pathophysiology, diagnosis, and treatment. Gastroenterol Clin North Am 1996;25(3):599–625.

el-Tahir MI, Omojola MF, Malatani T, et al. Hydatid disease of the liver: evaluation of ultrasound and computed tomography. Br J Radiol 1992;65(773):390–2.

Erdener A, Ozok G, Demircan M. Surgical treatment of hepatic hydatid disease in children. Eur J Pediatr Surg 1992;2(2):87–9.

Faberman RS, Mayo-Smith WW. Outcome of 17 patients with portal venous gas detected by CT. AJR 1997;169:1535–8.

Falkoff GE, Taylor KJW, Morse S. Hepatic artery pseudoaneurysm: diagnosis with real-time and pulsed Doppler US. Radiology 1986;158:155–6.

Farhi DC, Shikes RH, Murari PJ, et al. Hepatocellular carcinoma in young people. Cancer 1983;52:1516–25.

Farrant P, Meire HB, Karani J. Ultrasound diagnosis of portocaval anastomosis in infantsóa report of eight cases. Br J Radiol 1996;69(821):389–93.

Farrelly C, Lawrie BW. Diagnosis of intrabiliary rupture of hydatid cyst of the liver by fine- needle percutaneous transhepatic cholangiograhy. Br J Radiol 1982;55(653):372–4.

Farron F, Gudinchet F, Genton N. Hepatic trauma in children: long-term follow-up. Eur J Pediatr Surg 1996;6(6):347–9.

Fataar S, Bassiony H, Satyanath S, et al. Characteristic sonographic features of schistosomal periportal fibrosis. AJR 1984;143(1):69–71.

Fernandez MDP, Redvanly RD. Primary hepatic malignant neoplasms. Radiol Clin North Am 1998;36(2):333–48.

Ferrucci JT. Advances in abdominal MR imaging. Radiographics 1998;18(6):1569–86.

Filiatrault D, Garel L. Commentary: pediatric blunt abdominal traumaóto sound or not to sound? Pediatr Radiol 1995;25(5):329–31.

Filice C, Pirola F, Brunetti E, et al. A new therapeutic approach for hydatid liver cysts. Aspiration and alcohol injection under sonographic guidance. Gastroenterology 1990;98(5 Pt 1):1366–8.

Finlay JC, Speert DP. Sylvatic hydatid disease in children: case reports and review of endemic *Echinococcus granulosus* infection in Canada and Alaska. Pediatr Infect Dis J 1992;11(4):322–6.

Fischer A, Segal AW, Seger R, et al. The management of chronic granulomatous disease. Eur J Pediatr 1993;152(11):896–9.

Fishman LN, Jonas MM, Lavine JE. Update on viral hepatitis in children. Pediatr Clin North Am 1996;43(1):57–74.

Fitzgerald EJ, Coblentz C. Fungal microabscesses in immuno-suppressed patients' CT appearances. Can Assoc Radiol J 1988;39(1):10–2.

Fitzgerald R, Hale M, Williams CR. Case report: accessory lobe of the liver mimicking lesser omental lymphadenopathy. Br J Radiol 1993;66(789):839–41.

Foley WD, Jochem RJ. Computed tomography. Focal and diffuse liver disease. Radiol Clin North Am 1991;29(6):1213–33.

Forrest CB, Forehand JR, Axtell RA, et al. Clinical features and current management of chronic granulomatous disease. Hematol Oncol Clin North Am 1988;2(2):253–66.

Forsberg L, Floren CH, Hederstrom E, et al. Ultrasound examination in diffuse liver disease. Clinical significance of enlarged lymph nodes in the hepato-duodenal ligament. Acta Radiol 1987;28(3):281–4.

Foucor E, Williamson RA, Yiu-Chiu V, et al. Mesenchymal hamartoma of the liver identified by fetal sonography. AJR 1983;140:970–2.

Francis IR, Agha FP, Thompson NW, et al. Fibrolamellar hepatocarcinoma: clinical, radiologic, and pathologic features. Gastrointest Radiol 1986;11:67–72.

Francis IR, Glazer GM, Amendola MA, et al. Hepatic abscesses in the immunocompromised patient: role of CT in detection, diagnosis, management, and follow-up. Gastrointest Radiol 1986;11(3):257–62.

Franken EA, Smith WL, Cohen MD, et al. Hepatic imaging in stage N-S neuroblastoma. Pediatr Radiol 1986;16:107–9.

Frayha HH, Biggar WD. Chronic granulomatous disease of childhood: a changing pattern? J Clin Immunol 1983; 3(3):287–91.

Frider B, Marin AM, Goldberg A. Ultrasonographic diagnosis of portal vein cavernous transformation in children. J Ultrasound Med 1989;8(8):445–9.

Fried AM, Kreel L, Cosgrove DO. The hepatic interlobar fissure: combined in vitro and in vivo study. AJR 1984; 143:561–4.

Friedburg H, Kauffmann GW, Bohn N, et al. Sonographic and computed tomographic features of embryonal rhabdomyosarcoma of the biliary tract. Pediatr Radiol 1984;14:436–8.

Friedman A, Dachman A. Radiology of the liver, biliary tract and pancreas. St. Louis: Mosby Year Book; 1994.

Fujimoto M, Moriyasu F, Nishikawa K, et al. Color doppler sonography of hepatic tumors with a galactose-based contrast agent: correlation with angiographic findings. AJR 1994;163:1099–1104.

Furuse J, Matsutani S, Yoshikawa M, et al. Diagnosis of portal vein tumor thrombus by pulsed Doppler ultrasonography. J Clin Ultrasound 1992;20:439–46.

Gabaldon A, Mofidi C, Morishita K, et al. Control of aschariasis (report of a WHO expert committee). WHO Tech Rep Ser 1967;379:6–7.

Garden AS, Roberts N. Obstetrics: fetal and fetal organ volume estimations with magnetic resonance imaging. Am J Obstet Gynecol 1996;175(2):442–8.

Garel LA, Pariente DM, Nezelof C, et al. Liver involvement in chronic granulomatous disease: the role of ultrasound in diagnosis and treatment. Radiology 1984;153(1):117–21.

Gazelle G, Saini S, Mueller P. Hepatobiliary and pancreatic radiology: imaging and intervention. New York: Thieme Medical Publishers, Inc.; 1998.

Gazelle GS, Haaga JR. Hepatic neoplasms: surgically relevant segmental anatomy and imaging techniques. AJR 1992;158:1015–8.

Geoffray A, Couanet D, Montagne JP, et al. Ultrasonography and computed tomography for diagnosis and follow up of biliary duct rhabdomyosarcomas in children. Pediatr Radiol 1987;17:127–31.

George JC, Cohen MD, Tarver RD, et al. Ruptured cystic mesenchymal hamartoma: an unusual cause of neonatal ascites. Pediatr Radiol 1994;24:304–5.

Gharbi HA, Hassine W, Brauner MW, et al. Ultrasound examination of the hydatic liver. Radiology 1981;139(2): 459–63.

Gibney RG, Hendin AP, Cooperberg PL. Sonographically detected hepatic hemangiomas: Absence of change over time. AJR 1987;149:953–7.

Gillard J, Patel M, Abrahams P, et al. Riedel's lobe of the liver: fact or fiction? Clin Anat 1998;11:47–9.

Giorgio A, Tarantino L, Francica G, et al. Unilocular hydatid liver cysts: treatment with US-guided, double percutaneous aspiration and alcohol injection. Radiology 1992;184(3):705–10.

Giorgio A, Tarantino L, Mariniello N, et al. Pyogenic liver abscesses: 13 years of experience in percutaneous needle aspiration with US guidance. Radiology 1995;195(1):122–4.

Giovagnoni A, Gabrielli O, Coppa GV, et al. MRI appearances in amoebic granulomatous hepatitis: a case report. Pediatr Radiol 1993;23(7):536–7.

Goldberg MA, Hahn PF, Saini S, et al. Value of T1 and T2 relaxation times from echoplanar MR imaging in the characterization of focal hepatic lesions. AJR 1993;160:1011–17.

Goldenring JM, Flores M. Primary liver abscesses in children and adolescents. Review of 12 years clinical experience. Clin Pediatr (Phila) 1986;25(3):153–8.

Golli M, Tran Van Nhieu J, Mathieu D, et al. Hepatocellular adenoma: Color doppler US and pathologic correlations. Radiology 1994;190:741–4.

Gomori JM, Horev G, Tamary H, et al. Hepatic iron overload: quantitative MR imaging. Radiology 1991;179(2): 367–9.

Gorg C, Weide R, Schwerk WB, et al. Ultrasound evaluation of hepatic and splenic microabscesses in the immunocompromised patient: sonographic patterns, differential diagnosis, and follow-up. J Clin Ultrasound 1994;22(9):525–9.

Grandin C, Van Beers BE, Robert A, et al. Benign hepatocellular tumors: MRI after superparamagnetic iron oxide administration. J Comput Assist Tomogr 1995;19(3):412–18.

Griffin J, Jennings C, Owens A. Hepatic amoebic abscess communicating with the biliary tree. Br J Radiol 1983;56(671):887–90.

Griscom NT, Colodny AH, Rosenberg HK. Diagnostic aspects of neonatal ascites: report of 27 cases. AJR 1977;128:961–70.

Grumbach K, Coleman BG, Gal AA, et al. Hepatic and biliary tract abnormalities in patients with AIDS. Sonographic-pathologic correlation. J Ultrasound Med 1989;8(5):247–54.

Gupta RK, Pant CS, Prakash R, et al. Sonography in complicated hepatic amoebic abscess. Clin Radiol 1987;38(2):123–6.

Gurses N, Sungur R, Ozkan K. Ultrasound diagnosis of liver hydatid disease. Acta Radiol 1987;28(2):161–3.

Hackworth CA, Leef JA, Rosenblum JD, et al. Transjugular intrahepatic portosystemic shunt creation in children: initial clinical experience. Radiology 1998;206(1):109–14.

Hadidi A. Sonography of hepatic echinococcal cysts. Gastrointest Radiol 1982;7(4):349–54.

Haffar A, Boland FJ, Edwards MS. Amebic liver abscess in children. Pediatr Infect Dis 1982;1(5):322–7.

Hall TR, Mc Diarmid SV, Grant EG, et al. False-negative duplex doppler studies in children with hepatic artery thrombosis after liver transplantation. AJR 1990;154:573–5.

Halvorsen RA Jr, Foster WL Jr, Wilkinson RH Jr, et al. Hepatic abscess: sensitivity of imaging tests and clinical findings. Gastrointest Radiol 1988;13(2):135–41.

Halvorsen RA, Jones MA, Rice RP, et al. Anterior left subphrenic abscess: characteristic plain film and CT appearance. AJR 1982;139(2):283–9.

Halvorsen RA, Korobkin M, Foster WL, et al. The variable CT appearance of hepatic abscesses. AJR 1984;142(5):941–6.

Ham JM. Partial and complete atrophy affecting hepatic segments and lobes. Br J Surg 1979;66:333–7.

Hamrick-Turner JE, Shipkey FH, Cranston PE. Fibrolamellar hepatocellular carcinoma: MR appearance mimicking focal nodular hyperplasia. J Comput Assist Tomogr 1994;18(2):301–4.

Harada N, Ohshima I, Asano T, et al. Right hepatic lobe agenesis associated with bile duct carcinoma. Abdom Imaging 1995;20:456–8.

Harris KM, Morris DL, Tudor R, et al. Clinical and radiographic features of simple and hydatid cysts of the liver. Br J Surg 1986;73(10):835–8.

Hartleb M, Nowak A, Scieszka J. Hepatic pseudotumour - caudate lobe sparing in fatty liver. Eur J Ultrasound 1995;2:297–9.

Harty MP, Hebra A, Ruchelli ED, et al. Ciliated hepatic foregut cyst causing portal hypertension in an adolescent. AJR 1998;170(3):688–90.

Hasaart TH, Delarue MW, Bruine AP. Intra-partum fetal death due to thrombosis of the ductus venosus: a clinico-pathological case report. Eur J Obstet Gynecol Reprod Biol 1994;56:201–3.

Hashimoto L, Hermann R, Grundfest-Broniatowski S. Pyogenic hepatic abscess: results of current management. Am Surg 1995;61(5):407–11.

Hashimoto M, Oomachi K, Watarai J. Accessory lobe of the liver mimicking a mass in the left adrenal gland. Acta Radiol 1997;38:309–10.

Hayden CK Jr, Toups M, Swischuk LE, et al. Sonographic features of hepatic amebiasis in childhood. Can Assoc Radiol J 1984;35(3):279–82.

Hayes AM, Jaramillo D, Levy HL, et al. Neonatal hemochromatosis: diagnosis with MR imaging. AJR 1992;159(3):623–5.

Hazebroek FWJ, Tibboel D, Robben SGF, et al. Hepatic artery ligation for hepatic vascular tumors with arteriovenous and arterioportal venous shunts in the newborn: successful management of two cases and review of the literature. J Pediatr Surg 1995;30(8):1127–30.

Healey JE. Vascular anatomy of the liver. Ann N Y Acad Sci 1970;170:8–17.

Heaton ND, Davenport M, Karani J, et al. Congenital hepatoportal arteriovenous fistula. Surgery 1995;117(2):170–4.

Heiken JP, Lee JKT, Glazer HS, et al. Hepatic metastases studies with MR and CT. Radiology 1985;156:423–7.

Herman TE. Extensive hepatic calcification secondary to fulminant neonatal syphilitic hepatitis. Pediatr Radiol 1995;25(2):120–2.

Herman TE, Siegel MJ. Special imaging casebook. Neonatal hemochromatosis. J Perinatol 1995;15(4):338–40.

Hillman BJ, D' Orsi CJ, Smith EH, et al. Ultrasonic appearance of the falciform ligaments. AJR 1979;132:205–6.

Hochbergs P, Forsberg L, Hederstrom E, et al. Diagnosis and percutaneous treatment of pyogenic hepatic abscesses. Acta Radiol 1990;31(4):351–3.

Hoff FL, Aisen AM, Walden ME, et al. MR imaging in hydatid disease of the liver. Gastrointest Radiol 1987; 12(1):39–42.

Holbert BL, Campbell WL, Skolnick ML. Evaluation of the transplanted liver and postoperative complications. Radiol Clin North Am 1995;33(3):521–40.

Hopkins KL, Simoneaux SF, Patrick LE, et al. Imaging manifestations of cat-scratch disease. AJR 1996;166(2): 435–8.

Howard E. Aetiology of portal hypertension and anomalies of the portal venous system. In: Howard E, editor. Surgery of liver disease in children. Oxford: Butterworth Heinemann; 1991. p. 151–6.

Huang CJ, Pitt HA, Lipsett PA, et al. Pyogenic hepatic abscess. Changing trends over 42 years. Ann Surg 1996;223(5):600–9.

Hubbard A, Meyer J, Mahboubi S. Diagnosis of liver disease in children: value of MR angiography. AJR 1992; 159:617–21.

Hughes LA, Hartnell GG, Finn JP, et al. Time-of-flight MR angiography of the portal venous system: value compared with other imaging procedures. AJR 1996;166:375–8.

Hussain S. Diagnostic criteria of hydatid disease on hepatic sonography. J Ultrasound Med 1985;4(11):603–7.

Ikeda S, Yamaguchi Y, Sera Y, et al. Surgical corraction of patent ductus venosus in three brothers. Dig Dis Sci 1999;44(3):582–9.

Itai Y, Sekiyama K, Ahmadi T, et al. Fulminant hepatic failure: observation with serial CT. Radiology 1997; 202(2):379–82.

Itoh K, Nishimura K, Togashi K, et al. Hepatocellular carcinoma: MR imaging. Radiology 1987;164:21–5.

Jacobs JE, Birnbaum BA. Computed tomography imaging of focal hepatic lesions. Semin Roentgenol 1995;30(4): 308–23.

Jacobson AF, Teefey SA. Cavernous hemangiomas of the liver association of sonographic appearance and results of Tc-99m labeled red blood cell SPECT. Clin Nucl Med 1994;19(2):96–9.

Jeffrey RB Jr, Tolentino CS, Chang FC, et al. CT of small pyogenic hepatic abscesses: the cluster sign. AJR 1988; 151(3):487–9.

Johnson JL, Baird JS, Hulbert TV, et al. Amebic liver abscess in infancy: case report and review. Clin Infect Dis 1994;19(4):765–7.

Johnston RB, Newman SL. Chronic granulomatous disease. Pediatr Clin North Am 1977;24(2):365–76.

Juimo AG, Gervez F, Angwafo FF. Extraintestinal amebiasis. Radiology 1992;182(1):181–3.

Juul N, Sztuk FJ, Torp-Pedersen S, et al. Ultrasonically guided percutaneous treatment of liver abscesses. Acta Radiol 1990;31(3):275–7.

Kainberger FM, Vergesslich KA, Eilenberger M, et al. Color-coded Doppler evaluation of cholecystic varices in portal hypertension. Pediatr Radiol 1990;21(1):71–2.

Kakitsubata Y, Kakitsubata S, Asada K, et al. MR imaging of anomalous lobes of the liver. Acta Radiol 1993;34:417–9.

Kakitsubata Y, Kakitsubata S, Asada K, et al. Anomalous right lobe of the liver: CT appearance. Gastrointest Radiol 1991;16:326–8.

Kakitsubata Y, Kakitsubata S, Watanabe K. Hypoplasia of the right hepatic lobe with ectopy of the gallbladder. Clin Imaging 1995;19(2):85–7.

Kalovidouris A, Gouliamos A, Vlachos L, et al. MRI of abdominal hydatid disease. Abdom Imaging 1994;19(6): 489–94.

Kammerer WS, Schantz PM. Echinococcal disease. Infect Dis Clin North Am 1993;7(3):605–18.

Kanematsu M, Imaeda T, Yamawaki Y, et al. Agenesis of the right lobe of the liver: case report. Gastrointest Radiol 1991;16:320–2.

Kaplan SB, Zajko AB, Koneru B. Hepatic bilomas due to hepatic artery thrombosis in liver transplant recipients: percutaneous drainage and clinical outcome. Radiology 1990;174:1031–5.

Karp MP, Cooney DR, Pros GA, et al. The nonoperative management of pediatric hepatic trauma. J Pediatr Surg 1983;18(4):512–8.

Kays DW. Pediatric liver cysts and abscesses. Semin Pediatr Surg 1992;1(2):107–14.

Kelly DA. Pediatric liver transplantation. Curr Opin Pediatr 1998;10(5):493–8.

Kemmerer SR, Mortele KJ, Ross PR. CT scan of the liver. Radiol Clin North Am 1998;36(2):247–60.

Kerlan RK Jr, LaBerge JM, Gordon RL, et al. Transjugular intrahepatic portosystemic shunts: current status. AJR 1995;164(5):1059–66.

Keslar PJ, Buck JL, Selby DM. From the archives of the AFIP. Infantile hemangioendothelioma of the liver revisited. Radiographics 1993;13:657–70.

Khuroo MS, Wani NA, Javid G, et al. Percutaneous drainage compared with surgery for hepatic hydatid cysts. N Engl J Med 1997;337(13):881–7.

Kimura K, Stoopen M, Reeder MM, et al. Amebiasis: modern diagnostic imaging with pathological and clinical correlation. Semin Roentgenol 1997;32(4):250–75.

King S, Shuckett B. Sonographic diagnosis of portal venous gas in two pediatric liver transplant patients with benign pneumatosis intestinalis. Pediatr Radiol 1992;22:577–8.

Kinnard MF, Alavi A, Rubin RA, et al. Nuclear imaging of solid hepatic masses. Semin Roentgenol 1995;30(4):375–95.

Klotz HP, Flury R, Erhart P, et al. Magnetic resonance-guided laparoscopic interstitial laser therapy of the liver. Am J Surg 1997;174(4):448–51.

Kok T, Peeters PMJG, Hew JM, et al. Doppler ultrasound and angiography of the vasculature of the liver in children after orthotopic liver transplantation: a prospective study. Pediatr Radiol 1995;25:517–24.

Kressel HY, Filly RA. Ultrasonographic appearance of gas-containing abscesses in the abdomen. AJR 1978;130(1):71–3.

Kuligowska E, Connors SK, Shapiro JH. Liver abscess: sonography in diagnosis and treatment. AJR 1982;138(2):253–7.

Kuligowska E, Noble J. Sonography of hepatic abscesses. Semin Ultrasound 1983;4(2):102–16.

Kurtz AB, Rubin CS, Cooper HS, et al. Ultrasound findings in hepatitis. Radiology 1980;136(3):717–23.

Lafortune M, Madore F, Patriquin H, et al. Segmental anatomy of the liver: a sonographic approach to the Couinaud nomenclature. Radiology 1991;181:443–8.

Laing AD, Gibson RN. MRI of the liver. J Magn Reson Imaging 1998;8(2):337–45.

Lam WWM, Chan JHM, Hui Y, et al. Non-breath-hold gadolinium-enhanced MR angiography of the thoracoabdominal aorta: experience in 18 children. AJR 1998;170:478–80.

Landay MJ, Setiawan H, Hirsch G, et al. Hepatic and thoracic amaebiasis. AJR 1980;135(3):449–54.

Larsen CE, Patrick LE. Abdominal (liver, spleen) and bone manifestations of cat scratch disease. Pediatr Radiol 1992;22(5):353–5.

Larsen LR, Raffensperger J. Liver abscess. J Pediatr Surg 1979;14(3):329–31.

Larson RE, Semelka RC, Bagley AS, et al. Hypervascular malignant liver lesions: comparison of various MR imaging pulse sequences and dynamic CT. Radiology 1994;192:393–9.

Laucks S, Ballantine T, Boal D. Abscess of the falciform ligament in a child with a ventriculoperitoneal shunt. J Pediatr Surg 1986;21(11):979–80.

Laurin S, Kaude JV. Diagnosis of liver-spleen abscesses in childrenówith emphasis on ultrasound for the initial and follow-up examinations. Pediatr Radiol 1984;14(4):198–204.

Learch TJ, Ralls PW, Johnson MB, et al. Hepatic focal nodular hyperplasia: findings with color doppler sonography. J Ultrasound Med 1993;12:541–4.

Ledesma-Medina J, Dominguez R, Bowen A, et al. Pediatric liver transplantation. Part I. Standardization of preoperative diagnostic imaging. Radiology 1985;157(2):335–8.

Lee TY, Wan YL, Tsai CC. Gas-containing liver abscess: radiological findings and clinical significance. Abdom Imaging 1994;19(1):47–52.

Leslie DF, Johnson CD, Johnson CM, et al. Distinction between cavernous hemangiomas of the liver and hepatic metastases on CT: value of contrast enhancement patterns. AJR 1995;164:625–9.

Letourneau JG, Day DL, Frick MP, et al. Ultrasound and computed tomographic evaluation in hepatic transplantation. Radiol Clin North Am 1987;25(2):323–31.

Levin TL, Adam HM, van Hoeven KH, et al. Hepatic spindle cell tumors in HIV positive children. Pediatr Radiol 1994;24:78–9.

Lewall DB, McCorkell SJ. Hepatic echinococcal cysts: sonographic appearance and classification. Radiology 1985;155(3):773–5.

Lewall DB, McCorkell SJ. Rupture of echinococcal cysts: diagnosis, classification, and clinical implications. AJR 1986;146(2):391–4.

Li E, Stanley SL Jr. Protozoa. Amebiasis. Gastroenterol Clin North Am 1996;25(3):471–92.

Lim JH, Ko YT, Han MC, et al. The inferior accessory hepatic fissure: sonographic appearance. AJR 1987;149:495–7.

Liu KW, Fitzgerald RJ, Blake NS. An alternative approach to pyogenic hepatic abscess in childhood. J Paediatr Child Health 1990;26(2):92–4.

Liu LX, Harinasuta KT. Liver and intestinal flukes. Gastroenterol Clin North Am 1996;25(3):627–36.

Liu P, Daneman A, Stringer DA, et al. Percutaneous aspiration, drainage, and biopsy in children. J Pediatr Surg 1989;24(9):865–6.

Loberant N, Barak M, Gaitini D, et al. Closure of the ductus venosus in neonates: findings on real-time gray-scale, color-flow Doppler, and duplex Doppler sonography. AJR 1992;159:1083–5.

Love L, Demos TC, Reynes CJ. Visualization of the lateral edge of the liver in ascites. Radiology 1977;122:619–22.

Lubat E, Megibow AJ, Balthazar EJ, et al. Extrapulmonary Pneumocystis carinii infection in AIDS: CT findings. Radiology 1990;174(1):157–60.

Lucaya J, Enriquez G, Amat L, et al. Computed tomography of infantile hepatic hemangioendothelioma. AJR 1985;144:821–6.

Luks FI, Lemire A, St.-Vil D, et al. Blunt abdominal trauma in children: the practical value of ultrasonography. J Trauma 1993;34(5):607–11.

Lupetin AR, Dash N. Intrahepatic rupture of hydatid cyst: MR findings. AJR 1988;151(3):491–2.

Mahfouz AE, Hamm B, Taupitz M. Hepatic magnetic resonance imaging: new techniques and contrast agents. Endoscopy 1997;29(6):504–14.

Makanjuola D, Al-Smayer S, Al-Orainy I, et al. Radiographic features of lobar agenesis of the liver. Acta Radiol 1996;37:255–8.

Makler PT, Lewis E, Cantor R, et al. Nonvisualization of the left lobe of the liver due to atrophy or aplasia. Clin Nucl Med 1980;5(2):63–5.

Marani SA, Canossi GC, Nicoli FA, et al. Hydatid disease: MR imaging study. Radiology 1990;175(3):701–6.

Marino JM, Bueno J, Prieto C, et al. Residual cavities after surgery for hepatic hydatid cystsóan ultrasonographic evaluation. Eur J Pediatr Surg 1995;5(5):274–6.

Marn CS, Bree RL, Silver TM. Ultrasonography of liver. Technique and focal and diffuse disease. Radiol Clin North Am 1991;29(6):1151–70.

Marti-Bonmati L, Baamonde A, Poyatos CR, et al. Prenatal diagnosis of idiopathic neonatal hemochromatosis with MRI. Abdom Imaging 1994;19(1):55–6.

Marti-Bonmati L, Ferrer D, Menor F, et al. Hepatic mesenchymal sarcoma: MRI findings. Abdom Imaging 1993;176–9.

Marti-Bonmati L, Menor F, Ballesta A. Hydatid cyst of the liver: rupture into the biliary tree. AJR 1988;150(5):1051–3.

Marti-Bonmati L, Menor F, Vizcaino I, et al. Lipoma of the liver: US, CT and MRI appearance. Gastrointest Radiol 1989;14:155–7.

Marti-Bonmati L, Menor Serrano F. Complications of hepatic hydatid cysts: ultrasound, computed tomography, and magnetic resonance diagnosis. Gastrointest Radiol 1990;15(2):119–25.

Martinoli C, Cittadini G, Conzi R, et al. Sonographic characterization of an accessory fissure of the left hepatic lobe determined by omental infolding. J Ultrasound Med 1992;11(2):103–7.

Mathieu D, Rahmouni A, Anglade MC, et al. Focal nodular hyperplasia of the liver: assessment with contrast-enhanced turboFLASH MR imaging. Radiology 1991; 180:25–30.

Mathieu D, Vasile N, Fagniez PL, et al. Dynamic CT features of hepatic abscesses. Radiology 1985;154(3):749–52.

Maxwell AJ, Mamtora H. Fungal liver abscesses in acute leukaemiaóa report of two cases. Clin Radiol 1988;39(2):197–201.

McDiarmid SV, Millis MJ, Olthoff KM, et al. Indications for pediatric liver transplantation. Pediatr Transplant 1998;2(2):106–16.

McDonald KL, Davani M. The rim sign in hepatic abscess: case report and review of the literature. J Nucl Med 1997;38(8):1282–3.

McFadden S, Dunlop WE. Hepatic portal venous gas in adults: importance of ultrasonography in early diagnosis and survival. CJS 1989;32(4):297–8.

McFarland EG, Mayo-Smith WW, Saini S, et al. Hepatic hemangiomas and malignant tumors: improved differentiation with heavily T2-weighted conventional spin-echo MR imaging. Radiology 1994;193:43–7.

Mendez Montero JV, Arrazola Garcia J, Lopez Lafuente J, et al. Fat-fluid level in hepatic hydatid cyst: a new sign of rupture into the biliary tree? AJR 1996;167(1):91–4.

Mergo PJ, Ros PR. MR imaging of inflammatory disease of the liver. Magn Reson Imaging Clin N Am 1997;5(2):367–76.

Mergo PJ, Ros PR. Benign lesions of the liver. Radiol Clin North Am 1998a;36:319–31.

Mergo PJ, Ros PR. Imaging of diffuse liver disease. Radiol Clin North Am 1998b;36(2):365–75.

Merten DF, Kirks DR. Amebic liver abscess in children: the role of diagnostic imaging. AJR 1984;143(6):1325–9.

Michels NA. Blood supply and anatomy of the upper abdominal organs. Philadelphia: J. B. Lippincott; 1955.

Miller FJ, Ahola DT, Bretzman PA, et al. Percutaneous management of hepatic abscess: a perspective by interventional radiologists. J Vasc Interv Radiol 1997;8(2):241–7.

Miller JH, Greenfield LD, Wald BR. Candidiasis of the liver and spleen in childhood. Radiology 1982;142(2):375–80.

Miller JH, Greenspan BS. Integrated imaging of hepatic tumours in childhood. Part I. Malignant lesions (primary and metastatic). Radiology 1985;154:83–90.

Mills P, Saverymuttu S, Fallowfield M, et al. Ultrasound in the diagnosis of granulomatous liver disease. Clin Radiol 1990;41(2):113–5.

Monzawa S, Uchiyama G, Ohtomo K, et al. Schistosomiasis japonica of the liver: contrast-enhanced CT findings in 113 patients. AJR 1993;161(2):323–7.

Moon WK, Kim WS, Kim IO, et al. Hepatic choriocarcinoma in a neonate: MR appearance. J Comput Assist Tomogr 1993;17(4):653–5.

Moon WK, Kim WS, Kim IO, et al. Undifferentiated embryonal sarcoma of the liver: US and CT findings. Pediatr Radiol 1994;24:500–3.

Moore K, Persaud TVN. The developing human: clinically oriented embryology. 6th ed. Toronto: W.B. Saunders Co.; 1998.

Moreira VF, Merono E, Simon MA, et al. Endoscopic retrograde cholangiopancreatography in *Echinococcus* (hydatid) cysts of the liver. Gastrointest Radiol 1985; 10(2):123–8.

Morgan CL, Trought WS, Daffner RH. The use of CT scanning in resolving "pseudo" lesions of the liver. Comput Tomogr 1978;2(4):295–301.

Morgenstern L, Mazur M. Hypoplasia of the right hepatic lobe. Am J Surg 1959;98:628–30.

Morris DL, Buckley J, Gregson R, et al. Magnetic resonance imaging in hydatid disease. Clin Radiol 1987; 38(2):141–4.

Morris DL, Skene-Smith H, Haynes A, et al. Abdominal hydatid disease: computed tomographic and ultrasound changes during albendazole therapy. Clin Radiol 1984;35(4):297–300.

Moskovic E. Macronodular hepatic tuberculosis in a child: computed tomographic appearances. Br J Radiol 1990;63(752):656-8.

Mould R. An investigation of the variations in normal liver shape. Br J Radiol 1972;45:586–90.

Mowat AP. Liver disorders in childhood. 3rd ed. Toronto: Butterworth-Heinemann, Ltd.; 1994.

Mueller PR, Dawson SL, Ferrucci JT Jr, et al. Hepatic echinococcal cyst: successful percutaneous drainage. Radiology 1985;155(3):627–8.

Mueller PR, Simeone JF, Butch RJ, et al. Percutaneous drainage of subphrenic abscess: a review of 62 patients. AJR 1986;147(6):1237–40.

Mulliken JB, Glowacki J. Hemangiomas and vascular malformations in infants and children: a classification based on endothelial characteristics. Plast Reconstr Surg 1982;69:412–20.

Mungovan JA, Cronan JJ, Vacarro J. Hepatic cavernous hemangiomas: lack of enlargement over time. Radiology 1994;191:111–3.

Murakami T, Baron RL, Peterson MS, et al. Hepatocellular carcinoma: MR imaging with mangafodipir trisodium (Mn-DPDP). Radiology 1996;200:69–77.

Nakamura S, Tsuzuki T. Surgical anatomy of the hepatic veins and the inferior verna cava. Surg Gynecol Obstet 1981;152:43–50.

Nakhleh RE, Glock M, Snover DC. Hepatic pathology of chronic granulomatous disease of childhood. Arch Pathol Lab Med 1992;116(1):71–5.

Nazir Z, Moazam F. Amebic liver abscess in children. Pediatr Infect Dis J 1993;12(11):929–32.

Needleman L, Kurtz AB, Rifkin MD, et al. Sonography of diffuse benign liver disease: accuracy of pattern recognition and grading. AJR 1986;146(5):1011–5.

Netter F. Atlas of human anatomy. 2nd ed. New Jersey: Novartis Medical Education; 1997.

Newman B, Bowen A, Eggli KD. Recognition of malposition of the liver and spleen: CT, MRI, nuclear scan and fluoroscopic imaging. Pediatr Radiol 1994;24:274–9.

Newman KD, Schisgall R, Reaman G, et al. Malignant mesenchymoma of the liver in children. J Pediatr Surg 1989;24(8):781–3.

Nghiem HV. Imaging of hepatic transplantation. Radiol Clin North Am 1998;36(2):429–43.

Nghiem HV, Winter TC 3rd, Mountford MC, et al. Evaluation of the portal venous system before liver transplantation: value of phase-contrast MR angiography. AJR 1995;164(4):871–8.

Nino-Murcia M, Ralls PW, Jeffrey JRB, et al. Color flow doppler characterization of focal hepatic lesions. AJR 1992;159:1195–7.

Niron EA, Ozer H. Ultrasound appearances of liver hydatid disease. Br J Radiol 1981;54(640):335–8.

Nisenbaum HL, Rowling SE. Ultrasound of focal hepatic lesions. Semin Roentgenol 1995;30(4):324–46.

Numata K, Tanaka K, Mitsui K, et al. Flow characteristics of hepatic tumors at color doppler sonography: correlation with arteriographic findings. AJR 1993;160:515–21.

O' Hara SM. Pediatric gastrointestinal nuclear imaging. Radiol Clin North Am 1996;34(4):845–62.

Ohashi I, Ina H, Gomi N, et al. Hepatic pseudolesion in the left lobe around the falciform ligament at helical CT. Radiology 1995;196(1):245–9.

Okada Y, Yao YK, Yunoki M, et al. Lymph nodes in the hepatoduodenal ligament: US appearances with CT and MR correlation. Clin Radiol 1996;51(3):160–6.

Oleszczuk-Raszke K, Cremin BJ, Fisher RM, et al. Ultrasonic features of pyogenic and amoebic hepatic abscesses. Pediatr Radiol 1989;19(4):230–3.

O' Shea PA. Chronic granulomatous disease of childhood. Perspect Pediatr Pathol 1982;7:237–58.

Oubenaissa A, Perrault LP, Ridoux G, et al. Hepatodiaphragmatic interposition of the colonóan unusual case of combined anterior and posterior types treated with an original operative technique. Dis Colon Rectum 1999; 42(2):278–80.

Paley MR, Farrant P, Kane P, et al. Developmental intrahepatic shunts of childhood: radiological features and management. Eur Radiol 1997;7:1377–82.

Pant CS, Gupta RK. Diagnostic value of ultrasonography in hydatid disease in abdomen and chest. Acta Radiol 1987;28(6):743–5.

Papakonstantinou O, Kostaridou S, Maris T, et al. Quantification of liver iron overload by T2 quantitative magnetic resonance imaging in thalassemia: impact of chronic hepatitis C on measurements. J Pediatr Hematol Oncol 1999;21(2):142–8.

Parulekar SG. Ligaments and fissures of the liver: sonographic anatomy. Radiology 1979;130:409–11.

Pastakia B, Shawker TH, Thaler M, et al. Hepatosplenic candidiasis: wheels within wheels. Radiology 1988; 166(2):417–21.

Patrick LE, Ball TI, Atkinson GO, et al. Pediatric blunt abdominal trauma: periportal tracking at CT. Radiology 1992;183(3):689–91.

Paulson EK, Baker ME, Paine SS, et al. Detection of focal hepatic masses: STIR MR vs. CT during arterial portography. J Comput Assist Tomogr 1994;18(4):581–7.

Peh WCG, Ngan H, Fan ST, et al. Case report: variable imaging appearances of angiomyolipomas of the liver. Br J Radiol 1995;68:540–4.

Philips RL. Computed tomography and ultrasound in the diagnosis and treatment of liver abscesses. Australas Radiol 1994;38(3):165–9.

Pobiel RS, Bisset BS. Pictorial essay: imaging of liver tumors in the infant and child. Pediatr Radiol 1995; 25:495–506.

Porras-Ramirez G, Hernandez-Herrera MH, Porras-Hernandez JD. Amebic hepatic abscess in children. J Pediatr Surg 1995;30(5):662–4.

Port J, Leonidas JC. Granulomatous hepatitis in cat-scratch disease. Ultrasound and CT observations. Pediatr Radiol 1991;21(8):598–9.

Prando A, Goldstein HM, Bernardino ME, et al. Ultrasonic pseudolesions of the liver. Radiology 1979;130: 403–7.

Prassopoulos PK, Raissaki MT, Gourtsoyiannis NC. Hepatodiaphragmatic interposition of the colon in the upright and supine position. J Comput Assist Tomogr 1996;20(1):151–3.

Preimesberger KF, Goldberg ME. Acute liver abscess in chronic granulomatous disease of childhood. Radiology 1974;110(1):147–50.

Prince M, Grist T, Debatin J. 3D contrast MR angiography. 2nd ed. New York: Springer; 1999.

Puck J .Bacterial, parasitic, and other infections of the liver. In: Walker W, Durie P, Hamilton J, et al., editors. Pediatric gastrointestinal disease: pathophysiology, diagnosis, management. Toronto: B.C. Decker, Inc, 1991. 2: p. 890–7.

Radin DR, Baker EL, Klatt EC, et al. Visceral and nodal calcification in patients with AIDS-related *Pneumocystis carinii* infection. AJR 1990;154(1):27–31.

Radin DR, Colletti PM, Ralls PW, et al. Agenesis of the right lobe of the liver. Radiology 1987;164(3):639–42.

Rak K, Hopper KD, Parker SH. The "starry sky" liver with Burkitt's lymphoma. J Ultrasound Med 1988;7(5):279–81.

Ralls PW, Barnes PF, Johnson MB, et al. Medical treatment of hepatic amebic abscess: rare need for percutaneous drainage. Radiology 1987a;165(3):805–7.

Ralls PW, Colletti PM, Quinn MF, et al. Sonographic findings in hepatic amebic abscess. Radiology 1982a; 145(1):123–6.

Ralls PW, Henley DS, Colletti PM, et al. Amebic liver abscess: MR imaging. Radiology 1987b;165(3):801–4.

Ralls PW, Mikity VG, Colletti P, et al. Sonography in the diagnosis and management of hepatic amebic abscess in children. Pediatr Radiol 1982b;12(5):239–43.

Ralls PW, Quinn MF, Boswell WD Jr, et al. Patterns of resolution in successfully treated hepatic amebic abscess: sonographic evaluation. Radiology 1983;149(2):541–3.

Rappaport DC, Cumming WA, Ros PR. Disseminated hepatic and splenic lesions in cat-scratch disease: imaging features. AJR 1991;156(6):1227–8.

Reinhold C, Hammers L, Taylor CR, et al. Characterization of focal hepatic lesions with duplex sonography: findings in 198 patients. AJR 1995;164:1131–5.

Remedios PA, Colletti PM, Ralls PW. Hepatic amebic abscess: cholescintigraphic rim enhancement. Radiology 1986;160(2):395–8.

Richardson MC, Hollman AS, Davis CF. Comparison of computed tomography and ultrasonographic imaging in the assessment of blunt abdominal trauma in children. Br J Surg 1997;84(8):1144–6.

Rigauts HD, Selleslag DL, Van Eyken PL, et al. Erythromycin-induced hepatitis: simulator of malignancy. Radiology 1988;169(3):661–2.

Rintoul R, O'Riordain MG, Laurenson IF, et al. Changing management of pyogenic liver abscess. Br J Surg 1996; 83(9):1215–8.

Risaliti A, De Anna D, Terrosu G, et al. Chilaiditi's syndrome as a surgical and nonsurgical problem. Surg Gynecol Obstet 1993;176:55–8.

Roberts JL, Fishman EK, Hartman DS, et al. Lipomatous tumors of the liver: evaluation with CT and US. Radiology 1986;158:613–7.

Rodgers PM, Ward J, Baudouin CJ, et al. Dynamic contrast-enhanced MR imaging of the portal venous system: comparison with X-ray angiography. Radiology 1994; 191(3):741–5.

Rofsky NM, Fleishaker H. CT and MRI of diffuse liver disease. Semin Ultrasound CT MR 1995;16(1):16–33.

Rofsky NM, Yang BM, Schlossberg P, et al. MR-guided needle aspiration biopsies of hepatic masses using a closed bore magnet. J Comput Assist Tomogr 1998;22(4):633–7.

Rollins NK, Timmons C, Superina RA, et al. Hepatic artery thrombosis in children with liver transplants: false-positive findings at Doppler sonography and arteriography in four patients. AJR 1993;160:291–4.

Rollo FD, DeLand FH. The determination of liver mass from radionuclide images. Radiology 1968;91:1191–4.

Ros PR. Hepatic angiomyolipoma: is fat in the liver friend or foe? Abdom Imaging 1994;19:552–3.

Ros PR, Goodman ZD, Ishak KG, et al. Mesenchymal hamartoma of the liver: radiologic-pathologic correlation. Radiology 1986;158:619–24.

Routh WD, Keller FS, Cain WS, et al. Transcatheter embolization of a high-flow congenital intrahepatic arterial-portal venous malformation in an infant. J Pediatr Surg 1992;27(4):511–4.

Rubenstein W, Auh Y, Whalen J, et al. The perihepatic spaces: computed tomographic and ultrasound imaging. Radiology 1983;149(1):231–9.

Rubin E, Farber J. Pathology. 2nd ed. Philadelphia: J. B. Lippincott Co.; 1994.

Rubinson HA, Isikoff MB, Hill MC. Diagnostic imaging of hepatic abscesses: a retrospective analysis. AJR 1980; 135(4):735–45.

Ruess L, Sivit CJ, Eichelberger MR, et al. Blunt hepatic and splenic trauma in children: correlation of a CT injury severity scale with clinical outcome. Pediatr Radiol 1995; 25(5):321–5.

Sandrasegaran K, Kwo PW, DiGirolamo D, et al. Measurement of liver volume using spiral CT and the curved line and cubic spline algorithms: reproducibility and interobserver variation. Abdom Imaging 1999;24:61–5.

Saraswat VA, Agarwal DK, Baijal SS, et al. Percutaneous catheter drainage of amoebic liver abscess. Clin Radiol 1992;45(3):187–9.

Sarin SK, Bansal A, Sasan S, et al. Portal-vein obstruction in children leads to growth retardation. Hepatology 1992;15(2):229–33.

Sasaki F, Ohkawa Y, Sato N, et al. Imaging diagnosis of alveolar echinococcosis in young patients. Pediatr Radiol 1997;27(1):63–6.

Sashi R, Sato K, Hirano H, et al. Infantile choriocarcinoma: a case report with MRI, angiography and bone scintigraphy. Pediatr Radiol 1996;26:869–70.

Sato S, Watanabe M, Nagasawa S, et al. Laparoscopic observations of congenital anomalies of the liver. Gastrointest Endosc 1998;47(2):136–40.

Scherer U, Weinzierl M, Sturm R, et al. Computed tomography in hydatid disease of the liver: a report on 13 cases. J Comput Assist Tomogr 1978;2(5):612–7.

Schnall M. Magnetic resonance imaging of focal liver lesions. Semin Roentgenol 1995;30(4):347–61.

Schölmerich J, Volk BA, Gerok W. Value and limitations of abdominal ultrasound in tumour stagingóliver metastasis and lymphoma. Eur J Radiol 1987;7:243–5.

Schulman A. Non-western patterns of biliary stones and the role of ascariasis. Radiology 1987;162(2):425–30.

Schulman A. Intrahepatic biliary stones: imaging features and a possible relationship with ascaris lumbricoides. Clin Radiol 1993;47(5):325–32.

Schulman A, Loxton AJ, Heydenrych JJ, et al. Sonographic diagnosis of biliary ascariasis. AJR 1982;139(3):485–9.

Seeto RK, Rockey DC. Pyogenic liver abscess. Changes in etiology, management, and outcome. Medicine (Baltimore) 1996;75(2):99–113.

Segel MC, Zajko AB, Bowen A, et al. Doppler ultrasound as a screen for hepatic artery thrombosis after liver transplantation. Transplantation 1986;41:539–41.

Semelka RC, Brown ED, Ascher SM, et al. Hepatic hemangiomas: a multi-institutional study of appearance on T2-weighted and serial gadolinium-enhanced gradient-echo MR images. Radiology 1994;192:401–6.

Shamsi K, De Schepper A, Degryse H, et al. Focal nodular hyperplasia of the liver: radiologic findings. Abdom Imaging 1993;18:32–8.

Shanmuganathan K, Mirvis SE. CT scan evaluation of blunt hepatic trauma. Radiol Clin North Am 1998;36(2): 399–411.

Shapiro RS, Stancato-Pasik A, Glajchen N, et al. Color doppler applications in hepatic imaging. Clin Imaging 1998;22(4):272–9.

Sherlock S, Dooley J. The liver in infections. In: editors. Diseases of the liver and biliary system. Oxford and Cambridge (MA): Blackwell Science; 1997. p. 497–529.

Sheth S, Fishman EK, Sanders R. Actinomycosis involving the liver. Computed tomography/ultrasound correlation. J Ultrasound Med 1987;6(6):329–31.

Shirkhoda A. CT findings in hepatosplenic and renal candidiasis. J Comput Assist Tomogr 1987; 11(5):795–8.

Siegelman ES. MR imaging of diffuse liver disease. Hepatic fat and iron. Magn Reson Imaging Clin N Am 1997;5(2):347–65.

Siegelman ES, Mitchell DG, Outwater E, et al. Idiopathic hemochromatosis: MR imaging findings in cirrhotic and precirrhotic patients. Radiology 1993;188(3):637–41.

Siegelman ES, Outwater EK. MR imaging techniques of the liver. Radiol Clin North Am 1998;36(2):263–86.

Sigurdsson L, Reyes J, Kocoshis SA, et al. Neonatal hemochromatosis: outcomes of pharmacologic and surgical therapies. J Pediatr Gastroenterol Nutr 1998;26(1):85–9.

Silverman JM, Podesta L, Villamil F, et al. Portal vein patency in candidates for liver transplantation: MR angiographic analysis. Radiology 1995;197(1):147–52.

Simjee AE, Patel A, Gathiram V, et al. Serial ultrasound in amoebic liver abscess. Clin Radiol 1985;36(1):61–8.

Simonovsky V. The diagnosis of cirrhosis by high resolution ultrasound of the liver surface. Br J Radiol 1999; 72:29–34.

Singcharoen T, Mahanonda N, Powell LW, et al. Sonographic changes of hydatid cyst of the liver after treatment with mebendazole and albendazole. Br J Radiol 1985;58(693):905–7.

Singh Y, Winick AB, Tabbara SO. Multiloculated cystic liver lesions: radiologic-pathologic differential diagnosis. Radiographics 1997;17(1):219–24.

Sivit CJ, Taylor GA, Bulas DI, et al. Blunt trauma in children: significance of peritoneal fluid. Radiology 1991; 178(1):185–8.

Skibber JM, Lotze MT, Garra B, et al. Successful management of hepatic abscesses by percutaneous catheter drainage in chronic granulomatous disease. Surgery 1986;99(5):626–30.

Skolnick M, Dodd G. Doppler sonography in liver transplantation: pre- and post-transplant evaluation. In: Thrall J, editor. Current practice in radiology. Philadelphia: B.C. Decker, 1993. p. 161–72.

Slim MS, Khayat G, Nasr AT, et al. Hydatid disease in childhood. J Pediatr Surg 1971;6(4):440–8.

Slovis TL, Haller JO, Cohen HL, et al. Complicated appendiceal inflammatory disease in children: pylephlebitis and liver abscess. Radiology 1989;171(3):823–5.

Sollinger HW, D'Alessandro AM, Deierhoi MH, et al. Transplantation. In: Schwartz SI, editor. Principles of surgery. New York: McGraw-Hill Companies, Inc.; 1999. p. 361–439.

Soyer P, Roche A, Elias D, et al. Hepatic metastasis from colorectal cancer: influence of hepatic volumetric analysis on surgical decision making. Radiology 1992;184(3):695–7.

Soyer P, Van Beers B, Teillet-Thiebaud F, et al. Hodgkin's and non-Hodgkin's hepatic lymphoma: sonographic findings. Abdom Imaging 1993;18:339–43.

Stafford-Johnson DB, Hamilton BH, Dong Q, et al. Vascular complications of liver transplantation: evaluation with gadolinium-enhanced MR angiography. Radiology 1998;207:153–60.

Stalker H, Kaufman R, Towbin R. Patterns of liver injury in children: CT analysis. AJR 1986;147:1199–1205.

Stephenson NJH, Gibson RN. Hepatic focal nodular hyperplasia: colour doppler ultrasound can be diagnostic. Australas Radiology 1995;39:296–9.

Steventon DM, Kelly DA, McKiernan P, et al. Emergency transjugular intrahepatic portosystemic shunt prior to liver transplantation. Pediatr Radiol 1997;27(1):84–6.

Stöver B, Laubenberger J, Niemeyer C, et al. Haemangiomatosis in children: value of MRI during therapy. Pediatr Radiol 1995;25:123–6.

Stricof DD, Glazer GM, Amendola MA. Chronic granulomatous disease: value of the newer imaging modalities. Pediatr Radiol 1984;14(5):328–31.

Strouse PJ, Di Pietro MA. Persistent patency of the ductus venosus: consequence of portal hypertension in an infant? J Ultrasound Med 1997;16(8):559–61.

Suchy FJ. Liver disease in children. Toronto: Mosby-Year Book, Inc.; 1994.

Sukov RJ, Cohen LJ, Sample WF. Sonography of hepatic amebic abscesses. AJR 1980;134(5):911–5.

Swaim TJ, Gerald B. Hepatic portal venous gas in infants without subsequent death. Radiology 1970;94:343–5.

Taguchi T, Ikeda K, Yakabe S, et al. Percutaneous drainage for post-traumatic hepatic abscess in children under ultrasound imaging. Pediatr Radiol 1988;18(1):85–7.

Talenti E, Cesaro S, Scapinello A, et al. Disseminated hepatic and splenic calcifications following cat-scratch disease. Pediatr Radiol 1994;24(5):342–3.

Tanaka S, Kitamura T, Fugita M, et al. Colour doppler flow imaging of liver tumours. AJR 1990;154:509–14.

Tandon N, Karak PK, Mukhopadhyay S, et al. Amoebic liver abscess: rupture into retroperitoneum. Gastrointest Radiol 1991;16(3):240–2.

Taourel P, Marty-Ane B, Charasset S, et al. Hydatid cyst of the liver: comparison of CT and MRI. J Comput Assist Tomogr 1993;17(1):80–5.

Taylor GA. Imaging of pediatric blunt abdominal trauma: what have we learned in the past decade? [editorial; comment] Radiology 1995;195(3):600–1.

Taylor GA. Acute hepatic disease. Radiol Clin North Am 1997;35(4):799–814.

Taylor GA, O'Donnell R, Sivit CJ, et al. Abdominal injury score: a clinical score for the assignment of risk in children after blunt trauma. Radiology 1994;190(3):689–94.

Taylor KJW, Ramos I, Morse SS, et al. Focal liver masses: differential diagnosis with pulsed Doppler US. Radiology 1987;164:643–7.

Teefey SA, Stephens DH, Weiland LH. Calcification in hepatocellular carcinoma: not always an indication of fibrolamellar histology. AJR 1987;149:1173–4.

Teo ELHJ, Strouse PJ, Prince MR. Applications of magnetic resonance imaging and magnetic resonance angiography to evaluate the hepatic vasculature in the pediatric patient. Pediatr Radiol 1999;29(4):238–43.

Tonkin ILD, Wrenn JEL, Hollabaugh RS. The continued value of angiography in planning surgical resection of benign and malignant hepatic tumours in children. Pediatr Radiol 1988;18:35–44.

Toppet V, Souayah H, Delplace O, et al. Lymph node enlargement as a sign of acute hepatitis A in children. Pediatr Radiol 1990;20(4):249–52.

Treves S, Jones A, Markisz J. Liver and spleen. In: Treves S, editor. Pediatric nuclear medicine. New York: Springer-Verlag; 1995. p. 466–95.

Urban BA, Fishman EK, Kuhlman JE, et al. Detection of focal hepatic lesions with spiral CT: comparison of 4- and 8-mm interscan spacing. AJR 1993;160:783–5.

Van Way CW, Crane JM, Riddel DH, et al. Arteriovenous fistula in the portal circulation. Surgery 1971;70(6):876–90.

van Sonnenberg E, Mueller PR, Schiffman HR, et al. Intra-hepatic amebic abscesses: indications for and results of percutaneous catheter drainage. Radiology 1985;156(3):631–5.

Vassiliades VG, Bree RL, Korobkin M. Focal and diffuse benign hepatic disease: correlative imaging. Semin Ultrasound CT MR 1992;13(5):313–35.

Vock P, Kehrer B, Tschaeppeler H. Blunt liver trauma in children: the role of computed tomography in diagnosis and treatment. J Pediatr Surg 1986;21(5):413–8.

von Sinner W. Advanced medical imaging and treatment of human cystic echinococcosis. Semin Roentgenol 1997; 32(4):276–90.

von Sinner W, te Strake L, Clark D, et al. MR imaging in hydatid disease. AJR 1991;157(4):741–5.

von Sinner WN. New diagnostic signs in hydatid disease; radiography, ultrasound, CT and MRI correlated to pathology. Eur J Radiol 1991;12(2):150–9.

Waldman I, Berlin L, Fong JK, et al. Chilaiditi's syndrome—fact or fancy? JAMA 1966;198(9):168–9.

Wall SD, Fisher MR, Amparo EG, et al. Magnetic resonance imaging in the evaluation of abscesses. AJR 1985;144(6):1217–21.

Walsh TJ, Hiemenz JW, Anaissie E. Recent progress and current problems in treatment of invasive fungal infections in neutropenic patients. Infect Dis Clin North Am 1996;10(2):365–400.

Wang LY, Lin ZY, Change WY, et al. Duplex pulsed Doppler sonography of portal vein thrombosis in hepatocellular carcinoma. J Ultrasound Med 1991;10:265–9.

Ward J, Guthrie AJ, Hughes T, et al. Anatomy of the arterial supply to the liver demonstrated by MRI. Eur Radiol 1997;7(6):893–9.

Wechsler RJ, Munoz SJ, Needleman L, et al. The periportal collar: a CT sign of liver transplant rejection. Radiology 1987;165:57–60.

Weinstein JB, Heiken JP, Lee JKT, et al. High resolution CT of the porta hepatis and hepatoduodenal ligament. Radiographics 1986;6:55–74.

Weisleder R, Stark DD, Elizondo G, et al. MRI of hepatic lymphoma. Magn Reson Imaging 1988;6:675–81.

Welch TJ, Sheedy PF, Johnson CM, et al. Radiographic characteristics of benign liver tumours: focal nodular hyperplasia and hepatic adenoma. Radiographics 1985;5:673–82.

Welsh TJ, Sheedy PF, Johnson CM, et al. Focal nodular hyperplasia and hepatic adenoma: comparison of angiography, CT, Ultrasound and scintigraphy. Radiology 1985;150:593–5.

Westra SJ, Zaninovic AC, Hall TR, et al. Imaging in pediatric liver transplantation. Radiographics 1993;13(5):1081–99.

Westra SJ, Zaninovic AC, Vargas J, et al. The value of portal vein pulsatility on duplex sonograms as a sign of portal hypertension in children with liver disease. AJR 1995;165(1):167–72.

Wilde CC, Kueh YK. Case report: tuberculous hepatic and splenic abscess. Clin Radiol 1991;43(3):215–6.

Willemsen UF, Pfluger T, Zoller WG, et al. MRI of hepatic schistosomiasis mansoni. J Comput Assist Tomogr 1995;19(5):811–3.

Wilson SR, Arenson AM. Sonographic evaluation of hepatic abscesses. Can Assoc Radiol J 1984;35(2):174–7.

Witcombe JB. Ascaris perforation of the common bile duct demonstrated by intravenous cholangiography. Pediatr Radiol 1978;7(2):124–5.

Wojtasek DA, Teixidor HS. Echinococcal hepatic disease: magnetic resonance appearance. Gastrointest Radiol 1989;14(2):158–60.

Wolinski AP, Gall WJ, Dubbins PA. Hepatic artery aneurysm following pancreatitis diagnosed by ultrasound. Br J Radiol 1985;58:768–70.

Yamashita Y, Mitsuzaki K, Yi T, et al. Small hepatocellular carcinoma in patients with chronic liver damage: prospective comparison of detection with dynamic MR imaging and helical CT of the whole liver. Radiology 1996;200:79–84.

Zajko AB, Campbell WL, Bron KM, et al. Diagnostic and interventional radiology in liver transplantation. Gastroenterol Clin North Am 1988;17(1):105–43.

Zargar SA, Khuroo MS, Khan BA, et al. Intrabiliary rupture of hepatic hydatid cyst: sonographic and cholangiographic appearances. Gastrointest Radiol 1992;17(1):41–5.

Zirinsky K, Auh YH, Rubenstein WA, et al. The portacaval space: CT with MR correlation. Radiology 1985;156(2):453–60.

Zwiebel WJ. Sonographic diagnosis of diffuse liver disease. Semin Ultrasound CT MR 1995;16(1):8–15.

Zwiebel WJ, Mountford RA, Halliwell MJ, et al. Splanchnic blood flow in patients with cirrhosis and portal hypertension: investigation with duplex Doppler US. Radiology 1995;194(3):807–12

13

THE PANCREAS

Tara Williams, MD, and Paul S. Babyn, MDCM

THE NORMAL PANCREAS

Located in the anterior pararenal space of the retroperitoneum, the pancreas is typically shaped like a field hockey stick extending from the second portion of the duodenum to the splenic hilum. The splenic artery runs along the superior margin of the pancreas, while the splenic vein lies along the posterior border where it joins the superior mesenteric vein behind the pancreatic neck to form the portal vein. The pancreas is commonly divided into the head, neck, uncinate process, body, and tail. The uncinate process, a medial triangle-shaped extension of the head of the pancreas, lies posterior to the superior mesenteric vein (Semelka et al., 1997). The superior mesenteric artery lies behind the pancreatic body (Siegel and Sivit, 1997) (Figure 13–1).

The pancreatic parenchyma has both exocrine and endocrine functions. The exocrine portion of the pancreas is a compound tubuloacinar gland containing a highly branched collecting duct system. The endocrine portion of the pancreas consists of the pancreatic islets (islets of Langerhans) (Friedman and Dachman, 1994). Lacking a capsule, the pancreas is separated from the other retroperitoneal organs in the anterior pararenal space by a thin layer of connective tissue that forms the septa which separate the pancreatic lobules.

Pancreatic lobules consist mainly of acini but also contain ducts and pancreatic islets embedded in connective tissue containing blood vessels, lymphatics and nerves. The secretory acini are composed of pyramidal cells with a highly polarized internal structure arranged around a tiny lumen. The pancreatic enzymes are produced in the basal zone and stored in zymogen granules in the apical zone (Siegel et al., 1987). Tight junctions at the apical ends prevent the pancreatic enzymes expelled into the acinar lumen from reaching the intercellular spaces (Friedman and Dachman, 1994).

The size of the normal pancreas increases up to about eighteen years of age. The pancreas grows fastest in the first year of life, with slower growth between 1 and 18 years of age. In the first 2 decades, the pancreatic head and tail are similar in size whereas the neck and body are thinner. A study comparing the dimensions of the head, body, and tail of the pancreas with patient age, weight, height, and body surface area found the correlation between pancreatic dimensions and patient age as good as or better than that obtained with weight, height, and body surface area (Siegel et al., 1987). Mean pancreatic dimensions as a function of age are shown in Table 13–1.

Embryology

The pancreas develops at approximately 3 to 4 weeks' gestational age from two anlagen, dorsal and ventral, originating from the caudal portion of the foregut. The dorsal anlage arises first from duodenal epithelium and lies opposite the hepatic diverticulum. The ventral anlage develops later, has two separate buds (right and left), and lies caudal to the hepatic diverticulum (Figure 13–2A). The left ventral bud is usually smaller than the right bud and regresses while the right bud persists. During development the ventral anlage rotates clockwise 90 degrees to lie within the mesoduodenum along the posteroinferior margin of the dorsal pancreatic anlage (Figure 13–2B). The ventral anlage forms the uncinate process and a portion of the head of the pancreas, while the body, the tail, and the remainder of the

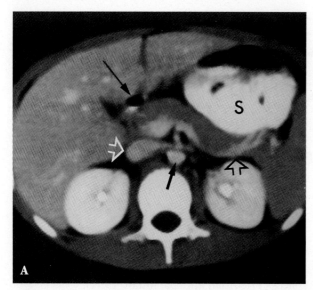 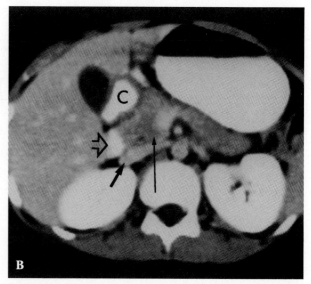

FIGURE 13–1. Normal pancreas (CT). *A,* The body and tail of the pancreas shown lying posterior to the stomach (S), anterior to the splenic vein (*open black arrow*), and posteromedial to the duodenum (*long black arrow*). The inferior vena cava (*open white arrow*), the aorta (*short black arrow*), and the superior mesenteric artery are useful posterior landmarks. *B,* A slightly lower cut in another patient shows the head of the pancreas lying anterior to the inferior vena cava (*short black arrow*) and medial to the duodenal cap (C) and the second part of the duodenum (*open black arrow*). The uncinate process (*long black arrow*) projects behind the superior mesenteric vein and separates it from the inferior vena cava and left renal vein.

head are formed from the larger dorsal anlage. At about 7 to 8 weeks of embryonic life, the dorsal and ventral anlagen fuse (Agha, 1987).

The ductal system of the pancreas arises from both dorsal and ventral anlagen. The dorsal anlage contains the duct of Santorini and the ventral anlage the duct of Wirsung. The distal portion of the duct of Santorini typically becomes the accessory duct, while the proximal portions of the duct of Santorini (from the dorsal anlage) and the duct of Wirsung (from the ventral analage) fuse to become the main pancreatic duct (Agha, 1987; Stringer, 1989). In 70% of cases, the main and accessory panceatic ducts retain their separate duodenal openings and join within the pancreatic head (Figure 13–3A). In 20%, however, the accessory pancreatic duct atrophies before it reaches the duodenum (Figure 13–3B). In the remaining 10%, both ducts keep their separate duodenal openings but are not united in the pancreatic head due to failure of the ducts of the ventral and dorsal anlagen to fuse or atrophy of a normally formed anastomosis during later fetal life (see Pancreas Divisum, below) (Figure 13–3C). Other, less prevalent, pancreatic duct variations include duplication of the main or accessory pancreatic ducts

(Figure 13–3D), crossing of the ducts (Figure 13–3E), and repeated anastomoses between the ducts (Figure 13–3F) (Friedman and Dachman, 1994).

Imaging

Echogenicity in ultrasonography (US) of the normal pancreas in children varies with age. The echogenicity of the pancreas is generally lower in children than in adults, likely related to lower fat content in children (Siegel et al., 1987). In premature infants and neonates less than 4 weeks of age, it is usually hyperechoic relative to the liver (Walsh et al., 1990) but with increasing age echogenicity becomes equal to or slightly greater than that of the adjacent liver. Uncommonly, the pancreas may be hypoechoic relative to the liver. Normal ductal diameter (if seen at all) should not be larger than 1 to 2 mm (Siegel and Sivit, 1997).

Computed tomography (CT) should be performed with oral and intravenous contrast. The typical dosage of intravenous contrast material is 2 mL per kg, administered manually as a bolus (Vaughn et al., 1998). On CT, the pancreas is a well-defined, homogeneously enhancing gland with a smooth or slightly irregular outer border (Herman and Siegel, 1991). The attenuation of the pancreas varies with

TABLE 13–1. Normal Dimensions of the Pancreas as a Function of Age

Patient Age	No. of Patients	Maximum Anteroposterior Dimensions (cm)		
		Head	Body	Tail
<1 mo	15	1.0 ± 0.4	0.6 ± 0.2	1.0 ± 0.4
1 mo–1 yr	23	1.5 ± 0.5	0.8 ± 0.3	1.2 ± 0.4
1–5 yr	49	1.7 ± 0.3	1.0 ± 0.2	1.8 ± 0.4
5–10 yr	69	1.6 ± 0.4	1.0 ± 0.3	1.8 ± 0.4
10–19 yr	117	2.0 ± 0.5	1.1 ± 0.3	2.0 ± 0.4

Data from Siegel et al., 1987; Ueda, 1989.

age and fat content but is normally similar to that of the liver before and after contrast. The transverse diameters of the pancreatic head (1.0–2.0 cm) and tail (0.8–2.2 cm) are usually similar whereas the pancreatic body is typically smaller (normal transverse diameter 0.4–1.0 cm) (Vaughn et al., 1998). The tail is usually cranially located relative to the head and body (Siegel and Sivit, 1997).

Magnetic resonance imaging (MR) of the pancreas is facilitated by higher field strengths, which allow improved signal-to-noise ratio and breath-hold imaging. The precise combination of sequences used to image the pancreas will vary depending on the indication for the study and the patient's ability to suspend respiration. A suggested standard MR protocol for imaging the pancreas in patients who are able to breath-hold includes T1-weighted spoiled gradient echo (SGE) and fat-suppressed SGE, T1-weighted non-fat-suppressed SGE, and postgadolinium imaging in the capillary phase (immediate after contrast) and interstitial phase (1 to 10 minutes after contrast). In patients who cannot breath-hold, T1-weighted fat-suppressed conventional spin echo (SE) should be substituted for SGE and fat-suppressed SGE sequences (Semelka et al., 1997). Although not always necessary, T2-weighted images are useful for demonstrating liver metastases and islet cell tumors and for providing information on the fluid in pancreatic pseudocysts, which may reflect complications such as infection or hemorrhage (Semelka and Ascher, 1993).

The normal pancreas is isointense relative to the liver on SGE images and hyperintense relative to the liver on fat-supressed spin echo images due to the presence of aqueous protein in the acini of the pancreas. The pancreas demonstrates uniform capillary blush on immediate after contrast images, rendering it higher in signal intensity than the liver and adjacent fat. The pancreas becomes isointense with fat by about 1 minute after contrast, and lower in signal intensity than background fat beyond 2 minutes (Semelka and Ascher, 1993). Studies of age-

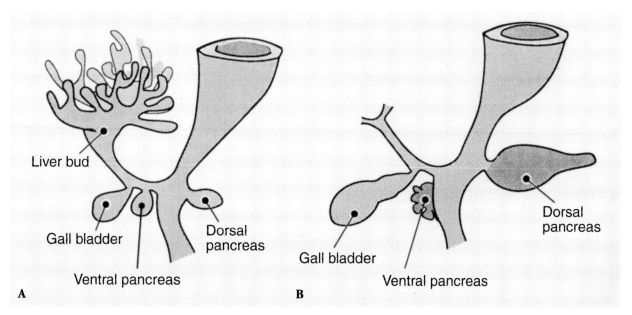

FIGURE 13–2. Embryology of the pancreas. At 35 days' gestation, frontal view shows the position of the gallbladder and ventral and dorsal pancreas (*A*). The ventral pancreas then rotates, posterior to the duodenum, so that by 50 days' gestation the ventral pancreas has come to reside anterior and inferior to the body of the dorsal pancreas (*B*).

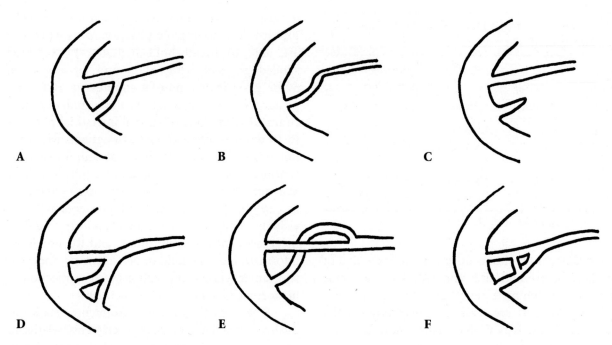

FIGURE 13–3. Pancreatic duct variations. *A*, Normal duct pattern. *B*, Absence of accessory pancreatic duct. *C*, Absence of communication between main and accessory pancreatic ducts. *D*, Duplication of main pancreatic duct. *E*, Crossing of duct. *F*, Multiple anastomoses between ducts.

related changes in the MR appearance of the pancreas in children have not been done.

In patients who are able to suspend respiration, T2-weighted echo-train spin echo sequences such as T2-weighted half-fourier acquisition snapshot turbo spin echo (HASTE) provide a sharp anatomic display of the common bile duct (CBD) on coronal plane images and of the pancreatic duct on transverse plane images. In patients who cannot suspend respiration, a breathing-independent sequence such as magnetization-prepared–rapid acquisition gradient echo (MP-RAGE) should be substituted (Semelka et al., 1997).

CONGENITAL AND DEVELOPMENTAL ANOMALIES OF THE PANCREAS

Pancreas Divisum

Pancreas divisum is the most common and clinically important major anatomic variant (Stringer, 1989). It results from the failure of the dorsal and ventral anlagen to fuse (Sugawa et al., 1987). Consequently, the pancreatic head is drained by the duct of Wirsung and the body by the duct of Santorini. Incomplete or partial divisum is defined as the com-

munication of the ventral and dorsal ducts by means of only a tiny branch. The reported incidence of pancreas divisum varies but is estimated to be 4 to 14% of the population, based on autopsy series (Soulen et al., 1989). Although not universally accepted, pancreas divisum may result in recurrent acute pancreatitis, as up to 25% of patients with recurrent pancreatitis have the anomaly (Sugawa et al., 1987). It is thought that partial obstruction to the passage of exocrine secretions from the dorsal pancreas through the narrow orifice at the duodenum results in leakage of secretions into the pancreatic tissue, causing pancreatitis (Semelka et al., 1997). Recurrent pancreatitis does not typically present until middle age. In children with pancreas divisum and recurrent pancreatitis there tends to be a female preponderance (Friedman and Dachman, 1994).

Ultrasonography may suggest a mass in the head and uncinate process of the pancreas in some patients with pancreas divisum. Typically the mass is isoechoic although it may be hypoechoic (Friedman and Dachman, 1994). Neither ultrasonography or CT reliably identify a cleavage plane between the dorsal and ventral anlagen although patients with pancreas divisum usually have an increased craniocaudal diameter of the pancreatic head, and the pancreatic duct is visualized more often (Lindstrom and Ihse, 1989). Changes of pancreatitis may be present in both dorsal and ventral aspects of the pancreas or be limited to the dorsal pancreas or less commonly the ventral pancreas (Friedman and Dachman, 1994). Until recently, endoscopic retrograde cholangiopancreatography (ERCP) was considered the gold standard for diagnosis, and with ERCP, noncommunication of the ducts of Wirsung and Santorini is demonstrated. The duct of Wirsung is short with early acinarization. Evidence of pancreatitis may be seen only in the duct of Santorini (Stringer, 1989). A recent study reported exact correlation between ERCP and magnetic resonance cholangio-pancreatography (MRCP) in the detection and exclusion of pancreas divisum. The ducts of Santorini and Wirsung were consistently shown to be separate entities due to the good conspicuity of the linear high-signal-intensity tubular structures (Bret et al., 1996).

Annular Pancreas

Annular pancreas, while infrequent, is the second most common congenital anomaly of the pancreas. In this anomaly the left side of the bilobed ventral anlage fails to degenerate. It grows around the left side of the duodenum and fuses with the remaining pancreatic segments, resulting in a ring of normal pancreatic tissue that encircles the second portion of the duodenum usually at or above the level of the ampulla of Vater (Orr et al., 1992; Eisenberg, 1990). In up to 75% of cases it is associated with other anomalies (Table 13–2). Patients often present with duodenal obstruction although this may not occur until adulthood (Figure 13–4).

Infants with symptomatic annular pancreas can present with the radiographic appearance of a double bubble sign. Unlike duodenal atresia, however, annular pancreas almost always results in an incomplete obstruction. A notchlike defect on the lateral duodenal wall may be evident on a barium examination but unlike a postbulbar ulcer or malignant tumor which may produce a similar deformity, the duodenal mucosal folds are intact without a discrete ulcer crater (Eisenberg, 1990). Ultrasonographically, annular pancreas appears as an echogenic band crossing the duodenum in the region of the pancreatic head. On CT, pancreatic tissue encircles the second portion of the duodenum. The T1-weighted fat-supressed images are particularly useful in showing this entity by MR due to the high signal

intensity of pancreatic tissue, easily distinguished from the lower signal intensity of the duodenum and adjacent tissue (Semelka et al., 1997).

Ectopic Pancreas

Ectopic pancreas is a relatively common anomaly with a reported incidence ranging from 0.55 to 14% at autopsy. It is most frequently seen in the duodenum, the stomach, or the jejunum and rarely in the ileum, ileal or jejunal diverticula, Meckel's diverticulum, the gallbladder or bile ducts, umbilicus, fallopian tube, or in a mediastinal teratoma. Microscopically, it consists of varying amounts of pancreatic ducts, acini, and islet cells (Rubesin et al., 1997; Lai and Tompkins, 1985).

Ectopic pancreas is an asymptomatic incidental finding in the majority of cases (Allison et al., 1995). In symptomatic patients, the lesions are usually in the stomach or duodenum (Rubesin et al., 1997). Problems related to ectopic pancreas include epigastric pain, gastrointestinal bleeding from the lesion itself, or associated gastric ulceration and pyloric obstruction caused by local spasm, edema, hypertrophy, or rarely gastroduodenal prolapse (Allison et al., 1995). Pancreatitis and pseudocyst formation may occur, also rarely. Pancreatic enzymes such as amylase or lipase may be elevated in some cases (Rubesin et al., 1997). Radiologic evaluation is generally helpful only when the lesion is located in the stomach. On an upper gastrointestinal series, ectopic pancreas appears as a small, 1- to 3-cm polypoid mass along

TABLE 13–2. Anomalies Associated with Annular Pancreas

Common Associations	Uncommon Associations or Concurrences
Esophageal atresia	Preduodenal portal vein
Tracheoesophageal fistula	Congenital absence of neck
Down syndrome (with	and tail of pancreas
or without congenital	Situs inversus viscerum
heart disease)	Hirschsprung's disease
Duodenal atresia	Hemivertebra
Duodenal stenosis	Lung agenesis
Duodenal diaphragm	Microcephaly
Malrotation with or	Absent radius
without Ladd's bands	Cornelia de Lange's
Imperforate anus	syndrome

Data from Stringer, 1989.

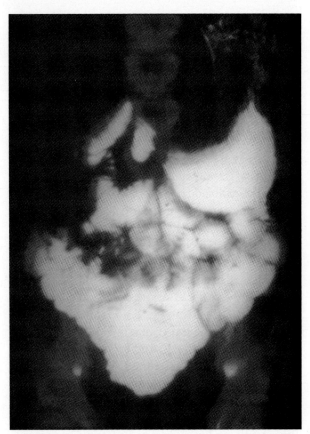

FIGURE 13–4. Annular pancreas. Upper GI demonstrates the circumferential narrowing of the mid second portion of the duodenum with dilatation of the proximal duodenum.

the distal greater curvature of the stomach with central umbilication representing a rudimentary duct (Stringer, 1989).

Congenital Cysts

True congenital cysts of the pancreas are rare and distinguishable from pancreatic pseudocysts by the presence of an epithelial lining. Cyst contents may or may not demonstrate elevated amylase levels (Baker et al., 1990). Cysts may be single or multiple and can be associated with hepatic and renal cysts as part of polycystic disease (Stringer, 1989). Most commonly asymptomatic, they may become symptomatic due to compression of adjacent viscera. They rarely present with pancreatitis (Casadei et al., 1996). Ultrasonography is useful in monitoring cyst growth, which may be rapid (Baker et al., 1990). Treatment of true congenital cysts depends on their location; cysts in the pancreatic body or tail are generally completely excised, whereas internal drainage

is recommended for those located in the pancreatic head (Casadei et al., 1996).

Aplasia and Hypoplasia

Complete agenesis of the pancreas is fatal. Partial agenesis of endocrine or exocrine tissue has been reported in Shwachman-Diamond syndrome, Johanson-Blizzard syndrome, and leprechaunism. Agenesis of the pancreas is generally seen only in its dorsal aspect, although there is one case report of agenesis of the ventral pancreas in an infant (Nishimori et al., 1990). Agenesis of the dorsal pancreas is rare and is typically diagnosed as an incidental finding in adulthood during investigation of abdominal pain. It is associated with diabetes mellitus but exocrine pancreatic dysfunction has not been reported. There is a reported association of dorsal agenesis with polysplenia (Deignan et al., 1996) (Figure 13–5). Recent reports have noted associated biliary dilatation and elevated ductal pressures, suggesting that dysfunction of Oddi's sphincter may play a role in the pathophysiology of this disorder (Nishimori et al., 1990; Wang et al., 1990). Computed tomography or MR is the technique of choice for demonstrating this abnormality as ultrasonographic visualization of the entire pancreas is not always possible due to technical limitations such as obesity or bowel gas (Deignan et al., 1996). With CT or MR, congenital absence of the dorsal pancreatic anlage is distinguished from surgical or post-traumatic absence of the distal pancreas by a rounded contour of the pancreatic head in the former in contrast to more squared-off or irregular terminations in the latter case (Semelka et al., 1997). Atrophy of the pancreas following an episode of acute pancreatitis (particularly when it spares the uncinate process) may resemble agenesis of the dorsal gland (Gold, 1993).

PANCREATITIS

Although uncommon, pancreatitis is associated with severe morbidity and mortality and is a cause of abdominal pain in children (Yeung et al., 1996). It has many causes, a poorly understood pathogenesis, few effective treatments, and an often unpredictable outcome (Lerner et al., 1996).

Acute Pancreatitis

A standardized terminology and clinically based classification system to facilitate interinstitutional comparison has been developed for acute pancreatitis. Acute pancreatitis is an acute inflammatory process of the pancreas characterized by edema and fat necrosis of the pancreatic parenchyma with variable involvement of other regional tissues or remote organ systems. It is classified as mild or severe based on the severity of pathologic and clinical changes (Bradley, 1993).

Etiology

In most series, accidental trauma, usually from motor vehicle accidents, causes most acute pancreatitis cases in children (Yeung et al., 1996; Lane et al., 1996; Siegel and Sivit, 1997). Other causes include nonaccidental injury (battered child syndrome), postsurgical trauma, systemic disease, structural disease, hereditary disease (cystic fibrosis, hereditary pancreatitis), drugs or toxins, and idiopathic causes. Systemic diseases include Reye's syndrome, lupus, hemolytic uremic syndrome, sepsis, shock, and viral infections (Siegel and Sivit, 1997; Yeung et al., 1996; Stringer, 1989; Tam et al., 1985; Ziegler et al., 1988; Weizman and Durie, 1988). Structural diseases include biliary tract disease (most often related to underlying hematologic disease such as sickle cell anemia) and congenital anomalies such as pancreas divisum. Patients with structural and systemic disease tend to present younger than patients with pancreatitis from other causes (Ziegler et al., 1988). Drugs commonly causing pancreatitis in children include steroids, L-asparaginase, and sulfasalazine (Stringer, 1989; Weizman and Durie, 1988).

Pathophysiology

The pathogenesis of acute pancreatitis is not well understood. Mechanisms that can initiate pancreatic inflammation include increased permeability of the pancreatic duct, overstimulation, obstruction to pancreatic flow, overdistention of the ductal system, toxin exposure, and metabolic abnormalities (Lerner et al., 1996).

One of several theories on the cause of acute pancreatitis is the common channel theory, suggested by Opie in 1901; according to which, obstruction of the ampulla of Vater leads to bile reflux into the pancreatic ducts, inducing pancreatitis. Numerous animal studies have failed to prove or disprove Opie's theory conclusively. Another theory is that pancreatitis results from duodenal regurgitation through an incompetent

Oddi's sphincter, which could explain pediatric cases of duodenal obstruction and pancreatitis.

Another possible cause of pancreatic inflammation is inappropriate activation of zymogen for unknown reasons. Upon such activation, the pancreatic acinar cell undergoes a cascade of events including edema, necrosis, hemorrhage, thrombosis, ischemia, and inflammation. The local process may spread into peripancreatic spaces with the release of toxins systemically into the peritoneal space, possibly leading to remote complications and multiorgan failure (Lerner et al., 1996).

Clinical Manifestations and Classification

Abdominal pain, typically epigastric pain, is the most common symptom in most pediatric series (Stringer, 1989; Yeung et al., 1996; Weizman and Durie, 1988). Other symptoms and signs include nausea and vomiting, fever, abdominal distension, epigastric tenderness (with rebound), and an abdominal mass.

Severe pancreatitis is characterized clinically by the presence of three or more of Ranson's criteria (Table 13–3) or eight or more Acute Physiology And Chronic Health Evaluation (APACHE II) points. Severe acute pancreatitis is associated with organ failure and/or local complications such as necrosis, abscess, or pseudocyst. The symptoms and signs of severe pancreatitis are typically the clinical expression of developing pancreatic necrosis. Although delayed progression from mild to severe acute pancreatitis can infrequently occur, the manifestations

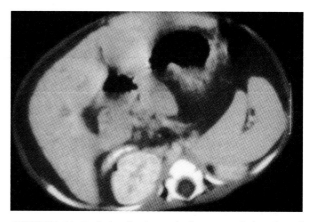

FIGURE 13–5. Polysplenia and absence of the dorsal pancreas. The body, tail, and a portion of the head of the pancreas are absent. Note the presence of two spleens in the left upper quadrant.

TABLE 13–3.   Ranson's Criteria for Severe Pancreatitis

Serum calcium	< 8 mg percent
Blood urea nitrogen	Rise > 5 mg percent
Hematocrit fall	> 10 percentage points
Base deficit	> 4 mEq/L
Arterial pO_2	< 60 mm Hg
Estimated fluid sequestration	> 6 L

Data from Ranson et al., 1975.

of severe acute pancreatitis are usually present shortly after the onset of initial symptoms.

Mild acute pancreatitis is asociated with minimal organ dysfunction and lacks the clinical features of severe acute pancreatitis. Patients typically improve within 48 to 72 hours after treatment is begun. The predominant macroscopic and histologic feature of mild acute pancreatitis is interstitial edema although microscopic areas of parenchymal necrosis and peripancreatic fat necrosis infrequently may be present (Bradley, 1993).

Diagnosis

The diagnosis of acute pancreatitis is usually based on combined clinical and biochemical findings. Imaging is generally required only when the diagnosis is in doubt, in patients with suspected complications, and for follow-up (Siegel and Sivit, 1997; Stringer, 1989). The most widely used test to support diagnosis of acute pancreatitis is total serum amylase (Yeung et al., 1996; Weizman and Durie, 1988). Unfortunately, this is a nonspecific test with falsely elevated values from other conditions. Although lipase assays are more specific their reported sensitivity is lower, ranging from 86.5 to 100% (Yeung et al., 1996). Other biochemical tests proposed as serum markers of pancreatic necrosis include C-reactive protein, polymorphonuclear neutrophil elastase, and trypsinogen activation peptide (TAP) (Uhl et al., 1991; Gudgeon et al., 1990). There has been limited clinical validation of these serum markers, however, and the enzyme levels have not been found to correlate with the severity or clinical course of the disease (Yeung et al., 1996).

Imaging

Of the variety of imaging techniques available to diagnose the presence and extent of pancreatitis, US

and CT are considered the primary means of evaluation (Siegel and Sivit, 1997).

The most common ultrasonographic finding of acute pancreatitis in children is focal (60% of children) or diffuse (46%) enlargement of the gland. Another useful ultrasonographic sign is dilatation of the pancreatic duct, reported to occur in 45% of patients (Figure 13–6). Decreased echogenicity of the gland may also be seen although not a reliable feature; in most children the echogenicity remains normal or occasionally increased (Siegel et al., 1987; Coleman et al., 1983).

Ultrasonography is less sensitive than CT in defining complex extrapancreatic spread of pancreatitis (Jeffrey et al., 1986). Peripancreatic fluid collections may be diagnosed by US and followed for the development of complications such as hemorrhage or infection (Siegel and Sivit, 1997).

Features of pancreatitis on CT include focal or diffuse enlargement, ductal dilatation, and intra- and peripancreatic fluid collections. The pancreas may show variable attenuation and enhancement characteristics (Figure 13–7). The reported false-negative rate for CT detection of pancreatitis in children ranges from 27 to 53% (Siegel et al., 1987; King et al., 1995). King and colleagues recently reviewed 28 children with acute pancreatitis and reported that only approximately 30% demonstrated pancreatic enlargement, while the pancreas was normal in the remainder. The major complications of acute pancreatitis are best demonstrated by CT. A relationship shown in adults between prognosis and the extent of morphologic changes in the pancreas at CT, particularly when extrapancreatic fluid collections are present, has not been demonstrated in children. However, the persistence of a fluid collection does suggest an underlying structural abnormality (King et al., 1995). Computed tomography is preferred over ultrasonography to guide percutaneous fine-needle aspiration and catheter drainage (Siegel and Sivit, 1997).

Although some studies suggest MR is more sensitive than CT for detecting subtle changes of acute pancreatitis (particularly minor peripancreatic inflammatory changes), its use in children has to date been limited (Semelka et al., 1997).

Early Complications of Acute Pancreatitis

Acute Fluid Collections.   Acute fluid collections in or near the pancreas occur early in acute pancreatitis.

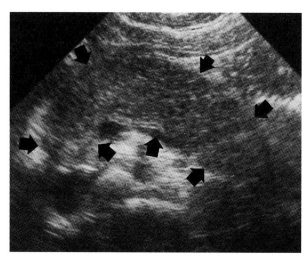

FIGURE 13–6. Acute pancreatitis. Transverse oblique ultrasonography shows diffuse enlargement of the pancreas.

Their precise composition is unknown (bacteria are variably present) but they lack a defined wall, thus distinguishing them from pseudocysts (Bradley, 1993). Intrapancreatic collections are less common in children than adults, occurring in less than 10% of children with acute pancreatitis but in approximately 30% of adult patients. Extrapancreatic fluid collections occur in about 40 to 50% of both children and adults with acute pancreatitis. Although extrapancreatic fluid collections tend to be more extensive in children than adults, they diminish spontaneously and most resolve within a few weeks (King et al., 1995; Siegel and Sivit, 1997). It is not known why some progress to become pseudocysts or abscesses. They occur mostly in the anterior pararenal space (71%), lesser sac (57%), lesser omentum (50%), and transverse mesocolon (50%). In adults, collections are most often in the lesser sac (59%), the anterior pararenal space (47%), and the small bowel mesentery (50%) (Stringer, 1989; King et al., 1995).

Ultrasonographically, most acute fluid collections are hypoechoic with enhanced through transmission. On CT, they are fluid attenuation structures without a definable wall, which distinguishes them from pseudocysts. Fluid collections may be complicated by hemorrhage, leading to increased echogenicity on US and increased attenuation on CT (Siegel and Sivit, 1997).

Pancreatic Necrosis. Pancreatic necrosis is defined as diffuse or focal areas of nonviable pancreatic parenchyma, commonly associated with peripan-

creatic fat necrosis. Pancreatic parenchymal necrosis rarely involves the entire gland and usually is confined to the periphery with preservation of the central core of the pancreas (Bradley, 1993). Necrosis develops early in severe acute pancreatitis and is usually well established by 96 hours after the onset of clinical symptoms (Balthazar et al., 1994).

Ultrasonography is not reliable for detecting pancreatic necrosis as the appearance of pancreatic necrosis on US does not differ significantly from that of pancreatitis without necrosis.

Computed tomography is currently considered the best imaging modality to diagnose pancreatic necrosis. A well-circumscribed zone of unenhancing parenchyma larger than 3 cm or involving more than 30% of the area of the pancreas is a reliable CT finding for the diagnosis of necrosis (Walsh et al., 1990). The overall accuracy of dynamic CT in detecting pancreatic necrosis is 80 to 90% although it is slightly less sensitive with lesser degrees of necrosis (less than 30%). Similarly, CT specificity is 100% when gland necrosis is more than 30% but drops considerably (50%) with less extensive necrosis. The presence and extent of peripancreatic necrosis, however, cannot be reliably determined with CT (Bradley, 1993; Bathazar et al., 1994).

Magnetic resonance imaging also may be used to detect pancreatic necrosis. Pancreatic necrosis is manifest on MR by the absence of enhancement on

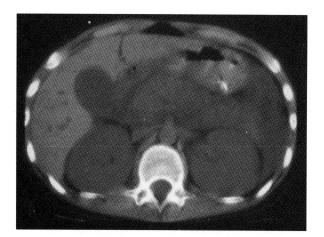

FIGURE 13–7. Acute pancreatitis. Computed tomography demonstrates diffuse enlargement, inhomogeneous attenuation, and poor definition of the pancreas. Peripancreatic fluid and fluid in both anterior pararenal spaces are present. Contrast was not administered because the patient was in renal failure.

dynamic gadolinium-enhanced SGE images. A study comparing immediate postgadolinium SGE images with dynamic contrast-enhanced CT images found both techniques comparable for detecting pancreatic necrosis (Semelka et al., 1997).

Infected necrosis is defined as a superinfection of necrotic pancreatic or peripancreatic tissue (Balthazar et al., 1990). As clinical and laboratory findings are often similar in patients with either sterile or infected necrosis, the distinction is made with cultures obtained by percutaneous needle aspiration. It is critical to identify the presence of infected necrosis as it is fatal without surgical drainage whereas sterile necrosis can be treated without surgery (Bradley, 1993).

Late Complications of Acute Pancreatitis
The late complications of pancreatitis include pseudocyst formation, abscesses, and vascular complications.

Pseudocysts. A pseudocyst is a fluid collection, usually rich in pancreatic enzymes, which has a wall of fibrous or granulation tissue. Formation of a pseudocyst requires 4 or more weeks and may result from acute or chronic pancreatitis or pancreatic trauma (Bradley, 1993). Pseudocysts are suspected clinically when there is persistent pain and hyperamylasemia.

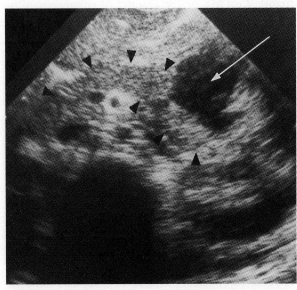

FIGURE 13–8. Acute pancreatic pseudocyst formation. Transverse ultrasonography shows a unilocular cystic mass (*white arrow*) adjacent to the tail of the pancreas. The pseudocyst arises from the pancreas and lies within the lesser sac.

They are usually located close to the pancreas although they may rupture into the adjacent gastrointestinal tract or peritoneal cavity, spleen, liver, or mediastinum. They may cause obstruction of the bowel or biliary system, hemorrhage, become infected, or leak slowly into the peritoneum, causing ascites (Freeny, 1989).

Pseudocysts resolve spontaneously in approximately one-third of patients. The remainder can usually be treated with percutaneous catheter drainage and in some cases, surgical drainage into the stomach or small bowel (Lerner et al., 1996; Freeny, 1989).

On ultrasonography, pseudocysts are encapsulated anechoic or hypoechoic collections with variable through transmission (Figure 13–8). However, CT is considered superior to ultrasonography for defining the extent of the lesion (Siegel and Sivit, 1997). Pseudocysts appear on CT as homogeneous fluid attenuation collections with a discernible wall. If complicated by hemorrhage or infection, there may be areas within them of increased attenuation (Figure 13–9).

On MR, simple pseudocysts are low in signal intensity or are signal void in a background of normal signal-intensity pancreatic tissue on both SGE and T1-weighted fat-suppressed images and relatively homogeneous and high in signal intensity on T2-weighted images. Breathing-independent T2-weighted sequences such as MP-RAGE are valuable in evaluating pseudocysts as these patients are often unable to breath-hold (Semelka et al., 1997). Pseudocysts complicated by necrotic debris, hemorrhage, or infection are heterogeneous in signal intensity on T1- and T2-weighted images.

Pancreatic Abscess. Pancreatic abscesses are collections of pus, usually in close proximity to the pancreas, typically occurring more than 4 weeks after the onset of acute pancreatitis or trauma. A pancreatic abscess is distinguished from infected necrosis by the absence of significant pancreatic necrosis. Infected necrosis requires surgical débridement and has twice the mortality risk of abscesses, which may be drained percutaneously (Bradley, 1993).

Vascular Complications. Vascular complications such as hemorrhage and pseudoaneurysm result from the leakage of proteolytic enzymes causing erosion of arterial walls. The splenic artery and branches of the pancreaticoduodenal arteries are most commonly affected. A pseudoaneurysm appears on US as a complex mass with enhanced through transmission which has turbulent arterial flow on duplex or color flow Doppler imaging. A pseudoaneurysm on CT is a fluid attenuation collection which demonstrates marked arterial enhancement. The treatment of choice for pseudoaneurysms is embolization (Freeny, 1989).

Venous complications of thrombosis or occlusion, typically of the splenic and superior mesenteric veins, are less common than arterial complications and are thought to be due to adjacent inflammation or extrinsic compression. Thrombosis is diagnosed by the presence of an intraluminal filling defect on US, CT, or MR, or as an abrupt cutoff on angiography. In the presence of chronic thromboses, collaterals may develop.

Endoscopic retrograde cholangiopancreatography can be performed in infants using a new, small endoscopic instrument. Pediatric indications for ERCP include evaluation of post-traumatic or

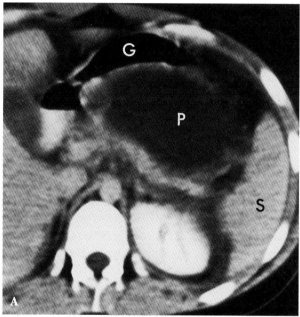

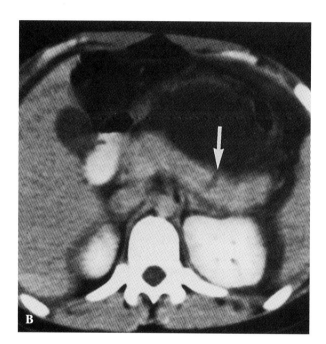

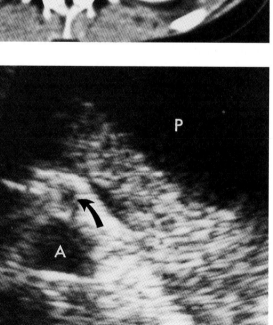

FIGURE 13–9. Pancreatic pseudocyst. *A*, Computed tomography demonstrates a pseudocyst (P) anterior to the tail of the pancreas, posterior to the air- and contrast-filled stomach (G), and medial to the spleen (S). *B*, The tail of the pancreas is demonstrated more clearly on a CT cut 1 cm lower. It also shows a linear streak of decreased attenuation (*arrow*), indicating a tear in the tail of the pancreas as a cause for the pancreatic pseudocyst. *C*, Detailed ultrasonography of the tail of the pancreas did not reveal the tear but did show the pseudocyst (P) anteriorly and the aorta (A) and superior mesenteric artery (*arrow*) posteriorly.

postpancreatitis complications, detection of underlying anatomic abnormalities associated with acute pancreatitis, and investigation of pancreatic ducts in chronic relapsing pancreatitis or hereditary pancreatitis. The reported incidence of pancreatitis following ERCP was 12% in the largest series done and 5% in the most recent series. In all cases it was self-limited (Lerner et al., 1996).

Management

Treatment of acute pancreatitis is mainly supportive. Specific clinical aims include removal of the cause (e.g., drugs or toxins), reduction of the autodigestive process in the pancreas, treatment of local and systemic complications, and removal of digestive enzymes or toxins from the peritoneal cavity or circulation (Lerner et al., 1996).

Indications for surgery include the following: exploration of an acute abdomen (in children, the most common preoperative diagnosis is acute appendicitis); drainage of pancreatic fluid collections (e.g., cysts and abscesses) refractory to percutaneous treatment; débridement of infected necrotic tissue; and removal of obstruction in the main pancreatic ducts or common bile duct. Adult data suggest that removal of impacted stones in severe gallstone-induced pancreatitis is best done not surgically but by endoscopy with sphincterotomy (Lerner et al., 1996).

CHRONIC PANCREATITIS

Chronic pancreatitis is a continuing inflammatory process of the pancreas characterized by irreversible morphologic change, typically causing pain and permanent loss of exocrine and endocrine function (Freeny, 1989).

Etiology

Acute pancreatitis rarely becomes chronic in children (Stringer, 1989). However, when it results from trauma, medication, or idiopathic causes it can sometimes become chronic. The two morphologic forms of chronic pancreatitis in children are calcific and noncalcific. Calcific chronic pancreatitis is more common and is usually due to juvenile tropical pancreatitis syndrome (the most common cause of chronic pancreatitis in children) or hereditary pancreatitis (the second most common cause) (Vaughn et al., 1998; Lerner et al., 1996). Noncalcific chronic pancreatitis is rare and may result from congenital

or acquired lesions of the pancreatic duct, trauma, dysfunction of Oddi's sphincter, sclerosing cholangitis, or idiopathic fibrosing pancreatitis (Vaughn et al., 1998).

Juvenile Tropical Pancreatitis Syndrome. Juvenile tropical pancreatitis syndrome is characterized by abdominal pain, diabetes, steatorrhea, and pancreatic calcification. The condition is due to blockage of the pancreatic ducts by laminated secretions or inspissated mucus plugs which later calcify. The plugs are thought to result from pancreatic stasis due to prolonged lack of food in the stomach and/or gastroenteritis and dehydration. The disease is prevalent in underdeveloped countries with low-protein diets and high rates of childhood infections. Imaging may show dilatation of the pancreatic duct and/or ductules which may contain calcifications. Evidence of parenchymal atrophy and fibrosis may be seen in chronic cases (Nwokolo and Oli, 1980).

Familial Hereditary Pancreatitis. Familial hereditary pancreatitis (HP) is an autosomal dominant disorder with variable (40 to 80%) penetrance, defined as recurrent inflammation of the pancreas that occurs in families over two or more generations and has no other known predisposing factors (Lerner et al., 1996). The mean age of onset is 10 years. The underlying genotypic or phenotypic abnormality is unknown, and the disorder has no specific pathologic features although the ducts are often markedly dilated (Stringer, 1989). Complications are more common with HP than with nonhereditary chronic pancreatitis. The most frequent complication is calcification, which occurs in 33 to 50% of HP patients, compared with about 25% of patients with nonhereditary chronic pancreatitis (Girard et al., 1981). The most significant complication is intra-abdominal carcinoma, especially of the pancreas (reported incidence 3 to 20%). Other complications include diabetes (3 to 30%, as a late complication), pseudocysts (5 to 17%), portal and splenic vein thrombosis, and exocrine pancreatic insufficiency (Lerner et al., 1996).

Fibrosing Pancreatitis. Chronic idiopathic fibrosing pancreatitis in childhood is a rare condition without distinctive clinical, laboratory, or histologic findings. In nonspecific fibrosis of the pancreas, division of the remaining glandular tissue into small islands is typically the only constant histologic feature. The diagnosis is one of exclusion. There may be associated duct abnormalities although stones are rarely seen in the pancreatic ducts (Lewin-Smith et al., 1996) (Figure 13–10).

Miscellaneous Causes of Chronic Pancreatitis. Rarer causes of chronic pancreatitis in children include hereditary hyperlipidemia and hyperparathyroidism. Although uncommon in North America, ascariasis can result in pancreatic calcification and chronic pancreatitis secondary to pancreatic duct obstruction and malnutrition (Stringer, 1989).

Pathophysiology

Chronic pancreatitis occurs either as a disease process distinct from acute pancreatitis or as a complication of repeated attacks of acute pancreatitis although this is less common in children than adults (Semelka et al., 1997; Stringer, 1989). It begins as a focal inflammatory process that spreads to other segments of the pancreas, becoming diffuse only in its end stage. An exception is chronic obstructive pancreatitis, a subtype of chronic pancreatitis characterized by homogeneous, diffuse, and steadily progressive fibrosis caused by benign or malignant obstruction of the main pancreatic duct (Freeny, 1989).

Clinical Manifestations

The first clinical sign of chronic pancreatitis usually is pain, which may be accompanied or followed by endocrine or exocrine functional impairment as the disease progresses. Pancreatic function tests or imaging may not detect chronic pancreatitis at its clinical onset, when pain is typically the only symptom (Freeny, 1989).

Imaging

Pancreatic calcification may be seen on plain-film radiography, ultrasonography, or CT (Figure 13–11). The pancreas appears echogenic on ultrasonography, and ductal dilatation may be seen. A review of the CT features of pancreatitis showed that 66% of cases had dilatation of the main pancreatic duct, 54% had parenchymal atrophy, 50% had pancreatic calcifications, 34% had pseudocysts, 32% had focal pancreatic enlargement, 29% had biliary ductal dilatation, and 16% had densities in the peri-

pancreatic fat or fascia. No abnormalities were detected in 7% of patients (Thompson et al., 1984). Magnetic resonance imaging may outperform CT in detecting changes of chronic pancreatitis because MR can detect not only morphologic changes but the presence of fibrosis. This appears as diminished signal intensity on T1-weighted fat-suppressed images and diminished heterogeneous enhancement on immediate postgadolinium gradient echo image (Ferroi et al., 1996). A recent study of 22 patients, including 13 with chronic calcifying pancreatitis and 9 with acute recurrent pancreatitis, found significant differences between these groups on T1-weighted, fat-suppressed and immediate postgadolinium MRs (Kelekis et al., 1995). All chronic pancreatitis patients with pancreatic calcifications on CT had decreased signal intensity of the pancreas on T1-weighted fat-suppressed images with abnormally low contrast enhancement on immediate postgadolinium gradient echo images whereas patients with acute recurrent pancreatitis had normal signal intensity of the pancreas. Since fibrosis occurs before calcification, MR may be able to detect chronic pancreatitis at an earlier stage than CT (Semelka et al., 1997).

PANCREATIC TRAUMA

Pancreatic trauma occurs in less than 10% of abdominal injury cases. The majority of injuries in children result from blunt abdominal trauma, most commonly from motor vehicle and bicycle accidents. Pancreatic trauma is the most common cause of acute pancreatitis in children. Early diagnosis is important as a delay of more than 24 hours is associated with increased morbidity (Bagi et al., 1996; Shilyansky et al., 1997; Lane et al., 1996; Wisner et al., 1990) (Table 13–4).

Clinical Presentation

The typical clinical presentation is initially nonspecific and worsens over time. The classic triad of upper abdominal pain, hyperamylasemia, and leukocytosis is present in only a minority of patients (Lane et al., 1996). False-negative amylase levels are present in approximately 70% of patients with penetrating, and 30% of patients with blunt, pancreatic injuries (Wisner et al., 1990; Olsen, 1973). Common associated injuries are liver, spleen, stomach, and

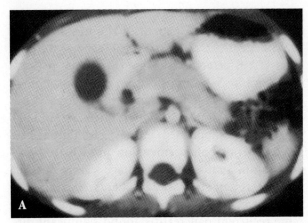
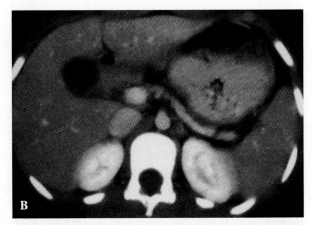

FIGURE 13–10. Fibrosing pancreatitis. *A*, Initial CT done at the time of onset of cholestasis shows diffuse enlargement of the pancreas, particularly the head. *B*, Follow-up CT 7 months later shows an atrophic pancreas partially replaced by fat.

colon injury, rupture of the diaphragm, and duodenal injury (Siegel and Sivit, 1997; Lane et al., 1996; Takishima et al., 1996). Isolated pancreatic injury and duodenal hematoma without perforation are more common in children than adults (Takishima et al., 1996). Out of 35 children who sustained pancreatic trauma at the Hospital for Sick Children (Toronto), 39 associated injuries were found in 22 children, including 12 duodenal, 6 splenic, and 2 lumbar spine injuries (Shilyansky et al., 1997).

Classification

Pancreatic injuries can be surgically classified by the Moore organ system, shown in Table 13–5. Severity of outcome is principally determined by the location of the injury and by the presence or absence of ductal disruption (Siegel and Sivit, 1997).

Most pancreatic injuries consist of contusions or lacerations without duct injury. Approximately 20% are more severe injuries with major ductal disruption or gland transection. The complication rate rises with the grade of injury. Mortality rates are highest when the head of the pancreas is injured and lowest when the tail is injured. The body is the part most frequently injured, due to its location in front of the lumbar spine (Siegel and Sivit, 1997; Lane et al., 1996).

Imaging

No single imaging modality is reliable for diagnosing all pancreatic injuries. Serial examinations may be necessary as pancreatic injuries evolve over time. Abdominal radiographs may demonstrate a sentinel loop or "ground glass" abdominal appearance

and separation of bowel loops from intraperitoneal fluid (Bagi et al., 1996; Akhrass et al., 1996; Wong et al., 1997).

Ultrasonography may demonstrate interruption of the pancreas, peripancreatic fluid collections, and altered pancreatic echogenicity. Often more time consuming and less sensitive than CT to pancreatic injury (Arkovitz et al., 1997), ultrasound is primarily used to follow known injuries, especially peripancreatic fluid collections (Siegel and Sivit, 1997) (Figure 13–12).

Computed tomography is the modality of choice for the investigation and initial evaluation of children with suspected pancreatic injury (Bagi et al., 1996; Akhrass et al., 1996; Wong et al., 1997). Findings of pancreatic injury on CT include direct visualization of pancreatic parenchymal injury with transection, fracture, contusion, hematoma, or enlargement. Pancreatic fracture or transection is shown on abdominal CT by a fracture line across the long axis of the pancreas. Indirect signs of injury include free fluid in the intra- and retroperitoneal spaces, fluid in the lesser sac, fluid separating the splenic vein and pancreatic body or surrounding the splenic and portal veins, and thickening of the left anterior renal fascia (Siegel and Sivit, 1997; Shilyansky et al., 1997; Lane et al., 1996; Sivit et al., 1992; Dodds et al., 1990; Lane et al., 1994; Van Steenbergen et al., 1987) (Figures 13–13, 13–14, 13–15). The most reliable indicators of pancreatic injury are lesser sac and focal peripancreatic fluid (Shilyansky et al., 1997; Sivit et al., 1992). Table 13–6 summarizes the direct and indirect CT findings in 25 children with pancreatic injuries at the Hospital for Sick Children.

Several studies have documented the insensitivity of CT to pancreatic injury at initial evaluation. The finding by Sivit et al. (1992) that approximately one-third of pancreatic injuries were missed by CT at initial evaluation has been corroborated by others (Akhrass et al., 1996; Rescorla et al., 1995). A recent review of 35 children with pancreatic injuries at the authors' institution gave similar results.

A CT-based grading system has recently been proposed for adults. Grade A injuries include pancreatitis and/or superficial (< 50% of parenchyma in anteroposterior dimension) lacerations at any site, grade B injuries are deep lacerations or transections distally, and grade C injuries are deep lacerations or transections proximally. Lacerations through more than 50% of the pancreas are considered deep and provide presumptive evidence of duct disruption. This grading system has been useful in predicting ductal integrity or disruption and the need for emergency ERCP or surgical exploration (Wong et al., 1997).

The role of MR in pediatric pancreatic injury remains to be established. Acute traumatic injury resulting in either transection or hemorrhagic pancreatitis shows increased signal intensity on T1-weighted images. Increased signal may also be noted on T2-weighted scans secondary to hemorrhage and pancreatic edema. Focal dilatation of the pancreatic duct may also be seen.

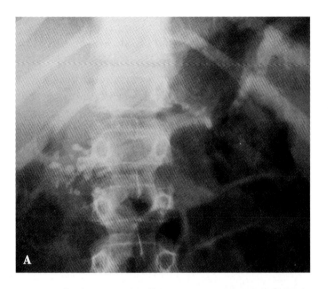

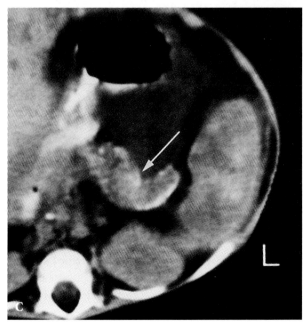

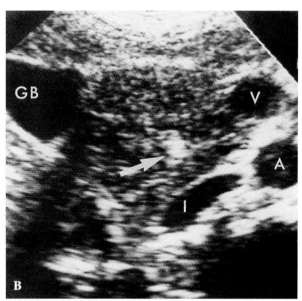

FIGURE 13–11. Chronic pancreatitis. *A,* Pancreatic calcification is visible on the plain-film radiograph of a 14-year-old boy with hereditary pancreatitis. *B,* Oblique ultrasonograph shows enlargement of the head of the pancreas and an echogenic focus of early calcification (*arrow*). The head of the pancreas lies medial to the gallbladder (GB), lateral to the aorta (A) and venous confluence (V) of the splenic and superior mesenteric vein, and anterior to the inferior vena cava (I). *C,* Computed tomography of a liver-transplant patient shows speckled calcification in the tail of the pancreas (*arrow*) and an anterior collection of fluid in the lesser sac.

TABLE 13–4.   Etiology of Pancreatic Trauma at the Hospital for Sick Children and Overall*

Etiology	HSC(%)	Overall(%)
Passenger in an automobile	7 (20)	39 (29)
Bicycle handlebars	7 (20)	38 (28)
Fall	6 (17.1)	15 (11)
Pedestrian vs. automobile	5 (14.3)	12 (9)
Recreational activity	5 (14.3)	3 (2.2)
Child abuse	3 (8.6)	13 (9.8)
Crush	2 (5.7)	1 (0.75)
Other	–	12 (9)
Total number of patients	35	133

*Bagi et al., 1996; Shilyanski et al., 1997; Lane et al., 1996; Wisner et al., 1990; Arkovitz et al., 1997; Akhrass et al., 1996. Data from Arkovitz et al., 1997; Akhrass et al., 1996; Tso et al., 1993; Takishima et al., 1996; McGahren, 1995; Bass et al., 1988; Keller et al., 1997; Smith et al., 1988; Grosfeld and Cooney, 1975.

Management

The management of pancreatic injuries is controversial. Most researchers agree that surgery is not required in the absence of pancreatic ductal disruption and that total parenteral nutrition and bowel rest is the standard of care (Siegel and Sivit, 1997; McGahren et al., 1995; Bass et al., 1988; Rescorla et al., 1990; Hilfer and Holgersen, 1995). For suspect-

TABLE 13–5.   Classification of Pancreatic Injury

Grade I	Superficial contusion or laceration without duct injury
Grade II	Major laceration without duct injury
Grade III	Distal parenchymal injury involving the distal main duct
Grade IV	Proximal parenchymal injury involving the proximal duct
Grade V	Combined pancreatic and duodenal injury

Data from Moore et al., 1990.

ed ductal disruption, however, some recommend ERCP while others advocate early surgical exploration and distal pancreatectomy (Shilyansky et al., 1997; McGahren et al., 1995; Van Steenbergen et al., 1987; Rescorla et al., 1990). The use of ERCP in pediatric pancreatic trauma has been limited as it requires experienced endoscopists and because of concerns of post-ERCP pancreatitis. Suggested indications for ERCP include a CT scan suggestive of deep pancreatic laceration, pancreatic swelling or heterogeneous pancreatic enhancement, elevated serum amylase levels, lesser-sac fluid collection, and persistent pancreatitis (McGahren et al., 1995; Wong et al., 1997; Sivit et al., 1992; Rescorla et al., 1995) (Figure 13–16).

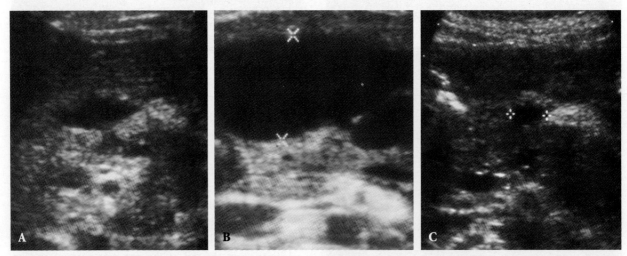

FIGURE 13–12. Pancreatic pseudocyst formation. *A,* Transverse ultrasonograph of the epigastrium in a 14-year-old male in a motor vehicle accident (MVA) obtained at the time of injury, demonstrates laceration of the pancreatic neck, inhomogeneity and enlargement of the pancreas, and peripancreatic fluid. *B,* Transverse ultrasonograph obtained 4 weeks later demonstrates the development of a multiloculated pseudocyst in the lesser sac. *C,* Transverse ultrasonograph obtained 8 weeks after the initial injury, without intervention, shows interval decrease in size of the pseudocyst. The fracture line is still visible.

A recent review of all children who sustained pancreatic injuries at the Hospital for Sick Children without associated injuries requiring surgery showed that all were treated successfully without surgery. Higher-grade injuries with apparent duct transection may heal spontaneously, possibly due to recanalization of the pancreatic duct (Shilyansky et al., 1997).

Complications

Common complications of pancreatic injury include pancreatitis and acute fluid collections, pseudocysts, abscesses, and fistulae. Most complications are well seen with either US or CT (Siegel and Sivit, 1997; Bagi et al., 1996; Akhrass et al., 1996) (Figures 13–17 and 13–18). In our study, the signs and symptoms of pancreatic trauma resolved spontaneously in 61% of patients. Pseudocysts developed in 10 out of 35 patients with other less frequent complications and resolved spontaneously in 4 patients. Percutaneous drainage was satisfactory in the remaining 6 cases, and no surgical intervention was needed in any patient. Pseudocysts should be suspected in the presence of continued abdominal pain or mass and should be monitored since hemorrhage, perforation, infection, and biliary or intestinal obstruction can occur (Siegel and Sivit, 1997). Pseudocysts larger than 6 cm causing persistent symptoms or not resolving should be considered for drainage. Most can be drained under ultrasonographic guidance, with surgery for those that persist despite attempted drainage. Pancreatic fistulae and abscesses may also need surgical management (Shilyansky et al., 1997; McGahren et al., 1995; Rescorla et al., 1990).

PANCREATIC NEOPLASMS

Pancreatic neoplasms are rare in children and have a different prognosis than in adults. Autopsy data suggest that pancreatic cancer causes less than 0.2% of deaths from malignant disease in children. A review of 92 cases of pancreatic disorders in infancy and childhood found only 10 cases of pancreatic tumors, of which only 40% were malignant. Insulinomas were the most common type. The rarity of these tumors makes them difficult to study (Jaksic et al., 1992; Vane et al., 1989). Table 13–7 (page 722) shows a simplified classification of pancreatic tumors (Vaughn et al., 1998; Cohen, 1992).

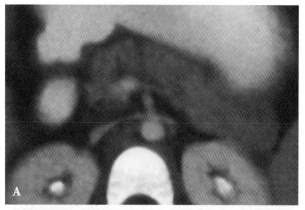
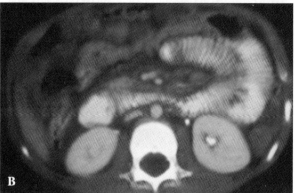
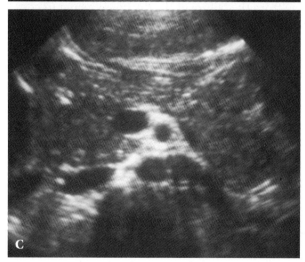

FIGURE 13–13. Pancreatic laceration. *A,* Contrast-enhanced axial CT scan in a 6-year-old male in an MVA shows a laceration of the pancreatic neck. *B,* An associated ileus of the duodenum and jejunum. *C,* Transverse US obtained 1 day later shows inhomogeneity and enlargement of the pancreatic neck, body, and tail but no definite laceration.

Pancreatoblastoma

Pancreatoblastoma most commonly occurs from ages 1 to 8 years although it can occur at any age and

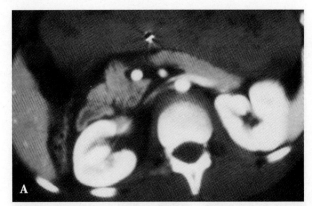 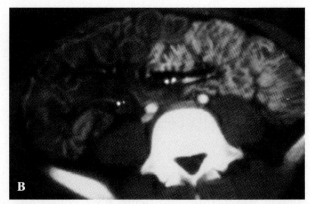

FIGURE 13–14. Axial contrast-enhanced CT scans in a 9-year-old male in an MVA. *A,* Laceration of the mid-body of the pancreas with peripancreatic fluid and distention of the stomach. There is air in the gallbladder fossa, indicating intestinal perforation. Note the slit-like inferior vena cava indicating volume depletion. *B,* Asymmetric enhancement of the small bowel, left greater than right, reflecting diffuse ischemia of the small bowel on the right.

has been reported in an infant aged 3 weeks, under the name infantile adenocarcinoma of the pancreas. It most often presents as an incidental large abdominal mass, one case also showing elevated alpha-fetoprotein (Cohen, 1992). The tumor is thought to be caused by a disturbance in organogenesis resulting from the failure of the duct of Wirsung to communicate with the duct of Santorini and the ampulla. There are two types of pancreatoblastoma: an encapsulated ventral type in the head of the pancreas and a nonencapsulated dorsal type in the remainder of the gland (Friedman and Dachman, 1994). Pancreatoblastomas are most common in the head of the pancreas. Metastases are common at diagnosis, most often to the liver and lymph nodes but also to the lungs and brain. A single case of bone

metastases has been described. Prognosis is favorable in the absence of metastases but poor when they are present (Siegel and Sivit, 1997; Cohen, 1992; Mergo et al., 1997).

Pancreatoblastomas are typically large (4 to 17 cm in greatest dimension) and sometimes encapsulated. Hemorrhage, necrosis, and cystic degeneration are common. Ultrasonographically, pancreatoblastomas are well-defined, large masses typically with a mixture of cystic and solid components. On CT scan these tumors are well-defined masses with inhomogeneous attenuation that may contain fine calcifications (Freeny, 1989; Cohen, 1992). On MR they are inhomogeneous low signal intensity on T1-weighted images and predominantly hyperintense on T2-weighted images with a heterogeneous appearance secondary to the hemorrhage and necrosis (Mergo et al., 1997).

Solid and Papillary Epithelial Neoplasm

Solid and papillary epithelial neoplasm (SPEN) is a rare low-grade malignancy occurring chiefly in young women (especially African American and East Asian women) at a mean age of about 24 years. One-third of cases occur in adolescents (Buetow et al., 1996; Friedman and Dachman, 1994). This tumor has also been called papillary epithelial neoplasm and solid and cystic acinar-cell tumor (Ohtomo et al., 1992). Patients may present with symptoms of abdominal discomfort and an enlarging abdominal mass or be asymptomatic and discovered incidentally following abdominal trauma. Sometimes they may also present with polyarthralgia or eosinophilia resulting from intravascu-

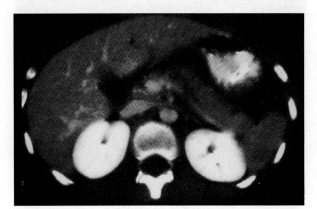

FIGURE 13–15. Unenhanced axial CT obtained in a 13-year-old male who fell 20 feet demonstrates transection of the pancreas. Note the presence of fluid between the splenic vein and pancreas.

TABLE 13–6. Direct and Indirect CT Findings in 25 Children with Pancreatic Injuries at the Hospital for Sick Children (Toronto)

Associated CT Findings	Children (n)
Intraperitoneal fluid	21
Lesser sac fluid	20
Focal peripancreatic fluid	20
Retroperitoneal fluid	20
Right anterior pararenal fluid	16
Thickened gerota's fascia (r&l)	16
Left anterior pararenal fluid	15
Mesenteric fluid or hematoma	13
Pancreatic contusion	10
Focal or diffuse pancreatic swelling	10
Left posterior pararenal fluid	9
Pancreatic fracture	7
Fluid separating splenic vein and pancreas	7
Fluid surrounding superior mesenteric vein and portal veins	7
Fluid separating pancreas and duodenum	6
Pancreatic transection	5

Data from Shilyansky et al., 1997.

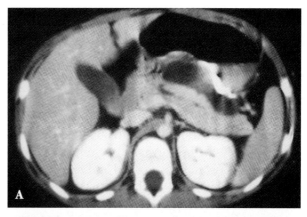

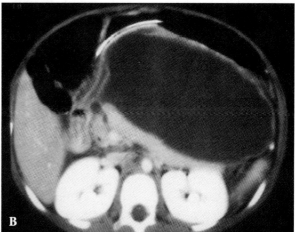

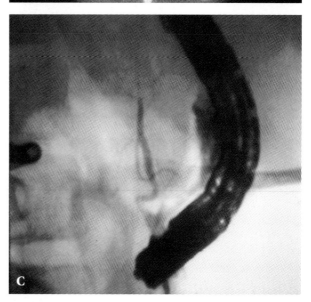

FIGURE 13–16. Pancreatic duct leak and pseudocyst. *A,B,* Enhanced axial CT scans in a 12-year-old male 4 weeks after an MVA demonstrates laceration of the neck of the pancreas, dilatation of the pancreatic duct in the body and tail of the pancreas, and a large pseudocyst in the lesser sac. *C,* Ductal disruption in the neck of the pancreas shown by ERCP.

lar release of lipase (Friedman and Dachman, 1994). Metastases are rare and most often seen in the liver (Ky et al., 1998). About one in six SPENs exhibit malignant behavior with local invasion or metastases. Treatment is resection; local invasion, recurrence, or limited metastases are not a contraindication for resection (Mao et al., 1995). In general, the survival rate is good, with patients who have unresectable tumors or hepatic metastases surviving for prolonged periods (Ky et al., 1998).

Solid and papillary epithelial neoplasms are usually large (mean diameter of 10 cm in largest review) well-encapsulated tumors most often in the body or tail of the pancreas (64%). Almost all have cystic components and internal areas of hemorrhage and calcification are common. They may be complicated by rupture of the capsule resulting in hemoperitoneum. There have been reports of papillary cystic and solid tumors developing outside the pancreas in the retroperitoneum, along the lesser curvature of the stomach, and in the liver (Mao et al., 1995; Buetow et al., 1996).

On US, these tumors are typically heterogeneous with isoechoic areas representing solid hemorrhagic or cystic hemorrhagic areas, and hypoechoic or anechoic areas corresponding to solid or cystic and hemorrhagic areas or solid and nonhemorrhagic areas. Anechoic and hypoechoic areas generally tend to be more centrally located (Ohtomo et al., 1992).

On CT scan the lesions are heterogeneously attenuated with variable enhancement (Figure 13–19). Pathologically, hyperattenuating areas correspond to solid hemorrhagic regions, soft tissue attenuation corresponds to solid and cystic hemorrhagic areas and solid nonhemorrhagic areas, and areas of attenuation equal to that of water represent cystic and hemorrhagic areas (Buetow et al., 1996).

Two review studies describing the MR appearance of these tumors found that all were well-demarcated lesions containing central high signal intensity on T1-weighted images. The central high signal intensity corresponded pathologically to areas of hemor-

rhagic necrosis. The tumors were heterogeneous on T2-weighted images, with areas of high signal intensity corresponding to solid or cystic hemorrhagic areas and solid areas without hemorrhage and areas of low signal intensity in solid and cystic hemorrhagic areas (Buetow et al., 1996; Ohtomo et al., 1992).

Although the differential diagnosis is broad, the most problematic differentiation is between SPEN and nonfunctioning islet cell tumors, as both may appear cystic, contain calcification, demonstrate areas of internal hemorrhage, and develop liver metastasis. Islet cell tumors tend to occur in a slightly older age group and do not have the female predominance seen in SPEN (Buetow et al., 1996).

Islet Cell (Endocrine) Tumors

Islet cell tumors are divided into those that are functioning and producing a clinically evident endocrine

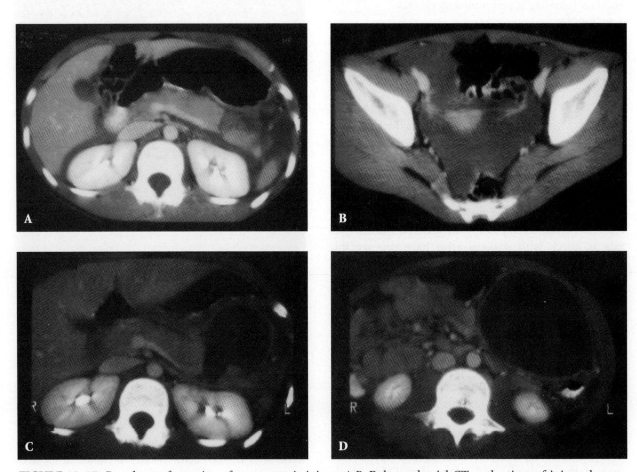

FIGURE 13–17. Pseudocyst formation after pancreatic injury. *A,B,* Enhanced axial CT at the time of injury demonstrates a laceration of the tail of the pancreas with peripancreatic, lesser sac, anterior pararenal, and intraperitoneal acute fluid collections. *C,D,* Enhanced axial CT 5 weeks after injury demonstrates the formation of a pseudocyst. This pseudocyst resolved spontaneously and did not require drainage.

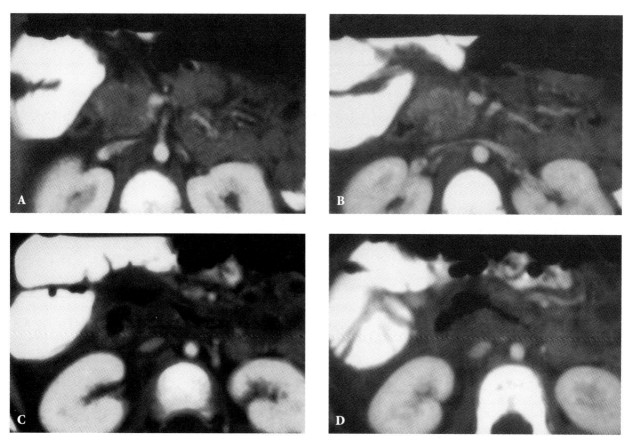

FIGURE 13–18. Post-traumatic pancreatitis. *A,B,C,D,* Enhanced axial CT scans obtained 1 week after a bicycle injury in a 4-year-old male with clinical pancreatitis demonstrate mild enlargement of the head of the pancreas and free fluid in Morison's pouch. The third segment of the duodenum is thickened due to a duodenal hematoma noted at the time of injury. The appearance of the pancreas was normal at initial presentation.

syndrome and those that are nonfunctioning and clinically silent. Functioning islet cell tumors tend to manifest earlier and are smaller at diagnosis than nonfunctioning tumors (Buetow et al., 1997). Nonfunctioning tumors account for approximately 15% of islet cell tumors (Semelka et al., 1997). Larger tumors are associated with cystic degeneration, necrosis, calcification, and more aggressive behavior (Buetow et al., 1997). Insulinomas are the most common endocrine tumor while glucagonomas almost never occur in children. Whereas the other endocrine tumors are more likely to be malignant (all over 50%), 90% of insulinomas are benign (Cohen, 1992). Islet cell tumors have no sex predilection (Friedman and Dachman, 1994). (See Table 13–2 for a classification of endocrine tumors of the pancreas.)

Islet cells probably arise from a single region of neuroendocrine-programmed ectoblast. These cells are characterized by cytochemical attributes of amine precursor uptake and decarboxylation, known as the APUD system. The potential for the secretion of multiple hormones, which occurs after neoplastic transformation, is common to APUD cells. Because some neuroendocrine cells do not fit the APUD concept, pancreatic endocrine neoplasms are called islet cell tumors. Clinical symptoms are uncommon in tumors less than 5 g; otherwise size does not correlate with severity of symptoms. The histologic diagnosis of malignancy in an islet cell tumor is difficult; only dissemination is unequivocal evidence of malignancy (Friedman and Dachman, 1994).

Insulinomas

Insulinomas manifest with inappropriately elevated plasma levels of insulin leading to symptomatic hypoglycemia with headaches, confusion, sweating, palpitations, and tremor. Because the clinical symptoms tend to appear early, these tumors are often

TABLE 13–7.   Classification of Pancreatic Tumors

Epithelial	*Nonepithelial*
Nonendocrine origin	Primary
Benign	Lymphoma
Adenoma	Primitive neuroectodermal tumor
Dermoid cyst	Sarcoma
Malignant	Metastatic
Pancreatoblastoma	Lymphoma
Solid and papillary neoplasm	Primitive neuroectodermal tumor
Endocrine origin*	Invading†
Insulinoma (beta cells)	Neuroblastoma
Gastrinoma (Zollinger-Ellison syndrome) (delta cells)	
VIPoma (PP cell)	
APUDoma	
ACTHoma (Cushing's syndrome)	

ACTH = adrenocorticotropic hormone; APUD = amine precursor uptake and decarboxylation; VIP = vasoactive intestinal polypeptide.
*Islet cell tumors (benign or malignant, functioning or nonfunctioning). Insulinomas are usually benign (90%); other endocrine tumors are more likely to be malignant (all over 50%) (Rossi et al., 1989).
†Direct invasion from the retroperitoneum.
Source: Semelka and Ascher, 1993.

small (< 2 cm in diameter) at presentation. Ninety percent of insulinomas are benign, and most are isolated neoplasms although they may be associated with multiple endocrine neoplasia type 1. Insulinomas so associated are much more likely to be multiple and recurrent (Mergo et al., 1997).

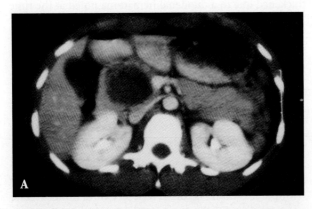

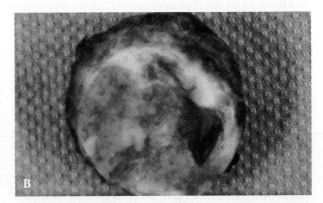

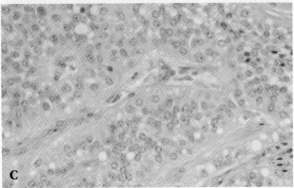

FIGURE 13–19. Solid and papillary epithelial neoplasm. *A,* Axial enhanced CT shows a spherical hypoattenuating mass in the head of the pancreas. *B,* Cut specimen shows an encapsulated mass with evidence of focal cystic change and hemorrhage. *C,* Microscopy demonstrates polygonal cells arranged in solid sheets and pseudopapillae.

Gastrinomas

Peptic ulcer disease is present in over 90% of patients with gastrinomas, due to elevated acid production. The ulcers may be multiple and are located typically in the postbulbar region of the duodenum or in the jejunum. Gastroesophageal reflux and esophagitis are also common (Buetow et al., 1997). This clinical picture is called the Zollinger-Ellison syndrome. The tumors are usually in the region of the head of the pancreas or the gastrinoma triangle, which includes the pancreatic head, duodenum, stomach, and lymph nodes (Higgins et al., 1997). The superior boundary of the triangle is the porta hepatis, and the second and third parts of the duodenum form the base. Gastrinomas are usually solitary.

Somatostatinoma, Vipoma, and ACTHoma

These islet cell tumors are much less common than insulinomas or gastrinomas. They are almost always malignant, often with liver metastases at diagnosis (Higgins et al., 1997). The classic symptoms of glucagonoma syndrome include diabetes mellitus, dermatitis, and painful glossitis. The characteristic rash, necrolytic migratory erythema, is present in more than 70% of patients. The hallmarks of the somatostatinoma syndrome are diabetes mellitus, gallbladder disease, and steatorrhea. Patients with vipomas may present with Verner-Morrison syndrome consisting of massive watery diarrhea, hypokalemia, and achlorhydria. Adrenocorticotropic hormone (ACTH)-producing tumors are a rare cause of Cushing's syndrome with the following symptoms in descending order of incidence: impaired glucose tolerance, central obesity, hypertension, oligomenorrhea, osteoporosis, purpura and striae, and muscle atrophy (Buetow et al., 1997).

IMAGING

Imaging larger islet cell tumors, such as nonfunctioning tumors, is different from that of small functioning tumors, typically insulinoma and gastrinoma. In the latter, the diagnosis has been made by the endocrinologist, and it is the radiologist's job to localize the lesion. In general, gastrinomas are more difficult to detect than insulinomas, even at surgery, partly because gastrinomas are often extrapancreatic and multiple. In contrast, over 90% of insulinomas are palpable at surgery (Buetow et al., 1997).

Ultrasonography

While ultrasonography is reliable in identifying larger islet cell tumors, its sensitivity drops considerably for tumors less than 2 cm in diameter. The sensitivity of US is approximately 20 to 75% for insulinomas and 20 to 35% for gastrinomas. These smaller lesions typically appear as hypoechoic round or oval, smoothly marginated masses. The appearance of larger tumors varies, depending on the degree of solid, cystic, hemorrhagic, and cystic components. Cystic areas are anechoic or hypoechoic with through transmission (Buetow et al., 1997).

Liver metastases may be hyper- or hypoechoic. Particularly in older patients, the presence of hyperechoic lesions helps in differentiating islet cell metastases from the typically hypoechoic metastases of pancreatic adenocarcinoma. An overall sensitivity of 77 to 94% is reported for endoscopic US. The sensitivity of intraoperative ultrasonography is between 75% and 100%, exceeding that of all other preoperative imaging methods. It is more sensitive for intrapancreatic than extrapancreatic lesions (Buetow et al., 1997).

Computed Tomography

Like ultrasonography, CT reliably detects larger islet cell tumors but is less sensitive to smaller tumors. The reported detection rates for gastrinomas and insulinomas vary between 30% and 75%. Dynamic imaging during the intra-arterial infusion of contrast has not improved overall sensitivity in detecting lesions. Larger lesions usually demonstrate hypervascular solid components, typically in the periphery, with central nonenhancing areas that correspond pathologically to areas of necrosis, fibrosis, or cystic degeneration. Smaller lesions tend to be hypervascular and of homogeneous soft tissue attenuation (Buetow et al., 1997).

Computed tomography is an effective means to detect liver metastases and vascular invasion. Although metastases from islet cell tumors are hypervascular, studies have found no significant difference in the detection of these metastases with the use of contrast-enhanced versus noncontrast CT images (Buetow et al., 1997).

Magnetic Resonance Imaging

Magnetic resonance imaging for islet cell tumors should include precontrast T1-weighted fat-suppressed images, immediate postgadolinium SGE images, and T1-weighted fat-suppressed or breath-hold images. Islet cell tumors are low in signal intensity on T1-weighted fat-suppressed images; demonstrate homogeneous, ring, or diffuse heterogeneous enhancement on immediate postgadolinium SGE; and are very high signal intensity on T2-weighted fat-suppresssed spin echo images (Higgins et al., 1997).

Gastrinomas are not as frequently hypervascular as insulinomas and tend to be slightly larger (mean size at presentation 4 cm versus insulinomas at less than 2 cm) (Higgins et al., 1997). Other conditions observable in gastrinomas by MR include gastric wall hypertrophy with intense mural enhancement on early postgadolinium SGE images, increased esophageal enhancement, and abnormal enhancement of thickness of proximal small bowel. These features are due to the effects of gastrin and reflect the inflammatory changes of peptic ulcer disease and gastic hyperplasia (Semelka et al., 1997). The ability of MR to distinguish islet cell tumors from other pancreatic neoplasms in children has not been assessed.

Scintigraphy

Octreotide, a somatostatin analogue, detects lesions that contain somatostatin receptors and can detect pancreatic endocrine tumors containing these receptors. However, only 60 to 70% of insulinomas are somatostatin receptor-positive; thus, for these tumors in particular octreotide receptor imaging is not reliable. Its reliability may be limited also by a relative paucity of receptors as opposed to the absolute size of the tumor. As a result, large tumors with few somatostatin receptors may be missed. However, octreotide-receptor imaging is more sensitive than CT, MR, US, and angiography in screening for metastatic disease, especially extrahepatic metastases (Buetow et al., 1997).

Arterial and Venous Sampling

Selective portal venous sampling (PVS) is sometimes used to detect islet cell tumors. The vein in which the highest concentration of hormone is detected indirectly identifies the location of the lesion. While PVS is accurate it is time consuming and technically difficult due to variations in venous drainage. As a result, selective arterial stimulation testing (SAST) has largely replaced PVS (Dubois et al., 1995; Buetow et al., 1997).

In SAST, secretagogues (drugs that stimulate hormone production by the specific islet cell tumor) are injected selectively into arterial branches that supply the pancreas or the liver. A twofold increase in the hormonal concentration in the hepatic vein after arterial injection identifies the artery supplying the tumor and thus the approximate location of the lesion. Different secretagogues are required for different tumors; for example, secretin is used for gastrinomas and calcium for insulinomas. This technique is generally used to detect small tumors not found with other modalities (Buetow et al., 1997).

CYSTIC PANCREATIC NEOPLASMS

Cystic pancreatic neoplasms are rare tumors. They account for less than 10 to 15% of pancreatic cysts and 1% of malignancies in adults and are far less prevalent in children. These tumors are classified into microcystic (serous) adenomas and mucinous cystic neoplasms. Microcystic adenomas are benign, without malignant potential, and thus require no treatment if asymptomatic whereas mucinous cystadenomas are thought to coexist with or develop into mucinous cystadenocarcinomas and should be removed (Johnson et al., 1988).

Microcystic adenomas typically contain over six cysts, each less than 2 cm in diameter, whereas mucinous cystadenomas and cystadenocarcinomas have six or fewer cysts, each greater than 2 cm in diameter. Calcification is seen in all types of cystic tumors but is more common in microcystic adenomas (38% versus 18% and 8% for mucinous cystadenomas and cystadenocarcinomas, respectively). A review of 12 cases comparing MR to CT found that cystic content was differentiated more easily with MR than CT. The cyst fluid is typically homogeneous in microcystic adenomas whereas it tends to vary more in signal intensity in mucinous cystadanomas and cystadenocarcinomas (Minami et al., 1989).

Cyst fluid analysis has been proposed as an aid to differential diagnosis of pancreatic cysts. Mucinous cysts are distinguished from nonmucinous cysts by a combination of cytologic findings, elevated carcinoembryonic antigen (CEA) levels, and high viscosity. Cytologic findings and elevated levels of CA15-3 and CA72-4 are useful in predicting malignancy. Pseudocysts can be identified by a combination of cytologic features, elevated levels of tumor markers including NB/70K, and elevated enzymes including amylase isoenzymes and leukocyte esterase. Serous tumors are a diagnosis of exclusion although in 50% of cases the cytologic findings will indicate a serous tumor (Lewandrowski et al., 1995).

Other Pancreatic Neoplasms

Mesenchymal Tumors
Benign mesenchymal tumors such as dermoid cyst, neurofibroma, hemangioma, and lymphangioma of the pancreas are rare. Their appearance is similar to lesions elsewhere (Friedman and Dachman, 1994). Although rare, rhabdomyosarcoma is the most common type of sarcoma seen in the pancreas (Vaughn et al., 1998).

Metastases
Metastases to the pancreas are rare and usually the result of direct extension from a contiguous organ, as in neuroblastoma, rather than a hematogenous spread. Additionally, metastases to peripancreatic nodes with secondary invasion of the pancreas are difficult to distinguish from direct metastases to the pancreas. Lymphoma has the highest incidence of metastatic spread to the pancreas in children. Other tumors reported to metastasize to the pancreas in children include ovarian, hepatocellular and renal carcinomas, and various sarcomas (Friedman and Dachman, 1994).

Clinical evidence of pancreatitis resulting from pancreatic metastases is present in only one-third to one-half of patients although the serum amylase level may be elevated in a greater proportion of patients (Friedman and Dachman, 1994). The radiologic appearance is variable and nonspecific (Figure 13–20). The diagnosis may be established by percutaneous or open biopsy.

Lymphoma
Intrinsic involvement of the pancreas occasionally occurs in non-Hodgkin's lymphoma (1% at staging laparotomy) but is rare in Hodgkin's disease. Because the pancreas lacks a well-defined capsule, it can be difficult to distinguish peripancreatic nodal disease from intrinsic pancreatic lymphoma. The incidence of both peripancreatic and pancreatic involvement is significantly higher in large-cell lymphoma (30 to 35%) and American Burkitt's lymphoma compared to other non-Hodgkin's lymphomas (Friedman and Dachman, 1994) (Figure 13–21).

Radiologic features favoring lymphoma over other pancreatic neoplasms include multifocality,

massive or widespread adenopathy, and one or more solid masses on CT that are homogeneous and very hypoechoic on ultrasonography. American Burkitt's lymphoma in particular can involve the pancreas diffusely and be impossible to distinguish from pancreatitis except by needle biopsy. Diagnosing pancreatic lymphoma with US or CT-guided biopsy is preferable as it may allow management without surgery (Friedman and Dachman, 1994).

MISCELLANEOUS PANCREATIC CONDITIONS

Cystic Fibrosis

General Considerations
Cystic fibrosis is a common multisystem disease characterized by dysfunction of exocrine glands, chronic bronchopulmonary infections, malabsorption secondary to pancreatic insufficiency, and a raised sweat sodium concentration. It occurs in approximately 1 in 2000 Caucasian children and 1 in 17,000 African American children in North America (Tham et al., 1991; McHugo et al., 1987). It is the most common life-threatening recessive genetic trait in Caucasians. Cystic fibrosis is caused by a variety of mutations in the cystic fibrosis transmembrane conductance regulator gene, most frequently F-508 (70% of cases). Patients with this genotype have a higher frequency of pancreatic insufficiency and earlier chronic airway

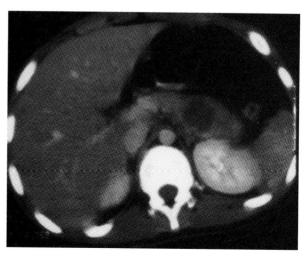

FIGURE 13–20. Ewing's sarcoma metastatic to the pancreas. Computed tomography shows a hypoattenuating mass in the body and tail of the pancreas, indistinguishable from a primary pancreatic tumor.

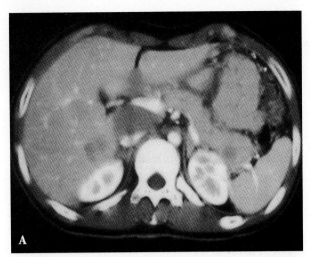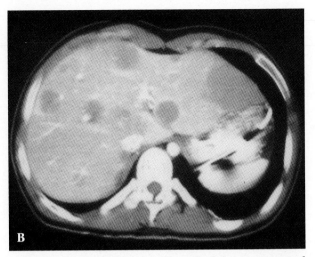

FIGURE 13–21. Lymphoblastic lymphoma of the pancreas. *A,* A hypoattenuating lesion in the tail of the pancreas and peripancreatic and periportal lymphadenopathy shown by CT. *B,* A higher image in the same patient demonstrates multiple liver lesions.

colonization by *Pseudomonas aeruginosa* than other patients (Ferrozzi et al., 1996).

Exocrine pancreatic insufficiency is present in most cystic fibrosis patients at or soon after birth although 10 to 15% of patients have sufficient pancreatic function to prevent steatorrhea. Although the course and prognosis of the disease are determined mainly by the progression of pulmonary obstruction and infection, assessment of pancreatic damage may be clinically relevant as a screen for patients at high risk of early pulmonary infection. It has been reported that patients with pancreatic insufficiency actually may have earlier colonization of the airway by *P. aeruginosa,* an event believed to be pivotal in the clinical development of the disease (Ferrozzi et al., 1996). Patients now live longer due to better management of their respiratory and pancreatic disease but the incidence of hepatobiliary complications has increased with this greater life span. In one study, approximately 47% of patients showed hepatic involvement post mortem (McHugo et al., 1987).

Imaging

Plain-Film Radiography. The pancreas rarely shows visible calcification on plain-film radiography, usually only in those patients with pancreatic insufficiency (Stringer, 1989). Calcification is seen earlier with US or CT. The calcification seen on plain-film radiographs can be fine and focal or more diffuse with large calcific foci (Figure 13–22).

Ultrasonography. The appearance of the pancreas depends on the stage and severity of disease. The pancreas is usually echogenic although in those patients lacking steatorrhea (approximately 15%) minimal or no changes may be seen (Figure 13–23). Patients with severe, long-standing symptoms of malabsorption may show marked fibrosis, fatty replacement, and cysts in the pancreas (McHugo et al., 1987; Daneman et al., 1983) (Figure 13–24). The pancreas is typically smaller than normal with increased echogenicity due to fat replacement and fibrosis although earlier it may be normal in size or occasionally enlarged. Pancreatic ductal dilatation and calcification may also be seen (Daneman et al., 1983).

Computed Tomography. Computed tomography is generally used only in those patients who present a diagnostic dilemma or in whom the pancreas is not visualized well by US. Appearances on CT generally reflect the pathologic changes of fatty replacement, fibrosis, calcifications, and cysts. Fatty replacement of the pancreas is manifested by focal or diffuse decreased attenuation of the pancreas in its normal shape whereas fibrotic replacement has normal or increased attenuation values (Daneman et al., 1983) (Figure 13–25).

Magnetic Resonance Imaging. Several studies have compared MR with US and CT for evaluating pancreatic involvement in cystic fibrosis patients.

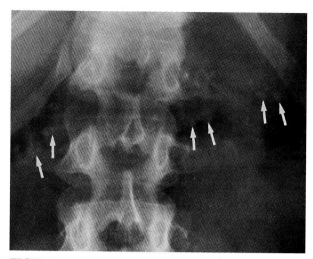

FIGURE 13–22. The pancreas in cystic fibrosis. There are multiple large calcifications (*arrows*) in the region of the pancreas.

These studies have found MR superior to US in detecting and quantitatively assessing morphologic changes in the pancreas (McHugo et al., 1987; Fiel et al., 1987). The sensitivity of MR is comparable to that of CT, ranging from 94 to 100%; however, CT requires the use of ionizing radiation (Tham et al., 1991). There are four main patterns of pancreatic involvement in cystic fibrosis patients seen on MR: a lobulated hyperintense pancreas on T1-weighted images, representing nearly complete lipomatous replacement; hyperintensity with focal areas of sparing, representing partial fatty replacement of the pancreas; no structural or signal intensity changes; and diffuse homogeneous hyperintensity without a residual lobular pattern. This last pattern has only recently been described and is thought to represent the last stage of lipomatous degeneration with destruction of the connective tissue stroma. For such patients, MR may be useful as a prognostic indicator of pancreatic insufficiency and pulmonary status (Ferrozzi et al., 1996).

Shwachman-Diamond Syndrome

Shwachman-Diamond syndrome is characterized by metaphyseal chondrodysplasia, neutropenia, and exocrine pancreatic insufficiency. Its etiology is unknown. The condition may be autosomal recessive although some cases are sporadic. Pathologically it is characterized by fatty infiltration of the pancreas, replacing the exocrine glands. Clinically it presents as shortening of the extremities, repeated

infections, and malabsorption with normal chloride levels in sweat (Berrocal et al., 1995).

Imaging

The most frequent abnormality is a delay in bone age with demineralization. Typically the carpus is more retarded than the phalanges. The typical appearance on US is diffuse increased echogenicity of a normal-sized pancreas due to fatty or fibrous infiltration. This is manifested as diffuse decreased attenutation of the pancreas on CT and increased signal on T1-weighted MR images. The differential diagnosis includes all processes causing fibrosis of the pancreas such as cystic fibrosis and chronic pancreatitis (typically resulting in a smaller-than-normal pancreas) or processes causing fat infiltration such as prolonged steroid treatment, Cushing's syndrome, or obesity and Johanson-Blizzard syndrome (Berrocal et al., 1995). Johanson-Blizzard syndrome is characterized by exocrine pancreatic insufficiency, nasal alar hypoplasia, deafness, dental abnormalities, ectodermal scalp defects, psychomotor retardation, short stature, hypothyroidism, and rectourogenital malformations (Barzilai et al., 1996).

Nesidioblastosis

Persistent hyperinsulinemic hypoglycemia of infancy (PHHI), or nesidioblastosis, is a rare heterogeneous

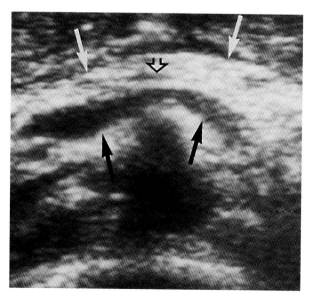

FIGURE 13–23. The pancreas in cystic fibrosis. Transverse ultrasonograph shows an echogenic pancreas (*white arrows*) just anterior to the splenic vein (*black arrows*). The pancreatic duct is dilated (*open black arrow*).

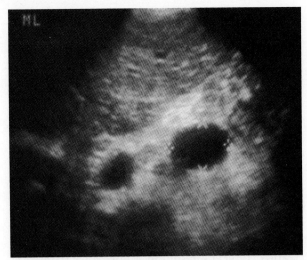

FIGURE 13–24. Pancreatic macrocyst in cystic fibrosis. Transverse ultrasonograph shows increased echogenicity of the pancreas containing a macrocyst.

disorder characterized by unregulated insulin secretion and profound hypoglycemia in the neonate due to focal or diffuse proliferation of the islet cells of the pancreas (de Lonay et al., 1997). It may be familial or sporadic and has been linked in some patients to mutations in the sulphonyl urea receptor gene (Macfarlane et al., 1997).

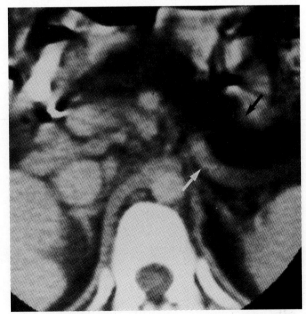

FIGURE 13–25. The pancreas in cystic fibrosis. Enhanced CT shows a small pancreas (*black arrow*) of markedly decreased attenuation due to fatty infiltration. It is just anterior to the splenic vein (*white arrow*).

It is important to distinguish patients with focal hyperplasia of islet cells of the pancreas (FoPHHI) from those with a diffuse abnormality of islets (DiPHHI) because management differs significantly. DiPHHI resistant to medical therapy is treated with a 95% pancreatectomy whereas FoPHHI is treated with a partial pancreatectomy of the affected area. This differentiation is difficult with preoperative imaging although selective venous sampling is used by some centers (Brunelle et al., 1989). Recently, a prospective review found specific loss of maternal alleles of the imprinted chromosome region 11p15 in the cells of the hyperplastic area of the pancreas in patients with focal but non-diffuse hyperplasia of pancreatic islet cells. This finding may prove useful in defining those patients with FoPHHI, thereby avoiding more extensive pancreatectomy and subsequent iatrogenic diabetes (de Lonay et al., 1997).

REFERENCES

Agha FP. Duplex ventral pancreas. Gastrointest Radiol 1987;12(1):23–5.

Akhrass R, Kim K, Brandt C. Computed tomography: an unreliable indicator of pancreatic trauma. Am Surg 1996;62(8):647–51.

Allison JW, Johnson JF III, Barr LL, et al. Induction of gastroduodenal prolapse by antral heterotopic pancreas. Pediatr Radiol 1995;25(1):50–1.

Arkovitz MS, Johnson N, Garcia VF. Pancreatic trauma in children: mechanisms of injury. J Trauma 1997;42(1): 49–53.

Bagi AE, Haddad MS, Harbi HA, Karawi MA. Delayed complications of pancreatic injury: role of CT in detection and management. Hepatogastroenterology 1996;43: 456–62.

Baker LL, Hartman GE, Northway WH. Sonographic detection of congenital pancreatic cysts in the newborn: report of a case and review of the literature. Pediatr Radiol 1990;20(6):488–90.

Balthazar EJ, Robinson DL, Megibow AJ, Ranson JH. Acute pancreatitis: value of CT in establishing prognosis. Radiology 1990;174(2):331–6.

Balthazar EJ, Freeny PC, van Sonnenberg E. Imaging and intervention in acute pancreatitis. Radiology 1994; 193(2):297–306.

Barzilai M, Lerner A, Branski D. Increased reflectivity of the pancreas in rare hereditary pancreatic insufficiency syndromes. Clin Radiol 1996;51(8):575–6.

Bass J, Di Lorenzo M, Desjardins JG, et al. Blunt pancreatic injuries in children: the role of percutaneous external drainage in the treatment of pancreatic pseudocysts. J Pediatr Surg 1988;23(8):721–4.

Berrocal T, Simon MJ, al-Assir I, et al. Shwachman-Diamond syndrome: clinical, radiological and sonographic findings. Pediatr Radiol 1995;25(5):356–9.

Bradley EL III. A clinically based classification system for acute pancreatitis. Ann Chir 1993;47(6):537–41.

Bret PM, Reinhold C, Taourel P, et al. Pancreas divisum: evaluation with MR cholangiopancreatography. Radiology 1996;199(1):99–103.

Brunelle F, Negre V, Barth MO, et al. Pancreatic venous samplings in infants and children with primary hyperinsulinism. Pediatr Radiol 1989;19(2):100–3.

Buetow PC, Buck JL, Pantongrag-Brown L, et al. Solid and papillary epithelial neoplasm of the pancreas: imaging-pathologic correlation on 56 cases. Radiology 1996;199(3):707–11.

Buetow PC, Miller DL, Parrino TV, Buck JL. Islet cell tumors of the pancreas: clinical, radiologic, and pathologic correlation in diagnosis and localization [published erratum appears in Radiographics 1997 Jul–Aug;17(4):1010]. Radiographics 1997; 17(2):453–72.

Casadei R, Campione O, Greco VM, Marrano D. Congenital true pancreatic cysts in young adults: case report and literature review [letter]. Pancreas 1996;12(4):419–21.

Cohen MD. Imaging of children with cancer. 1st ed. St. Louis: Mosby Year Book; 1992. p. 389.

Coleman BG, Rosenberg HK, Arger PH. Grayscale sonographic assessment of pancreatitis in children. Radiology 1983;146:145–50.

Daneman A, Gaskin K, Martin DJ, Cutz E. Pancreatic changes in cystic fibrosis: CT and sonographic appearances. AJR 1983;141(4):653–5.

Deignan RW, Nizzero A, Malone DE. Case report: agenesis of the dorsal pancreas: a cause of diagnostic error on abdominal sonography. Clin Radiol 1996;51(2):145–7.

de Lonlay P, Fournet JC, Rahier J, et al. Somatic deletion of the imprinted 11p15 region in sporadic persistent hyperinsulinemic hypoglycemia of infancy is specific of focal adenomatous hyperplasia and endorses partial pancreatectomy. J Clin Invest 1997;100(4):802–7.

Dodds WJ, Taylor AJ, Erickson SJ, Lawson TL. Traumatic fracture of the pancreas: CT characteristics. J Comput Assist Tomogr 1990;14(3):375–8.

Dubois J, Brunelle F, Touati G, et al. Hyperinsulinism in children: diagnostic value of pancreatic venous sampling correlated with clinical, pathological and surgical outcome in 25 cases. Pediatr Radiol 1995;25(7):512–6.

Eisenberg RL. Gastrointestinal radiology: a pattern approach. 2nd ed. Philadelphia: JB Lippincott; 1990. p. 1053.

Ferrozzi F, Bova D, Campodonico F, et al. Cystic fibrosis: MR assessment of pancreatic damage. Radiology 1996; 198(3):875–9.

Fiel SB, Friedman AC, Caroline DF, et al. Magnetic resonance imaging in young adults with cystic fibrosis. Chest 1987;91(2):181–4.

Freeny PC. Radiology of the pancreas. Radiol Clin North Am 1989;27(1):193.

Friedman ARC, Dachman AH. Radiology of the liver, biliary tract, and pancreas. St. Louis: Mosby Year Book; 1994. p. 957.

Girard RM, Dube S, Archambault AP. Hereditary pancreatitis: report of an affected Canadian kindred and review of the disease. Can Med Assoc J 1981;125(6):576–80.

Gold RP. Agenesis and pseudo-agenesis of the dorsal pancreas. Abdom Imaging 1993;18:141–4.

Grosfeld JL, Cooney DR. Pediatric and gastrointestinal trauma in children. Pediatr Clin North Am 1975;22(2):365–6.

Gudgeon AM, Heath DI, Hurley PR, et al. Trypsinogen activation peptides assay in the early prediction of severity of acute pancreatitis. Lancet 1990;335:4–8.

Herman TE, Siegel MJ. CT of the pancreas in children. AJR 1991;157:375–9.

Higgins CB, Hricak H, Helms CA. Magnetic resonance imaging of the body. 3rd ed. Philadelphia: Lippincott-Raven Publishers; 1997. p. 1588.

Hilfer CL, Holgersen LO. Massive chylous ascites and transected pancreas secondary to child abuse: successful non-surgical management. Pediatr Radiol 1995;25:117–19.

Jaksic T, Yaman M, Thorner P, et al. A 20-year review of pediatric pancreatic tumors. J Pediatr Surg 1992;27(10): 1315–7.

Jeffrey RB, Laing FC, Wing VW. Extrapancreatic spread of acute pancreatitis: new observations with real-time US. Radiology 1986;159:707–11.

Johnson CD, Stephens DH, Charboneau JW, et al. Cystic pancreatic tumors: CT and sonographic assessment. AJR 1988;151(6):1133–8.

Kelekis NL, Semelka RC, Moline PL, Doerr ME. ACTH-secreting islet cell tumor: appearances on dynamic gadolinium-enhanced MRI. Magn Reson Imaging 1995;13:641–4.

Keller MS, Stafford PW, Vane DW. Conservative management of pancreatic trauma in children. J Pediatr Surg 1997;1097–1100.

King LR, Siegel MJ, Balfe DM. Acute pancreatitis in children: CT findings of intra- and extrapancreatic fluid collections. Radiology 1995;195(1):196–200.

Ky A, Shilyansky J, Gerstle J, et al. Experience with papillary and solid epithelial neoplasms of the pancreas in children. J Pediatr Surg 1998;33(1):42–4.

Lai EC, Tompkins RK. Heterotopic pancreas. Review of a 26 year experience. Am J Surg 1985;151:697–700.

Lane MJ, Mindelzun RE, Sandhu JS, et al. CT diagnosis of blunt pancreatic trauma: importance of detecting fluid between the pancreas and the splenic vein. AJR 1994;163: 833–5.

Lane MJ, Mindelzun RE, Jeffrey RB. Diagnosis of pancreatic injury after blunt abdominal trauma. Semin Ultrasound CT MR 1996;17(2):177–82.

Lerner AD, Branski D, Lebenthal E. Pancreatic diseases in children. Pediatr Clin North Am 1996;43(1):125–56.

Lewandrowski K, Lee J, Southern J, et al. Cyst fluid analysis in the differential diagnosis of pancreatic cysts: a new approach to the preoperative assessment of pancreatic cystic lesions [see comments]. AJR 1995;164(4):815–9.

Lewin-Smith MR, Dipalma JS, Hoy GR, et al. Chronic fibrosing pancreatitis in childhood: report of a case and literature review. Pediatr Pathol Lab Med 1996;16: 681–90.

Lindstrom E, Ihse I. Computed tomography findings in pancreas divisum. Acta Radiol 1989;30(6):609–13.

Macfarlane WM, Cragg H, Docherty HM, et al. Impaired expression of transcription factor IUF1 in a pancreatic beta-cell line derived from a patient with persistent hyperinsulinaemic hypoglycaemia of infancy (nesidioblastosis). FEBS Lett 1997;413(2):304–8.

Mao C, Guvendi M, Domenico DR, et al. Papillary cystic and solid tumors of the pancreas: a pancreatic embryonic tumor? Studies of three cases and cumulative review of the world's literature. Surgery 1995;118(5):821–8.

McGahren ED, Magnuson D, Schaller RT, Tapper D. Management of the transected pancreas in children. Austr N Z J Surg 1995;65:242–6.

McHugo JM, McKeown C, Brown MT, et al. Ultrasound findings in children with cystic fibrosis. Br J Radiol 1987;60(710):137–41.

Mergo PJ, Helmberger TK, Buetow PC, et al. Pancreatic neoplasms: MR imaging and pathologic correlation. Radiographics 1997;17(2):281–301.

Minami M, Itai Y, Ohtomo K, et al. Cystic neoplasms of the pancreas: comparison of MR imaging with CT. Radiology 1989;171(1):53–6.

Moore EE, Cogbill TH, Malangoni MA. Organ injury scaling: pancreas, duodenum, small bowel, colon, and rectum. J Trauma 1990;30:1427–9.

Nishimori I, Okazaki K, Morita M, et al. Congenital hypoplasia of the dorsal pancreas: with special reference to duodenal papillary dysfunction. Am J Gastroenterol 1990;85(8):1029–33.

Nwokolo C, Oli J. Pathogenesis of juvenile tropical pancreatitis syndrome. Lancet 1980;1(8166):456–9.

Ohtomo K, Furui S, Onoue M, et al. Solid and papillary epithelial neoplasm of the pancreas: MR imaging and pathologic correlation. Radiology 1992;184(2):567–70.

Olsen WR. The serum analysis in blunt abdominal trauma. Trauma 1973;13:200–4.

Orr LA, Powell RW, Melhem RE. Sonographic demonstration of annular pancreas in the newborn. Ultrasound Med 1992;11:373–5.

Ranson JHC, Rifkind RM, Roses DF. Prognostic signs and the role of operative management in acute pancreatitis. Surg Gynecol Obstet 1975;139:69–80.

Rescorla FJ, Cory D, Vane DW, et al. Failure of percutaneous drainage in children with traumatic pancreatic pseudocysts. J Pediatr Surg 1990;25(10):1038–42.

Rescorla FJ, Plumley DA, Sherman S, et al. The efficacy of early ERCP in pediatric trauma. J Pediatr Surg 1995; 30(2):336–40.

Rossi P, Allison DJ, Bezzi M. Endocrine tumors of the pancreas. Radiol Clin North Am 1989;27:127–61.

Rubesin SE, Furth EE, Birnbaum BA, et al. Ectopic pancreas complicated by pancreatitis and pseudocyst formation mimicking jejunal diverticulitis. Br J Radiol 1997; 70:311–13.

Semelka RC, Ascher SM. MR imaging of the pancreas. Radiology 1993;188:593–602.

Semelka RC, Reinholdt C, Ascher SM. MRI of the abdomen and pelvis. New York: John Wiley & Sons; 1997.

Shilyansky J, Sena LM, Kreller M, et al. Non-operative management of pancreatic injuries in children. 1997. [Submitted]

Siegel MJ, Martin KW, Worthington JL. Normal and abnormal pancreas in children: US studies. Radiology 1987;165:15–8.

Siegel MJ, Sivit CJ. Pancreatic emergencies. Radiol Clin North Am 1997;35(4):815–30.

Sivit CJ, Eichlberger MR, Taylor GA, et al. Blunt pancreatic trauma in children: CT diagnosis. AJR 1992;158: 1097–1100.

Smith SD, Nakayama DK, Gantt N, et al. Pancreatic injuries in childhood due to blunt trauma. J Pediatr Surg 1988;23(7):610–4.

Soulen MC, Zerhouni EA, Fishman EK, et al. Enlargement of the pancreatic head in patients with pancreas divisum. Clin Imaging 1989;13(1):51–7.

Stringer DA. Pediatric gastrointestinal imaging. Burlington, Philadelphia: BC Decker;1989. p. 654.

Sugawa C, Walt AJ, Nunez DC, Masuyama H. Pancreas divisum: is it a normal anatomic variant? Am J Surg 1987; 153(1):62–7.

Takishima T, Sugimoto K, Asari Y, et al. Characteristics of pancreatic injury in children: a comparison with such injury in adults. J Pediatr Surg 1996;31(7):896–900.

Tam PK, Saing H, Irving IM, Lister J. Acute pancreatitis in children. J Pediatr Surg 1985;20(1):58–60.

Tham RT, Heyerman Hg, Falke TH, et al. Cystic fibrosis: MR imaging of the pancreas. Radiology 1991;179(1): 183–6.

Thompson NW, Eckhauser FE, Vinik AI, et al. Cystic neuroendocrine neoplasms of the pancreas and liver. Ann Surg 1984;199:158–64.

Tso EL, Beaver BL, Haller JA. Abdominal injuries in restrained pediatric passengers. J Pediatr Surg 1993;28(7): 915–9.

Ueda D. Sonographic measurement of the pancreas in children. J Clin Ultrasound 1989;17:417–23.

Uhl W, Buchler M, Malfertheiner P, et al. PMN elastase in comparison with CRP, antiproteases, and LDH as indicators of necrosis in human acute pancreatitis. Pancreas 1991;6:243–59.

Vane DW, Grosfeld JL, West KW, Rescorla FJ. Pancreatic disorders in infancy and childhood: experience with 92 cases. J Pediatr Surg 1989;24(8):771–6.

Van Steenbergen W, Samain H, Pouillon M. Transection of the pancreas demonstrated by ultrasound and CT. Gastrointest Radiol 1987;12:128–30.

Vaughn DD, Jabra AA, Fishman EK. Pancreatic disease in children and young adults: evaluation with CT. Radiographics 1998;18:1171–87.

Walsh E, Cramer B, Pushpanathan C. Pancreatic echogenicity in premature and newborn infants. Pediatr Radiol 1990;20(5):323–5.

Wang JT, Lin JT, Chuang CN, et al. Complete agenesis of the dorsal pancreas—a case report and review of the literature. Pancreas 1990;5(4):493–7.

Weizman Z, Durie PR. Acute pancreatitis in childhood. J Pediatr 1988;113(1 Pt 1):24–9.

Wisner DH, Wold RL, Frey CF. Diagnosis and treatment of pancreatic injuries. Arch Surg 1990;125:1109–13.

Wong Y-C, Wang L-J, Lin B-C, et al. CT grading of blunt pancreatic injuries: prediction of ductal disruption and surgical correlation. J Comput Assist Tomogr 1997;21(2): 246–50.

Yeung CY, Lee HC, Huang FY, et al. Pancreatitis in children—experience with 43 cases. Eur J Pediatr 1996; 155(6):458–63.

Ziegler DW, Long JA, Philippart AI, Klein MD. Pancreatitis in childhood. Experience with 49 patients. Ann Surg 1988;207(3):257–61.

14

THE SPLEEN

Paul S. Babyn, MDCM, and David A. Stringer, BSc, MBBS, FRCR, FRCPC

EMBRYOGENESIS AND NORMAL FUNCTION

The spleen is the body's largest lymphatic organ. Derived from the fusion of vascularized, isolated mesenchymal cells in the layers of the left dorsal mesogastrium, the spleen begins development during the fifth week of gestation (Dodds et al., 1990; Skandalakis et al., 1993). It develops rapidly, acquiring its characteristic triangular shape early in fetal life. In the fetus, the spleen has a lobulated outline that usually disappears by birth but occasionally may persist postnatally. A splenic lobule that remains completely separate is termed a succenturiate lobe (Hine and Wilson, 1989).

Histologic study shows that the spleen has two major components: red and white pulp. The reticuloendothelial cells are organized into lymphoid follicles collectively known as white pulp. Interspersed between these follicles are vascular sinusoids referred to as red pulp. The splenic microcirculation is important as it accounts for a variety of imaging appearances, especially following contrast injection. In the closed or fast system, blood initially flows through the white and red pulps in series with direct connection of capillaries to the venous sinuses. A smaller proportion of blood flows in the open system through the reticular meshwork of the red pulp, where direct vascular connections do not exist. The open system is slower and is associated with the sequestration of damaged erythrocytes (Miles et al., 1995).

The spleen has many functions, several of which are exploited in its imaging. It acts as a reservoir of concentrated blood and can contract following adrenergic stimulation, releasing blood into the circulation (Aoki et al., 1992). Early in fetal life, the spleen is an important site of hematopoiesis, with maximal erythropoiesis evident at 20 weeks of ges-

tation. It is also involved in the sequestration and destruction of senescent red blood cells and platelets and plays a significant part in the body's immune system through phagocytosis.

NORMAL ANATOMY AND VARIANTS

Position, Shape, and Size

Normally, the spleen lies between the fundus of the stomach and the left hemidiaphragm. Almost completely enveloped by firmly adherent peritoneum, the spleen is usually attached to the stomach by the gastrosplenic ligament and to the kidney by the splenorenal ligament (Dodds et al., 1990; Skandalakis et al., 1993). These ligaments contain fine vessels that are important potential channels for collaterals if portal hypertension develops. The spleen can be ectopic if its attachments are incomplete (see Wandering Spleen in this chapter).

The spleen has a variety of shapes and sizes. In adults, it is approximately 12 cm long, 7 cm wide, and 3 cm thick, and is correspondingly smaller in children, depending on their age. Clinical evaluation of splenic enlargement is often difficult, especially when it is mild. Many nomograms for normal splenic size and volume in children as a function of body weight and age have been proposed, using ultrasonography (US), computed tomography (CT), or scintigraphy. Most nomograms use either maximal spleen length or a simplified index of splenic volume (Schlesinger et al., 1993; Prassopoulos and Cavouras, 1994; Rosenberg et al., 1991; Markisz et al., 1987; Koga and Morikawa, 1975). Splenic weight is an almost linear function of body weight: the spleen weighs approximately 15 g at birth and usually reaches maximal weight at puberty.

Splenic variants arise primarily from excessive splenogenesis and fusion anomalies. Clefts and lobulations are irregularities of the splenic outline that may be mistaken for lacerations. Lobules tend to be situated anteriorly or inferiorly and arise from fusion anomalies (Hine and Wilson, 1989). Marked lobulation can occur with deep intralobar fissures present (Hine and Wilson, 1989; Kasales et al., 1994). Splenic clefts usually lie adjacent to the diaphragm (Dodds et al., 1990).

Imaging of the Normal Spleen

On plain-film radiography, the normal spleen is usually seen in the left upper quadrant of the abdomen as a soft-tissue mass that may indent the gastric air bubble. It is particularly well visualized by US, scintigraphy, CT, and magnetic resonance imaging (MR). The spleen has a smooth, convex outer margin bounded laterally by the left hemidiaphragm and abdominal wall, and has a concave border medially where it borders the left kidney. Usually, the spleen does not extend beyond the left kidney (Freeman et al., 1993). Along its inferior border, the spleen may occasionally have prominent clefts that mimic laceration (Kasales et al., 1994).

For evaluation of the spleen in children, US is the preferred initial imaging modality. The spleen normally has a homogeneous echotexture similar to that of the liver. It may occasionally be difficult to separate the two organs in imaging, particularly in the neonate, where the left lobe of the liver may extend far across the abdomen (Figure 14–1). Transverse scans are helpful in such cases.

The largest lymphoid organ in the body, the spleen contains numerous reticuloendothelial cells, which (along with any accessory spleens) take up technetium Tc 99m sulfur colloid, showing the functioning spleen(s) as a region of radionuclide uptake.

On unenhanced CT imaging, the spleen has a homogeneous attenuation of approximately 35 to 40 Hounsfield units, higher than the renal cortex but slightly lower than the liver. With rapid scanning following contrast enhancement, the spleen initially shows heterogeneous enhancement, (Figure 14–2) reflecting uneven perfusion within the parenchyma (Miles et al., 1995; Kasales et al., 1994; Taylor et al., 1991). Shortly afterwards, the spleen displays a more homogeneous enhancement pattern (Figure 14–3) (Freeman et al., 1993).

Magnetic resonance imaging of the older child and adult typically shows the normal spleen as hypointense to liver on T1-weighted images and hyperintense on T2-weighted images (Donnelly et al., 1996; Adler, Glazer et al., 1986). The spleen typically shows similar signal intensity as the paravertebral muscles on T1-weighted images and as subcutaneous fat and the kidney on T2-weighted images (Donnelly et al., 1996). Several artifacts may be encountered on MR of the spleen, including flow and magnetic susceptibility artifacts that can mimic pathology (Ito et al., 1996). Magnetic resonance angiography can be used to show the major splenic and abdominal vessels (Johnson et al., 1991; Niwa et al., 1994).

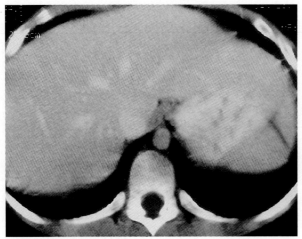

FIGURE 14–1. Axial enhanced CT scan showing left lobe of liver extending across the upper abdomen to the left side of the spleen.

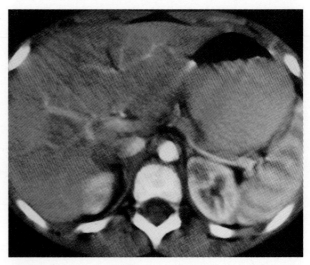

FIGURE 14–2. Axial CT scan showing normal variation in pattern of splenic enhancement.

In the neonate, particularly in the first week of life, the signal intensity of the spleen is equal to or slightly less than that of the liver on T2-weighted images. On T1-weighting, its intensity is similar to the liver, gradually decreasing by 1 month of age. By 8 months, the adult pattern has been reached for both T1- and T2-weighted images. The reason for this variation in signal intensity may be the fact that lymphoid follicles (white pulp) are small and immature in neonates, lacking active germinal matrices. The relative increased amount of vascular space in the neonate may give rise to the relatively low signal intensity observed (Donnelly et al., 1996).

Dynamic imaging after gadolinium enhancement improves detection and characterization of splenic lesions, decreasing the T1 relaxation time in tissues in which the agent accumulates. The normal spleen may show different enhancement patterns on MR, as it does on CT. These patterns are attributed to variable rates of blood flow through the red and white pulp (Miles et al., 1995; Ito et al., 1996; Mirowitz, Brown et al., 1991; Mirowitz, Gutierrez et al., 1991; Hamed et al., 1992; Semelka et al., 1992a). Splenic enhancement may be arciform, mottled, peripheral, or uniform. Uniform enhancement may occasionally be abnormal. These normal enhancement patterns seen on arterial phase imaging become homogeneous with delayed imaging (by 1 minute), helping to exclude other splenic lesions (Semelka et al., 1992a). Fat suppression may aid in defining the upper abdominal viscera by reducing image noise and improving the signal-to-noise and contrast-to-noise ratios of the spleen (Lu et al., 1994).

Other MR contrast agents are being developed but further clinical research into their effectiveness is required. Superparamagnetic iron oxide (SPIO) is a tissue-specific contrast agent that causes preferential T2 shortening and may improve detection of splenic lesions (Schwartz et al., 1994; Ferrucci and Stark, 1990). It is cleared primarily by the reticuloendothelial system of the liver and spleen, localizing in the Kupffer's cells. Iron oxide enhances contrast-to-noise ratios between normal splenic parenchyma and tumor. Since neoplastic tumor nodules do not contain phagocytic Kupffer's cells, they do not sequester SPIO. In lymphoma patients, splenomegaly by itself is an unreliable indicator of active neoplastic infiltrate. Superparamagnetic iron oxide can demonstrate diffuse lymphomatous involvement because lymphomatous spleens retain

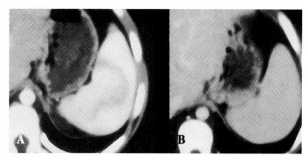

FIGURE 14–3. Normal variation in splenic enhancement. *A*, Early enhanced axial CT image demonstrates unusual splenic parenchymal attenuation, which was normal on more delayed axial image (*B*).

their diffuse bright signal after its use (Ferrucci and Stark, 1990).

Accessory Spleen

Accessory spleens, also known as splenules or splenunculi, may be single or multiple (Dodds et al., 1990; Skandalakis et al., 1993) and are found in 10 to 30% of cases at autopsy (Freeman et al., 1993), most often in the splenic hilum. They appear as round or oval opacities with imaging characteristics identical to those of the adjacent spleen (Subramanyam et al., 1984). Although not often a diagnostic problem, splenules may occasionally cause diagnostic confusion by mimicking lymphadenopathy (Figure 14–4). In rare cases, accessory spleens may be found in other locations, including the pancreas, pelvis, or wall of the stomach or intestines (Takayama et al., 1994; Barrett et al., 1996). The presence of ectopic functioning splenic tissue can be confirmed by technetium Tc 99m sulfur colloid scans (Dodds et al., 1990).

After splenectomy, accessory spleens may hypertrophy and even assume the normal configuration and function of the removed spleen (Hine and Wilson, 1989). This condition and splenosis are discussed further in this chapter under Trauma to the Spleen.

CONGENITAL AND DEVELOPMENTAL ANOMALIES

Anomalies of Situs and Heterotaxy Syndromes

Description of Syndromes
Splenic agenesis is most often associated with severe congenital cardiac defects and abnormalities of

situs although isolated agenesis is occasionally found. As abnormalities of situs and heterotaxy syndromes are complex and confusing, they are discussed in detail here.

The term situs is used to define the position of the atria and viscera relative to the sagittal midline plane. Situs solitus is the normal differentiation and placement of these asymmetric body organs with a right-sided inferior vena cava, liver, gallbladder, and trilobed lung and left-sided aorta, stomach, spleen, and bilobed lung. Situs inversus is the mirror image of situs solitus. Abnormalities occasionally occur in the arrangement of body parts, including discordance between visceral and atrial situs, variable anatomic symmetry, and dysmorphism of asymmetric structures. This condition is known as heterotaxy or situs ambiguus; it is occasionally termed partial situs inversus (Figure 14–5).

The heterotaxy syndromes represent a complex set of abnormalities of the heart, lungs, and abdominal viscera that are often associated with anomalies of situs. These syndromes are commonly categorized as polysplenia (left atrial isomerism or bilateral left-sidedness), where left-sided structures predominate, and asplenia (right isomerism or bilateral right-sidedness), where right-sided structures tend to dominate (Figures 14–5, 14–6) (Peoples et al., 1984). A wide variation in presence and

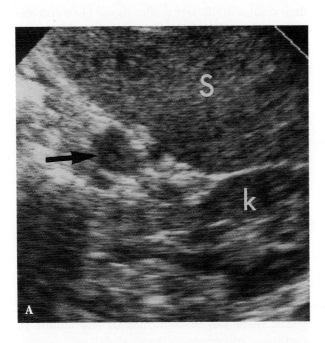

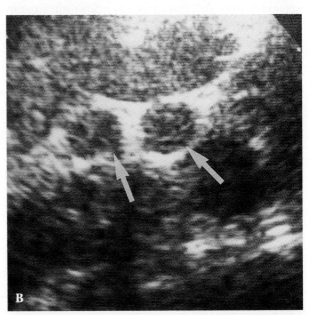

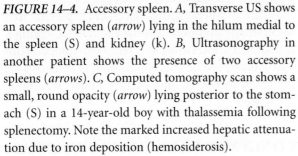

FIGURE 14–4. Accessory spleen. *A,* Transverse US shows an accessory spleen (*arrow*) lying in the hilum medial to the spleen (S) and kidney (k). *B,* Ultrasonography in another patient shows the presence of two accessory spleens (*arrows*). *C,* Computed tomography scan shows a small, round opacity (*arrow*) lying posterior to the stomach (S) in a 14-year-old boy with thalassemia following splenectomy. Note the marked increased hepatic attenuation due to iron deposition (hemosiderosis).

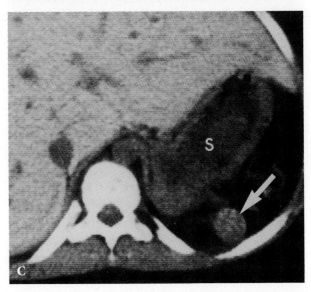

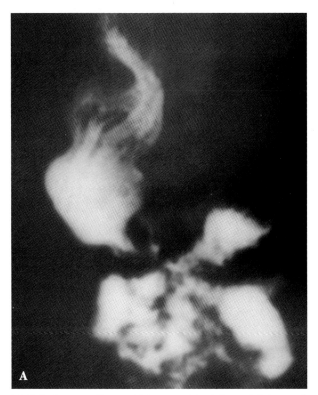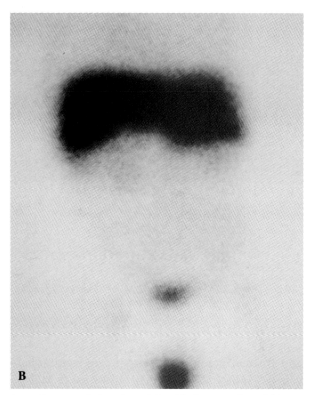

FIGURE 14–5. Situs ambiguus with right atrial isomerism. *A,* Barium meal showing right-sided stomach and hiatus hernia. *B,* Poorly functioning spleen is evident on liver/spleen scan.

type of underlying anomalies exists, and individual cases may display few of the so-called typical features (Table 14–1). Animal and human pedigree studies suggest that heterotaxy syndromes are not discrete but constitute a continuum; the unifying term "polyasplenia" has therefore been introduced to describe their overlap (Hernanz-Schulman et al., 1990). Heterotaxy syndromes should not be confused with isolated situs inversus, which is not associated with other abnormalities.

Although the exact causes are not fully understood, heterotaxy and situs abnormalities likely result from an abnormal folding of the embryo during its early development at the same time as the primitive heart and venous connections are developing. Arrested development at this stage helps explain the preponderance of cardiac abnormalities, including common atria, ventricles, abnormal venous connections, and cono-truncal anomalies (Pierce et al., 1997).

Asplenia is the absence of a spleen. Associated typical features include bilateral morphologic right lungs (trilobed, bilateral eparterial bronchi), bilateral right atrial appendages, other cardiac anomalies, midline liver, and other visceral abnormalities (Majeski and Upshur, 1978; Phoon and Neill, 1994).

By definition, multiple spleens are present in polysplenia. Polysplenia must be distinguished from a normal spleen with several accessory spleens. From 2 to 16 splenic masses of roughly equal size are generally found. Occasionally, one or two large spleens with several smaller spleens may be seen. In rare cases, a single bilobed spleen may be present, associated with all the other anomalies of polysplenia. The spleens always lie behind the stomach within the left or right upper quadrant, depending on the situs (Peoples et al., 1984). Typical features of polysplenia include bilateral morphologic left lungs (bilobed, bilateral hyparterial bronchi), absent minor fissure, bilateral morphologic left atrial appendages, and abnormal venous anatomy. Visceral abnormalities include polysplenia and malposition or absence of various organs. The stomach may be midline or left-sided. Most often the liver is midline but it may lie on either the right or left (Gagner et al., 1991).

Asplenia and polysplenia are often associated with numerous cardiac anomalies, including atrioventricular canal defects, cono-truncal anomalies,

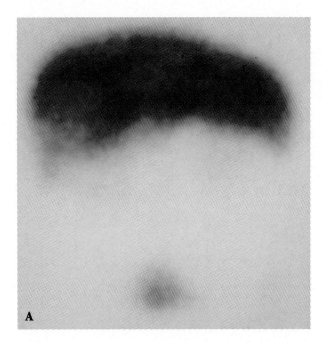

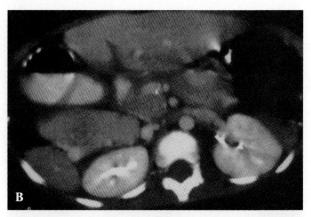

FIGURE 14–6. Polysplenia. Multiple spleens lie posterior to a right-sided stomach. *A,* Liver/spleen scintigraph shows midline liver. *B,* Axial enhanced CT shows central liver, right-sided stomach, polysplenia, and prominent azygous vein.

and frequent anomalous systemic and pulmonary venous connections (Peoples et al., 1984; Majeski and Upshur, 1978; Phoon and Neill, 1994; Sener and Alper, 1994; Sheley et al., 1995; Soler et al., 1992; Vaughn et al., 1971). Prognosis is usually determined by the severity of the anomalies. Patients with polysplenia usually have less severe or no cardiac anomalies and a better prognosis (Figure 14–7) (Peoples et al., 1984); those with asplenia have greater morbidity and mortality because of more severe anomalies as well as a predisposition to sepsis. Numerous extracardiac anomalies of the pulmonary system, gastrointestinal tract, biliary system, and vascular system, among others, have been associated with both asplenia and polysplenia. The more common of these are listed in Table 14–1.

A segmental or individualized approach to the heterotaxy syndromes has been proposed to take account of the significant variation in anatomic findings (Hernanz-Schulman et al., 1990; Pierce et al., 1997). For each patient, the exact anatomy should be described, e.g., heterotaxy syndrome: bilateral bilobed lungs, levocardia, stomach-left, malrotated, spleens-left. This description may serve as a reminder of the variability in anatomy and may thereby enhance patient care (Pierce et al., 1997).

Abnormalities of the gastrointestinal tract are common, especially malrotation (Peoples et al., 1984; Moller et al., 1971). Indeed, the presence of congenital heart disease and malrotation suggests the diagnosis of heterotaxy. Incomplete rotation or nonrotation, reversed rotation, and midgut volvulus may be found (Peoples et al., 1984). Intestinal obstruction may be seen from intraluminal membrane, annular pancreas, duodenal or jejunal atresia, or preduodenal portal vein (Peoples et al., 1984; Phoon and Neill, 1994).

Anomalies of the stomach, including hiatal hernia, tubular stomach, and gastric volvulus, have been reported with asplenia. Recurrent pneumonia or bronchiolitis in patients with asplenia should prompt evaluation for the presence of hiatal hernia and gastroesophageal reflux (Wang et al., 1993).

Biliary anomalies including biliary atresia are frequently associated with heterotaxy, most commonly polysplenia (Peoples et al., 1984; Abramson et al., 1987; Davenport et al., 1993). Other biliary anomalies reported include gallbladder agenesis or hypoplasia, choledochal cyst, and quadruplication of the intrahepatic biliary system. Biliary atresia is associated with asplenia in rare instances (Davenport et al., 1993).

Vascular anomalies are generally associated with heterotaxy syndromes (Peoples et al., 1984; Sheley et al., 1995). One of the most common vascular anomalies is interruption of the inferior vena cava with absence of its hepatic segment. The hepatic veins enter directly into the right atrium, and the azygos and hemiazygos veins enlarge to drain the lower extremities. This condition can be diagnosed prenatally if two vessels of similar size are seen posterior to the heart; normally, only the aorta is present posterior to the heart (Sheley et al., 1995). In either polysplenia or asplenia, the inferior vena cava may cross the midline anterior to the aorta in piggyback fashion to enter the common atrium. A preduodenal portal vein can also be seen in asplenia but is more common in polysplenia (Peoples et al., 1984; Tsuda et al., 1991).

Pancreatic anomalies include intraperitoneal location of the pancreas, annular pancreas, semiannular shape, and a short pancreas composed of a normal-appearing head with absent body and tail (Sener and Alper, 1994; Soler et al., 1992; Herman and Siegel, 1991a; Hadar et al., 1991). This short pancreas can simulate pathologic enlargement of the pancreatic head similar to annular pancreas or pan-

TABLE 14–1. Anomalies Associated with Heterotaxy Syndrome*

Anomalies Associated with Asplenia	Percentage of Cases Where Anomalies are Present
Cardiac	
Levocardia	53
Bilateral SVC (superior vena cava)	46
Absent coronary sinus	32
Atrial septal defect	50
Total atrioventricular canal	92
Transposition of the great arteries	62
Total anomalous venous return	51
Extracardiac	
Pulmonary	
Right isomerism	65
Left isomerism	2
Normal lobation	5
Midline liver	25
Malrotation of gut	9
Dextroposition of stomach	2
Genitourinary defects	11
Musculoskeletal	8

Anomalies Associated with Polysplenia†

Anomalies	Percentage of Cases with Polysplenia Who Do Not Have Lung or Other Abnormalities	Most Common Anomaly
Lungs	18	Bilateral bilobed lungs (58%)
Gastrointestinal tract	21	Heterotaxia (56%)
Superior vena cava	30	Bilateral superior vena cava (47%)
Inferior vena cava	18	Azygos continuation of inferior vena cava (65%)
Pulmonary veins	48	Partial anomalous pulmonary venous connection (39%)
Atrial septum	22	Ostium primum defect or variant (63%)
Ventricular septum	30	Ventricular septal defect (63%)
Great arteries	70	Transposition of the great arteries or double outlet right ventricle (each 13%)
Aortic valve	85	Subaortic stenosis (8%), atresia (5%)
Pulmonary valve	65	Valvular stenosis (23%)

*Sources: Peoples et al., 1984; Majeski and Upshur, 1978; Phoon and Neill, 1994; Sener and Alper, 1994; Vaughn et al., 1971.
†Source: Peoples et al., 1984.

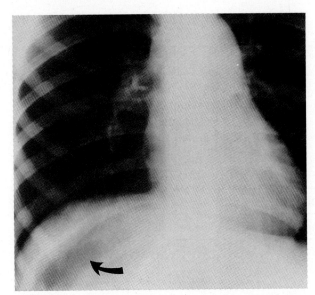

FIGURE 14–7. Polysplenia. There is levocardia and situs inversus with the stomach gas bubble on the right side (*arrow*).

creas divisum. Its presumed cause is agenesis of the dorsal pancreas or dysgenesis of pancreatic buds.

Diagnosis and Imaging of Heterotaxy Syndromes

The presence of Howell-Jolly bodies in the blood strongly suggests asplenia. These bodies can occasionally be seen in normal infants during the first week of life and in conditions of polysplenia, megaloblastic and hemolytic anemia, thalassemia, and leukemia. Absence of the spleen can then be inferred by its absence on cross-sectional imaging or radionuclide scintigraphy (Figure 14–8).

The exact form of heterotaxy is determined by evaluating numerous thoracic and abdominal structures. The evaluation should include a combination of radiologic studies: chest radiography, echocardiography, abdominal US, and upper gastrointestinal series (Pierce et al., 1997; Moller et al., 1971). Computed tomography, MR, and/or angiocardiography may also be indicated.

Chest radiography helps in evaluating the thoracic structures, showing enlargement of the azygos vein and the presence of bilobed or trilobed lungs. Lobation of the lungs can be assessed by a high kilo voltage (KV) film of the tracheal bifurcation, using a copper, tin, or aluminum filter (Deanfield and Chrispin, 1981). Plain films also help show the location of the cardiac apex and stomach bubble (see Figure 14–7).

Abdominal structures such as infradiaphragmatic venous drainage, position of the aorta relative to the midline, stomach location, liver position, and presence of the gallbladder can be evaluated with US. Barium studies (Moller et al., 1971) can show associated malrotation of the gastrointestinal tract (Figure 14–9).

All cross-sectional modalities can detect abnormal positions of the intra-abdominal vessels and liver and other associated anomalies of the viscera (Tonkin and Tonkin, 1982). Computed tomography and MR add little to the findings of US in diagnosing polysplenia or asplenia. However, MR is safe and effective for evaluating cardiac anomalies, systemic venous anomalies, and anomalies of the viscera, tracheobronchial tree, and abdomen. It should be reserved for cases that require further investigation following US (Hernanz-Schulman et al., 1990; Pierce et al., 1997).

Radionuclide scanning with technetium Tc 99m labeled and denatured red blood cells may also be useful in diagnosing heterotaxy, especially in assessing the presence of a spleen (Figure 14–10) (Bakir et al., 1994; Oates et al., 1995). A symmetric midline location of the liver may present diagnostic pitfalls, however, and lead to difficulty in separating the overlapping signals of liver and spleen. In some patients with polysplenia, the scintigraphic images take the form of a single spleen. Adjunctive single photon emission computed tomography (SPECT) in suspected polysplenia/asplenia syndromes strengthens the diagnosis when planar imaging is inconclusive, improving the identification and localization of functioning splenic tissue (Oates et al., 1995).

Despite radionuclide uptake, Howell-Jolly bodies are occasionally found in patients with cyanotic heart disease. This condition has been termed "functional splenic hypoplasia." Asplenic and hyposplenic patients need immunization and antibiotics to prevent overwhelming sepsis.

Angiography was formerly used to diagnose polysplenia (Vaughn et al., 1971). The diagnosis of numerous splenules could be made since splenic parenchyma opacifies before liver parenchyma becomes apparent. Angiography is now generally reserved for investigating associated cardiac lesions.

Wandering Spleen

Causes and Implications

A wandering or ectopic spleen is a rare condition in which the spleen migrates from its normal position

(Allen et al., 1992; Rodkey and Macknin, 1992; Broker et al., 1978). It generally originates from the failure of the dorsal mesogastrium to fuse during fetal development. This leads to a congenital deficiency of suspensory ligaments, especially the splenorenal and gastrosplenic ligaments, and predisposes the spleen to hypermobility and (often) torsion (Allen et al., 1992; Rodkey and Macknin, 1992; Herman and Siegel, 1991b; Gordon et al., 1977; Allen and Andrews, 1989). Other possible causes include acquired conditions such as splenomegaly, abdominal wall laxity (e.g., prune-belly syndrome), and the

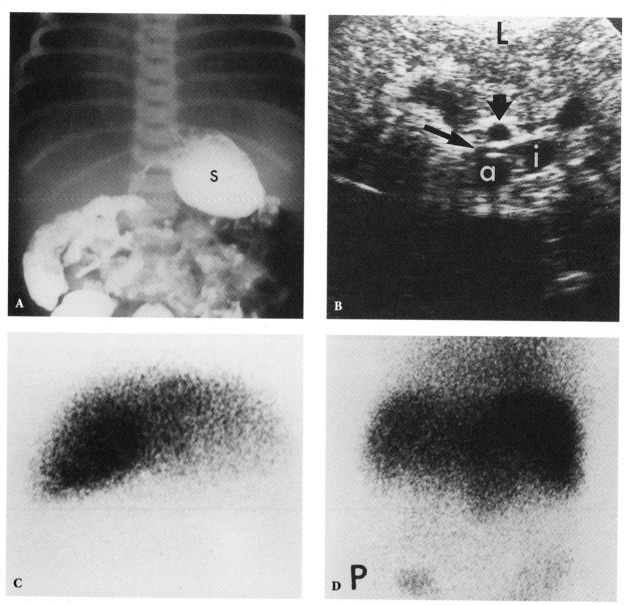

FIGURE 14–8. Asplenia. *A,* Barium meal study shows the stomach (S) on the left side. Lateral to the stomach, a soft-tissue shadow looks like the spleen but in fact is part of a symmetrical liver extending across both sides of the midline. Malrotation was confirmed during the early part of the barium meal study. In the chest, the heart is positioned on the right (dextrocardia). *B,* Transverse US shows a central liver (L) and the aorta (a) lying on the right, with the inferior vena cava (i) on the left. The right renal vein (*long black arrow*) passes between the superior mesenteric artery (*short black arrow*) and the aorta. *C,* Technetium Tc 99m sulfur colloid scintigraphy shows a centrally positioned liver and the absence of a spleen. *D,* The absence of the spleen is confirmed by a technetium Tc 99m labeled heat-damaged red-blood-cell scan that showed no functioning splenic tissue.

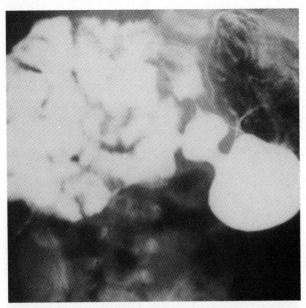

FIGURE 14–9. Polysplenia. Barium meal study demonstrates a malrotation with the small bowel on the right side.

hormonal effects of pregnancy (Rodkey and Macknin, 1992; Garcia et al., 1994).

Splenic malposition and torsion may be associated with omphaloceles or with Morgagni's and Bochdalek's diaphragmatic hernias (Phillpott and Cumming, 1994; Williams et al., 1987). Herniation

of the spleen is rarely isolated, usually occurring with other viscera (Fairhurst et al., 1992). Torsion of an intrathoracic spleen may lead to bloody pleural fluid (Phillpott and Cumming, 1994). Given the deficiency of supporting ligaments in the left upper quadrant, it is not surprising that gastric volvulus may occasionally be associated with wandering spleen (Garcia et al., 1994).

Wandering spleens are rare in childhood, and most cases occur in the first year of life or after the age of 10 years (Allen et al., 1992; Rodkey and Macknin, 1992; Allen and Andrews, 1989). Most affected children present with acute abdominal pain from torsion of the vascular pedicle. Chronic or intermittent pain or an incidental discovery of a malpositioned spleen or abdominal mass occur less frequently (Broker et al., 1978; Allen and Andrews, 1989; Shiels et al., 1989). In rare cases, gastrointestinal bleeding from varices or bowel obstruction may be the initial sign (Garcia et al., 1994).

Splenic torsion may lead to splenomegaly, hypersplenism, or splenic infarction (Rodkey and Macknin, 1992; Herman and Siegel, 1991b). Constant pain may arise from splenic congestion alone; intermittent pain may arise from intermittent torsion and spontaneous derotation of the splenic pedicle (Herman and Siegel, 1991b). More severe

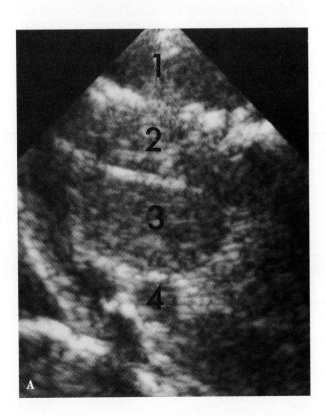

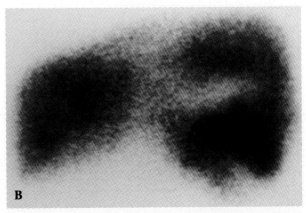

FIGURE 14–10. Polysplenia. *A,* Longitudinal US demonstrates at least four spleens (1 to 4) on the left side of the abdomen. *B,* Technetium Tc 99m sulfur colloid liver/spleen scan shows several areas of activity in the region of the spleen on the left side of the abdomen, compatible with multiple spleens. The clinical history aids differentiation between this condition and trauma, abscesses, or tumors. All these conditions can mimic polysplenia on scintigraphy with defects within a large spleen.

vascular obstruction with ischemia or infarction causes acute abdominal pain (Rodkey and Macknin, 1992). Other clinical signs and symptoms of splenic torsion are nonspecific; they include fever, nausea and vomiting, abdominal tenderness, peritoneal signs, and mild leukocytosis. Clinical diagnosis of splenic torsion is often challenging because the condition often mimics more common causes of acute abdominal pain, such as appendicitis or torsion of the ovary (Rodkey and Macknin, 1992; Herman and Siegel, 1991b).

An intraperitoneal and caudally positioned pancreatic tail may occasionally be associated with wandering spleen. If the tail is involved in the torsion, pancreatitis may occur (Sheflin et al., 1984). Other complications of splenic torsion include gangrene, abscess, localized peritonitis, and necrosis of the pancreatic tail (Herman and Siegel, 1991b).

Imaging of Wandering Spleen

Plain films may show the absence of a normally positioned spleen and the presence of a mass in the mid- or lower left abdomen (Broker et al., 1978; Allen and Andrews, 1989; Berkenblit et al., 1994). Barium enema tests may indicate displacement of the left colon by an extrinsic mass or compression of the colon from the splenic pedicle (Broker et al., 1978). Occasionally, one can see the splenic flexure interposed posteriorly between the left hemidiaphragm and the ectopic spleen (Allen et al., 1992; Rodkey and Macknin, 1992).

Ultrasonography is the initial investigation of choice. It can show the absence of a normally placed spleen and detect a mobile mass with a notched border, typically in the mid- or left abdomen. The homogeneous parenchymal echogenicity and vasculature of the spleen can be recognized. The splenic hilum often will be malpositioned and not directed medially (Kinare et al., 1990). Gastric distension alone rarely causes ultrasonographically detectable splenic displacement (Vick et al., 1985).

With torsion, US may demonstrate splenomegaly, often of rapid onset, and abnormalities of parenchymal echogenicity (Masamune et al., 1994; Bollinger and Lorentzen, 1990). Splenic parenchymal echogenicity may be coarse and diffusely hypoechoic (Shiels et al., 1989). However, a complex cystic appearance or patchy areas of increased echogenicity have been reported along with subcapsular hematomas (Kinare et al., 1990). Once the

spleen has been displaced from the left upper quadrant, bowel contents or hemorrhage in the left upper quadrant have been reported to mimic normal splenic echogenicity in rare cases. Careful assessment by US is therefore necessary (Herman, Friedwald et al., 1991). Color duplex Doppler ultrasonography helps show diminished or absent blood flow to the spleen and associated thrombosis of the splenic vein and artery if present (Berkenblit et al., 1994; Nemcek et al., 1991).

Intrasplenic dilation of the splenic vein not extending to the confluence of the portal vein is a helpful sign in the uncommon situation where the torsed spleen is still in the left upper quadrant. Involvement of the pancreatic tail with pancreatitis may give rise to abnormal echogenicity of the pancreas and peripancreatic fluid. There may be perisplenic ascites (Masamune et al., 1994).

Computed tomographic scans may show a homogeneous or heterogeneous soft-tissue mass in the lower abdomen, often with lower attenuation than normal splenic parenchyma, depending on the presence or absence of torsion (Herman and Siegel, 1991b; Berkenblit et al., 1994; Nemcek et al., 1991). After contrast administration, limited or no enhancement will be seen with torsion (Franic et al., 1988). A thick peripheral enhancing rind may be present as a result of residual capsular or subcapsular blood flow or, less likely, of adhesions (Herman and Siegel, 1991b; Shiels et al., 1989). A helpful sign of torsion on CT scan is a whorled appearance of the twisted splenic vessels and adjacent fat (Fujiwara et al., 1995; Swischuk et al., 1993).

The abnormal location of the spleen can also be confirmed by liver/spleen technetium Tc 99m sulfur colloid scintigraphy (Broker et al., 1978; Berkenblit et al., 1994). However, absence of the spleen on scintigraphy does not necessarily indicate torsion since absence can also be seen in asplenia and functional asplenia (Figure 14–11). Angiography can demonstrate the abnormal course and/or twisting of the splenic artery but is almost never needed for diagnosis (Broker et al., 1978). Angiography shows that the splenic vein is typically obstructed and not visualized, and collateral veins may be evident (Broker et al., 1978; Gordon et al., 1977).

Splenic infarction is generally treated by splenectomy. However, conservative management should be considered for patients with asymptomatic malposition and at low risk of rupture (Rodkey and Macknin, 1992; Allen and Andrews, 1989). Splenoplexy with fixation of the spleen in the left upper quadrant should be considered for children who demonstrate return of blood flow following detorsion and for those with isolated ectopia (Allen and Andrews, 1989).

Torsion of accessory spleens occurs more rarely, with similar signs and symptoms (Seo et al., 1994). Diagnosing torsion in an accessory spleen can be difficult as there is usually a normally positioned spleen (Seo et al., 1994; Erden et al., 1995).

Splenogonadal and Other Splenovisceral Fusions

Splenogonadal Fusion

Splenogonadal fusion is a rare congenital anomaly that nearly always affects males (Karaman and Gonzales, 1996; Cortes et al., 1996; Balaji et al., 1996; Miceli, 1994; Knorr and Borden, 1994; Halvorsen and Stray, 1978). The fusion occurs between the spleen and gonad, epididymis, or vas. The ectopic splenic tissue usually is contained within the tunica albuginea, with a surrounding capsule separating

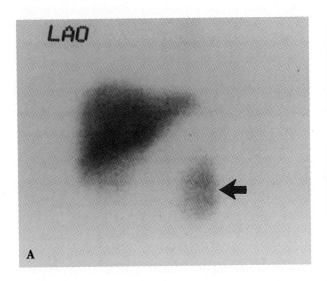

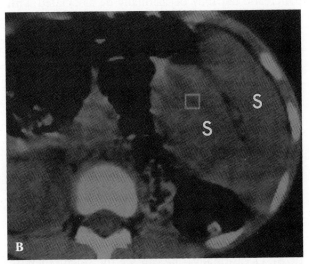

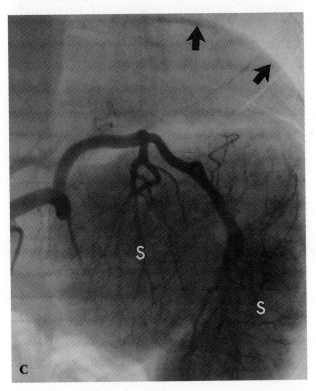

FIGURE 14–11. Ectopic spleen. *A,* The spleen is low in position as shown by the inferior location of the splenic scintigram on technetium Tc 99m sulfur colloid scan (*arrow*). *B,* Computed tomography also shows an inferiorly displaced bilobed spleen (S) inferior to the left kidney, which was seen only on more superior CT slices. Note the abnormally directed splenic hilum directed more anteriorly than normal. *C,* Angiography shows a splenic artery curling inferiorly to reach the bilobed ectopic spleen (S), which is some distance from the left hemidiaphragm (*arrows*). (Reprinted with permission from Liu et al. J Can Assoc Radiol 1985;36:163–5.)

the splenic and testicular tissue. The fusion is almost always on the left side and may be continuous or discontinuous (Karaman and Gonzales, 1996).

The slightly more common continuous type is marked by the presence of a long band of splenic or fibrous tissue that may contain splenic nodules (Karaman and Gonzales, 1996) (Figure 14–12). This band, which may be a remnant of the diaphragmatic testicular ligament, connects the normally positioned spleen to the testis and epididymis or to the ovary and mesovarium (Cortes et al., 1996). The continuous type is frequently associated with cryptorchidism and limb deformities such as amelia or peromelia. Other rare associations include anal atresia, skull asymmetry, and abnormal lung and liver fissures (Balaji et al., 1996). In the discontinuous type, ectopic splenic tissue is attached to the gonad but separated from the normally positioned spleen (Barrett et al., 1996). This condition probably occurs before the eighth week of gestation, when the mesonephros and spleen separate (Cortes et al., 1996). Associated congenital anomalies are less frequent with the discontinuous type (Walther et al., 1988).

Splenogonadal fusion is usually discovered in early childhood during the surgical repair of cryptorchidism as this anomaly often simulates a testicular mass or an inguinal hernia (Balaji et al., 1996). It can be accompanied by acute scrotal pain from acute scrotal/splenic enlargement, torsion, or rupture (Karaman and Gonzales, 1996; Balaji et al., 1996).

Ultrasonography and radionuclide scans may help diagnose this condition. Scintigraphy is specific and may show the ectopic splenic tissue and a tail of tissue extending down from the spleen (see Figure 14–12) (Miceli, 1994). Ultrasonography is not specific and may show only a homogeneous hypoechoic intratesticular or adjacent soft-tissue mass (Henderson et al., 1991). Magnetic resonance imaging may detect the lesion during investigation of the associated limb anomalies but is rarely carried out before surgery (Figure 14–13).

Other Splenovisceral Fusions

Rare anomalies are found in which splenic tissue is fused to the kidney or liver (Gonzalez-Giussi et al., 1977; Cotelingam and Saito, 1978). Intrarenal splenic tissue may mimic more ominous renal lesions such as Wilms' tumor (Gonzalez-Giussi et al., 1977).

SPLENIC INFECTION AND ABSCESS

General Considerations

The spleen may be infected by a variety of organisms including bacteria, fungi, and viruses. With viral infections, whether due to Epstein-Barr virus, *Varicellavirus*, or *Cytomegalovirus*, the spleen may be enlarged but focal abnormalities are not generally seen.

Although bacterial splenic abscesses are uncommon, the mortality rate in those patients affected may be high if the diagnosis is delayed. The clinical presentation is nonspecific and includes fever, left upper-quadrant pain and tenderness, and leukocytosis. Most of these abscesses are solitary and can be quite large especially in immunocompromised children. Common organisms include *Staphylococcus*, *Streptococcus*, *Enterobacter*, *Enterococcus*, and *Bacteroides* (Lawhorne and Zuidema, 1976; Robinson et al., 1992; Balthazar et al., 1985; Schwerk et al., 1994; Tikkakoski et al., 1992). Impaired host resistance predisposes patients to

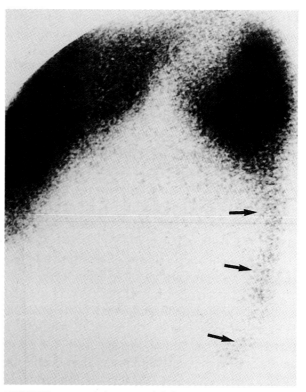

FIGURE 14–12. Splenogonadal fusion. A technetium Tc 99m sulfur colloid liver/spleen scan shows an abnormal extension of splenic activity inferiorly into the lower abdomen (*arrows*).

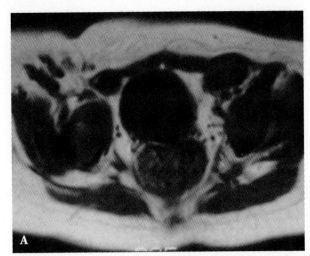

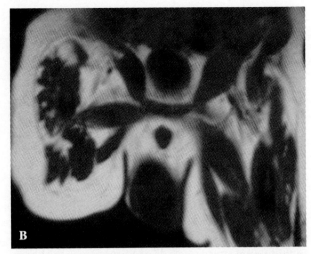

FIGURE 14–13. Splenogonadal fusion. T1-weighted axial (*A*) and coronal (*B*) imaging demonstrate soft-tissue mass anteriorly on the left, just subjacent to the anterior abdominal muscle. This child was being evaluated for extensive musculoskeletal anomalies present.

splenic infection. Abscesses occur more often in septic patients as circulating bacteria are deposited in splenic sinusoids, frequently leading to multiorgan abscesses (Balthazar et al., 1985; Tikkakoski et al., 1992). They also occur more frequently with diseases in which splenic parenchyma are damaged, such as splenic infarction, trauma, sickle cell disease, malaria, and leukemia (Lawhorne and Zuidema, 1976; Balthazar et al., 1985; Tikkakoski et al., 1992). In foci of infection such as endocarditis (Figure 14–14), symptoms of abscesses may be masked by the primary infection; in these cases, directed examination to exclude splenic abscesses may prove valuable (Lawhorne and Zuidema, 1976; Robinson et al., 1992; Balthazar et al., 1985; Ralls et al., 1982). In patients refractory to antibiotic therapy, any splenic abnormality should be considered an abscess, and appropriate therapy should be initiated (Robinson et al., 1992; Balthazar et al., 1985).

Most nonbacterial splenic abscesses are multiple and occur as complications of systemic sepsis. They are usually small, often microscopic (Lawhorne and Zuidema, 1976), and difficult to detect with imaging. Fungal infections, most commonly hepatosplenic *Candida* infections, are a frequent cause of small abscesses (Helton et al., 1986; Fitzgerald and Coblentz, 1988; Goerg et al., 1994). In immunocompromised patients, especially those receiving myelosuppressive agents for hematologic malignancies, fungal infection is often fatal (Helton et al., 1986; Miller et al., 1982; Shirkhoda et al., 1986; Flynn et al., 1995). Prolonged

antibiotic therapy can lead to changes in intestinal flora, overgrowth of *Candida* species, and ultimately to intestinal mucosal damage with resultant portal fungemia. As most fungi are filtered from the blood by the reticuloendothelial system, there may be hepatosplenic spread. Ineffective cellular immunity allows *Candida* to proliferate and leads to development of abscesses, with fungi in its central hypoechoic regions within the abscesses (Helton et al., 1986). Fungal infection is difficult to diagnose because symptoms can be nonspecific, with fever, pain, and hepatosplenomegaly often present (Helton et al., 1986; Fitzgerald and Coblentz, 1988; Goerg et al., 1994; Shirkhoda et al., 1986; Flynn et al., 1995; Semelka et al., 1992b; Schmidt et al., 1986; Vasquez et al., 1987; Schmidt et al., 1987; Chew et al., 1991).

The radiologic appearance of splenic abscesses may not be specific. Correlation with clinical history is therefore important in differentiating patients with infection from those with trauma, infarction, splenic lymphoma, or metastatic disease (Balthazar et al., 1985; Goerg et al., 1994). Diagnosis may need to be established by fine-needle aspirate (Goerg et al., 1994). The standard treatment for pyogenic abscesses has been surgery, with the addition of chemotherapy for fungal infections. Needle aspiration with instillation of antibiotics and/or placement of a drainage catheter for small pyogenic lesions may be successful. Splenectomy may still be required for larger abscesses (Schwerk et al., 1994; Tikkakoski et al., 1992). Complications of percuta-

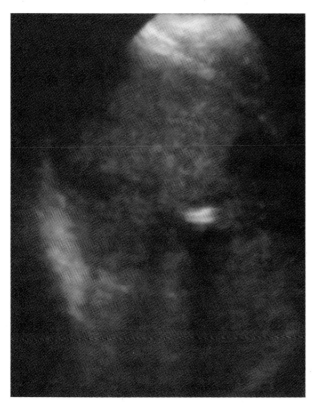

FIGURE 14–14. Inhomogeneous splenic echogenicity in this child with splenic abscess and endocarditis.

neous drainage include transgression of the pleural space, bleeding, pneumothorax, and leakage of contents along the drainage route (Schwerk et al., 1994).

Imaging of Splenic Abscesses and Specific Organisms

Splenic Abscesses

With splenic abscesses, plain films of the chest may show pleural effusion, elevation of the left hemidiaphragm, left basilar infiltrate, or extraluminal gas collection in the left upper quadrant (Paris et al., 1994). However, US is the preferred initial diagnostic modality. On US, the appearance reflects the underlying organism and its virulence, the age of the abscess, and the immunologic status of the host (Goerg et al., 1994). The abscess may be difficult to see at first and may show up only as a minor irregularity or hypoechoic area in the splenic parenchyma (Figure 14–15). Later, it typically appears as an irregular, poorly defined, hypoechoic or anechoic mass, with varying sonolucency (Figure 14–16) (Pawar et al., 1982). Internal echogenicity from debris or gas, often with distal acoustic shadowing, may be present. Associated

splenomegaly is common (Tikkakoski et al., 1992; Ralls et al., 1982; Goerg et al., 1991a). Spontaneous rupture and perisplenic extension may be seen (Pawar et al., 1982).

Computed tomography is also effective in delineating bacterial abscesses and detecting the presence of a perisplenic collection (Balthazar et al., 1985; Tikkakoski et al., 1992). Scans show the lesions with variably decreased attenuation and variable rim enhancement without central enhancement (Figure 14–17). Well-defined, wedge-shaped, peripherally situated defects most likely represent splenic infarcts. Centrally located, larger, and/or multiple lesions that are round or irregularly shaped should raise suspicions of a developing abscess (Balthazar et al., 1985).

Scans with technetium Tc 99m sulfur colloid may also detect abscesses. Nonspecific splenomegaly or focal photon-deficient areas may be present; however, false-negative studies are not uncommon (Tikkakoski et al., 1992; Miller et al., 1982; Pawar et al., 1982). Gallium-67-citrate scans are useful in showing an inflammatory mass, which appears as an area of increased activity or decreased regions, but cannot reliably distinguigh an abscess from a neoplastic mass (Miller et al., 1982).

Fungal infection can be identified on ultrasonography, especially if higher-frequency linear-

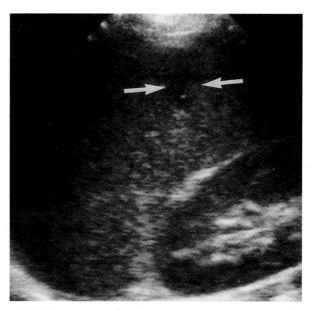

FIGURE 14–15. Early splenic abscess. Longitudinal US demonstrates a small, ill-defined hypoechoic area in the spleen (*between arrows*).

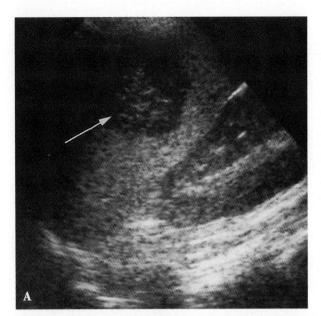

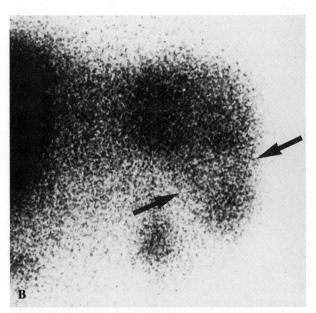

FIGURE 14–16. Later splenic abscess. *A,* Longitudinal US shows a large, well-defined hypoechoic area that contains some hyperechoic debris (*arrow*). *B,* A technetium Tc 99m sulphur colloid liver/spleen scan shows an area of decreased activity in the lower portion of the spleen (*between arrows*) at the site of the defect seen on ultrasonography.

array transducers are used (Murray et al., 1995). Candidiasis and other fungal infections consist of pus, necrotic tissue, and fungus surrounded by layers of histiocytes, chronic inflammatory cells, and fibrosis (Chew et al., 1991). Ultrasonographic changes are usually detected only when the absolute neutrophil count is higher than 1000. Fungal infection has a variable appearance on US that most likely depends on the host's inflammatory response (Figure 14–18) (Goerg et al., 1994; Pastakia et al., 1988). Computed tomography and perhaps MR may be more helpful in establishing the diagnosis of fungal infection (Figure 14–19) (Fitzgerald and Coblentz, 1988). Despite the addition of a variety of cross-sectional imaging modalities, however, many splenic abscesses remain undetected because of their small size.

Four patterns of hepatosplenic candidiasis have been described: wheel-within-a-wheel, bull's-eye, hypoechoic foci, and echogenic foci. The most common pattern consists of uniformly hypoechoic lesions. The wheel-within-a-wheel pattern consists of three concentric rings of altering echogenicity: a peripheral hypoechoic zone corresponding to a ring of fibrosis, an echogenic wheel of inflammatory cells, and a central hypoechoic nidus marked by necrosis. Fewer concentric rings are seen with the bull's-eye pattern. Any of these patterns or a combination can be found in any given patient (Pastakia et al., 1988). As healing occurs, lesions show fibrosis without a central inflammatory mass (Chew et al., 1991). This process accounts for the final pattern of echogenic foci, in which variable degrees of posterior acoustic shadowing are seen, especially after therapy. Ultrasonography may continue to show fungal lesions for many weeks (Goerg et al., 1994).

FIGURE 14–17. Extensive inhomogeneous splenic parenchyma in this child with splenic abscess.

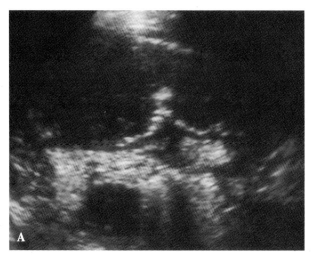
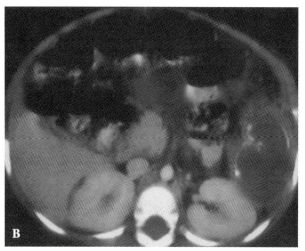

FIGURE 14–18. Splenic necrosis with fungal infection. *A,* Longitudinal US shows coarse splenic parenchyma and echogenic splenic parenchyma. *B,* Hypodense splenic parenchyma with calcified periphery.

Another ultrasonographic pattern, identified in immunocompromised patients, consists of highly echogenic foci with or without shadowing—the so-called snowstorm pattern. This is seen in many opportunistic infections, including *Pneumocystis carinii,* and likely results from calcification and/or fibrosis and fibrinous exudate (Keane et al., 1995).

Computed tomography can be used to determine the extent of visceral involvement, monitor response to therapy, and guide the progress of antifungal therapy. As with US results, however, a normal appearance on CT scan does not exclude fungal disease. The reason, as shown by histologic study, is that

during the period of low absolute neutrophil counts, little inflammatory response will be present. Findings on CT include splenomegaly, typically with multiple small (1 to 2 cm), round, hypodense, nonenhancing or minimally enhancing lesions in the liver, spleen, and kidney (Flynn et al., 1995). A bull's-eye pattern can be seen infrequently on CT; however, uniform hypodense lesions are more commonly encountered, and the wheel-within-a-wheel pattern is not observed. Areas of increased attenuation can be seen late in the course representing foci of calcification. In addition, periportal areas of increased density are evident, representing fibrosis (Pastakia et al., 1988). Both

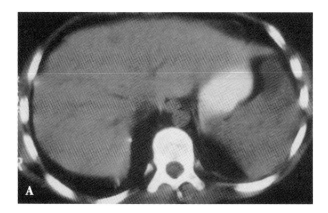
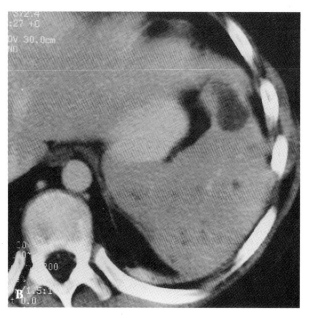

FIGURE 14–19. Fungal disease. Hypodense lesion at the anterior tip of the spleen on both (*A*) unenhanced and (*B*) enhanced CT images. Note only one splenic lesion seen on the unenhanced image, with an increased number following contrast administration.

US and CT have produced false-negative studies when compared with each other and with laparotomy (Fitzgerald and Coblentz, 1988; Pastakia et al., 1988). When CT is used, both pre- and postcontrast studies are necessary.

The differential diagnosis of multiple small lesions within the spleen includes leukemic infiltrates, fungal lesions, and pyogenic abscesses. Lesions caused by cryptococcosis, aspergillosis, or fusariosis may have a similar appearance on CT scans or US. Presumptive diagnosis of disseminated fungal disease based on clinical features and characteristic CT findings may be a reasonable approach as most fungal infections are due to *Candida* (Flynn et al., 1995). To confirm the diagnosis, however, needle or open biopsy may be needed.

Antifungal therapy may include amphotericin B. This drug can be attached to liposomes, which are selectively taken up by the reticuloendothelial system, thereby decreasing its general toxicity. Most fungal lesions will resolve within a few months but can persist for much longer. Increased calcification may be seen after treatment, and the number of lesions may remain stable or decrease. Some clinicians continue therapy until CT shows that all lesions have resolved or have become calcified. However, since most of them likely become sterile much sooner, therapy can be safely terminated when symptoms have disappeared and CT demonstrates that lesions have stabilized or decreased in number (Flynn et al., 1995). Development of new lesions on therapy, although not often seen, may represent active disease or fibrosis. Biopsy results must therefore be carefully correlated with CT findings in assessing response to therapy (Shirkhoda et al., 1986).

Magnetic resonance imaging can detect lesions in the acute, subacute, or chronic phases. These lesions are usually small foci that show high-signal intensity on fat-suppressed T2-weighted or Short Tau Inversion Recovery (STIR) images. Lesions are not usually seen on precontrast SGE T1-weighted images but are evident after contrast enhancement (Semelka et al., 1992b). Increased signal intensity may show on T1-weighted images. The appearance of bacterial infection is not well described on MR. These infections tend to be larger than fungal abscesses and more likely to have a high signal on T2-weighted images. They should have substantial perilesional enhancement after contrast injection.

Specific Organisms

Hydatid Cysts. Caused by the larval form of the genus *Echinococcus*, splenic hydatid cysts are rare but should be suspected in areas where the disease is endemic (von Sinner and Stridbeck, 1992; Franquet et al., 1990). The cysts are usually not primary but rather are encountered with cysts elsewhere, especially in the liver, a tendency that may help in diagnosis. The clinical manifestations of splenic hydatidosis are nonspecific and include abdominal pain, splenomegaly, and fever. Several immunologic tests are diagnostic for the disease (Franquet et al., 1990).

The radiographic appearance is influenced by cyst age and location along with the presence of associated complications such as secondary rupture or infection. Hydatid cysts may calcify and show up on plain films (Franquet et al., 1990). Since their appearance may be nonspecific, other cystic lesions need to be considered, including tumors, metastases, pseudocysts, abscesses, hematomas, and hemangiomas.

The germinal matrix within a hydatid cyst often produces a variety of distinctive appearances on cross-sectional imaging (Zancar et al., 1992). The presence of daughter cysts, separation of a laminated membrane from the cyst wall, and water-lily sign are characteristic of hydatid disease. A fluid debris level (caused by hydatid sand) and mural calcification are typical findings (Zancar et al., 1992; Pant and Gupta, 1987). A bull's-eye appearance on US or MR is another distinctive but uncommon finding (Zancar et al., 1992). In rare cases, cysts may have an echogenic pattern from infolded intracystic membranes and hydatid sand. Degenerated or damaged cysts may demonstrate calcification in the collapsed membranes on US, CT, or MR. Computed tomographic scans typically show hydatid cysts as sharply defined, nonenhancing lesions with homogeneous fluid water attenuation. Linear calcification or multiple daughter cysts also can be seen (Franquet et al., 1990).

Typhoid Fever. Typhoid fever patients with persistent or recurrent symptoms of deep left upper-quadrant abdominal pain, fever, or splenomegaly should be examined for splenic abscess. The *Salmonella typhi* abscess may be central or subcapsular, single or multiple, and may range from 16 mm to 6 cm in size. Splenic rupture may occur, leading to peritonitis and its high mortality rate (Allal et al., 1993).

Cat-Scratch Fever. Cat-scratch fever, a common cause of regional subacute or chronic lymphadenopathy in children and adults, is most likely due to *Rochalimaea* (Talenti et al., 1994; Larsen and Patrick, 1992). It is usually initiated by a cat scratch. When disseminated, the disease may lead to fever of unknown origin, weight loss, and visceral involvement simulating malignancy. Its effects on the spleen include enlargement and abscesses. Multiple small, round, well-defined hypoechoic lesions may be seen on ultrasonographs, or the spleen may have inhomogeneous echogenicity. Computed tomography may show hypodense lesions with peripheral or homogeneous contrast enhancement (Talenti et al., 1994; Larsen and Patrick, 1992). Splenic and liver lesions may appear similar in cat-scratch fever, with decreased attenuation both before and after contrast administration. Some lesions may be isodense after contrast. Splenic lesions may develop thick walls and demonstrate posterior wall enhancement similar to abscesses (Larsen and Patrick, 1992), and calcifications may develop with time (Talenti et al., 1994; Larsen and Patrick, 1992).

Chronic Granulomatous Disease. Chronic granulomatous disease is a rare inherited disorder of leukocyte bactericidal function, characterized by chronic infections with widespread granulomatous lesions and recurrent abscess formation. Early diagnosis and management are crucial since the mortality rate is high. Splenomegaly is common. Granulomas with hypoechoic lesions without distal acoustic enhancement suggestive of abscesses are evident in rare cases (Figures 14–20, 14–21) (Atlas et al., 1990; Orduna et al., 1989).

MASS LESIONS

Splenic Cysts

General Considerations

Cysts are among the most common focal lesions of the spleen in childhood. They may be classified as parasitic, true, or false cysts (Urrutia et al., 1996). Although the hydatid cyst is the most common cyst worldwide, post-traumatic false and true cysts are seen much more frequently in North America (Dachman et al., 1986). True cysts are developmental in origin in that they have a lining formed from an infolding of peritoneal mesothelium (Urrutia et al., 1996). This lining may undergo metaplasia, with squamous epithelium present. False cysts or pseudocysts are more common, have no lining, and are most often post-traumatic in origin (Shirkhoda et al., 1995).

True cysts are referred to as epidermoid, epithelial, or congenital (Dachman et al., 1986; Shirkhoda et al., 1995). They can show up within the fetal or neonatal periods as small or large masses (Griscom et al., 1977; Daneman and Martin, 1982; Garel and Hassan, 1995) but usually develop in later childhood or adult life. Familial cases have been described (Ragozzino et al., 1990). Most true cysts are unilocular, solitary, and lacking in rim calcification (Daneman and Martin, 1982; Musy et al., 1992). The cyst fluid may contain bilirubin, iron, cholesterol crystals, or fat (Daneman and Martin, 1982).

The clinical presentation of true and false cysts is similar: pain or splenomegaly may be noted, or a mass may be found incidentally (Dachman et al., 1986). Congenital cysts are usually asymptomatic left upper-quadrant masses although mild epigastric discomfort occasionally occurs. Less common presentations include post-traumatic splenic rupture and infection (Shirkhoda et al., 1995).

Imaging of Splenic Cysts

Differentiation between true and false cysts is not generally possible by radiologic modalities and sometimes not even by histologic analysis since both types can be affected by trauma (Dachman et al., 1986). The epithelial lining of true cysts may be deficient in parts because of pressure effects. The differential

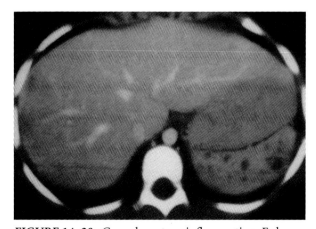

FIGURE 14–20. Granulomatous inflammation. Enhanced CT scan showing multiple small hypodense lesions within the spleen in this child with granulomatous inflammation.

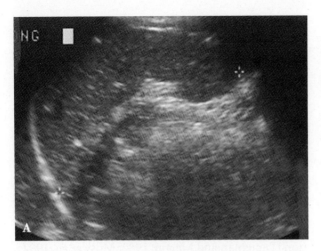

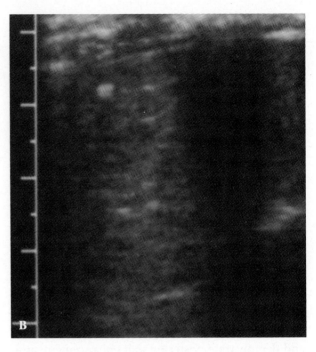

FIGURE 14–21. Prior miliary tuberculosis. *A* and *B*, Longitudinal ultrasonograph showing multiple small echogenic foci within the spleen with minimal distal acoustic shadowing from tuberculous granulomatous disease.

diagnosis includes cystic neoplasms, abscesses, and vascular lesions (see Hemangiomas in this chapter).

Plain films may show splenomegaly or evidence of a large, round soft-tissue mass (Figure 14–22), with the colon displaced inferiorly and the stomach to the

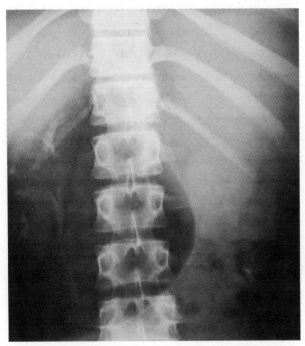

FIGURE 14–22. Splenic cyst appearing as a left upper-quadrant mass. A large cyst displaces the stomach to the right and the colon inferiorly.

right (Griscom et al., 1977). The mass may be mobile and lie in the pelvis, attached to the spleen by a narrow pedicle (Daneman and Martin, 1982).

Ultrasonography is the diagnostic modality of choice when focal splenic disease such as a cyst is suspected (Urrutia et al., 1996; Daneman and Martin, 1982; Goerg et al., 1991b). Congenital cysts usually appear as unilocular, smooth-walled anechoic lesions with enhanced through transmission (Figure 14–23). Septations and wall calcifications are infrequently present (Shirkhoda et al., 1995). Internal echogenicity, likely due to cholesterol crystals, lipid droplets, or prior hemorrhage, may be evident (Figure 14–24) (Shirkhoda et al., 1995; Daneman and Martin, 1982). Ultrasonography is particularly useful in detecting internal complex echoes, a fluid-fluid level indicating hematoma (Figure 14–25) (Dachman et al., 1986) or (in rare cases) an infection.

Scintigraphy or CT is usually not indicated after US. On technetium Tc 99m sulfur colloid liver/spleen scan, splenic cysts will appear as an area of decreased or absent uptake but the appearance will depend on their exact size and site (Dachman et al., 1986). A cyst arising superiorly may displace functioning tissue inferiorly, mimicking an ectopic spleen (Figure 14–26). The technetium Tc 99m sulfur colloid liver/spleen scan is more specific when splenic tissue surrounds a defect (Figure 14–27) or forms a claw at the cyst margin (Figure 14–28).

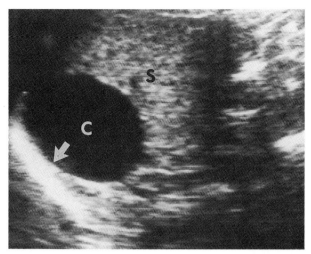

FIGURE 14–23. Splenic cyst in a 2-day-old neonate. Longitudinal US through the spleen (S) shows a unilocular, smooth-walled, well-defined cyst (C) with no internal echoes and increased through transmission (*arrow*).

Computed tomography will show a cystic appearance similar to that seen on ultrasonography (see Figure 14–26). The cysts appear as smooth-walled structures containing material near water density (Figure 14–29) that do not enhance following intravenous contrast injection. Septations and rim calcification may be better detected on CT but rarely are encountered (Dachman et al., 1986).

Angiography may be helpful in unusual cases. It shows the lesions as an avascular area (Dachman et al., 1986).

Magnetic resonance imaging of splenic cysts shows sharp lesion margination. Signal intensity is low on T1-weighted images and very high on T2-weighted images (Urrutia et al., 1996). Complicated cysts or pseudocysts with protein or hemorrhage within them can have higher signal intensity on T1-weighted images and/or heterogeneous signal on T2-weighted sequences. Cysts do not enhance after gadolinium administration.

Treatment
Large cysts are in danger of rupture or hemorrhage secondary to trauma and can cause pain. Infection is rare. Total or partial splenectomy including marsupialization has been advocated (Musy et al., 1992).

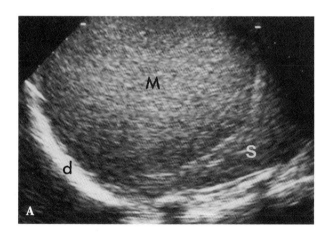

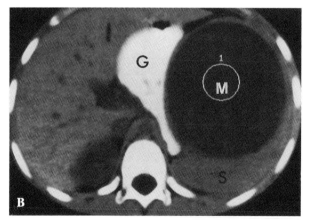

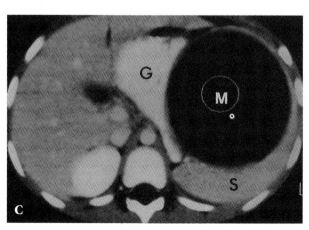

FIGURE 14–24. Splenic cyst. *A,* Longitudinal ultrasonography. *B,* Axial unenhanced CT. *C,* Ultrasonography through an abdominal mass in the left upper quadrant showed an echogenic lesion with fine echoes throughout the mass (M). It appeared less echogenic than the more normal portion of spleen (S) seen inferiorly. The diaphragm (d) was shown superior to the mass. On CT, the mass was uniformly hypodense without enhancement. The echoes were found on pathologic analysis to be cholesterol crystals. Reprinted with permission from Daneman A et al. Pediatr Radiol 1982;12:119–25.

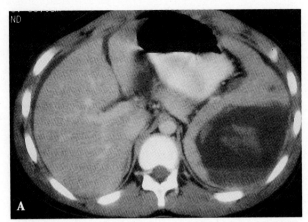

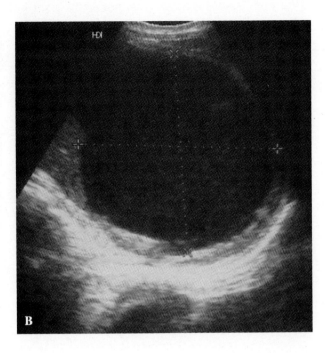

FIGURE 14–25. Post-traumatic hemorrhage within a large splenic cyst. *A,* Axial CT scan showing heterogeneous density and fluid-fluid level. *B,* At 2 weeks, US shows hypoechoic cyst fluid and irregular cyst outline. Reprinted from Daneman et al. Congenital Epithelial Splenic Cysts in Children. Pediatric Radiolgy 1982:12;119–125.

Ideally, a cyst should be removed or opened, leaving the spleen intact, as splenectomy in children runs the risk of overwhelming sepsis (Griscom et al., 1977). Spontaneous regression of apparent cysts discovered in utero or during the neonatal period has been noted. The exact cause is not known (Garel and Hassan, 1995), however, so conservative management of asymptomatic cysts may be warranted.

Percutaneous aspiration or drainage of cysts has been attempted as well as injection of a sclerosing agent; however, recurrence appears to be common (Jequier et al., 1987; Jequier et al., 1989).

Benign Tumors

Benign tumors other than splenic cysts are rare. Hemangiomas, lymphangiomas, and hamartomas

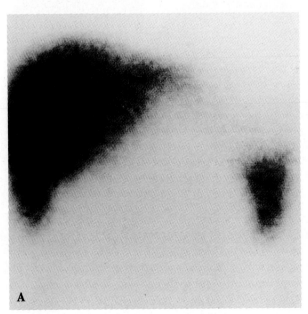

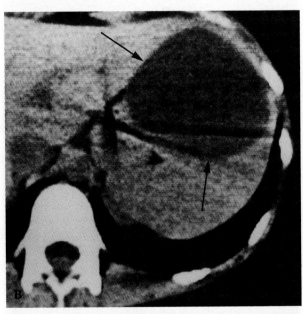

FIGURE 14–26. Splenic cyst. *A,* A splenic cyst appears as an area of absent uptake in the superior part of the spleen on technetium Tc 99m sulfur colloid liver/spleen scan. This could be mistaken for an ectopic spleen (see Figure 14–11). *B,* On CT, there is a round mass of decreased attenuation (*arrows*).

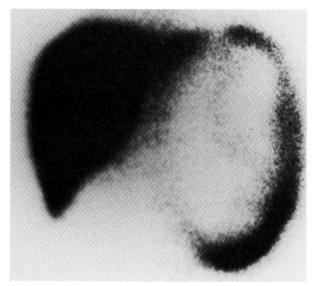

FIGURE 14–27. Splenic cyst. technetium Tc 99m sulfur colloid liver/spleen scan shows a large photon-deficient area surrounded by functioning splenic tissue.

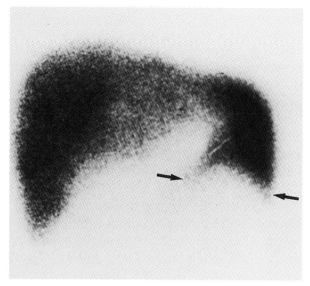

FIGURE 14–28. Splenic cyst. technetium Tc 99m sulfur colloid liver/spleen scan shows a claw of splenic tissue (*between arrows*) at the superior margin of the cyst.

are most common. Other tumors have occasionally been reported (Wadsworth et al., 1997).

Hemangiomas

Although hemangiomas are the commonest primary neoplasm of the spleen (Ros et al., 1987), they are rarely encountered in childhood (Panuel et al., 1992). Splenic hemangiomas are believed to be congenital, arising from sinusoidal epithelium (Ramani et al., 1997). They are slow-growing, may be wholly intrasplenic or exophytic, may be small or large, and can (rarely) replace the entire splenic parenchyma (Panuel et al., 1992). Generally not encapsulated, hemangiomas may appear solid or may show cystic areas of variable size (Urrutia et al., 1996; Panuel et al., 1992). Larger lesions may appear heterogeneous as a result of associated infarction, fibrosis, calcification, or pseudocystic degeneration from necrosis. Splenomegaly, portal hypertension, or rupture may also be present, particularly in adults. Hemangiomas may occasionally be multiple, either within the spleen or elsewhere, and may be associated with the Klippel-Trénaunay syndrome (Panuel et al., 1992).

Most hemangiomas are discovered incidentally as asymptomatic masses in the left upper quadrant although pain or congestive heart failure is sometimes present (Panuel et al., 1992). With splenic hemangiomatosis, the parenchyma may appear to be spongelike. Hematologic disorders

such as anemia, thrombocytopenia, and consumptive coagulopathy, features of the Kasabach-Merritt syndrome, may occur (Ros et al., 1987).

Plain films of splenic masses are usually unrewarding. Large masses with splenomegaly may dis-

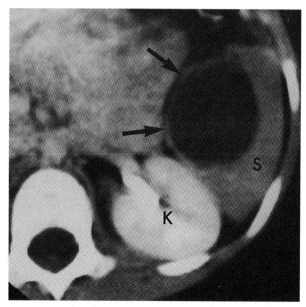

FIGURE 14–29. Splenic cyst. Contrast-enhanced CT scan shows a round mass of material of near water density arising from the spleen (S) anterior to the kidney (K). A thin enhancing rim (*arrows*) is visible around the medial aspect of the cyst.

place surrounding organs and bowel. On ultrasonographs and CT scans, hemangiomas, especially the cavernous type, may appear nonspecific and demonstrate a solid and/or cystic pattern. When US is used, the solid regions are echogenic while the cystic areas may be anechoic or show internal echogenicity from hemorrhage or necrotic material (Panuel et al., 1992). Use of compression with disappearance of vascular flow on color Doppler US suggests that the lesion is soft, in keeping with splenic hemangioma (Niizawa et al., 1991) (Figure 14–30).

Unenhanced CT images may show a hypodense or isodense mass compared with the normal spleen. After contrast enhancement, the solid parts progressively fill in from the periphery (Figure 14–31) (Panuel et al., 1992). Cavernous hemangiomas may appear more cystic (Taylor et al., 1991) and are difficult to distinguish from splenic lymphangiomas (Panuel et al., 1992). Mottled or curvilinear calcification may be present; however, calcification can be seen in other splenic masses such as cysts, hamartomas, lymphangiomas, and inflammatory pseudotumors.

Magnetic resonance imaging shows the margins of hemangiomas as well defined or slightly ill defined. The tumors are predominantly hypointense or isointense with a normal spleen on T1-weighted imaging, and mildly to strongly hyperintense on T2-weighted imaging (Panuel et al., 1992; Ros et al.,

1987; Niizawa et al., 1991). The hyperintensity is generally homogeneous although small central scars may be present. When sclerosed, hemangiomas may be isointense with a normal spleen or hypointense on T2-weighted imaging. Dynamic enhancement with gadolinium shows peripheral enhancement with centripetal progression in most hemangiomas, a pattern like that of hepatic hemangiomas. Later, on postcontrast enhancement, most of these tumors will show uniform homogeneous enhancement, hyperintense compared with the spleen, with an occasional small central scar (Ramani et al., 1997).

Technetium Tc 99m scans may show single or multiple filling defects within the spleen or increased uptake. Angiograms of hemangiomas may show an enlarged splenic artery with hypervascular or hypovascular nodule(s).

Hamartomas

Hamartomas are well-circumscribed, solid, nodular tumors composed of an anomalous mixture of unorganized vascular channels (Ohtomo et al., 1992; Thompson et al., 1996). They are extremely rare in childhood. They consist of an aberrant mixture of normal splenic constituents, predominantly red pulp elements and occasionally lymphoid (white pulp) elements (Ramani et al., 1997; Thompson et al., 1996). Rarely, hamartomas of the spleen are associated with hamartomas elsewhere, as in tuberous sclero-

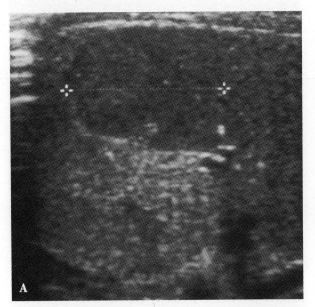
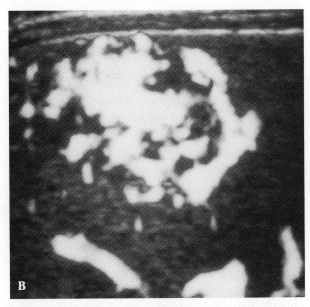

FIGURE 14–30. Splenic hemangioma. *A,* Ultrasonograph showing a well-defined hypoechoic splenic lesion outlined by Xs at the periphery of the spleen. *B,* Color Doppler shows intense flow within lesion, in keeping with hemangioma.

sis or Wiskott-Aldrich syndrome. Most hamartomas are smaller than 3 cm in size, are asymptomatic, and are discovered incidentally. However, they may cause left upper-quadrant pain, fatigue, recurrent infections, lymphadenopathy, and anemia (Thompson et al., 1996). Splenomegaly may be present. These symptoms may disappear after splenectomy.

Ultrasonography may show hamartomas as homogeneous or of mixed echogenicity. Punctate areas suggestive of calcification may be present; however, pathologic analysis may show these as hyalinized nodules (Thompson et al., 1996). On CT, hamartomas appear as solid masses of mixed attenuation that may show moderate and heterogeneous contrast enhancement (Thompson et al., 1996; Ferrozzi et al., 1996).

Magnetic resonance imaging shows hamartomas with smooth, well-defined borders, isointense with a normal spleen on T1-weighted imaging and heterogeneously hyperintense on T2-weighted imaging (Ramani et al., 1997; Ohtomo et al., 1992; Thompson et al., 1996). Hamartomas may not be as hyperintense on prolonged T2-weighted sequences as cerebrospinal fluid, a finding that may help distinguish them from splenic hemangiomas in some cases (Ramani et al., 1997; Thompson et al., 1996). After contrast administration, hamartomas show diffuse heterogeneous enhancement rather than the peripheral enhancement typically seen in hemangiomas (Ohtomo et al., 1992). On delayed imaging, however, both types of lesion enhance more uniformly. Prolonged enhancement with gadolinium has been demonstrated (Ohtomo et al., 1992).

Lymphangiomas

Splenic lymphangiomas are rare slow-growing malformations composed of thin, endothelial-lined cystic spaces characteristic of lymphatic vessels. They contain proteinaceous fluid resembling lymph rather than the erythrocytes found in hemangiomas (Ferrozzi et al., 1996). They may be isolated or part of diffuse lymphangiomatosis. The term "systemic cystic angiomatosis" has been proposed to describe the association of hemangiomas and lymphangiomas seen throughout the body, involving bones, soft tissues, and other viscera. The characteristic appearance of splenic lymphangiomas can help diagnose a more diffuse lymphangiomatous disorder. Lymphangiomas are usually discovered incidentally during investigation of other abdominal or

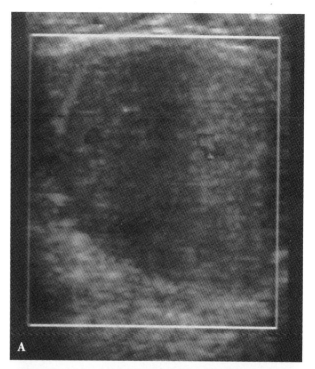

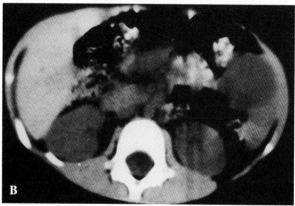

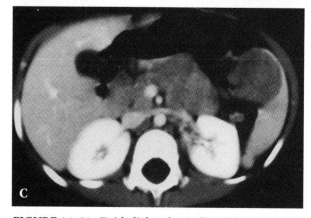

FIGURE 14–31. Epithelial and spindle cell hemangioendothelioma. *A,* Transverse US showing hypoechoic well-defined lesion with flow present on Doppler examination. Lesion confirmed on axial unenhanced (*B*) and enhanced (*C*) CT.

pelvic disorders. Symptoms may include anemia, thrombocytopenia, and moderate splenomegaly. The prognosis for splenic lymphangiomas was thought to be poor but a recent report suggests otherwise (Wadsworth et al., 1997).

Ultrasonography shows multiple well-defined anechoic or hypoechoic lesions throughout the spleen (Wadsworth et al., 1997). Internal echogenicity may be evident from proteinaceous debris (Pistoia and Markowitz, 1988). Unenhanced CT scans show hypodense, typically well-defined lesions, usually less than 1 cm in size but sometimes extending to 2 to 3 cm. These lesions typically do not enhance following contrast or fill in on delayed imaging. Punctate or curvilinear calcifications may be present (Ferrozzi et al., 1996). Magnetic resonance imaging shows multiple well-defined cysts, with signal inten-

sity decreased on T1-weighted images and increased on T2-weighted images (Figure 14–32) (Wadsworth et al., 1997; Ito et al., 1995). The septations are seen as low-signal-intensity bands on T2-weighted images (Ito et al., 1995). Angiography, which typically reveals a Swiss-cheese appearance, is rarely indicated for diagnosis.

Leiomyoma

Splenic leiomyomas are rare benign tumors originating from smooth-muscle cells, most commonly those of the renal capsule and the esophagus (Figure 14–33). In a case of splenic leiomyoma that has been reported in association with ataxia telangiectasia (Coskun et al., 1995), the tumor was a solid one that appeared minimally hyperechoic on US. On unenhanced CT, it was heterogeneous without calcifica-

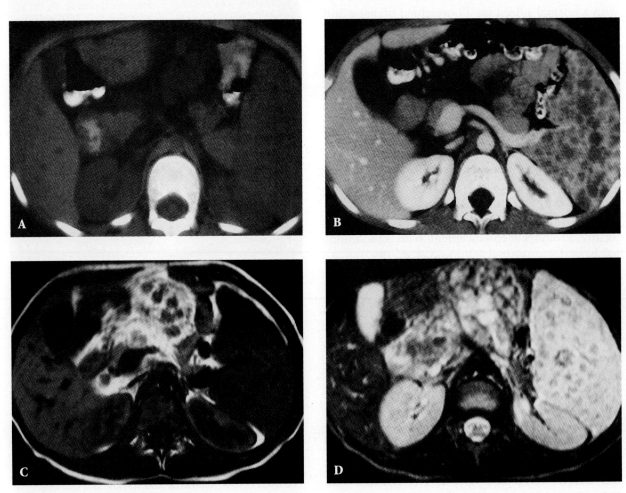

FIGURE 14–32. Splenic angiomatosis. *A,* Axial unenhanced CT scan. *B,* Enhanced CT scan. Both scans (*A and B*) show diffuse inhomogeneous splenic parenchyma with diffuse involvement in diffuse angiomatosis. *C,* Corresponding axial T1-weighted MR. *D,* Axial T2-weighted MR. Both scans show diffuse inhomogeneous T1 and T2 splenic parenchyma.

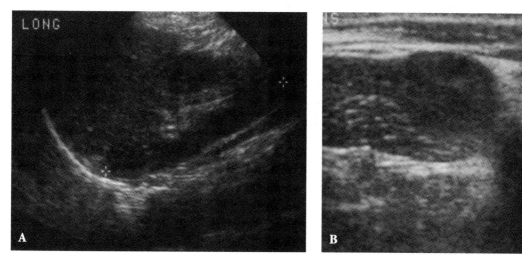

FIGURE 14–33. EBV (Epstein-Barr virus)-related smooth-muscle tumor. Initial longitudinal US showed normal splenic echogenicity (*A*). Subsequent examination 6 months later showed coarsening of splenic echogenicity with a focal hypoechoic lesion evident with bulging of the splenic capsule in this immunocompromised child (*B*).

tion; following contrast, it showed enhancement at the periphery but not in the central area. On MR, the leiomyoma was hypointense on both T1- and T2-weighted imaging compared with normal splenic parenchyma, with a central hyperintense area. On both CT and MR, the appearance of splenic hamartoma and hemangioma may mimic leiomyoma (Coskun et al., 1995).

Langerhans' Cell Histiocytosis
In this type of histiocytosis, Langerhans' cells normally present in the skin and in the buccal,

esophageal, and vaginal mucosa proliferate in the spleen. Multiple hypoechoic lesions of varying size can be observed on US (Figure 14–34) (Muwakkit et al., 1994). These lesions resolve following therapy.

Inflammatory Myofibroblastic Tumor
Inflammatory myofibroblastic tumor, also known as plasma cell granuloma or inflammatory pseudotumor (Herman et al., 1994; Glazer et al., 1992; Franquet et al., 1989; Irie et al., 1996), is uncommon in childhood. It is rarely found in the spleen, arising most often in the lungs (Herman et al., 1994). The

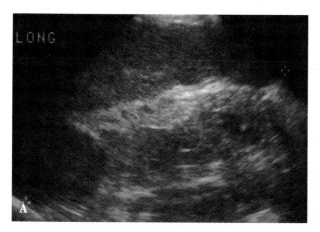
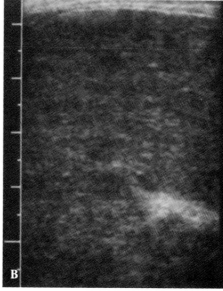

FIGURE 14–34. Langerhans' cell histiocytosis. *A*, Longitudinal ultrasonograph showing splenomegaly with multiple small hypoechoic nodules, and better demonstration on detail view (*B*).

tumor consists of mature plasma cells and lympho-cytes in a hyoid stoma and is always localized, well defined, and unencapsulated (Herman et al., 1994; Glazer et al., 1992; Franquet et al., 1989; Irie et al., 1996). Stellate calcification can be seen. The cause of the tumor remains unclear. This tumor has been considered a reparative process of an inflammatory disorder or a neoplasm (Glazer et al., 1992; Franquet et al., 1989; Irie et al., 1996). The lesion may be asymptomatic or associated with clinical symptoms of anemia, growth failure, and weight loss (Herman et al., 1994).

Ultrasonography shows this tumor as a lesion of mixed echogenicity hypoechoic to the normal spleen. It is well defined and hypodense compared with surrounding normal spleen on CT (Herman et al., 1994), which also may show a stellate central area corresponding to a fibrous area, suggestive of inflam-matory pseudotumor (Herman et al., 1994; Irie et al., 1996). The tumor's appearance on MR in adults has been reported to be isointense on T1-weighted images and to show heterogeneous low to increased signal intensity on T2-weighted sequences (Glazer et al., 1992). The T2-weighted appearance probably depends on the relative amounts of fibrous and cel-lular material present. Enhancement with gadolini-um produces a mild to moderate increase in signal intensity with delayed enhancement, particularly in the central stellate region (Glazer et al., 1992; Irie et al., 1996).

Malignant Tumors

General Considerations

Other than leukemia and lymphoma, malignant tumors affecting the spleen in childhood are uncom-mon. Angiosarcoma is the one most often reported (Falk et al., 1994; Davey and Cohen, 1996). Metas-tases from melanoma or direct extension from Wilms' tumor or neuroblastoma occur rarely. Patho-logic study shows that leukemic spleens are firm and enlarged, with focal and diffuse infiltrates of leukemic cells (Figure 14–35). Often infarcts are present.

Lymphomatous involvement of the spleen occurs in up to one-third of patients with either Hodgkin's or non-Hodgkin's lymphoma, generally reflecting systemic disease rather than isolated splenic involvement (Taylor et al., 1991). Pathologic study may show an enlarged spleen, with or without gross-ly evident masses (Freeman et al., 1993; Urrutia et al., 1996). Single or multiple small or large masses may be present but usually only small foci (less than 1 cm) of tumor cells are present (Freeman et al., 1993; Tay-lor et al., 1991; Urrutia et al., 1996). Splenomegaly caused by reactive hyperplasia or congestion may occur without lymphomatous involvement; at the same time, a normal-sized spleen does not exclude it (Freeman et al., 1993; Taylor et al., 1991). Internal necrosis with cystic degeneration may occur (Urrutia et al., 1996). Associated adenopathy elsewhere, partic-ularly in the splenic hilum, suggests lymphomatous

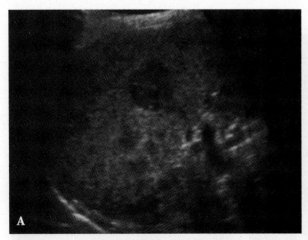
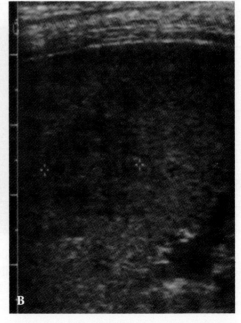

FIGURE 14–35. Acute myelogenous leukemia. *A,* Longi-tudinal ultrasonograph showing multiple varying-sized hypoechoic nodules scattered throughout the spleen without increased flow centrally. *B,* The lesions are better shown on detailed view.

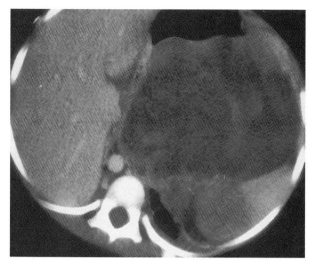

FIGURE 14–36. Neuroblastoma metastasis. Axial enhanced CT scan with large left-sided neuroblastoma which invades the spleen posteromedially.

involvement (Freeman et al., 1993). Metastases to the spleen may result from direct extension or hematogeneous spread (Figure 14–36).

Imaging of Tumors

Conventional imaging modalities are generally unreliable in determining splenic involvement (Weiss-leder et al., 1989). Plain films may show a large spleen (Figure 14–37). Ultrasonography may also demonstrate splenomegaly and, less commonly, focal disease. Diffuse infiltration can result in a patchy echo pattern, while discrete larger lesions usually produce hypoechoic areas with ill-defined margins (Goerg, Schwerk et al., 1990). Although improvements in equipment are aiding the detection of small lesions (Figure 14–38), US still does not reliably exclude them (Siniluoto et al., 1991; King et al., 1985). Focal malignant lesions are predominantly hypoechoic and infrequently hyperechoic (Goerg, Schwerk et al., 1990). Occasionally, a target appearance with central echogenicity, bulging of the capsule, or diffuse heterogeneity may be present (Goerg, Schwerk et al., 1990; Siniluoto et al., 1991; Wernecke et al., 1987). Hypoechoic splenic lesions in patients with malignant lymphoma are virtually certain to be neoplastic (Goerg, Schwerk et al., 1990).

Computed tomography has limitations similar to those of US (King et al., 1985): it does not reliably detect limited disease (Figure 14–39) and may be less dependable than US (Siniluoto et al., 1994). Lymphomatous lesions are typically hypodense compared with normal enhanced parenchyma (Freeman et al., 1993). Although lesions larger than

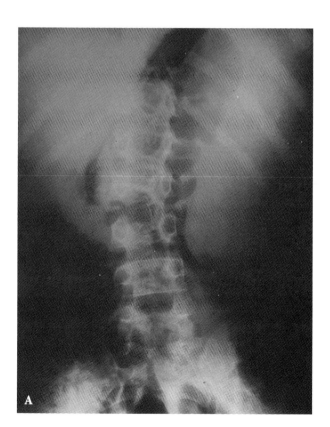

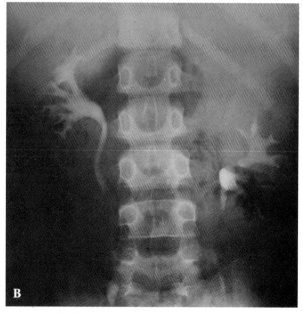

FIGURE 14–37. Splenic lymphoma. *A,* Plain film shows an enlarged spleen displacing the stomach and large bowel medially and inferiorly. *B,* Intravenous urography shows the left kidney displaced inferiorly by the spleen.

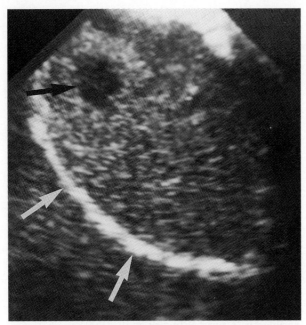

FIGURE 14–38. Splenic lymphoma. Longitudinal US shows a slightly ill-defined hypoechoic lesion (*black arrow*) in the superior portion of the spleen near the left hemidiaphragm (*white arrows*).

1 cm can be reliably detected as low-attenuation areas (see Figure 14–39) (Strijk et al., 1987), lesions of this size are unusual. The greatest value of CT lies

in its ability to demonstrate associated lymphadenopathy and assess splenic weight (Freeman et al., 1993; Hancock et al., 1994). Spleens with elevated weight are more likely to be involved with Hodgkin's disease (Hancock et al., 1994).

On conventional unenhanced T1- and T2-weighted sequences in MR, lymphomatous tissue has a signal intensity almost undistinguishable from that of normal parenchyma (Weissleder et al., 1989). Focal lymphomatous involvement may be detected when tissue heterogeneity is present, as occurs with necrosis (Hahn et al., 1988). Magnetic resonance imaging done immediately after gadolinium enhancement appears to be more sensitive than CT for evaluating splenic lymphoma. Immediate imaging is crucial, as rapid re-equilibration may lead to the disappearance of the lesions from images (Semelka et al., 1992a). Splenic involvement takes on a variety of appearances after gadolinium enhancement. Large, irregularly enhancing regions of low and high signal intensity may be noted. Multifocal involvement, which is common, appears as focal low signal intensity scattered throughout the spleen. Focal involvement appears as a spherical mass in contrast to the wavy tubular pattern of arciform enhancement of the uninvolved spleen (Semelka et al., 1992a).

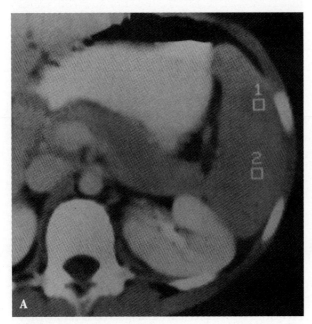
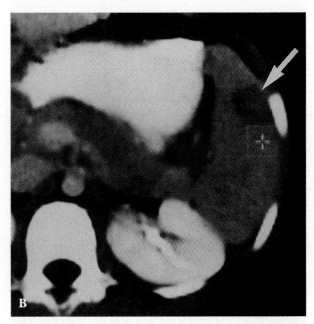

FIGURE 14–39. Splenic lymphoma. *A,* Computed tomography scan at wide window settings shows an ill-defined area of slightly decreased attenuation (*square cursor #1*) in an otherwise normal spleen (*square cursor #2*). *B,* This lesion appears much better defined and is easier to see (*arrow*) in the same CT cut in which the window width is narrower.

Use of superparamagnetic particles can sharpen the contrast between the normal spleen and lymphoma by decreasing the signal intensity of normal spleen on T2-weighted imaging (Weissleder et al., 1989).

Biopsy of suspicious areas under ultrasonographic control is possible but not usually necessary (Lindgren et al., 1985). Histologic confirmation is recommended for echogenic lesions, as these may be malignant. Melanoma may have paramagnetic properties, allowing for its detection on T1- and T2-weighted sequences, typically with mixed high- and low-signal-intensity regions as a result of hemorrhage (Hahn et al., 1988).

TRAUMA TO THE SPLEEN

Clinical Features

General Considerations
The spleen is the second most frequently injured abdominal organ in childhood, after the liver (Bond et al., 1996; Yoo et al., 1996; Benya and Bulas, 1996). Splenic injury is due most often to blunt trauma, chiefly from motor vehicle accidents but also from falls and child abuse (Benya and Bulas, 1996). The presence of mild shock, signs of left upper-quadrant peritoneal irritation, or left shoulder-tip pain suggests splenic trauma; however, mild shock alone is nonspecific. Abdominal tenderness and distension are other cardinal signs of intraperitoneal

bleeding from splenic rupture. In 10 to 20% of patients, the diagnosis of rupture is not obvious. Splenic injuries are commonly associated with injuries to the lung, kidney, liver, and pancreas (Benya and Bulas, 1996; Rescorla and Grossfield, 1989). Multiple injuries, particularly when they include the head, may obscure the clinical signs of splenic trauma (Coburn et al., 1995). Rupture may occasionally be delayed, causing more diagnostic confusion (Yoo et al., 1996).

Splenic rupture from birth trauma is uncommon and is associated with hemoperitoneum (Figure 14–40) (Cywes and Cremin, 1969). It may occur immediately after birth but more often happens between the second and fifth days of life. It may be suspected if a child experiences a sudden onset of pallor, followed by grunting, respiration, and circulatory collapse. The apparent cause is minor trauma in the presence of a hemorrhagic tendency due to a vitamin K–dependent coagulation defect. Autotransplantation of the spleen may be considered if splenectomy is thought necessary (Yamataka et al., 1996).

Treatment
Historically, blunt splenic injuries were generally operated on directly. At the time of laparotomy, however, many of these injuries were not marked by active hemorrhage and thus required no treatment. Total splenectomy in children may be followed by overwhelming sepsis (Balfanz et al., 1976), so con-

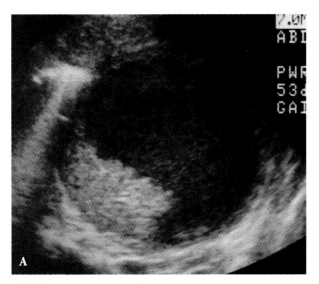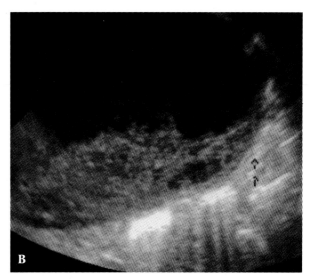

FIGURE 14–40. A and B, sonography showingSplenic rupture following post-traumatic delivery and in association with Erb's palsy.

servative treatment, limited resection, or repair is preferable to total resection (Ein et al., 1977; Ein et al., 1978; Sherman and Asch, 1978).

Most children suffering from blunt abdominal trauma can be stabilized through administration of crystalloid or blood products. Once a child is stable, contrast-enhanced CT or other imaging techniques can be carried out. Imaging can help determine the severity of injury and thereby the length of bed rest and the restriction of activities required. Serial clinical examinations should be performed to ensure that bowel injury or continued visceral bleeding have not been overlooked.

The majority of pediatric splenic injuries can be managed without an operation. This holds true for a child with many injuries even though the presence of multiple injuries complicates assessment of blood loss and vital signs (Coburn et al., 1995). Selective expectant therapy based on the child's physiologic status is now common practice, preserving splenic function. Failure of nonsurgical management is uncommon in children (Bond et al., 1996; Benya and Bulas, 1996; Coburn et al., 1995; Pearl et al., 1989).

Surgery is generally reserved for patients with massive continued bleeding: either splenorrhaphy or splenectomy is considered (Wesson et al., 1981). When splenectomy is necessary, vaccine and antibiotics must be administered. Antibiotic prophylaxis should be continued for at least several months after surgery and even indefinitely. Complications of surgical management of splenic injuries include hemorrhage, infection, bowel obstruction, pancreatitis, atelectasis, and pneumonia.

Imaging of Splenic Trauma

Preferred Methods

The imaging method used in the initial investigation of splenic injury depends on the clinical status of the patient and the practice of individual clinicians. At most North American centers, CT is the primary technique used to diagnose significant splenic and intra-abdominal trauma (Wolfman et al., 1992); at other centers, particularly in Europe, US is often the first modality used (Taylor, 1995). Computed tomography is generally preferred because of its superior diagnostic capabilities for injury to the spleen and other intra-abdominal organs, including bowel, pancreas, and bone (Benya and Bulas, 1996; Roche et al., 1992). However, CT is costly and not needed with

many patients whose injuries are limited. The advantage of US is that it can be performed at the bedside (Adler, Blane et al., 1986; Filiatrault et al., 1987).

Computed Tomography

Traumatic splenic lesions are all clearly shown by CT. They include lacerations, fractures, devascularization of tissue, and intrasplenic, subcapsular, and perisplenic hematomas (Benya and Bulas, 1996; Do and Cronan, 1991). Computed tomography is especially valuable with children suffering trauma to the head, spine, and intra-abdominal organs other than the spleen (Coburn et al., 1995). It is sensitive to and specific for splenic trauma although false-positive and false-negative results occasionally occur (Thomas and Dubbins, 1991; Federle et al., 1987).

Lacerations or hematomas appear as irregular low-attenuation areas in an otherwise enhanced spleen (Benya and Bulas, 1996). Purely intrasplenic hematomas without transcapsular extension are rare. Hematomas vary in density, often appearing isodense or hyperdense compared with the spleen at first, then showing reduced attenuation with time (Korobkin et al., 1978). Contrast enhancement may make the hematoma relatively hypodense (Figure 14–41) or isodense with normal spleen.

The presence around the spleen of unenhanced fluid within or outside the splenic capsule is seen with subcapsular and perisplenic hematomas, respectively (Figure 14–42) (Benya and Bulas, 1996). Subcapsular hematomas are typically lenticular, low-density fluid collections that flatten or indent the lateral aspect of the spleen. A perisplenic hematoma signals the presence of an intrasplenic laceration or hematoma. Since the splenic capsule is not normally identified, it can be difficult to distinguish subcapsular from perisplenic hematoma; indeed, often a mixture of injuries is present. Regions of devascularization may be seen as regions of nonperfusion (Benya and Bulas, 1996).

With splenic injury, hemorrhage can extend from the left upper quadrant into the perihepatic and paracolic gutters or pelvis, necessitating routine pelvic imaging. Hemorrhage may also be seen in the gastrosplenic ligament, Morison's pouch, and lesser sac (Balachandran et al., 1994). Fluid is sometimes seen in the left pararenal space, likely a result of injury at the splenic hilum extending along the splenorenal ligament. Free fluid suggests that the splenic capsule is torn. High-density contrast

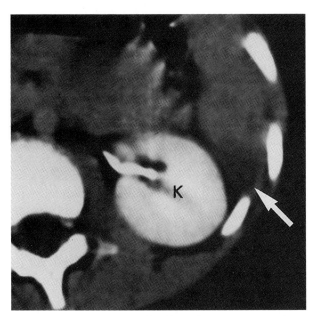

FIGURE 14–41. Ruptured spleen due to trauma. Contrast-enhanced CT scan showed a small area of decreased attenuation (*arrow*) adjacent to the left kidney (K) resulting from trauma. This abnormality was not seen on the unenhanced scan.

enhancement around the spleen may represent hemorrhage, and if adjacent to a nonenhancing spleen, vascular injury (Figure 14–43). The presence and amount of hemoperitoneum shown on CT may predict transfusion requirements. In most patients, however, even large amounts of hemoperitoneum can be compensated for without transfusion.

Several grading systems for splenic injuries have been proposed to facilitate clinical investigation and research into outcomes (Bond et al., 1996; Kohn et al., 1994; Ruess et al., 1995; Benya et al., 1995; Sugrue et al., 1991; Mirvis et al., 1989; Scatamacchia et al., 1989). Grading systems for CT are based primarily on morphologic demonstrations of injury and do not necessarily equate with physiologic status. Higher-grade injuries show more extensive parenchymal involvement. Grading of injuries on CT is challenging: subcapsular hematomas are difficult to distinguish from subphrenic intraperitoneal blood around the spleen, and splenic hematoma is hard to separate from laceration. In addition, hemorrhage from the diaphragm or tail of the pancreas can mimic acute splenic bleeding.

Grading is not useful in determining the need for initial surgery as this decision is primarily clinical (Pearl et al., 1989; Wesson et al., 1981). Grading systems may help guide long-term management, as the severity of injury influences the time required for healing (Benya et al., 1995). Although gradations on a CT injury scale correlate with increased requirements for blood transfusion for adult liver injuries, a similar correlation has not been demonstrated for pediatric splenic injuries (Ruess et al., 1995).

Ultrasonography
Ultrasonography offers a practical alternative to CT in the initial investigation of splenic injury, particularly if CT is difficult to obtain (Filiatrault et al., 1987;

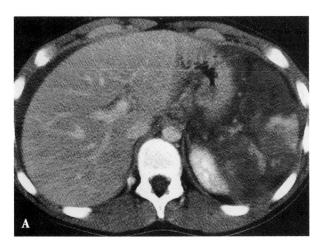
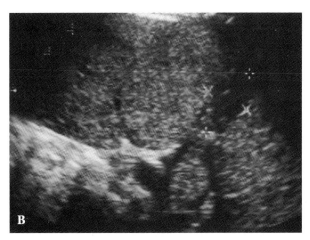

FIGURE 14–42. Splenic injury. *A,* Axial enhanced CT scan with extensive splenic disruption and splenic and perisplenic hematoma. *B,* Follow-up transverse ultrasonograph 5 months later shows a hypoechoic central region at the site of injury, with irregular periphery and absent flow in this region. (Courtesy of Dr. Douglas Jamieson, B.C. Children's Hospital Vancouver, British Columbia.)

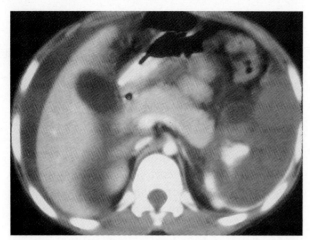

FIGURE 14–43. Splenic trauma. Extensive splenic trauma in a child involved in a pedestrian–motor vehicle accident. Extensive perisplenic blood and active extravasation of contrast is evident on enhanced axial CT scans.

Thomas and Dubbins, 1991; Asher et al., 1976; Siniluoto et al., 1992). The ability of US to detect the full spectrum of retroperitoneal and bowel injuries, however, has not been established. With US, traumatic splenic lesions typically demonstrate abnormal heterogeneous echogenicity, with or without hemoperitoneum (Asher et al., 1976; Siniluoto et al., 1992).

Regions of both increased and decreased echogenicity may be evident, as may intrasplenic fluid from hematoma (Benya and Bulas, 1996; Asher et al., 1976). Splenic hematomas are typically hyperechoic at first and become hypoechoic with time. Splenic echogenicity may initially appear normal (Siniluoto et al., 1992; Booth et al., 1987). This may be due to several factors: the echogenicity of early hematoma may be similar to that of normal spleen for the first 24 hours; interval bleeding may occur; or scanning may prove technically difficult because of abdominal tenderness or limited visualization (Filiatrault et al., 1987; Siniluoto et al., 1992; Booth et al., 1987). Injury adjacent to the diaphragm, especially subcapsular hematoma or splenic laceration, may be difficult to visualize. Repeating US in 2 to 3 days may reveal areas of echolucency caused by hematoma at the site of splenic injury areas that at first appeared normal.

Perisplenic fluid is seen with subcapsular hematoma formation (see Figure 14–44) (Lupien and Sauerbrei, 1984), and adjacent hematomas will be seen as hypoechoic fluid collections (Siniluoto et al., 1992). Other fluid collections, such as free intraperitoneal fluid or pleural effusion, can be readily identified. The presence of intraperitoneal fluid alone does not specifically indicate splenic

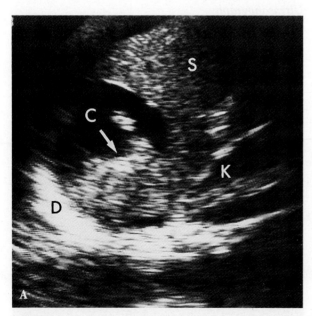

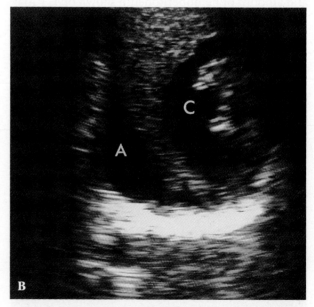

FIGURE 14–44. Hemorrhage into a splenic cyst as a result of trauma. *A,* Longitudinal US shows the spleen (S) containing a cystic structure (C) that contains highly echogenic material (*arrow*). This lesion lies adjacent to the hemidiaphragm (D) and above the left kidney (K). *B,* Transverse US also demonstrated the splenic lesion (C) and showed some perisplenic ascites (A). The cystic lesion was a congenital cyst into which there was hemorrhage as the result of a motor vehicle accident.

injury but is suggestive in cases in which the injury is not identified (Booth et al., 1987). Splenic fracture appears as a more extensive plane of fluid traversing the entire thickness of the pulp. Other ultrasonographic signs of splenic injury include enlargement, irregular border, change in contour or position, progressive enlargement on sequential scans, and free intraperitoneal fluid (Asher et al., 1976). Underlying abnormalities such as cysts may produce a less typical appearance marked by echogenic hemorrhage into anechoic lesions (Figure 14–44).

Aneurysms of the splenic artery rarely occur after blunt abdominal trauma in childhood, and intraparenchymal pseudoaneurysms are even less common (Oguzkurt et al., 1996; Goletti et al., 1996). Color Doppler ultrasonography can confirm the diagnosis of intrasplenic aneurysm by demonstrating flow within parahilar anechoic lesions next to the subcapsular hematoma. Color Doppler evaluation has been recommended as a follow-up procedure to detect post-traumatic (pseudo) aneurysms, as they may be delayed in presentation (Goletti et al., 1996).

Other Modalities

Plain films (often taken in emergency departments) may show evidence of free fluid in the peritoneal cavity, as shown by homogeneous grayness of the abdomen and a tendency for bowel gas to localize in the midline (Cywes and Cremin, 1976). The distended abdomen may have separated bowel loops (Figure 14–45) and full flanks. Rib fractures are seen less frequently in children than in adults.

Although barium studies are not generally indicated, they may show evidence of bowel trauma or indentations from extrinsic hemorrhage (Figure 14–46). Intravenous urography is also not generally indicated but may demonstrate lucency in the splenic region during the body opacification phase (Marquis et al., 1976).

Historically, scintigraphy was often used to evaluate splenic trauma both initially and in follow-up but it has been supplanted by CT and US. In isolated hepatic or splenic trauma, technetium Tc 99m sulfur colloid liver/spleen scans may show a defect in the scintigraph (Figure 14–47), a bandlike defect being the most common (Erasmie et al., 1988). Subcapsular concave and irregular defects are nonspecific and less frequent (Bethel et al., 1992). Scintigraphy cannot assess the presence of hemorrhage in the pleural or peritoneal space.

Angiography has also been used to diagnose splenic trauma, showing rupture, subcapsular hematomas, and arteriovenous fistulae (Oguzkurt et al., 1996; Love et al., 1968). Although this technique is rarely indicated, it can be used to control splenic hemorrhage primarily and in embolization of (pseudo)aneurysms (Hagiwara et al., 1996).

Follow-Up

In planning the long-term management of children with splenic injury, some physicians recommend restricting activity until complete healing is documented by CT or US or at least until serial examinations show that the patient has been stabilized (Yoo et al., 1996; Benya et al., 1995; Pranikoff et al., 1994). Others suggest restricting activity for 6 to 12 weeks and performing follow-up imaging only if new

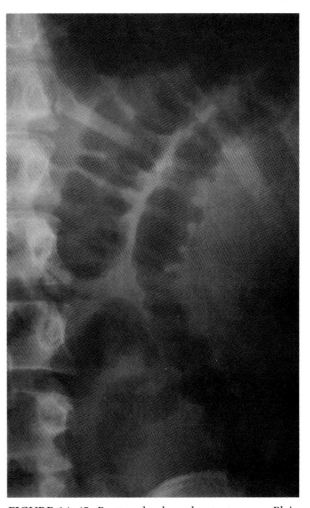

FIGURE 14–45. Ruptured spleen due to trauma. Plain films show displacement of the splenic flexure medially by a large soft-tissue mass.

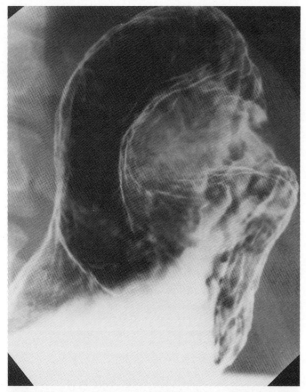

FIGURE 14–46. Ruptured spleen due to trauma. Barium meal study shows an indentation of the greater curvature from an extrinsic mass lesion.

symptoms or signs develop. Surgery is not indicated unless the initial injuries worsen or the patient's clinical status deteriorates.

After abdominal trauma, the spleen may increase in size during the initial follow-up period (Goodman and Aprahamian, 1990). This progressive enlargement is a sign not of deterioration but of a return of the spleen to normal size after the physiologic contraction and decreased blood volume resulting from the injury. This change is similar to the transient decrease in spleen size following vaginal delivery (Aoki et al., 1992).

Ultrasonography and CT are the modalities most used in follow-up studies (Figures 14–42, 14–48). Intraperitoneal fluid and pleural effusions disappear in 2 to 4 weeks whereas splenic contusion and hematomas can take up to a year to resolve. Ultrasonography may show a spleen returned to normal or a spleen containing linear echogenic foci or possibly calcifications. Echogenic scar tissue may remain at the site of the trauma (Lupien and Sauerbrei, 1984). Persistent abnormalities should not be mistaken for failure to heal or for repeat hemorrhage. Less severe injuries usually heal in 4 months; more severe injuries can take from 6 to 11 months. Lesions remain less attenuated on CT than normal splenic parenchyma and may show sharp margins as they decrease in size. The contour of the spleen may appear normal or distorted. Occasionally, cyst formation or calcification is seen at the site of injury (Benya et al., 1995).

Complications of splenic trauma include abscess, artery aneurysm or pseudoaneurysm, infarction, and delayed bleeding (Yoo et al., 1996; Benya

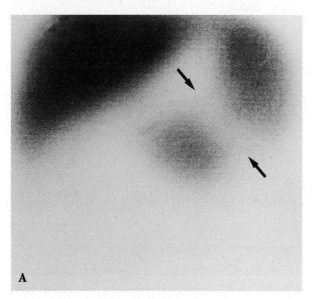

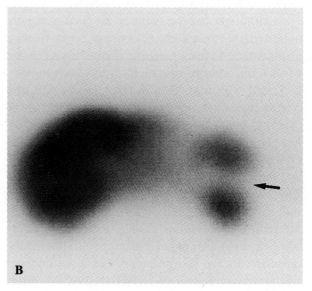

FIGURE 14–47. Ruptured spleen due to trauma. *A,* Filling defect (*arrows*) is present in the scintigraph of the spleen on a technetium Tc 99m sulfur colloid liver/spleen scan. *B,* Axial reconstruction scintigraph also shows the defect (*arrow*).

and Bulas, 1996; Oguzkurt et al., 1996; Goletti et al., 1996). Splenic infarcts appear as wedge-shaped, nonenhancing areas of parenchyma with apices directed to the hilum. Maturation of hematomas leads to a decrease in attenuation values and to the development of sharp splenic margins. Some patients may be left with a chronic pseudocyst containing serous fluid but this condition is rare in children (Pachter et al., 1993). Delayed rupture of the spleen is also uncommon in childhood (Pearl et al., 1989).

Scintigraphy is no longer used in follow-up imaging of splenic trauma. It shows injury typically as wedge-shaped defects involving a focal or diffuse portion of the spleen (Bethel et al., 1992). Magnetic resonance imaging is little used and generally is not required in splenic trauma. Magnetic resonance images of trauma reflect the time course of blood degradation and changes in signal intensity due to the paramagnetic effects of the degradation products of hemoglobin. Subacute blood is particularly evident by its high signal on T1- and T2-weighted sequences. Traumatized devascularized regions are well shown following gadolinium enhancement, with areas of persistent low signal intensity.

Children who have undergone splenectomy for trauma are generally at less risk of infection than those who have had splenectomy for other reasons. The reduced risk of infection is probably due to splenic spill of tissue into the peritoneum. In some children, despite splenectomy, splenic function may be present, with nodules of recurrent splenic tissue evident (Pearson et al., 1978), a phenomenon referred to as the "born again spleen." These ectopic nodules show up clearly on a technetium Tc 99m sulfur colloid liver/spleen scan (Gunes et al., 1994) or on MR following injection of superparamagnetic iron oxide (Storm et al., 1992). The presence of multiple implants of splenic tissue in the peritoneum is called splenosis. This condition is primarily intraperitoneal but may in rare cases be found in subcutaneous tissues or in the thorax after combined diaphragmatic and splenic disruption (Moncada et al., 1985; Maillard et al., 1989). It may be noted in abdominal viscera such as the liver but such cases are rarer (Yoshimitsu et al., 1993). Although splenosis is usually asymptomatic, there may be abdominal pain, recurrent splenic disease, or an intrathoracic or peritoneal mass (Gunes et al., 1994). Since its imaged appearance is similar to that of accessory spleens, it can be confused with lymphadenopathy.

MISCELLANEOUS DISORDERS

Splenomegaly

Causes
The spleen may be enlarged by hematologic disorders, infections (see Splenic Infection and Abscess, earlier), portal hypertension (see Chapter 12, The Liver), cystic or neoplastic infiltration (see Mass Lesions, earlier), and the collagenoses. These various causes of splenomegaly are listed in detail in Table 14–2. Splenomegaly has also been noted in extracorporeal membrane oxygenation, probably the result of sequestration of damaged red blood cells sustained from the apparatus used in this process (Klippenstein et al., 1994).

Marked splenic enlargement, although easy to assess by radiologic methods, is obvious clinically. Slight increases in spleen size, however, are difficult to assess radiologically unless the volume is carefully measured. Usually the enlarged spleen has a nonspecific appearance and maintains a homogeneous parenchymal pattern. Rarely does the spleen exhibit specific imaging features unless focal lesions are present, as in abscess or neoplasms. In portal hypertension, suggestive features

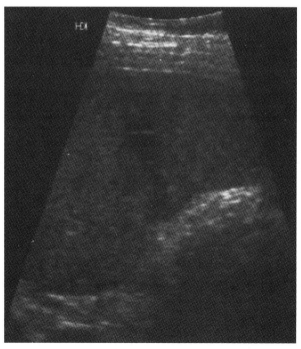

FIGURE 14–48. A healing splenic injury with a residual irregular hypoechoic area within the center of the spleen, mimicking a splenic cyst.

TABLE 14–2. Some Causes of Splenomegaly in Children

Hematologic disorders
　Hemolytic anemias
　Hemoglobinopathies
　Thalassemia

Infections
　Focal—abscess
　Diffuse
　　Septicemia
　　Malaria
　　Toxoplasmosis
　　Typhoid
　　Cytomegalovirus
　　Epstein-Barr virus

Portal hypertension
　Extrahepatic
　Intrahepatic
　Budd-Chiari
　Hyperkinetic
　Congestive cardiac failure

Infiltrations
　Lipoidosis – Gaucher's disease
　Mucopolysaccharidosis
　Langerhans' cell histiocytosis

Cysts or tumors
　Congenital cysts
　Leukemia
　Lymphoma
　Hemangioma
　Lymphangioma

Collagenoses
　Lupus erythematosus
　Rheumatoid arthritis

can occasionally be seen, including collateral vessels in the hilum, Gamna-Gandy bodies, and multiple reflective parallel lines on ultrasonography. These reflective lines or channels probably result from periarterial fibrosis and dilatation of venous sinuses, with increased collagen in their walls from chronically raised venous pressure (Kedar et al., 1994). Gamna-Gandy bodies represent organized foci of hemorrhage within the spleen, usually caused by portal hypertension and rarely observed

in children. However, they can be seen in other disorders, such as sickle cell disease. A Gamna-Gandy body contains fibrous tissue, hemosiderin, and calcium. Ultrasonography may reveal diffuse hyperechoic spots within the spleen (Minami et al., 1989). Foci of iron deposition are infrequently seen in the spleen of patients with cirrhosis and portal hypertension or in those who have had a blood transfusion. Multiple low-intensity nodules, possibly related to hemosiderin deposition, may show on MR. These nodules are especially evident on gradient-echo imaging with their susceptibility artifact (Minami et al., 1989; Sagoh et al., 1989).

Hypersplenism
Hypersplenism is characterized by increased destruction or storage of blood components in an enlarged spleen, leading to a reduction in one or more cellular blood elements, generally platelets. Imaging of the spleen in this condition demonstrates only an enlarged spleen (Figure 14–49). Therapy is indicated not only for thrombocytopenia and pancytopenia but also for the mechanical and infectious complications of hypersplenism (Hickman et al., 1992). Hypersplenism can occur with splenomegaly from a variety of causes, the most common of which are portal hypertension and hematologic disorders such as thalassemia, leukemia, and lymphoma (Israel et al., 1994). Splenectomy reverses the process but carries a lifetime risk of infection (see Trauma to the Spleen in this chapter). Embolization may be of value before splenectomy (Hickman et al., 1992). Following splenectomy, splenic and portal vein thrombosis may occur, especially in patients with thalassemia (Figure 14–50).

　Partial embolization has been advocated to reduce splenic bulk (Israel et al., 1994; Spigos et al., 1979; Kumpe et al., 1985; Becker et al., 1995; Stanley and Shen, 1995; Watanabe et al., 1996). It can lower the need for tranfusions in patients with thalassemia and reduce the risk of variceal hemorrhage in cases of portal hypertension (Hickman et al., 1992; Israel et al., 1994; Stanley and Shen, 1995). Various embolic agents have been used, such as Gelfoam, polyvinyl alcohol particles, and intra-arterial irradiation with yttrium-90 in adults (Becker et al., 1995; Stanley and Shen, 1995). Few complications after partial embolization from splenic infarction have been reported in children. They

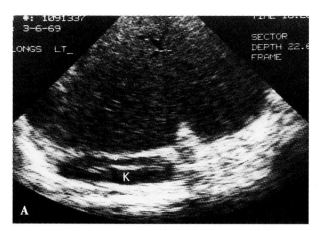
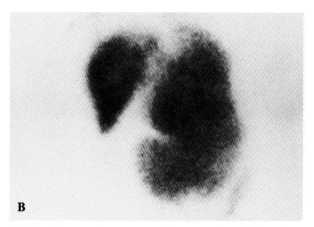

FIGURE 14–49. Splenomegaly in a 15-year-old boy with cystic fibrosis secondary to portal hypertension. *A*, Longitudinal US shows a large spleen that is isoechoic relative to the compressed left kidney (K). *B*, A technetium Tc 99m sulfur colloid liver/spleen scan shows a greatly enlarged spleen on the right and a smaller liver on the left. The spleen shows patchy activity due to the cirrhosis, which has resulted in hypersplenism.

happen more frequently in cases of extensive infarction of the spleen. Complications include atelectasis, rupture, abscess, and pancreatitis (Israel et al., 1994; Spigos et al., 1979; Kumpe et al., 1985; Stanley and Shen, 1995). Acutely wedge-shaped hypoechoic regions may be evident on ultrasonographs, along with a further increase in spleen size (Watanabe et al., 1996; Weingarten et al., 1984).

Gaucher's Disease

Gaucher's disease is an inherited lysosomal storage disorder characterized by enzymatic deficiency of glucocerebrosidase. Glucocerebroside accumulates in reticuloendothelial cells, affecting the liver, spleen, bone marrow, and lymph nodes. This accumulation usually causes hepatosplenomegaly and may be associated with hypersplenism, sympto-

matic or asymptomatic splenic infarction, and sub capsular fluid in a few cases (Hill et al., 1992; Hill et al., 1986). Clusters of Gaucher's cells are often present in the spleen, causing focal lesions (Hill et al., 1986). Patients with the disease often have left upper-quadrant abdominal pain that necessitates radiologic examination.

Ultrasonography typically shows splenomegaly often associated with multiple splenic lesions of varying size. These lesions usually are hypoechoic but can occasionally be hyperechoic. They may contain fibrosis or infarction (Hill et al., 1986). However, lesions of mixed echogenicity without either condition have been described (McLennan and Withers, 1992). Less common is a geographic pattern of irregular areas of Gaucher's cell infiltration (Hill et al., 1986).

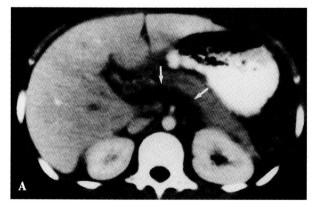
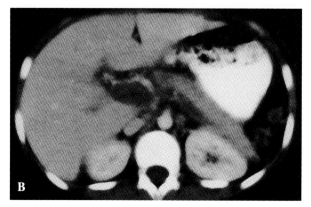

FIGURE 14–50. Splenic vein thrombosis. *A* and *B*, selected axial enhanced CT images showing thrombosis of the splenic vein extending into the portal vein following splenectomy (*arrows*).

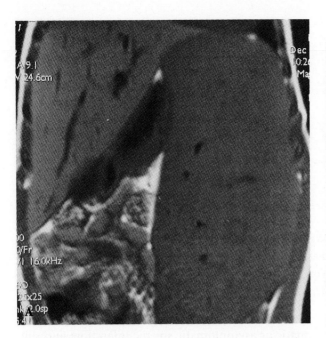

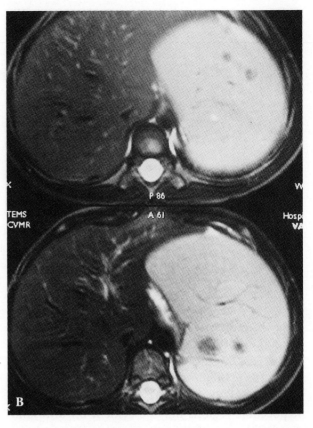

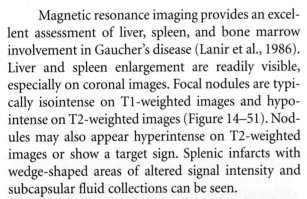

FIGURE 14–51. Splenomegaly in an 8-year-old boy with Gaucher's disease. *A,* A T1-weighted coronal image demonstrates massive splenomegaly. *B,* Selected fast spin echo T2-weighted axial images showing focal hypointense nodules within the enlarged spleen.

Magnetic resonance imaging provides an excellent assessment of liver, spleen, and bone marrow involvement in Gaucher's disease (Lanir et al., 1986). Liver and spleen enlargement are readily visible, especially on coronal images. Focal nodules are typically isointense on T1-weighted images and hypointense on T2-weighted images (Figure 14–51). Nodules may also appear hyperintense on T2-weighted images or show a target sign. Splenic infarcts with wedge-shaped areas of altered signal intensity and subcapsular fluid collections can be seen.

Treatment of Gaucher's disease with enzyme replacement may reduce the size of the spleen. Follow-up of both liver and spleen size may be important in management (Terk et al., 1995).

Hereditary Spherocytosis

Hereditary spherocytosis is an autosomal dominant disorder resulting in splenomegaly, bone marrow expansion, and extramedullary hematopoiesis in some cases. Ultrasonography will show the enlarged spleen, usually with homogeneous, increased echogenicity (Figure 14–52) (Mittelstaedt and Partain, 1980). Areas of infarction can be seen. Focal hyper-echoic deposits of intrasplenic hematopoiesis have been described in an adult (Gupta and Woodham, 1986).

Sickle Cell Disease

Abnormalities of the spleen are commonly observed in homozygous sickle cell disease (SCD) and the various sickle cell syndromes such as sickle cell thalassemia. The disease causes focal areas of infarction resulting from the blockage of small vessels by abnormal red blood cells. Microscopic perivascular and parenchymal calcification are found along with iron deposition in areas of infarction (Adler, Glazer et al., 1986). Initially, SCD can cause an enlarged spleen; however, if the blockages recur, autosplenectomy occurs and the spleen is obliterated. Sickle cell disease usually leads to impaired splenic function and functional asplenia from repeated infarction by the age of 5 to 10 years. In homozygous SCD, the spleen generally becomes small and densely calcified whereas in the heterozygous form of the disease, it is usually enlarged, with subcapsular calcification. Radiography may show the spleen as enlarged but more often it appears small and dense from calcifi-

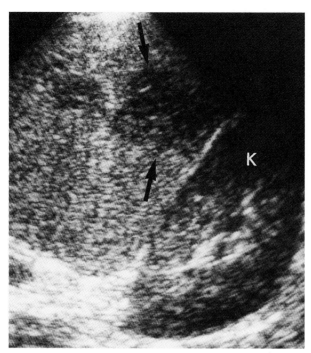

FIGURE 14–52. Splenomegaly in a 12-year-old girl with spherocytosis. Longitudinal US shows a very large spleen that is hyperechoic relative to the left kidney (K). An ill-defined hypoechoic lesion (*between arrows*) in the spleen represents a focal infarct.

cation and iron deposition. These characteristics are more frequently recognized with CT and MR.

In sickle cell disease, US, CT, and MR show focal round masses that can simulate abscess or infarct, especially in the setting of sickle cell crisis

with abdominal pain and fever (Adler, Glazer et al., 1986; Walker and Serjeant, 1993; Magid et al., 1987; Levin et al., 1996). These masses probably represent focal regions of spared splenic parenchyma or extramedullary hematopoiesis. They are hypoechoic on US and hypodense on CT within a spleen marked by calcification and increased density (Figures 14–53, 14–54) (Magid et al., 1987; Levin et al., 1996). Magnetic resonance imaging shows them as focal islands of normal intensity (intermediate on T1-weighted images and high on T2-weighted images) within a spleen of diminished intensity (Magid et al., 1987; Levin et al., 1996). With bone scanning, the surrounding calcified spleen demonstrates increased uptake but no residual normal parenchyma. A diagnosis of functioning splenic tissue can be made with technetium Tc 99m sulfur colloid scanning (Levin et al., 1996). The presence of these focal regions does not imply adequate protection against infection. Additional findings in SCD include abscesses, patchy or more diffuse areas of infarction, acute sequestration, hemorrhage, and Gamna-Gandy bodies. In some patients, benign hyperechoic masses have been noted (Figure 14–55) but this is without published pathologic confirmation (Walker and Serjeant, 1993).

Splenic Iron Deposition

An increase in body iron stores, termed "iron overload," can occur in the spleen. Iron can be deposited in either the parenchymal cells or the reticuloendothelial system, especially in the spleen, bone mar-

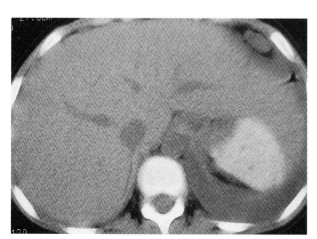

FIGURE 14–53. Sickle cell disease. Axial CT showing calcified spleen in this child with sickle cell disease. Left pleural effusion is also present.

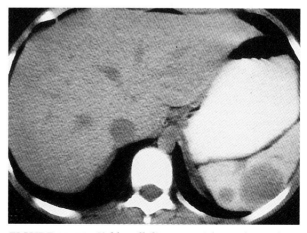

FIGURE 14–54. Sickle cell disease. Axial unenhanced CT image showing multiple well-defined hypodense areas within the spleen that is of increased attenuation overall.

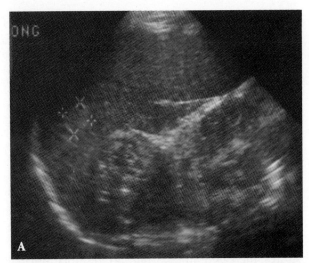

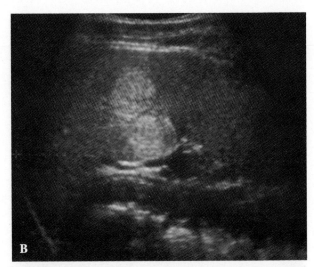

FIGURE 14–55. Sickle cell disease. *A,* Initial longitudinal ultrasonograph showing several small hyperechoic foci in this child with sickle cell disease. *B,* The lesions are larger and more distinct on subsequent study 8 months later.

row, and liver (Arrive et al., 1990). Prior blood transfusions may decrease the spleen's normal intensity from hemosiderosis (Querfeld et al., 1988). In the spleen, reticuloendothelial iron is chiefly in the form of hemosiderin (Arrive et al., 1990).

The iron deposition that occurs in SCD and hemochromatosis affects the appearance of the spleen on both CT and MR and on US to a lesser extent (Figure 14–56). The best imaging modality to assess iron overload is MR. With moderate overload,

there is a decrease on T2-weighted imaging compared with that of subcutaneous fat or the renal cortex (Arrive et al., 1990). With more severe overload, lower signal intensity is evident on both T1-weighted images (lower than fat, renal cortex, and muscle) and T2-weighted images (Adler, Glazer et al., 1986; Arrive et al., 1990; Querfeld et al., 1988). Magnetic resonance imagining is not sensitive to mild overload (Arrive et al., 1990).

Splenic Vascular Disorders and Infarction

Aneurysms of the splenic artery are rare, as are fistulas between the artery and vein. An aneurysm may infrequently develop with communication into the splenic vein as a result of trauma. This condition can be demonstrated by color Doppler US (Oguzkurt et al., 1996). An aneurysm may be congenital, mycotic, or traumatic in origin or it may arise following pancreatitis. Rupture is seen in 6 to 9% of patients. Although splenic artery aneurysms can be asymptomatic, clinical features include a pulsatile mass, continuous bruit and thrill, abdominal pain, diarrhea due to congestion of mesenteric veins, and ascites in rare cases (Oguzkurt et al., 1996). Splenic artery aneurysms may lead to splenomegaly and portal hypertension. The conventional surgical treatment is ligation or excision of the artery with or without splenectomy. Nonsurgical intra-arterial embolization can also be performed.

Splenic infarction may be either arterial or venous in origin. Arterial infarcts are typically

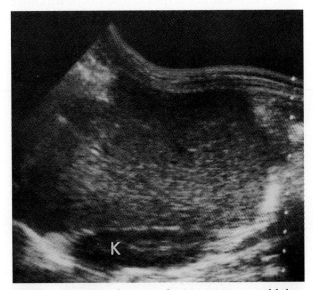

FIGURE 14–56. Splenomegaly in an 11-year-old boy with thalassemia. Longitudinal US shows a large spleen that is hyperechoic relative to the compressed left kidney (K) as a result of hemochromatosis (iron deposition).

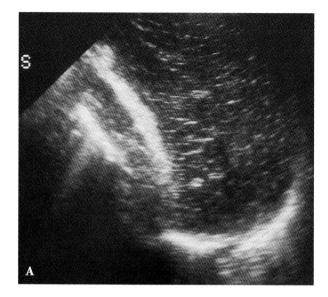

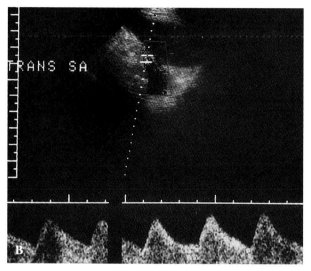

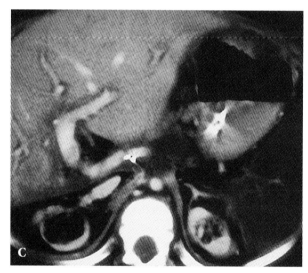

FIGURE 14–57. Liver transplant recipient with splenic vein thrombosis and splenic infarction. *A,* Transverse ultrasonograph showing coarse splenic echogenicity with small bright echoes evident. *B,* Doppler evaluation of the splenic artery shows high diastolic flow. *C,* Axial enhanced CT showing diffuse hypodensity of the splenic parenchyma, in keeping with infarction.

ischemic, and venous infarcts are hemorrhagic. Venous infarction is caused by thrombosis of splenic sinusoids and occurs in patients with massive splenomegaly (Urrutia et al., 1996). Splenic infarcts can be found in patients with hematologic disorders, including myeloproliferative disorders, hemolytic anemia, sickle cell disease, and sepsis (Goerg and Schwerk, 1990; Alvarado et al., 1988; Jaroch et al., 1986). Other reported causes include Wegener's granulomatosis (McHugh et al., 1991) and complications of liver transplantation (Figure 14–57) (Lehar et al., 1990). Clinical features include left upper abdominal pain, painful restriction of respiration, and local pain on palpation (Goerg and Schwerk, 1990). Splenic infarction can be managed medically unless complications develop.

The appearance of infarction on US depends on whether edema, bleeding, necrosis, and/or inflammation are present (Goerg and Schwerk, 1990). Acute infarction typically appears as a round or wedge-shaped focal lesion that may be hypoechoic or anechoic (Figure 14–58) (Goerg and Schwerk, 1990; Shirkhoda et al., 1985). A true cystic appearance is not present (Urrutia et al., 1996). Complications such as subcapsular hemorrhage or superinfection may occur and can be recognized with US, with increasing liquefaction, subcapsular hemorrhage, flow phenomena in the area of infarction, or development of hemoperitoneum. The presence of arterial signals in a region of liquefied infarction has been suggested as representing superinfection (Goerg and Schwerk, 1990). Spontaneous rupture may occur as a result of

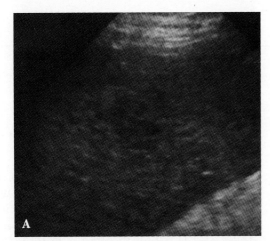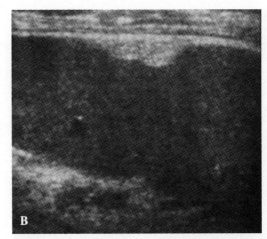

FIGURE 14–58. Splenic infarction in a child with lupus erythematosus. *A*, Longitudinal US. *B*, Transverse US. Both sonograms show splenomegaly with an ill-defined region of decreased echogenicity centrally and a peripheral hyperechoic region evident from focal splenic infarctions.

increasing subcapsular hemorrhage and infection. Follow-up examinations during the healing process show gradual shrinkage of infarct and progressive normalization of echogenicity or development of echogenic foci (Goerg and Schwerk, 1990; Wetton and Tran, 1995).

The appearance of splenic infarction on CT scans varies with the age of the infarct and the presence of hemorrhage (Urrutia et al., 1996). In acute cases, infarcts show decreased attenuation on unenhanced scans and a mottled pattern after contrast enhancement; however, focal hyperdense lesions from hemorrhage may be present.

With time, infarcts become progressively better defined without contrast enhancement and are usually wedge-shaped or irregular. Chronic infarcts gradually decrease in size and attenuation. They may return to normal appearance on both unenhanced and enhanced scans or leave the spleen with a lobulated outline from scarring. Calcification may be evident within the spleen (typical in sickle cell disease). Similarly, the appearance of infarction on MR varies with the stage of the infarct and the presence of hemorrhage. The appearance of venous infarction depends on the phase of evolution of the blood products (Urrutia et al., 1996). Subacute or chronic arterial infarcts may show signal characteristics similar to those of a cyst.

Atrophic Spleen

A small spleen is associated with a variety of conditions: familial splenic hypoplasia, Fanconi's aplastic anemia, ulcerative colitis, Crohn's disease, dermatitis herpetiformis, thyrotoxicosis, and sickle cell disease.

REFERENCES

Abramson SJ, Berdon WE, Altman RP, et al. Biliary atresia and noncardiac polysplenic syndrome: US and surgical considerations. Radiology 1987;163(2):377–9.

Adler DD, Blane CE, Coran AG, Silver TM. Splenic trauma in the pediatric patient: the integrated roles of ultrasound and computed tomography. Pediatrics 1986;78(4): 576–80.

Adler D, Glazer G, Aisen A. MRI of the spleen: normal appearance and findings in sickle cell anemia. AJR 1986;147:843–5.

Allal R, Kastler B, Gangi A, et al. Splenic abscesses in typhoid fever: US and CT studies. J Comput Assist Tomogr 1993;17(1):90–3.

Allen KB, Andrews G. Pediatric wandering spleen—the case for splenopexy: review of 35 reported cases in the literature. J Pediatr Surg 1989;24(5):432–5.

Allen KB, Gay B Jr, Skandalakis JE. Wandering spleen: anatomic and radiologic considerations. South Med J 1992;85(10):976–84.

Alvarado CS, Wyly B, Buchanan I, Fajman WA. Splenic infarction at low altitude in a child with hemoglobin S-C disease. Clin Pediatr 1988;27(8):396–9.

Aoki S, Hata T, Kitao M. Ultrasonographic assessment of fetal and neonatal spleen. Am J Perinatol 1992;9(5-6): 361–7.

Arrive L, Thurnher S, Hricak H, Price DC. Magnetic resonance imaging of splenic iron overload. Eur J Radiol 1990;10(2):98–104.

Asher W, Parvin S, Virgilio R, Haber K. Echographic evaluation of splenic injury after blunt trauma. Radiol 1976;118:411–5.

Atlas AB, Manthei U, Zutter MM, Polmar SH. Necrotizing granulomatosis of the spleen in chronic granulomatous disease [letter]. Am J Dis Child 1990;144(1):14–5.

Bakir M, Bilgic A, Ozmen M, Caglar M. The value of radionuclide splenic scanning in the evaluation of asplenia in patients with heterotaxy. Pediatr Radiol 1994; 24(1):25–8.

Balachandran S, Leonard M Jr, Kumar D, Goodman P. Patterns of fluid accumulation in splenic trauma: demonstration by CT. Abdom Imaging 1994;19(6):515–20.

Balaji KC, Caldamone AA, Rabinowitz R, et al. Splenogonadal fusion. J Urol 1996;156(2 Pt 2):854–6.

Balfanz J, Nesbit MJ, Jarvis C, Krivit W. Overwhelming sepsis following splenectomy for trauma. J Pediatrics 1976;88(3):458–60.

Balthazar E, Hilton S, Naidich D, et al. CT of splenic and perisplenic abnormalities in septic patients. AJR 1985; 144:53–6.

Barrett RL, Daniels AL, Mogil RA. Intrascrotal paratesticular accessory spleen. J Ultrasound Med 1996;15(2):173–4.

Becker CD, Rosler H, Biasiutti FD, Baer HU. Congestive hypersplenism: treatment by means of radioembolization of the spleen with Y-90. Radiology 1995;195(1):183–6.

Benya EC, Bulas DI, Eichelberger MR, Sivit CJ. Splenic injury from blunt abdominal trauma in children: follow-up evaluation with CT. Radiology 1995;195(3):685–8.

Benya EC, Bulas DL. Splenic injuries in children after blunt abdominal trauma. Semin Ultrasound CT MR 1996;17(2):170–6.

Berkenblit RG, Mohan S, Bhatt GM, et al. Wandering spleen with torsion: appearance on CT and ultrasound. Abdom Imaging 1994;19(5):459–60.

Bethel CA, Touloukian RJ, Seashore JH, Rosenfield NS. Outcome of nonoperative management of splenic injury with nuclear scanning. Clinical significance of persistent abnormalities. Am J Dis Child 1992;146(2):198–200.

Bollinger B, Lorentzen T. Torsion of a wandering spleen: ultrasonographic findings. J Clin Ultrasound 1990;18(6): 510–1.

Bond SJ, Eichelberger MR, Gotschall CS, et al. Nonoperative management of blunt hepatic and splenic injury in children. Ann Surg 1996;223(3):286–9.

Booth AJ, Bruce DI, Steiner GM. Ultrasound diagnosis of splenic injuries in children—the importance of free peritoneal fluid. Clin Radiol 1987;38(4):395–8.

Broker F, Fellows K, Treves S. Wandering spleen in three children. Pediatr Radiol 1978;6:211–4.

Chew FS, Smith PL, Barboriak D. Candidal splenic abscesses [clinical conference]. AJR 1991;156(3):474.

Coburn MC, Pfeifer J, De Luca FG. Nonoperative management of splenic and hepatic trauma in the multiply injured pediatric and adolescent patient. Arch Surg 1995;130(3):332–8.

Cortes D, Thorup JM, Visfeldt J. The pathogenesis of cryptorchidism and splenogonadal fusion: a new hypothcsis. Br J Urol 1996;77(2):285–90.

Coskun M, Aydingoz U, Tacal T, et al. CT and MR imaging of splenic leiomyoma in a child with ataxia telangiectasia. Pediatr Radiol 1995;25(1):45–7.

Cotelingam JD, Saito R. Hepatolienal fusion: case report of an unusual lesion. Hum Pathol 1978;9(2):234–6.

Cywes S, Cremin B. The roentgenologic features of hemoperitoneum in the newborn. AJR 1969;106:193–9.

Dachman A, Ros P, Murari J, et al. Nonparasitic splenic cysts: a report of 52 cases with radiologic-pathologic correlation. AJR 1986;147:537–42.

Daneman A, Martin D. Congenital epithelial splenic cysts in children: emphasis on sonographic appearances and some unusual features. Pediatr Radiol 1982;12:119–25.

Davenport M, Savage M, Mowat AP, Howard ER. Biliary atresia splenic malformation syndrome: an etiologic and prognostic subgroup. Surgery 1993;113(6):662–8.

Davey MS, Cohen MD. Imaging of gastrointestinal malignancy in childhood. Radiol Clin North Am 1996;34(4): 717–42.

Deanfield J, Chrispin A. The investigation of chest disease in children by high kilovoltage filtered beam radiography. Br J Radiol 1981;54:856–60.

Do HM, Cronan JJ. CT appearance of splenic injuries managed nonoperatively. AJR 1991;157(4):757–60.

Dodds WJ, Taylor AJ, Erickson SJ, et al. Radiologic imaging of splenic anomalies. AJR 1990;155(4):805–10.

Donnelly LF, Emery KH, Bove KE, Bissett GS 3rd. Normal changes in the MR appearance of the spleen during early childhood. AJR 1996;166(3):635–9.

Ein S, Shandling B, Simpson J, et al. The morbidity and mortality of splenectomy in childhood. Ann Surg 1977; 185:307–10.

Ein S, Shandling B, Simpson J, et al. Nonoperative management of traumatized spleen in children: how and why. J Pediatr Surg 1978;13:117–9.

Erasmie U, Mortensson W, Persson U, Lannergren K. Scintigraphic evaluation of traumatic splenic lesions in children. Acta Radiol 1988;29(1):121–5.

Erden A, Karaalp G, Ozcan H, Cumhur T. Wandering accessory spleen. Surg Radiol Anat 1995;17(1):89–91.

Fairhurst JJ, Christensen SL, Kuhn JP, Brody AS. Isolated intrathoracic spleen presenting as an enlarging chest mass. CT and MRI findings. Pediatr Radiol 1992;22(4):305–6.

Falk S, Krishnan J, Meis JM. Primary angiosarcoma of the spleen: clinicopathologic study of 40 cases (ab). Radiology 1994;191:292.

Federle M, Griffiths B, Minagi H, et al. Splenic trauma: evaluation with CT. Radiology 1987;162:69–71.

Ferrozzi F, Bova D, Draghi F, Garlaschi G. CT findings in primary vascular tumors of the spleen. AJR 1996;166(5): 1097–101.

Ferrucci JT, Stark DD. Iron oxide-enhanced MR imaging of the liver and spleen: review of the first 5 years. AJR 1990;155(5):943–50.

Filiatrault D, Longpre D, Patriquin H, et al. Investigation of childhood blunt trauma: a practical approach using ultrasound as the initial diagnostic modality. Pediatr Radiol 1987;17:373–9.

Fitzgerald EJ, Coblentz C. Fungal microabscesses in immuno-suppressed patients—CT appearances. J Can Assoc Radiol 1988;39(1):10–2.

Flynn PM, Shenep JL, Crawford R, Hughes WT. Use of abdominal computed tomography for identifying disseminated fungal infection in pediatric cancer patients. Clin Infect Dis 1995;20(4):964–70.

Franic S, Pirani M, Stevenson GW. Torsion of a wandering spleen. J Can Assoc Radiol 1988;39(3):232–4.

Franquet T, Montes M, Aizcorbe M, et al. Inflammatory pseudotumor of the spleen: ultrasound and computed tomographic findings. Gastrointest Radiol 1989;14(2): 181–3.

Franquet T, Montes M, Lecumberri FJ, et al. Hydatid disease of the spleen: imaging findings in nine patients. AJR 1990;154(3):525–8.

Freeman JL, Jafri SZ, Roberts JL, et al. CT of congenital and acquired abnormalities of the spleen. Radiographics 1993;13(3):597–610.

Fujiwara T, Takehara Y, Isoda H, et al. Torsion of the wandering spleen: CT and angiographic appearance. J Comput Assist Tomogr 1995;19(1):84–6.

Gagner M, Munson JL, Scholz FJ. Hepatobiliary anomalies associated with polysplenia syndrome. Gastrointest Radiol 1991;16(2):167–71.

Garcia JA, Garcia-Fernandez M, Romance A, Sanchez JC. Wandering spleen and gastric volvulus. Pediatr Radiol 1994;24(7):535–6.

Garel C, Hassan M. Foetal and neonatal splenic cyst-like lesions. US follow-up of seven cases. Pediatr Radiol 1995; 25(5):360–2.

Glazer M, Lally J, Kanzer M. Inflammatory pseudotumor of the spleen: MR findings. J Comput Assist Tomogr 1992;16(6):980–3.

Goerg C, Schwerk WB, Goerg K, Havemann K. Sonographic patterns of the affected spleen in malignant lymphoma. J Clin Ultrasound 1990;18(7):569–74.

Goerg C, Schwerk WB. Splenic infarction: sonographic patterns, diagnosis, follow-up, and complications. Radiology 1990;174(3 Pt 1):803–7.

Goerg C, Schwerk WB, Goerg K. Splenic lesions: sonographic patterns, follow-up, differential diagnosis. Eur J Radiol 1991a;13(1):59–66.

Goerg C, Schwerk WB, Goerg K. Sonography of focal lesions of the spleen. AJR 1991b;156(5):949–53.

Goerg C, Weide R, Schwerk WB, et al. Ultrasound evaluation of hepatic and splenic microabscesses in the immunocompromised patient: sonographic patterns, differential diagnosis, and follow-up. J Clin Ultrasound 1994;22(9):525–9.

Goletti O, Ghiselli G, Lippolis PV, et al. Intrasplenic posttraumatic pseudoaneurysm: echo color doppler diagnosis. J Trauma 1996;41(3):542–5.

Gonzalez-Giussi F, Raibley S, Ballantine T, et al. Splenorenal fusion: heterotopia simulating a primary renal neoplasm. Am J Dis Child 1977;131:994–6.

Goodman LR, Aprahamian C. Changes in splenic size after abdominal trauma. Radiology 1990;176(3):629–32.

Gordon D, Burrell M, Levin D, et al. Wandering spleen—the radiological and clinical spectrum. Radiology 1977;125:39–46.

Griscom N, Hargreaves H, Schwartz M, et al. Huge splenic cyst in a newborn: comparison with 10 cases in later childhood and adolescence. AJR 1977;129:889–91.

Gunes I, Yilmazlar T, Sarikaya I, et al. Scintigraphic detection of splenosis: superiority of tomographic selective spleen scintigraphy. Clin Radiol 1994;49(2):115–7.

Gupta R, Woodham C. Unusual ultrasound appearance of the spleen—a case of hereditary spherocytosis. Br J Radiol 1986;59:284–5.

Hadar H, Gadoth N, Herskovitz P, Heifetz M. Short pancreas in polysplenia syndrome. Acta Radiol 1991;32(4):299–301.

Hagiwara A, Yukioka T, Ohta S, et al. Nonsurgical management of patients with blunt splenic injury: efficacy of transcatheter arterial embolization. AJR 1996;167:159–66.

Hahn PF, Weissleder R, Stark DD, et al. MR imaging of focal splenic tumors. AJR 1988;150(4):823–7.

Halvorsen J, Stray O. Splenogonadal fusion. Acta Pediatr Scand 1978;67:379–81.

Hamed MM, Hamm B, Ibrahim ME, et al. Dynamic MR imaging of the abdomen with gadopentetate dimeglumine: normal enhancement patterns of the liver, spleen, stomach, and pancreas. AJR 1992;158(2):303–7.

Hancock SL, Scidmore NS, Hopkins KL, et al. Computed tomography assessment of splenic size as a predictor of splenic weight and disease involvement in laparotomy staged Hodgkin's disease. Int J Radiat Oncol Biol Phys 1994;28(1):93–9.

Helton WS, Carrico CJ, Zaveruha PA, Schaller R. Diagnosis and treatment of splenic fungal abscesses in the immune-suppressed patient. Arch Surg 1986;121(5):580–6.

Henderson RG, Henderson DC, Reid IN, Atkinson PM. Case report: splenic-gonadal fusion—the ultrasound appearances. Clin Radiol 1991;44(2):117–8.

Herman TE, Siegel MJ. Polysplenia syndrome with con-

genital short pancreas. AJR 1991a;156(4):799–800.

Herman TE, Siegel MJ. CT of acute splenic torsion in children with wandering spleen. AJR 1991b;156(1):151–3.

Herman ZW, Friedwald JP, Donovan C, Scuesa D. Torsion of a wandering spleen in a one month old, with a confusing ultrasound examination. Pediatr Radiol 1991;21(6):442–3.

Herman TE, Shackelford GD, Ternberg JL, Dehner LP. Inflammatory myofibroblastic tumor of the spleen: report of a case in an adolescent. Pediatr Radiol 1994;24(4):280–2.

Hernanz-Schulman M, Ambrosino MM, Genieser NB, et al. Pictorial essay. Current evaluation of the patient with abnormal visceroatrial situs. AJR 1990;154(4):797–802.

Hickman MP, Lucas D, Novak Z, et al. Preoperative embolization of the spleen in children with hypersplenism. J Vasc Interv Radiol 1992;3(4):647–52.

Hill SC, Reinig JW, Barranger JA, et al. Gaucher disease: sonographic appearance of the spleen. Radiology 1986;160(3):631–4.

Hill SC, Damaska BM, Ling A, et al. Gaucher disease: abdominal MR imaging findings in 46 patients. Radiology 1992;184(2):561–6.

Hine AL, Wilson SR. Ultrasonography of splenic variants. J Can Assoc Radiol 1989;40(1):25–7.

Irie H, Honda H, Kaneko K, et al. Inflammatory pseudotumors of the spleen: CT and MRI findings. J Comput Assist Tomogr 1996;20(2):244–8.

Israel DM, Hassall E, Culham JA, Phillips RR. Partial splenic embolization in children with hypersplenism. J Pediatr 1994;124(1):95–100.

Ito K, Murata T, Nakanishi, T. Cystic lymphangioma of the spleen: MR findings with pathologic correlation. Abdom Imaging 1995;20(1):82–4.

Ito K, Mitchell DG, Honjo K, et al. Gadolinium-enhanced MR imaging of the spleen: artifacts and potential pitfalls. AJR 1996;167(5):1147–51.

Jaroch MT, Broughan TA, Hermann RE. The natural history of splenic infarction. Surgery 1986;100(4):743–50.

Jequier S, Guttman F, Lafortune M. Non-surgical treatment of a congenital splenic cyst. Pediatr Radiol 1987;17(3):248–9.

Jequier S, Guttman F, Lafortune M. Non-surgical treatment of a congenital splenic cyst [letter]. Pediatr Radiol 1989;19(5):346–7.

Johnson CD, Ehman RL, Rakela J, Ilstrup DM. MR angiography in portal hypertension: detection of varices and imaging techniques. J Comput Assist Tomogr 1991; 15(4):578–84.

Karaman MI, Gonzales ET Jr. Splenogonadal fusion: report of 2 cases and review of the literature. J Urol 1996;155(1):309–11.

Kasales CJ, Patel S, Hopper KD, et al. Imaging variants of the liver, pancreas, and spleen. Crit Rev Diagn Imaging 1994;35(6):485–543.

Keane MA, Finlayson C, Joseph AE. A histological basis for the 'sonographic snowstorm' in opportunistic infection of the liver and spleen. Clin Radiol 1995;50(4):220–2.

Kedar RP, Merchant SA, Malde HH, Patel VH. Multiple reflective channels in the spleen: a sonographic sign of portal hypertension. Abdom Imaging 1994;19(5):453–8.

Kinare AS, Ambardekar ST, Pande SA. Sonographic diagnosis of splenic torsion in a spleen situated in the left upper quadrant. J Clin Ultrasound 1990;18(7):586–8.

King D, Dawson A, Bayliss A. The value of ultrasonic scanning of the spleen in lymphoma. Clin Radiol 1985; 36:473–4.

Klippenstein DL, Zerin JM, Hirschl RB, Donn SM. Splenic enlargement in neonates during ECMO. Radiology 1994;190(2):411–2.

Knorr PA, Borden TA. Splenogonadal fusion. Urology 1994;44(1):136–8.

Koga T, Morikawa Y. Ultrasonographic determination of the splenic size and its clinical usefulness in various liver diseases. Radiology 1975;115:157–61.

Kohn JS, Clark DE, Isler RJ, Pope CF. Is computed tomographic grading of splenic injury useful in the nonsurgical management of blunt trauma? J Trauma 1994;36(3): 385–9.

Korobkin M, Moss A, Callen P, et al. Computed tomography of subcapsular splenic hematoma. Radiology 1978; 129:441–5.

Kumpe D, Rumack C, Pretorius D, et al. Partial splenic embolization in children with hypersplenism. Radiology 1985;155:357–62.

Lanir A, Hadar H, Cohen I, et al. Gaucher disease: assessment with MR imaging. Radiology 1986;161(1):239–44.

Larsen CE, Patrick LE. Abdominal (liver, spleen) and bone manifestations of cat scratch disease. Pediatr Radiol 1992;22(5):353–5.

Lawhorne T, Zuidema G. Splenic abscesses. Surgery 1976; 79:686–9.

Lehar SC, Zajko AB, Koneru B, et al. Splenic infarction complicating pediatric liver transplantation: incidence and CT appearance. J Comput Assist Tomogr 1990;14(3):362–5.

Levin TL, Berdon WE, Haller JO, et al. Intrasplenic masses of "preserved" functioning splenic tissue in sickle cell disease: correlation of imaging findings (CT, ultrasound, MRI, and nuclear scintigraphy). Pediatr Radiol 1996; 26(9):646–9.

Lindgren PG, Hagberg H, Eriksson B, et al. Excision biopsy of the spleen by ultrasonic guidance. Br J Radiol 1985;58(693):853–7.

Love L, Greenfield G, Braun T, et al. Arteriography of splenic trauma. Radiology 1968;91:96–102.

Lu DS, Saini S, Hahn PF, et al. T2-weighted MR imaging of the upper part of the abdomen: should fat suppression be used routinely? AJR 1994;162(5):1095–100.

Lupien C, Sauerbrei E. Healing in the traumatized spleen: sonographic investigation. Radiology 1984;151:181–5.

Magid D, Fishman EK, Charache S, Siegelman SS. Abdominal pain in sickle cell disease: the role of CT. Radiology 1987;163(2):325–8.

Maillard JC, Menu Y, Scherrer A, et al. Intraperitoneal splenosis: diagnosis by ultrasound and computed tomography. Gastrointest Radiol 1989;14(2):179–80.

Majeski J, Upshur J. Asplenia syndrome. A study of congenital anomalies in 16 cases. JAMA 1978;240:1508–10.

Markisz JA, Treves ST, Davis RT. Normal hepatic and splenic size in children: scintigraphic determination. Pediatr Radiol 1987;17(4):273–6.

Marquis J, Sun S, Verasestakul S. Rupture of the spleen in a newborn infant: report of a new roentgen sign. Radiology 1976;119:177–8.

Masamune A, Okano T, Satake K, Toyota T. Ultrasonic diagnosis of torsion of the wandering spleen. J Clin Ultrasound 1994;22(2):126–8.

McHugh K, Manson D, Eberhard BA, et al. Splenic necrosis in Wegener's granulomatosis. Pediatr Radiol 1991; 21(8):588–9.

McLennan MK, Withers CE. Gaucher's disease involving the spleen. J Can Assoc Radiol 1992;43(1):45–8.

Miceli AB. Splenogonadal fusion: a rare cause of a scrotal mass. Br J Urol 1994;74(2):250.

Miles KA, McPherson SJ, Hayball MP. Transient splenic inhomogeneity with contrast-enhanced CT: mechanism and effect of liver disease. Radiology 1995;194(1):91–5.

Miller J, Greenfield L, Wald B. Candidiasis of the liver and spleen in childhood. Radiology 1982;142:375–80.

Minami M, Itai Y, Ohtomo K, et al. Siderotic nodules in the spleen: MR imaging of portal hypertension. Radiology 1989;172(3):681–4.

Mirowitz SA, Brown JJ, Lee JK, Heiken JP. Dynamic gadolinium-enhanced MR imaging of the spleen: normal enhancement patterns and evaluation of splenic lesions. Radiology 1991;179(3):681–6.

Mirowitz SA, Gutierrez E, Lee JK, et al. Normal abdominal enhancement patterns with dynamic gadolinium-enhanced MR imaging. Radiology 1991;180(3):637–40.

Mirvis SE, Whitley NO, Gens DR. Blunt splenic trauma in adults: CT-based classification and correlation with prognosis and treatment. Radiology 1989;171(1):33–9.

Mittelstaedt C, Partain C. Ultrasonic-pathologic classification of splenic abnormalities: gray-scale patterns. Radiology 1980;134:697–705.

Moller J, Amplatz K, Wolfson J. Malrotation of the bowel in patients with congenital heart disease associated with splenic anomalies. Radiology 1971;99:393–8.

Moncada R, Williams V, Fareed J, et al. Thoracic splenosis. AJR 1985;144:705–6.

Murray JG, Patel MD, Lee S, et al. Microabscesses of the liver and spleen in AIDS: detection with 5-MHz sonography. Radiology 1995;197(3):723–7.

Musy PA, Roche B, Belli D, et al. Splenic cysts in pediatric patients—a report on 8 cases and review of the literature. Eur J Pediatr Surg 1992;2(3):137–40.

Muwakkit S, Gharagozloo A, Souid AK, Spirt BA. The sonographic appearance of lesions of the spleen and pancreas in an infant with Langerhans' cell histiocytosis. Pediatr Radiol 1994;24(3):222–3.

Nemcek AA Jr, Miller FH, Fitzgerald SW. Acute torsion of a wandering spleen: diagnosis by CT and duplex Doppler and color flow sonography. AJR 1991;157(2):307–9.

Niizawa M, Ishida H, Morikawa P, et al. Color Doppler sonography in a case of splenic hemangioma: value of compressing the tumor. AJR 1991;157(5):965–6.

Niwa K, Uchishiba M, Aotsuka H, et al. Magnetic resonance imaging of heterotaxia in infants. J Am Coll Cardiol 1994;23(1):177–83.

Oates E, Austin JM, Becker JL. Technetium-99m-sulfur colloid SPECT imaging in infants with suspected heterotaxy syndrome. J Nucl Med 1995;36(8):1368–71.

Oguzkurt L, Balkanci F, Ariyurek M, Demirkazik FB. Traumatic aneurysm and arteriovenous fistula of the splenic artery. Pediatr Radiol 1996;26(3):195–7.

Ohtomo K, Fukuda H, Mori K, et al. CT and MR appearances of splenic hamartoma. J Comput Assist Tomogr 1992;16(3):425–8.

Orduna M, Gonzalez de Orbe G, Gordillo MI, et al. Chronic granulomatous disease of childhood. Report of two cases with unusual involvement of the gastric antrum and spleen. Eur J Radiol 1989;9(1):67–70.

Pachter HL, Hofstetter SR, Elkowitz A, et al. Traumatic cysts of the spleen—the role of cystectomy and splenic preservation: experience with seven consecutive patients. J Trauma 1993;35(3):430–6.

Pant CS, Gupta RK. Diagnostic value of ultrasonography in hydatid disease in abdomen and chest. Acta Radiol 1987;28(6):743–5.

Panuel M, Ternier F, Michel G, et al. Splenic hemangioma—report of three pediatric cases with pathologic correlation. Pediatr Radiol 1992;22(3):213–6.

Paris S, Weiss SM, Ayers W Jr, Clarke LE. Splenic abscess. Am Surg 1994;60(5):358–61.

Pastakia B, Shawker TH, Thaler M, et al. Hepatosplenic candidiasis: wheels within wheels. Radiology 1988; 166(2):417–21.

Pawar S, Kay C, Gonzalez R, et al. Sonography of splenic abscess. AJR 1982;138:259–62.

Pearl RH, Wesson DE, Spence LJ, et al. Splenic injury: a 5-year update with improved results and changing criteria for conservative management. J Pediatr Surg 1989;24(5): 428–31.

Pearson H, Johnston D, Smith K, et al. The born-again

spleen. Return of splenic function after splenectomy for trauma. N Engl J Med 1978;298(25):1389–92.

Peoples W, Moller J, Edwards J. Polysplenia: a review of 146 cases. Pediatr Cardiol 1983;Apr–Jun;4(2):129–37.

Phillpott JW, Cumming WA. Torsion of the spleen: an unusual presentation of congenital diaphragmatic hernia. Pediatr Radiol 1994;24(2):150–1.

Phoon CK, Neill CA. Asplenia syndrome: insight into embryology through an analysis of cardiac and extracardiac anomalies. Am J Cardiol 1994;73(8):581–7.

Pierce G, Applegate K, Goske M, Murphy D. Situs revisited: chest X-ray recognition, embryology and imaging of heterotaxy syndrome. At RSNA, scientific exhibition, Chicago, 1997 in Radio Graphics, Sitis Revisited: Imaging of the heterotaxy syndrome, Volume 19, July/August 1999, IV: 837–53, K. Applegate, M. Goske, G. Pierce, and D. Murphy.

Pistoia F, Markowitz SK. Splenic lymphangiomatosis: CT diagnosis. AJR 1988;150(1):121–2.

Pranikoff T, Hirschl RB, Schlesinger AE, et al. Resolution of splenic injury after nonoperative management. J Pediatr Surg 1994;29(10):1366–9.

Prassopoulos P, Cavouras D. CT assessment of normal splenic size in children. Acta Radiol 1994;35(2):152–4.

Querfeld U, Dietrich R, Taira RK, et al. Magnetic resonance imaging of iron overload in children treated with peritoneal dialysis. Nephron 1988;50(3):220–4.

Ragozzino MW, Singletary H, Patrick, R. Familial splenic epidermoid cyst. AJR 1990;155(6):1233–4.

Ralls P, Quinn M, Colletti P, et al. Sonography of pyogenic splenic abscess. AJR 1982;138:523–5.

Ramani M, Reinhold C, Semelka RC, et al. Splenic hemangiomas and hamartomas: MR imaging characteristics of 28 lesions. Radiology 1997;202(1):166–72.

Rescorla FJ, Grosfeld JL. Splenic and liver trauma in children. Indiana Med 1989;82(7):516–20.

Robinson SL, Saxe JM, Lucas CE, et al. Splenic abscess associated with endocarditis. Surgery 1992;112(4):781–7.

Roche BG, Bugmann P, Le Coultre C. Blunt injuries to liver, spleen, kidney and pancreas in pediatric patients. Eur J Pediatr Surg 1992;2(3):154–6.

Rodkey ML, Macknin ML. Pediatric wandering spleen: case report and review of literature. Clin Pediatr 1992; 31(5):289–94.

Ros P, Moser R, Dachman A, et al. Hemangioma of the spleen: radiologic-pathologic correlation in ten cases. Radiology 1987;162:73–7.

Rosenberg HK, Markowitz RI, Kolberg H, et al. Normal splenic size in infants and children: sonographic measurements. AJR 1991;157(1):119–21.

Ruess L, Sivit CJ, Eichelberger MR, et al. Blunt hepatic and splenic trauma in children: correlation of a CT injury severity scale with clinical outcome. Pediatr Radiol 1995;25(5):321–5.

Sagoh T, Itoh K, Togashi K, et al. Gamna-Gandy bodies of the spleen: evaluation with MR imaging. Radiology 1989;172(3):685–7.

Scatamacchia SA, Raptopoulos V, Fink MP, Silva WE. Splenic trauma in adults: impact of CT grading on management. Radiology 1989;171(3):725–9.

Schlesinger AE, Edgar KA, Boxer LA. Volume of the spleen in children as measured on CT scans: normal standards as a function of body weight. AJR 1993;160(5): 1107–9.

Schmidt H, Fischedick AR, Peters PE, von Lengerke HJ. [Candida abscesses in the liver and spleen. The sonographic and computed tomographic morphology.] Dtsch Med Wochenschr 1986;111(21):816–20.

Schmidt H, Peters PE, von Lengerke HJ, et al. [Microabscesses of the spleen in patients with acute leukemia.] Radiologe 1987;27(1):20–4.

Schwartz LH, Seltzer SE, Adams DF, et al. Effects of superparamagnetic iron oxide (AMI-25) on liver and spleen imaging using spin-echo and fast spin-echo magnetic resonance pulse sequences. Invest Radiol 1994;29(2):S21–3.

Schwerk WB, Gorg C, Gorg K, Restrepo I. Ultrasound-guided percutaneous drainage of pyogenic splenic abscesses. J Clin Ultrasound 1994;22(3):161–6.

Semelka RC, Shoenut JP, Lawrence PH, et al. Spleen: dynamic enhancement patterns on gradient-echo MR images enhanced with gadopentetate dimeglumine. Radiology 1992a;185(2):479–82.

Semelka RC, Shoenut JP, Greenberg HM, Bow EJ. Detection of acute and treated lesions of hepatosplenic candidiasis: comparison of dynamic contrast-enhanced CT and MR imaging. J Magn Reson Imaging 1992b;2(3):341–5.

Sener RN, Alper H. Polysplenia syndrome: a case associated with transhepatic portal vein, short pancreas, and left inferior vena cava with hemiazygous continuation. Abdom Imaging 1994;19(1):64–6.

Seo T, Ito T, Watanabe Y, Umeda T. Torsion of an accessory spleen presenting as an acute abdomen with an inflammatory mass. US, CT, and MRI findings. Pediatr Radiol 1994;24(7):532–4.

Sheflin J, Lee C, Kretchmar K. Torsion of wandering spleen and distal pancreas. AJR 1984;142:100–1.

Sheley RC, Nyberg DA, Kapur R. Azygous continuation of the interrupted inferior vena cava: a clue to prenatal diagnosis of the cardiosplenic syndromes. J Ultrasound Med 1995;14(5):381–7.

Sherman N, Asch M. Conservative surgery for splenic injuries. Pediatrics 1978;61:267–71.

Shiels WE, Johnson JF, Stephenson SR, Huang YC. Chronic torsion of the wandering spleen. Pediatr Radiol 1989;19(6–7):465–7.

Shirkhoda A, Lopez-Berestein G, Holbert JM, Luna MA. Hepatosplenic fungal infection: CT and pathologic evaluation after treatment with liposomal amphotericin B. Radiology 1986;159(2):349–53.

Shirkhoda A, Freeman J, Armin AR, et al. Imaging features of splenic epidermoid cyst with pathologic correlation. Abdom Imaging 1995;20(5):449–51.

Shirkhoda A, Wallace S, Sokhandan M. Computed tomography and ultrasonography in splenic infarction. J Can Assoc Radiol 1985;36(1):29–33.

Siniluoto T, Paivansalo M, Alavaikko M. Ultrasonography of spleen and liver in staging Hodgkin's disease. Eur J Radiol 1991;13(3):181–6.

Siniluoto TM, Paivansalo MJ, Lanning FP, et al. Ultrasonography in traumatic splenic rupture. Clin Radiol 1992;46(6):391–6.

Siniluoto TM, Tikkakoski TA, Lahde ST, et al. Ultrasound or CT in splenic diseases? Acta Radiol 1994;35(6):597–605.

Skandalakis PN, Colborn GL, Skandalakis LJ, et al. The surgical anatomy of the spleen. Surg Clin North Am 1993;73(4):747–68.

Soler R, Rodriguez E, Comesana ML, et al. Agenesis of the dorsal pancreas with polysplenia syndrome: CT features. J Comput Assist Tomogr 1992;16(6):921–3.

Spigos D, Jonasson O, Mozes M. Partial splenic embolization in the treatment of hypersplenism. AJR 1979;132:777–82.

Stanley P, Shen TC. Partial embolization of the spleen in patients with thalassemia. J Vasc Interv Radiol 1995;6(1):137–42.

Storm BL, Abbitt PL, Allen DA, Ros PR. Splenosis: superparamagnetic iron oxide-enhanced MR imaging. AJR 1992;159(2):333–5.

Strijk SP, Boetes C, Bogman MJ, et al. The spleen in non-Hodgkin lymphoma. Diagnostic value of computed tomography. Acta Radiol 1987;28(2):139–44.

Subramanyam B, Balthazar E, Horii S. Sonography of the accessory spleen. AJR 1984;143:47–9.

Sugrue M, Knox A, Sarre R, et al. Management of splenic trauma: a new CT-guided splenic injury grading system. Aust N Z J Surg 1991;61(5):349–53.

Swischuk LE, Williams JB, John SD. Torsion of wandering spleen: the whorled appearance of the splenic pedicle on CT. Pediatr Radiol 1993;23(6):476–7.

Takayama T, Shimada K, Inoue K, et al. Intrapancreatic accessory spleen [letter]. Lancet 1994;344(8927):957–8.

Talenti E, Cesaro S, Scapinello A, et al. Disseminated hepatic and splenic calcifications following cat-scratch disease. Pediatr Radiol 1994;24(5):342–3.

Taylor AJ, Dodds WJ, Erickson SJ, Stewart ET. CT of acquired abnormalities of the spleen. AJR 1991;157(6):1213–9.

Taylor GA. Imaging of pediatric blunt abdominal trauma: what have we learned in the past decade? [editorial]. Radiology 1995;195(3):600–1.

Terk MR, Esplin J, Lee K, et al. MR imaging of patients with type 1 Gaucher's disease: relationship between bone and visceral changes. AJR 1995;165(3):599–604.

Thomas EA, Dubbins PA. Diagnosing splenic trauma. Clin Radiol 1991;43(5):297–300.

Thompson SE, Walsh EA, Cramer BC, et al. Radiological features of a symptomatic splenic hamartoma. Pediatr Radiol 1996;26(9):657–60.

Tikkakoski T, Siniluoto T, Paivansalo M, et al. Splenic abscess. Imaging and intervention. Acta Radiol 1992;33(6):561–5.

Tonkin I, Tonkin A. Visceroatrial situs abnormalities: sonographic and computed tomographic appearance. AJR 1982;138:509–15.

Tsuda Y, Nishimura K, Kawakami S, et al. Preduodenal portal vein and anomalous continuation of inferior vena cava: CT findings. J Comput Assist Tomogr 1991;15(4):585–8.

Urrutia M, Mergo P, Ros L, et al. Cystic masses of the spleen: radiologic-pathologic correlation. Radiographics 1996;16:107–29.

Vasquez TE, Evans DG, Schiffman H, Ashburn WL. Fungal splenic abscesses in the immunosuppressed patient. Correlation of imaging modalities. Clin Nucl Med 1987; 12(1):36–8.

Vaughan T, Hawkins I, Elliott L. Diagnosis of polysplenia syndrome. Radiology 1971;101:511–8.

Vick CW, Hartenberg MA, Allen HA, Haynes JW. Abdominal pseudotumor caused by gastric displacement of the spleen: sonographic demonstration. Pediatr Radiol 1985;15(4):253–4.

von Sinner WN, Stridbeck H. Hydatid disease of the spleen. Ultrasonography, CT and MR imaging. Acta Radiol 1992;33(5):459–61.

Wadsworth D, Newman B, Abramson S, et al. Splenic lymphangiomatosis in children. Radiology 1997;202:173–6.

Walker TM, Serjeant GR. Focal echogenic lesions in the spleen in sickle cell disease. Clin Radiol 1993;47(2): 114–6.

Walther MM, Trulock TS, Finnerty DP, Woodard J. Splenic gonadal fusion. Urology 1988;32(6):521–4.

Wang JK, Chang MH, Li YW, et al. Association of hiatus hernia with asplenia syndrome. Eur J Pediatr 1993; 152(5):418–20.

Watanabe Y, Todani T, Noda T. Changes in splenic volume after partial splenic embolization in children. J Pediatr Surg 1996;31(2):241–4.

Weingarten MJ, Fakhry J, McCarthy J, et al. Sonography after splenic embolization: the wedge-shaped acute infarct. AJR 1984;142(5):957–9.

Weissleder R, Elizondo G, Stark DD, et al. The diagnosis of splenic lymphoma by MR imaging: value of superparamagnetic iron oxide. AJR 1989;152(1):175–80.

Wernecke K, Peters PE, Kruger KG. Ultrasonographic patterns of focal hepatic and splenic lesions in Hodgkin's and non-Hodgkin's lymphoma. Br J Radiol 1987;60(715): 655–60.

Wesson D, Filler R, Ein S, et al. Ruptured spleen - when to operate? J Pediatr Surg 1981;16:324–6.

Wetton CW, Tran TL. Case report: splenic infarct in sickle cell disease. Clin Radiol 1995;50(8):573–4.

Williams JL, Bush D, Wright PG. Omphalocele and ectopic spleen. J Clin Ultrasound 1987;15(6):409–11.

Wolfman NT, Bechtold RE, Scharling ES, Meredith JW. Blunt upper abdominal trauma: evaluation by CT. AJR 1992;158(3):493–501.

Yamataka A, Fujiwara T, Tsuchioka T, et al. Heterotopic splenic autotransplantation in a neonate with splenic rupture, leading to normal splenic function. J Pediatr Surg 1996;31(2):239–40.

Yoo SY, Lim KS, Kang SJ, Kim CS. Pitfalls of nonoperative management of blunt abdominal trauma in children in Korea. J Pediatr Surg 1996;31(2):263–6.

Yoshimitsu K, Aibe H, Nobe T, et al. Intrahepatic splenosis mimicking a liver tumor. Abdom Imaging 1993;18(2): 156–8.

Zankar R, Malde HM, Soni M, Chadha D. Hydatid cyst of spleen with bull's-eye appearance on imaging [letter]. AJR 1992;159(6):1347.

APPENDIX

Development of the Gastrointestinal Tract Up To 5 Weeks of Gestational Age

By 4 weeks, cephalocaudal growth of the embryo with lateral folding results in the formation of the primitive gut and two extra-embryonic portions—the yolk sac and allantois (Figs. 1A, 1B). The buccopharyngeal membrane between the stomadeum and foregut ruptures in the fourth week.

Henceforth, there is free communication between the foregut and the amniotic cavity. By 28 days, a primitive liver bud and a tracheobronchial diverticulum have started to develop (Fig. 1C).

During the fourth and fifth weeks, the pharyngeal pouches and branchial arches begin to develop and the liver enlarges (Fig. 1D). The primitive gut can be divided into three parts at this stage. The further development of these three parts is discussed in the following chapters:

Foregut From buccopharyngeal membrane to just distal to pancreatic and liver buds.
• Branchial arches – chapter 6

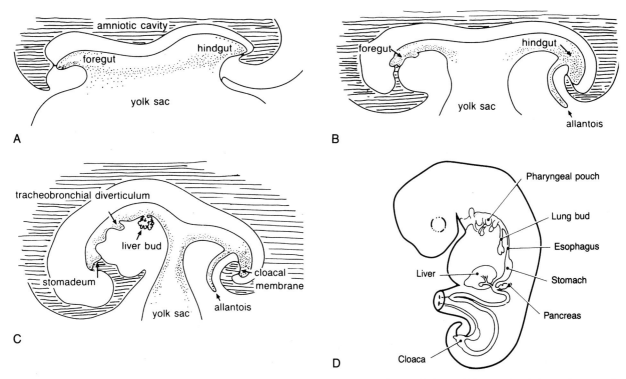

FIGURE 1. Development of the gastrointestinal tract: *A* and *B,* By 4 weeks, cephalocaudal growth of the embryo with lateral folding results in the formation of the primitive gut and two extra-embryonic portions—the yolk sac and allantois. *C,* By 28 days, a primitive liver bud and a tracheobronchial diverticulum have started to develop. *D,* During the fourth and fifth weeks, the pharyngeal pouches and branchial arches begin to develop and the liver is enlarging. The primitive gut can be divided into three parts at this stage.

- Trachea and esophagus – chapter 6
- Stomach – chapter 8

Development of vascular arches is considered on Chapter 6.

Midgut   From end of foregut to distal transverse colon
- General development and rotation – chapter 9
- Portal vein development – chapter 9

- Vitelline duct – chapter 9
- Anterior abdominal wall – chapter 9

Hindgut   From distal transverse colon to cloacal membrane
- General – chapter 10
- Cloaca – chapter 10
- Ganglion development – chapter 10

The development of the liver, pancreas, and spleen is considered in chapters 12, 13 and 14.

INDEX